D1710519

FOUNDATIONS IN SOCIAL NEUROSCIENCE

Social Neuroscience Series
Series Editors:
John T. Cacioppo and Gary Berntson
Series Editorial Board:
Sue Carter, Richard J. Davidson, Martha McClintock, Bruce McEwen, Daniel L. Schacter, Esther Sternberg, Steve Suomi, Shelley Taylor

Foundations in Social Neuroscience, edited by John T. Cacioppo, Gary G. Berntson, Ralph Adolphs, C. Sue Carter, Richard J. Davidson, Martha K. McClintock, Bruce S. McEwen, Michael J. Meaney, Daniel L. Schacter, Esther M. Sternberg, Steve S. Suomi, and Shelley E. Taylor

FOUNDATIONS IN SOCIAL NEUROSCIENCE

edited by
John T. Cacioppo, Gary G. Berntson, Ralph Adolphs, C. Sue Carter, Richard J.
Davidson, Martha K. McClintock, Bruce S. McEwen, Michael J. Meaney, Daniel
L. Schacter, Esther M. Sternberg, Steve S. Suomi, and Shelley E. Taylor

A Bradford Book

The MIT Press
Cambridge, Massachusetts
London, England

© 2002 Massachusetts Institute of Technology

All rights reserved. No part of this book may be reproduced in any form by any electronic or mechanical means (including photocopying, recording, or information storage and retrieval) without permission in writing from the publisher.

This book was set in Times New Roman on 3B2 by Asco Typesetters, Hong Kong, and was printed and bound in the United States of America.

Library of Congress Cataloging-in-Publication Data

Foundations in social neuroscience / edited by John T. Cacioppo ... [et al.].
    p.   cm. — (Social neuroscience series)
"A Bradford book."
Includes bibliographical references and index.
ISBN 0-262-03291-0 (alk. paper) — ISBN 0-262-53195-X (pbk. : alk. paper)
1. Neurosciences—Social aspects. I. Cacioppo, John T. II. Series.
RC343 .F635   2002
612.8—dc21   2001044754

Contents

I GENERAL INTRODUCTION

1 Social Neuroscience

John T. Cacioppo and Gary G. Berntson

Social neuroscience addresses fundamental questions about the mind and its dynamic interactions with the biological systems of the brain and the social world in which it resides (Cacioppo & Berntson, 1992; Cacioppo, 1994). This field studies the relationship between neural and social processes, including the intervening information-processing components and operations at both the neural and the computational levels of analysis. As such, work in social neuroscience builds on work in the neurosciences, cognitive sciences, and social sciences. Neuroscientists and cognitive scientists have collaborated for more than a decade with the common goal of understanding how the mind works. The premise underlying this book is that the study of complex aspects of the mind and behavior will benefit from yet a broader collaboration of neuroscientists, cognitive scientists, and social scientists.

Collaborations between cognitive scientists and neuroscientists have helped solve puzzles of the mind including aspects of perception, imagery, attention, and memory (Churchland & Sejnowski, 1988; Kosslyn & Andersen, 1992). Many aspects of the mind, however, require a more comprehensive approach to reveal the mystery of mind-brain connections. Attraction, altruism, aggression, affiliation, attachment, attitudes, identification, cooperation, competition, empathy, sexuality, communication, dominance, persuasion, obedience, and nurturance are just a few examples. Humans are fundamentally social animals who can exist only in a web of relationships. To simplify their study of the mind, many scientists have ignored social aspects. As discussed in chapter 3,

Not long ago, it was thought that a set of master genes activated the DNA necessary to produce the appropriate proteins for development and behavior (Crick, 1970). The architects of this construction were conceived as the forces of evolution operating over millennia; the builders were conceived as encapsulated within each living cell far from the reach of personal ties or sociocultural influences. Human biology, however, has evolved within a fiercely social world, provides potentials and constraints for representation and behavior attuned to this social world, and is shaped profoundly by the social world. The papers in this book call into question this fundamental assumption.

The notion that the nervous, endocrine, and immune systems operate outside the reach of sociocultural influences had advantages, to be sure. This approach allowed focused study of isolated anatomical systems with a resulting specification of component structures and processes. As scientists began applying neuroscientific approaches to more complex questions, however, what they thought to be basic principles came into question. For instance, researchers knew that the phenotypic expression (e.g., behavior) of strains of mice with specific genes inactivated (i.e., knockout mice) depends on the genetic background (e.g., Gerlai, 1996); the effects of the social context, on the other hand, they thought to be unimportant. Crabbe, Wahlsten, and Dudek (1999) demonstrated that the specific behavioral effects associated with a given knockout could vary dramatically across environmental contexts (e.g., experimenters, testing environments, laboratories). In parallel, the social and psychological scientific community realized that behavioral data alone were often insufficient to characterize underlying processes, and that social processes are products of brain operations (e.g., Anderson, 1978; Cacioppo, Gardner, & Berntson, 1999; Fazio, Zanna, & Cooper, 1977). As in the cognitive sciences (cf. Kosslyn & Andersen, 1992), this led some scientists interested in social phenomena to consider more seriously the neural substrates of behavior. That is, both sides had something to gain by expanding their traditional approach to include multi-level integrative analyses of social influences and behavior.

Humans Are Social Animals

Why might social factors be so important to an understanding of the brain and mind? The human brain and biology have evolved within a fiercely social world; individuals who live in isolation are unlikely to survive and less likely yet to reproduce. As Spiegel (2000) noted:

We are fundamentally social organisms, our mythic rugged individualism notwithstanding. We are born to the most prolonged period of abject dependency of any mammal. For the species to survive, human infants must instantly engage their parents in protective behavior, and the parents must care enough about their offspring to nurture and protect them. Even once grown we are not particularly splendid physical specimens. Other animals can run faster, see and smell better, and fight more effectively than we can. Our major evolutionary advantage is our brain and ability to communicate, remember, plan, and work together. Our survival depends on our collective abilities, not our individual might. Thus, it makes sense that our health may also depend on our interactions with one another.

Epidemiological research has indeed established that even relative social isolation is as important a risk factor for broad-based morbidity and mortality as cigarette smoking or high blood pressure (House, Landis, & Umberson 1988). More than health is affected by the social world, of course. The human mind constructs the meaning of events in the context of people, relationships, families, alliances and competitors, societies, cultures, and history. Memory makes possible not only the formation of stimulus associations and learning but of social connections, alliances, norms, traditions, culture, and histories that link us to minds of others present and past. This makes possible actions, thoughts, and feelings exceeding anything that could be accomplished by any individual alone. Social relationships subtly embrace us in the warmth of self-affirmation, the whispers of encouragement, and the meaningfulness of belonging. Disruptions or the absence of stable social relationships,

in contrast, disturb our minds and biology as few other events can. Individuals are often plunged into deep, emotionally troubling pains when an important social connection or relationship is disrupted, as by an unexpected departure or loss of a loved one (Panksepp, 1998).

Selective brain injuries and imaging studies also reveal important links between the brain and social context (cf. Adolphs, 1999; Klein & Kihlstrom, 1998). Individuals with damage to the amygdala and associated inferior portions of the temporal cortex exhibit features of the Klüver-Bucy syndrome, which is characterized by blunted affect and increased and inappropriate sexual activity (Trimble, Mendez, & Cummings, 1997). Prosopagnosics, who typically have bilateral lesions in the occipital lobes near the temporal lobes, do not undergo a change in personality but have another disturbing problem that alters their social behavior: they no longer recognize the faces of those they once knew (e.g., spouses), even though larger skin conductance responses to familiar faces shows that—at some level—the brain still recognizes these individuals (Tranel & Damasio, 1985). With Capgras syndrome, typically associated with bilateral lesions in the temporal and right fronto-parietal cortices (Benson, 1994; Signer, 1994), an individual insists that others who are emotionally close to them have been replaced by physically identical imposters. In the Fregoli syndrome, typically associated with right hemisphere dysfunction, the individual perceives strangers as familiar individuals—that is, people are perceived as physically different but psychologically identical to familiar individuals (e.g., Mojtabai, 1994; Oyebode & Sargeant, 1996).

In addition to the impact of the brain on social behavior, social behavior can have a substantial impact on the brain. Early social interactions, for instance, are important in normal brain and behavioral development. Tactile contact is a stronger determinant of mother-infant attachment in monkeys than feeding (Harlow & Harlow, 1973). Early tactile deprivation reduces the number of glucocorticoid receptors (stress monitoring and dampening) binding sites in the hippocampus and frontal cortex. These changes are permanent; as a consequence, the negative feedback to stress hormones is diminished, and stress reactivity as a rat pup and as an adult is elevated (Meaney, Sapolsky, & McEwen, 1985). Attachment and communication are so important that infants respond to faces and try to gain a response soon after birth; even in rare instances in which language is neither modeled nor taught, a form of language develops nevertheless (Goldin-Meadow & Mylander, 1983, 1984).

The findings outlined above document reciprocal interactions between brain and social behavior. Human biology is anchored in concrete anatomy and genetics, providing fundamental elements from which to draw interconnections and with which to construct theory. The social world, in contrast, is a complex set of abstractions representing the actions and influences of and the relationships among individuals, groups, societies, and cultures. The differences in levels of analysis have resulted in distinct histories, research traditions, and technical demands, leaving what some regard as an impassable abyss between social and biological approaches. The assumptions in social neuroscience, in contrast, are that the abyss can and must be bridged, that the mechanisms underlying mind and behavior will not be fully explicable by a biological or a social approach alone, that a multi-level integrative analysis may be required, and that a common scientific language—grounded in the structure and function of the brain and biology—can contribute to this goal. All human behavior, at some level, is biological; this does not mean that biological reductionism yields a simple, singular, or satisfactory explanation for complex behaviors, or that molecular forms of representation provide the only or best level of analysis for understanding human behavior. Molar constructs such as those developed by the social sciences provide a means of understanding highly complex activity

without needing to specify each individual action of the simplest components, thereby providing an efficient means of describing the behavior of a complex system. Chemists who work with the periodic table on a daily basis nevertheless use recipes rather than the periodic table to cook, not because food preparation cannot be reduced to chemical expressions but because it is not cognitively efficient to do so.

Organizing Principles

The papers constituting this volume reveal numerous findings, principles, and mechanisms. Three important principles have served as general heuristics for organizing research in the field of social neuroscience (Cacioppo & Berntson, 1992) and health (Anderson, 1998). The principle of *multiple determinism* specifies that a target event at one level of organization, but especially at molar (e.g., social) levels of organization, can have multiple antecedents within or across levels of organization. On the biological level, for instance, researchers identified the contribution of individual differences in the endogenous opiod receptor system in drug use while on the social level investigators have noted the important role of social context. Both operate, and our understanding of drug abuse is incomplete if either perspective is excluded. Similarly, while scientists once considered immune functions reflective of specific and nonspecific physiological responses to pathogens or tissue damage, it is now clear that immune responses are heavily influenced by central nervous processes affected by social interactions and processes. For instance, the effects of social context now appear to be powerful determinants of the expression of immune reactions. Of course, an understanding of immunocompetence will be inadequate without a consideration of psychosocial factors. Major advances in the neurosciences can derive from increasing the scope of the analysis to include the contributions of social factors and processes.

A corollary to this principle is that the mapping between elements across levels of organization becomes more complex (e.g., many-to-many) as the number of intervening levels of organization increases. One implication is that the likelihood of complex and potentially obscure mappings increases as one skips levels of organizations. Cognitive neuroscience, therefore, is an important companion to social neuroscience because it bridges intervening levels of organization.

The principle of *nonadditive determinism* specifies that properties of the whole are not always readily predictable from the properties of the parts. Consider an illustrative study by Haber and Barchas (1983), who investigated the effects of amphetamine on primate behavior. They examined the behavior of nonhuman primates following the administration of amphetamine or placebo. No clear pattern emerged between the drug and placebo conditions until each primate's position in the social hierarchy was considered. When this social factor was taken into account, the amphetamine was found to increase dominant behavior in primates high in the social hierarchy and to increase submissive behavior in primates low in the social hierarchy. This study clearly demonstrates how the effects of physiological changes on social behavior can appear unreliable until the analysis is extended across levels of organization. A strictly physiological (or social) analysis, regardless of the sophistication of the measurement technology, may not have revealed the orderly relationship that existed.

The principle of *reciprocal determinism* specifies that there can be mutual influences between microscopic (e.g., biological) and macroscopic (e.g., social) factors in determining behavior. For example, research has revealed that while testosterone levels in nonhuman male primates promote sexual behavior, the availability of receptive females influences this level of testosterone (Bernstein, Gordon, & Rose, 1983; Rose, Gordon, & Bernstein, 1972). Within social psychology, Zillmann (1984) has demonstrated that exposure to violent and erotic materials influences the level of physiological arousal in males, and that this level of physiological arousal has a reciprocal influence on the perceptions of and tendencies toward sex and aggression. Accordingly, comprehensive accounts of these behaviors cannot exist if scientists consider the biological or the social level of organization unnecessary or irrelevant.

Structure of the Book

A social neuroscience perspective requires multilevel analyses spanning neural and social levels of organization. The contributors to this book represent disciplines ranging from molecular biology; neurology; zoology; endocrinology; immunology; and biological psychology to cognitive, clinical, and social psychology; ethology; and anthropology. The selection of chapters does not present a monolithic position on a particular topic—indeed this would be premature in such a young field. Instead, the chapters represent a survey of the immense breadth of the field, raise questions about and challenges to traditional ways of thinking, provoke and stimulate some new ways of thinking, highlight methodologies and controversies, and illustrate newly discovered connections. In short, this book aims to rouse interest rather than to provide definitive answers.

The first group of chapters, "Multilevel Integrative Analyses of Social Behavior," includes specific analyses or general reviews that suggest the potential of multilevel integrative analyses of social behavior. These chapters, each of which presents a very different approach, serves to illustrate the breadth of social neuroscience and to demonstrate how such an approach might contribute to more comprehensive accounts of the mind, health, and social processes.

The second group, "Social Cognition and the Brain," deals with some of the most elemental mental processes underlying social behavior. Initially, studies of the neural structures and processes associated with psychological and social events used only animal models, postmortem examinations, multiply determined peripheral assessments, and observations of the occasional unfortunate individual who suffered trauma to or disorders of localized areas of the brain. Developments in electrophysiological recording, functional brain imaging, neurochemical techniques, neuroimmunologic measures, and ambulatory recording procedures have increasingly made it possible to investigate the role of neural systems and processes in intact humans. These developments have fostered multilevel integrative analyses of the relationship between neural and social processes. The initial set of papers in this section covers basic processes including consciousness, cognition, memory systems, and automatic and controlled mental processes. The succeeding papers in this section build on these component processes, covering new conceptualizations and methods for studying the self, perceiving others, and social information processing (e.g., reasoning about or influenced by others).

The social world has especially large effects on motivation and emotion, which in turn govern the selection of the specific information-processing mechanisms that are invoked. The focus of the third major group of papers, therefore, is "Social Neuroscience of Motivation, Emotion, and Attitudes." Evaluative categorizations and response dispositions—criterial attributes of attitudes, affect, and emotion—are fundamental and ubiquitous in behavior. All organisms have rudimentary biological mechanisms for approaching, acquiring, or ingesting certain classes of stimuli and withdrawing from, avoiding, or rejecting others. Knowledge of the organization and operating characteristics of these rudimentary mechanisms may therefore lay down, at least in broad strokes, the rules by which rudimentary biological and social factors alter evaluative categorizations and evaluative response dispositions. Decerebrate organisms, for example, display stereotyped orofacial ingestion/ejection reflexes to relevant gustatory stimuli. Furthermore, reflexive responses demonstrate a sensitivity to social and motiva-

tional variables. These inherent dispositions allow an organism, even at early stages of development and without previous experience, to respond adaptively to important classes of environmental stimuli. These reflexes also represent only a single level in what appears to be a continuum of evaluative mechanisms. With the involvement of additional subcortical structures, the reactions of the decorticate organism evidence greater directedness, integration, serial coherence, goal seeking, and contextual adaptability. Thus, evaluative mechanisms are not localized to specific neuraxial levels but evidence a hierarchy or representation throughout the central nervous system. With progressively higher organizational levels in evaluative mechanisms, there is a general expansion in the range and relational complexity of contextual controls and in the breadth and flexibility of adaptive response. The chapters in this section therefore challenge the notion that affect operates in a linear, unidimensional fashion and underscore the close connections between affect and social behavior. As throughout, the initial chapters in this section survey selected formulations of the neural or conceptual substrates of motivation and emotion. The subsequent chapters in this section focus on specific studies of motivation, affect, preferences, and decision making from various levels of analysis.

Coverage of work on social emotions is deferred until the fourth group of chapters, the section "Biology of Social Relationships and Interpersonal Processes." The decade of the brain led to a realization that a comprehensive understanding of the brain cannot be achieved by focusing on neural mechanisms alone. The human brain, the organ of the mind, is a fundamental component of a social species. Indeed, humans are such social animals that a basic "need to belong" has been posited (Baumeister & Leary, 1995; Gardner, Gabriel, & Diekman, 2000). People form associations and connections with others from the moment they are born. The very survival of newborns depends on their attachment to and nurturance by others over extended periods of time. Accordingly, evolution has sculpted the human genome to be sensitive to and succoring of contact and relationships with others. For instance, caregiving and attachment have hormonal and neurophysiological substrates. The reciprocal influences between social and biological levels of organization do not stop at infancy. Affiliation and nurturant social relationships, for instance, are essential for physical and psychological well-being across the lifespan. Disruptions of social connections, whether through ridicule, separation, divorce, or bereavement, are among the most stressful events people endure. The initial chapters in this section provide overviews of basic processes ranging from the development of autism to gender differences in stress responses. The remaining chapters cover the processes and consequences of attachment, personal ties, affiliation, sexuality, aggression, social hierarchies, and individual differences.

The final section features work on "Social Influences on Biology and Health." The United States is undergoing social changes that rival in magnitude and impact the technological changes in medicine, genetics, and computer science. The overall population in the United States is over 273 million, an increase of 7% over the preceding decade (U.S. Census Bureau, 1999). The number of persons under the age of sixty-five tripled during the twentieth century while the number of persons sixty-five and over increased by a factor of 11. In older adults, chronic diseases have become the most frequent source of complaints and the largest causes of morbidity and mortality. The costs of medical care continue to rise more rapidly than inflation or the gross national product, and a disproportionate amount of medical costs goes to the treatment of aging-related disorders. By the early 1990s, for instance, individuals sixty-five and over accounted for approximately 36% of all hospital stays and 48% of total days of doctor care (Luskin & Newell, 1997). Furthermore, changes in marital and childbearing patterns and in the age structure of U.S. society are projected to produce in the twenty-

first century a steady increase in the number of older people who lack spouses or children. By the end of the current decade, the number of people living alone is projected to reach almost 31 million—a 40% increase since 1980. This confluence of sociodemographic currents is important because social isolation predicts morbidity and mortality from broad-based causes in later life, even after controlling for health behaviors and biological risk factors (House, Landis, & Umberson, 1988). Understanding the mechanisms by which social factors influence the mind, biology, and health is particularly important for the continued health and prosperity of society. The initial chapters in this section survey basic processes and underscore the reciprocal influences across anatomical systems and levels of organization; the subsequent chapters outline the deleterious and salubrious effects of social contact.

Summary

Collectively, the chapters illustrate that: (1) theory and research in the neurosciences are helping to illuminate the mechanisms underlying social phenomena; (2) the study of social processes challenge existing theories in the neurosciences, resulting in refinements, extensions, or complete revolutions in neuroscientific theory and research; (3) more complex aspects of the mind are tractable by considering or pursuing jointly macro-level and microlevel analyses; (4) deciphering the structure and function of the brain is fostered by sophisticated conceptual models in which the elementary operations underlying complex social phenomena are explicated, and by experimental paradigms which allow these elementary operations to be studied in isolation and in specific combinations using neuroscientific methods; and (5) the social environment shapes neural structures and processes, and vice versa.

Given the importance of social context, much is left to learn about the brain, mind, and biology through truly collaborative efforts that bring together multiple levels of analysis of complex behaviors. This premise formed the impetus for this book—a collection of articles defining the breadth, substance, and value of work in the field of social neuroscience. Information is processed at multiple levels of the neuraxis, and reactions to that information may be quite divergent across levels. Because priority in the control of behavior may shift among these levels, important research directions include the characterization of the operations of these multiple levels, the interactions among levels, and the determinants of their expression. If this is the case, then a multilevel approach will be necessary to achieve a comprehensive understanding of complex social phenomena. Collective interdisciplinary teams have forged fresh, exciting hypotheses about the mind that researchers are testing using a wide array of new techniques. The secrets of the complex human mind have never been more tractable.

References

Adolphs, R. (1999). Social cognition and the human brain. *Trends in Cognitive Sciences, 3*, 469–479.

Anderson, J. R. (1978). Arguments concerning representations for mental imagery. *Psychological Review, 85*, 249–277.

Anderson, N. B. (1998). Levels of analysis in health science: A framework for integrating sociobehavioral and biomedical research. *Annals of the New York Academy of Sciences, 840*, 563–576.

Baumeister, R. F., & Leary, M. R. (1995). The need to belong: Desire for interpersonal attachment as a fundamental human motivation. *Psychological Bulletin, 117*, 497–529.

Benson, D. F. (1994). *The neurology of thinking.* New York: Oxford University Press.

Bernstein, I. S., Gordon, T. P., & Rose, R. M. (1983). The interaction of hormones, behavior, and social context in nonhuman primates. In B. B. Svare (Ed.), *Hormones and aggressive behavior* (pp. 535–561). New York: Plenum Press.

Cacioppo, J. T. (1994). Social neuroscience: Autonomic, neuroendocrine, and immune responses to stress. *Psychophysiology, 31*, 113–128.

Cacioppo, J. T., & Berntson, G. G. (1992). Social psychological contributions to the decade of the brain: The doctrine of multilevel analysis. *American Psychologist, 47*, 1019–1028.

Cacioppo, J. T., Gardner, W. L., & Berntson, G. G. (1999). The affect system has parallel and integrative processing components: Form follows function. *Journal of Personality and Social Psychology, 76*, 839–855.

Churchland, P. S., & Sejnowski, T. J. (1988). Perspectives on cognitive neuroscience. *Science, 242*, 741–745.

Crabbe, J. C., Wahlsten, D., & Dudek, B. C. (1999). Genetics of mouse behavior: Interactions with laboratory environment. *Science, 284*, 1670–1672.

Crick, F. (1970). Central dogma of molecular biology. *Nature, 227*, 561–563.

Fazio, R. H., Zanna, M. P., & Cooper, J. (1977). Dissonance and self perception: An integrative view of each theory's proper domain of application. *Journal of Experimental Social Psychology, 13*, 464–479.

Gardner, W. L., Gabriel, S., & Diekman, A. B. (2000). Interpersonal processes. In J. T. Cacioppo, L. G. Tassinary, & G. G. Berntson (Eds.), *Handbook of psychophysiology* (pp. 643–664). New York: Cambridge University Press.

Gerlai, R. (1996). Gene-targeting studies of mammalian behavior: Is it the mutation or the background genotype? *Trends in Neurosciences, 19*, 177–181.

Goldin-Meadow, S., & Mylander, C. (1983). Gestural communication in deaf children: Noneffect of parental input on language development. *Science, 221*, 372–374.

Goldin-Meadow, S., & Mylander, C. (1984). Gestural communication in deaf children: The effects and noneffects of parental input on early language development. *Monographs of the Society for Research in Child Development, 49*, 1–121.

Haber, S. N., & Barchas, P. R. (1983). The regulatory effect of social rank on behavior after amphetamine administration. In P. R. Barchas (Ed.), *Social hierarchies: Essays toward a sociophysiological perspective* (pp. 119–132). Westport, CT: Greenwood Press.

Harlow, H. F., & Harlow, M. K. (1973). Social deprivation in monkeys. In *Readings from the Scientific American: The nature and nurture of behavior* (pp. 108–116). San Francisco: W. H. Freeman.

House, J. S., Landis, K. R., & Umberson, D. (1988). Social relationships and health. *Science, 241*, 540–545.

Klein, S. B., & Kihlstrom, J. F. (1998). On bridging the gap between social-personality psychology and neuropsychology. *Personality and Social Psychology Review,* 2, 228–242.

Kosslyn, S. M., & Andersen, R. A. (1992). *Frontiers in cognitive neuroscience.* Cambridge, MA: MIT Press.

Luskin, F., & Newell, K. (1997). Mind-body approaches to successful aging (pp. 251–268). In A. Watkins (Ed.), *Mind-body medicine: A clinician's guide to psychoneuroimmunology.* New York: Churchill Livingstone.

Meaney, M. J., Sapolsky, R. M., & McEwen, B. S. (1985). The development of the glucocorticoid receptor system in the rat limbic brain: II. An autoradiographic study. *Developmental Brain Research,* 18, 159–164.

Mojtabai, R. (1994). Fregoli syndrome. *Australian and New Zealand Journal of Psychiatry,* 28, 458–462.

Oyebode, F., & Sargeant, R. (1996). Delusional misidentification syndromes: A descriptive study. *Psychopathology,* 29, 209–214.

Panksepp, J. (1998). *Affective neuroscience.* New York: Oxford University Press.

Rose, R. M., Gordon, T. P., & Bernstein, I. S. (1972). Plasma testosterone levels in the male rhesus: Influences of sexual and social stimuli. *Science,* 178, 643–645.

Scott, T. R. (1991). A personal view of the future of psychology departments. *American Psychologist,* 46, 975–976.

Signer, S. F. (1994). Localization and lateralization in the delusion of substitution. *Psychopathology,* 27, 168–176.

Spiegel, D. (2000). *Social support and health.* Unpublished manuscript, Stanford University, Stanford, California.

Tranel, D., & Damasio, A. R. (1985). Knowledge without awareness: An autonomic index of facial recognition by prosopagnosics. *Science,* 228, 1453–1454.

Trimble, M. R., Mendez, M. F., & Cummings, J. L. (1997). Neuropsychiatric symptoms from the temporolimbic lobes. *Journal of Neuropsychiatry and Clinical Neurosciences,* 9, 429–438.

Zillmann, D. (1984). *Connections between sex and aggression.* Hillsdale, NJ: Erlbaum.

II MULTILEVEL INTEGRATIVE ANALYSES OF SOCIAL BEHAVIOR

2 Genetics of Mouse Behavior: Interactions with Laboratory Environment

John C. Crabbe, Douglas Wahlsten, and Bruce C. Dudek

Targeted and chemically induced mutations in mice are valuable tools in biomedical research, especially in the neurosciences and psychopharmacology. Phenotypic effects of a knockout often depend on the genetic background of the mouse strain carrying the mutation (1), but the effects of environmental background are not generally known.

Different laboratories commonly employ their own idiosyncratic versions of behavioral test apparatus and protocols, and any laboratory environment also has many unique features. These variations have sometimes led to discrepancies in the outcomes reported by different labs testing the same genotypes for ostensibly the same behaviors (2). Previous studies could not distinguish between interactions arising from variations in the test situation itself and those arising from subtle environmental differences among labs. Usually, such differences are eventually resolved by repetition of tests in multiple labs. However, null mutants and transgenic mice are often scarce and tend to be behaviorally characterized in a single laboratory with a limited array of available tests.

We addressed this problem by testing six mouse behaviors simultaneously in three laboratories (Albany, New York; Edmonton, Alberta, Canada; and Portland, Oregon) using exactly the same inbred strains and one null mutant strain (3). We went to extraordinary lengths to equate test apparatus, testing protocols, and all possible features of animal husbandry (4). One potentially important feature was varied systematically. Because many believe that mice tested after shipping from a supplier behave differently from those reared in-house, we compared mice either shipped or bred locally at the same age (77 days) starting at the same time (0830 to 0900 hours local time on 20 April 1998) in all three labs (5). Each mouse was given the same order of tests [Day 1: locomotor activity in an open field; Day 2: an anxiety test, exploration of two enclosed and two open arms of an elevated plus maze; Day 3: walking and balancing on a rotating rod; Day 4: learning to swim to a visible platform; Day 5: locomotor activation after cocaine injection; Days 6 to 11: preference for drinking ethanol versus tap water (6)].

Despite our efforts to equate laboratory environments, significant and, in some cases, large effects of site were found for nearly all variables (Table 2.1). Furthermore, the pattern of strain differences varied substantially among the sites for several tests. Sex differences were only occasionally detected, and, much to our surprise, there were almost no effects of shipping animals before testing. Large genetic effects on all behaviors were confirmed, which is not surprising because we chose strains known to differ markedly on these tasks.

Results for locomotor activity and the effect of a subsequent cocaine injection on locomotion are shown in Fig. 2.1. Expected strain differences in undrugged activity were found: A/J mice were relatively inactive at all three sites, whereas C57BL/6J mice were very active. An effect of laboratory was also found: mice tested in Edmonton were, on average, more active than those tested in Albany or Portland. In addition, the pattern of genetic differences depended on site. For example, 129/SvEvTac mice tested in Albany were very inactive compared to their counterparts in other labs. Similar results were seen for sensitivity to cocaine stimulation. For example, B6D2F2 mice were very responsive (and A/J mice quite insensitive) to cocaine in Portland, but not at other sites.

In the elevated plus maze, a very similar pattern was seen: strong effects of genotype, site, and their interaction. This was true both for activity measures and for time spent in open arms, the putative index of anxiety (Fig. 2.2). For total arm entries, the testing laboratory was particularly

Table 2.1
Statistical significance and effect sizes for selected variables in the multisite trial

Task	Measure	Eight genotypes	Three sites	Two sexes	Local vs. shipped	Genotype × site	Genotype × sex	Genotype × ship	Multiple R^2
Open field	Distance in 15 min	.600	.157	—	—	.059	.045	—	.604
Open field	# vertical movements	.788	.281	.039	—	—	—	—	.772
Cocaine	Difference from Day 1	.338	.053	—	—	.086	—	—	.342
Plus maze	Total arm entries	.385	.327	—	—	.210	—	—	.660
Plus maze	Time in open arms	.082	.212	—	—	.066	—	—	.266
Water maze	Mean escape latency	.221	—	—	.026	—	—	—	.177
Alcohol preference	Alcohol consumed (g/kg)	.483	—	.043	—	—	—	—	.451
Body size	Weight (g)	.408	.204	.637	—	.071	.070	—	.698

Color of cell depicts Type I error probability or significance of main effects and two-way interactions from $8 \times 2 \times 3 \times 2$ analyses of variance: blue, $P < 0.00001$; purple, $P < 0.001$; gold, $P < 0.01$; dashes with no shading, $P > 0.01$. Cell entries are effect sizes, expressed as partial omega squared, the proportion of variance accounted for by the factor or interaction if only that factor were in the experimental design ($r = 0-1.0$). Multiple R^2 (unbiased estimate) gives the proportion of the variance accounted for by all factors. For the water escape task, results are based on only seven strains because most A/J mice never escaped because of wall-hugging. We recognize that the issue of appropriate alpha level correction for multiple comparisons is contentious. Details of the statistical analyses are available on the Web site,[4] including a discussion of our rationale for presenting uncorrected values in this table.

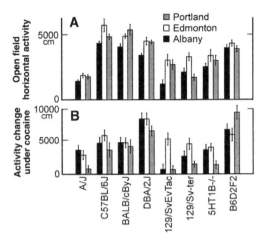

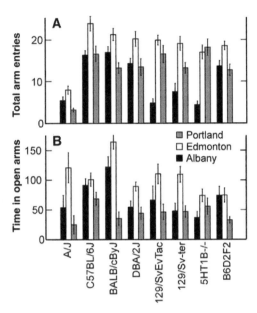

Figure 2.1
Group means ($\pm$ SEM for $n = 16$ mice) for activity in
a 40 cm $\times$ 40 cm open field for eight strains tested at
the same time of day in identical apparatus in three
laboratories. (A) Horizontal distance (centimeters)
traveled in 15 min on the first test on day 1. (B)
Cocaine-induced activation, expressed as the difference
between horizontal activity (centimeters in 15 min)
after cocaine (20 mg/kg) on day 5 minus the score on
day 1.

Figure 2.2
Group means ($\pm$ SEM for $n = 16$ mice) for behavior
videotape for 5 min on elevated plus mazes having two
open and two enclosed arms. (A) Total number of
entries into any arm (defined as all four limbs in the
arm). (B) Time (seconds) spent in the two open arms
during the 300-s test. Smaller amounts of time indicate
higher levels of anxiety.

important for the 5-HT$_{1B}$ knockout mice versus
their wild-type 129/Sv-ter background controls.
Knockout mice had greater activity than wild
types in Portland and tended to have less activity
in Albany, while not differing in Edmonton.
Edmonton mice of all strains spent more time
in open arms (lower anxiety). Portland mice also
spent less time in open arms, but this was especially true for strains A/J, BALB/cByJ, and the
B6D2F2 mice.

Although the testing laboratory was an important variable, there was a good deal of consistency to the genetic results as well. For example,
comparison of the genotype means (averaged
over sites) for the initial 5 min of the activity test
on Day 1 with the total arm entry scores from
the plus maze yielded a high correlation between
strains ($r = 0.91$, $P < 0.002$). This indicates that

a strain's characteristic activity in novel apparatus is robust and occurs in different apparatus as
well as different labs (7).

For some behaviors, laboratory environment
was not critical. For example, ethanol drinking
scores were closely comparable across all three
labs, and genotypes alone accounted for 48%
of the variance (Table 2.1 and Fig. 2.3). The genetic differences showed the well-known pattern
of C57BL/6J mice strongly preferring and DBA/
2J mice avoiding ethanol (8). Females drank
more, as is also well known (8), but there were no
significant effects of site, shipping, or any other
interactions. Unlike the other five tests, ethanol
preference testing extended over 6 days in the

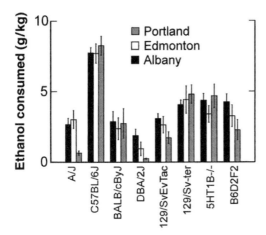

Figure 2.3
Mean ($\pm$ SEM) ethanol consumed per day, expressed as grams per kilogram body weight, over 4 days of an ethanol preference test where each mouse had free access to two drinking bottles, one with local tap water and the other with 6% ethanol in tap water.

home cage and involved a bare minimum of handling mice by the experimenter.

For some measures, the difference between 5-HT$_{1B}$ null mutant and wild-type mice depended on the specific laboratory environment. In Edmonton, for example, no difference was observed between $+/+$ and $-/-$ mice in distance traveled in the activity monitor, whereas there was greater activity in the knockouts at the other two sites, especially Portland ($P = 0.002$). In the elevated plus maze, knockouts were considerably more active than wild types only in Portland (Fig. 2.2A; $P = 0.02$).

The numbers of mice we tested made formal statistical assessment of reliability infeasible, but it would be important to know whether each laboratory would obtain essentially the same strain-specific results if this experiment were repeated. Because our experiment included an internal replication, we estimated the lower bounds of reliability for each site separately by correlating the

mean scores for each strain (collapsed over sex and shipping group) obtained during the two replicates of the experiment. These correlations differed depending upon the behavior, and were consonant with the relative importance of genotype in the overall analysis. For example, for locomotor activity, the correlations were 0.97, 0.74, and 0.87 for the three sites. For open-arm time on the plus maze, possibly the most intrinsically unstable task we employed, the correlations were lower (0.32, 0.52, and 0.26). These can be compared to correlations for body weight, which can serve as a type of control variable not influenced by idiosyncratic dynamics of the test situation (0.83, 0.74, and 0.90). No site had generally higher or lower reliability than the others, and formal analyses of replication in analyses of variance indicated no strong interactions of strain by replication. We conclude that reasonable estimates of strain-specific scores are highly dependent on behavioral endpoint, and that some behaviors are highly stable.

Several sources of these laboratory-specific behavioral differences could be ruled out by the rigor of the experimental design. For example, Edmonton mice might have been more sensitive to cocaine-induced locomotion because the source of cocaine differed from the other two sites (4), but this could not explain the relatively marked response of the three 129-derived strains in Edmonton only. However, specific experimenters performing the testing were unique to each laboratory and could have influenced behavior of the mice. The experimenter in Edmonton, for example, was highly allergic to mice and performed all tests while wearing a respirator—a laboratory-specific (and uncontrolled) variable.

Whether animals were bred in each laboratory or shipped as adults 5 weeks before testing had no consistent influence on results in this experiment. Shipped animals took routes of varying duration and difficulty. For example, some Taconic mice were trucked to Albany from nearby Germantown, New York, whereas others spent 2 days in transit during a flight in midwinter to Edmonton. At least in this experiment, allowing animals a lengthy period of acclimation to new quarters was sufficient to overcome any strong effects of putative shipping stress on subsequent behavior.

These results support both optimistic and pessimistic interpretations. Seen optimistically, genotype was highly significant for all behaviors studied, accounting for 30 to 80% of the total variability, and several historically documented strain differences were also seen here. In general, we conclude that very large strain differences are robust and are unlikely to be influenced in a major way by site-specific interactions. However, a more cautious reading suggests that for behaviors with smaller genetic effects (such as those likely to characterize most effects of a gene knockout), there can be important influences of environmental conditions specific to individual laboratories, and specific behavioral effects should not be uncritically attributed to genetic manipulations such as targeted gene deletions.

When studying mutant mice, relatively small genetic effects should first be replicated locally before drawing conclusions (9). We further recommend that, if possible, genotypes should be tested in multiple labs and evaluated with multiple tests of a single behavioral domain (such as several tests of anxiety-related behavior) before concluding that a specific gene influences a specific behavioral domain. We also suggest the possibility that laboratory-specific effects on genetic differences will affect phenotypes other than behaviors to an extent similar to that we report.

It is not clear whether standardization of behavioral assays would markedly improve future replicability of results across laboratories. Standardization will be difficult to achieve because most behaviorists seem to have differing opinions about the "best" way to assay a behavioral domain. For example, two of us typically test behavior during the light phase of the animals' cycle, whereas the third typically tests during the

dark phase (but switched to the light phase for this study). Which apparatus specifications or test protocol to employ is also a subject of differing opinion. There is a risk of prematurely limiting the "recommended" tests in a domain to those deemed "industry standard," because this may constrain the intrinsic richness of a domain and obscure interesting interactions. On the other hand, increased communication and collaboration between the molecular biologists creating mutations and behavioral scientists interested in the psychological aspects of behavioral testing will benefit both groups.

References and Notes

1. M. Sibilia and E. F. Wagner, *Science* 269, 234 (1995); R. Gerlai, *Trends Neurosci.* 19, 177 (1996); M. Nguyen et al., *Nature* 390, 78 (1997).

2. It has been known for some time that comparisons of multiple genotypes on learning-related tests do not always yield consistent results across laboratories [D. Wahlsten, in *Psychopharmacology of Aversively Motivated Behavior,* H. Anisman and G. Bignami, Eds. (Plenum, New York, 1978), pp. 63–118]. For another example, the Crabbe laboratory has reported that C57BL/6 mice show a small enhancement of locomotor activity after low doses of ethanol, while the Dudek laboratory finds no such stimulant response [J. C. Crabbe et al., *J. Comp. Physiol. Psychol.* 96, 440 (1982); B. C. Dudek and T. J. Phillips, *Psychopharmacology* 101, 93 (1990)]. Similar variation has been reported in other measures of activity in various laboratories and apparatus [J. M. LaSalle and D. Wahlsten, in *Techniques for the Genetic Analysis of Brain and Behavior: Focus on the Mouse,* D. Goldowitz, D. Wahlsten, R. E. Wimer, Eds. (Elsevier, Amsterdam, 1992), pp. 391–406].

3. We tested males and females from the inbred strains: A/J, BALB/cByJ, C57BL/6J, DBA/2J, 129/Sv-ter, and 129/SvEvTac; the F_2 hybrid cross of C57BL/6J and DBA/2J (B6D2F2); and the serotonin receptor subtype null mutant, 5-HT$_{1B}^{-/-}$, which is maintained on the 129/Sv-ter background. Mice were obtained from the Jackson Laboratory (Bar Harbor, ME), Taconic Farms (Germantown, NY), or the colonies of R. Hen

(Columbia University, New York, NY). Because many targeted deletions are placed on the 129/SvEvTac background, we included this close relative of 129/Sv-ter. The genealogy of many 129 substrains has recently been discussed [E. M. Simpson et al., *Nature Genet.* 16, 19 (1997); D. W. Threadgill, D. Yee, A. Matin, J. H. Nadeau, T. Magnuson, *Mamm. Genome* 8, 390 (1997)].

4. Details of procedures and test protocols are given in the Web site for this study (www.albany.edu/psy/obssr). Variables explicitly equated across laboratories included apparatus, exact testing protocols, age of shipped and laboratory-reared mice, method and time of marking before testing, food (Purina 5001; Purina 5000 for breeders), bedding (Bed-o-cob, 1/4 inch; Animal Specialties, Inc., Hubbard, OR), stainless steel cage tops, four to five mice per cage, light/dark cycle, cage changing frequency and specific days, male left in cage after births, culling only of obvious runts, postpartum pregnancy allowed, weaned at 21 days, specific days of body weight recording, and gloved handling without use of forceps. Unmatched variables included local tap water, requirement of filters over cage tops in Portland only, variation of physical arrangement of colonies and testing rooms across sites, different air handling and humidity, and different sources of batches of cocaine and alcohol.

5. All breeding stock was shipped on 2 or 3 December 1997, and mating pairs were set simultaneously on 13 January 1998 in all labs to provide "unshipped" mice for testing. On 15 to 17 March 1998, a second batch of mice from each genotype was shipped to each laboratory. These "shipped" mice, age matched with the unshipped cohort already in place, were allowed to acclimate to the laboratory for 5 weeks before testing commenced. We tested 128 mice in each lab, in two groups of 64 separated by 1 week. With an $n = 4$ mice in each genotype/shipping condition/sex/laboratory condition, we had 16 mice per group for the crucial genotype × laboratory comparisons. This sample size gave us statistical power of 90% to detect modest interactions of genotype × laboratory when Type I error probability was set at 0.01 [J. Cohen, *Statistical Power Analysis* (Erlbaum, Hillsdale, NJ, 1988); D. Wahlsten, *Behav. Brain. Sci.* 13, 109 (1990)]. For results of analysis of variance, we report only effects significant at $P < 0.01$. The Web site in (4) provides detailed protocols used for each test, descriptions of the laboratory conditions rigorously equated across labs, and

raw data that may be examined for other interesting patterns.

6. AccuScan Digiscan monitors (AccuScan Instruments, Columbus, OH) were generously loaned to D. Wahlsten by R. H. Kant to match those available in the other two laboratories. AccuScan also provided all sites with rotarod apparatus. Mouse-scaled water mazes and elevated plus mazes were constructed by D. Wahlsten and shipped to the other two labs. On the first test day, each mouse was tested for 15 min in a Digiscan open-field monitor in a dark, sound-attenuated chamber. On Day 2, each mouse was videotaped for 5 min in an elevated plus maze. On Day 3, mice were given 10 trials on a rotarod set to accelerate from 0 to 100 rpm in 75 s. After all mice had been tested on the rotarod, mice were pretrained briefly to escape from the water maze. On Day 4, mice were given eight massed trials of escape learning to a visible platform in the water maze. On Day 5, the activity test was repeated immediately following an ip injection of 20 mg of cocaine per kilogram. After 2 days of rest, mice were individually housed, given only tap water for 2 days, and then tested for 4 days for drinking of 6% ethanol in tap water versus tap water alone.

7. J. Flint et al., *Science* 269, 1432 (1995); S. R. Mitchell, J. K. Belknap, J. C. Crabbe, unpublished observations.

8. G. E. McClearn and D. A. Rodgers, *Q. J. Stud. Alcohol* 20, 691 (1959); J. K. Belknap, J. C. Crabbe, E. R. Young, *Psychopharmacology* 112, 503 (1993); L. A. Rodriguez et al., *Alcohol. Clin. Exp. Res.* 19, 367 (1995).

9. It was previously reported that 5-HT$_{1B}$ null mutant mice drank much more alcohol than the 129/Sv-ter wild-type strain [J. C. Crabbe et al., *Nature Genet.* 14, 98 (1996)]. In the experiments here, no site detected this difference (Fig. 2.3 and Table 2.1). The original outcome was replicated four times (J. C. Crabbe et al., unpublished data). It is possible that residual polymorphisms for genes segregating in the 129/SvPas substrain that served as the original source of the embryonic stem cell line and in the 129/Sv-ter substrain to which the null mutant was crossed have subsequently been fixed differentially in the 5-HT$_{1B}$ +/+ and −/− strains maintained at Columbia University (3). If so, these genes must exert very large epistatic effects on the 1B gene deletion's phenotypic effects on drinking (1). Alternatively, some undetected variable (for example, a

change in animal care personnel) may have occurred specifically at the Portland site between the original (1995–96) observations and the current experiments.

Supported by the Office of Behavioral and Social Sciences Research, NIH, as supplements to grants AA10760 (J.C.C.) and DA10731 (J. Marley and B.C.D., co-principal investigators), and by the Natural Sciences and Engineering Research Council of Canada Grant # 45825 (D.W.), the Department of Veterans Affairs (J.C.C.), and a K02 Award to B.C.D. AA00170. We thank R. H. Kant at AccuScan for the generous loan of equipment and R. Hen for providing the serotonin receptor mutants. We appreciate the comments of C. Cunningham, R. A. Harris, J. Janowsky, and G. Westbrook on a draft of this manuscript. We also thank S. Boehm II, S. Burkhart-Kasch, J. Dorow, S. Doerksen, C. Downing, J. Fogarty, K. Henricks, C. McKinnon, C. Merrill, P. Metten, C. Nolte, T. Phillips, M. Schalomon, J. Schlumbohm, J. Sibert, J. Singh, and C. Wenger for valuable assistance.

3 Multilevel Integrative Analyses of Human Behavior: Social Neuroscience and the Complementing Nature of Social and Biological Approaches

John T. Cacioppo, Gary G. Berntson, John F. Sheridan, and Martha K. McClintock

Social and biological approaches to human behavior have traditionally been contrasted as if the two were antagonistic or mutually exclusive. Consider the conclusion in the following news report, an interpretational bias that can also be found in the scientific literature:

Just five days after President Clinton announced in his State of the Union address, that the Justice Department is preparing to sue tobacco companies to recover money that Medicaid spends treating smoking-related diseases, scientists have given the companies a possible out. In papers published this week, geneticists report that a specific gene can affect whether or not someone starts smoking—and, if he does, whether he becomes addicted. People who have one particular gene, which is involved in the brain's use of the molecule dopamine, are less likely to smoke than those without the gene; if they do smoke, they start later and have an easier time quitting. So maybe it's not those Joe Camel ads after all. (Howard, O'Donnell, Stevenson, & Oxfeld, 1999, p. 6)

The thesis of this article is that the mechanisms underlying mind and behavior are not fully explicable by a biological or a social approach alone but rather that a multilevel integrative analysis may be required. All human behavior, at some level, is biological, but this is not to say that biological reductionism yields a simple, singular, or satisfactory explanation for complex behaviors or that molecular forms of representation provide the only or best level of analysis for understanding human behavior (Cacioppo & Berntson, 1992b; Gottlieb, 1998). Molar constructs such as those developed by the social sciences provide a means of understanding highly complex activity without needing to specify each individual action of the simplest components, thereby offering an efficient means of describing the behavior of a complex system (Cacioppo & Berntson, 1992a; Turkheimer, 1998).

Within the discipline of psychology, the tensions between biological and social approaches surface in biopsychology/behavioral neuroscience and social psychology. Biopsychology focuses on neural substrates and production mechanisms for behavior, whereas social psychology emphasizes multivariate systems and situational influences in studies of the impact of human association on mind and behavior. Human biology is anchored in concrete anatomy and genetics, providing fundamental elements from which to draw interconnections and with which to construct theory. The social world, in contrast, is a complex set of abstractions representing the actions and influences of and the relationships among individuals, groups, societies, and cultures. The differences in levels of analysis have resulted in distinct histories, research traditions, and technical demands, leaving what some regard both as an impassable abyss between social and biological approaches and as evidence of the impending demise of psychology as a discipline.

Psychology lacks a clear identity.... Some of the vectors along which the subdisciplines have matured ... have developed at obtuse angles to one another, and as the distance between them grows, they strain against the departmental membrane and are irritated by the requirements of common membership in a distended administrative unit. Social and biopsychology are an example. Most biopsychology students consider a core course in social psychology to be an impediment.... I assume that our students in social psychology reflect that sentiment about their core experience in biopsychology.... The centrifugal forces in psychology departments today far exceed the centripetal force of the departmental membrane. (Scott, 1991, p. 975)

The abyss between biological and social levels of organization is a human construction, however, one that must be bridged to achieve a complete understanding of human behavior.

Not long ago, it was thought that a set of master genes activated the DNA necessary to produce the appropriate proteins for development and behavior (Crick, 1970). The architects of this construction were conceived as the forces of evolution operating over millennia; the builders were conceived as encapsulated within each living cell far from the reach of personal ties or sociocultural influences. Human biology, however, has evolved within a fiercely social world, provides potentials and constraints for representation and behavior attuned to this social world, and is shaped profoundly by the social world.

The full complement of DNA is in each cell of the newborn, but evidence is mounting that signals from the internal and external environment play an important role in the constitution and transcription of DNA and in the translation of RNA to proteins (see, e.g., Bronfenbrenner & Ceci, 1994; Gottlieb, 1998). A distinction between genotype and phenotype that is situationally determined is evident in infants born with phenylketonuria (PKU). These infants lack the appropriate gene for an enzyme critical for protein metabolism (McClintock, 1979). This results in the inability to digest a particular amino acid present in certain foods (e.g., milk, dairy products), which in turn leads to the accrual of this amino acid and its metabolites, which can be toxic. When the levels of these compounds are high, normal neurological development is disrupted, and severe, irreversible mental retardation results. In most cases, however, it is possible to greatly attenuate this mental retardation by changing the diet of these infants until the critical period of neurological development has passed. Thus, PKU is an inherited behavioral trait that is innate in a genetic sense but not innate in the developmental sense because its occurrence can be diminished by modifying what the infant is fed (McClintock, 1979).

Early life experiences have also been shown to affect phenotypic expression in animals. Rats raised in enriched environments show more dendritic branching (Greenough, Juraska, & Volkmar, 1979), more postsynaptic dendritic spines (Globus, Rosenzweig, Bennett, & Diamond, 1973), and larger and more numerous synapses per neuron (Turner & Greenough, 1985). When a restricted sector of somatosensory cortex is deprived of its normal pattern of activation, the affected cortex becomes largely reactivated by inputs from adjoining and nearby skin fields (Kaas, Merzenich, & Killackey, 1983). Maternal stimulation during rearing affects the number of fibers in the corpus callosum and related areas in the central nervous system (see, e.g., Juraska & Kopik, 1988). Although the generalization of these findings from animals to humans needs to be demonstrated, they suggest clear connections rather than an impassable abyss between biological and social levels of organization. Studies that span biological and sociocultural levels of analysis are needed to examine these connections in humans and to plumb causal (including possible reciprocal) relationships and underlying mechanisms.

The nervous, endocrine, and immune systems were also once thought to function independently, outside the reach of the personal ties and cultural influences. Both of these simplifying assumptions are understandable given the complexities involved, and studies guided by these assumptions have led to impressive advances in knowledge. An inherent limitation in such studies, however, is that they are blind to linkages across these systems and to the mechanisms underlying these interactions. Research on the molecular aspects of neuroimmunomodulation, for instance, has revealed these to be integrative systems that communicate by a common biochemical language (i.e., shared ligands— compounds, such as cytokines, hormones, and neurotransmitters, that bind to receptors and exert functional actions). The discovery of adrenergic (see Madden, Thyagarajan, & Felton, 1998) and glucocorticoid (see, e.g., Bauer, 1983; Glaser, Kutz, MacCallum, & Malarkey, 1995) receptors on immune cells provided avenues through which the nervous and endocrine systems could exert their influence on immune function (see McCann et al., 1998). The immune system also acts on the central nervous system, as illustrated by studies of a peripheral immune cytokine (lymphocyte secretion) that is transduced into a neuronal signal and conveyed to the brain by means of afferent fibers in the vagus nerve (Maier & Watkins, 1998).

The assumption that nervous, endocrine, and immune systems operate outside the reach of sociocultural influences allowed focused study of isolated anatomical systems. The advances resulting from such studies do not imply logically that social psychological or behavioral approaches have been eclipsed or are obsolete, however. Research that considers contextual and social factors has uncovered new effects that challenge some of the existing conceptualizations in the neurosciences. For instance, strains of mice with specific genes inactivated (i.e., knockout mice) have become important tools in biomedical research. Although the phenotypic expression of a knockout has been known to depend on the genetic background (see, e.g., Gerlai, 1996), the effects of the environmental context were thought to be unimportant. Crabbe, Wahlsten, and Dudek (1999), however, demonstrated that the specific behavioral effects associated with a given knockout varied across testing environments within and across laboratories. Crabbe et al. noted that the specific experimenters performing the testing were unique to each laboratory and could have influenced the behavior of the mice, concluding that

for behaviors with smaller genetic effects (such as those likely to characterize most effects of a gene knockout), there can be important influences of environmental conditions specific to individual laboratories, and specific behavioral effects should not be uncritically attributed to genetic manipulations such as targeted gene deletions. (p. 1672)

As discussed below, the effects of social context also appear to be powerful determinants of the expression of autonomic, neuroendocrine, and immune reactions.

The documentation of associations between social and biological events does not prove that these events are causally linked, nor does it speak to the mechanisms underlying such effects. These are essential questions that need to be addressed, and we return to this issue in a later section. Generally speaking, however, the field is in a relatively embryonic stage with current knowledge about underlying mechanisms woefully inadequate. As the 21st century begins, specialization is increasing within the biological and social sciences. Some in the neurosciences contend that psychological/behavioral approaches have been eclipsed, whereas some in the social sciences contend that biological approaches are irrelevant to an understanding of society and culture (see Berntson & Cacioppo, in press). It is not surprising in this context that some departments have become fractionated and that alternative organizations to the discipline of psychology have been offered (cf. Gazzaniga, 1998; Scott, 1991). One aim here is to review evidence for the importance of adopting complementary social and biological levels of analysis in the study of complex biobehavioral phenomena.

We focus on a few relatively well-developed fields of research in the area of health and disease. Within the normal range of human behaviors, social and biological approaches are also beginning to advance understanding of affect and emotions, attraction and sexuality, social development, and altruism and aggression. By way of background, however, we start with a brief discussion of why the social world could conceivably be central to understanding the biology of the mind and behavior.

The Centrality of Personal Ties and Social Interactions

Evolution has sculpted the human genome to be sensitive to and succoring of contact and relationships with others. People form associations and connections with others from the moment they are born. The very survival of newborns depends on their attachment to and nurturance by others over an extended period of time (see Baumeister & Leary, 1995). The human brain may have evolved to recognize human faces holistically (Farah, Wilson, Drain, & Tanaka, 1998). Distress vocalization, a signaling mechanism designed to solicit and sustain care, is one of the most primitive forms of audiovocal communication (Carden & Hofer, 1990; Panksepp, Herman, Conner, Bishop, & Scott, 1978). Language, the bedrock of complex social interaction, is universal and ubiquitous in humans. Even in the rare instances in which language is not modeled or taught to nonhearing children, a language system nevertheless develops (see, e.g., Goldin-Meadow & Mylander, 1983, 1984).

The need to belong does not stop at infancy; rather, affiliation and nurturant social relationships are essential for physical and for psychological well-being across the life span (see, e.g., Cohen & Syme, 1985; Gardner, Gabriel, & Diekman, 2000; Seeman, 1996). The handling of rat pups alters maternal behavior toward the pups and affects the structure and reactivity of the hypothalamic pituitary adrenocortical system (Meaney, Sapolsky, & McEwen, 1985). These early influences on the stress-hormone system, in turn, affect the pups' reactions to stressors and possibly their susceptibility to disease in later life (King & Edwards, 1999; Meaney et al., 1996). If these results generalize to humans, their theoretical and clinical implications are of significant import.

In humans, hormonal (see, e.g., Uvns-Mosberg, 1997) and neurophysiological substrates of caregiving and attachment have been identified (see Carter, Lederhendler, & Kirkpatrick, 1997). Consistent with animal research, the restriction of social contact during infancy and childhood has dramatic effects on psychopathology across the life span (Carlson & Earls, 1997). People who report having contact with intimate friends not only are more likely to report that their lives are very happy as compared with those who do not report such contact (Burt, 1986) but also tend to have lower blood pres-

sure (see Uchino, Cacioppo & Kiecolt-Glaser, 1996). Disruptions of personal ties, whether through ridicule, discrimination, separation, divorce, or bereavement, are among the most stressful events people must endure (see Gardner et al., 2000).

The motivational potency of the absence of personal ties and social acceptance is reminiscent of more basic needs such as hunger. Solitary confinement is one of humankind's most severe punishments (Felthous, 1997). Ostracism, the exclusion by general consent from common privileges or social acceptance, is universal in its aversive and deleterious effects (Williams, 1997). Positively, tactile contact is a stronger determinant of mother–infant attachment than feeding (Harlow & Harlow, 1973). Subtle cultural influences can also rival more basic drives in governing feeding behavior and body weight (Becker, 1999).

Social and cultural influences not only cause behavior but alter biological processes as well. In such instances, a strictly physiological (or social) analysis is not sufficient to reveal the orderly relationships that exist, regardless of the sophistication of the measurement technology. For example, when Haber and Barchas (1983) investigated the effects of amphetamine on male Rhesus macaques, no clear contrast between the drug and placebo conditions was detected until each male's role in the social group was considered. When this social factor was taken into account, amphetamines were found to increase dominant behavior in males high in the social rank and to increase submissive behavior in low-ranking animals. Although, in retrospect, this pattern of data fits Hull-Spence drive theory in which arousal enhances habitual modes of response, the pattern became apparent only when considering the social and the biological contexts in which the behavior unfolds. The mechanisms underlying mind and behavior may therefore not be fully explicable by a biological or social approach alone; rather, a multilevel integrative analysis may be essential.

Social Influences on Genetic Constitution

In biology, the environment is seen as the agent of natural selection (Gottlieb, 1998). The notion that physical and social forces modulate gene frequency may therefore be regarded as uncontroversial. Mechanisms of selection may help explain otherwise perplexing demographic differences. For instance, the prevalence and incidence rates of hypertension, obesity, and Type 2 diabetes in immigrants from developing countries are substantially higher than in the majority population. Neel (1962) proposed the "thrifty gene" hypothesis—that across generations, individuals who were most likely to survive the hardship and food and water deprivation of developing countries inherited a gene (or set of genes) that conserved energy. Those who were constitutionally characterized by high insulin levels, low metabolism, high fat storage, and insulin resistance were more likely to survive these severe conditions. Migration from traditional lifestyles and environments to more sedentary lifestyles and calorie-dense environments has, therefore, been posited to increase the likelihood of obesity, Type 2 diabetes, and related diseases (see review by Osei, 1999). Such outcomes might be thought of as natural social (i.e., migratory patterns, lifestyle) and environmental (e.g., caloric density of the diet) influences on gene frequency in a population. The social forces operating as the agents of selection are not always so natural, however.

Wilson and Grim (1991) examined the historical record of the transatlantic slave trade and New World slavery from the 16th to 19th centuries to determine the circumstantial evidence for this reasoning (see also Anderson & Scott, 1999). More than 12 million young men and women were imported to the western hemisphere from Africa during the centuries of slave trade. Wilson and Grim estimated that the average mortality from capture to delivery on the West African coast was about 10%, mortality during confinement on the coast was about 12%, and

mortality during the transatlantic passage was about 12%–15%. Of those who made it to the western hemisphere, 10%–30% were estimated to not have survived the first 3 years of slavery, and mortality rates remained high thereafter. Fertility rates of the survivors were low, and infant mortality rates may have been as high as 50%. It is at least plausible, therefore, that the transatlantic slave trade, which continued for centuries, imposed a strong selection pressure favoring specific biological mechanisms enabling survival and reproduction under the harsh conditions of slave trading.

Wilson and Grim (1991) further hypothesized that the specific biological mechanism underlying these effects was the set-point for salt regulation. The combined hardships of food and water deprivation and intense physical demands, Wilson and Grim suggested on the basis of historical records, resulted in a high proportion of deaths by volume depletion. Cholera pandemics also swept through the New World, killing thousands of slaves. This led Wilson and Grim to conclude that

salt-depleting conditions and diseases seemed to be ubiquitous throughout the slavery period.... Individuals with an enhanced genetic-based ability to conserve salt (Na^+ conservers) would have a decided advantage over others under the severe salt-depletive conditions of slavery. (p. 1126)

Wilson and Grim's (1991) hypothesis is untestable, there is some uncertainty about the accuracy of their specific estimates, and the physical environment in West Africa during the 16th to 19th centuries may have been an important factor as well (see, e.g., Weder & Schork, 1994). It is nevertheless a provocative theory that has helped organize and explain some of the contemporary research on ethnic differences in hypertension (Anderson & Scott, 1999). Sodium intake results in cardiovascular volume expansion and an associated increase in arterial blood pressure, which triggers the kidney to increase sodium excretion until a new steady state is reached. If the kidneys retain more salt, a steady state is ultimately reached at a higher than normal blood pressure (Blaustein & Grim, 1991). If the high and nonrandom mortality rates that characterized the slave trade over 3 centuries resulted in a change in frequencies of specific genes—an increase in those favoring an elevated regulatory set-point for sodium balance—this could help explain why African Americans, relative to Whites, have higher rates of hypertension (see Anderson & Scott, 1999), greater sensitivity to increases in dietary salt (Luft, Rankin, et al., 1979), greater retention of an intravenous sodium load (Luft, Grim, Fineberg, & Weinberger, 1979), and better de-pressor responses to diuretics (Freis, Reda, & Materson, 1988).

Even here, though, the phenotypic expression of blood pressure is sensitive to social and environmental factors (Anderson & Scott, 1999; Grim et al., 1990; Light et al., 1995; Saab et al., 1997; Wilson, Hollifield, & Grim, 1991). In a study of 10,014 African Americans in Nigeria, Cameroon, Jamaica, St. Lucia, Barbados, and Chicago, for instance, Cooper et al. (1997) found that the prevalence of hypertension rose with urbanization. Specifically, mean arterial pressure was similar among young adults (aged 25–34), but the increase in hypertension prevalence with age was significantly steeper in the United States than in the Caribbean and twice as steep in the United States as in Africa. Stress on the job and lack of control in everyday life—features of urbanization—have been found to covary with elevated ambulatory blood pressure, increased left ventricular mass index, increased progression of atherosclerosis, and increased risk of coronary heart disease (Bosma et al., 1997; Schnall, Schwartz, Landsbergis, Warren, & Pickering, 1992).

As suggestive as these studies might be, none prove any necessary or causal influence between social factors and cardiovascular function. We therefore turn to the experimental literature on social factors and cardiovascular function.

Social Influences on Cardiovascular Function

Animal studies provide among the best experimental evidence for social influences on autonomic function and cardiovascular disease. In a series of studies in cynomolgus monkeys, for instance, Manuck, Kaplan and colleagues (e.g., Manuck, Marsland, Kaplan, & Williams, 1995; Skantze et al., 1998) demonstrated that social disruptions and instability promote coronary atherogenesis. Specifically, animals exhibiting a heightened cardiac reactivity to stress were found to develop the most extensive coronary lesions, whereas beta-adrenergic blockade—a pharmacological intervention that blocks the sympathetic activation of the heart—was found to prevent the behavioral exacerbation of atherosclerosis. To study the effects of a stressful social environment, social groups were repeatedly reorganized. Macaque males respond antagonistically to the presence of strangers and reassert their hierarchic relationships (Kaplan et al., 1982). Disruptions of social connections increased the formation of endothelial lesions even in the absence of an atherosclerosis-inducing diet (Kaplan et al., 1983), an effect that was again eliminated by beta-adrenergic blockade (see, e.g., Skantze et al., 1998). These results implicate the sympathetic nervous system in the etiology of behaviorally induced atherosclerosis.

The incidence of atherosclerosis is lower for premenopausal females than for similarly aged males, an effect found in humans and monkeys (cynomolgus macaques). Kaplan et al. (1984) found that premenopausal female monkeys developed significantly less coronary artery atherosclerosis than similarly housed males but only if the females were socially dominant. The mechanism underlying this effect is different for females than for males, however (Kaplan et al., 1996). Subordinate monkeys were found to have fewer ovulatory cycles, reduced levels of circulating estradiol, and altered luteal phase plasma progesterone concentrations. Ovariectomized females fed an atherogenic diet resulted in endothelial lesions in dominant females that were comparable to those found in reproductively intact subordinate females (Adams, Kaplan, Koritnik, & Clarkson, 1987). These results suggest that estrogen serves a protective function against atherosclerosis. In a subsequent study, subordinate premenopausal females and dominant females developed comparably low levels of atherosclerosis when fed an atherogenic diet and an oral contraceptive containing estrogen (ethinyl estradiol and levonorgestrel), relative to subordinate females fed an atherogenic diet (Kaplan et al., 1995). These results suggest that social subordination impairs ovarian function, thereby potentiating atherosclerosis.

In both males and females in this research, high cardiovascular reactivity has been associated with increased risk for atherosclerosis. Light and colleagues have similarly focused on cardiovascular reactivity but have examined its relationship to hypertension and predisease indicators of hypertension such as left ventricular mass—essentially, the size of the muscle of the left ventricle of the heart (Hinderliter, Light, Girdler, Willis, & Sherwood, 1996; Light, Girdler, & Hinderliter, 2000). For instance, Hinderliter et al. (1996) found that the magnitude of blood pressure responses during laboratory stressors and natural life demands was a stronger predictor of left ventricular mass index and relative vascular wall thickness than either clinical blood pressure or baseline blood pressure. These and related studies by Light and colleagues indicate that cardiovascular responses to the demands of everyday life add prognostic information to that which can be obtained from clinical blood pressure levels (Light et al., 2000).

The risk of hypertension varies with family history. To test whether stress reactivity to the demands of everyday life would increase the risk of later blood pressure elevation in those individuals with a genetic susceptibility to develop hypertension, Light et al. (1999) conducted a 10-year follow-up study of 103 young men. Results revealed that men with a positive family history of hypertension had a twofold increase in risk of elevated blood pressure over 10 years as compared with men with a negative family history. However, men with a positive family history who also were in the top quartile in cardiovascular reactivity—as measured 10 years earlier—had a sevenfold increase in risk. In addition, high exposure to stress fostered increases in blood pressure at the follow-up in the high reactors. Importantly, it tends to be social stressors, not postural changes and exercise, that elicit these damaging cardiovascular reactions (Light et al., 1999).

The generalizability of the animal studies to humans can be questioned, and longitudinal research on the development or exacerbation of hypertension in humans has tended to use samples of convenience, is generally correlational, and typically relies on predisease markers or risk factors rather than disease end points. Rather than looking for increased blood pressure following social disruption, a handful of intervention studies exist with a complementing aim— to foster social support in an attempt to lower blood pressure in hypertensives. In a classic study, Levine et al. (1979) identified 400 hypertensive patients and assigned them to interventions consisting of an exit interview, family support, small group, various combinations of these three, or a control condition. In the family support intervention, for instance, patients identified an individual with whom they had frequent contact (e.g., spouse), and these individuals were trained to increase understanding, support, and reinforcement about the positive management of the patient's hypertension. Assessment at an 18-month follow-up indicated that family support was associated with an 11% decrease in diastolic blood pressure, and all of the interventions combined produced a 28% decrease. Subsequent follow-ups revealed that there were long-term benefits in blood pressure regulation as well (Morisky, DeMuth, Field-Fass, Green, & Levine, 1985). Meta-analyses of this and related studies confirmed that increases in social support resulted in decreased blood pressure in hypertensive patients (Uchino, Cacioppo, & Kiecolt-Glaser, 1996). Together, studies of social influences on cardiovascular function suggest substantial plasticity in the relationship between genetic factors and the development of cardiovascular disease.

Social Influences on Genetic Expression

As noted above, a central precept of molecular biology is that all the information needed to construct a mammalian body, whether human or mouse, is contained in the approximately 100,000 genes of mammalian DNA and that a set of master genes activates the DNA necessary to produce the appropriate proteins for development and behavior (Crick, 1970; Panksepp, 1998). Our thesis in this article is that the social world, as well as the organization and operation of the brain, shapes and modulates genetic and biological processes, and accordingly, knowledge of biological and social domains is necessary to develop comprehensive theories in either domain. In this section, we review evidence that some aspects of genetic expression that had been thought to be encapsulated within each living cell far from the reach of personal ties or social influences are in fact subject to modulation by the social environment (see Gottlieb, 1998).

In broad brush strokes, DNA encodes the sequence of amino acids in proteins and peptides by the sequence of nucleotides in the gene. By means of the process of transcription, involving RNA polymerases (enzymes), this sequential code is transferred to messenger RNA (mRNA), followed by translation to polypeptide chains and proteins. Recent research on the control of the secretion of lymphocyte growth hormone (L-GH) by peripheral blood mononuclear cells indicates that the social world can modulate transcription processes (as reflected in differences in mRNA levels). Briefly, Wu, Devi, and Malarkey (1996) localized (by in situ hybridization) growth hormone messenger RNA (GH mRNA)

in human immune organs, including the thymus, lymph nodes, spleen, and peripheral blood, as well as in thymomas and lymphomas. The extant literature on growth hormone suggests that it can influence cellular immunity by altering the efficacy of lymphocytes in responding to antigens (Wu et al., in press). The genetic transcriptions responsible for the production of L-GH are in part predetermined, as evidenced by the robust finding that L-GH secretion decreases with aging. However, Malarkey et al. (1996; Wu et al., in press) also found evidence for the modulation of L-GH levels by social stressors. Specifically, caregivers of spouses with Alzheimer's disease were found to have markedly suppressed L-GH concentrations compared with age- and gender-matched controls. Although more research is needed to specify the mechanism by which the social world modulates GH mRNA, stress hormones such as adrenocorticotropic hormone, cortisol, and catecholamines appear to play a role through their regulatory effects on lymphocytes.

The social influence on phenotypic expression is also illustrated in recent research on early nurturance. Suomi (1999) selectively bred Rhesus monkeys to produce offspring who, on the basis of their genetic pedigree, were either normally or highly reactive to stressors. These selectively bred infants were then cross-fostered to unrelated multiparous females who were either normally or unusually nurturant with respect to attachment-related behavior. The infants were reared by their foster mothers for the first 6 months of life and were then placed in a larger social group containing age-mates who were cross-fostered or were raised by their biological mothers (Suomi, 1987). Genetically high-reactive infants raised by normal (i.e., highly reactive) females showed the typical deficits in early exploration and accentuated responses to mild stressors, relative to genetically high-reactive infants raised by especially nurturant females. These latter infants explored their environments more and showed as little disturbance to mild stressors as, or lower levels than, their genetically high-reactive counterparts who were fostered by normal rather than nurturant mothers. Behavioral differences among these groups persisted when these monkeys were permanently separated from their foster mothers and were placed into a larger social group at 6 months of age (Suomi, 1991). Although the results are preliminary, Suomi (1999) reported that the serotonin transporter gene (5-HTTT)—and specifically, a 5-HTTT polymorphism, LS (short) vs. LL (long) 5-HTT allele—may be involved. Bennett et al. suggested that relatively nurturant mothering may buffer the deleterious developmental effects of the LS allele on serotonin metabolism and aggression.

Studies of rodents and monkeys have found that genetically highly reactive females also exhibit aberrant patterns of maternal care. For instance, Fischer rats are characterized by high hypothalamic–pituitary–adrenal (HPA) reactivity to stressors, whereas Lewis rats are characterized by low HPA reactivity. Accordingly, the Fischer rats have a lower threshold for stress reactions and show larger responses to stressors than Lewis rats. Fischer and Lewis dams also differ in their attention to and nurturance of their pups, with Fischer dams being much less attentive and nurturant even in the absence of an explicit stressor (Gomez, Riley, & Sternberg, 1997). A similar difference in maternal care has been observed in Rhesus monkeys (see, e.g., Suomi & Levine, 1998). Early nurturance appears capable of modifying this genetic predisposition, however. Suomi (1999), for instance, reported that genetically reactive females raised the first 6 months of life by an unusually nurturant mother "adopted the general maternal style of their foster mothers, independent of both their own original reactivity profile and the type of maternal style shown by their biological mothers" (p. 193).

Research on rats further suggests that early tactile deprivation reduces the number of glucocorticoid receptor binding sites in the hippocampus and frontal cortex by means of an action on gene expression (Meaney et al., 1985). Studies of rat pups indicate that transient early-life stress (e.g., brief handling) attenuates the behavioral and neuroendocrine responses to stressors encountered in adulthood, whereas early-life exposure to more severe stressors (e.g., protracted separation from the dam) accentuates responses to stressors in adulthood (Anisman, Zaharia, Meaney, & Merali, 1998). These effects appear to be mediated by variations in maternal care. Specifically, the brief handling of rat pups leads to greater maternal nurturance, increased glucocorticoid receptor binding sites in the hippocampus and frontal cortex, and lowered HPA reactivity in adulthood, whereas severe early-life stress has the opposite effects (Anisman et al., 1998; Meaney et al., 1993). Interestingly, as adult rats, the offspring of mothers that exhibited more licking and grooming and nurturance of pups during the first 10 days of life were not only characterized by reduced adrenocorticotropic hormone and corticosterone responses to acute stress but also, as mothers, tended to lick and groom their pups more (Liu et al., 1997).

Additional studies on the social influence of genetic expression are reviewed in the next section on psychoneuroimmunology. Together, these studies clearly illustrate synergistic influences between the social and biological levels of organization. The specific genes or social factors that interact may differ across species, but given the importance and complexities of genotypes and social factors in humans, the short-term and long-term modulation of genetic expression by social factors is almost certainly important to consider if a comprehensive model of human nature is to be developed. In monkeys, rats, mice, and humans, developmental processes and long-term health are not fully comprehensible if limited solely to either the social or the biological level of analysis.

Social Influences on Immune Activity

Empirical observations of social influences on autonomic activity date back more than 2,000 years (Mesulam & Perry, 1972). Until recently, however, immune functions were thought to reflect specific and nonspecific physiological responses to pathogens or tissue damage. It is now clear that the immune system is tightly regulated and integrated with the nervous and endocrine systems and that social events influence immune function through these systems. As noted above, a bidirectional communication network composed of soluble ligands and cellular receptors links both afferent and efferent limbs of the immune system to the nervous and endocrine systems. Thus, a stimulus within the nervous system that activates the sympathetic adrenomedullary (SAM) and HPA axis results in peripheral release of catecholamines and adrenal steroids, respectively, that have immunoregulatory potential. Similarly, a challenge within host tissue that induces an inflammatory response (e.g., an infection or a wound) results in the release of cytokines that stimulate peripheral and central circuits of the nervous system. This communication provides an important link through which the neuroendocrine response modulates the development of an inflammatory response at a site of challenge (Kusnecov, Liang, & Shurin, 1999; Maier & Watkins, 1998).

This communication system appears to be tuned, presumably by direct sympathetic innervation and circulating neuroendocrines, to social interactions, as well as to pathogens and tissue damage. Persons in marital conflict (see, e.g., Kiecolt-Glaser et al., 1987), taking important examinations (see, e.g., Kiecolt-Glaser, Garner, Speicher, Penn, & Glaser, 1984), and living near the site of a serious nuclear-power plant accident (McKinnon, Weisse, Reynolds, Bowles, & Baum, 1989) have been found to show diminished immune function on quantitative and functional measures. Clinical depression (Herbert & Cohen, 1993a) and psychological distress (Herbert & Cohen, 1993b) have also been associated with decreased immune function. Small immunological decrements do not necessarily indicate poorer health status or risk for disease among young

and healthy adults, however. Studies of the effects of psychosocial stress on vaccine responses have therefore been conducted to help address this criticism (see Glaser, Rabin, Chesney, Cohen, & Natelson, 2000). Using the stress of taking a university examination (Glaser et al., 1992) or the chronic stress of being a caregiver (Glaser, Kiecolt-Glaser, Malarkey, & Sheridan, 1998; Kiecolt-Glaser, Glaser, Gravenstein, Malarkey, & Sheridan, 1996), Glaser and colleagues found that the response to vaccination was diminished in high- compared with low-stress conditions. Because respiratory and viral infections remain a major cause of morbidity and mortality among older adults (McGlone & Arden, 1987), the differences in immune response to influenza virus vaccination in the elderly were thought to have health significance (Glaser et al., in press).

Another arena of research that has emerged in part to improve experimental control and in part to address the health relevance of the changes in immune function found in psychoneuroimmunological studies is wound healing. An individual is protected from infection following wounding by the rapid reestablishment of the barrier provided by intact mucosal surfaces or skin. This process is orchestrated by early inflammatory responses that include proinflammatory cytokines (e.g., IL-1 and TNF), chemokines (e.g., IL-8, MCP-1, and MIP-1α), and growth factors (e.g., keratinocyte growth factor and vascular endothelial growth factor). Consequently, the speed and completeness of wound healing has health relevance (Marucha, Kiecolt-Glaser, & Favagehi, 1998). Perhaps more importantly, the wound-healing paradigm affords greater experimental control over individual differences and spurious behavioral and contextual factors in human studies. For instance, Kiecolt-Glaser and colleagues examined wound healing and the immunological responses contributing to this end point in spousal caregivers of patients with Alzheimer's disease and age- and gender-matched controls (Kiecolt-Glaser, Marucha, Malarkey, Mercado, & Glaser, 1995) and in dental school students when they were or were not undergoing exams (Kiecolt-Glaser, Page, Marucha, MacCallum, & Glaser, 1998; Marucha et al., 1998). In both models, higher levels of stress were associated with delayed wound healing.

If social disruptions are transduced to the level of regulation of gene expression, it is conceivable that the expression of host resistance genes (encoded within the cells of the immune system) can also be modulated by social disruption. To test this hypothesis, Padgett and Sheridan (1999) developed an experimental model in which they explored the biological effects of reorganizing established murine (mouse) hierarchies during a respiratory viral infection. Results revealed that social disruption led to significantly higher mortality due to viral infection than found in home-cage control animals (Padgett & Sheridan, 1999). Further analyses revealed that the increased severity of the infection leading to mortality was associated with the development of hyper-inflammatory responses due to overexpression of key cytokine genes. The increased cell trafficking and accumulation in the lungs of infected animals led to tissue consolidation or congestion and, consequently, to diminished lung function. Importantly, a different result was found for nonsocial stress (i.e., physical restraint). The physical restraint paradigm is devoid of social interactions but activates the HPA axis in a fashion similar to the psychosocial stressor. Thus, physical restraint is as stressful to the animal as social disruption, but the stressor is centered on the animal's interaction with the physical rather than the social world. In physical restraint, hypo-inflammatory (rather than hyper-inflammatory) responses were observed during respiratory viral infection in these animals, due to suppression of cytokine responses by glucocorticoid hormones. Consequently, the observed rate of mortality was much lower in these infected animals than in those who were infected and exposed to social disruptions.

The social ordering within social hierarchies may also play a role in the individual responses to psychosocial stress and susceptibility to in-fectious disease. For instance, in the social disruption paradigm, dominant male mice, when latently infected in the trigeminal ganglia with herpes simplex virus (HSV; a model for recurrent herpes labialis in humans), were twice as likely as subordinate animals to reactivate and shed infectious virus when their social environment was disrupted by reorganization (Padgett, Sheridan, et al., 1998). The psychosocial nature of the stressor was again important, as simply stressing latently infected mice by physical restraint did not cause reactivation (Padgett, Sheridan, et al., 1998).

The key finding of these experimental studies is that social interactions influenced physiological signals that modulate the expression of individual host/pathogen genes. In the model of latent HSV infection, the inactive viral genome represents an environmental (or foreign) gene that has parasitized the host. It resides in the neurons of the trigeminal ganglia and remains latent or inactive until an appropriate set of physiological signals is received. Although the reason is not entirely understood yet, psychosocial stress provided the appropriate set of signals for reactivation of the viral genes leading to recurrent infection and the shedding of infectious virus (Padgett, Sheridan, et al., 1998).

The focus in these studies is on the immuno-suppressive effects of stress, but acute stressors can also facilitate the development of localized immunity by causing cells of the immune system, such as lymphocytes and macrophages, to redistribute throughout the body (Dhabhar & McEwen, 1997; Dhabhar, Miller, McEwen, & Spencer, 1995; see also Uchino, Cacioppo, Malarkey, & Glaser, 1995). Immune cells marginate on blood vessel walls and traffic or localize within the skin, lymph nodes, and bone marrow (Dhabhar et al., 1995). It has been suggested that the regional positioning of these immunocytes (in response to acute stress) may provide the host with a selective advantage should aggressive behavioral interactions lead to cutaneous wounding and the possibility of infection

(Dhabhar & McEwen, 1997). The selective advantage that may accompany acute stress does not extend to chronic forms of stress, however, as the prolonged activation of the HPA axis and sympathetic nervous system seen in chronic stress tends to suppress cellular immunity (Lupien & McEwen, 1997; Sheridan, 1998), reduce response to vaccination (Kiecolt-Glaser et al., 1996), and slow the healing of experimental cutaneous and mucosal wounds (Kiecolt-Glaser et al., 1995; Marucha et al., 1998; Padgett, Marucha, & Sheridan, 1998). Accordingly, it is the prolonged activation of the HPA axis and sympathetic nervous system that is thought to underlie the disruption of normal immune functioning by chronic family or job strain, although this is almost certainly an incomplete answer.

Social Influences on Disease

One implication of the research reviewed thus far is that the development and progression of disease, once bastions of the biological approach, may be influenced dramatically by social factors (Anderson, 1998). Epidemiological research has indeed marshaled evidence for a strong relationship between health and various social circumstances (see, e.g., Adler et al., 1994; Carroll & Sheffield, 1998; Kitagava & Hauser, 1973; Rogot, Sorlie, Johnson, & Schmit, 1993; Townshend & Davidson, 1982). In a classic study, Berkman and Syme (1979) operationalized social connections as marriage, contacts with friends and extended family members, church membership, and other group affiliations. They found that adults with fewer social connections suffered higher rates of mortality over the succeeding 9 years even after accounting for self-reports of physical health, socioeconomic status, smoking, alcohol consumption, obesity, race, life satisfaction, physical activity, and preventive health-service usage.

House, Robbins, and Metzner (1982) replicated these findings using physical examinations to assess health status. In their review of five prospective studies, House, Landis, and Umberson (1988) concluded that social isolation was a major risk factor for morbidity and mortality from widely varying causes. This relationship was evident even after statistically controlling for known biological risk factors, social status, and baseline measures of health. The negative health consequences of social isolation were particularly strong among some of the fastest growing segments of the population: the elderly, the poor, and minorities such as African Americans. The strength of social isolation as a risk factor was comparable to high blood pressure, obesity, sedentary lifestyles, and possibly even smoking. House et al. (1988) concluded that

the mere presence of, or sense of relatedness with, another organism may have relatively direct motivational, emotional, or neuroendocrinal effects that promote health either directly or in the face of stress or other health hazards but that operate independently of cognitive appraisal or behavioral coping and adaptation. (p. 544)

A meta-analytic review of the experimental literature revealed that perceived social isolation was associated with physiological adjustments, with the most reliable effects found for blood pressure, catecholamines, and aspects of both cellular and humoral immune function (Uchino et al., 1996; see also Seeman & McEwen, 1996). These results could not be explained entirely in terms of existing individual differences because intervention studies designed to reduce social isolation improved physiological functioning (Uchino et al., 1996). People's perceptions of others in light of their desire for affiliation appear to be important, too, as subjective indices of social isolation/support have been found to be more powerful predictors of stress and health than objective indices (see Seeman, 1996; Uchino et al., 1996).

Although individual differences and differences in health behaviors may contribute to health outcomes, social isolation and stress appear to diminish health by means that are not yet fully understood. Cohen, Tyrrell, and Smith (1991), for instance, tested 420 healthy volunteers, measured their level of stress (e.g., perceived stress, major life events), and exposed them to saline or one of five different strains of Rhinoviruses, to a strain of coronavirus, and to respiratory syncytial virus. Following inoculation, participants were quarantined and monitored for the development of disease. After 7 days of quarantine, each participant was classified as not infected, infected but not ill, or infected and ill. No participant who was exposed to saline became ill, and about a third of the participants exposed to the cold viruses became ill.

Three measures of stress were related to disease onset: a stressful-life-event scale to measure the cumulative event load, a perceived-stress scale to assess perceptions of overload-induced stress, and a measure of negative affect. For each measure, participants were categorized as under high or low stress according to whether their score on each scale fell above or below the median score. For all three measures, participants who reported high stress were more likely to develop an infectious disease than those who reported low stress. In a follow-up study, Cohen et al. (1998) used an interview to determine the type of stressors that increased susceptibility for disease. Results revealed that risk was increased most by stressors lasting over a month, especially social conflicts, unemployment, and underemployment. The effect appears to be replicable; more research is now needed to delineate the mechanism underlying these findings.

The research by Cohen and colleagues also suggests that close relationships are not uniformly positive or salubrious. Indeed, results from the Terman Life Cycle Study indicate that past negative behaviors in social relationships are associated with greater mortality (Friedman et al., 1995; Tucker, Friedman, Wingard, & Schwartz, 1996). Laboratory research has found that negative or hostile behaviors during a marital conflict produce greater and/or more persistent alterations in autonomic activation (Gottman & Lev-

enson, 1992; Levenson, Cartensen, & Gottman, 1994) and circulating stress hormones (Kiecolt-Glaser, Malarkey, Cacioppo, & Glaser, 1994; Kiecolt-Glaser et al., 1997). Moreover, couples characterized by high, relative to low, negative behaviors during a marital conflict also showed greater decrements in cellular immune function over the 24 hours of study (e.g., natural killer-cell lysis, the blastogenic response to two mitogens, the proliferative response to a monoclonal antibody to the T3 receptor; Kiecolt-Glaser et al., 1994). In a cross-sectional study of young and older adults, Uchino, Holt-Lunstad, Uno, and Flinders (1999) found that high ambivalence was associated with increasing levels of depression and cardiovascular reactivity as a function of age. As in the animal studies, studies of humans suggest that feeling embattled or feeling isolated can have deleterious health consequences. Sympathetic hyper-reactivity (see, e.g., Uchino et al., 1996) and elevated HPA activation (see, e.g., Cacioppo et al., in press) may be especially fruitful candidates for study as mediators between social disruptions and disease.

Multilevel Integrative Analyses

The Decade of the Brain has led to a realization that a comprehensive understanding of the brain cannot be achieved by a focus on neural mechanisms alone, and advances in molecular biology have made it clear that genetic expressions are not entirely encapsulated, that heritable does not mean predetermined. A social or behavioral level of analysis is also insufficient, of course. Social processes and behavior are profoundly affected by brain injury, as documented in cases such as that of Phineas Gage (Damasio, 1994; Macmillan, 1986). Phineas Gage was a railway worker who was described as an exemplary citizen, energetic, shrewd in personal and financial affairs, and persistent. At work one day, he accidentally ignited an explosive charge, driving his tamping iron through his skull and ravaging the ventromedial aspects of the most anterior portions of the frontal cortex in the left and right hemispheres. Gage's personality changed permanently and profoundly following the accident. He became profane, impatient, capricious, and impulsive, as well as given to outbursts of anger and rage. The social relationships that existed prior to the accident deteriorated thereafter.

Individuals who lose the amygdala and associated inferior portions of the temporal cortex exhibit another disruption of social propriety known as the Kluver-Bucy syndrome (Kluver & Bucy, 1939). These individuals are characterized by a loss of fear and increased and inappropriate sexual activity. Prosopagnosics, who typically have bilateral lesions in the occipital lobes near the temporal lobes, do not undergo a change in personality but have another disturbing problem that alters their social behavior: They no longer recognize the faces of those they once knew (e.g., spouses) even though they show larger skin conductance responses to familiar faces (Tranel, Fowles, & Damasio, 1985). Interested readers should see Klein and Kihlstrom (1998) for a recent review of this literature, but the examples here illustrate that everyday social behaviors such as sexuality, decorum, aggression, altruism, conformity, and social influence are quintessentially social and neurophysiological processes.

Several general principles may help organize research in this area (Anderson, 1998; Cacioppo & Berntson, 1992b). First, the principle of multiple determinism specifies that a target event at one level of organization—particularly at molar (e.g., social) levels of organization—may have multiple antecedents within or across levels of organization. Eating, for instance, is influenced by both hunger and social cues (Cornell, Rodin, & Weingarten, 1989).

The principle of nonadditive determinism specifies that properties of the whole are not always readily predictable from the properties of the parts (Cacioppo & Berntson, 1992b). This principle is evident in a study of male mice

infected intranasally with a respiratory virus (Padgett & Sheridan, 1999). One group was left in their home cage (five mice per cage), a second group was exposed to 12 hrs of daily restraint stress, and a third group underwent social reorganization (dominant animal shifted to new cage on Days −3, −1, +1, and +3 of infection). Corticosterone levels were equally elevated in the stressed groups, relative to the control group. Within 8 days of the infection, however, approximately 8% of the control group died, 15% of the restraint stressed group died, and 70% of the socially stressed group died (Padgett & Sheridan, 1999). The order in these data is not fully comprehensible at any one level of organization but instead emerges when viewed across social and biological levels of analysis.

Associations do not imply causation, but often, the causal direction that is tested depends on one's disciplinary level of analysis. The principle of reciprocal determinism specifies that there can be mutual influences between microscopic (e.g., biological) and macroscopic (e.g., social) factors in determining behavior (Cacioppo & Berntson, 1992b). For example, not only has the level of testosterone in nonhuman male primates been shown to promote sexual behavior but also the availability of receptive females influences the level of testosterone (Bernstein, Gordon, & Rose, 1983; Rose, Gordon, & Bernstein, 1972). Zillmann (1984) has demonstrated that exposure to violent and erotic materials influences the level of sympathetic arousal in male humans, and that the level of arousal has a reciprocal influence on the perceptions of and tendencies toward sex and aggression. A low-reactive HPA system produces an adult rat who is low in stress reactivity, who is attentive to offspring, and who frequently licks and grooms the offspring. Licking and grooming, however, are essential for the offspring to develop into a low-reactive adult who frequently licks and grooms offspring (Liu et al., 1997). Given the reciprocal influences between social and biological processes, comprehensive accounts of these behaviors will remain elusive as long as either biological or social levels of organization are considered unnecessary or irrelevant.

In writing about unhealthy environments, Taylor, Repetti, and Seeman (1997) articulated a general framework for thinking about how social factors penetrate the skin. Although Taylor et al. focused on the effects of race and social class on health, the routes are applicable generally to the question of how other social factors get under the skin. These routes, although distinguishable, are not mutually exclusive.

The first route emphasizes the cumulative effects of chronic or repeated stressors. Primary caregivers for spouses with dementia, who are subject to years of daily physical and social stressors, also show poorer immunosurveillance (Kiecolt-Glaser, Dura, Speicher, Trask, & Glaser, 1991) and elevated sympathetic cardiac tonus (Cacioppo et al., 1998) than matched controls. Studies of the cumulative effects of stressors on biology and health have led to the concept of allostatic load (McEwen & Stellar, 1993). Sterling and Eyer (1988) introduced the term allostasis to capture the complexities of visceral regulation, particularly the effort required to maintain a highly regulated state in a complex system. Like Selye (1973), these authors recognized that regulatory levels are not fixed but may be flexibly adjusted to meet changing demands. The allostatic concept recognizes that many visceral dimensions are regulated by multiple, interacting mechanisms and that these mechanisms are subject to a broader range of modulatory influences, whether derived from exogenous challenges or natural endogenous processes. These adjustments are seen as reflecting the adaptive readjustment of regulatory levels, given changing physiological demands (Berntson & Cacioppo, in press). Over time, however, the physiological costs of these adjustments (i.e., the allostatic load) build up, culminating in cumulative identifiable damage that results in increased pathology (Seeman, Singer, Rowe, Horwitz, & McEwen, 1997). The

heightened, repeated, or extended activation of the SAM and HPA axes and the concept of allostatic load are thought to play a role in several of the routes outlined below, as well.

A second route by which social factors may affect biology and health is by means of their impact on affective processes (e.g., distress) and mental health (Taylor et al., 1997). The anxiety, hostility, and depression that characterize lonely individuals, for instance, represent a constellation of psychological traits that has been linked to maladaptive coping, increased stress reactivity, and all-cause mortality (see, e.g., Booth-Kewley & Friedman, 1987; Martin et al., 1995). Hostility, distress, depression, and negativity more generally have been linked to alterations in the activation of both the SAM and the HPA systems, with consequent effects on cardiovascular disease (see, e.g., Krantz & Manuck, 1984; Manuck et al., 1995; Troxler, Sprague, Albanese, Fuchs, & Thompson, 1977) and immune function (see, e.g., Cohen & Herbert, 1996).

A third route by which social factors may have adverse health effects is through their impact on beliefs and attitudes about oneself (e.g., self-esteem), one's life (e.g., life satisfaction), one's future (e.g., hopefulness), or one's purpose in life (e.g., religiosity). In a remarkable study of the power of beliefs on health, Phillips, Ruth, and Wagner (1993) compared the deaths of 28,169 adult Chinese Americans with those of 412,632 randomly selected, matched Caucasian controls. Chinese astrology specifies that a person's fate is influenced by his or her year of birth. When people who believe in Chinese astrology contract a disease that is associated with the phase of their birth year, they are more likely than others to feel helpless, hopeless, or stoic. Phillips et al. reasoned, therefore, that if these beliefs influenced biological processes and health, then Chinese Americans who have a combination of a disease and a birth year that Chinese astrology regards as ill-fated should be more likely to die significantly earlier than matched Caucasians.

Results confirmed this prediction and further revealed that the more strongly a group was attached to Chinese traditions, the more years of life were lost. These effects were found for nearly all major causes of death.

A fourth and related route is the effects of coping strategies (Taylor et al., 1997). Research by Scheier et al. (1989) on recovery from coronary artery bypass surgery, for instance, demonstrated that optimism was associated with better coping efforts and surgical outcomes. Specifically, optimism was associated with more problem-focused coping and less denial, as well as faster rates of physical recovery during hospitalization and faster returns to normal activities following discharge. In a related line of research, Greenberg, Wortman, and Stone (1996) conducted a follow-up to research by Pennebaker and colleagues (e.g., Pennebaker, Kiecolt-Glaser, & Glaser, 1988) on the health benefits of personal disclosures and demonstrated that disclosing imaginary traumas had comparable health benefits to personal disclosures, a result they attributed to the enhancement of self-efficacy from the imaginal enactment of competent coping efforts.

Fifth, social factors may have an impact on biology and health through their influence on health habits and behaviors. Taylor et al. (1997; see also Adler & Matthews, 1994) reviewed recent evidence linking smoking, substance abuse, diet, exercise, adherence to treatment recommendations, and the use of preventive and secondary health services to the development of chronic diseases. Social isolation may be associated with higher rates of morbidity and mortality (House et al., 1988), for instance, because lonely individuals perform more health-endangering behaviors (smoking, alcohol or drug abuse, risk-taking actions; Cohen, 1988), engage in less frequent or effective recreational or restorative activities that counteract the typical effects of daily hassles and stresses (e.g., exercise, sleep, relaxation, eating nutritious meals; see, e.g., Umberson, 1987), or

benefit less from salubrious behaviors such as sleep (Cacioppo et al., 2000).

A sixth and related route, and one that can clearly coexist with others, is individual differences (cf. Uchino et al., 1996). Intelligent, optimistic, attractive people may tend to make better career and life decisions, have more options, and enjoy better health. Individuals high on hostility or neuroticism, in contrast, may have relatively negative social interactions, higher allostatic load, and poorer health. Indeed, personality factors such as neuroticism and extraversion appear to have large (and contrary) effects especially on subjective measures of health, such as self-reported symptomatology (Watson & Pennebaker, 1989). Schmidt et al. (1997) found that children who, at 4 months of age, displayed a high frequency of motor activity and negative affect (i.e., behaviorally inhibited temperamental pattern of behavior), in contrast to other 4-month-old infants, were described at 4 years of age by their mothers as being more shy. In addition, 4-year-olds who were characterized by a higher frequency of wary behavior during peer play also exhibited relatively high morning salivary cortisol, were reported as contemporaneously shy by their mothers, and had been behaviorally inhibited at 14 months of age. Schmidt et al. suggested that high levels of cortisol in these children may induce changes in the amygdala, exacerbating their fearfulness. Research is needed to examine the interface between social and personal factors, especially in reference to biology and health (McGonigle, Smith, Benjamin, & Turner, 1993; Uchino et al., 1996).

Finally, social isolation can lay the initial groundwork for a direct health effect (Taylor et al., 1997). Gurley, Lum, Sande, Lo, and Katz (1996), for instance, conducted a population-based study of patients who were found in their homes either helpless or dead. The median age of such persons was 73 years (51% women), with the frequency of such incidents rising sharply with age, in large part because these individuals were more likely to be living alone and, hence, were more vulnerable when a health problem arose.

These mechanisms have been difficult to examine for various reasons. First, these explanations, although distinguishable, are not mutually exclusive. Social behavior is multiply determined, as is likely are the means by which social factors have an impact on biology and health. Investigations of individual mechanisms in isolation, therefore, may hinder discovery of associations and interactions among these mechanisms. Furthermore, the routes outlined above need not be orthogonal. For example, an individual's beliefs and expectations may shape his or her appraisals, which in turn may influence the individual's affective reactions or health behaviors. Parsing the relative influence of these mechanisms requires multidisciplinary research drawing from expertise across multiple levels of organization. Traditionally, most laboratories and funding opportunities have supported single or very limited levels of analysis.

Second, the effect of social relationships on physiological responses has typically been studied in the laboratory. This makes it possible to rigorously examine specific constructs such as differential reactivity—the differences in the magnitude of a response to a given stimulus as a function of social processes (e.g., cardiovascular responses in individuals low vs. high in hostility). The extent to which these laboratory snapshots generalize to what people do or how they actually respond in their daily lives is an open question, however, one that advances in ambulatory recording procedures and experience sampling methods now make it possible to address (cf. Guyll & Contrada, 1998). The problem is not simply one of generalizability, either. The reactivity measured in the laboratory may generalize to everyday life, yet the effect may manifest not in differential reactivity but rather in differential exposure. Hostile individuals, for instance, may

differ in the situations (e.g., social stressors or conflicts) they encounter or create rather than in the magnitude of their reactivity to a given stressor. Thus, both laboratory and field research may contribute to our understanding of the means by which the social world gets under the skin.

Third, cross-sectional studies in the area have relied primarily on self-reports to assess people's social construals and activities. It is imperative to consider the extent to which these data are reliable and valid descriptions of their social world, mean the same thing across groups of individuals (e.g., gender, ethnicity), and capture the important states of mind (see, e.g., Bradburn, Rips, & Shevell, 1987). Specific distortions in the retrospective verbal reports of stressful or emotional events, for instance, have been documented (Redelmeier & Kahneman, 1996).

Fourth, the prior research that has been conducted in the field has been almost exclusively correlational, leaving open the question of causal factors. Animal studies offer a valuable complement, although the generalizability of the results to humans is an issue that must be considered. Nevertheless, one of the greatest challenges is to go beyond correlational data to reveal the psychological and physiological mechanisms involved. Longitudinal studies that span several levels of analysis may contribute to this end.

Finally, scientific inquiries require that individual investigators specialize and focus. Interdisciplinary research teams provide a means of overcoming this limitation, but disciplinary training and departmental reward contingencies tend to foster parochialism and work against the establishment of such teams. Parochialism, however, ignores the distinction between levels of explanation, the organization in the data that may become evident from research across levels of organization, the theoretical insights about the nature and timing of the relationships among variables that can be derived from descriptions of phenomena from multiple scales or perspectives, and the economy of thought that can be gained by using the form of representation most appropriate for the task. It also alienates scientists working at a different level of organization who might otherwise contribute relevant theory and data and renders it acceptable to ignore relevant research simply because it was not born from one's own level of analysis. Given that there are phenomena deriving from events at one level of analysis that are only or distinctly observable at other or broader levels of analysis, multilevel integrative analyses may contribute to the empirical data and theoretical insight needed for a comprehensive understanding of human behavior.

Conclusion

The complementarity of biological and social approaches to human behavior were not readily apparent when research methods were limited primarily to descriptions of the behavior of animals far removed from their ecological or evolutionary context, observations of patients who suffered trauma to or disorders of localized areas of the brain, and postmortem examinations. As a consequence, biological approaches tended to be viewed by social psychologists as uselessly reductionistic, whereas social approaches tended to be viewed by biopsychologists as more literary than scientific, more a history of human experience than a rigorous, robust, and replicable body of scientific knowledge (see Allport, 1947). Technical and methodological developments now enable biological measures of ongoing human behavior, including electrophysiological recording, functional brain imaging, and neurochemical techniques. Conversely, social methods for studying behavior and ambulatory recordings of biological function can now be applied to animals and humans living in complex environments, providing a more fruitful model for the dynamic interaction between biological mechanisms and social context. New disciplines have also emerged—genetics, molecular biology, neu-

roendocrinology, social neuroscience, and psychoneuroimmunology—along with techniques sufficiently refined that they can now be used together to elucidate the reciprocal interactions between neural and social processes. Changes in medical science, worldwide health problems (e.g., AIDS, chronic disease), and U.S. demographics have helped fuel basic social and biological research on societal problems. With both means and motive now available, there is growing evidence that a more comprehensive understanding of the mind and behavior will be fostered by integrative, theoretical analyses that span the biological and social levels of organization.

In sum, social and biological approaches are complementary rather than antagonistic. Together, these perspectives are helping to illuminate questions ranging from the social sciences to the neurosciences by examining how organismic processes are shaped, modulated, and modified by social factors and vice versa. Rather than viewing social psychology and biological psychology as generating inevitably oppositional forces that are ripping apart psychology departments (Scott, 1991), we see the potential for strong centripetal forces generated by research cutting across these distinct but equally important levels of organization.

Acknowledgments

Research and scholarly activities for this article were supported by the John D. and Catherine T. MacArthur Foundation Network on Mind–Body Interactions.

References

Adams, M. R., Kaplan, J. R., Kovitnik, D. R., & Clarkson, T. B. (1987). Pregnancy-associated inhibition of coronary artery atherosclerosis in monkeys: Evidence of a relationship with endogenous estrogen. *Arteriosclerosis, 7,* 378–384.

Adler, N. E., Boyce, T., Chesney, M. A., Cohen, S., Folkman, S., Kahn, R. L., & Syme, S. L. (1994). Socioeconomic status and health: The challenge of the gradient. *American Psychologist,* 49, 15–24.

Adler, N. E., & Matthews, K. A. (1994). Health and psychology: Why do some people get sick and some stay well? *Annual Review of Psychology,* 45, 229–259.

Allport, G. W. (1947). Scientific models and human morals. *Psychological Review,* 54, 182–192.

Anderson, N. B. (1998). Levels of analysis in health science: A framework for integrating sociobehavioral and biomedical research. *Annals of the New York Academy of Sciences,* 840, 563–576.

Anderson, N. B., & Scott, P. A. (1999). Making the case for psychophysiology during the era of molecular biology. *Psychophysiology,* 36, 1–13.

Anisman, H., Zaharia, M. D., Meaney, M. J., & Merali, Z. (1998). Do early-life events permanently alter behavioral and hormonal responses to stressors? *International Journal of Developmental Neuroscience,* 16, 149–164.

Bauer, G. (1983). Induction of Epstein-Barr virus early antigens by corticosteroids: Inhibition by TPA and retinoic acid. *International Journal of Cancer,* 31, 291–295.

Baumeister, R. F., & Leary, M. R. (1995). The need to belong: Desire for interpersonal attachment as a fundamental human motivation. *Psychological Bulletin,* 117, 497–529.

Becker, A. (1999, May). *Acculturation and disordered eating in Fiji.* Paper presented at the annual meeting of the American Psychiatric Association, Washington, DC.

Berkman, L. F., & Syme, S. L. (1979). Social networks, host resistance, and mortality: A nine-year follow-up study of Alameda County residents. *American Journal of Epidemiology,* 109, 186–204.

Bernstein, I. S., Gordon, T. P., & Rose, R. M. (1983). The interaction of hormones, behavior, and social context in nonhuman primates. In B. B. Svare (Ed.), *Hormones and aggressive behavior* (pp. 535–561). New York: Plenum.

Berntson, G. G., & Cacioppo, J. T. (2000). From homeostasis to allodynamic regulation. In J. T. Cacioppo, L. G. Tassinary, & G. G. Berntson (Eds.), *Handbook of psychophysiology,* 2nd edition (pp. 459–481). New York: Cambridge University Press.

Blaustein, M. P., & Grim, C. E. (1991). The pathogenesis of hypertension: Black–White differences. *Cardiovascular Clinics,* 21, 97–114.

Booth-Kewley, S., & Friedman, H. S. (1987). Psychological predictors of heart disease: A quantitative review. *Psychological Bulletin,* 101, 343–362.

Bosma, H., Marmot, M. G., Hemingway, H., Nicholson, A. C., Brunner, E., & Stansfeld, S. A. (1997). Low job control and risk of coronary heart disease in Whitehall II (prospective cohort) study. *British Medical Journal (Clinical Research Edition),* 314, 558–565.

Bradburn, N., Rips, L. J., & Shevell, S. K. (1987, April 10). Answering autobiographical questions: The impact of memory and inference on surveys. *Science,* 236, 157–161.

Bronfenbrenner, U., & Ceci, S. J. (1994). Nature–nurture reconceptualized in developmental perspective: A bioecological model. *Psychological Review,* 101, 568–586.

Burt, R. S. (1986). *Strangers, friends, and happiness* (GSS Tech. Rep. No. 72). Chicago: National Opinion Research Center, University of Chicago.

Cacioppo, J. T., & Berntson, G. G. (1992a). The principles of multiple, nonadditive, and reciprocal determinism: Implications for social psychological research and levels of analysis. In D. Ruble, P. Costanzo, & M. Oliveri (Eds.), *The social psychology of mental health* (pp. 328–349). New York: Guilford Press.

Cacioppo, J. T., & Berntson, G. G. (1992b). Social psychological contributions to the decade of the brain: The doctrine of multilevel analysis. *American Psychologist,* 47, 1019–1028.

Cacioppo, J. T., Berntson, G. G., Malarkey, W. B., Kiecolt-Glaser, J. K., Sheridan, J. F., Poehlmann, K. M., Burleson, M. H., Ernst, J. M., Hawkley, L. C., & Glaser, R. (1998). Autonomic, neuroendocrine, and immune responses to psychological stress: The reactivity hypothesis. *Annals of the New York Academy of Sciences,* 840, 664–673.

Cacioppo, J. T., Ernst, J. M., Burleson, M. H., McClintock, M. K., Malarkey, W. B., Hawkley, L. C., Kowalewski, R. B., Paulsen, A., Hobson, J. A., Hugdahl, K., Spiegel, D., & Berntson, G. G. (2000). Lonely traits and concomitant physiological processes: The MacArthur Social Neuroscience Studies. *International Journal of Psychophysiology,* 35, 143–154.

Carden, S. E., & Hofer, M. A. (1990). Independence of benzodiazepine and opiate actions in the suppression of isolation and distress in rat pups. *Behavioral Neuroscience, 104,* 160–166.

Carlson, M., & Earls, F. (1997). Psychological and neuroendocrinological sequelae of early social deprivation in institutionalized children in Romania. In C. S. Carter, I. I. Lederhendler, & B. Kirkpatrick (Eds.), *The integrative neurobiology of affiliation* (pp. 419–428). New York: New York Academy of Sciences.

Carroll, D., & Sheffield, D. (1998). Social psychophysiology, social circumstances, and health. *Annals of Behavioral Medicine, 20,* 333–337.

Carter, C. S., Lederhendler, I. I., & Kirkpatrick, B. (1997). *The integrative neurobiology of affiliation.* New York: New York Academy of Sciences.

Cohen, S. (1988). Psychosocial models of the role of social support in the etiology of disease. *Health Psychology, 7,* 269–297.

Cohen, S., Frank, E., Doyle, W. J., Skoner, D. P., Rabin, B. S., & Gwaltney, J. M., Jr. (1998). Types of stressors that increase susceptibility to the common cold in adults. *Health Psychology, 17,* 214–223.

Cohen, S., & Herbert, T. B. (1996). Health psychology: Psychological factors and physical disease from the perspective of human psychoneuroimmunology. *Annual Review of Psychology, 47,* 113–142.

Cohen, S., & Syme, S. L. (1985). *Social support and health.* Orlando, FL: Academic Press.

Cohen, S., Tyrrell, D. A. J., & Smith, A. P. (1991). Psychological stress in humans and susceptibility to the common cold. *New England Journal of Medicine, 325,* 606–612.

Cooper, R., Rotimi, C., Ataman, S., McGee, D., Osotimehin, B., Kadiri, S., Muna, W., Kingue, S., Fraser, H., Forrester, T., Bennett, F., & Wilks, R. (1997). The prevalence of hypertension in seven populations of west African origin. *American Journal of Public Health, 87,* 160–168.

Cornell, C. E., Rodin, J., & Weingarten, H. P. (1989). Stimulus-induced eating when satiated. *Physiology and Behavior, 45,* 695–704.

Crabbe, J. C., Wahlsten, D., & Dudek, B. C. (1999, June 4). Genetics of mouse behavior: Interactions with laboratory environment. *Science, 284,* 1670–1672.

Crick, F. (1970, August 8). Central dogma of molecular biology. *Nature, 227,* 561–563.

Damasio, A. R. (1994). *Descartes' error: Emotion, reason, and the human brain.* New York: Grosset/Putnam.

Dhabhar, F. S., & McEwen, B. S. (1997). Acute stress enhances while chronic stress suppresses cell-mediated immunity in vivo: A potential role for leukocyte trafficking. *Brain, Behavior, and Immunity, 11,* 286–306.

Dhabhar, F. S., Miller, A. H., McEwen, B. S., & Spencer, R. L. (1995). Effects of stress on immune cell distribution. *Journal of Immunology, 154,* 5511–5527.

Farah, M. J., Wilson, K. D., Drain, M., & Tanaka, J. N. (1998). What is "special" about face perception? *Psychological Review, 105,* 482–498.

Felthous, A. R. (1997). Does "isolation" cause jail suicides? *Journal of the American Academy of Psychiatry and the Law, 25,* 285–294.

Freis, E. D., Reda, D. J., & Materson, B. J. (1988). Volume (weight) loss and blood pressure response following thiazide diuretics. *Hypertension, 12,* 244–250.

Friedman, H. S., Tucker, J. S., Schwartz, J. E., Tomlinson-Keasey, C., Martin, L. R., Wingard, D. L., & Criqui, M. H. (1995). Psychosocial and behavioral predictors of longevity: The aging and death of the "Termites." *American Psychologist, 50,* 69–78.

Gardner, W. L., Gabriel, S., & Diekman, A. B. (2000). Interpersonal processes. In J. T. Cacioppo, L. G. Tassinary, & G. G. Berntson (Eds.), *Handbook of psychophysiology* (2nd ed., pp. 643–664). New York: Cambridge University Press.

Gazzaniga, M. S. (1998, October 9). How to change the university. *Science, 282,* 237.

Gerlai, R. (1996). Gene-targeting studies of mammalian behavior: Is it the mutation or the background genotype? *Trends in Neurosciences, 19,* 177–181.

Glaser, R., Kiecolt-Glaser, J. K., Bonneau, R. H., Malarkey, W. B., Kennedy, S., & Hughes, J. (1992). Stress-induced modulation of the immune response to recombinant Hepatitis B vaccine. *Psychosomatic Medicine, 54,* 22–29.

Glaser, R., Kiecolt-Glaser, J. K., Malarkey, W. B., & Sheridan, J. F. (1998). The influence of psychological stress on the immune response to vaccines. *Annals of the New York Academy of Sciences, 840,* 649–655.

Glaser, R., Kutz, L. A., MacCallum, R. C., & Malarkey, W. B. (1995). Hormonal modulation of Epstein-Barr virus replication. *Neuroendocrinology, 62,* 356–361.

Glaser, R., Rabin, B., Chesney, M., Cohen, S., & Natelson, B. (2000). Stress-induced immunomodulation: Are there implications for infectious diseases? *JAMA, 281,* 2268–2270.

Globus, A., Rosenzweig, M. R., Bennett, E. L., & Diamond, M. C. (1973). Effects of differential experience on dendritic spine counts in rat cerebral cortex. *Journal of Comparative and Physiological Psychology, 82,* 175–181.

Goldin-Meadow, S., & Mylander, C. (1983, July 22). Gestural communication in deaf children: Noneffect of parental input on language development. *Science, 221,* 372–374.

Goldin-Meadow, S., & Mylander, C. (1984). Gestural communication in deaf children: The effects and noneffects of parental input on early language development. *Monographs of the Society for Research in Child Development, 49,* 1–121.

Gomez, M. A., Riley, A. L., & Sternberg, E. M. (1997). Maternal differences between Lewis and Fischer rat strains. *Society for Neuroscience 1997 Abstracts, 20,* 204.

Gottlieb, G. (1998). Normally occurring environmental and behavioral influences on gene activity: From central dogma to probabilistic epigenesis. *Psychological Review, 105,* 792–802.

Gottman, J. M., & Levenson, R. W. (1992). Marital processes predictive of later dissolution: Behavior, physiology, and health. *Journal of Personality and Social Psychology, 63,* 221–233.

Greenberg, M. A., Wortman, C. B., & Stone, A. A. (1996). Emotional expression and physical health: Revising traumatic memories or fostering self-regulation? *Journal of Personality and Social Psychology, 71,* 588–602.

Greenough, W. T., Juraska, J. M., & Volkmar, F. R. (1979). Maze training effects on dendritic branching in the occipital complex of adult rats. *Behavioral and Neural Biology, 26,* 287–297.

Grim, C. E., Wilson, T. W., Nicholson, G. D., Hassell, T. A., Fraser, H. S., Grim, C. M., & Wilson, D. M. (1990). Blood pressure in Blacks: Twin studies in Barbados. *Hypertension, 15,* 803–809.

Gurley, R. J., Lum, N., Sande, M., Lo, B., & Katz, M. H. (1996). Persons found in their homes helpless or dead. *New England Journal of Medicine, 334,* 1710–1716.

Guyll, M., & Contrada, R. J. (1998). Trait hostility and ambulatory cardiovascular activity: Responses to social interaction. *Health Psychology, 17,* 30–39.

Haber, S. N., & Barchas, P. R. (1983). The regulatory effect of social rank on behavior after amphetamine administration. In P. R. Barchas (Ed.), *Social hierarchies: Essays toward a sociophysiological perspective* (pp. 119–132). Westport, CT: Greenwood Press.

Harlow, H. F., & Harlow, M. K. (1973). Social deprivation in monkeys. In W. T. Greenough (Compiler), *The nature and nurture of behavior: Readings from the Scientific American* (pp. 108–116). San Francisco: Freeman.

Herbert, T. B., & Cohen, S. (1993a). Depression and immunity: A meta-analytic review. *Psychological Bulletin, 113,* 472–486.

Herbert, T. B., & Cohen, S. (1993b). Stress and immunity in humans: A meta-analytic review. *Psychosomatic Medicine, 55,* 364–379.

Hinderliter, A. L., Light, K. C., Girdler, S. S., Willis, P. W., & Sherwood, A. (1996). Blood pressure responses to stress: Relation to left ventricular structure and function. *Annals of Behavioral Medicine, 18,* 61–66.

House, J. S., Landis, K. R., & Umberson, D. (1988, July 29). Social relationships and health. *Science, 241,* 540–545.

House, J. S., Robbins, C., & Metzner, H. L. (1982). The association of social relationships and activities with mortality: Prospective evidence from the Tecumseh Community Health Study. *American Journal of Epidemiology, 116,* 123–140.

Howard, L., O'Donnell, P., Stevenson, S., & Oxfeld, O. (1999, February 1). An out for big tobacco. *Newsweek,* 6.

Juraska, J. M., & Kopcik, J. R. (1988). Sex and environmental influences on the size and ultrastructure of the rat corpus callosum. *Brain Research, 450,* 1–8.

Kaas, J. H., Merzenich, M. M., & Killackey, H. (1983). The reorganization of somatosensory cortex following peripheral nerve damage in adult and developing mammals. *Annual Review of Neuroscience, 6,* 325–356.

Kaplan, J. R., Adams, M. R., Anthony, M. S., Morgan, T. M., Manuck, S. B., & Clarkson, T. B. (1995). Dominant social status and contraceptive hormone treatment inhibit atherogenesis in premenopausal monkeys. *Arteriosclerosis, Thrombosis, and Vascular Biology,* 15, 2094–2100.

Kaplan, J. R., Adams, M. R., Clarkson, T. B., & Koritnik, D. R. (1984). Psychosocial influences on female "protection" among cynomolgus macaques. *Atherosclerosis,* 53, 283–295.

Kaplan, J. R., Adams, M. R., Clarkson, T. B., Manuck, S. B., Shively, C. A., & Williams, J. K. (1996). Psychosocial factors, sex differences, and atherosclerosis: Lessons from animal models. *Psychosomatic Medicine,* 58, 598–611.

Kaplan, J. R., Manuck, S. B., Clarkson, T. B., Lusso, F. M., & Taub, D. M. (1982). Social status, environment and atherosclerosis in cynomolgus monkeys. *Arteriosclerosis,* 2, 359–368.

Kaplan, J. R., Manuck, S. B., Clarkson, T. B., Lusso, F. M., Taub, D. M., & Miller, E. W. (1983, May 13). Social stress and atherosclerosis in normocholesterolemic monkeys. *Science,* 220, 733–735.

Kiecolt-Glaser, J. K., Dura, J. R., Speicher, C. E., Trask, O. J., & Glaser, R. G. (1991). Spousal caregivers of dementia victims: Longitudinal changes in immunity and health. *Psychosomatic Medicine,* 53, 345–362.

Kiecolt-Glaser, J. K., Fisher, L., Ogrocki, P., Stout, J. C., Speicher, C. E., & Glaser, R. (1987). Marital quality, marital disruption, and immune function. *Psychosomatic Medicine,* 49, 13–34.

Kiecolt-Glaser, J. K., Garner, W., Speicher, C. E., Penn, G., & Glaser, R. (1984). Psychosocial modifiers of immunocompetence in medical students. *Psychosomatic Medicine,* 46, 7–14.

Kiecolt-Glaser, J. K., Glaser, R., Cacioppo, J. T., MacCallum, R. C., Snydersmith, M., Kim, C., & Malarkey, W. B. (1997). Marital conflict in older adults: Endocrinological and immunological correlates. *Psychosomatic Medicine,* 59, 339–349.

Kiecolt-Glaser, J. K., Glaser, R., Gravenstein, S., Malarkey, W. B., & Sheridan, J. (1996). Chronic stress alters the immune response to influenza virus vaccine in older adults. *Proceedings of the National Academy of Sciences, USA,* 93, 3043–3047.

Kiecolt-Glaser, J. K., Malarkey, W., Cacioppo, J. T., & Glaser, R. (1994). Stressful personal relationships: Endocrine and immune function. In R. Glaser & J. K. Kiecolt-Glaser (Eds.), *Handbook of human stress and immunity* (pp. 321–339). San Diego, CA: Academic Press.

Kiecolt-Glaser, J. K., Marucha, P. T., Malarkey, W. B., Mercado, A. M., & Glaser, R. (1995). Slowing of wound healing by psychological stress. *Lancet,* 346, 1194–1196.

Kiecolt-Glaser, J. K., Page, G. G., Marucha, P. T., MacCallum, R. C., & Glaser, R. (1998). Psychological influences on surgical recovery: Perspectives from psychoneuroimmunology. *American Psychologist,* 11, 1209–1218.

King, J. A., & Edwards, E. (1999). Early stress and genetic influences on hypothalamic–pituitary–adrenal axis functioning in adulthood. *Hormones and Behavior,* 36, 79–85.

Kitagava, E. M., & Hauser, P. M. (1973). *Differential mortality in the United States: A study of socioeconomic epidemiology.* Cambridge, MA: Harvard University Press.

Klein, S. B., & Kihlstrom, J. F. (1998). On bridging the gap between social-personality psychology and neuropsychology. *Personality and Social Psychology Review,* 2, 228–242.

Kluver, H., & Bucy, P. C. (1939). Preliminary analysis of the functions of the temporal lobes in monkeys. *Archives of Neurology and Psychiatry,* 42, 979–1000.

Krantz, D. S., & Manuck, S. B. (1984). Acute psychophysiologic reactivity and risk of cardiovascular disease: A review and methodologic critique. *Psychological Bulletin,* 96, 435–464.

Kusnecov, A. W., Liang, R., & Shurin, G. (1999). T-lymphocyte activation increases hypothalamic and amygdaloid expression of CRH mRNA and emotional reactivity to novelty. *Journal of Neuroscience,* 19, 4533–4543.

Levenson, R. W., Cartensen, L. L., & Gottman, J. M. (1994). Influence of age and gender on affect, physiology, and their interrelationships: A study of long-term marriages. *Journal of Personality and Social Psychology,* 67, 56–68.

Levine, D. M., Green, L. W., Deeds, S. G., Chwalow, J., Russell, R. P., & Finlay, J. (1979). Health education for hypertensive patients. *JAMA,* 241, 1700–1703.

Light, K. C., Brownley, K. A., Turner, J. R., Hinderliter, A. L., Girdler, S. S., Sherwood, A., & Anderson, N. B. (1995). Job status and high-effort coping influence work blood pressure in women and Blacks. *Hypertension,* 25, 554–559.

Light, K. C., Girdler, S. S., & Hinderliter, A. L. (2000). *Genetic and behavioral factors in combination influence risk of hypertensive heart disease.* Manuscript submitted for publication.

Light, K. C., Girdler, S. S., Sherwood, A., Bragdon, E. E., Brownley, K. A., West, S. G., & Hinderliter, A. L. (1999). High stress responsivity predicts later blood pressure only in combination with positive family history and high life stress. *Hypertension,* 33, 1458–1464.

Liu, D., Diorio, J., Tannenbaum, B., Caldji, C., Francis, D., Freedman, A., Sharma, S., Pearson, D., Plotsky, P. M., & Meaney, M. J. (1997, September 12). Maternal care, hippocampal glucocorticoid receptors, and hypothalamic–pituitary–adrenal responses to stress. *Science,* 277, 1659–1662.

Luft, F. C., Grim, C. E., Fineberg, N., & Weinberger, M. C. (1979). Effects of volume expansion and contraction in normotensive Whites, Blacks, and subjects of different ages. *Circulation,* 59, 643–650.

Luft, F. C., Rankin, L. I., Bloch, R., Weyman, A. E., Willis, L. R., Murray, R. H., Grim, C. E., & Weinberger, M. H. (1979). Cardiovascular and humoral responses to extremes of sodium intake in normal Black and White men. *Circulation,* 60, 697–706.

Lupien, S. J., & McEwen, B. S. (1997). The acute effects of corticosteroids on cognition: Integration of animal and human model studies. *Brain Research Reviews,* 24, 1–27.

Macmillan, M. B. (1986). A wonderful journey through skull and brains: The travels of Mr. Gage's tamping iron. *Brain and Cognition,* 5, 67–107.

Madden, K. S., Thyagarajan, S., & Felten, D. L. (1998). Alterations in sympathetic noradrenergic innervation in lymphoid organs with age. In S. M. McCann, E. M. Sternberg, J. M. Lipton, G. P. Chrousos, P. W. Gold, & C. C. Smith (Eds.), *Neuroimmunomodulation: Molecular aspects, integrative systems, and clinical advances* (pp. 262–268). New York: New York Academy of Sciences.

Maier, S. F., & Watkins, L. R. (1998). Cytokines for psychologists: Implications for bidirectional immune-to-brain communication for understanding behavior, mood, and cognition. *Psychological Review,* 105, 83–107.

Malarkey, W. B., Wu, H., Cacioppo, J. T., Malarkey, K. L., Poehlmann, K. M., Glaser, R., & Kiecolt-Glaser, J. K. (1996). Chronic stress down-regulates growth hormone gene expression in peripheral blood mononuclear cells of older adults. *Endocrine,* 5, 33–39.

Manuck, S. B., Marsland, A. L., Kaplan, J. R., & Williams, J. K. (1995). The pathogenicity of behavior and its neuroendocrine mediation: An example from coronary artery disease. *Psychosomatic Medicine,* 57, 275–283.

Martin, L. R., Friedman, H. S., Tucker, J. S., Schwartz, J. E., Criqui, M. H., Wingard, D. L., & Tomlinson-Keasey, C. (1995). An archival prospective study of mental health and longevity. *Health Psychology,* 14, 381–387.

Marucha, P. T., Kiecolt-Glaser, J. K., & Favagehi, M. (1998). Mucosal wound healing is impaired by examination stress. *Psychosomatic Medicine,* 60, 362–365.

McCann, S. M., Sternberg, E. M., Lipton, J. M., Chrousos, G. P., Gold, P. W., & Smith, C. C. (Eds.). (1998). *Neuroimmunomodulation: Molecular aspects, integrative systems, and clinical advances.* New York: New York Academy of Sciences.

McClintock, M. K. (1979). Innate behavior is not innate. *Signs,* 4, 703–710.

McEwen, B. S., & Stellar, E. (1993). Stress and the individual: Mechanisms leading to disease. *Archives of Internal Medicine,* 153, 2093–2101.

McGlone, F. B., & Arden, N. H. (1987). Impact of influenza in geriatrics and an action plan for prevention and treatment. *American Journal of Medicine,* 82, 55–57.

McGonigle, M. M., Smith, T. W., Benjamin, L. S., & Turner, C. W. (1993). Hostility and nonshared family environment: A study of monozygotic twins. *Journal of Research in Personality,* 27, 23–34.

McKinnon, W., Weisse, C. S., Reynolds, C. P., Bowles, C. A., & Baum, A. (1989). Chronic stress, leukocyte subpopulations, and humoral response to latent viruses. *Health Psychology,* 8, 389–402.

Meaney, M. J., Bhatnagar, S., Diorio, J., Larocque, S., Francis, D., O'Donnell, D., Shanks, N., Sharma, S., Smythe, J., & Viau, V. (1993). *Cellular and Molecular Neurobiology,* 13, 321–347.

Meaney, M. J., Bhatnagar, S., Larocque, S., McCormick, C. M., Shanks, N., Sharma, S., Smythe, J., Viau, V., & Plotsky, P. M. (1996). Early environment and the development of individual differences in the hypothalamic–pituitary–adrenal stress response. In C. R. Pfeffer (Ed.), *Severe stress and mental distur-*

bance in children (pp. 85–127). Washington, DC: American Psychiatric Press.

Meaney, M. J., Sapolsky, R. M., & McEwen, B. S. (1985). The development of the glucocorticoid receptor system in the rat limbic brain: II. An autoradiographic study. Developmental Brain Research, 18, 159–164.

Mesulam, M., & Perry, J. (1972). The diagnosis of lovesickness: Experimental psychophysiology without the polygraph. Psychophysiology, 9, 546–551.

Morisky, D. E., DeMuth, N. M., Field-Fass, M., Green, L. W., & Levine, D. M. (1985). Evaluation of family health education to build social support for long-term control of high blood pressure. Health Education Quarterly, 12, 35–50.

Neel, J. V. (1962). Diabetes mellitus: A thrifty genotype rendered detrimental by progress. American Journal of Human Genetics, 14, 353–362.

Osei, K. (1999). Metabolic consequences of the west African diaspora: Lessons from the thrifty gene. Journal of Laboratory and Clinical Medicine, 133, 98–111.

Padgett, D. A., Marucha, P. T., & Sheridan, J. F. (1998). Restraint stress slows cutaneous wound healing in mice. Brain, Behavior and Immunity, 12, 64–73.

Padgett, D. A., & Sheridan, J. F. (1999). Social stress, dominance, and increased mortality from an influenza viral infection. Manuscript submitted for publication.

Padgett, D. A., Sheridan, J. F., Dorne, J., Berntson, G. G., Candelora, J., & Glaser, R. (1998). Social stress and the reactivation of latent herpes simplex virus-type 1. Proceedings of the National Academy of Sciences, USA, 95, 7231–7235.

Panksepp, J. (1998). Affective neuroscience. New York: Oxford University Press.

Panksepp, J., Herman, B. H., Conner, R., Bishop, P., & Scott, J. P. (1978). The biology of social attachments: Opiates alleviate separation distress. Biological Psychiatry, 13, 607–613.

Pennebaker, J. W., Kiecolt-Glaser, J. K., & Glaser, R. (1988). Disclosure of traumas and immune function: Health implications for psychotherapy. Journal of Consulting and Clinical Psychology, 56, 239–254.

Phillips, D. P., Ruth, T. E., & Wagner, L. M. (1993). Psychology and survival. Lancet, 342, 1142–1145.

Redelmeier, D. A., & Kahneman, D. (1996). Patients' memories of painful medical treatments: Real-time and retrospective evaluations of two minimally invasive procedures. Pain, 66, 3–8.

Rogot, E., Sorlie, P. D., Johnson, N. J., & Schmit, C. (1993). A mortality study of 1.3 million persons by demographic, social, and economic factors: 1979–1985 follow-up U.S. National Longitudinal Mortality Study. Washington, DC: National Institutes of Health.

Rose, R. M., Gordon, T. P., & Bernstein, I. S. (1972, November 10). Plasma testosterone levels in the male Rhesus: Influences of sexual and social stimuli. Science, 178, 643–645.

Saab, P. G., Llabre, M. M., Schneiderman, N., Hurwitz, B. E., McDonald, P. G., Evans, J., Wohlgemuth, W., Hayashi, P., & Klein, B. (1997). Influence of ethnicity and gender on cardiovascular responses to active coping and inhibitory-passive coping challenges. Psychosomatic Medicine, 59, 434–446.

Scheier, M. F., Matthews, K. A., Owens, J. F., Magovern, G. J., Sr., Lefebvre, R. C., Abbott, R. A., & Carver, C. S. (1989). Dispositional optimism and recovery from coronary artery bypass surgery: The beneficial effects on physical and psychological well-being. Journal of Personality and Social Psychology, 57, 1024–1040.

Schmidt, L. A., Fox, N. A., Rubin, K. H., Sternberg, E. M., Gold, P. W., Smith, C. C., & Schulkin, J. (1997). Behavioral and neuroendocrine responses in shy children. Developmental Psychobiology, 30, 127–140.

Schnall, P. L., Schwartz, J. E., Landsbergis, P. A., Warren, K., & Pickering, T. G. (1992). Relation between job strain, alcohol, and ambulatory blood pressure. Hypertension, 19, 488–494.

Scott, T. R. (1991). A personal view of the future of psychology departments. American Psychologist, 46, 975–976.

Seeman, T. E. (1996). Social ties and health: The benefits of social integration. Annals of Epidemiology, 6, 442–451.

Seeman, T. E., & McEwen, B. S. (1996). Impact of social environment characteristics on neuroendocrine regulation. Psychosomatic Medicine, 58, 459–471.

Seeman, T. E., Singer, B., Rowe, J. W., Horwitz, R., & McEwen, B. (1997). The price of adaptation: Allostatic load and its health consequences. Archives of Internal Medicine, 157, 2259–2268.

Selye, H. (1973). Homeostasis and heterostasis. Perspectives in Biology and Medicine, 16, 441–445.

Sheridan, J. F. (1998). Stress-induced modulation of anti-viral immunity. *Brain, Behavior and Immunity,* 12, 1–6.

Skantze, H. B., Kaplan, J., Pettersson, K., Manuck, S., Blomqvist, N., Kyes, R., Williams, K., & Bondjers, G. (1998). Psychosocial stress causes endothelial injury in cynomolgus monkeys via betal-adrenoceptor activation. *Atherosclerosis,* 136, 153–161.

Sterling, P., & Eyer, J. (1988). Allostasis: A new paradigm to explain arousal pathology. In S. Fisher & J. Reason (Eds.), *Handbook of life stress, cognition and health* (pp. 629–649). New York: Wiley.

Suomi, S. (1987). Genetic and maternal contributions to individual differences in Rhesus monkeys' biobehavioral development. In N. A. Krasnagor, E. M. Blass, M. A. Hofer, & W. P. Smotherman (Eds.), *Perinatal development: A psychobiological perspective* (pp. 397–420). New York: Academic Press.

Suomi, S. (1991). Up-tight and laid-back monkeys: Individual differences in the response to social challenges. In S. Brauth, W. Hall, & R. Dooling (Eds.), *Plasticity of development* (pp. 27–56). Cambridge, MA: MIT Press.

Suomi, S. (1999). Attachment in Rhesus monkeys. In J. Cassidy & P. R. Shaver (Eds.), *Handbook of attachment* (pp. 181–197). New York: Guilford Press.

Suomi, S., & Levine, S. (1998). Psychobiology of intergenerational effects of trauma: Evidence from animal studies. In Y. Danieli (Ed.), *International handbook of multigenerational legacies of trauma* (pp. 623–637). New York: Plenum.

Taylor, S. E., Repetti, R. L., & Seeman, T. E. (1997). Health psychology: What is an unhealthy environment and how does it get under the skin? *Annual Review of Psychology,* 48, 411–447.

Townshend, P., & Davidson, N. (1982). *The Black report.* Harmondsworth, England: Penguin.

Tranel, D., Fowles, D. C., & Damasio, A. R. (1985). Electrodermal discrimination of familiar and unfamiliar faces: A methodology. *Psychophysiology,* 22, 403–408.

Troxler, R. G., Sprague, E. A., Albanese, R. A., Fuchs, R., & Thompson, A. J. (1977). The association of elevated plasma cortisol and early atherosclerosis as demonstrated by coronary angiography. *Atherosclerosis,* 26, 151–162.

Tucker, J. S., Friedman, H. S., Wingard, D. L., & Schwartz, J. E. (1996). Marital history at midlife as a predictor of longevity: Alternative explanations to the protective effects of marriage. *Health Psychology,* 15, 94–101.

Turkheimer, E. (1998). Heritability and biological explanation. *Psychological Review,* 105, 782–791.

Turner, A. M., & Greenough, W. T. (1985). Differential rearing effects on rat visual cortex synapses: I. Synaptic and neuronal density and synapses per neuron. *Brain Research,* 329, 195–203.

Uchino, B. N., Cacioppo, J. T., & Kiecolt-Glaser, J. K. (1996). The relationship between social support and physiological process: A review with emphasis on underlying mechanisms and implications for health. *Psychological Bulletin,* 119, 488–531.

Uchino, B. N., Cacioppo, J. T., Malarkey, W. B., & Glaser, R. (1995). Individual differences in cardiac sympathetic control predict endocrine and immune responses to acute psychological stress. *Journal of Personality and Social Psychology,* 69, 736–741.

Uchino, B. N., Holt-Lunstad, J., Uno, D., & Flinders, J. B. (1999, June). *Understanding the health effects of social relationships: An examination of positivity and negativity (ambivalence) in the social networks of young and older adults.* Paper presented at the annual meeting of the Society for Behavioral Medicine, San Diego, CA.

Umberson, D. (1987). Family status and health behaviors: Social control as a dimension of social integration. *Journal of Health and Social Behavior,* 28, 306–319.

Uvns-Mosberg, K. (1997). Physiological and endocrine effects of social contact. *Annals of the New York Academy of Sciences,* 807, 146–163.

Watson, D., & Pennebaker, J. W. (1989). Health complaints, stress, and distress: Exploring the central role of negative affectivity. *Psychological Review,* 96, 234–254.

Weder, A. B., & Schork, N. J. (1994). Adaptation, allometry, and hypertension. *Hypertension,* 24, 145–156.

Williams, K. D. (1997). Social ostracism. In R. M. Kowalski (Ed.), *Aversive interpersonal behaviors* (pp. 133–170). New York: Plenum.

Wilson, T. W., & Grim, C. E. (1991). Biohistory of slavery and blood pressure differences in Blacks today. *Hypertension,* 17(Suppl I), I122–I128.

Wilson, T. W., Hollifield, L. R., & Grim, C. E. (1991). Systolic blood pressure levels in Black populations in sub-Sahara Africa, the West Indies, and the United States: A meta-analysis. *Hypertension,* 18, 187–191.

Wu, H., Devi, R., & Malarkey, W. B. (1996). Localization of growth hormone messenger ribonucleic acid in the human immune system: A clinical research center study. *Journal of Clinical Endocrinology and Metabolism,* 81, 1278–1282.

Wu, H., Wang, J., Cacioppo, J. T., Glaser, R., Kiecolt-Glaser, J. K., & Malarkey, W. B. (in press). Chronic stress associated with spousal caregiving of patients with dementia is associated with downregulation of B-lymphocyte GH mRNA. *Journal of Gerontology: Medical Sciences.*

Zillmann, D. (1984). *Connections between sex and aggression.* Hillsdale, NJ: Erlbaum.

4 On Bridging the Gap between Social-Personality Psychology and Neuropsychology

Stanley B. Klein and John F. Kihlstrom

For a very long time psychology thought it could get along without looking at the brain. Skinner and other functional behaviorists treated the organism as a "black box" that connected stimuli with responses but whose internal workings could safely be ignored. Classic cognitive psychology and artificial intelligence also endorsed a version of the doctrine of "empty organism" by focusing on the analogy between mind and software and embracing the notion of a Turing machine that could be made out of neurons, silicon chips, or even old radio parts—thus making the biological substrates of mind irrelevant (for a review, see Gardner, 1985).

All that began to change in the mid-1950s, when theory oriented psychologists began to take notice of patients being seen in the neurological clinic and realized that experimental studies of such cases might provide evidence for theories about how the mind is organized (for comprehensive coverage of the neuropsychological syndromes, see Ellis & Young, 1988; Gazzaniga, Ivry, & Mangun, 1998; Heilman & Valenstein, 1993; Kolb & Whishaw, 1996; McCarthy & Warrington, 1990). The most famous case, of course, is the patient known as H. M., who underwent a bilateral resection of the medial portion of the temporal lobes, including the hippocampus and mammillary bodies, in a desperate attempt to ameliorate intractable epilepsy (e.g., Milner, Corkin, & Teuber, 1968; Scoville & Milner, 1957), H. M. emerged from surgery greatly relieved of his epileptic symptoms; the down side was that he now suffered a profound anterograde amnesia, which prevented him from remembering anything that happened to him from the day of surgery until the present.

Studies of H. M., and patients like him, have provided evidence for a *medial temporal lobe memory system* (e.g., Squire & Zola-Morgan, 1991) that seems to be critical for encoding lasting representations of new experiences. That much is

clear, but what exactly do these neural structures do? This, of course, is a question for psychological theory, and over the years various theories about memory structure and processing have been proposed to explain the behavior of H. M. and others like him.

Initially, amnesic patients were thought to lack a capacity for transferring information from short-term to long-term memory (e.g., Baddeley & Warrington, 1970; Cermak, 1972; Milner, 1966; Wickelgren, 1973). This view, however, soon ran into problems. Consider, for example, what happens when amnesic patient K. C.[1] is tutored in the basics of computer operation (e.g., Glisky, Schacter, & Tulving, 1986b). A few minutes following completion of a lesson, K. C. has no conscious recollections of what he was taught or even that he had a lesson. Nonetheless, he shows clear evidence of having acquired complex knowledge about the programming and operation of a computer; he can understand computer related vocabulary (e.g., *software, modem, save, print*), can perform disk storage and retrieval operations, and even can be taught to write simple programs (e.g., Glisky, 1995; Glisky, Schacter, & Tulving, 1986a; Glisky et al., 1986b). Yet, if asked how he knows the procedure for downloading a file or writing a program, K. C. is likely to respond that these are just ordinary facts about the world that everyone knows (cf. Tulving, Hayman, & Macdonald, 1991).

Observations such as these (for related findings, see Brooks & Baddeley, 1976; Graf, Squire, & Mandler, 1984; Warrington & Weiskrantz, 1970) suggest that amnesic patients show a dissociation between two forms of long-term memory: *Episodic memory*, which enables people to become consciously aware of specific past events from their life, is impaired, whereas *semantic memory*, which enables people to retrieve knowledge abstracted from events but does not entail recollection of the events themselves, is intact (e.g., Cermak, 1984; Evans, Wilson, Wraight, & Hodges, 1993; Kinsbourne & Wood, 1975; Klein, Loftus, & Kihlstrom, 1996; Schacter & Tulving, 1982; Tulving, 1983, 1993; Van der Linden, Bredart, Depoorter, & Coyette, 1996).[2] Characterizing the difference between types or systems of memories is a major growth industry within contemporary cognitive psychology (see, for example, Foster & Jelicic, in press; Schacter & Tulving, 1994), but cognitive psychologists didn't really start asking questions about multiple memory systems until they started contemplating evidence from brain damaged patients (for a review, see Polster, Nadel, & Schacter, 1991). In this way, a great advance in psychological theory began with data from the neurological clinic.

Cognitive psychologists now agree on the value of neurological evidence. For example, psycholinguists are interested in syndromes like Broca's and Wernicke's aphasias for the insights they can provide into the nature of language processing (e.g., Berndt & Caramazza, 1980; Brown, 1972; Goodglass, 1993; Pinker, 1994). Vision scientists are interested in phenomena like blindsight, prosopagnosia, and visual neglect for what they can tell us about perceptual processes (e.g., Coslett, 1997; Prigatano & Schacter, 1991; Weiskrantz, 1997).

The central question addressed in this article is whether the study of patients with neuropsychological impairments should interest personality and social psychologists. We believe the answer to this question is "yes" and hope the arguments we present will challenge our colleagues to join us in considering neuropsychological evidence in theorizing about personality and social processes. Brain damage isn't just for cognitive psychologists anymore; it has a great deal to tell personality and social psychologists about the things we're interested in. However, before that happens, we have to ask the appropriate questions. In the following sections we suggest ways in which neuropsychological evidence can provide important new insights into the role of cognition in personality and social interaction.

H. M., Amnesias, and Knowledge of Self

Reading a case like H. M. can be extremely frustrating to personality and social psychologists because there is so much we want to know, yet so few answers. For example, H. M.'s surgery was in 1953, when he was 27 years old. So what happens now, 45 years later, when H. M. goes into the bathroom to shave in the morning: Does he look in the mirror and say: "Who the hell are you?" What can the self-concept of a person who lacks episodic memory for the past 45 years be like? Can a person preserve a sense of identity, including changes in identity over a long period of time, without also preserving an autobiography? More generally, to what extent is our knowledge of what we are like dependent on our ability to remember the behavioral evidence on which that knowledge is based? Unfortunately, with rare exceptions (e.g., Klein, Loftus, et al., 1996; O'Connor, Cermak, & Seidman, 1995; Tulving, 1993), neuropsychological investigations of the amnesic syndrome seldom have considered the impact of catastrophic memory loss on the patient's personal identity.

In the last few years, however, this situation has begun to change as psychologists come to appreciate the ways in which theoretical issues surrounding the self can be addressed with neurological data. Consider, as an example, the case of W. J. (Klein, Loftus, et al., 1996), an 18-year-old undergraduate who suffered a concussive blow to the head shortly after completing her first quarter in college. Brain scans revealed no neurological abnormalities, but she complained of memory and concentration difficulties and testing revealed that she had, in fact, forgotten much of what had happened in her life during the preceding 6 to 7 months—a period of time covering approximately her first quarter at college. Over the next month, W. J.'s amnesia remitted completely.

W. J.'s amnesic deficit in episodic memory was documented by the Galton (1879) memory cueing procedure popularized by J. A. Robinson (1976) and Crovitz (e.g., Crovitz & Quina-Holland, 1976; Crovitz & Schiffman, 1974). In this task, participants are read cue words (representing affects, objects, and activities) one at a time and for each are asked to recall a specific personal event from any time in the past and provide as precise a date as possible for that event. When tested 5 days after her accident, W. J. showed little episodic memory for personal events from recent years. Four weeks later her performance had improved considerably and was indistinguishable from that of three neurologically healthy women who served as controls.

W. J. was also asked both during her amnesia and after its resolution to provide personality ratings describing what she was like during her first term at college. In contrast to the change in her episodic memory performance over the month following her accident, W. J.'s personality ratings of herself at college did not change at all over the same period of time; her trait ratings made during her amnesic period agreed with those she made afterward. Thus, although she was amnesic, W. J. knew what she had been like in college despite the fact that she couldn't recall anything from her time in college.

Of course, it is conceivable that W. J.'s personality didn't change much between high school and college. If so, then she could have achieved reasonably reliable ratings of her personality simply on the basis of her memories from high school, without accessing any information from her college years. To check this possibility, W. J. was asked during her amnesia to rate how she saw herself during high school. Statistical analyses revealed that the correlation between her ratings of herself at high school and ratings of herself at college was reliable ($r = .53$), meaning that some degree of reliability in W. J.'s ratings of her college self could have been achieved by reliance on her memories of her precollege behaviors and experiences. However, this figure was significantly lower than the correlation obtained between W. J.'s two ratings of herself at college,

taken during and after her amnesia ($r = .74$, $p < .05$). So, there is reliable variability in her college self which is not accounted for by her high school self. Put another way, although she was amnesic, W. J. knew something about what she was like in college, which was different from what she was like in high school; she knew this despite the fact that she could not recall any personally experienced events from her time in college.

To explain these findings, Klein, Loftus, et al. (1996; see also Kihlstrom & Klein, 1994, 1997; Klein, 1993, in press; Klein, Babey, & Sherman, 1997; Klein & Loftus, 1993; Klein, Sherman, & Loftus, 1996) proposed that knowledge of personality traits and recollections of specific personal events involving those traits reflect the operations of two distinct, neurally dissociable types of personal memory: semantic personal memory and episodic personal memory (see also Brewer, 1986; Cermak & O'Connor, 1983; Kihlstrom et al., 1988; Tulving, 1993; Wheeler, Stuss, & Tulving, 1996). *Episodic personal memory* stores the specific details of personally experienced events, whereas *semantic personal memory* stores generalizations about the self abstracted from those experiences. The fact that during her amnesia W. J. had access to trait abstractions about herself, but not the particular episodes on which that knowledge was based, was taken as evidence that these two types of self-knowledge are served by different neural systems, one of which had become dysfunctional as a result of her concussion, whereas the other remained unimpaired (e.g., Kihlstrom & Klein, 1994, 1997; Klein & Loftus, 1993; Klein et al., 1997).[3]

Admittedly, Klein, Loftus, et al.'s (1996) conclusion could be questioned on the basis of W. J.'s continued access to episodic memories that were not covered by her amnesia and the possibility that she drew on those memories, not her semantic personal knowledge, for her ratings of self-at-college. However, there is other evidence indicating that accurate self-description can occur even with total episodic memory loss. Tulving (1993), for example, found that patient

K. C., who lost his entire fund of episodic memory (and underwent a marked personality change) following a motorcycle accident, was able to describe his postmorbid personality with considerable accuracy. Tulving asked K. C. to judge a list of trait adjectives for self-descriptiveness. Tulving also asked K. C.'s mother on two separate occasions to rate K. C. on the same traits, the first time rating K. C. as he currently was and the second time rating him as he was before his accident. K. C.'s choices were highly correlated with his mother's judgments of his postmorbid personality, but not with her judgments of his premorbid personality. Thus, K. C. was able to acquire accurate knowledge of his new personality (with his mother's ratings serving as the criterion) without being able to retain any episodic knowledge of the specific actions and experiences on which that knowledge was based.

Although theorists differ concerning the precise interpretation of the findings just discussed (e.g., Schneider, Roediger, & Kahn, 1993), this much is clear: Neurally impaired individuals who have lost the ability to recall personal experiences show no obvious impairment in the ability to make accurate personality judgments about themselves, and (in the case of K. C.) even maintain the ability to revise those judgments based on new episodes that they cannot remember. Apparently you do not need to remember how you behaved in the past to know what you are like.

Additional support for this conclusion recently was presented by Craik et al. (in press). Using positron emission tomography (PET), these investigators discovered that requiring participants to judge trait adjectives for self-descriptiveness produced activation of cortical areas associated with semantic memory retrieval (left frontal regions) but not those associated with episodic memory retrieval (right frontal regions).[4]

The dissociations between episodic and semantic self-knowledge have made several things clear. First, contrary to long-held beliefs about the memorial basis of self (e.g., Grice, 1941; James, 1890; Keenan, 1993; Locke, 1690/1731;

Quinton, 1962; Tulving, 1984), episodic memory is not the sole repository of self-knowledge. The fact that a loss of episodic memory does not lead to a complete loss of self-knowledge has led theorists to expand the basis of self-knowledge to include both episodic and semantic memory (e.g., Cermak & O'Connor, 1983; Conway, 1992; Evans et al., 1993; Klein & Loftus, 1993; Klein, Loftus, et al., 1996; Tulving, 1993; Tulving, Schacter, McLachlan, & Moscovitch, 1988). Second, the finding that individuals can have accurate and detailed knowledge of their personalities despite having no conscious access to behavioral episodes suggests these two types of self-knowledge are represented independently in memory and perhaps mediated by separate cognitive systems.

Over and above these specific issues, the analysis of cases like W. J. and K. C. shows a little of what is possible when neurological disorders are approached with personality and social theories in mind. We hope that these studies stimulate other self-theorists to consider the theoretical promise of patients with neuropsychological impairments, for it would seem there is much such patients can teach us about the representation and function of knowledge about the self.

Autism, Theory of Mind, and Theory of Self

An interesting implication of the proposal that episodic and semantic self-knowledge are served by different cognitive systems is that a person could, in principle, have complete access to his or her episodic self-knowledge yet be unable to know whether a particular trait adjective was descriptive of self. Although this question has not been addressed empirically, some intriguing hints at an answer are found from a rather unusual source—the study of patients with autism (Klein, 1996).

In a series of publications, Baron-Cohen, Leslie, U. Frith, and colleagues (e.g., Baron-Cohen, 1989, 1990, 1991, 1995; Baron-Cohen,

Leslie, & Frith, 1985; Baron-Cohen, Tager-Flusberg, & Cohen, 1993; U. Frith, 1989; Leslie, 1987, 1991; Leslie & Frith, 1988; Leslie & Thaiss, 1992) have argued that a defining feature of the autistic syndrome is the failure of autistic individuals to develop what Premack and Woodruff (1978) termed *a theory of mind*—a capacity to attribute mental states (e.g., intentions, desires, thoughts, beliefs) to other persons in order to make sense of their behavior (see also, Flavell, Green, & Flavell, 1995; Gopnik & Metzloff, 1997; Wellman, 1990).

Leslie (1987), in a pioneering paper on the topic, suggested that the failure of autistic individuals to explain behavior in terms of mental states (i.e., to mentalize) stemmed from their inability to form "second order representations." By this account, autistic individuals are able to form "first order representations" of people, things, and events based directly on perceptual experience (e.g., "Robert smiled when he got the candy bar"). They are, however, deficient in forming second order representations—that is, representations of first order representations (e.g., "Robert smiled because he thought [or knew, or hoped, or believed] he would get the candy bar"). The capacity to represent representations, Leslie argued, is the essence of a theory of mind and is a capacity that fails to fully develop in autistic individuals (a recent review can be found in Baron-Cohen, 1995).

What about the autistic individual's awareness of his or her own mental states? If autism involves a dysfunction of the neural structures necessary for forming a theory of other minds, it is reasonable to wonder whether these individuals might also show an impaired ability to reflect on their own mental states—to know about their own knowing.[5]

Surprisingly, the question of whether the problems autistic patients experience in understanding and recognizing mental states in others extend to their understanding of their own mental states has been largely overlooked (for a recent discussion, see Carruthers, 1996). However, the few empirical findings that are available do suggest that autistic patients have trouble reflecting on their own mental states (e.g., Baron-Cohen, 1989, 1991; Baron-Cohen, Ring, Moriarty, Schmitz, Costa, & Ell, 1994; Jordan, 1989; Tager-Flusberg, 1992). For example, several recent studies reported that compared to normally developing children, autistic children have problems in acquiring a normal grasp of the personal pronouns *I* and *me* (e.g., Fay, 1979; Jordan, 1989; Lee, Hobson, & Chiat, 1994). Tager-Flusberg (1992) showed that autistic individuals use significantly less spontaneous speech than matched controls when referring to their own cognitive mental states (e.g., beliefs, desires, traits). Along similar lines, Baron-Cohen (1991) found that autistic individuals have as much trouble attributing beliefs to themselves as they do in attributing beliefs to others. Finally, clinical descriptions of autistic individuals often make reference to their inability to self-reflect or to self-monitor (e.g., Baron-Cohen, 1989; Bishop, 1993).

Admittedly, the evidence that autistic individuals may be lacking in awareness of their own mental states is small, indirect, and often anecdotal. Nonetheless, if this hypothesis is correct, it suggests the interesting possibility that an autistic individual, although capable of recalling trait-relevant personal behaviors (e.g., "I remember getting a high score on a math test"), may be unable to make trait-based generalizations about the self on the basis of those behaviors (e.g., "I know [or think, or hope, or believe] that I am an intelligent person"). If such an outcome were obtained, it would provide strong converging evidence in support of the proposed independence between episodic and semantic self-knowledge.

Self-Awareness and the Brain: Locating the Jamesian Self-as-Knower

In light of the previous discussion, it is interesting to wonder whether we know enough about the neural correlates of mentalizing to identify where in the brain such capacity resides. Although a definitive answer is not yet available, some fascinating clues can be found. For example, neuroimaging studies conducted on individuals engaged in theory of mind tasks (e.g., tasks requiring inferences about mental states) report evidence for selective activation of the frontal lobes during task performance, suggesting a role for these structures in the capacity to mentalize (e.g., Baron-Cohen et al., 1994; Fletcher et al., 1995; Goel, Grafman, Sadato, & Hallett, 1995). This possibility receives support from two additional sources. First, there is some evidence that patients with frontal lobe damage show deficits on theory of mind tasks (e.g., Price, Daffner, Stowe, & Mesulam, 1990; Stone, Baron-Cohen, & Knight, 1996). Second, a number of investigators have noted strong parallels between the behavior of autistic individuals and that of patients suffering frontal lobe damage (e.g., Bishop, 1993; Damasio & Maurer, 1987; C. D. Frith & U. Frith, 1991; Ozonoff, Pennington, & Rogers, 1991; Prior & Hoffman, 1990). Specifically, both groups show (a) limited ability to plan for the future, or to anticipate the long-term consequences of their behavior, (b) deficits in the capacity to self-reflect or self-monitor, and (c) difficulties learning from mistakes, persevering with maladaptive strategies even when repeatedly made aware of their errors (for comprehensive reviews, see Damasio, 1985, and Fuster, 1997).

Interestingly, the psychological processes compromised in patients with frontal lobe dysfunction—the capacity to monitor and reflect on one's mental states—are defining features of James's (1890) *self-as-knower,* the subjective experience of self as a thinking, feeling, wanting, doing being. Although there is much we do not understand about this self-reflective aspect of self (for discussions, see Greenwald & Pratkanis, 1984; Kihlstrom & Klein, 1994; Stuss, 1991), we are perhaps a step closer to knowing where in the brain such a capacity resides. By capitalizing on what we know about frontal lobe function in

both normal and brain damaged individuals, we may come to a better understanding of the structure and function of this most elusive of Jamesian concepts.

Anosognosia and Attribution Theory

H. M. is aware of his memory deficit (he describes it as "like waking from a dream"), and he knows that there are things that he can't remember. However, there are other patients suffering from a variety of problems with memory, language, perception, or voluntary movement who appear to have no awareness of their deficits. This lack of awareness of a mental deficit was named *anosagnosia* by Babinski (1914, 1918; for recent reviews, see McGlynn & Schacter, 1989; Prigatano & Schacter. 1991). Anosognosic patients may acknowledge some difficulty in their impaired domains, but they attribute their problems to something besides their own deficits. It should be understood that these patients' behavior is not mere denial of deficit or indifference to it (when a patient acknowledges deficit but seems unconcerned about it, the syndrome is called *anosodiaphoria*).

Most of the classical descriptions of anosognosia are in cases of acute hemiplegia, hemianesthesia, and hemianopia (Bisiach & Geminiani, 1991). In *hemiplegia,* the person is paralyzed on one side of the body, due to damage to the contralateral hemisphere; in *hemianopia,* the person has a loss of sight in one side of the visual field. Interestingly, anosognosia is more likely to occur when the loss is localized on the left side of the body, implying that it is caused by damage to structures in the right cerebral hemisphere. However, the syndrome also occurs in cases of left-hemisphere damage, as for example in aphasia (e.g., Rubens & Garrett, 1991). Many aphasics, both expressive and receptive, attempt to correct their faulty speech production; by virtue of hesitations, pauses, and self-corrections they show clearly that they know that what they have intended to say hasn't come out as planned. However, many do not realize this, a failure that is common in cases of *jargon aphasia,* a special form of receptive aphasia in which the patient's speech is freely littered with meaningless utterances and phonemic and semantic paraphasias (using the wrong sounds or words). Such patients do not seem to realize that they are not communicating with their listeners, and, furthermore, they do not seem to realize that they don't understand what is being said to them. Interestingly, jargon aphasia seems to be more common in cases of bilateral damage; again, this implies that the right hemisphere plays a special role in awareness of deficits.

Anosognosia is a real danger to the patient, of course. People who don't realize that they are paralyzed on one side are headed for disaster if they should try to get up; those who don't realize they are blind on one side are unlikely to take special steps to avoid obstacles and oncoming objects on the affected side. In the dementing disorders, such as Alzheimer's disease and even schizophrenia, anosognosia is particularly insidious because it occurs in the late stages of illness (e.g., McGlynn & Kaszniak, 1991), when the patient is most impaired. Interestingly, however, anosognosics sometimes implicitly acknowledge their difficulties. The hemiplegic may not complain about being confined to a hospital bed or attempt some task that must be performed with both hands, and the hemianopic may actively ignore the affected portion of the environmental field. Neurological patients who are unaware of their deficits are poorly motivated for rehabilitation.

From a social-psychological view one wants to know what these patients make of their own behavior, given that they don't acknowledge their deficits. Some patients attribute their inability to move to arthritis or rheumatism rather than paralysis; others, when asked to move the affected limb, appear distracted or move the unaffected limb or respond that they have moved the affected limb, when in fact they have not (this even

happens when patients look at the affected limb during the examination). The explanations can sometimes become bizarre or delusional.

For example, the patient may claim that the affected limb is not his or her own, but rather belongs to someone else—forgotten by a previous patient or belonging to someone else lying at their side (often doing something naughty). One woman studied by Bisiach and Geminiani (1991) was anosognosic for her hemiplegia. She claimed that her left hand did not belong to her, but rather had been forgotten in the ambulance by another patient. She acknowledged that her left shoulder was her own and agreed with the inference that her left arm and elbow were also her own, because they were attached to her shoulder, but this inference did not extend to her left hand (she could not explain why that hand carried her wedding ring). Another hemiplegic patient stated that his own left arm was the examiner's. When the examiner placed the patient's left hand between his own two hands, the patient continued to deny that his arm hand was his own and attributed three arms and three hands to the examiner.

What we're seeing here, of course, are phenomena of attribution; the patients are trying to make sense of their experiences, given their beliefs about themselves and the world at large. These attributions may be convenient laboratory models for other kinds of beliefs, including those that are frankly delusional (for a review of attributional accounts of delusions, see Kihlstrom & Hoyt, 1988). Consider the following scenario: A hemiplegic patient is unaware of the loss of function on his left side and denies that his left arm and hand are his. Then what's he doing in bed? Why is someone else wearing his wedding ring? Where is the rest of that person, anyway? If he's forgotten his left hand, doesn't he miss it? Why doesn't the patient retrieve his wedding ring and put it back on his own left hand? Anomalous perceptual experiences arouse anxiety until they are satisfactorily explained, and in the course of formulating acceptable explanations, the patient must go through the sorts of processes studied by attribution theory. Accordingly, cases of anosognosia can provide an interesting proving ground for testing and refining theories about causal attributions, self–other differences, and other aspects of social judgment and inference.

Split Brains and Self-Perception

Few neuropsychological syndromes have generated greater interest among neuroscientists (e.g., Gazzaniga, 1970; Sperry, 1968, 1974; Springer & Deutsch, 1998) and philosophers (e.g., Marks, 1981; Nagel, 1971; Puccetti, 1973) than that of the commissurotomized (colloquially referred to as *split-brain*) patient. These patients have suffered from severe and uncontrollable epileptic seizures, much like those experienced by H. M., but their treatment is quite different. In an effort to alleviate the effects of otherwise intractable epilepsy, a procedure known as a complete cerebral commissurotomy is performed (e.g., Bogen, Fisher, & Vogel, 1965; Bogen & Vogel, 1962) in which the *corpus callosum,*[6] a large transverse band of approximately 200 million nerve fibers that directly connect the left and right cerebral hemispheres, is surgically cut.[7] Because epileptic seizures, which originate as electrical outbursts at a particular cortical site, tend to spread from one cerebral hemisphere to the other (thereby increasing the magnitude of the disturbance), cutting the corpus callosum is seen as a way of limiting the disturbance to one hemisphere, thereby decreasing its magnitude (e.g., Gazzaniga & LeDoux, 1978; Kolb & Whishaw, 1996; Sperry, 1974).

Medically, complete cerebral commissurotomy proved quite successful; confined to a single hemisphere, patients' epileptic seizures became less frequent or disappeared entirely (e.g., Kolb & Whishaw, 1996; Springer & Deutsch, 1998). Moreover, initial reports revealed no obvious postsurgical changes in their perceptual, cognitive, or everyday behavior (e.g., Akelaitis, 1941a, 1941b, 1944; Bogen, 1985).

However, extensive psychological testing by Roger Sperry and his colleagues (e.g., Franco & Sperry, 1977; Levy-Agresti & Sperry, 1968; Sperry, 1968) eventually uncovered some peculiar psychological consequences of hemispheric disconnection. Sperry's approach to testing split-brain patients depended on two key assumptions. First, that under suitable experimental control, it is possible to confine input presented to a split-brain patient to a single hemisphere (e.g., Sperry, 1968, 1974). Second, that in the vast majority of people, verbal reports issue from the left cerebral hemisphere. By contrast, the right hemisphere, although capable of limited linguistic analyses, lacks access to the speech mechanisms of the left hemisphere and thus is unable to initiate speech (e.g., Corballis, 1991; Kolb & Whishaw, 1996; Springer & Deutsch, 1998).

Using several subtle experimental techniques, Sperry and his colleagues were able to direct input exclusively to a single hemisphere and request a response of it (e.g., Franco & Sperry, 1977; Gordon & Sperry, 1969; Levy, Trevarthen, & Sperry, 1972; Levy-Agresti & Sperry, 1968; Sperry, 1968, 1974; Sperry, Gazzaniga, & Bogen, 1969; Zaidel, 1975). For example, when an object was visually presented to the left hemisphere, split-brain patients reported seeing it and could identify it verbally. However, when the same object was presented to the nonspeaking right hemisphere, patients claimed they saw nothing at all. Nevertheless, the right hemisphere could demonstrate nonverbally what it had seen by pointing at the correct object with the left hand (which is controlled by the right hemisphere). Similar findings were obtained using olfactory stimuli. When a clove of garlic was presented to a split-brain patient's right nostril (which stimulates the right hemisphere), he verbally denied smelling anything. However, when asked to point with his left hand to the object corresponding to the odor he smelled, he correctly selected the clove from among a set of smell related objects, at the same time verbally protesting that he didn't smell anything!

Findings such as these led Sperry to propose that surgery had left split-brain patients with two separate minds, each with its own separate sphere of consciousness (e.g., Sperry, 1966, 1968, 1974). In Sperry's (1968) words:

Each hemisphere seems to have its own separate and private sensations; its own perceptions; its own concepts; and its own impulses to act, with related volitional, cognitive, and learning experiences. Following surgery, each hemisphere also has thereafter its own separate chain of memories that are rendered inaccessible to the recall processes of the other. (p. 724)

A particularly intriguing case is that of patient P. S. (e.g., Gazzaniga & LeDoux, 1978; LeDoux, 1985; LeDoux, Wilson, & Gazzaniga, 1977). P. S. is unique among split-brain patients in that his right hemisphere, although unable to generate speech, has extensive linguistic abilities, enabling it to respond to a wide variety of verbal commands. For example, when the experimenters asked his right hemisphere to "laugh," it did as told and P. S. laughed aloud. Interestingly, however, when asked why he was laughing, the left hemisphere replied "Oh you guys are really something" (Gazzaniga & LeDoux, 1978, p. 146). In another study the experimenters simultaneously flashed an image of a snow scene to P. S.'s right hemisphere and an image of a chicken claw to his left hemisphere. Each hemisphere then was shown a set of pictures and instructed to select the one most closely associated with the image it had seen. The right responded by choosing (with his left hand) a picture of a shovel, and the left selected (with the right hand) a picture of a chicken to match the claw. When asked why he chose these particular pictures, his left hemisphere responded "I saw a claw and I picked a chicken, and you have to clean out the chicken shed with a shovel" (Gazzaniga & LeDoux, 1978, p. 148).

In each of these examples, P. S.'s left hemisphere was faced with a problem—it had observed a response but did not know why the response was performed. When asked "Why are you doing that?", the talking left hemisphere had to come up with a plausible explanation for a behavior performed in response to a command directed to the mute right hemisphere. As Gazzaniga and LeDoux (1978) noted, the left hemisphere proved quite adept at this task, interpreting the actions of the right as though it had insight into the cause of the behavior (when in fact it did not). On the basis of these findings, Gazzaniga and LeDoux concluded that the left hemisphere acts as the interpreter of action, attempting to provide as plausible an account as possible for the individual's behavior (for related views, see Jaynes, 1976; Popper & Eccles, 1977; Sperry, 1974).

Gazzaniga and LeDoux (1978; see also LeDoux, 1985) go on to suggest that the left hemisphere plays a similar role in individuals with intact brains. A considerable body of evidence suggests that we are not consciously aware of the causes of all the behaviors we produce or feelings we experience (for reviews, see Gazzaniga, 1998; Kihlstrom, 1987, in press-a, in press-b, Nisbett & Wilson, 1977; Oakley & Eames, 1985; Velmans, 1996). When an activity is initiated by a neural system whose motives are not consciously accessible, the verbal left hemisphere finds itself confronted with behavior carried out for unknown reasons. Under these circumstances, it attempts to attribute a cause to the action, thereby integrating the action into a coherent personal narrative (e.g., Gazzaniga, 1998; LeDoux, 1985). As Gazzaniga and LeDoux (1978) remarked, "It is as if the verbal self [i.e., left hemisphere] looks out to see what the person is doing, and from that knowledge it interprets reality" (p. 150).[8]

What Gazzaniga and LeDoux have provided us with, of course, is a neuropsychological model of Bem's (1967, 1972) influential theory of self-perception—the idea that people "come to know their own attitudes, emotions, and other internal states partially by inferring them from observations of their own overt behavior and/or the circumstances in which this behavior occurs" (Bem,

1972, p. 5). We believe that such a model can contribute in important ways to our understanding of the process involved in self-perception. The relation between lateralization and hemispheric specialization is becoming increasingly well-mapped experimentally (for a recent review, see Springer & Deutsch, 1998). By drawing on that knowledge, self-perception theorists may gain an understanding of the functional properties of the neural system responsible for drawing inferences about behavior whose origins are outside conscious awareness—an understanding that ultimately may lead to a better appreciation of the ways in which individuals attempt to construct a coherent story of self. And, by learning which of a person's behaviors are likely to be initiated by the nonverbal right hemisphere, theorists may be better able to identify the types of behaviors whose explanation require the inference-making capacities of the left hemisphere. Although the contributions of these particular neuropsychological perspectives on self-perception theory remain to be determined, it seems clear to us that, in the long run, research and theory both will benefit from a greater understanding of the neuropsychological mechanisms that make self-perception possible.

Phineas Gage and the Question of Cognition and Emotion

The relevance of neuropsychology for personality and social psychology is also illustrated by the classic case of Phineas Gage (e.g., Macmillan, 1986). In 1848, this young railway worker was preparing some explosive charges for use in an excavation. In so doing, he accidentally set off a spark that exploded the gunpowder, driving his custom-made tamping iron right through his skull—entering under his left eye socket, traveling behind his eye (severing the optic nerve), and emerging from the top of his head. Gage lived for a dozen more years, which is extraordinary in itself, but he also showed a marked change in personality. Whereas before the accident he had been described as shrewd, smart, energetic, and persistent, he now was described as fitful, irreverent, grossly profane, lacking in deference, impatient, obstinate, capricious and vacillating, childlike in his intellectual capacity, and with strong animal passions—in short, as the physician who attended his wounds put it, he was "no longer Gage" (Harlow, 1868).

The significance of the Gage case was not lost on the phrenologists. Nelson Sizer (1882), an American disciple of Gall and Spurzheim, concluded that the injury had obviously destroyed brain tissue "in the neighborhood of Benevolence and the front part of Veneration" (pp. 193–194). Even after the abandonment of phrenology, the Gage case was used, along with Broca's and Wernicke's cases of expressive and receptive aphasia, as a primary example of specialization of function in the cerebral cortex—in particular, for the localization of faculties relating to personality, social relationships, and emotion in the frontal lobe.[9] Modern neuropsychology has generally confirmed this conclusion, although we now know that the frontal lobes support cognitive as well as emotional and interpersonal functions (for a review of other cases of frontal lobe damage, see Damasio, 1985).

Neuropsychological evidence also can be brought to bear on the vexatious question of the relation between emotion and cognition. Is emotion a cognitive construction or an independent mental faculty? Although cognitive processing undoubtedly plays a role in emotion (e.g., Clark & Fiske, 1982), neuropsychological evidence does seem to show that some brain structures are specialized for emotion and for the processing of emotional as opposed to nonemotional memories. Consider, for example, the Kluver-Bucy syndrome (Kluver & Bucy, 1939), resulting from bilateral destruction of the amygdala and associated inferior portions of the temporal cortex. Humans and nonhuman animals with such lesions show a loss of fear and other emotional responses and increased and inappropriate sexual activity, among other symptoms. Such outcomes suggest that the amygdala plays a special role in emotion, a hypothesis that has been supported by LeDoux's (1987, 1996) finding that bilateral amygdalectomy impairs classical fear conditioning. Of course, cortical structures also are involved in emotion; patients with lesions in the right hemisphere, and in particular the temporal-parietal regions of the right hemisphere, have special difficulties in judging the mood of others from vocal or facial cues, choosing which uncaptioned cartoons are funny, selecting the correct punchlines to joke set-ups, and matching scenes for emotional valence. Cognition and emotion are certainly related, but the neuropsychological evidence seems to indicate that there are certain brain systems that are specialized for emotional processing, suggesting that cognition and emotion are also different mental faculties.

Prosopagnosia and Face Recognition

Neuropsychological evidence would seem to be especially relevant to understanding a basic social-cognitive process: how one person recognizes the face of another. The face is the fundamental social stimulus. It is the point of contact in the infant's very earliest social interactions; the smiles exchanged between infant and caregiver are the beginnings of life-long social bonds. Perceiving, identifying, and comprehending faces is absolutely basic to social interaction. We have to know who we are dealing with, what they are like, and how we relate to them, before we can interpret their behavior or plan our own. Even when dealing with strangers, the face provides cues to the emotional state of the other person, as well as hints of other things, like deception, that are important in negotiating an interaction. If we want to understand how we come to know another person, we have to understand how we read the face.

As it happens, neuropsychology has been very interested in the face, and, in fact, there is a specific form of visual agnosia involving the face. In general, *visual agnosia*—a term coined by Sigmund Freud (1891/1953) before he turned from neurology to psychoanalysis—refers to the inability to recognize objects (or pictures of objects). A person with visual object agnosia can describe an object, but cannot name it, recognize it as familiar, or demonstrate how it is used. Visual agnosia specific to the face is called *prosopagnosia,* a term coined by Bodamer (1947; for a recent review, see Damasio, Damasio, & Van Hoesen, 1982), and refers to the inability to recognize faces. Prosopagnosic patients can describe the physical features of faces, but they cannot name the individuals to whom they belong; interestingly, they are able to identify people from such characteristics as their voice, dress, posture, or gait. However, given the face alone, these patients have no idea who the person is or what to expect from them. This deficit is linked to bilateral damage in the occipital lobe, especially those areas adjacent to the temporal lobe. As social animals, we seem to have been built by evolution with brain structures specifically tuned to that most social of stimuli, the face (e.g., Brothers, 1997).

Prosopagnosia has been taken as evidence that there is a particular brain system specialized for the identification of faces (e.g., Farah, 1990; Farah, Wilson, Drain, & Tanaka, 1998). This proposal is not unreasonable, given our status as social animals and the obvious evolutionary advantages of being able to identify faces and discriminate among them, quickly and reliably. However, there is an interesting controversy here. It has been suggested that prosopagnosics have difficulty identifying any particular visual stimulus, not just faces. Unfortunately, the clinical evidence is equivocal. One prosopagnosic farmer was unable to recognize his own cows, as well as members of his own family (Bornstein, Sroka, & Munitz, 1969), whereas another prosopagnosic farmer—What's the chance of that?—lost the ability to recognize both his family members and his cows, but eventually recovered the former but not the latter (Assal, Favre, & Anderes, 1984). However, case studies are always difficult to interpret, and recent experimental and neuro-imaging studies of both prosopagnosic patients and intact participants strongly suggest that the "face area" damaged in prosopagnosia is actually specialized for expert recognition of objects at subordinate levels of categorization—objects which include, but are not limited to, faces (Gauthier, 1998).

Although prosopagnosia is dramatic, it turns out that there are many different forms of facial agnosia, each reflecting the selective impairment of some functions and the sparing of others. In general, the finding that two functions are dissociable from each other supports the hypothesis that the functions in question are qualitatively different. For example, some prosopagnosics are able to interpret the emotional meaning of facial expressions without being able to recognize the faces themselves, and others recover the ability to identify familiar faces but not the ability to interpret facial expressions. Interestingly, single-unit analyses of face perception in monkeys find separate neurons (or, more likely, separate clusters of neurons) that are responsive to identity and expression.

In an attempt to summarize the neuropsychological evidence, Bruce and Young (1986) proposed that facial perception involves several different processes that are carried out in parallel. According to their view, input from a facial stimulus is first processed by a structural encoding system that creates two different descriptions of the face—one which is view-centered (e.g., full-face or profile) and one that is independent of the particular expression on the face. Output from this structural encoding system then passes to other systems specialized for analysis of facial expressions, speech (actually, lip-reading), sameness or difference (as between full-face or profile views), and facial recognition. These functions are performed by separate systems, as indicated by the fact that they are dissociable. For example, prosopagnosic patients can identify facial expressions even though they do not recognize the faces as familiar, and there is at least one patient who has lost the ability to analyze facial expressions of emotion, but who retains the ability to lip-read.

In addition, among brain-damaged patients performance on a test of memory for unfamiliar faces is essentially unrelated to the ability to recognize famous faces. All of these results indicate that remembering unfamiliar faces and recognizing familiar faces are mediated by separate systems. The face recognition system is a sort of visual lexicon containing template representations of familiar faces. Information processed by the face recognition system then contacts associated information pertaining to the identity of the person whose face has been recognized and by this route retrieves the name associated with the familiar face. Thereafter, other information about the person is retrieved through the generic cognitive system. Note that the general cognitive system can influence some facial processing systems (e.g., expression analysis, facial speech analysis, and directed visual processing), but it cannot directly influence facial recognition. That influence must be mediated by cognitive activation of the person–identity nodes.

A model like this makes some interesting predictions about face processing that should interest social psychologists. For example, priming with the name attached to a face should influence face recognition, but not expression analysis; priming with the label of an emotional state should influence expression analysis, but not face recognition. We don't know yet whether this is true. A prediction that has been tested, however, is that familiarity should influence identity matching but not expression analysis. In an experiment performed by Young, Ellis, and their colleagues (e.g., Young, McWeeny, Hay, & Ellis, 1986), intact participants were asked whether two photographs showed the same type of facial expression or whether they showed the same person. Half the photographs were of individuals who were familiar from the news or entertainment media, the other half were mere mortals. In terms of response latencies, familiarity affected identity matching but not expression matching. This is especially interesting, insofar as other research indicates that facial expression analysis and face recognition rely on the same facial features. Although these features may be analyzed by a single structural encoding system, the output from this module appears to be passed to different task-specific systems operating in parallel.

We don't mean to imply that the Bruce–Ellis model has been tested and proven in every respect; it hasn't, and it might be wrong in significant ways. The point is only to show how neuropsychological evidence can contribute to social-psychological theory: First, by providing empirical evidence of a sort that would be difficult or impossible to obtain in laboratory studies of college sophomores or interviews of people in airports and laundromats; second, by providing specific theoretical models of cognitive processes that can be tested in laboratory studies of the sort that we do.

Toward a Social Neuropsychology

One of the most exciting trends in cognitive psychology over the past 20 years has been the increasing application of data and conceptual tools derived from the study of patients with neuropsychological syndromes. To date, however, social and personality psychologists have rarely considered neuropsychological case material when developing theories about social and personality processes. We hope this situation changes, for we believe the domain of clinical neuropsychology holds considerable untapped potential for formulating and testing models within personality and social psychology.

In this article we have described some of the ways in which questions of interest to social and personality psychologists can be addressed with neuropsychological data. For example, we have shown (a) how studying both the preserved and impaired capacities of patients suffering amnesia and autism can provide important new insights into the mental representation of self, (b) how understanding the ways in which anosognosic patients attempt to make sense of their disabilities can shed new light on the process of causal attribution, and (c) how consideration of the data from frontal lobe patients can help address questions concerning the relation between cognition and emotion. As we hope our review shows, there clearly is much social and personality psychologists can learn from the study of patients with neuropsychological syndromes.

Although our focus in this article has been on ways in which personality and social psychology can benefit from a consideration of neuropsychological case material, we also are convinced that neuropsychological theory and research can benefit from insights derived from personality and social psychology. To date, almost all of the work on patients with neuropsychological impairments has been done within the confines of cognitive psychology and cognitive neuropsychology, with relatively little attention paid to the interpersonal, emotional, and motivational lives of these individuals. Yet, the syndromes described in this article invariably are accompanied by profound changes in the individual's personal, social, and professional life (e.g., Blumer & Benson, 1975; Damasio, 1994; Hilts, 1995; Luria, 1972; O'Connor et al., 1995; M. F. Robinson & Freeman, 1954; Sacks, 1985), changes that have important implications for the way we approach treatment, conduct research, and formulate theory. Thus, it would seem that an important agenda item for the near future would be the adoption by cognitive neuropsychologists of the concepts and principles that have served their social and personality colleagues so well and the systematic extension of research on neuropsychological impairment beyond the purely cognitive to include the personal and social.

The study of the interpersonal and emotional lives of patients with neuropsychological syndromes promises to provide new perspectives on the relation between cognitive neuropsychology and social-personality psychology. However, this will not happen until psychologists interested in social and personality issues start considering neuropsychological case material and psychologists interested in neuropsychology begin to inquire into their patients' personal and social lives. Such an interdisciplinary approach is exciting because it would represent the beginning of a collaboration that ultimately might bridge a gap between social-personality psychology and cognitive neuropsychology.

Notes

1. Patient K. C. (e.g., Tulving, 1989, 1993) receives more detailed treatment in the next section of this article.

2. More recently, documentation of spared priming effects, coupled with the observation that amnesic patients can acquire new semantic knowledge and procedural knowledge that does not depend on episodic memory for their performance, has led cognitive scientists to draw a distinction between two expressions of memory: Explicit memory entails conscious recollection of past events, whereas implicit memory reflects the influence of past events on ongoing experience, thought, and action independent of conscious recollection (e.g., Schacter, 1987; see also Squire & Knowlton, 1995). The dissociation between explicit and implicit cognition is now a major research enterprise within cognitive psychology (e.g., Kihlstrom, in press-a), but it is not relevant to the present context.

3. The finding that one function is impaired and another one is spared reveals the basic methodology of cognitive neuropsychology: the *functional dissociation* (e.g., Shallice, 1988; Teuber, 1955; Weiskrantz, 1989). This term is rather confusing, because to most psychologists the term *dissociation* refers to the isolation of some percepts, memories, thoughts, or actions from conscious awareness (Kihlstrom, 1993). What neuropsychologists mean by dissociation, social psychologists recognize as the *interaction:* An independent variable (reflecting a state, condition, or experimental manipulation) affects one dependent variable but not another.

The dissociations that interest neuropsychologists come in four types (e.g., Dunn & Kirsner, 1988; Kelley & Lindsay, 1996; Neely, 1989). In the case of a *single dissociation,* a single independent variable, A, selectively affects performance on one task, X, but not on another, Y. In the *double dissociation,* one independent variable, A, affects dependent variable X but not dependent variable Y, whereas another independent variable, B, affects Y but not X. The double dissociation can be uncrossed or crossed: *Crossed* double interactions are especially interesting to neuropsychologists, because they are especially good evidence that two different processes are involved in the two tasks. Otherwise one would worry about artifacts like differential task difficulty. Even better evidence is provided by the *reversed association,* in which there is a positive correlation between dependent variables X and Y under conditions of independent variable A, but a negative correlation between these same variables under conditions of independent variable B. Reversed associations are particularly difficult to account for in terms of task difficulty (e.g., Dunn & Kirsner, 1988; Klein et al., 1997; Neely, 1989).

4. Craik et al. (in press) also concluded that the cognitive processes involved in self-reference were no different from those involved in referring to other individuals or in performing nonsocial semantic analyses. Thus, the neuroscience method of brain imaging confirmed conclusions that already had been reached on the basis of traditional experimental procedures employing behavioral measures (e.g., Kihlstrom et al., 1988; Klein & Kihlstrom, 1986).

5. Nicholas Humphrey's (1984, 1986, 1990) recent writings on the evolution of self-awareness in humans are suggestive of such a possibility. According to Humphrey, self-awareness, having been designed by natural selection, must contribute to our biological success. However, what selective advantage is provided by an ability to reflect on one's own mental states?

Humphrey proposed that the answer is to be found in the social challenges faced by our ancestors. From their initial appearance approximately 150,000 years ago (e.g., Dunbar, 1996), modern humans lived in a highly complex interpersonal milieu; accordingly, their survival depended on their being able to explain, predict, and manipulate the behavior of others. Self-reflective awareness served this function: By showing us how our own mind works, it provided us, by analogy, with a tool for understanding the minds of others like ourselves (for a related view, see Sedikides &

Skowronski, 1997). Thus, a necessary precondition for developing a theory of other minds is the possession of a theory of one's own mind. By implication, the absence of a theory of other minds may be diagnostic of a failure to develop a theory of self.

6. In addition to sectioning the corpus callosum, the Bogen and Vogel (1962) procedure also involved complete sectioning of the anterior and hippocampal commissures. It is via these three links that direct interhemispheric communication and integration take place.

7. Strictly speaking, the designation *split-brain surgery* is somewhat of a misnomer—although the corpus callosum and minor commissures are surgically severed, the subcortical regions linking the two hemispheres are left untouched by the surgery.

8. Additional support for this idea comes from studies of normal participants showing that the right hemisphere is greatly inferior to the left at drawing inferences and making decisions nonverbally (e.g., Gazzaniga & Smylie, 1984; Phelps & Gazzaniga, 1992; Vallar, Bisiach, Cerizza, & Rusconi, 1988).

9. Incidentally, despite appearances, the Gage case did not lay the foundation for prefrontal lobotomy (originally called *prefrontal leucotomy*) as treatment for mental illness. The inventor of psychosurgery, Egas Moniz (who won the 1949 Nobel Prize in Physiology or Medicine for his efforts), was much more influenced by the case of Joe A., reported by Brickner (1936). However, Freeman and Watts (1950), who were chiefly responsible for importing prefrontal lobotomies into the United States, made much of the Gage case (for a critical review of psychosurgery, see Valenstein, 1973). Why they did so is not at all clear, insofar as damage to Gage's frontal lobes seem to have made him very much worse as a person. Perhaps they were reassured by the preliminary reports of Harlow (1849) and Bigelow (1850), which suggested that Gage had suffered no mental impairment. However, by the time of Harlow's final reports (1868, 1869), it was clear that Gage had suffered a serious disorder of the emotions.

References

Akelaitis, A. J. (1941a). Psychobiological studies following section of the corpus callosum: A preliminary report. *American Journal of Psychiatry,* 97, 1147–1157.

Akelaitis, A. J. (1941b). Studies on the corpus callosum: II. The higher visual functions in each homonymous field following complete section of the corpus callosum. *Archives of Neurology and Psychiatry,* 45, 788–796.

Akelaitis, A. J. (1944). The study of gnosis, praxis and language following section of the corpus callosum and anterior commissure. *Journal of Neurosurgery,* 1, 94–102.

Assal, G., Favre, C., & Anderes, J. P. (1984). Non-reconnaissance d'animaux familiers chez un paysan: Zooagnosie ou prosopagnosie pour les animaux [Non-recognition of familiar animals by a peasant: Zooagnosia or Prosopagnosia for animals]. *Revue Neurologique,* 140, 580–584.

Babinski, J. (1914). Contribution a l'etude des troubles mentaux dans l'hemiplegie organique cerebrale (anosognosie) [Contribution to the study of mental disturbance in organic cerebral hemiplegia (anosognosia)]. *Revue Neurologie,* 1, 845–848.

Babinski, J. (1918). Anosognosie [Anosognosia]. *Revue Neurologie,* 31, 365–367.

Baddeley, A. D., & Warrington, E. K. (1970). Amnesia and the distinction between long- and short-term memory. *Journal of Verbal Learning and Verbal Behavior,* 9, 176–189.

Baron-Cohen, S. (1989). Are autistic children "behaviorists"? An examination of their mental–physical and appearance–reality distinctions. *Journal of Autism and Developmental Disorders,* 19, 579–600.

Baron-Cohen, S. (1990). Autism: A specific cognitive disorder of "mind-blindness." *International Review of Psychiatry,* 2, 79–88.

Baron-Cohen, S. (1991). The development of a theory of mind in autism: Deviance or delay? *Psychiatric Clinics of North America,* 14, 33–51.

Baron-Cohen, S. (1995). *Mindblindness: An essay on autism and theory of mind.* Cambridge, MA: MIT Press.

Baron-Cohen, S., Leslie, A. M., & Frith, U. (1985). Does the autistic child have a "theory of mind"? *Cognition,* 21, 37–46.

Baron-Cohen, S., Ring, H., Moriarty, J., Schmitz, B., Costa, D., & Ell, P. (1994). Recognition of mental state terms: Clinical findings in children with autism and a functional neuroimaging study in normal adults. *British Journal of Psychiatry,* 165, 640–649.

Baron-Cohen, S., Tager-Flusberg, H., & Cohen, D. (Eds.). (1993). *Understanding other minds: Perspectives from autism.* Oxford, England: Oxford University Press.

Bem, D. J. (1967). Self-perception: An alternative interpretation of cognitive dissonance phenomena. *Psychological Review, 74,* 183–200.

Bem, D. J. (1972). Self-perception theory. In L. Berkowitz (Ed.), *Advances in experimental social psychology* (Vol. 6, pp. 1–62). New York: Academic.

Berndt, R. S., & Caramazza, A. (1980). A redefinition of the syndrome of Broca's aphasia: Implications for a neuropsychological model of language. *Applied Linguistics, 1,* 225–278.

Bigelow, H. J. (1850). Dr. Harlow's case of recovery from the passage of an iron bar through the head. *American Journal of Medical Sciences, 19,* 13–22.

Bishop, D. V. M. (1993). Annotation: Autism, executive functions and theory of mind: A neuropsychological perspective. *Journal of Child Psychology and Psychiatry, 34,* 279–293.

Bisiach, E., & Geminiani, G. (1991). Anosognosia related to hemiplegia and hemianopia. In G. P. Prigatano & D. L. Schacter (Eds.), *Awareness of deficit after brain injury: Clinical and theoretical issues* (pp. 17–39). New York: Oxford University Press.

Blumer, D., & Benson, D. F. (1975). Personality changes with frontal and temporal lobe lesions. In D. F. Benson & D. Blumer (Eds.), *Psychiatric aspects of neurological disease* (pp. 151–169). New York: Grune & Stratton.

Bodamer, J. (1947). Die prosopagnosia [Prosopagnosia]. *Archiv fur Psychiatrie und Zeitschrift fur Neurologie, 179,* 6–54.

Bogen, J. E. (1985). The callosal syndromes. In K. M. Heilman & E. Valenstein (Eds.), *Clinical neuropsychology* (2nd ed., pp. 295–338). Oxford, England: Oxford University Press.

Bogen, J. E., Fisher, E. D., & Vogel, P. J. (1965). Cerebral commissurrotomy: A second case report. *Journal of the American Medical Association, 194,* 1328–1329.

Bogen, J. E., & Vogel, P. J. (1962). Cerebral commissurotomy in man: Preliminary case report. *Bulletin of the Los Angeles Neurological Societies, 27,* 169–172.

Bornstein, B., Sroka, M., & Munitz, H. (1969). Prosopagnosia with animal face agnosia. *Cortex, 5,* 164–169.

Brewer, W. F. (1986). What is autobiographical memory? In D. C. Rubin (Ed.), *Autobiographical memory* (pp. 25–49). Cambridge, England: Cambridge University Press.

Brickner, R. M. (1936). *The intellectual functions of the frontal lobes.* New York: Macmillan.

Brooks, D. N., & Baddeley, A. D. (1976). What can amnesic patients learn? *Neuropsychologia, 14,* 111–122.

Brothers, L. (1997). *Friday's footprint: How society shapes the human mind.* New York: Oxford University Press.

Brown, J. W. (1972). *Aphasia, apraxia, agnosia.* Springfield, IL: Thomas.

Bruce, V., & Young, A. (1986). Understanding face recognition. *British Journal of Psychology, 77,* 305–327.

Carruthers, P. (1996). Autism as mind-blindness: An elaboration and partial defence. In P. Carruthers & P. K. Smith (Eds.), *Theories of theories of mind* (pp. 257–273). Cambridge, England: Cambridge University Press.

Cermak, L. S. (1972). *Human memory: Theory and research.* New York: Ronald Press Company.

Cermak, L. S. (1984). The episodic–semantic distinction in amnesia. In R. L. Squire & N. Butters (Eds.), *Neuropsychology of memory* (pp. 45–54), New York: Guilford.

Cermak, L. S., & O'Connor, M. (1983). The anterograde and retrograde retrieval ability of a patient with amnesia due to encephalitis. *Neuropsychologia, 21,* 213–234.

Clark, M. S., & Fiske, S. T. (1982). *Affect and cognition: The seventeenth annual Carnegie symposium on cognition.* Hillsdale, NJ: Lawrence Erlbaum Associates, Inc.

Conway, M. A. (1992). A structural model of autobiographical memory. In M. A. Conway, D. C. Rubin, H. Spinnler, & W. A. Wagenaar (Eds.), *Theoretical perspectives on autobiographical memory* (pp. 167–194). Amsterdam: Kluwer.

Corballis, M. C. (1991). *The lopsided ape: Evolution of the generative mind.* New York: Oxford University Press.

Coslett, H. B. (1997). Neglect in vision and visual imagery: A double dissociation. *Brain, 120,* 1163–1171.

Craik, F. I. M., Moroz, T. M., Moscovitch, M., Stuss, D. T., Winocur, G., Tulving, E., & Kapur, S. (in press). In search of the self: A PET investigation of self-referential information. *Psychological Science.*

Crovitz, H. F., & Quina-Holland, K. (1976). Proportion of episodic memories from early childhood by years of age. *Bulletin of the Psychonomic Society, 7,* 61–62.

Crovitz, H. F., & Schiffman, H. (1974). Frequency of episodic memories as a function of their age. *Bulletin of the Psychonomic Society, 4,* 517–518.

Damasio, A. R. (1985). The frontal lobes. In K. M. Heilman & E. Valenstein (Eds.), *Clinical neuropsychology* (pp. 339–375). New York: Oxford University Press.

Damasio, A. R. (1994). *Descartes' error: Emotion, reason, and the human brain.* New York: Grosset/Putnam.

Damasio, A. R., Damasio, H., & Van Hoesen, G. W. (1982). Prosopagnosia: Anatomic basis and behavioral mechanisms. *Neurology, 32,* 331–341.

Damasio, A. R., & Maurer, R. G. (1987). A neurological model for childhood autism. *Archives of Neurology, 35,* 777–786.

Dunbar, R. (1996). *Grooming, gossip, and the evolution of language.* Cambridge, MA: Harvard University Press.

Dunn, J. C., & Kirsner, K. (1988). Discovering functionally independent mental processes: The principle of reversed association. *Psychological Review, 95,* 91–101.

Ellis, A. W., & Young, A. W. (1988). *Human cognitive neuropsychology.* London: Lawrence Erlbaum Associates, Inc.

Evans, J., Wilson, B., Wraight, E. P., & Hodges, J. R. (1993). Neuropsychological and SPECT scan findings during and after transient global amnesia: Evidence for the differential impairment of remote episodic memory. *Journal of Neurology, Neurosurgery, and Psychiatry, 56,* 1227–1230.

Farah, M. (1990). *Visual agnosia: Disorders of object recognition and what they tell us about normal vision.* Cambridge, MA: MIT Press.

Farah, M. J., Wilson, K. D., Drain, M., & Tanaka, J. N. (1998). What is "special" about face perception? *Psychological Review, 105,* 482–498.

Fay, W. H. (1979). Personal pronouns and the autistic child. *Journal of Autism and Developmental Disorders, 9,* 247–260.

Flavell, J. H., Green, F. L., & Flavell, E. R. (1995). Young children's knowledge about thinking. *Monographs of the Society for Research in Child Development, 60*(1, Serial No. 243).

Fletcher, P. C., Happe, F., Frith, U., Baker, S. C., Dolan, R. J., Frackowiak, R. S. J., & Frith, C. D. (1995). Other minds in the brain: A functional imaging study of "theory of mind" in story comprehension. *Cognition, 57,* 109–128.

Foster, J. K., & Jelicic, M. (Eds.). (in press). *Unitary and multiple system accounts of memory.* New York: Oxford University Press.

Franco, L., & Sperry, R. W. (1977). Hemisphere lateralization for cognitive processing of geometry. *Neuropsychologia, 15,* 107–113.

Freeman, W., & Watts, J. W. (1950). *Psychosurgery in the treatment of mental disorders and intractable pain.* Springfield, IL: Charles C. Thomas.

Freud, S. (1953). *On aphasia.* New York: International Universities Press. (Original work published 1891)

Frith, C. D., & Frith, U. (1991). Elective affinities in schizophrenia and childhood autism. In P. Bebbington (Ed.), *Social psychiatry: Theory, methodology and practice* (pp. 66–88). New Brunswick, NJ: Transactions.

Frith, U. (1989). *Autism: Explaining the enigma.* Oxford, England: Blackwell.

Fuster, J. M. (1997). *The prefrontal cortex: Anatomy, physiology, and neuropsychology of the frontal lobe.* Philadelphia: Lippincott-Raven.

Galton, F. (1879). Psychometric experiments. *Brain, 2,* 149–162.

Gardner, H. (1985). *The mind's new science: A history of the cognitive revolution.* New York: Basic Books.

Gauthier, I. (1998). *Dissecting face recognition: The role of categorization level and expertise in visual object recognition.* Unpublished doctoral dissertation, Yale University, New Haven, CT.

Gazzaniga, M. S. (1970). *The bisected brain.* New York: Appleton-Century-Crofts.

Gazzaniga, M. S. (1998). *The mind's past.* Berkeley, CA: University of California Press.

Gazzaniga, M. S., Ivry, R. B., & Mangun, G. R. (1998). *Cognitive neuroscience: The biology of the mind.* New York: Norton.

Gazzaniga, M. S., & LeDoux, J. E. (1978). *The integrated mind.* New York: Plenum.

Gazzaniga, M. S., & Smylie, C. S. (1984). Dissociation of language and cognition: A psychological profile of two disconnected right hemispheres. *Brain,* 107, 145–153.

Glisky, E. L. (1995). Computers in memory rehabilitation. In A. D. Baddeley, R. A. Wilson, & F. N. Watts (Eds.), *Handbook of memory disorders* (pp. 557–575). Chichester, England: Wiley.

Glisky, E. L., Schacter, D. L., & Tulving, E. (1986a). Computer learning by memory-impaired patients: Acquisition and retention of complex knowledge. *Neuropsychologia,* 24, 313–328.

Glisky, E. L., Schacter, D. L., & Tulving, E. (1986b). Learning and retention of computer-related vocabulary in memory-impaired patients: Method of vanishing cues. *Journal of Clinical and Experimental Neuropsychology,* 8, 292–312.

Goel, V., Grafman, J., Sadato, N., & Hallett, M. (1995). Modeling other minds. *Neuroreport,* 6, 1741–1746.

Goodglass, H. (1993). *Understanding aphasia.* San Diego, CA: Academic.

Gopnik, A., & Metzloff, A. N. (1997). *Words, thoughts, and theories.* Cambridge, MA: MIT Press.

Gordon, H. W., & Sperry, R. W. (1969). Lateralization of olfactory perception in the surgically separated hemispheres in man. *Neuropsychologia,* 12, 111–120.

Graf, P., Squire, L., & Mandler, G. (1984). The information that amnesic patients do not forget. *Journal of Experimental Psychology: Learning, Memory, and Cognition,* 10, 164–178.

Greenwald, A. G., & Pratkanis, A. R. (1984). The self. In R. S. Wyer & T. K. Srull (Eds.), *Handbook of social cognition* (Vol. 3, pp. 129–178). Hillsdale, NJ: Lawrence Erlbaum Associates, Inc.

Grice, H. P. (1941). Personal identity. *Mind,* 50, 330–350.

Harlow, J. M. (1849). Letter in "Medical miscellany." *Boston Medical and Surgical Journal,* 39, 506–507.

Harlow, J. M. (1868). Recovery from the passage of an iron bar through the head. *Publications of the Massachusetts Medical Society,* 2, 327–347.

Harlow, J. M. (1869). *Recovery from the passage of an iron bar through the head.* Boston: Clapp.

Heilman, K. M., & Valenstein, E. (1993). *Clinical neuropsychology* (3rd ed.). New York: Oxford University Press.

Hilts, P. J. (1995). *Memory's ghost: The strange tale of Mr. M. and the nature of memory.* New York: Simon & Schuster.

Humphrey, N. (1984). *Consciousness regained: Chapters in the development of mind.* Oxford, England: Oxford University Press.

Humphrey, N. (1986). *The inner eye.* London: Faber & Faber.

Humphrey, N. (1990). The uses of consciousness. In J. Brockman (Ed.), *Speculations: The reality club* (pp. 67–84). New York: Prentice Hall.

James, W. (1890). *The principles of psychology* (Vol. 1). New York: Holt.

Jaynes, J. (1976). *The origin of consciousness in the breakdown of the bicamarel mind.* Boston: Houghton Mifflin.

Jordan, R. R. (1989). An experimental comparison of the understanding and use of speaker–addressee personal pronouns in autistic children. *British Journal of Disorders of Communication,* 24, 169–179.

Keenan, J. M. (1993). An exemplar model can explain Klein and Loftus' results. In T. K. Srull & R. S. Wyer (Eds.), *Advances in social cognition* (Vol. 5, pp. 69–77). Hillsdale, NJ: Lawrence Erlbaum Associates, Inc.

Kelley, C. M., & Lindsay, D. S. (1996). Conscious and unconscious forms of memory. In E. L. Bjork & R. A. Bjork (Eds.), *Memory* (pp. 31–63). New York: Academic.

Kihlstrom, J. F. (1987). The cognitive unconscious. *Science,* 237, 1445–1452.

Kihlstrom, J. F. (1993, October). *Toward a neuropsychology of social cognition.* Paper presented at the Annual Meeting for the Society for Experimental Social Psychology, Santa Barbara, CA.

Kihlstrom, J. F. (in press-a). Conscious and unconscious cognition. In R. J. Sternberg (Ed.), *The concept of cognition.* New York: Oxford University Press.

Kihlstrom, J. F. (in press-b). The psychological unconscious. In L. Pervin (Ed.), *Handbook of personality: Theory and research* (2nd ed.). New York: Guilford.

Kihlstrom, J. F., Cantor, N., Albright, J. S., Chew, B. R., Klein, S. B., & Niedenthal, P. M. (1988). Information processing and the study of the self. In L. Berkowitz (Ed.), *Advances in experimental social psychology* (Vol. 21, pp. 145–178). San Diego, CA: Academic.

Kihlstrom, J. F., & Hoyt, E. P. (1988). Hypnosis and the psychology of delusions. In T. F. Oltmanns & B. A.

Maher (Eds.), *Delusional beliefs* (pp. 66–109). New York: Wiley-Interscience.

Kihlstrom, J. F., & Klein, S. B. (1994). The self as a knowledge structure. In R. S. Wyer & T. K. Srull (Eds.), *Handbook of social cognition* (Vol. 1, pp. 153–208). Hillsdale, NJ: Lawrence Erlbaum Associates, Inc.

Kihlstrom, J. F., & Klein, S. B. (1997). Self-knowledge and self-awareness. In J. G. Snodgrass & R. L. Thompson (Eds.), *Annals of the New York Academy of Sciences: Vol. 818. The self across psychology: Self-awareness, self-recognition, and the self-concept* (pp. 5–17). New York: New York Academy of Science.

Kinsbourne, M., & Wood, F. (1975). Short-term memory processes and the amnesic syndrome. In D. Deutsch & J. A. Deutsch (Eds.), *Short-term memory* (pp. 257–291). New York: Academic.

Klein, S. B. (1993, October). *The mental representation of self-knowledge: Evidence from clinical amnesia.* Paper presented at the Annual Meeting for the Society for Experimental Social Psychology, Santa Barbara, CA.

Klein, S. B. (1996, October). *The self and cognition.* Paper presented at the 1st Annual SELF Preconference at the Annual Meeting for the Society for Experimental Social Psychology, Sturbridge, MA.

Klein, S. B. (in press). Memory and the self. *McGraw-Hill 1999 yearbook of science and technology.* New York: McGraw-Hill.

Klein, S. B., Babey, S. H., & Sherman, J. W. (1997). The functional independence of trait and behavioral self-knowledge: Methodological considerations and new empirical findings. *Social Cognition,* 15, 183–203.

Klein, S. B., & Kihlstrom, J. F. (1986). Elaboration, organization, and the self-reference effect in memory. *Journal of Experimental Psychology: General,* 115, 26–38.

Klein, S. B., & Loftus, J. (1993). The mental representation of trait and autobiographical knowledge about the self. In T. K. Srull & R. S. Wyer (Eds.), *Advances in social cognition* (Vol. 5, pp. 1–49). Hillsdale, NJ: Lawrence Erlbaum Associates, Inc.

Klein, S. B., & Loftus, J., & Kihlstrom, J. F. (1996). Self-knowledge of an amnesic patient: Toward a neuropsychology of personality and social psychology. *Journal of Experimental Psychology: General,* 125, 250–260.

Klein, S. B., Scherman, J. W., & Loftus, J. (1996). The role of episodic and semantic memory in the development of trait self-knowledge. *Social Cognition,* 14, 227–291.

Kluver, H., & Bucy, P. C. (1939). Preliminary analysis of the functions of the temporal lobes in monkeys. *Archives of Neurology and Psychiatry,* 42, 979–1000.

Kolb, B., & Whishaw, I. Q. (1996). *Fundamentals of human neuropsychology* (4th ed.). New York: Freeman.

LeDoux, J. E. (1985). Brain, mind and language. In D. A. Oakley (Ed.), *Brain and mind* (pp. 197–216). London: Methuen.

LeDoux, J. E. (1987). Emotion. In F. Plum (Ed.), *Handbook of physiology: Section 1. The nervous system; Vol. 5. Higher functions of the brain* (pp. 419–460). Bethesda, MD: American Physiological Society.

LeDoux, J. E. (1996). *The emotional brain: The mysterious underpinnings of emotional life.* New York: Simon & Schuster.

LeDoux, J. E., Wilson, D. H., & Gazzaniga, M. S. (1977). A divided mind: Observations on the conscious properties of the separated hemispheres. *Annals of Neurology,* 2, 417–421.

Lee, A., Hobson, R. P., & Chiat, S. (1994). I, you, me, and autism: An experimental study. *Journal of Autism and Developmental Disorders,* 24, 155–176.

Leslie, A. M. (1987). Pretense and representation: The origins of "theory of mind." *Psychological Review,* 94, 412–426.

Leslie, A. M. (1991). The theory of mind impairment in autism: Evidence for a modular mechanism of development. In A. Whiten (Ed.), *Natural theories of mind* (pp. 63–78). Oxford, England: Blackwell.

Leslie, A. M., & Frith, U. (1988). Autistic children's understanding of seeing, knowing and believing. *British Journal of Developmental Psychology,* 6, 315–324.

Leslie, A. M., & Thaiss, L. (1992). Domain specificity in conceptual development: Neuropsychological evidence from autism. *Cognition,* 43, 225–251.

Levy, J., Trevarthen, C., & Sperry, R. W. (1972). Perception of bilateral chimeric figures following hemispheric disconnection. *Brain,* 92, 61–78.

Levy-Agresti, J., & Sperry, R. W. (1968). Differential perceptual capacities in major and minor hemispheres. *Proceedings of the National Academy of Science,* 61, 1151.

Locke, J. (1731). *An essay concerning human understanding.* London: Edmund Parker. (Original work published 1690)

Luria, A. R. (1972). *The man with a shattered world: The history of a brain wound.* Cambridge, MA: Harvard University Press.

Macmillan, M. B. (1986). A wonderful journey through skull and brains: The travels of Mr. Gage's tamping iron. *Brain & Cognition, 5,* 67–107.

Marks, C. E. (1981). *Commissurotomy consciousness and unity of mind.* Cambridge, MA: MIT Press.

McCarthy, R. A., & Warrington, E. K. (1990). *Cognitive neuropsychology: A clinical introduction.* San Diego, CA: Academic.

McGlynn, S. M., & Kaszniak, A. W. (1991). Unawareness of deficits in dementia and schizophrenia. In G. P. Prigatano & D. L. Schacter (Eds.), *Awareness of deficit after brain injury: Clinical and theoretical perspectives* (pp. 84–110). New York: Oxford University Press.

McGlynn, S. M., & Schacter, D. L. (1989). Unawareness of deficits in neuropsychological syndromes. *Journal of Clinical & Experimental Neuropsychology, 11,* 143–205.

Milner, B. (1966). Amnesia following operations on the temporal lobes. In C. W. M. Whitty & O. L. Zangwill (Eds.), *Amnesia.* London: Butterworth.

Milner, B., Corkin, S., & Teuber, H.-L. (1968). Further analysis of the hippocampal amnesic syndrome: 14-year follow up study of H. M. *Neuropsychologia, 6,* 215–234.

Nagel, T. (1971). Brain bisection and the unity of consciousness. *Synthese, 22,* 396–413.

Neely, J. H. (1989). Experimental dissociations and the episodic/semantic memory distinction. In H. L. Roediger & F. I. M. Craik (Eds.), *Varieties of memory and consciousness: Essays in honor of Endel Tulving* (pp. 229–270). Hillsdale, NJ: Lawrence Erlbaum Associates, Inc.

Nisbett, R. E., & Wilson, T. D. (1977). Telling more than we can know: Verbal reports on mental processes. *Psychological Review, 84,* 231–236.

Oakley, D. A., & Eames, L. C. (1985). The plurality of consciousness. In D. A. Oakley (Ed.), *Brain and mind* (pp. 217–251). London: Methuen.

O'Connor, M. G., Cermak, L. S., & Seidman, L. J. (1995). Social and emotional characteristics of a profoundly amnesic postencephalitic patient. In R. Camp-

bell & M. A. Conway (Eds.), *Broken memories: Case studies in memory impairment* (pp. 45–53). Oxford, England: Blackwell.

Ozonoff, S., Pennington, B. F., & Rogers, S. J. (1991). Executive function deficits in high-functioning autistic individuals: Relationship to theory of mind. *Journal of Child Psychology and Psychiatry, 32,* 1081–1105.

Phelps, E. A., & Gazzaniga, M. S. (1992). Hemispheric differences in mnemonic processing: The effects of left hemisphere interpretation. *Neuropsychologia, 30,* 293–297.

Pinker, S. (1994). *The language instinct: How the mind creates language.* New York: HarperCollins.

Polster, M. R., Nadel, L., & Schacter, D. L. (1991). Cognitive neuroscience analyses of memory: A historical perspective. *Journal of Cognitive Neuroscience, 3,* 95–116.

Popper, K. R., & Eccles, J. C. (1977). *The self and its brain.* Berlin, Germany: Springer-Verlag.

Premack, D., & Woodruff, G. (1978). Does the chimpanzee have a theory of mind? *The Brain and Behavioral Sciences, 4,* 515–526.

Price, B., Daffner, K., Stowe, R., & Mesulam, M. (1990). The compartmental learning disabilities of early frontal lobe damage. *Brain, 113,* 1383–1393.

Prigatano, G. P., & Schacter, D. L. (Eds.). (1991). *Awareness of deficit after brain injury: Clinical and theoretical issues.* New York: Oxford University Press.

Prior, M. R., & Hoffman, W. (1990). Brief report: Neuropsychological testing of autistic children through an exploration with frontal lobe tests. *Journal of Autism and Developmental Disorders, 20,* 581–590.

Puccetti, R. (1973). Brain bisection and personal identity. *British Journal for the Philosophy of Science, 24,* 339–355.

Quinton, A. (1962). The soul. *Journal of Philosophy, 59,* 393–409.

Robinson, J. A. (1976). Sampling autobiographical memory. *Cognitive Psychology, 8,* 578–595.

Robinson, M. F., & Freeman, W. (1954). *Psychosurgery and the self.* New York: Grune & Stratton.

Rubens, A. B., & Garrett, M. F. (1991). Anosognosia of linguistic deficits in patients with neurological deficits. In G. P. Prigatano & D. L. Schacter (Eds.), *Awareness of deficit after brain injury: Clinical and theoretical issues* (pp. 40–52). New York: Oxford University Press.

Sacks, O. (1985). *The man who mistook his wife for a hat*. New York: Doubleday.

Schacter, D. L. (1987). Implicit memory: History and current status. *Journal of Experimental Psychology: Learning, Memory, and Cognition,* 13, 501–518.

Schacter, D. L., & Tulving, E. (1982). Memory, amnesia, and the episodic/semantic memory distinction. In R. L. Isaacson & N. E. Spear (Eds.), *The expression of knowledge* (pp. 33–65). New York: Plenum.

Schacter, D. L., & Tulving, E. (Eds.). (1994). *Memory systems 1994*. Cambridge, MA: MIT Press.

Schneider, D. J., Roediger, H. L., & Khan, M. (1993). Diverse ways of accessing self-knowledge: Comment on Klein and Loftus. In T. K. Srull & R. S. Wyer (Eds.), *Advances in social cognition* (Vol. 5, pp. 123–136). Hillsdale, NJ: Lawrence Erlbaum Associates, Inc.

Scoville, W. B., & Milner, B. (1957). Loss of recent memory after bilateral hippocampal lesions. *Journal of Neurology, Neurosurgery, & Psychiatry,* 20, 11–21.

Sedikides, C., & Skowronski, J. J. (1997). The symbolic self in evolutionary context. *Personality and Social Psychology Review,* 1, 80–102.

Shallice, T. (1988). *From neuropsychology to mental structure*. New York: Cambridge University Press.

Sizer, N. (1882). *Forty years in phrenology: Embracing recollections of history, anecdote, and experience*. New York: Fowler & Wells.

Sperry, R. W. (1966). Brain bisection and the mechanisms of consciousness. In J. C. Eccles (Ed.), *Brain and conscious experience* (pp. 298–313). Heidelberg, Germany: Springer-Verlag.

Sperry, R. W. (1968). Hemisphere deconnection and unity in conscious awarencess. *American Psychologist,* 23, 723–733.

Sperry, R. W. (1974). Lateral specialization in the surgically separated hemispheres. In F. O. Schmitt & F. G. Worden (Eds.), *The neurosciences third study program* (pp. 5–19). Cambridge, MA: MIT Press.

Sperry, R. W., Gazzaniga, M. S., & Bogen, J. E. (1969). Interhemispheric relationships: The neocortical commissures: Syndromes of hemisphere disconnection. In P. J. Vinken & G. W. Bruyn (Eds.), *Handbook of clinical neurology* (Vol. 4, pp. 273–290). New York: North Holland.

Springer, S. P., & Deutsch, G. (1998). *Left brain right brain: Perspective from cognitive neuroscience*. New York: Freeman.

Squire, L. R., & Knowlton, B. J. (1995). Memory, hippocampus, and brain systems. In M. S. Gazzaniga (Ed.), *The cognitive neurosciences* (pp. 825–837). Cambridge, MA: MIT Press.

Squire, L. R., & Zola-Morgan, S. (1991). The medial temporal lobe memory system. *Science,* 253, 1380–1386.

Stone, V. E., Baron-Cohen, S., & Knight, R. T. (1996). Frontal lobe contributions to theory of mind. *Journal of Cognitive Neuroscience,* 10, 640–656.

Stuss, D. T. (1991). Self-awareness, and the frontal lobes: A neuropsychological perspective. In J. Strauss & G. R. Goethals (Eds.), *The self: Interdisciplinary approaches* (pp. 255–278). New York: Springer-Verlag.

Tager-Flusberg, H. (1992). Autistic children's talk about psychological states: Deficits in the early acquisition of a theory of mind. *Child Development,* 63, 161–172.

Teuber, H.-L. (1955). Physiological psychology. *Annual Review of Psychology,* 9, 267–296.

Tulving, E. (1983). *Elements of episodic memory*. New York: Oxford University Press.

Tulving, E. (1984). Precis of elements of episodic memory. *The Behavioral and Brain Sciences,* 7, 223–268.

Tulving, E. (1989). Remembering and knowing. *American Scientist,* 77, 361–367.

Tulving, E. (1993). Self-knowledge of an amnesic patient is represented abstractly. In T. K. Srull & R. S. Wyer (Eds.), *Advances in social cognition* (Vol. 5, pp. 147–156). Hillsdale, NJ: Lawrence Erlbaum Associates, Inc.

Tulving, E., Hayman, C. A. G., & Macdonald, C. A. (1991). Long-lasting perceptual priming and semantic learning in amnesia: A case experiment. *Journal of Experimental Psychology: Learning, Memory, and Cognition,* 17, 595–617.

Tulving, E., Schacter, D. L., McLachlan, D. R., & Moscovitch, M. (1988). Priming of semantic autobiographical knowledge: A case study of retrograde amnesia. *Brain and Cognition,* 8, 3–20.

Vallar, G., Bisiach, E., Cerizza, M., & Rusconi, M. L. (1988). The role of the left hemisphere in decision making. *Cortex,* 24, 399–410.

Valenstein, E. S. (1973). *Brain control: A critical examination of brain stimulation and psychosurgery*. New York: Wiley.

Van der Linden, M., Bredart, S., Depoorter, N., & Coyette, F. (1996). Semantic memory and amnesia: A case study. *Cognitive Neuropsychology,* 13, 391–413.

Velmans, M. (1996). *The science of consciousness: Psychological, neuropsychological and clinical reviews.* London: Routledge.

Warrington, E. K., & Weiskrantz, L. (1970). Amnesic syndrome: Consolidation or retrieval? *Nature,* 228, 628–630.

Weiskrantz, L. (1989). Remembering dissociations. In H. L. Roediger & F. I. M. Craik (Eds.), *Varieties of memory and consciousness: Essays in honor of Endel Tulving* (pp. 101–120). Hillsdale, NJ: Lawrence Erlbaum Associates, Inc.

Weiskrantz, L. (1997). *Consciousness lost and found.* New York: Oxford University Press.

Wellman, H. M. (1990). *The child's theory of mind.* Cambridge, MA: MIT Press.

Wheeler, M. A., Stuss, D. T., & Tulving, E. (1996). Toward a theory of episodic memory: The frontal lobes and autonoetic consciousness. *Psychological Bulletin,* 121, 331–354.

Wickelgren, W. A. (1973). The long and the short of memory. *Psychological Bulletin,* 80, 425–438.

Young, A. W., McWeeny, K. H., Hay, D. C., & Ellis, A. W. (1986). Matching familiar and unfamiliar faces on identity and expression. *Psychological Research,* 48, 63–68.

Zaidel, E. (1975). A technique for presenting lateralized visual input with prolonged exposure. *Vision Research,* 15, 283–289.

5   The Social Brain Hypothesis

Robin I. M. Dunbar

The consensus view has traditionally been that brains evolved to process information of ecological relevance. This view, however, ignores an important consideration: Brains are exceedingly expensive both to evolve and to maintain. The adult human brain weighs about 2% of body weight but consumes about 20% of total energy intake.[1] In the light of this, it is difficult to justify the claim that primates, and especially humans, need larger brains than other species merely to do the same ecological job. Claims that primate ecological strategies involve more complex problem-solving[2,3] are plausible when applied to the behaviors of particular species, such as termite-extraction by chimpanzees and nut-cracking by *Cebus* monkeys, but fail to explain why all primates, including those that are conventional folivores, require larger brains than those of all other mammals.

An alternative hypothesis offered during the late 1980s was that primates' large brains reflect the computational demands of the complex social systems that characterize the order.[4,5] Prima facie, this suggestion seems plausible: There is ample evidence that primate social systems are more complex than those of other species. These systems can be shown to involve processes such as tactical deception[4] and coalition-formation,[6,7] which are rare or occur only in simpler forms in other taxonomic groups. Because of this, the suggestion was rapidly dubbed the Machiavellian intelligence hypothesis, although there is a growing preference to call it the social brain hypothesis.[8,9]

Plausible as it seems, the social brain hypothesis faced a problem that was recognized at an early date. Specifically, what quantitative empirical evidence there was tended to favor one or the other of the ecological hypotheses,[10] whereas the evidence adduced in favor of the social brain hypothesis was, at best, anecdotal.[5] In this article, I shall first show how we can test between the competing hypotheses more conclusively and then consider some of the implications of the social brain hypothesis for humans. Finally, I shall briefly consider some of the underlying cognitive mechanisms that might be involved.

Testing between Alternative Hypotheses

To test between the competing hypotheses, we need to force the hypotheses into conflict in such a way that their predictions are mutually contradictory. This allows the data to discriminate unequivocally between them. In the present case, we can do this by asking which hypothesis best predicts the differences in brain size across the primate order. To do so, we need to identify the specific quantitative predictions made by each hypothesis and to determine an appropriate measure of brain size.

The four classes of hypotheses that have been put forward to explain primate brain evolution are epiphenomenal, developmental, ecological, and social in orientation (table 5.1). The epiphenomenal and developmental hypotheses share the assumption that evolution of the brain (or brain part) is not a consequence of external selection pressures but rather simply a consequence of something to do with the way biological growth processes are organized. The epiphenomenal hypotheses thus argue that brain evolution is a mere byproduct of body size evolution, and that brain part size is, in turn, a byproduct of total brain evolution.[11]

The developmental versions differ only in that they provide a more specific mechanism by presuming that maternal metabolic input is the critical factor influencing brain development. This claim is given credibility by the fact that the bulk of brain growth in mammals occurs prenatally. Indeed, it appears to be the completion of brain development that precipitates birth in mammals,

Table 5.1
Hypotheses used to explain the evolution of large brains in primates

Hypothesis	Sources
A. Epiphenomenal hypotheses	
1. Large brains (or brain parts) are an unavoidable consequence of having a large body (or brain)	11, 70
B. Ecological hypotheses	
2. Frugivory imposes higher cognitive demands than folivory does	10, 65
3. Brain size constrains the size of the mental map:	10
(a) constraint on size of home range	
(b) constraint on inertial navigation (day journey length)	
4. Extractive foraging hypothesis	2, 3
C. Social hypotheses	
5. Brain size constrains size of social network (group size):	5, 71, 72
(a) constraint on memory for relationships	
(b) constraint on social skills to manage relationships	
D. Developmental hypotheses	
6. Maternal energy constraints determine energy capacity for fetal brain growth	12, 13, 46, 55, 73

with what little postnatal brain growth occurs being completed by the time an infant is weaned. From this, the conclusion is drawn that brain evolution must be constrained by the spare energy, over and above her basal metabolic requirements, that the mother has to channel into fetal development.[12-14] Some evidence in support of this claim comes from the fact that frugivorous primates have larger adult brains relative to body size than do folivorous primates.[10] This has been interpreted as implying that frugivores have a richer diet than folivores do and thus have more spare energy to divert into fetal growth.

Large brains are thus seen as a kind of emergent epigenetic effect of spare capacity in the system.

Both kinds of explanations suffer from the problem that they ignore a fundamental principle of evolutionary theory, which is that evolution is the outcome of the balance between costs and benefits. Because the cost of maintaining a large brain is so great, it is intrinsically unlikely that large brains will evolve merely because they can. Large brains will evolve only when the selection factor in their favor is sufficient to overcome the steep cost gradient. Developmental constraints are undoubtedly important, but rather than being causal their role is that of a constraint that must be overcome if larger brains are to evolve. In addition, Pagel and Harvey[15] have shown that the energetic arguments do not add up: Precocial mammals do not have higher metabolic rates than do altricial mammals despite the fact that they have neonatal brain sizes that are, on average, twice as large. We therefore do not need to consider either epiphenomenal or developmental hypotheses any further in the context of this article.

This does not necessarily mean that these explanations are wrong. Both kinds of explanation may be true in the sense that they correctly identify developmental constraints on brain growth, but they do not tell us why brains actually evolved as they did. They may tell us that if you want to evolve a large brain, then you must evolve a large body in order to carry the energetic costs of doing so or a diet that ensures sufficient energy to provide for fetal brain development. No such allometric argument can ever imply that you have to evolve a large brain or a large body. The large brain or brain part is a cost that animals must factor into their calculations when considering whether or not a large body or a large brain is a sensible solution to a particular ecological problem. Shifts to more energy-rich or more easily processed diets may be essential precursors of significant increases in brain or brain part size.[1] This would explain why frugivores have larger brains than folivores do and why hominids have larger brains than great apes do.

This leaves us with just two classes of hypotheses, the ecological and the social. At least three versions of the former can be identified, which I will term the dietary, mental maps, and extractive foraging hypotheses. In essence, these argue, respectively, that primate species will need larger brains if (i) they are frugivorous because fruits are more ephemeral and patchy in their distribution than leaves are, and hence require more memory to find; (ii) they have larger ranges because of the greater memory requirements of large-scale mental maps; or (iii) their diet requires them to extract resources from a matrix in which they are embedded (e.g., they must remove fruit pulp from a case, stimulate gum flow from a tree, extract termites from a termitarium, or hunt species that are cryptic or behave evasively).

For obvious reasons, I used the percentage of fruit in the diet as an appropriate index for the dietary hypothesis. I used the size of the range area and the length of the day journey as alternative indices for the mental mapping hypothesis, though I present the data only for the first of these here. The first index corresponds to the case in which animals have to be able to manipulate information about the locations of resources relative to themselves in a Euclidean space (an example would be the nut-cracking activities of the Taï chimpanzees[16]); the second corresponds to the possibility that the constraint lies in the needs of some aspect of inertial navigation. The extractive foraging hypothesis is less easy to characterize in quantitative terms because there is no objective measure of the degree to which diets vary in their extractiveness. However, Gibson[3] provided a classification of primate species into four categories of diet that differ in their degree of extractiveness. We can test this hypothesis by asking whether there is a consistent variation in brain size among these four categories, with the species having the more extractive diets having larger brains than those with the less extractive diets.

Finally, we need an index of social complexity. In my original analyses, I used social group size as a simple measure of social complexity. Although at best rather crude, this measure nonetheless captures one aspect of the complexity of social groups, the fact that information-processing demands can be expected to increase as the number of relationships involved increases. More importantly, perhaps, this measure has the distinct merit of being easily quantified and widely available. Although it is possible to conceive of a number of better measures of social complexity, the appropriate data are rarely available for more than one or two species.

The second problem concerns the most appropriate measure of brain evolution. Hitherto, most studies have considered the brain as a single functional unit. This view has been reinforced by Finlay and Darlington,[11] who argued that the evolution in brain part size closely correlates with the evolution of total brain size and can be explained simply in terms of allometric consequences of increases in total brain size. However, Finlay and Darlington failed to consider the possibility that changes in brain size might actually be driven by changes in its parts rather than in the whole brain. This is especially true of the neocortex, for its volume accounts for 50% to 80% of total brain volume in primates. Thus, changes in the volume of the neocortex inevitably have a large direct effect on apparent change in brain volume that may be quite unrelated to changes in other brain components. This point is given weight by the fact that Finlay and Darlington themselves showed that neocortex size is an exponential function of brain size, whereas other brain components are not.

Finlay and Darlington[11] notwithstanding, there is evidence that brain evolution has not been a history of simple expansion in total volume. Rather, brain evolution has been mosaic in character, with both the rate and the extent of evolution having varied between components of the system. MacLean[17] pointed out many years ago that primate brain evolution can be viewed

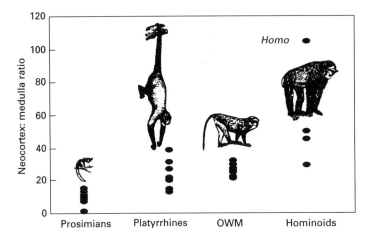

Figure 5.1
Neocortex volume as a ratio of medulla volume in different groups of primates (after Passingham[19]). (From: Stephan et al.[29])

in terms of three major systems (his concept of the triune brain). These systems correspond to the basic reptilian brain (hind- and midbrain systems), the mammalian brain (palaeocortex, subcortical systems), and the primate brain (broadly, the neocortex). A more important point, perhaps, is that variations can be found within these broad categories in the rates at which different components expanded, which, in at least some cases, have been shown to correlate with ecological factors.[9] Partialling out the effects of body size on the size of brain components suggests that the story may be more complex than Finlay and Darlington[11] supposed, with some remodeling of brain growth patterns occurring in the transitions between insectivores, prosimians, and anthropoids.[18]

The important point in the present context is that, as Passingham[19] noted, relative to the more primitive parts of the brain such as the medulla, the neocortex shows dramatic and increasing expansion across the range of primates (figure 5.1). The neocortex is approximately the same size as the medulla in insectivores; however, it is about

10 times larger than the medulla in prosimians and 20–50 times larger in the anthropoids, with the human neocortex being as much as 105 times the size of the medulla.

This suggests that rather than looking at total brain size, as previous studies have done, we should in fact be considering the brain system, namely the neocortex, that has been mainly responsible for the expansion of the primate brain. From the point of view of all the hypotheses of primate brain evolution, this makes sense: The neocortex is generally regarded as being the seat of those cognitive processes that we associate with reasoning and consciousness, and therefore may be expected to be under the most intense selection from the need to increase or improve the effectiveness of these processes.

One additional problem needs to be resolved. In his seminal study of brain evolution, Jerison[20] argued that brain size can be expected to vary with body size for no other reason than fundamental allometric relationships associated with the need to manage the physiological machinery of the body. What is of interest, he suggested, is not absolute brain size, but the spare brain capacity over and above that needed to manage body mechanisms. For this reason, Jerison derived his encephalization quotient. All subsequent studies have used body size as the appropriate baseline against which to measure relative deviations in brain size. However, a problem has since emerged: Brain size is determined early in development and, compared to many other body systems, appears to be highly conservative in evolutionary terms. As a result, body size can often change dramatically both ontogenetically across populations in response to local environmental conditions[21] and phylogenetically[22,23] without corresponding changes in brain size. This is particularly conspicuous in the case of phyletic dwarfs (e.g., callitrichids and perhaps modern humans and hylobatids[22]) and species in which body size may have increased in response to predation pressure following the occupation of more open terrestrial habitats (e.g., papionids[24]).

The lability of body size therefore makes it a poor baseline, though one that probably is adequate for analyses on the mouse-elephant scale. Consequently, it is necessary to find an internally more consistent baseline for taxonomically fine-grained analyses. Willner[22] suggested that either molar tooth size or brain size may be suitable because both are developmentally conservative. Because we are concerned with brain part size, some aspect of brain size seems the most appropriate.

At this point, three options are available. One is to compare the neocortex, the brain part of interest, with the whole brain; the second is to use the rest of the brain other than the part of interest; the third is to use some less variable primitive component of the brain, such as the medulla, as a baseline. Two options are in turn available as mechanisms for controlling for brain size in each of these cases. One is to use residuals from a common regression line against the baseline (e.g., the residual of neocortex volume on total brain volume or medulla volume). The other choice is to use ratios.

We have considered and tested all these options[9,24] (see box 5.1). The results are virtually identical irrespective of which measure is used. One explanation for this may be that all these measures actually index the same thing, absolute neocortex size, mainly because the neocortex is such a large component of the primate brain. Indeed, the use of absolute neocortex size produces results that are similar to those obtained from relativized indices of neocortex volume.[24,25] This makes some sense in computational terms: As Byrne[26] has pointed out, a 10% increase in the processing capacity of a small computer is worth a great deal less in information-processing terms than is a 10% increase in a large computer. Although residuals from a common regression line would conventionally be considered the safest measure, and have been used in many recent analyses,[27,28] I shall continue to use my original ratio index because it provides the best predictor (see box 5.1).

Finally, it is now widely appreciated that comparative analyses need to control for the effects of phylogenetic inertia. Closely related species can be expected to have similar values for many anatomical and behavioral dimensions merely by virtue of having inherited them from a recent common ancestor. In such cases, plotting raw data would result in pseudoreplication, artificially inflating the sample size by assuming that closely related species are actually independent evolutionary events. The ways of dealing with this problem include plotting means for higher taxonomic units, performing nested analyses of variance using phylogenetic levels as factors, comparing matched pairs of species, and making independent contrasts that control directly for phylogeny. Each method has its own advantages and disadvantages, but the first and third procedures are particularly associated with loss of information and small sample sizes. I shall use the first and last method, the last because it allows individual species to be compared, but the first because it allows grade shifts within data sets to be identified (a problem that independent-

Box 5.1
How to measure brains

R. Dunbar and Tracey H. Joffe

The different ways of measuring relative brain size have raised doubts as to the most appropriate technique to use.[65] Many researchers have preferred to use residuals from the common regression line of best fit for the data set concerned. This provides a measure of the extent to which brain (or brain part) volume deviates from what would be expected for an average member of the relevant taxon of the appropriate size. Although ratios have been used to compare the relative size of brain components,[29,66] this has been criticized on the grounds that trade-offs within the brain may mean that a given index simply measures total brain size (or the size of a brain part) and thus does not remove the effects of absolute size. Ratios may also be prone to autocorrelation effects, especially when the baseline is taken to be the whole brain and, as in the case of the neocortex, the part in question is a major volumetric component of the brain.

Although there are likely to be some trade-offs of this kind within the brain, the fact that neocortex volume increases progressively across the primate order suggests that such constraints are less likely to have a significant effect on a ratio measure. Of course the residuals procedure is itself a ratio: Encephalization-type indices are calculated as actual volume divided by predicted volume (which, when data are logged, becomes the conventional actual minus predicted values). Thus, ratio measures per se may not be the problem. Rather, the substantive objection is whether or not a ratio partials out the allometric effects of body size. In fact, it seems that neocortex ratios are not correlated with the basal brain (i.e., brain volume excluding the neocortex) within major taxonomic groups (unpublished analyses). Consequently, this criticism has less force than it might appear to have on first sight. Moreover, any index that uses the whole brain as its base is likely to suffer from autocorrelation effects. Because the neocortex is such a large proportion of the brain in primates, residuals of neocortex from total brain size may simply be a measure of neocortex plotted against itself.

To consider the problem in more detail, we ran a stepwise regression analysis on the 24 species of anthropoid primates, including humans, on the data base of Stephan, Frahm, and Baron,[29] with group size as the dependent variable and nine indices of relative brain or brain-part volume as independent variables. In addition to neocortex ratio, these included total brain volume as well as telencephalon and neocortex volume, each taken as absolute volume and as a residual from both body mass and brain volume. All variables were $\log_{10}$-transformed for analysis. In both cases, neocortex ratio was selected as the variable of first choice. We carried out both regressions on generic plots and independent contrast analyses. For the contrasts analysis, the best fit least-squares regression equation through the origin was:

Contrast in $\log_{10}$(group size) = 3.834
* Contrast in $\log_{10}$(neocortex ratio)
($r^2 = 0.395, F_{1,22} = 15.39, P = 0.001$).

Table 5.2
Stepwise regression analysis of indices of brain component volume as predictors of group size in anthropoid primates, based on independent contrasts analysis*

Independent variable	t	P
Absolute brain volume	-1.69	0.107
Residual of brain volume on body mass	-0.91	0.371
Absolute telencephalon volume	-1.72	0.101
Residual of telencephalon volume on body mass	0.61	0.546
Residual of telencephalon volume on brain volume	1.69	0.107
Absolute neocortex volume	-1.70	0.104
Residual of neocortex volume on body mass	0.56	0.583
Residual of neocortex volume on brain volume	1.60	0.136
Neocortex ratio (against rest of brain)	3.79	0.001

*Sample: 24 species of anthropoid primates from Stephan, Frahm, and Baron.[29]

Box 5.1
(continued)

With all other variables held constant, none of the other eight indices made a significant contribution to the variability in group size in either analysis. Table 5.2 gives the results for the independent contrasts analysis.

Neocortex ratio is thus the single most powerful predictor of group size in these species. While the biological significance of this variable remains open to interpretation, the fact that it provides the best predictor, independently of all other confounding measures, suggests that more detailed consideration needs to be given to its significance and meaning. It may be, for example, that body size, rather than being a determinant[20] is simply a constraint on neocortex size: A species can evolve a large neocortex only if its body is large enough to provide the spare energy capacity through Kleiber's relationship for basal metabolic rate to allow for a larger than average brain. This interpretation is implied by the Aiello and Wheeler[1] "expensive tissue hypothesis." It would also be in line with Finlay and Darlington's[11] claim that in mammals the evolution of brain-part size is driven, developmentally at least, by the evolution of the whole brain, thus generating very tight correlations between brain-part size and total brain size.

contrasts methods have difficulty dealing with). I shall take the genus as a suitable basis for analysis because genera typically represent different reproductive or ecological radiations and thus are more likely to constitute independent evolutionary events.

The resulting analyses are relatively straightforward: figure 5.2 presents the data for neocortex ratio for the anthropoid primate species in the data base of Stephan, Frahm, and Baron.[29] Neocortex size, however measured, does not correlate with any index of the ecological hypotheses, but does correlate with social group size. Similar findings were reported by Sawaguchi and Kudo,[30] who found that neocortex size correlated with mating system in primates. Barton and Purvis[31] have confirmed that using both residuals of neocortex volume on total brain volume and the method of independent contrasts yields the same result. Both Barton[9] and T. Joffe (unpublished) have repeated the analyses using the medulla as the baseline for comparison. More importantly, Barton and Purvis[31] have shown that while relative neocortex volume correlates with group size but not the size of the ranging area, the reverse is true of relative hippocampus size. A correlation between range area and hippocampus size is to be expected because of hippocampal involvement in spatial memory.[32,33] This correlation demonstrates that it is not simply total brain size that is important (a potential problem, given the overwhelming size of the primate neocortex). Moreover, it points to the specific involvement of the neocortex.

The validity of this relationship could be tested directly by using it to predict group sizes in a sample of species for which brain volumetric data were not available in the original sample of Stephan, Frahm, and Baron.[29] I did this by exploiting the fact that neocortex ratios can be predicted from total brain volume,[34] a result that, in fact, follows directly from the Finlay and Darlington[11] findings. The result was a significant fit between predicted neocortex ratio and observed mean group size for a sample of 15 New and Old World monkey species.[35]

Barton[27] noted that the original analyses of Dunbar[24] seemed to imply that variation in neocortex size was much greater than variation in group size in the prosimians. Using Dunbar's[24] data on group size, Barton suggested that the relationship between neocortex and group size did not apply in the case of prosimians. However, the data on prosimian group sizes in this sample suffered from a paucity of data, particularly for the nocturnal species. Because many of these are

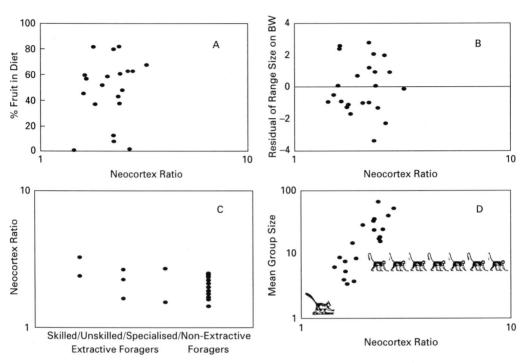

Figure 5.2
Relative neocortex size in anthropoid primates plotted against (a) percentage of fruit in the diet, (b) mean home-range size scaled as the residual of range size regressed on body weight (after Dunbar[24]), (c) types of extractive foraging (after Gibson[3]), and (d) mean group size. (Panels a, b, and d are redrawn from Dunbar,[24] figures 6, 2, and 1, respectively; panel c is from Dunbar,[35] figure 2.)

described as semi-solitary, it was conservatively assumed in the Dunbar[24] database that their group size was one. More recent field studies have produced markedly improved estimates of the sizes of social groups and, in the case of the semi-solitary species, daytime nest groups.[36] Re-analysis of the data for prosimians using these improved estimates of social group size suggests that these species do in fact adhere to the same relationship between neocortex and group size as that which pertains for other primates.[25] More importantly, the regression line for this taxon is parallel to, but shifted to the left of, that for other anthropoid primates (figure 5.3).

This relationship has now been shown to hold for at least four other mammalian orders: bats,[9] carnivores and insectivores,[37,38] and odontocete cetaceans.[39,40] In the case of the insectivores, the data points are shifted far to the left of those for the primates, as might be expected of a taxonomic group that is considered to be broadly representative of the ancestral mammals.[37] However, the relationship is weak in this case, probably because estimates of group size are particularly uncertain for insectivores.

Surprisingly, the data for the carnivores map directly onto those for the simian primates, that is, the regression lines for the two data sets do

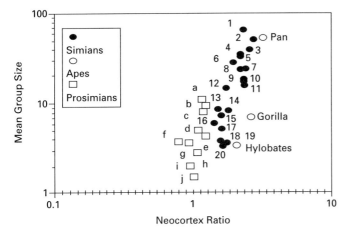

Figure 5.3

Mean group size plotted against neocortex ratio for individual genera, shown separately for prosimian, simian, and hominoid primates. Prosimian group size data, from Dunbar and Joffe,[25] include species for which neocortex ratio is estimated from total brain volume. Anthropoid data are from Dunbar.[24] Simians: 1, *Miopithecus;* 2, *Papio;* 3, *Macaca;* 4, *Procolobus;* 5, *Saimiri;* 6, *Erythrocebus;* 7, *Cercopithecus;* 8, *Lagothrix;* 9, *Cebus;* 10, *Ateles;* 11, *Cercocebus;* 12, *Nasalis;* 13, *Callicebus;* 14, *Alouatta;* 15, *Callimico;* 16, *Cebuella;* 17, *Saguinius;* 18, *Aotus;* 19, *Pithecia;* 20, *Callicebus.* Prosimians: a, *Lemur;* b, *Varecia;* c, *Eulemur;* d, *Propithecus;* e, *Indri;* f, *Microcebus;* g, *Galago;* h, *Hapalemur;* i, *Avahi;* j, *Perodictus.*

not differ significantly. However, the carnivores do not exhibit as wide a range of neocortex ratios or group sizes as do anthropoid primates. The fact that the prosimians lie to the left of both these taxonomic groups implies that the carnivores represent an independent evolutionary development along the same principles as the anthropoid primates, the difference being that they just have not taken it as far as primates have. One reason for this may be that the carnivore social world is olfaction-dominated rather than vision-dominated, as in the case of the primates. Barton[9,27,41] has pointed out that the shift to a diurnal lifestyle based on color vision, perhaps initially diet-driven, but leading to a shift into vision-based communication, may be the key feature that has spurred on the dramatic development of the primate neocortex.

Refining the Relationship

The social brain hypothesis implies that constraints on group size arise from the information-processing capacity of the primate brain, and that the neocortex plays a major role in this. However, even this proposal is open to several interpretations as to how the relationship is mediated. At least five possibilities can be usefully considered. The constraint on group size could be a result of the ability to recognize and interpret visual signals for identifying either individuals or their behavior; limitations on memory for faces; the ability to remember who has a relationship with whom (e.g., all dyadic relationships within the group as a whole); the ability to manipulate information about a set of relationships; and the

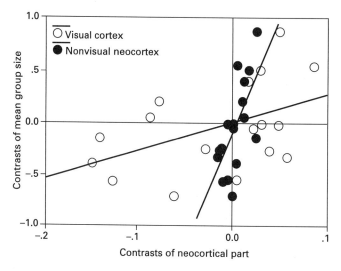

Figure 5.4

Independent contrasts in mean group size plotted against contrasts in the visual cortex and the volume of the rest of the neocortex (nonvisual neocortex) for individual anthropoid species. Note that the visual cortex is here defined as visual area V1; the nonvisual cortex is the non-V1 volume of the neocortex and thus includes some higher order visual processing components (e.g., visual area V2). Unfortunately, the data base of Stephan, Frahm, and Baron[29] does not allow us to define our measure of the nonvisual area any more finely than this. (Reprinted from Joffe and Dunbar,[28] figure 1.)

capacity to process emotional information, particularly with respect to recognizing and acting on cues to other animals' emotional states. These are not all necessarily mutually exclusive, but they do identify different points in the cognitive mechanism that might be the crucial information-processing bottleneck.

Although visual mechanisms are likely to be important for social interaction, and may well have been the initial kick for the evolution of large brains in primates,[9] it seems intrinsically unlikely that the ultimate constraint lies in the mechanisms of the visual system itself.[28] Although there is a correlation between the relative size of the visual cortex and group size in anthropoid primates, the fit is much poorer, and the slope significantly shallower than that between the nonvisual neocortex and group size ($r^2 = 0.31$ vs $r^2 = 0.61$, respectively) (figure 5.4). Partial

correlation analysis indicates that only the correlation for the nonvisual relationship remains significant when the other component is held constant[28] (though this is not true for prosimians[25]). A more important point is that the volume of the lateral geniculate nucleus, a major subcortical way station in visual processing, does not correlate with group size at all, indicating that pattern recognition per se is unlikely to be the issue.[28] It may be of some significance that the absolute size of the visual cortex seems to reach an asymptotic value in the great ape clade, whereas the nonvisual neocortex continues to increase in size. One interpretation of this is that visual processing does not necessarily continue to improve indefinitely as the size of the cortical processing machinery increases, at least relative to the opportunity cost of taking cortical neurons away from other cognitive processes.

It seems equally unlikely that the problem lies with a pure memory constraint, though memory capacity obviously must impose some kind of upper limit on the number of relationships that an animal can have. There are three reasons for this claim. First, in humans at least, memory for faces is an order of magnitude larger than the predicted cognitive group size: Humans are said to be able to attach names to around 2,000 faces but have a cognitive group size of only about 150. Second, there is no intrinsic reason to suppose that memory per se is the issue. The social brain hypothesis is about the ability to manipulate information, not simply to remember it. Third, and perhaps most significantly, memories appear to be stored mainly in the temporal lobes,[42] whereas recent PET scan studies implicate the prefrontal neocortex, notably Brodman area 8, as the area for social skills and, specifically, theory of mind.[43] Frith[44] has suggested that memories and representations for objects or events may involve interactions between several levels of the neocortex depending on the kinds of operations involved. These interactions could occur between the sensory and association cortices (perceiving an object), between the association and frontal cortices (remembering an object), and among all three (being aware of perceiving an object). It is worth noting in this context that although social skills are commonly disrupted by damage to the prefrontal cortex, memory for events and people is not.[42]

It seems unlikely that emotional responses per se are the substantive constraint. Although the correct emission and interpretation of emotional cues is of singular importance in the management of social relationship,[45] there is little evidence that the subcortical areas principally associated with emotional cuing (for example, the amygdala in the limbic system) correlate in any way with social group size.[28] Indeed, Keverne, Martel, and Nevison[46] point out that there has been progressive reduction in the relative sizes of the "emotional" centers in the brain (the hypothalamus and septum) in favor of the "executive" centers

(the neocortex and striate cortex) during primate evolution. They interpret this in terms of a shift away from emotional control of behavior to more conscious, deliberate control.

The only remaining alternative is that the mechanisms involved lie in the ability to manipulate information about social relationships themselves. This claim is supported by six additional lines of evidence that point to the fundamental importance of social skills in the detailed management of social relationships.

One is the fact that close analysis of the data on group size and neocortex volume suggests that there are, in fact, distinct grades even within the anthropoid primates (figure 5.3). Apes seem to lie on a separate grade from the monkeys, which in turn lie on a separate grade from the prosimians. The slope coefficients on these separate regression lines do not differ significantly, but the intercepts do. It is as if apes require more computing power to manage the same number of relationships that monkeys do, and monkeys in turn require more than prosimians do. This gradation corresponds closely to the perceived scaling of social complexity.

The second line of evidence is that the rates with which tactical deception are used correlate with neocortex size.[26] Species with large neocortex ratios make significantly more use of tactical deception, even when the differential frequencies with which these large-brained species have been studied are taken into account.

Third, Pawlowski, Dunbar, and Lowen[47] have shown that among polygamous primates the male rank correlation with mating success is negatively related to neocortex size (figure 5.5). This is just what we would predict if the lower ranking males of species with larger neocortices were able to use their greater computational capacities to deploy more sophisticated social skills, such as the use of coalitions and capitalizing on female mate choice, to undermine or circumvent the power-based strategies of the dominant animals.

The fourth line of evidence is Joffe's[48] demonstration that adult neocortex size in primates

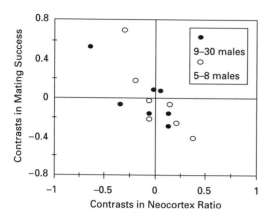

Figure 5.5
Independent contrasts in the Spearman rank correlation (r_s) between male rank and mating success plotted against contrasts in neocortex size for two different male cohort sizes (4–8, and 9–30 males) for individual species. The regression equations for the two cohort sizes are significantly different from $b = 0$. The species sampled are *C. apella*, *P. entellus*, *C. aethiops*, *M. fuscata*, *M. mulatta*, *M. radiata*, *M. arctoides*, *P. cynocephalus*, *P. anubis*, *P. ursinus*, and *P. troglodytes*. (Redrawn from Pawlowski, Dunbar, and Lowen,[47] figure 1.)

correlates with the length of the juvenile period, but not with the length of gestation, lactation, or the reproductive life span, even though total brain size in mammals correlates with the length of the gestation period.[49,50] This suggests that what is most important in the development of a large neocortex in primates is not the embryological development of brain tissue per se, which is associated mainly with gestation length, but rather the "software programming" that occurs during the period of social learning between weaning and adulthood.

Fifth, Kudo, Lowen, and Dunbar[51] have shown that grooming clique size, a surrogate variable that indexes alliance size, correlates rather tightly with relative neocortex and social group size in primates, including humans (figure 5.6). The human data derive from two samples: hair-care networks among female bushmen[52] and support cliques among adults in the United Kingdom.[53] What is remarkable is how closely the human data fit with the data from other primate species. Grooming cliques of this kind in-

variably function as coalitions in primate groups. Coalitions are functionally crucial to individuals within these groups because they enable the animals to minimize the levels of harassment and competition that they inevitably suffer when living in close proximity to others.[54] Coalitions essentially allow primates to manage a fine balancing act between keeping other individuals off their backs while at the same time avoiding driving them away altogether and thereby losing the benefits for which the groups formed in the first place. These results can thus probably be interpreted as a direct cognitive limitation on the number of individuals with which an animal can simultaneously maintain a relationship of sufficient depth that they can be relied on to provide unstinting mutual support when one of them is under attack. Because this is the core process that gives primate social groups their internal structure and coherence, this can be seen as a crucial basis for primate sociality.

Finally, Keverne, Martel, and Nevison[46] have suggested that the neocortex and striate cortex,

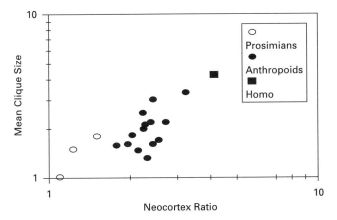

Figure 5.6
Mean grooming clique size plotted against mean neocortex ratio for individual primate genera. The square is *Homo sapiens*. Species sampled are *L. catta, L. fulvus, Propithecus, Indri, S. sciureus, C. apella, C. torquatus, A. geoffroyi, A. fusciceps, P. badius, P. entellus, P. pileata, P. johnii, C. cambelli, C. diana, C. aethiops, C. mitis, E. patas, M. mulatta, M. fuscata, M. arctoides, M. sylvana, M. radiata, P. anubis, P. ursinus, P. cynocephalus, P. hamadryas, T. gelada, P. troglodytes, P. paniscus*. (Redrawn from Kudo, Lowen, and Dunbar,[51] figure 4a.)

those areas of the primate brain that are responsible for executive function, are under maternally rather than paternally imprinted genes (i.e., genes that "know" which parent they came from), whereas the converse is true for the limbic system, those parts of the brain most closely associated with emotional behavior. They interpret this in relation to the cognitive demands of the more intense social life of females in matrilineal female-bonded societies.

Implications for Human Groups

The fact that the relationship between neocortex size and what I will term the cognitive group size holds up so well in so many different taxonomic groups raises the obvious question of whether or not it also applies to humans. We can easily predict a value for group size in humans. Doing so, which is simply a matter of using the human neocortex volume to extrapolate a value for group size from the primate equation, produces a value

in the order of 150. The real issue is whether humans really do go around in groups of this size.

Identifying the relevant level of grouping to measure in humans is difficult because most humans live in a series of hierarchically inclusive groups. This, in itself, is not especially unusual: Hierarchically structured groups of this kind are characteristic of primates[54] and may be typical of many mammals and birds.[55] At least in the case of the diurnal primates, it seems that, with a few notable exceptions, the various species' grouping patterns exhibit an overt level of stability at roughly the same position in the hierarchy across a wide range of taxa. Moreover, because the various layers of this hierarchy appear to be intimately related to each other, probably through being part of a series of cause-and-consequence chains,[51] it would not matter which particular grouping level (for example, stable social group, network, or grooming clique) was taken to be the grouping criterion.

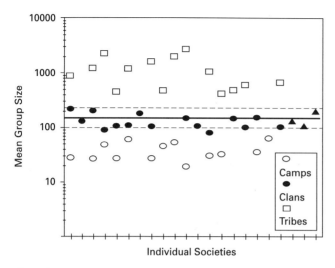

Figure 5.7
Mean sizes for different types of groups in traditional human societies. Individual societies are ordered along the bottom, with data for three main types of social groups (overnight camps, clans or villages, and tribes). Societies include hunter-gatherer and settled horticulturalists from Australia, Africa, Asia, and North and South America. The triangles give mean group sizes for three contemporary United States samples: mean network size from small-worlds experiments (N = 2),[67] mean Hutterite community size,[68] and the size of an East Tennessee mountain community.[69] The value of 150 predicted by the primate neocortex size relationship (from figure 2d) is indicated by the horizontal line, with 95% confidence intervals shown as dashed lines.

The problem with respect to humans is that it is difficult to identify which of the many potential grouping levels is functionally or cognitively equivalent to the particular level of grouping that I happened to use for primates. This difficulty is particularly intrusive in this case because humans live in a dispersed social system sometimes referred to as a fission-fusion system. In order to get around this problem, I adopted the converse strategy in my original analysis,[56] asking whether there was any group size consistently characteristic of humans that was of about the requisite size and, if so, whether its intrinsic psychological characteristics were similar to those found in primate groups.

Because of the structural complexity of postagricultural societies, I considered only traditional hunter-gatherer and small-scale horti-cultural societies. Although census data on such societies are limited, those that are available suggest that there is indeed a consistent group size in the region of 150 individuals (figure 5.7). Except among settled horticulturalists, where the village seems to be the relevant unit, this typically involves the set of individuals from whom overnight camps are easily and regularly formed. Such groups are not often conspicuous as physical entities (they do not often appear together in one place at one time), but they do invariably have important ritual functions for the individuals concerned. Among Australian aboriginals, for example, the relevant group is the clan, which meets from time to time in jamborees where the rituals of life (marriages and rites of passage) are enacted and tales of the old times are rehearsed to remind everyone who they are and why they hold a particular relationship to each other. Indeed, this genuinely seems to be the largest group of people who know everyone in the group as individuals at the level of personal relationships. This is essentially the definition that holds in the case of primates.

A more extensive exploration of human groups in other contexts suggests that groupings of this size are widespread and form an important component of all human social systems, being present in structures that range from business organizations to the arrangement of farming communities.[56] Estimates of community size for two traditional farming communities in the United States, Hutterites and an East Tennessee mountain community, and of actual social network sizes (from small-worlds experiments) (shown as triangles on the right side of figure 5.7) fit very closely within the relevant range of group sizes.

It is easy, of course, to play the numerologist in this context by finding groups that fit whatever group size one wishes to promote. The important feature to note here, however, is that the various human groups that can be identified in any society seem to cluster rather tightly around a series of values (5, 12, 35, 150, 500, and 2,000) with virtually no overlap in the variance around these characteristic values. They seem to represent points of stability or clustering in the degrees of familiarity within the broad range of human relationships, from the most intimate to the most tenuous.

Cognitive Mechanisms

The suggestion that the mechanisms involved in these processes may be concerned with social skills raises the issue alluded to by the original Machiavellian intelligence hypothesis, namely to what extent cognitively sophisticated mechanisms conferring the ability to "mind-read" might be involved. Tactical deception, in its strong sense, implies the ability to hold false beliefs and, thus, the presence of the ability known as "theory of mind" (ToM). Of course, tactical deception as practiced by primates on a daily basis may not, as Byrne[26] himself has pointed out, be quite as sophisticated as first impressions suggest. A more conventional behaviorist account based on simple associative learning can invariably be given for almost all examples reported in the literature.

Nonetheless, convincing evidence suggests that humans at least do use ToM in executing some of their more manipulative social activities. And while we may not wish to attribute full ToM to all primates, at least circumstantial evidence suggests that basic ToM is present in great apes and that monkeys may aspire to a level that Byrne[26] has described as level 1.5 intentionality (full ToM being level 2 intentionality) (see box 5.2). The difference has been summed up rather graphically by Cheney and Seyfarth's[57] observation that apes seem to be good psychologists in that they are good at reading minds, whereas monkeys are good ethologists in that they are good at reading behavior—or at least at making inferences about intentions in the everyday sense, even if not in the philosophical sense of belief states.

Evidence that chimpanzees aspire to at least a basic form of ToM is provided by their performance on experimental false-belief tasks.[58–61] These studies have attempted to develop analogues of the classic false-belief tasks used with children.[62] Though it is clear that chimpanzees do not perform to the level at which fully competent children perform, O'Connell's[61] experiments at least suggest that they can perform at the level of children who stand on the threshold of acquiring ToM. More importantly, chimpanzees do better than autistic adults, one of whose defining features is the lack of ToM, on the same tests.

That mind-reading, the basis of ToM, is difficult to do has been shown by experiments on normal adults tested on "advanced" ToM tasks, up to fifth-order intentionality.[62] These data suggest that normal humans find tasks of greater than fourth-order intentionality exceedingly hard

Box 5.2
A beginner's guide to intensionality

Computers can be said to know things because their memories contain information; however, it seems unlikely that they know that they know these things, in that we have no evidence that they can reflect on their states of "mind." In the jargon of the philosophy of mind, computers are zero-order intensional machines. Intensionality (with an −s) is the term that philosophers of mind use to refer to the state of having a state of mind (knowing, believing, thinking, wanting, understanding, intending, etc.).

Most vertebrates are probably capable of reflecting on their states of mind, at least in some crude sense: they know that they know. Organisms of this kind are first-order intensional. By extension, second-order intensional organisms know that someone else knows something, and third-order intensional organisms know that someone else knows

that someone else knows something. In principle, the sequence can be extended reflexively indefinitely, although, in practice, humans rarely engage in more than fourth-order intensionality in everyday life and probably face an upper limit at sixth-order ("Peter knows that Jane believes that Mark thinks that Paula wants Jake to suppose that Amelia intends to do something").

A minimum of fourth-order intensionality is required for literature that goes beyond the merely narrative ("the writer wants the reader to believe that character A thinks that character B intends to do something"). Similar abilities may be required for science, since doing science requires us to ask whether the world can be other than it is (a second-order problem at the very least) and then ask someone else to do the same (an additional order of intensionality).

to do. The high error rates at these levels do not reflect a memory retention problem: All subjects pass the tests that assess memory for the story line. Moreover, the same subjects show considerable competence on reasoning tasks that involve causal chains of up to the sixth order. The difficulty seems genuinely to be something to do with operating with deeply embedded mental states.

One possibly significant observation in this context is that the visual and nonvisual components of the primate neocortex do not increase isometrically. Although initially there is a more or less linear increase in the visual area V1 with increasing size of the rest of the neocortex, this drops off within the great ape clade. From gorillas through humans, increases in the size of the visual area progress more slowly than do increases in the size of the rest of the neocortex.[28] We interpret this as implying that beyond a certain point the acuity of the visual system does not increase linearly with size. Because the total size of the neocortex is limited by embryological and energetic factors, this means that disproportionately

more capacity can be dedicated to nonvisual areas of the neocortex once the volume is above the crucial threshold. This might explain why apes appear to be capable of the additional cognitive processing associated with mind reading, whereas monkeys are not. It might also explain why humans are better at it than apes.

For humans, one important aspect of ToM concerns its relevance to language, a communication medium that crucially depends on understanding interlocutors' mental states or intentions. The kinds of metaphorical uses of language that characterize not only our rather telegraphic everyday exchanges (in which "you know what I mean?" is a common terminal clause) but also lies at the very heart of the metaphorical features of language. As studies of pragmatics have amply demonstrated,[63] a great deal of linguistic communication is based on metaphor: Understanding the intentions behind a metaphor is crucial to successful communication. Failure to understand these intentions commonly results in confusion or inappropriate responses.

Indeed, without these abilities it is doubtful whether literature, notably poetry, would be possible. Our conversations would be confined to the banally factual; those fine nuances of meaning that create both the ambiguities of politeness and the subtleties of public relations would not be possible.[64]

References

1. Aiello LC, Wheeler P (1995) The expensive tissue hypothesis. Curr Anthropol 36:184–193.
2. Parker ST, Gibson KR (1977) Object manipulation, tool use and sensorimotor intelligence as feeding adaptations in great apes and cebus monkeys. J Hum Evol 6:623–641.
3. Gibson KR (1986) Cognition, brain size and the extraction of embedded food resources. In Else J, Lee PC (eds), Primate Ontogeny, Cognition and Social Behaviour, pp 93–104. Cambridge: Cambridge University Press.
4. Whiten A, Byrne R (1988) Tactical deception in primates. Behav Brain Sci 12:233–273.
5. Byrne R, Whiten A (eds) (1988) *Machiavellian Intelligence.* Oxford: Oxford University Press.
6. Harcourt AH (1988) Alliances in contests and social intelligence. In Byrne R, Whiten A (eds), *Machiavellian Intelligence,* pp 142–152. Oxford: Oxford University Press.
7. Harcourt AH (1989) Sociality and competition in primates and non-primates. In Standen V, Foley R (eds), Comparative Socioecology, pp 223–242. Oxford: Blackwell Scientific.
8. Brothers L (1990) The social brain: A project for integrating primate behaviour and neurophysiology in a new domain. Concepts Neurosci 1:27–251.
9. Barton RA, Dunbar RLM (1997) Evolution of the social brain. In Whiten A, Byrne R (eds), *Machiavellian Intelligence,* Vol. II. Cambridge: Cambridge University Press.
10. Clutton-Brock TH, Harvey PH (1980) Primates, brains and ecology. J Zool Lond 190:309–323.
11. Finlay BL, Darlington RB (1995) Linked regularities in the development and evolution of mammalian brains. Science 268:1678–1684.
12. Martin RD (1981) Relative brain size and metabolic rate in terrestrial vertebrates. Nature Lond 293:57–60.
13. Martin RD (1983) Human brain evolution in an ecological context. 52nd James Arthur Lecture, American Museum of Natural History, New York.
14. Hofman MA (1983) Evolution of the brain in neonatal and adult placental mammals: A theoretical approach. J Theoret Biol 105:317–322.
15. Pagel M, Harvey PH (1988) How mammals produce large-brained offspring. Evolution 42:948–957.
16. Boesch C, Boesch H (1984) Mental map in chimpanzees. Primates 25:110–170.
17. MacLean PD (1982) On the origin and progressive evolution of the triune brain. In Armstrong E, Falk D (eds), *Primate Brain Evolution,* pp 291–310. New York: Plenum Press.
18. Joffe T, Dunbar RIM (n.d.). Primate brain system evolution. Brain Behav Evol, submitted for publication.
19. Passingham RE (1982) *The Human Primate.* San Francisco: Freeman.
20. Jerison HJ (1973) *Evolution of the Brain and Intelligence.* New York: Academic Press.
21. Dunbar RIM (1989) Environmental determinants of intraspecific variation in body weight in baboons. J Zool London 220:167–169.
22. Willner LA (1989) Sexual Dimorphism in Primates. Ph.D. thesis, University of London.
23. Deacon TW (1990) Fallacies of progression indices in theories of brain-size evolution. Int J Primatol 12:193–236.
24. Dunbar RIM (1992) Neocortex size as a constraint on group size in primates. J Hum Evol 20:469–493.
25. Dunbar RIM, Joffe TH (n.d.). Neocortex size and social group size in prosimians. Primates, submitted for publication.
26. Byrne RB (1995) *The Thinking Primate.* Oxford: Oxford University Press.
27. Barton RA (1995) Neocortex size and behavioural ecology in primates. Proc R Soc London B, 263:173–177.
28. Joffe TH, Dunbar RIM (1997) Visual and sociocognitive information processing in primate brain evolution. Proc R Soc London B, 264:1303–1307.

29. Stephan H, Frahm H, Baron G (1981) New and revised data on volumes of brain structures in insectivores and primates. Folia Primatol 35:1–29.

30. Sawaguchi T, Kudo H (1990) Neocortical development and social structure in primates. Primates 31: 283–290.

31. Barton RA, Purvis A (1994) Primate brains and ecology: Looking beneath the surface. In Anderson JR, Thierry B, Herrenschmidt N (eds), *Current Primatology*, pp 1–12. Strasbourg: University of Strasbourg Press.

32. O'Keefe J, Nadel L (1978) *The Hippocampus as a Cognitive Map*. Oxford: Oxford University Press.

33. Krebs JH, Sherry DF, Healy SD, Perry VH, Vaccarino AL (1989) Hippocampal specialisation of food-storing birds. Proc Natl Acad Sci USA 86:1488–1492.

34. Aiello LC, Dunbar RIM (1993) Neocortex size, group size and the evolution of language. Curr Anthropol 34:184–193.

35. Dunbar RIM (1995) Neocortex size and group size in primates: A test of the hypothesis. J Hum Evol 28:287–296.

36. Bearder SK (1987) Lorises, bushbabies and tarsiers: Diverse societies in solitary foragers. In Smuts B, Cheney D, Seyfarth R, Wrangham R, Struhsaker T (eds), *Primate Societies,* pp 12–24. Chicago: Chicago University Press.

37. Dunbar RIM, Bever J (n.d.) Neocortex size determines group size in carnivores and insectivores. Ethology, in press.

38. Gittleman JH (1986) Carnivore brain size, behavioural ecology and phylogeny. J Mammal 67:23–36.

39. Marino L (1996) What can dolphins tell us about primate evolution? Evol Anthropol 5:81–86.

40. Tschudin A (1996) The Use of Neuroimaging in the Assessment of Brain Size and Structure in Odontocetes. MSc thesis, University of Natal (Durban).

41. Barton RA, Purvis A, Harvey PH (1995) Evolutionary radiation of visual and olfactory brain systems in primates, bats and insectivores. Philos Trans R Soc B 348:381–392.

42. Kolb B, Wishaw LO (1996) *Fundamentals of Human Neuropsychology*. San Francisco: Freeman.

43. Fletcher P, Happé F, Frith U, Baker SC, Dolan RJ, Frakowiak RSJ, Frith CD (1996) Other minds in the brain: A functional imaging study of "theory of mind" in story comprehension. Cognition.

44. Frith C (1996) Brain mechanisms for "having a theory of mind." J Psychopharmacol 10:9–16.

45. Armstrong E, Clarke MR, Hill EM (1987) Relative size of the anterior thalamic nuclei differentiates anthropoids by social system. Brain Behav Evol 30: 263–271.

46. Keverne EB, Martel FL, Nevison CM (1996) Primate brain evolution: Genetic and functional considerations. Proc R Soc Lond B 262:689–696.

47. Pawlowski B, Dunbar R, Lowen C (n.d.) Neocortex size, social skills and mating success in primates. Behaviour, in press.

48. Joffe TH (1997) Social pressures have selected for an extended juvenile period in primates. J Hum Evol, in press.

49. Bennett PM, Harvey PH (1985) Brain size, development and metabolism in birds and mammals. J Zool London 207:491–509.

50. Marino L (1997) The relationship between gestation length, encephalisation and body weight in odontocetes. Marine Mammal Sci 14:143–148.

51. Kudo H, Lowen S, Dunbar RIM (n.d.) Neocortex size and social network size in primates. Behaviour, submitted for publication.

52. Sugawara K (1984) Spatial proximity and bodily contact among the central Kalahari San. Afr Studies Monogr 3.

53. Dunbar RIM, Spoor M (1995) Social networks, support cliques and kinship. Hum Nature 6:273–290.

54. Dunbar RIM (1988) *Primate Social Systems*. London: Chapman & Hall.

55. Dunbar RIM (1989) Social systems as optimal strategy sets. In Standen V, Foley R (eds), *Comparative Socioecology,* pp 141–149. Oxford: Blackwell Scientific.

56. Dunbar RIM (1993) Coevolution of neocortical size, group size and language in humans. Behav Brain Sci 11:681–735.

57. Cheney DL, Seyfarth RM (1990) *How Monkeys See the World*. Chicago: Chicago University Press.

58. Povinelli DJ, Nelson KE (1990) Inferences about guessing and knowing in chimpanzees. J Comp Psychol 104:203–210.

59. Povinelli DJ (1994) What chimpanzees (might) know about the mind. In Wrangham R, McGrew W, de Waal F, Heltne P (eds), *Chimpanzee Cultures,* pp 285–300. Cambridge: Harvard University Press.

60. O'Connell SM (1996) Theory of Mind in Chimpanzees. Ph.D. thesis, University of Liverpool.

61. Perner J, Wimmer D (1985) "John thinks that Mary thinks that...." Attribution of second-order beliefs by 5 and 10 year-old children. J Exp Child Psychol 39:437–471.

62. Kinderman P, Dunbar RIM, Bentall RP (n.d.) Theory of mind deficits and causal attributions. Br J Psychol, in press.

63. Desalles J-L (n.d.) Altruism, status and the origin of relevance. In Hurford JR, Studdert-Kennedy M, Knight C (eds), *Evolution of Language.* Cambridge: Cambridge University Press.

64. Dunbar RIM (1997) *Grooming, Gossip and the Evolution of Language.* Cambridge: Harvard University Press.

65. Harvey PH, Krebs JR (1990) Comparing brains. Science 249:150–156.

66. Stephan H (1972) Evolution of primate brains: A comparative anatomical investigation. In Tuttle R (ed), *Functional and Evolutionary Biology of Primates,* pp 165–174. Chicago: Aldine-Atherton.

67. Killworth PD, Bernard HR, McCarty C (1984) Measuring patterns of acquaintanceship. Curr Anthropol 25:391–397.

68. Mange A, Mange E (1980) *Genetics: Human Aspects.* W.B. Saunders.

69. Bryant FC (1981) *We're All Kin: A Cultural Study of a Mountain Neighbourhood.* Knoxville: University of Tennessee Press.

70. Gould SJ (1975) Allometry in primates, with emphasis on scaling and the evolution of the brain. Contrib Primatol 5:244–292.

71. Jolly A (1969) Lemur social behaviour and primate intelligence. Science 163:501–506.

72. Humphrey NK (1976) The social function of intellect. In Bateson PPG, Hinde RA (eds), *Growing Points in Ethology,* pp 303–317. Cambridge: Cambridge University Press.

73. Armstrong E (1985) Relative brain size in monkeys and prosimians. Am J Phys Anthropol 66:263–273.

6 Levels of Analysis in Health Science: A Framework for Integrating Sociobehavioral and Biomedical Research

Norman B. Anderson

The Office of Behavioral and Social Sciences Research (OBSSR) was created by Congress to focus greater attention on the behavioral and social sciences as they relate to health research. This chapter provides a brief overview of the OBSSR and highlights the importance of one of its principal goals: the fostering of interdisciplinary research between sociobehavioral and biomedical scientists. A framework for this type of interdisciplinary research is outlined, with examples of research that support this approach. Finally, a summary is provided of the OBSSR activities that will further interdisciplinary research.

The OBSSR officially opened on July 1, 1995. Some of the major responsibilities of the office and its director, as mandated by Congress, are to provide leadership and direction in the development, refinement, and implementation of a trans-NIH plan to increase the scope of and support for behavioral and social sciences research; to develop funding initiatives designed to stimulate research in the behavioral and social sciences; to promote cross-cutting, interdisciplinary research; to integrate a biobehavioral perspective into research on the promotion of good health, and the prevention, treatment, and cure of diseases; and to ensure that findings from behavioral and social sciences research are disseminated to the public. Further information about the OBSSR and its mission may be found in Anderson[1] or the OBSSR home page (http://wwwl.od.nih.gov/obssr/obssr.htm).

Integrating Sociobehavioral and Biomedical Research

One of the principal goals of the OBSSR is to integrate sociobehavioral and biomedical research across the NIH through the stimulation of cross-disciplinary research. But why is such an integration between these vast fields warranted or desirable? In other words, is cross-disciplinary research necessary or valuable? These questions are relevant because behavioral, social, and biomedical research, and the various disciplines they represent, have attained extraordinary records of accomplishments in the understanding, treatment, and prevention of disease. Most of these accomplishments resulted from research occurring within separate disciplines, such as the subfields of both biomedicine (e.g., molecular biology, endocrinology, neurology, immunology, virology) and sociobehavioral sciences (e.g., psychology, sociology, public health, social epidemiology).

However, although the success of single-discipline research is evident, this approach may also be seen as somewhat limiting. The limitations exist because, while the disciplines concerned with health research may be separated conceptually, methodologically, and administratively, the processes about which they are concerned are inextricably linked. In other words, the social, behavioral, and biological processes that affect health are interdependent. Failure to conduct research across disciplinary lines precludes the discovery of these interdependent processes. The formation and success of the International Society of Neuroimmunomodulation, as demonstrated by the other chapters in this volume, is a recognition of the connections between the nervous system and the immune system. Despite these and other interconnections, the distinctions between scientific disciplines have been reified as if the compartmentalization of the health sciences reflects a corresponding compartmentalization of the origins of human illness. A substantial body of research exists that demonstrates the manifold connections across what might be termed "levels of analysis" of health science, of which research on neuroimmune interactions is exemplary. Research that integrates the various levels of analysis represents one of the next great frontiers in the health sciences, with the potential to accelerate advances in both basic and clinical research and in public health. The hallmark of such integrated, multilevel research is interdisciplinary collaborations, which use the expertise of several disciplines to address complex health issues. The next two sections provide an outline of the notion of multilevel research and some of the principles on which it is based.

The Concept of Levels of Analysis

The notion of levels of analysis is not new to the health sciences. For example, it has been applied quite productively to cognitive and behavioral neuroscience, where both theoretical models and empirical findings have emerged.[2-4] Cacioppo and Berntson[5] have provided one of the most detailed overviews of the concept of multilevel analyses in their discussion of the interdependence of social psychological and neuroscience research. The success of this approach in neuroscience research suggests that it might be a useful heuristic in other areas of the health science enterprise. In fact, an integrated, multilevel approach to research may represent a unifying framework for all of the health sciences.

Figure 6.1 illustrates one potentially useful way of categorizing the various levels of analysis in health research: the social/environmental, behavioral/psychological, organ systems, cellular, and molecular. Each of these levels contains a large number of indices that have been used to study specific health outcomes or pathogenic sociobehavioral or biological processes. Some of these indices are shown in table 6.1. The social/environmental level includes such variables as stressful life events, social support, economic resources, neighborhood characteristics, and environmental hazards. The behavioral/psychological level may include emotion, cognition, memory, dietary practices, stress coping styles, and tobacco use. The organ systems level of analysis includes

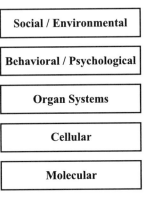

Figure 6.1
Levels of analysis in health research.

the cardiovascular, endocrine, immune, and central nervous systems and their outputs. On the cellular level, variables include receptor number and sensitivity, dendritic branches, synapse number, and electrical conductance. Finally, the molecular or genetic level includes such variables as DNA structure, proteins, mRNA, and transcription factors.

The determination of which indices fall within which levels of analysis is admittedly somewhat arbitrary (e.g., do stressful life events fall in the social/environmental or behavioral/psychological levels?). The point, however, is that the majority of research in the health sciences occurs within a single level of analysis, closely tied to specific disciplines. Even when interdisciplinary research occurs in an area, where scientists from different disciplines are working together on the same problem, it is not always *multilevel* research. This type of interdisciplinary research focuses on a single level of analysis, with no exploration of influences from higher or lower levels on the problem of interest. As mentioned, the single-level approach clearly has been successful, with important contributions made from each level. At the same time, knowledge produced at one level has not always been used to inform research at other levels. Moreover, the science in

Table 6.1
Some indices of various levels of analysis

Social/ environmental	Behavioral/ psychological	Organ systems	Cellular	Molecular
Stressful life events	Emotion	Cardiovascular	Receptor number	DNA structure
Social support	Memory	Blood pressure	Receptor sensitivity	Proteins
Sociocultural groupings	Learning	Heart rate	Cell number	mRNA
	Diet	Ejection fraction	Dendritic branches	tRNA
Economic resources	Exercise	Occlusion	Synapse number	rRNA
Family environment	Smoking	Endocrine	Cortical reorganization	Protooncogenes
	Alcohol intake	Catecholamines		Transcription factors
Neighborhood characteristics	Drug abuse	Cortisol	Electrical conductance (e.g., cell firing)	Second messengers
	Perception	ACTH		Translation factors
Environmental stimulation and enrichment	Stress appraisal and coping	GH		
		Insulin		
Environmental hazards	Language	Immune		
	Personality	Lymphocytes		
	Aggression	Phagocytes		
		Cytokines		
		CNS		
		Evoked potentials		
		Cortical weight		
		Blood flow		
		Metabolic rate		
		ANS		
		SNS		
		PNS		

some areas has progressed to a point where a more integrated, multilevel approach to research design and analysis could pay dividends.

Processes and Principles of Integrated, Multilevel Research

In their discussion of an integrated, multilevel approach to social psychological and neuroscience research, Cacioppo and Berntson[5] state that "analysis of a phenomenon at one level of organization can inform, refine, or constrain inferences based on observations at another level of analysis and, therefore, can foster comprehensive accounts and general theories of complex psychological phenomena." That is, the *interpretation* of findings from single-level research might benefit from the consideration of relevant factors from other levels. Applied to health sciences research more generally, an integrated, multilevel approach involves two types of processes. The first, following from Cacioppo and

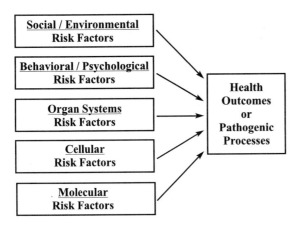

Figure 6.2
Parallel causation.

Berntson, involves the use of findings from one level of analysis to inform, refine, and constrain inferences from observations at another level of analysis. This process might be thought of as "multilevel model or hypothesis development." Here, the objective is a more complete conceptualization of the phenomenon of interest by developing multilevel models or hypotheses, which necessitates the incorporation of findings from other levels. The researcher is asking the question, "What are the variables at higher or lower levels of analysis that might influence or be influenced by the phenomenon that I am studying?" The second process logically follows the first and involves the simultaneous study of a phenomenon across levels of analysis to foster a more comprehensive understanding of the determinants of health outcomes or pathogenic processes. This second process is epitomized by integrated, multilevel, cross-disciplinary research designed to test well-articulated multilevel models or hypotheses.

Several principles and a corollary of multilevel research have been proposed[5] that may be adapted for the broader domain of health re-search. These include the principle of parallel causation, the principle of convergent causation, the principle of reciprocal causation, and the corollary of proximity. Each of these concepts is defined in the following.

The Principle of Parallel Causation

The principle of parallel causation holds that each level of analysis may contain risk factors for a single health outcome or pathogenic process (figure 6.2). Each of these risk factors may be sufficient, but not necessary, for the prediction of outcomes or processes. For example, in the prediction of coronary heart disease (CHD), social level risk factors include socioeconomic status and social support; behavioral level risk factors include physical inactivity and smoking; and organ systems level risk factors include low-density lipoproteins and hypertension. Each level of analysis contains variables that alone are sufficient to account for a significant proportion of the variance in CHD, though no particular level is necessary for the prediction of CHD.

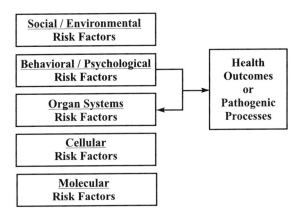

Figure 6.3
Convergent causation.

The Principles of Convergent and Reciprocal Causation

With convergent causation, a convergence or interaction of variables from at least two levels of analysis lead to a health outcome or pathogenic process (figure 6.3). Thus, variables within a single level may be necessary, but not sufficient, to produce an outcome. Here, factors from one level of analysis affect factors at another level, and this cross-level causation ultimately influences outcomes. The principle of reciprocal causation is similar to convergent causation, but posits bidirectional influences across levels, involving negative and positive feedback loops (figure 6.4). For example, the initiation of cigarette smoking (behavioral level) in adolescents may be strongly tied to such social and environmental factors as peer influences and advertising (convergent causation); smoking behavior in turn could later affect biological processes leading to a biological addiction (convergent causation); and this biological addiction contributes to the maintenance smoking behavior (reciprocal causation). Thus, the behavior of smoking leads to biological changes that further serve to maintain this behavior. The principles of convergent and re-

ciprocal causation are the foundations of integrated, multilevel research in that they highlight the critical importance of interactions across levels of analysis in fostering more complete accounts of health phenomena.

The Corollary of Proximity

This corollary holds that the mapping of elements or variables across levels of organization increases in complexity as the number of intervening levels increases.[5] That is, research aimed at exploring interactions between variables at adjacent levels of analysis will typically be less complex than that examining variables at non-adjacent levels. This is because events at any level of analysis (e.g., the cellular level) can be influenced by events within the same or at adjacent levels (e.g., organ systems level), which in turn may be affected by events at the next level of organization (e.g., behavioral level). This added complexity does not preclude research across multiple levels, but suggests that an incremental approach may be the most useful one.[5] Churchland and Sejnowski[2] voiced a similar perspective, stating that: "The ultimate goal of a unified account does not require that it be a single model

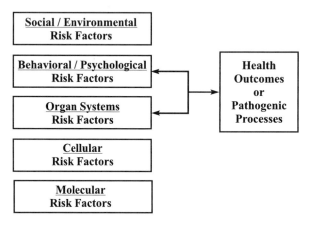

Figure 6.4
Reciprocal causation.

that spans all levels of organization. Instead, the integration will probably consist of a chain of models linking adjacent levels. When one level is explained in terms of a lower level, this does not mean that the higher level theory is useless or that high-level phenomena no longer exist. On the contrary, explanations will coexist at all levels. . . ."

Examples of Convergent and Reciprocal Causation

A number of examples are available to illustrate the principles of convergent and reciprocal causation. Although some of the clearest examples of this type of research come from the field of psychoneuroimmunology,[6,7] those will not be discussed here because that literature is summarized in other papers in this issue. Furthermore, the examples provided will focus on sociobehavioral influences on the "biological" levels of analysis. However, it is also clear that the biological variables significantly affect behavioral and social functioning,[8] and that behavioral and social functioning are also interdependent.[9,10]

Sociobehavioral Effects on Organ Systems

A number of researchers have examined the importance of social and behavioral influences on organ systems. There is a large body of research on the effects of early life stressors on activity of neuroendocrine processes—especially those associated with the hypothalamic-pituitary-adrenal (HPA) axis[11-13]—thought to mediate mood and anxiety disorders. For example, it has been shown that monkeys exposed to adverse early rearing conditions (reared by mothers foraging under unpredictable conditions) exhibit elevations in corticotropin-releasing factor (CRF) as adults.[11] Interestingly, CRF is also elevated in patients with major depression and anxiety disorders,[12] in whom childhood experiences with abuse and neglect and adult experiences with untoward life events may increase risk for these disorders.[14,15]

In a series of elegant studies, Schanberg and colleagues have examined the neuroendocrine effects of maternal separation in rat neonates.[16,17] These studies have demonstrated that after separation of rat pups from their mother for as little as one hour, there is a decrease in the basal activity of ornithine decarboxylase

(ODC)—an important growth-related enzyme—and a suppression of ODC response to trophic stimuli in several tissues, including the brain and the heart.[16,17] Furthermore, separation-induced ODC suppression can be prevented or reversed by tactile stimulation that mimics maternal licking patterns (firm stocking with a moist brush).[57] Importantly, this discovery resulted in development of tactile interventions for preterm infants, resulting in improved growth and earlier hospital discharge.[18]

A variety of studies on coronary heart disease (CHD) highlight convergent causation. Studies by Kaplan, Manuck, and associates exposed male cynomolgus monkeys to "stable" and "unstable" social groupings.[19] For animals in the unstable condition, group membership was reorganized regularly such that animals had to reestablish their dominance and affiliative relationships periodically. Animals in the stable condition had an undisrupted social grouping. Regardless of social grouping, the monkeys who were initially either dominant or subordinate maintained their social positions. It was found that neither living in an unstable environment nor social position alone predicted atherosclerosis. However, monkeys who were consistently behaviorally dominant *and* were housed in the unstable condition showed twice the amount of coronary atherosclerosis as those housed in the stable environment.[19] This interaction of social environment and behavior on atherosclerosis was later found to be mediated by heightened sympathetic nervous system arousal.[20] Recently, it has been found that in patients with a history of heart disease, those who show the largest increases in myocardial ischemia in response to an acute psychological stressor are the greatest risk for cardiac events years later.[21]

Several studies have demonstrated the influence of sociobehavioral factors on the central nervous system (CNS). In particular, various forms of behavioral and environmental experience have been shown to alter cortical organization of the brain in animals and humans.[22–25] A consistent finding over the last several decades is that young and adult rodents exposed to enriched or stimulating living environments (e.g., housed with a variety of "toys" and objects with which to interact) exhibit increased cortical weight compared to animals not similarly housed.[24,25]

Research suggests that some disorders characterized by impaired brain functioning may be treated using behavioral methods. Children with impairments in language-learning are believed to have phonological processing deficits characterized by difficulties in processing rapidly changing sensory inputs[26,27] Tallal and associates have found that language–learning-impaired children provided with daily training with temporarily modified speech sounds show significant improvements in speech discrimination, language comprehension, and temporal processing of *unmodified* speech sounds.[26,27] For patients diagnosed with obsessive-compulsive disorder—a problem characterized by recurrent, unwanted thoughts (obsessions) and conscious, ritualized acts (compulsions)—both behavioral and pharmacological approaches have proven effective.[28,29] Brain-imaging studies have linked this disorder to a number of brain regions, especially the caudate nucleus.[30] Baxter and colleagues have determined that behavior therapy, using principles of stimulus exposure and response prevention, results in a decreased glucose metabolic rate in the caudate nucleus—the same changes that result from drug therapy.[31]

Sociobehavioral Effects on the Cellular Level

Perhaps the most striking and consistent illustrations of the effects of sociobehavioral factors on the cellular level come from studies of environmental enrichment. It is now well recognized that exposure to relatively enriched, complex, or stimulating environments can produce substantial changes on the cellular level. Compared to rats housed in standard or "impoverished" conditions, those in enriched environments show more dendritic branches,[32] more postsynaptic dendritic spines,[33] larger and more numerous synapses,[34] and more synapses per neuron.[34] Interestingly, these findings have been extended to human populations, where intensive, preschool educational interventions are demonstrated to significantly improve later intellectual functioning and lower rates of mental retardation.[35]

In crayfish, social status may modify the effects of serotonin on the neural circuit for tailflip escape behavior.[36] In animals who were socially dominant, serotonin reversibly enhanced the response of the lateral giant (LG) tailflip command neuron to sensory stimuli. However, in subordinate animals, the serotonin response was reversibly inhibited and was persistently enhanced in socially isolated crayfish. In fact, subordinate animals who were later placed in situations that elevated their dominance behavior showed an enhancement of the LG neuron response. Thus, social experience can modulate neural circuit function by altering the effect of a neuromodulator (serotonin) on the response of an identified neuron.[36]

Sociobehavioral Effects on the Molecular Level

Research on the molecular level of analysis, especially the identification of genetic risk factors, is one of the fastest growing fields of health research. What is less often recognized is that nongenetic factors participate in eliciting gene expression. For example, monozygotic twins, who have identical genotypes, vary widely in: heir susceptibility to diseases such as breast cancer, heart disease, Alzheimer's disease, schizophrenia, Parkinson's disease, manic depressive illness, rheumatoid arthritis, and hypertension.[37] Animal studies have shown that sociobehavioral and environmental factors may produce phenotypic differences in animals with the same genotype. In these studies, genetically identical animals are exposed to different behavioral or environmental experiences, and differences in phenotypic characteristics are assessed. This paradigm has been used with animal models of both Type I and Type II diabetes. Surwit and colleagues[38] have examined insulin and glucose status in the obese mouse (ob/ob), a commonly used genetic model of non–insulin-dependent (Type II) diabetes. Although these animals were found to exhibit the characteristic hyperinsulinemia, they did not exhibit hyperglycemia in the resting state relative to lean animals. However, after exposure to repeated daily stress (immobilization and vibration), both the lean and obese mice became hyperglycemic, but the magnitude of hyperglycemia was exaggerated in the obese mice.[38] The obese animals also showed a corresponding exaggeration in glucose response following the injection of epinephrine. The increase in plasma glucose following both stress and epinephrine was accompanied by a decrease in the plasma insulin responses. Stress has also been found to affect diabetes expression in the BB rat, a genetic model of Type I diabetes.[39]

A body of research is now emerging on the impact of behavior and the environment on protein synthesis and the process of gene transcription and translation.[40–50] As described in the previous section, studies have shown that exposure to enriched environments may alter the structure and function of cells. Investigations have recently been undertaken to determine the molecular basis for these cellular alterations. It has now been demonstrated that rats exposed to complex living environments exhibit significantly higher levels of mRNA for the immediate early gene transcription factor NGFI-A (also known as ZENK, zif/268, egr-1, and Krox 24) than animals not similarly housed.[40] Importantly this study determined that the expression of NGFI-A mRNA was most pronounced in brain regions previously shown to have the greatest experience-based morphological plasticity on the cellular level and was highly correlated with such changes.[40]

Another line of research has investigated more directly the role of learning and motor activity in gene expression. Kleim et al.[43] reported that rats trained to traverse a complex series of obstacles exhibited a significantly higher expression of the c-*fos* protein than control animals. The increase in c-*fos* was not simply a function of increased motor activity, but was directly associated with motor *learning*. Similarly, Paylor et al.[44] have reported that brief exposure to an enriched environment improves learning and memory and produces increases in hippocampal protein kinase C (PKC), which is believed to be an important biological substrate learning and memory.[45] It has also been shown that classical conditioning may induce activation of PKC in rabbit hippocampal CA1 neurons[45] and that physical activity enhances special learning accompanied by increases in hippocampal PKC and NGFI-A.[46,47]

Recently, studies have begun to explore the genetic mechanism underlying previously observed associations of sociobehavioral factors with pathogenic processes or health outcomes. As discussed earlier, neonatal material deprivation in rat pups suppresses ODC, an effect due to lack of tactile stimulation. More recently, researchers have determined that maternal touch deprivation affects certain hepatic protooncogenes—such as c-*myc, max,* c-*fos,* c-*jun,* and others—whose protein products are known to interact with the regulatory region of the ODC gene.[51,52] Specifically, it has been demonstrated that maternal separation not only suppresses ODC enzyme activity, but may do so by the suppression of prolactin-induced increases in c-*myc, max,* and ODC mRNAs.[51] Finally, human research has for some time demonstrated a link between cigarette smoking and lung cancer[53] and that a key carcinogen in cigarette smoke is benzo[*a*]pyrene diol epoxide (BPDE).[54] It has also been recognized that mutations in the p53 tumor suppression gene are also associated with increased risk for lung cancer.[55] A recent study has now demonstrated that BPDE binds or joins the p53 gene at the same points where mutations are associated with lung cancer.[56] Thus, it appears that the behavior of cigarette smoking, and a chemical associated with it, may induce specific changes on the genetic level that increase risk for lung cancer.

Stimulating Integrated, Multilevel Research: Activities of the OBSSR

From the above examples, it is clear that an integrated, multilevel approach has the potential to answer critical scientific questions that cannot be adequately addressed with single-level research. The OBSSR Strategic Plan includes a number of goals, strategies, and actions designed to facilitate a growth in integrated, multilevel research. In particular, three key approaches will be used. First, the OBSSR will work to foster funding initiatives such as Request for Applications (RFA) or Program Announcements (PA) that address important basic or clinical research questions for which a multilevel approach would be beneficial. Second, the office will take a leadership role in the training of a generation of social, behavioral, and biomedical scientists who are broadly equipped to think across levels of analysis, and to develop cross-disciplinary collaborations. One plan already underway is for an RFA to fund summer training workshops where graduate students, post-doctoral fellows, and faculty can be immersed in the methods and findings from a level of analysis about which they are less familiar. For example, biomedically trained neuroscientists may learn about the latest procedures for assessing cognitive or behavioral functioning, or behaviorally trained stress researchers may learn about important indices of immune or neuroendocrine functioning that may be relevant to their research. Finally, the OBSSR will work to increase communication and cooperation between sociobehavioral and biomedical researchers. This will be accomplished through the sponsorship of workshops at the NIH and at professional meetings on interdisciplinary research; the creation of internet-based forums for cross-disciplinary exchanges; the commission of literature reviews that integrate research across levels of analysis; and the establishment of an NIH-wide steering committee to promote cross-disciplinary research. It is hoped that these and other activities will stimulate integrated, multi-level research, which will ultimately accelerate our understanding of the etiology of illness, and aid in the development of better treatment and prevention approaches.

References

1. Anderson, N. B. 1995. Integrating behavioral and social sciences research at the NIH. *Acad. Med.* 70: 1106–1107.

2. Churchland, P. S. & T. J. Sejnowski. 1988. Perspectives on cognitive neuroscience. *Science* 242:741–745.

3. Koob, G. F. & F. E. Bloom. 1988. Cellular and molecular mechanisms of drug dependence. *Science* 242:715–723.

4. Fodor, J. A. 1968. *Psychological Explanation*. Random House. New York.

5. Cacioppo, J. T. & G. G. Berntson. 1992. Social psychological contributions to the decade of the brain: The doctrine of multilevel analysis. *Am. Psychol.* 47(8):1019–1028.

6. Kiecolt-Glaser, J. K. & R. Glaser. 1995. Psychoneuroimmunology and health consequences: Data and shared mechanisms. *Psychosom. Med.* 57:269–274.

7. Sheridan, J. F., N. Feng, R. H. Bonneau, et al. 1991. Restraint stress differentially affects antiviral cellular and humoral immune responses in mice. *J. Neuroimmunol.* 31:245–255.

8. Plomin, R., M. J. Owen & P. McGuffin. 1994. The genetic basis of complex human behaviors. *Science* 264:1733–1739.

9. Wyer, R. S. 1989. *Memory and Cognition in Its Social Context*. L. Earlbaum. Hillsdale, NJ.

10. Cialdini, R. B. 1984. *Influence: How and Why People Agree on Things*. William Morrow. New York.

11. Coplan, J. D., M. W. Andrews, L. A. Rosenblum, M. J. Owens, S. Friedman, J. M. Gorman & C. B. Nemeroff. 1996. Persistent elevations of cerebrospinal fluid concentrations of corticotropin-releasing factor in adult nonhuman primates exposed to early-life stressors: Implications for the pathophysiology of mood and anxiety disorders. *Proc. Natl. Acad. Sci. USA* 93:1619–1623.

12. Nemeroff, C. B. The corticotropin-releasing factor (CRF) hypothesis of depression: New findings and new directions. *Mol. Psychiatry,* in press.

13. Meaney, M. J., B. Tannenbaum, D. Francis, S. Bhatnagar, N. Shanks, V. Viau, D. O'Donnell & P. M. Plotsky. 1994. Early environmental programming of hypothalamic-pituitary-adrenal responses to stress. *Neurosciences* 6:247–259.

14. Hammen, C., J. Davila, G. Brown, A. Ellicott & M. Gitlin. 1992. Psychiatric history and stress: Predictors of severity of unipolar depression. *J. Abnorm. Psych.* 101:45–52.

15. Kendler, K. S., R. C. Kessler, M. C. Neale, A. C. Heath & L. J. Eaves. 1993. The prediction of major depression in women: Toward an integrated etiologic model. *Am. J. Psychiatry* 150:1139–1148.

16. Butler, S. R., M. R. Suskind & S. M. Schanberg. 1978. Maternal behavior as regulator of polyamine biosynthesis in brain and heart of the developing rat pup. *Science* 199:445–446.

17. Schanberg, S. M. & C. M. Kuhn. 1980. Maternal deprivation: An animal model of psychosocial dwarfism. In *Enzymes and Neurotransmitters in Mental Disease*. E. Usdin & T. Sourkes, Eds.: 373–395. John Wiley. Chichester, England.

18. Field, T. M., S. M. Schanberg, F. Scafidi, C. R. Bauer, N. Vega-Lahr, R. Garcia, J. Nystrom & C. M. Kuhn. 1986. Effect of tactile/kinesthetic stimulation on preterm neonates. *Pediatrics* 77:654–658.

19. Kaplan, J. R., S. B. Manuck, T. B. Clarkson, et al. 1982. Social status environment and atherosclerosis in cynomolgus monkeys. *Arteriosclerosis* 2:359–368.

20. Kaplan, J. R., S. B. Manuck, M. R. Adams, et al. 1987. Inhibition coronary atherosclerosis by propranolol in behaviorally predisposed monkeys fed an atherogenic diet. *Circulation* 76:1364–1372.

21. Jiang, W., M. Babyak, D. S. Krantz, R. A. Waugh, R. E. Coleman, M. M. Hanson, D. J. Frid, S. McNulty, J. J. Morris, C. M. O'Connor & J. A. Blumenthal. 1996. Mental stress-induced myocardial ischemia and cardiac events. *JAMA* 275(21):1651–1655.

22. Elbert, T., C. Pantev, C. Wienbruch, B. Rockstroth & E. Taub. 1995. Increased cortical representation of the fingers of the left hand in string players. *Science* 270:305–307.

23. Bennett, E. L., M. C. Diamond, D. Krech & M. R. Rosenzweig. 1964. Chemical and anatomical plasticity of brain. Changes in brain through experience, demanded by learning theories, are found in experiments with rats. *Science* 146:610–619.

24. Ferchmin, P. A. & V. A. Eterovic. 1986. Forty minutes of experience increase the weight and RNA content of cerebral cortex in periadolescent rats. *Dev. Psychobiol.* 19(6):511–519.

25. Bennett, E. L., M. R. Rosenzweig & M. C. Diamond. 1969. Rat brain: Effects of environmental enrichment on wet and dry weights. *Science* 163:825–826.

26. Tallal, P., S. L. Miller, G. Bedi, G. Byma, X. Wang, S. S. Nagarajan, C. Schreiner, W. M. Jenkins & M. M. Merzenich. 1996. Language comprehension in language-learning impaired children improved with acoustically modified speech. *Science* 271:81–84.

27. Merzenich, M. M., W. M. Jenkins, P. Johnston, C. Schreiner, S. L. Miller & P. Tallal. 1996. Temporal processing deficits of language-learning impaired children ameliorated by training. *Science* 271:77–81.

28. Baer, L. & W. E. Minichiello. 1990. Behavior therapy for obsessive-compulsive disorder. In *Obsessive-Compulsive Disorders: Theory and Management.* Second ed. M. A. Jenike, L. Baer & W. E. Minichiello, Eds.: 203–232. Mosby-Year Book. St. Louis, MO.

29. DeVeaugh-Geiss, J. 1991. Pharmacologic treatment of obsessive-compulsive disorder. In *The Psychobiology of Obsessive-Compulsive Disorder.* J. Zohar, T. Insel & S. Rasmussen, Eds.: 187–207. Springer. New York.

30. Baxter, L. R., Jr., S. Saxena, A. L. Brody, R. F. Ackermann, M. Colgan, J. M. Schwartz, Z. Allen-Martinez, J. M. Fuster & M. E. Phelps. 1996. Brain mediation of obsessive-compulsive disorder symptoms: Evidence from functional brain imaging studies in the human and nonhuman primate. Semin. Clin. *Neuropsychiatry* 1(1):32–47.

31. Baxter, L. R., Jr., J. M. Schwartz, K. S. Bergman, M. P. Szuba, B. H. Guze, J. C. Mazziotta, A. Alazraki, C. E. Selin, H. K. Ferng, P. Munford & M. E. Phelps. 1992. Caudate glucose metabolic rate changes with both drug and behavior therapy for obsessive-compulsive disorder. *Arch. Gen. Psychiatry* 49:681–689.

32. Greenough, W. T., J. M. Juraska & F. R. Volkmar. 1979. Maze training effects on dendritic branching in occipital cortex of adult rats. *Behav. Neurobiol.* 26:287–297.

33. Globus, A., M. R. Rosenzweig, E. L. Bennett & M. C. Diamond. 1973. Effects of differential experience on dendritic spine counts in rat cerebral cortex. *J. Comp. Physiol. Psychol.* 82:175–181.

34. Turner, A. M. & W. T. Greenough. 1985. Differential rearing effects on rat visual cortex synapses. I. Synaptic and neuronal density and synapses per neuron. *Brain Res.* 329:195–203.

35. Campbell, F. A. & C. T. Ramey. 1994. Effects of early intervention on intellectual and academic achievement: A follow-up study of children from low-income families. *Child Dev.* 65:684–698.

36. Yeh, S. R., R. A. Fricke & D. H. Edwards. 1996. The effect of social experience on serotonergic modulation of the escape circuit of crayfish. *Science* 271:366–369.

37. King, R. A., J. Rotter & A. G. Motulsky, Eds. 1992. *The Genetic Basis of Common Diseases.* Oxford University Press. New York. pp. 775–791.

38. Surwit, R. S., M. N. Feinglos, E. G. Livingston, C. M. Kuhn & J. A. McCubbin. 1984. Behavioral manipulation of the diabetic phenotype in ob/ob mice. *Diabetes* 33:616–618.

39. Lehman, C. D., J. Rodin, B. McEwen & R. Brinton. 1991. Impact of environmental stress on the expression of insulin-dependent diabetes mellitus. *Behav. Neurosci.* 105(2):241–245.

40. Wallace, C. S., G. S. Withers, I. J. Weiler, J. M. George, D. F. Clayton & W. T. Greenough. 1995. Correspondence between sites of NGFI-A induction and sites of morphological plasticity following exposure to environmental complexity. *Mol. Brain Res.* 32:211–220.

41. Mack, K. J. & P. A. Mack. 1992. Induction of transcription factors in somatosensory cortex after tactile stimulation. *Mol. Brain Res.* 12:141–147.

42. Nikolaev, E., B. Kaminska, W. Tishmeyer, H. Matthies & L. Kaczmarek. 1992. Induction factors in the rat brain elicited by behavioral training. *Brain Res. Bull.* 28:479–484.

43. Kleim, J. A., E. Lussnig, E. R. Schwarz, T. A. Comery & W. T. Greenough. 1996. Synaptogenesis and FOS expression in the motor cortex of the adult rat after motor skill learning. *J. Neurosci.* 16(14):4529–4535.

44. Paylor, R., S. K. Morrison, J. W. Rudy, L. T. Waltrip & J. M. Wehner. 1992. Brief exposure to an enriched environment improves performance on the Morris water task and increases hippocampal cytosolic protein kinase C activity in young rats. *Behav. Brain Res.* 52:49–59.

45. Alkon, D. L. 1988. Classical conditioning induces long-term translocation of protein kinase C in rabbit hippocampal CA1 cells. *Proc. Natl. Acad. Sci. USA* 85:1988–1992.

46. Fordyce, D. E. & J. M. Wehner. 1993. Physical activity enhances spatial learning performance with an associated alteration in hippocampal protein kinase C activity in C57BL/6 and DBA/2 mice. *Brain Res.* 619:111–119.

47. Fordyce, D. E., R. V. Bhat, J. M. Baraban & J. M. Wehner. 1994. Genetic and activity-dependent regulation of Zif268 expression: Association with spatial learning. *Hippocampus* 4(5):559–568.

48. Bank, B., J. J. LoTurco & D. L. Alkon. 1989. Learning-induced activation of protein kinase C. A molecular memory trace. *Mol. Neurobiol.* 3:55–70.

49. Plotsky, P. M. & M. J. Meaney. 1993. Early, postnatal experience alters hypothalamic corticotropin-releasing factor (CRF) mRNA, median eminence CRF content and stress-induced release in adult rats. *Mol. Brain Res.* 18:195–200.

50. Meaney, M. J., S. Bhatnagar, J. Diorio, S. La-rocque, D. Francis, D. O'Donnell, N. Shanks, S. Sharma, J. Smythe & V. Viau. 1993. Molecular basis for the development of individual differences in the hypothalamic-pituitary-adrenal stress response. *Cell. Mol. Neurobiol.* 13(4):321–347.

51. Wang, S., J. V. Bartolome & S. M. Schnaberg. Neonatal deprivation of maternal touch may suppress ornithine decarboxylase via down regulation of the protooncogenes C-MYC and MAX. *J. Neurosci.*

52. Schanberg, S. M. 1995. The genetic basis for touch effects. In *Touch in Early Development.* T. M. Field, Ed.: 67–79. Lawrence Erlbaum Associates.

53. U.S. Department of Health and Human Services. 1982. *The Health Consequences of Smoking: Cancer.* DHHS Pub. No. (PHS) 82-50179. A Report of the Surgeon General. Washington, DC.

54. Singer, B. & D. Grunberger. 1983. *Molecular Biology of Mutagens and Carcinogens.* Plenum. New York.

55. Hollstein, M., D. Sidransky, B. Vogelstein & C. C. Harris. 1991. P53 mutations in human cancers. *Science* 253(5015):49–53.

56. Denissenko, M. F., A. Pao, M. S. Tang & G. P. Pfeifer. 1996. Preferential formation of benozo[a]pyrene adducts at lung cancer mutational hotspots in P53. *Science* 274:430–432.

57. Pauk, J., C. M. Kuhn, T. M. Field & S. M. Schanberg. 1986. Positive effects of tactile versus kinesthetic or vestibular stimulation on neuroendocrine and ODC activity in maternally-deprived rat pups. *Life Sci.* 39:2081–2087.

III SOCIAL COGNITION AND THE BRAIN

A. Basic Processes

7   The Role of the Anterior Prefrontal Cortex in Human Cognition

Etienne Koechlin, Gianpaolo Basso, Pietro Pietrini, Seth Panzer, and Jordan Grafman

Complex problem-solving and planning involve the most anterior part of the frontal lobes including the fronto-polar prefrontal cortex (FPPC),[1-6] which is especially well developed in humans compared with other primates.[7,8] The specific role of this region in human cognition, however, is poorly understood. Here we show, using functional magnetic resonance imaging, that bilateral regions in the FPPC alone are selectively activated when subjects have to keep in mind a main goal while performing concurrent (sub)goals. Neither keeping in mind a goal over time (working memory) nor successively allocating attentional resources between alternative goals (dual-task performance) could by themselves activate these regions. Our results indicate that the FPPC selectively mediates the human ability to hold in mind goals while exploring and processing secondary goals, a process generally required in planning and reasoning.

This process of integrating working memory with attentional resource allocation is referred to as branching. In everyday life, branching is frequently required: for example, if a person is interrupted with a question while reading. As in dual-task performance, branching successively allocates processing resources between concurrent tasks (such as listening and reading). As in delayed-response performance, branching keeps relevant information in working memory to allow a return to the main task after completing a secondary task (in our example, remembering and returning to where you left off reading). Knowing that problem-solving and planning involve the FPPC[1-6] and generally involve branching, whenever goal-tree sequences are processed we proposed that only fronto-polar regions would be selectively engaged by the integration of working memory and attentional-resource allocation.

Using functional magnetic resonance imaging (fMRI), we employed a 2×2 factorial design

crossing delayed-response and dual-task performance (table 7.1), so that subjects performed an online letter-matching task in four conditions including a control, a delay, a dual-task and a branching condition (see figures 7.1 and 7.2). Accordingly, specific branching activations were specified as an interaction between delayed-response and dual-task performance and were expected to be found only in fronto-polar regions.

The fMRI results confirm our prediction (table 7.2 and figures 7.3–7.5). First, we tested for regions selectively involved in either dual- or delayed-task performance (see Methods). The main effect of dual-task performance was found to involve, selectively and bilaterally, the posterior dorsolateral prefrontal cortex (BA (Brodman's area) 9, middle frontal gyrus, close to the pre-central gyrus and BA 8) and the lateral parietal cortex (inferior parietal lobule, BA 40). In accordance with previous studies, this confirms that this network of brain areas is involved in allocating attentional resources between successively alternating tasks or stimuli.[9,10] In contrast, the main effect of delayed performance involved no specific brain region even at low statistical thresholds. This indicates that the duration of delay during which information is maintained online in this task is not in itself a main factor triggering the activation of specific cortical regions.

Our main aim was to identify brain regions involved in both delayed-response and dual-task performance. Those regions fall into one of two categories: regions that exhibit additive effects, where the evoked response is simply explained by the activation due to utilizing working memory or attention allocation independently; and regions that show an interaction, where there is a super-additive component that is attributable to the cognitive integration of working memory and attentional allocation (in our framework, a branching process).

Table 7.1
Factorial design of the experiment

Attentional resource allocation	Working memory	
	No delayed response	Delayed response
Single-task performance	Control	Delay
Dual-task performance	Dual task	Branching

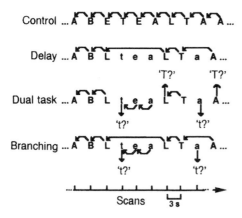

Figure 7.1
Behavioural tasks. Stimuli were pseudorandom sequences of upper- or lower-case letters from the word 'tablet'. Control condition: subjects had to decide whether two successively presented letters were also in immediate succession in the word 'tablet' (only upper-case letters were presented). Delay condition: subjects had to ignore lower-case letters which were used to occasionally delay the response required by the control condition. Dual-task condition: subjects had to respond as in the control condition for both upper- and lower-case letter series with one exception. Subjects had to decide whether every first letter indicating a case change was the letter T (or t). Branching condition: subjects had to respond to upper-case letters exactly as in the delay condition and to lower-case letters exactly as in the dual-task condition.

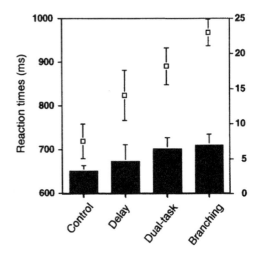

Figure 7.2
Behavioural performance. Symbols: increases in reaction times (mean $\pm$ SE in ms) across conditions ($F(3, 15) = 14.6$, $P < 0.0001$), confirming that additional processes and regions are engaged successively in the control, delay, dual-task and branching conditions. Bars: error rates (mean $\pm$ SE in percentage) remained very similar across conditions ($F(3, 15) = 1.2, P > 0.34$) with virtually no difference between the dual-task and branching conditions.

Additive activations were obtained by selecting the regions engaged in all experimental conditions compared with baseline (see Methods). No interaction was observed *post hoc* in those regions ($P > 0.05$), namely the right anterior dorsolateral prefrontal cortex (BA 9/46, middle frontal gyrus), the right superior frontal gyrus (BA 10) and the right precuneus (BA 7) (figures 7.3 and 7.5). When compared to the control condition, the MR signal change recorded in these brain regions during the branching condition co-varied with the sum of the signal changes in the delay and dual-task conditions. This cortical network is involved in episodic memory tasks, becoming activated when the circumstances in which events occurred are retrieved.[11–16] In ac-

Table 7.2
Coordinates and Z-score for maxima of activations

Regions Brodman's area*	Talairach coordinates†	Statistical effects (Z-value)‡						
		BR-CR	DE-CT	DT-CT	BR-DE	BR-DT	DE-DT	DT-DE
Interaction								
Right, BA 10, GFp	36, 66, 21	8.2	n.s.	n.s.	6.8	6.8	n.s.	n.s.
Left, BA 10, GFp	−36, 57, 9	8.1	n.s.	n.s.	6.2	7.3	n.s.	n.s.
Additivity								
Right, BA 10, GFs	30, 75, 12	8.5	6.8	7.6	7.0	5.2	n.s.	n.s.
Right, BA9/46, GFm	54, 36, 30	8.5	6.5	7.9	7.1	3.9	n.s.	n.s.§
Right, BA 7, Pcu	6, −60, 48	8.3	6.1	7.5	6.1	3.6	n.s.	n.s.
Main effects (dual task)								
Right, BA 9/8, GFm	45, 21, 36	8.3	5.3	8.1	6.8	n.s.	n.s.	5.6
Right, BA 40, LPi	48, −39, 48	7.7	n.s.	8.0	6.5	n.s.	n.s.	7.3
Left, BA 9/8, GFm	−45, 27, 36	7.9	n.s.	7.3	7.2	n.s.	n.s.	5.6
Left, BA 7, LPs	−42, −51, 54	8.3	n.s.§	8.2	7.7	n.s.	n.s.	7.3

Data relate to maxima of activations shown in Fig. 7.3.
*BA, Brodman's area; GF, frontal gyrus; LP, parietal lobule; i, inferior; m, middle; s, superior; p, polar; Pcu, precuneus.
† Talairach coordinates of maxima in contrast branching minus control conditions.
‡ BR, branching; DE, delay; DT, dual-task; CT, control; n.s. not significant ($P > 0.9$, corrected).
§ $P > 0.5$, corrected.

cordance with these results, all but the control conditions in our experiment share the common feature that subject performance depends upon processing and retrieving the context in which a stimulus occurs (either its lower/upper case status on a given trial or the task rules on a given experimental block). Performance in the branching condition required subjects to combine the previously independent contextual information used in the delay and dual-task conditions, which may explain the additivity effect found in these regions.

Super-additive, or branching-specific, activation was obtained by selecting regions which were engaged in the branching condition compared with baseline and, in addition, showed a significant interaction between working memory and attentional allocation factors (see Methods).

As predicted, this revealed only two regions, located symmetrically in the left and right dorsal FPPC (BA 10, fronto-polar gyrus; figures 7.3 and 7.4). In both regions, the MR signal increased significantly in the branching condition, but was quantitatively similar in all other conditions (figure 7.5). As neither the delayed nor dual-task performance alone significantly activated these regions, these results indicate that these fronto-polar regions are crucial only when branching processes are engaged. The activated foci differed slightly in the left and right fronto-polar regions, which may result from variations in the anatomy or the functional mapping between the two frontal lobes.[17]

Behavioural data show that these fronto-polar activations were not related to variations in mental effort alone. If that had been the case,

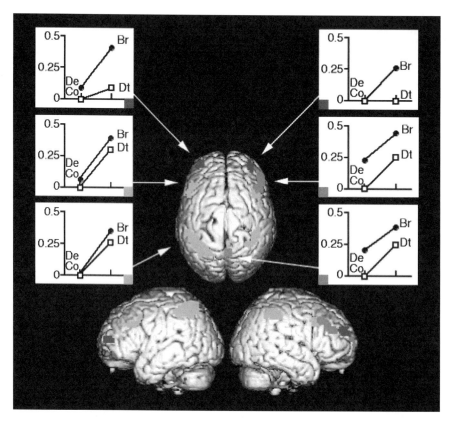

Figure 7.3

Topography of brain regions with distinct activation profiles. Yellow, main effects of dual-task performance. Green, additivity of the dual-task and delayed-response performance effects. Red, interaction of dual-task and delayed performance effects or branching-specific activations. See Methods for details and table 7.2 for coordinates of activation foci. Inserts, data points are the mean signal changes (vertical axis, percentage) in the delay (De), dual-task (Dt) and branching (Br) conditions (measured in the stationary state, that is, in the second half-block) relative to the adjusted signal mean in the control condition (Co).

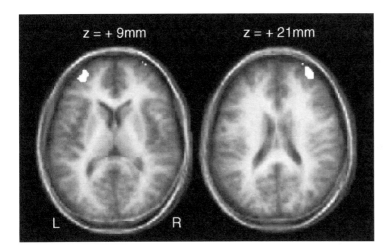

Figure 7.4
Branching-specific activations (Z-maps thresholded at $Z > 4.5$, $P < 0.05$, corrected) superimposed on anatomical axial slices averaged across subjects (Talairach coordinates $Z = 9$ and 21 mm). See figure 7.3 for details.

a gradual increase in MR signal, associated with the gradual increase in difficulty of the tasks from the control to the delayed-task, dual-task and branching conditions (figure 7.2), would have been observed.[18] Instead, no difference in brain activation was found in these regions between conditions with different behavioural performances (for example, the control and dual-task conditions), whereas significant activation differences were observed between the dual-task and branching conditions despite very similar behavioural performance. Moreover, six more normal right-handed subjects (three males and three females, aged 20–28) performed the dual-task condition under more difficult constraints using degraded letters. Although subjects could still identify all letters, the task was significantly more difficult than the branching condition. Response times increased by 112 ms from the regular to the difficult dual-task condition ($P < 0.02$), and mean accuracy fell from 96.2 to 87.7%. As expected, increasing difficulty resulted in increased frontal activations in the posterior dorsolateral prefrontal cortex and the anterior cingulate cortex, but not in the FPPC ($Z < 1.0$, $P > 0.15$) in contrast to the results predicted by a mental effort interpretation of our data.

In summary, distinct dorsal fronto-polar regions were selectively engaged in branching processes when compared with other executive processes including working memory,[19–22] attentional resource allocation[9,10] and processing episodic information.[11–16] This finding may clarify why the FPPC was found to be engaged in complex problem-solving[1–6] and, incidentally, in working-memory tasks performed in dual-task contexts.[2,3,23,24] These branching-specific regions may have a key role in processing goal-tree sequences, which frequently requires the temporary interruption of a current plan to achieve subgoals, or to respond to new environmental demands or intrusive thoughts, and may help to mediate a range of human behaviours including planning and reasoning.

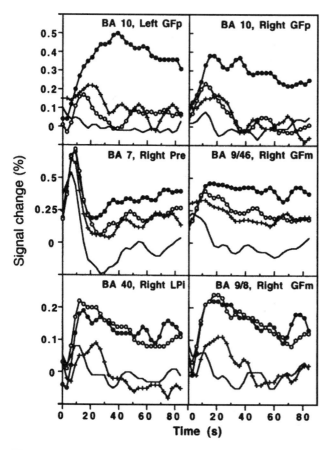

Figure 7.5

Dynamics of activation profiles. Plots are related to the regions shown in figure 7.3 and table 7.2; x-axis, time measured from experimental block onsets. Stimulus onsets occur every 3 s, starting from time 3. Data points are relative signal changes averaged in every region during branching (filled circle), delay (cross), dual-task (circle) and control (no symbol) conditions. Signal changes (in per cent) are measured from the adjusted signal mean in the control condition.

Methods

Behavioural Protocol

Subjects responded to visually presented letters (500 ms duration, 3,000 ms stimulus-onset-asynchrony (SOA)) by pressing response buttons with their right (match) or left (no match) hand, respectively. Matching proportions were maintained between 40 and 43% of trials in each condition. In all but the control conditions lower-case letters were pseudorandomly presented in 64% of trials and the mean SOA between two successive upper-case letters was strictly maintained at 6.3 s. In the delay condition, subjects were asked to ignore lower-case letters by always pressing the no-match button (see figure 7.1 legend for details). The task was administered in six scanning runs using the Expe software package.[25] Each condition was included once in each run as a block of 28 trials. The resulting 24 blocks were pseudo-randomly ordered so that each condition appears at all serial positions within a run and two conditions appeared once or twice in immediate succession to prevent confounding order effects. Subjects were given standard instructions to respond quickly and accurately. Behavioural and fMRI data were recorded simultaneously from six right-handed subjects (three females and three males, aged 20–28 years) who were trained and reached a threshold accuracy ($> 70\%$) in all conditions before and during scanning. Three additional subjects were excluded because they did not reach this threshold during scanning. Subjects provided written informed consent approved by the NIH.

Image Acquisition and Analysis

A standard 1.5 GE signa scanner whole-body and RF coil scanner were used to perform a high-resolution structural scan for each subject followed by six runs of 120 functional axial scans (TR 3 s, TE 40 ms, flip angle 90°; FOV 24 cm, acquisition matrix 64×64, number of slices 18, thickness 6 mm) synchronized with stimulus presentation. All fMRI data were processed using the SPM96 software package (http://www.fil.ion.ucl.ac.uk/spm/)[26] with modified memory-mapping procedures. Standard linear image realignment, linear normalization to the stereotaxic Talairach atlas (MNI template),[27] spatial (3D gaussian kernel: 10 mm) and temporal smoothing, and mean MR-signal normalization across scans were successively performed for each subject. Then, all subjects were pooled together and statistical parametric maps (SPM) were computed from local MR signals using a linear multiple regression with conditions (modelled as two temporal basis functions) and runs as co-variates.[26] Only regions formed by more than 12 contiguous active voxels ($P < 0.05$) were analysed. The main effect of dual-task (and delayed-response, respectively) performance was computed by selecting the regions which were co-jointly significantly activated in the dual-task (delay) and branching conditions compared with the control and delay (dual-task) conditions ($Z > 5.4$, $P < 0.0005$, corrected for multiple comparisons). The additive effect of delay and dual-task performance was observed in the regions co-jointly and significantly activated in all conditions compared with the baseline ($Z > 5.4$, $P < 0.0005$, corrected). No interaction between those factors ($P > 0.05$, uncorrected) was observed in those regions. Branching-specific activations were computed as the regions with significant activations in the branching condition compared with the control ($Z > 5.4$, $P < 0.0005$, corrected) and with a significant interaction between the delayed-response and dual-task factors (branching and control compared to delay and dual-task conditions; $P < 0.0005$, uncorrected). The same branching-specific activation was found *post hoc* by computing the voxels co-jointly activated in the branching condition compared separately with all other conditions (fronto-polar: $Z > 5.4$, $P < 0.0005$, corrected; elsewhere

$P > 0.05$, corrected). Branching-specific activations were confirmed in five single-subject analyses. They were located bilaterally in the superior fronto-polar gyrus at the crossing of the middle frontal gyrus (two subjects) or in the middle fronto-polar gyrus (three subjects).[28] Moreover, bilateral fronto-polar activations were replicated in six additional normal right-handed subjects performing the branching and two additional control tasks.

References

1. Grafman, J. in *Structure and Function of the Human Prefrontal Cortex* (eds Grafman, J., Holyoak, K. J. & Boller, F.) 337–368 (Annals of the New York Academy of Sciences, New York, 1995).
2. Baker, S. C. et al. Neural system engaged by planning: A PET study of the Tower of London task. *Neuropsychologia* 34, 515–526 (1996).
3. Owen, A. M., Doyon, J., Petrides, M. & Evans, A. C. Planning and spatial working memory: a positron emission tomography study in human. *Eur. J. Neurosci.* 8, 353–564 (1996).
4. Sirigu, A. et al. Planning and script analysis following prefrontal lobe lesions. *Ann. NY Acad. Sci.* 769, 277–288 (1995).
5. Spector, L. & Grafman, J. in *Handbook of Neuropsychology* (eds Boller, F. & Grafman, J.) 377–392 (Elsevier, Amsterdam, 1994).
6. Wharton, C. & Grafman, J. Reasoning and the human brain. *Trends Cogn. Sci.* 2, 54–59 (1998).
7. Stuss, D. T. & Benson, D. F. *The Frontal Lobes* (Raven, New York, 1986).
8. Fuster, J. M. *The Prefrontal Cortex. Anatomy, Physiology, and Neuropsychology of the Frontal Lobe* (Raven, New York, 1989).
9. D'Esposito, M. et al. The neural basis of the central executive system of working memory. *Nature* 378, 279–281 (1995).
10. Corbetta, M. Frontoparietal cortical networks for directing attention and the eye to visual locations: identical, independent, or overlapping neural systems? *Proc. Natl Acad. Sci. USA* 95, 831–838 (1998).
11. Squire, L. R. et al. Activation of the hippocampus in normal humans: a functional anatomical study of memory. *Proc. Natl Acad. Sci. USA* 89, 1837–1841 (1992).
12. Buckner, R. L. et al. Functional anatomical studies of explicit and implicit memory retrieval tasks. *J. Neurosci.* 15, 12–29 (1995).
13. Shallice, T. et al. Brain regions associated with acquisition and retrieval of verbal episodic memory. *Nature* 368, 633–635 (1994).
14. Grady, C. L. et al. Age-related reductions in human recognition memory due to impaired encoding. *Science* 269, 218–221 (1995).
15. Tulving, E. et al. Neuroanatomical correlates of retrieval in episodic memory: auditory sentence recognition. *Proc. Natl Acad. Sci. USA* 91, 2012–2015 (1994).
16. Tulving, E. *Elements of Episodic Memory* (Oxford Science, Oxford, 1983).
17. Galaburda, A. M., LeMay, M., Kemper, T. L. & Geschwind, N. Right-left asymmetries in the brain. *Science* 199, 852–856 (1978).
18. Furey, M. L. et al. Cholinergic stimulation alters performance and task-specific regional cerebral blood flow during working memory. *Proc. Natl Acad. Sci. USA* 94, 6512–6516 (1997).
19. Goldman-Rakic, P. C. in *Handbook of Physiology, The Nervous System* (eds Plum, F. & Mountcastle, V.) 373–417 (American Physiological Society, Bethesda, MD, 1987).
20. Petrides, M. in *Handbook of Neuropsychology* (eds Boller, F. & Grafman, J.) 59–82 (Elsevier, Amsterdam, 1994).
21. Jonides, J. et al. Spatial working memory in humans as revealed by PET. *Nature* 363, 623–625 (1993).
22. Courtney, S. M., Ungerleider, L. G., Keil, K. & Haxby, J. V. Transient and sustained activity in a distributed neural system for human working memory. *Nature* 386, 608–611 (1997).
23. MacLeod, A. K., Buckner, R. L., Miezin, F. M., Petersen, S. E. & Raichle, M. E. Right anterior prefrontal cortex activation during semantic monitoring and working memory. *NeuroImage* 7, 41–48 (1998).
24. Grafton, S. T., Hazeltine, E. & Ivry, R. Functional mapping of sequence learning in normal humans. *J. Cogn. Neurosci.* 7, 497–510 (1995).
25. Pallier, C., Dupoux, E. & Jeannin, X. EXPE: an expandable programing language for on-line psycho-

logical experiments. *Behav. Res. Methods Instrum. Comput.* 29, 322–327 (1997).

26. Friston, K. J., Frith, C. D., Liddle, P. F. & Frackowiak, R. S. J. Comparing functional (PET) images: The assessment of significant change. *J. Cereb. Blood Flow Metab.* 11, 690–699 (1991).

27. Talairach, J. & Tournoux, P. *Co-planar Stereo-taxic Atlas of the Human Brain* (Thieme Medical, New York, 1988).

28. Duvernoy, H. *The Human Brain. Surface, Three Dimensional Sectional Anatomy and MRI* (Springer, Wien, 1991).

8 The Seven Sins of Memory: Insights from Psychology and Cognitive Neuroscience

Daniel L. Schacter

Question: If Vernon Jordan has told us that you have an extraordinary memory, one of the greatest memories he has ever seen in a politician, would that be something you would care to dispute?

Clinton: No. I do have a good memory. At least I have had a good memory in my life ... It's also—if I could say one thing about my memory—I have been blessed and advantaged in my life with a good memory. I have been shocked and so have members of my family and friends of mine at how many things that I have forgotten in the last six years—I think because of the pressure and the pace and the volume of events in a president's life, compounded by the pressure of your four-year inquiry, and all the other things that have happened.

When President Clinton testified before Kenneth Starr's grand jury, his numerous lapses of memory prompted investigators to query him about his reputation for prodigious recall. The logic implicit in their question, later articulated explicitly by Starr in his own testimony to the House committee investigating impeachment charges, seems clear: How could someone with such a seemingly exceptional memory forget as much as Clinton did about the details of his encounters with Monica Lewinsky? Starr's lawyers were, to put it mildly, suspicious about the self-serving aspects of Clinton's failures to recall potentially damning incidents and statements. Although their skepticism may indeed be warranted, the contrast between Clinton's reputation for extraordinary memory on the one hand, and his claims of sketchy recollections for his encounters with Lewinsky on the other, also illustrates a fundamental duality of memory.

I have previously referred to this duality as memory's "fragile power" (Schacter, 1996). The power of memory is evident when one contemplates what the various forms of memory make possible in our everyday lives: a sense of personal history, knowledge of facts and concepts, and learning of complex skills. Because of memory's importance in everyday life, it is easy to see why

Vernon Jordan would be struck by Clinton's "extraordinary memory" and how that ability would enhance Clinton's prospects as a politician. But, as Clinton professed to have learned during his term as President, memory also has a darker, more fragile side. People may forget events rapidly or gradually, distort the past in surprising ways, and sometimes experience intrusive recollections of events that they wish they could forget.

This darker side of memory has occupied center stage in recent scientific, clinical, and popular discussions. As most psychologists are acutely aware, a bitter controversy has raged throughout the 1990s concerning the accuracy of recovered memories of childhood sexual abuse (see, for instance, Conway, 1997; Freyd, 1996; Herman, 1992; Kihlstrom, 1995; Lindsay & Read, 1994; Loftus, 1993; Pope, 1996; Poole, Lindsay, Memon, & Bull, 1995; Read & Lindsay, 1997; Schacter, Norman, & Koutstaal, 1997). Some recovered memories have been corroborated and appear to be accurate, but there are also good reasons to believe that many such memories are inaccurate (e.g., Lindsay & Read, 1994; Schacter, 1996; J. W. Schooler, 1994). False memories of childhood sexual abuse are associated with devastating psychological consequences for accusers and their families (Loftus & Ketcham, 1994; Pendergrast, 1995). As the debate concerning recovered memories has raged, memory researchers have focused increasingly on developing experimental paradigms to explore illusory or false memories in which people confidently claim to recollect events that never happened (for review and discussion, see Estes, 1997; Roediger, 1996; Schacter, Norman, & Koutstaal, 1998).

Although false memories have been discussed intensively in recent years, forgetting is perhaps the most familiar of memory's indiscretions. Psychologists and neuroscientists have studied forgetting ever since Ebbinghaus (1885) applied experimental methods to the study of memory and provided quantitative estimates of forgetting. The general public, too, has become increasingly concerned with forgetting, even prior to the release of Clinton's forgetting-filled grand jury testimony. As highlighted by a recent cover story concerning memory in *Newsweek* (Cowley & Underwood, 1998), millions of aging baby-boomers in addition to Clinton are trying to understand why they now forget more frequently than in the past and what, if anything, they can do about it (e.g., Crook & Adderly, 1998).

We are all affected by memory's shortcomings in our everyday lives, and scientists have studied them for decades. But there have been few attempts to systematically organize or classify the various ways in which memory can lead us astray and to assess the state of the scientific evidence concerning them. Given the scientific attention paid recently to the fallibility of memory, and the important real-world consequences that are sometimes associated with forgetting and distortion, such an undertaking would appear to be both timely and potentially useful.

I suggest that memory's transgressions can be divided into seven basic "sins." I call them transience, absent-mindedness, blocking, misattribution, suggestibility, bias, and persistence. The first three sins reflect different types of forgetting. *Transience* involves decreasing accessibility of information over time, *absent-mindedness* entails inattentive or shallow processing that contributes to weak memories of ongoing events or forgetting to do things in the future, and *blocking* refers to the temporary inaccessibility of information that is stored in memory. The next three sins all involve distortion or inaccuracy. *Misattribution* involves attributing a recollection or idea to the wrong source, *suggestibility* refers to memories that are implanted as a result of leading questions or comments during attempts to recall past experiences, and *bias* involves retrospective distortions and unconscious influences that are related to current knowledge and beliefs. The seventh and final sin, *persistence*, refers to patho-

logical remembrances: information or events that we cannot forget, even though we wish we could.

Like the biblical seven deadly sins—pride, anger, envy, greed, gluttony, lust, and sloth—the seven sins of memory occur frequently in human affairs. The biblical sins, however, can also be seen as exaggerations of human traits that are in many respects useful and even necessary for survival. So, too, is the case for the seven sins of memory. As annoying and occasionally dangerous as they may be, I suggest later in this article that memory's sins should not be viewed as flaws in system design or unfortunate errors made by Mother Nature during the course of evolution. Instead, the seven sins are more usefully conceptualized as by-products of otherwise desirable features of human memory (cf. J. R. Anderson & Schooler, 1991; Bjork & Bjork, 1988). Perhaps paradoxically, then, the seven sins can provide insights into the very operations of memory that make it such a valuable resource in numerous aspects of our everyday lives.

In the body of this chapter, I summarize two major types of evidence and ideas concerning each of the seven sins. First, much of what is known about the seven sins comes from work in cognitive, social, and clinical psychology; I summarize recent research from each of these domains. Second, I consider what we have learned about the seven sins from the perspective of contemporary cognitive neuroscience. During the past 20 years, cognitive neuroscience analyses of human memory have become increasingly influential (for general summaries, see Gabrieli, 1998; Gazzaniga, 1995; Schacter, 1992, 1996). The cognitive neuroscience approach has relied heavily on studies of patients with brain lesions that selectively affect particular forms of memory and, more recently, on studies using functional neuroimaging techniques, such as positron emission tomography (PET) and functional magnetic resonance imaging (fMRI). PET and fMRI measure local changes in hemodynamic responses that are correlated with changes in neuronal activity: PET is sensitive to changes in blood flow, whereas fMRI is sensitive to oxygenation-level-dependent changes in the magnetic properties of blood, usually referred to as BOLD contrast. Both techniques allow relatively precise localization of the observed changes in hemodynamic response. To make inferences about the activation of particular brain regions during performance of behavioral tasks, investigators generally measure changes in blood flow or blood oxygenation level in one experimental condition relative to another condition. Estimates of blood flow or oxygenation level can then be subtracted from one another, or assessed with various other analysis strategies (for further discussion of the nature and logic of neuroimaging approaches, see Posner & Raichle, 1994). The neuroimaging of human memory has progressed rapidly during the past five years (for reviews, see Buckner & Koutstaal, 1998; Cabeza & Nyberg, 1997; Schacter & Wagner, in press; Ungerleider, 1995).

In the sections that follow, I ask what (if anything) cognitive neuroscience approaches have taught us about each of the seven sins. I then conclude by considering the sense in which, and the extent to which, the seven sins reflect the operation of otherwise adaptive features of memory.

Understanding the Seven Sins: Evidence from Mind and Brain

Transience

Memory for facts and events typically becomes less accessible over time. Gradual forgetting was first documented in Ebbinghaus's (1885) well-known studies, where he attempted to learn and remember nonsense syllables. He assessed his own memory at various delays after initial learning and observed a rapid drop-off in retention at the early delays, followed by a more gradual drop-off at later delays. Cognitive psychologists continue to investigate and characterize the form of the forgetting function. Although the basic characteristics of the forgetting curve described

by Ebbinghaus have been observed in numerous situations, recent evidence indicates that forgetting over time is best described mathematically with a power function: the rate of forgetting is slowed down by the passage of time (e.g., Wixted & Ebbesen, 1997).

Discussions about the cause of long-term forgetting have focused on whether forgetting is attributable to actual loss of information from memory storage, to retrieval failure that can be reversed by provision of appropriate cues, or both (e.g., Loftus & Loftus, 1980; Schacter, 1996; Squire, 1987). There is no doubt that retrieval failure plays an important role in forgetting. Some experiences may be rendered temporarily inaccessible because of interference from related experiences (Postman & Underwood, 1973), and it is well-established that cues and hints can elicit recall of seemingly forgotten memories (e.g., Tulving & Pearlstone, 1966; for a recent review, see Koutstaal & Schacter, 1997b). Nonetheless, such findings need not indicate that all forgetting is attributable to access failure. The view that experiences are recorded permanently, with all forgetting attributable to access failure, is surprisingly common—even among psychologists (Loftus & Loftus, 1980). However, it seems likely that information is also lost from storage over time (Schacter, 1996; Squire, 1987). Loss of information over time may be particularly likely to occur when people do not "use" a memory. It is known, for instance, that retrieving and rehearsing experiences plays an important role in determining whether those experiences will be remembered or forgotten (e.g., Bjork, 1988; Koutstaal, Schacter, Johnson, Angell, & Gross, 1998) and in determining what aspects of those experiences will be retained (e.g., Suengas & Johnson, 1988). Memories that are not retrieved and rehearsed may slowly dissipate over time. Although there is no direct evidence for such dissipation in studies of humans, neurobiological evidence from invertebrate organisms has revealed loss of synaptic connectivity over time (e.g., Bailey & Chen, 1989).

It has also been established that forgetting can occur quite rapidly—on a time scale of seconds, rather than minutes, hours, or days. Beginning with the classic studies of J. Brown (1958) and Peterson and Peterson (1959), rapid forgetting has been attributed to the operation of a short-term or working memory system (Baddeley, 1986). Working memory is necessary for holding information "on-line," usually for brief periods of time, while other cognitive activities are carried out. The exact cause of rapid forgetting within working memory has long been debated (for a discussion of alternative views, see Crowder, 1989) but, as noted below, the evidence suggests that it involves different mechanisms than long-term forgetting.

Cognitive neuroscience analyses have been instrumental in providing insights into the underlying bases of both gradual (i.e., long-term) and rapid (i.e., short-term) transience. Beginning with the pioneering studies of Scoville and Milner (1957), studies of brain-damaged amnesic patients have shown that damage to the medial temporal lobes, including the hippocampus and related structures, produces profound long-term forgetting. Such patients perform reasonably well on tasks that tap short-term or working memory (e.g., digit span) and can maintain information in working memory if they are not distracted (Parkin & Leng, 1993; Squire, 1987). However, once distraction or delay are introduced, amnesic patients forget experiences rapidly (anterograde amnesia). They also exhibit varying degrees of forgetting for experiences that occurred prior to the injury (retrograde amnesia; for alternative perspectives, see Nadel & Moscovitch, 1997; Squire & Alvarez, 1995). However, studies with amnesic patients have not been highly successful in pinpointing the exact source of the pathological forgetting that patients exhibit. Thus, for instance, investigations of anterograde amnesia have not yet resolved whether forgetting is attributable specifically to problems in encoding, storage, or retrieval of information, or some com-

bination of these processes (for a recent discussion, see Mayes & Downes, 1997).

Neuroimaging studies are also limited with respect to the kinds of insights they can provide concerning the neural bases of transience. Current neuroimaging techniques do not permit direct study of the storage or consolidation processes that intervene between encoding and retrieval and that are directly related to the occurrence of transience. However, neuroimaging techniques do allow a separation between encoding and retrieval processes. Thus, studies using fMRI and PET have provided some initial insights into the role of medial temporal lobes in encoding and retrieval processes that has not been possible to obtain in studies of amnesic patients (for review and discussion, see Lepage, Habib, & Tulving, 1998; Schacter & Wagner, 1999).

Two recent fMRI studies illuminate an important source of transience: initial encoding of information into memory. Both studies used "event-related" fMRI procedures, which make it possible to track encoding processes on a trial-by-trial basis. Responses can be sorted later according to whether an item is remembered or forgotten, much in the manner that data from studies using electrophysiological measures, such as event-related potentials, can be selectively sorted and averaged (for discussion of event-related fMRI methods, see Dale & Buckner, 1997).

Wagner, Schacter, et al. (1998) used event-related fMRI to determine whether responses to individual words during encoding predict subsequent remembering and forgetting of those words. During the scanning period, participants viewed a long list of words and decided whether each word was abstract or concrete. This encoding phase was followed by a nonscanned recognition test in which participants made old–new judgments indicating whether or not they remembered having encountered an item in the study phase and also indicated their degree of confidence in their judgment. Analysis of the fMRI data revealed that two regions of the brain were more active during the encoding phase of the experiment for words that were subsequently remembered with high confidence than for words that were subsequently forgotten. One of these regions was in the posterior (i.e., back) portions of the left temporal lobe (the left parahippocampal gyrus), and the other was in the lower portion of the left frontal lobe (the left inferior frontal gyrus). Thus, level of activity in these two regions at the time of encoding predicted whether an individual word was later remembered or forgotten.

Brewer, Zhao, Desmond, Glover, and Gabrieli (1998) carried out a similar event-related fMRI encoding study, using pictures of everyday scenes instead of words. Their results converged nicely with those of Wagner, Schacter, et al. (1998). Brewer et al. found that degree of activity during encoding in parahippocampal regions of both the left and right hemispheres, and inferior frontal regions in the right hemisphere, predicted subsequent remembering and forgetting: There was greater parahippocampal and right prefrontal activity during encoding for subsequently remembered than forgotten pictures. The fact that right hemisphere regions predicted subsequent remembering and forgetting of pictures, whereas only left hemisphere regions predicted subsequent memory for words, fits with other neuroimaging data linking the left hemisphere with verbal encoding and the right hemisphere with nonverbal encoding (Kelley et al., 1998; Wagner, Poldrack, et al., 1998). Gradual forgetting of different types of information thus appears to be attributable, at least in part, to initial levels of activity in regions involved with encoding verbal and nonverbal experiences.

Turning from long-term to short-term transience, neuropsychological studies of brain-damaged patients have illuminated the nature of short-term forgetting by demonstrating a pattern opposite to that observed in amnesic patients.

Specifically, a number of studies have described patients who show relatively intact long-term memory—they can remember the ongoing experiences of everyday life and perform well on tests of memory that amnesic patients fail—but have severe problems with immediate retention (for a review, see Vallar & Shallice, 1990). Such patients may exhibit entirely normal performance on such long-term memory tasks as learning pairs of associated words, yet exhibit virtually instant forgetting on such immediate memory tasks as digit span.

These patients have problems within the working memory system. According to Baddeley (1986), this system contains a number of interrelated components. In many cases of short-term memory loss, the observed deficit can be attributed to a specific component of working memory known as the phonological loop (see Baddeley, Gathercole, & Papagano, 1998). The phonological loop is necessary for holding small amounts of speech-based information. It is the type of memory one would rely on when attempting to hold on to a telephone number as one races from the phone book to the telephone. Patients with damage to the phonological loop usually have a lesion in the lower part of the left parietal lobe, and they exhibit rapid forgetting of speech-based information. It is important to note that patients with damage to the phonological loop also have difficulty with long-term retention of phonological information, such as learning new vocabulary (Baddeley et al., 1998). Developmental studies have shown that performance on working memory tasks that require the phonological loop is closely associated with long-term vocabulary acquisition and related aspects of language learning (Gathercole & Baddeley, 1994). Thus, when the phonological loop does not operate normally (as in cases of left parietal damage or some children with developmental disabilities), problems with short-term forgetting arise that have important consequences for such fundamental abilities as language learning.

Neuroimaging studies have also begun to illuminate some of the neural systems that are relevant to short-term transience by revealing the
component structures of working memory (for
reviews, see Awh & Jonides, 1998; Schacter,
Wagner, & Buckner, in press; E. E. Smith &
Jonides, 1997). To take just one example, neuropsychological studies suggest that two key
components of the phonological loop—a phonological store and a rehearsal mechanism that
maintains the contents of this store—are based
on distinct neural substrates, because storage and
rehearsal processes can be impaired selectively
(e.g., Vallar & Baddeley, 1984). Neuroimaging studies support this distinction: A number
of studies suggest that regions within the left
(posterior) parietal lobe subserve phonological
storage, whereas portions of left (inferior) prefrontal cortex (Broca's area) are important for
phonological rehearsal (e.g., Paulesu, Frith, &
Frackowiak, 1993). Short-term forgetting can
result from a failure of rehearsal processes, storage processes, or both.

Absent-Mindedness

Transience—forgetting over time—can occur
even when an event or fact is initially well-
encoded and remembered immediately and can
occur even when we deliberately search memory
in an attempt to recall a specific event or fact.
However, a good deal of forgetting likely occurs
because insufficient attention is devoted to a
stimulus at the time of encoding or retrieval or
because attended information is processed super-
ficially. Such incidents of forgetting associated
with lapses of attention during encoding or during attempted retrieval can be described as errors
of absent-mindedness (e.g., Reason & Mycielska,
1982).

Absent-mindedness during encoding is a likely
source of common everyday memory failures,
such as forgetting where one recently placed an
object (e.g., car keys). Such absent-minded encoding failures occur when actions are carried out

automatically and attention is focused elsewhere
(Reason & Mycielska, 1982). Consistent with this
observation, cognitive studies have established
that dividing attention at the time of encoding results in poor subsequent memory for target information (e.g., Craik, Govoni, Naveh-Benjamin,
& Anderson, 1996). Likewise, even when attention is nominally devoted to a target item, subsequent memory suffers when that item is initially
encoded at a shallow level. This effect was firmly
established in cognitive studies demonstrating the
well-known "depth of processing" effect (Craik
& Lockhart, 1972). When people are induced to
carry out "shallow" encoding of target information by making judgments about low-level, nonsemantic features of target information (e.g., Is
TABLE printed in upper- or lowercase letters?),
they later have considerably worse memory for
the target (TABLE) than when they are induced
to carry out "deep" encoding by making judgments about semantic features of the target item
(e.g., Is TABLE a type of furniture?; Craik &
Tulving, 1975).

A form of shallow encoding also plays a role in
recent demonstrations of an intriguing phenomenon termed "change blindness" (for a review,
see Simons & Levin, 1997). In studies of change
blindness, people observe objects or scenes in
which various features are changed over time.
Change blindness occurs when people fail to
detect these changes. For example, Levin and
Simons (1997) showed participants a movie in
which an actor carried out a simple action. Unknown to the observers, the actor was replaced
by a different person during the course of the
scene. Only one third of observers noticed the
change. Even more striking, Simons and Levin
(1998) described a naturalistic study in which one
of the experimenters asked a person on a college
campus for directions. While they were talking,
two men walked between them holding a door
that hid the second experimenter. Behind the
door, the two experimenters traded places, so
that when the men carrying the door moved on,
a different person was asking for directions than

the one who had been there just a second or two earlier. Remarkably, only 7 of 15 participants reported noticing this change!

One explanation for change blindness is that people typically encode features of a scene at an extremely shallow level, recording the general gist of the scene but few of the specific details (Simons & Levin, 1997). As Simons and Levin (1998) noted, "successful change detection probably requires effortful encoding of precisely those features or properties that will distinguish the original from the changed object" (p. 648). Support for this explanation is provided by a follow-up to the "door study." Simons and Levin (1998) noted that the people who failed to notice that a different person emerged from behind the door were middle-aged and older adults; college students tended to notice the change. They hypothesized that the older individuals might have encoded the initial (young) experimenter categorically as a "college student," whereas the college students (for whom the person asking directions was a peer) encoded the experimenter at a more specific level. To determine whether college students would be more susceptible to change blindness when induced to encode at a categorical or generic level, Simons and Levin repeated the "door study," but now attired as construction workers. They reasoned that college students now might tend to encode them categorically as "construction workers" and, hence, show higher levels of change blindness. Results supported the hypothesis: Only 4 of 12 students noticed when a different construction worker emerged from behind the door to ask instructions. Thus, shallow encoding that does not proceed beyond a categorical level results in poor recollection of the details of a scene and consequent vulnerability to change blindness.

Some of the neural bases of absent-minded encoding have been elucidated in neuroimaging studies that have compared "deep" and "shallow" encoding tasks. Several early studies revealed greater activation in the lower (i.e., inferior) regions of the left frontal cortex during semantic encoding trials than during nonsemantic encoding trials (e.g., Demb et al., 1995; Kapur et al., 1994), thereby indicating that level of left prefrontal activation is related to semantic encoding processes. More recent work has indicated that the left parahippocampal region discussed earlier also shows greater activation during semantic than nonsemantic encoding tasks (Wagner, Schacter, et al., 1998). Thus, we can tentatively infer that "absent-minded" encoding operations (at least within a verbal domain) are those that involve relatively little recruitment of left inferior prefrontal and parahippocampal regions. These observations are consistent with the previously discussed event-related fMRI data showing that level of activation in inferior prefrontal and parahippocampal regions predicts subsequent remembering and forgetting.

Absent-mindedness also occurs at the time of retrieval, when people may forget to carry out a particular task or function. Because such absent-minded lapses involve forgetting to execute a planned action at some point in the future, they are typically referred to as failures of prospective memory (e.g., Brandimonte, Einstein, & McDaniel, 1996; Cohen, 1989). Absent-minded errors of prospective memory can have important everyday consequences, as when elderly patients forget to take prescribed medications (Park & Kidder, 1996) or when air traffic controllers cannot execute a control action immediately and subsequently forget that they need to take deferred action in the near future (Vortac, Edwards, & Manning, 1995). Prospective memory researchers have found it useful to distinguish between "event-based" and "time-based" prospective memory tasks. Event-based tasks involve remembering to perform a future action when a specified event occurs, such as remembering to deliver a message to a friend the next time you see her. Time-based tasks, in contrast, involve remembering to perform an action at a specified time, such as remembering to take one's medicine at 11:00 p.m. or remembering to turn off the burner on the stove five minutes from now. Event-based prospective memory tasks are externally cued, so forgetting tends to occur when a cue is not recognized. Time-based prospective memory tasks, in contrast, depend more on generating appropriate cues at the time an intended action needs to be carried out (McDaniel & Einstein, 1993; Vortac et al., 1995). Absent-minded forgetting in time-based tasks thus tends to occur because people fail to prospectively generate retrieval cues ahead of time, and then spontaneously fail to do so at the time the intended action needs to be performed. This distinction appears to be particularly relevant to studies of aging memory, which indicate that older adults often perform well on event-based prospective tasks and more poorly on time-based tasks (for a review, see Einstein & McDaniel, 1996; Maylor, 1996).

Cognitive neuroscience has so far contributed relatively little to understanding absent-minded errors of prospective forgetting. Shallice and Burgess (1991) have demonstrated that failures to carry out future tasks in patients with frontal lobe lesions are associated with level of planning skills and executive functions. Cockburn (1995) investigated a variety of prospective memory tasks in a patient with bilateral frontal lobe damage. The patient performed well on each of five event-based prospective tasks, but performed poorly on several time-based prospective tasks, particularly those tasks that required interrupting one action to perform an unrelated one. In a recent PET study, Okuda et al. (1998) investigated the neural correlates of event-based prospective remembering. They required participants to perform a routine task (repeating spoken words) during scanning. In a condition that required prospective memory, participants were also required to retain a planned action (to tap when prespecified words were presented) while carrying out other activities. Prospective remembering was associated with activation in a number of brain regions, most notably the surface of the right frontal lobe (dorsolateral and ventrolateral re-

gions), the front of the left frontal lobe (frontal pole), and inner parts of the frontal lobe near the midline. Taken together, the patient studies and neuroimaging experiment implicate prefrontal cortex in aspects of both event-based and time-based prospective memory (note, however, that Cockburn's [1995] patient performed well on event-related prospective tasks; it would be important to determine whether this patient performed well on the exact task that produced prefrontal activation in the PET study). This apparent link between prospective memory and frontal lobe function makes sense in view of the role that frontal regions play in allowing "mental time travel" into both the past and the future (Wheeler, Stuss, & Tulving, 1997). Failure to activate appropriate frontal regions, either at the time of planning a future action or at the moment when it needs to be carried out, may be implicated in absent-minded errors of prospective memory, such as forgetting to keep an appointment or to take a prescribed medicine.

Blocking

Even when a fact or event has been encoded deeply, and has not been lost over time, it may sometimes be temporarily inaccessible (Koutstaal & Schacter, 1997b; Tulving & Pearlstone, 1966). When people are provided with cues that are related to a sought-after item, but are nonetheless unable to elicit it, a retrieval block has occurred (Roediger & Neely, 1982). Such blocks occur in both episodic memory (i.e., memory for specific personal experiences) and semantic memory (i.e., general knowledge of the world). Blocking constitutes one of the most subjectively compelling of memory's seven sins, in the sense that people are acutely aware of the block at the time it occurs. When blocking occurs at an inopportune moment under high stress—such as with actors who suddenly cannot recall their lines—the accompanying subjective awareness can be overwhelming (Reason & Mycielska, 1982).

The most thoroughly investigated example of blocking is the tip-of-the-tongue (TOT) state. In a TOT state, people are unable to produce a word or a name, but they have a powerful subjective conviction that the item is available in memory. Further, they can sometimes produce partial phonological or semantic information about the item (R. Brown & McNeil, 1966; for review, see A. S. Brown, 1991). TOT retrieval blocks are often resolved quickly: Several studies have shown that roughly half of the sought-after target items are retrieved within a minute or so after the onset of blocking, although some items may not be retrieved until days later (see A. S. Brown, 1991, pp. 211–213). TOT blocks appear to be partly attributable to the retrieval of similar but incorrect items that interfere with access to the target (see Harley & Brown, 1998, for other relevant factors). For example, in a diary study, Reason and Lucas (1984) found that over half of naturally occurring TOT states were characterized by the presence of what they termed "ugly sisters," referring to Cinderella's undesirable but dominating older sisters. Ugly sisters are incorrect items that are related to the sought-after target and that recur intrusively during the retrieval attempt. Consistent with this observation, when Jones and Langford (1987) induced TOT states by giving definitions of low frequency words, they found that providing phonologically or semantically related cues along with the definitions resulted in more TOT states than when unrelated words were given (see also Smith & Tindell, 1997).

Blocking appears to be especially pronounced in old age. The incidence of TOT states increases with aging (A. S. Brown & Nix, 1996; Maylor, 1990), although it remains unclear as to whether older adults are more susceptible to interference from "ugly sisters" than are younger adults (cf. Burke, MacKay, Worthley, & Wade, 1991; A. S. Brown & Nix, 1996). The age-related increase in TOT states may be particularly pronounced when people attempt to retrieve names (Maylor, 1990). This observation is consistent with other evidence indicating that name retrieval failure is a frequent subjective complaint by older adults and that older adults exhibit difficulties retrieving proper names. However, it is unclear whether these problems are disproportionately worse than age-related retrieval problems for other kinds of information (for review and discussion, see Cohen & Burke, 1993; Maylor, 1997).

The foregoing observations concerning the role of "ugly sisters" in the TOT state resemble a curious phenomenon known as the "part-set cueing" effect, which has been documented in laboratory studies of episodic memory in which participants encode and retrieve lists of words. In part-set cueing, provision of some retrieval cues that are related to a previously studied word can block or inhibit, rather than enhance, retrieval of the target item (e.g., Roediger, 1974; Slamecka, 1968; Sloman, Bower, & Rohrer, 1991). In a similar vein, several studies have shown that retrieving and reviewing an item or event is sometimes associated with decreased memory for related but nonretrieved items, perhaps because the nonretrieved items become inhibited as a result of retrieving related items (e.g., M. C. Anderson, Bjork, & Bjork, 1994; M. C. Anderson & Spellman, 1995). Although most such evidence comes from word-list learning studies, Shaw, Bjork, and Handal (1995) reported inhibitory effects of retrieval in an eyewitness memory paradigm involving more complex events. Participants first viewed color slides of a crime scene (a student's room where a theft had occurred). The experimenters then questioned them repeatedly about certain categories of objects in the scene (e.g., some of the college sweatshirts that were present), resulting in retrieval and review of these objects. No questions were asked about other categories of objects (e.g., college schoolbooks). Compared with objects about which no questions were asked (schoolbooks), participants recalled fewer of the nonretrieved and nonreviewed objects from the categories that had been repeatedly probed. Thus, access to these nonretrieved items seemed to be blocked by successful retrieval of related items (for similar results in a paradigm involving review of photographs depicting events that participants themselves had performed, see Koutstaal, Schacter, Johnson, & Galluccio, in press).

Cognitive neuroscience has so far provided some relevant observations concerning retrieval blocks in semantic memory and relatively little information concerning blocking in episodic memory. Within the domain of semantic memory, a variety of studies have examined anomic patients who have difficulties with retrieval of common names of objects or with retrieval of proper names. Some patients have difficulty retrieving proper names but not common names, and still others exhibit a selective deficit in retrieving one type of proper name (e.g., names of people; for recent reviews, see Hanley & Kay, 1998; Semenza, Mondini, & Zettin, 1995). Semenza et al. (1995) observed that proper name retrieval deficits are typically associated with the most anterior regions of the left temporal lobe (temporal pole). Consistent with the neuropsychological evidence, a PET study by Damasio, Grabowski, Tranel, Hichwa, and Damasio (1996) revealed activation of the left temporal pole during proper name production. A more posterior temporal region showed increased activation during animal naming, and an even more posterior region showed increased activation during naming of tools. These observations raise the intriguing possibility that retrieval blocks associated with attempts to name different kinds of items (e.g., individual persons, animals, tools) may reflect inhibition of slightly different left temporal regions. Although no neuroimaging studies of TOT states have yet been reported (and may be difficult to carry out because of the relative infrequency of the TOT phenomenon), such studies could provide novel insights into the neural correlates of retrieval blocking.

Numerous neuroimaging studies of episodic memory retrieval have been reported (for review and discussion, see Buckner & Koutstaal, 1998; Lepage et al., 1998; Schacter & Wagner, 1999),

but none have specifically examined episodic retrieval blocks. Perhaps the most relevant data have been reported by Nyberg et al. (1996), who uncovered evidence of what they termed "ensemble inhibition." Nyberg et al. (1996) reported that regions that showed increased activity during a retrieval task appeared to actively inhibit other regions showing decreased activity. These observations suggest that, consistent with psychological observations (e.g., M. C. Anderson, Bjork, & Bjork, 1994; M. C. Anderson & Spellman, 1995), inhibitory processes may be a normal and perhaps necessary component of episodic retrieval. Whether and to what extent ensemble inhibition processes are related to retrieval blocks remains to be elucidated.

Misattribution

Transience, absent-mindedness, and blocking can all be thought of as sins of omission: At a moment when individuals need to remember, the desired information is inaccessible or unavailable. However, memory is also characterized by sins of commission: Situations in which some form of memory is present, but is misattributed to an incorrect time, place, or person (e.g., Jacoby, Kelley, & Dywan, 1989; Johnson, Hashtroudi, & Lindsay, 1993; Roediger, 1996: Schacter, Norman, et al., 1998). I find it useful to distinguish among three closely related forms of misattribution.

First, people may remember correctly an item or fact from a past experience but misattribute the fact to an incorrect source. For instance, individuals sometimes recall encountering a bit of trivia in the newspaper that, in fact, they acquired from an experimenter (Schacter, Harbluk, & McLachlan, 1984). Similarly, people may assert that they saw a face in one context when they encountered it in another (e.g., Read, 1994) or that they perceived an event that they only imagined (e.g., Garry, Manning, Loftus, & Sherman, 1996; Goff & Roediger, 1998; Johnson, Raye, Wang, & Taylor, 1979; for review, see Johnson et al., 1993). Source confusions of this kind can be particularly pronounced in older adults (McIntyre & Craik, 1987). In a recent study, for example, Schacter, Koutstaal, Johnson, Gross, and Angell (1997) found that older adults often confused whether they had seen an everyday action in a videotape or only in a photograph that they viewed several days later, whereas younger adults had little difficulty remembering the correct source.

Source confusions can have important implications in everyday life, as exemplified by cases of erroneous eyewitness identifications in which a person seen in one context is mistakenly "transferred" to another (D. F. Ross, Ceci, Dunning, & Toglia, 1994). A particularly dramatic example involved the psychologist Donald Thomson, a respected memory researcher who was accused of rape on the basis of the victim's detailed recollection of the rapist (Thomson, 1988). Fortunately for Thomson, he had an airtight alibi: He was giving a live television interview (ironically, concerning memory distortion) at the moment that the rape occurred. The victim had been watching that interview just prior to being raped. She had confused the source of her vivid memory of Thomson, misattributing the television image to the rapist. Thomson's alibi led to his immediate vindication, but others have not been so fortunate. Recent investigations into cases of wrongful imprisonment, where innocence was established by DNA evidence, provide sobering evidence. In a sample of 40 such cases, 36 (90%) involved false identification of the perpetrator by one or more eyewitnesses (Wells et al., in press; this finding is also relevant to the discussion of suggestibility in the next section).

In the foregoing examples of misattribution, recall of the item or fact is accompanied by a subjective experience of remembering a past event. A second type of misattribution is characterized by an absence of any subjective experience of remembering. People sometimes misattribute a spontaneous thought or idea to their own imagination, when in fact they are retrieving it— without awareness of doing so—from a specific prior experience (e.g., Schacter, 1987). This phenomenon of cryptomnesia is exemplified in everyday life by instances of unintentional plagiarism and has been studied recently in the laboratory (e.g., A. S. Brown & Murphy, 1989; Ceci, 1995; Marsh & Landau, 1995). A related type of misattribution has been dubbed the "false fame effect" by Jacoby and colleagues (e.g., Jacoby, Kelley, Brown, & Jasechko, 1989). In Jacoby et al.'s experiments, participants first studied lists including famous names (e.g., Ronald Reagan) and nonfamous names (e.g., Sebastian Weisdorf). Either immediately or one day after studying the names, participants were given a "fame judgment" task in which they made famous-nonfamous judgments about previously studied names and new names. On the one-day delayed test, participants frequently classified nonfamous names they had studied a day earlier as "famous," but they hardly ever made the false fame error on an immediate test. During the delayed test, having forgotten that they studied a nonfamous name such as "Sebastian Weisdorf," participants misattributed the familiarity of the name to the "fame" of the nonfamous individual. Older adults are sometimes more susceptible to the false fame effect than are younger adults (cf. Dywan & Jacoby, 1990; Multhaup, 1995).

A third type of misattribution occurs when individuals falsely recall or recognize items or events that never happened. During the 1960s and 1970s, a number of researchers produced laboratory demonstrations of false recall and recognition in which people claimed to have seen or heard sentences (Bransford & Franks, 1971), words (Underwood, 1965), or dot patterns (e.g., Posner & Keele, 1968) that had not been previously presented. Although a number of researchers have since produced impressive demonstrations of similar kinds of misattributions (e.g., Hintzman, 1988), the most striking such finding was reported recently by Roediger and McDermott (1995). They revived and modified a paradigm that was originally devised by Deese

(1959). Deese had reported that when people studied lists of semantically associated words and later tried to recall them, they frequently intruded or falsely recalled a strongly associated word that had not been previously presented.

Roediger and McDermott (1995) replicated this false-recall effect and extended it to recognition. In Roediger and McDermott's extension of the Deese task, participants initially studied 15 semantic associates that were all related to a nonpresented "theme word." After studying a number of such 15-word sets, they were then asked to recall words from the list or to recognize them. For instance, participants might study a list containing the words candy, sour, sugar, bitter, good, taste, tooth, and other related words. They would later receive a recognition test that includes studied words (e.g., taste), nonstudied words that are unrelated to words that had appeared on the study list (e.g., point) and, most important, new theme words (e.g., sweet) that are associatively related to words from the study list. Roediger and McDermott (1995) reported that participants made false alarms to approximately 65–80% of the nonpresented theme words in various conditions; indeed, false alarm rates to the theme words were indistinguishable from hit rates to words that were actually presented. Participants expressed as much confidence in these false memories as they did in accurate recollections of previously studied words. Roediger and McDermott also asked participants whether they possessed a specific, detailed recollection of having encountered a word on the list (a "remember" response; cf. Gardiner & Java, 1993; Tulving, 1985), or whether they thought it was on the list because it just seemed familiar to them (a "know" response). Participants provided as many "remember" responses to nonstudied theme words as they did to studied words. This striking false-recognition effect has been replicated and explored in a number of other laboratories (e.g., Mather, Henkel, & Johnson, 1997; Norman & Schacter, 1997; Payne, Elie, Black-

well, & Neuschatz, 1996; Seamon, Luo, & Gallo, 1998).

One explanation for this kind of misattribution is that participants are relying on their memory for the general semantic features or "gist" of the items that they studied (cf. Payne et al., 1996; Reyna & Brainerd, 1995; Schacter, Norman, et al., 1998). Participants may bind together studied items and generated associates, thereby forming and retaining a well-organized representation of the semantic gist of the study list (for discussion of alternative theoretical accounts of false recognition, see Roediger, McDermott, & Robinson, 1998; Schacter, Norman, et al., 1998). Theme words that match this semantic representation, such as "sweet," are likely to be falsely recognized; unrelated words that do not match it are likely to be correctly rejected (for additional evidence on this point, see Mather et al., 1997; Norman & Schacter, 1997).

Consistent with this explanation, recent studies have shown that it is possible to reduce or suppress the false-recognition effect when study conditions are created that encourage participants to focus on distinctive properties of individual items. For example, Israel and Schacter (1997) reported that when participants study Roediger-McDermott (1995) lists along with pictures that represent each word, the false-recognition effect is reduced significantly compared with a word-only study condition. Schacter, Israel, and Racine (1999) have provided evidence that this reduction of false recognition involves the use of a "distinctiveness heuristic"—a mode of responding based on participants' expectation that recognition of studied items should be accompanied by recollection of distinctive details (i.e., pictorial information). After studying lists of words that are all accompanied by pictures, participants are less likely to rely solely on semantic gist when making a recognition decision. Instead, they demand access to distinctive perceptual information before they are willing to call an item "old" (for other studies on reducing false recognition of semantic associates, see Gallo, Roberts, & Seamon, 1997; McDermott & Roediger, 1998).

As with previous examples of source misattributions, older adults appear to be especially vulnerable to the kinds of misattributions involved in false recall and recognition. For example, several studies have demonstrated that older adults show disproportionately high levels of false recall and recognition in the Deese/Roediger-McDermott paradigm (Balota et al., in press; Kensinger & Schacter, in press; Norman & Schacter, 1997; Tun, Wingfield, Rosen, & Blanchard, 1998). Koutstaal and Schacter (1997a) provided a particularly striking demonstration of age differences in false recognition. In their paradigm, younger and older adults studied detailed colored pictures from various categories. When given a recognition test after a three-day delay, older adults showed considerably higher levels of false recognition to nonpresented pictures from studied categories than did younger adults. The age differences were most pronounced when participants studied large numbers of pictures (18) from a given category, with older adults showing approximately twice as many false alarms (60–70%) as younger adults (e.g., 25–35%). These observations contrast with other studies in which older adults exhibit high levels of picture recognition accuracy that do not differ substantially from that of younger adults (e.g., Park, Puglisi, & Smith, 1986). In Koutstaal and Schacter's (1997a) paradigm, presentation of numerous perceptually and conceptually similar pictures likely increased reliance on memory for the general features or gist of target items in the older adults compared with younger adults (for further relevant evidence and discussion, see Balota et al., in press; Kensinger & Schacter, in press; Norman & Schacter, 1997; Tun et al., 1998).

Cognitive neuroscience analyses have begun to explore aspects of misattribution. Studies of brain-injured patients have revealed that damage to the frontal lobes is often associated with a selective increase in source memory errors (e.g.,

Janowsky, Shimamura, & Squire, 1989; Schacter et al., 1984). More recent experiments have also linked frontal lobe damage with increased susceptibility to false recognition (Parkin, Bindschaedler, Harsent, & Metzler, 1996; Rapcsak, Reminger, Glisky, Kaszniak, & Comer, in press; Schacter, Curran, Galluccio, Milberg, & Bates, 1996).

By contrast, several studies of amnesic patients with damage to the medial temporal lobes and related structures have revealed decreased susceptibility to certain forms of false recognition. For instance, several experiments using the Deese/Roediger-McDermott paradigm and similar procedures have shown that amnesic patients exhibit reduced levels of false recognition compared with nonamnesic controls (e.g., Koutstaal, Schacter, Verfaellie, Brenner, & Jackson, in press; Schacter, Verfaellie, & Pradere, 1996; Schacter, Verfaellie, Anes, & Racine, 1998). Balota et al. (in press) reported similar findings in patients with memory deficits attributable to Alzheimer's disease. Thus, false recognition in these paradigms depends on the same or similar brain regions that are usually associated with veridical recollection. Medial temporal regions appear to be involved in encoding and retrieving the kinds of semantic gist or similarity information that can support both true and false memories.

Several neuroimaging investigations of false recognition have also been reported. Using a modified version of the Deese/Roediger-McDermott paradigm, Schacter, Reiman, et al. (1996) investigated true and false recognition with PET, and Schacter, Buckner, Koutstaal, Dale, and Rosen (1997) did so with fMRI. The main finding from the two studies is that patterns of brain activity were highly similar during the two forms of recognition, including some evidence of medial temporal lobe activation during both true and false recognition. Differences in brain activity during true and false recognition were relatively small and appeared to depend on specific characteristics of recognition testing procedures (for a discussion, see Schacter, Buckner, et al., 1997; see also Johnson et al., 1997). Frontal lobe activation was quite prominent in each of the PET and fMRI studies of false recognition. Indeed, both studies reported some evidence suggesting that frontal regions may be involved in strategic monitoring processes that are invoked as participants struggle to determine whether a related lure word was actually presented earlier in a study list (for elaboration and further relevant evidence, see Johnson et al., 1997). Such findings fit well with the previously mentioned observation that damage to regions within the frontal lobe is sometimes associated with heightened false recognition (Parkin et al., 1996; Rapcsak et al., in press; Schacter, Curran, et al., 1996). Thus, activity in the frontal lobes may signal an attempt to monitor or scrutinize the output of medial temporal lobe structures. As noted earlier, although medial temporal activity often provides a basis for accurate remembering, it is also implicated in the encoding and retrieval of the gist or general similarity information that sometimes produces false recollections (for further discussion, see Schacter, Norman, et al., 1998).

Suggestibility

The foregoing material indicates that false memories can occur spontaneously when a current situation or test item is conceptually or perceptually similar to a previous one. But such illusory memories may also occur in response to suggestions that are made when one is attempting to recall an experience that may or may not have occurred. Suggestibility in memory refers to the tendency to incorporate information provided by others, such as misleading questions (Loftus, Miller, & Burns, 1978), into one's own recollections (note that this definition corresponds closely to Gudjonsson's [1992] notion of "interrogative suggestibility," which he distinguishes from various other forms of suggestibility). Suggestibility is closely related to misattribution in the sense

that the conversion of suggestions into false recollections must involve misattribution. However, misattribution can occur in the absence of overt suggestion. Thus, suggestibility seems appropriately viewed as a distinct sin of memory.

Suggestion can influence memory in several different ways. Perhaps the most familiar example to experimental psychologists comes from the work of Loftus and colleagues concerning memory distortions produced by misleading postevent information (e.g., Loftus, Miller, & Burns, 1978). When people are asked suggestive and misleading questions about a previous event, their recollections of the original event may be altered by the provision of erroneous postevent information. In the classic studies of Loftus and colleagues (for a review see Loftus, Feldman, & Dashiell, 1995), experimental participants viewed a slide sequence involving an automobile accident in which a car stopped at a stop sign; some were later asked what the car did after it passed the yield sign. Compared with a control group that did not receive any misleading questions, participants in the misleading information group more often mistakenly claimed that they had seen a yield sign. Loftus et al. (1978) argued that misleading suggestions "overwrite" the original memory, but this interpretation has been convincingly challenged (e.g., Bekerian & Bowers, 1983; McCloskey & Zaragoza, 1985). Recent studies indicate that source misattributions—confusing whether target information had been previously perceived or only suggested—play an important role in misleading-information effects (e.g., Belli, Windschitl, McCarthy, & Winfrey, 1992; Lindsay, 1990; Zaragoza & Lane, 1994).

The work of Loftus et al. (1978) on misleading information was motivated initially by concerns about the potentially damaging effects of suggestion on eyewitness testimony. Wells and Bradfield (1998) have recently provided a dramatic example of a form of suggestion involving misleading feedback to eyewitnesses. In their experiments, participants viewed a videotape of a crime and were later asked to identify the gunman from a set of photos. The actual gunman was not present in the photos. After making their choice, some participants were given confirming feedback (i.e., they were told that they were correct), whereas others were given no feedback. All participants were later asked to remember various aspects of the crime. Compared with those given no feedback, participants who were given the confirming feedback indicated higher confidence and trust in their recollection, a clearer view of the gunman, and increased memory for facial details.

Suggestibility is also closely related to the controversy concerning false and recovered memories of childhood sexual abuse. Some of this work has been conducted with young children, inspired by concerns about suggestive procedures used in investigations of alleged abuses in day care settings (Ceci & Bruck, 1995). A growing body of evidence from controlled studies with preschoolers indicates that although their memories are often accurate, suggestive procedures can lead to the creation of subjectively compelling false recollections of autobiographical episodes in a substantial proportion of preschool children (for a review, see Ceci, 1995; Ceci & Bruck, 1995).

In studies of adults, the idea that many recovered memories are the products of suggestion during psychotherapy (e.g., Lindsay & Read, 1994; Loftus, 1993) has spurred controlled research investigating whether it is possible to implant false memories of entire autobiographical episodes by using various kinds of suggestive procedures. A number of studies using hypnosis have shown that sizeable proportions (e.g., 50%) of highly hypnotizable individuals will sometimes claim, following hypnotic suggestions, to remember such illusory events as hearing loud noises at night (e.g., Laurence & Perry, 1983). However, hypnotic "pseudomemories" of this kind are determined by a complex interaction of social, situational, and subject variables (for thorough reviews, see Lynn & Nash, 1994; McConkey, Barnier, & Sheehan, 1998) and may

have limited relevance to questions concerning false memory creation outside of the hypnotic context.

Loftus (1993, p. 532) described preliminary observations from what has since come to be known as the "lost in the mall" study. Loftus focused on the case of 14-year-old Chris, who had been asked by his older brother, Jim, to try to remember an event that, according to Jim and other family members, had never occurred: The time Chris had been lost in a shopping mall at age five. He initially recalled nothing, but after several days of attempted recall, Chris produced a detailed recollection of an event that had never occurred. Loftus and Pickrell (1995) reported a more extensive study of 24 participants who were asked to respond to descriptions by close relatives of four different events. Three of the events were actual episodes from the individual's past, and one was the "false episode" of being lost in a shopping mall or similar public place. Participants were given booklets containing the descriptions, were told to write down what they recalled from the event, and were also instructed that if they did not remember the event described they should indicate so. Two additional interviews were conduced to further probe participants' recall of both the true and false events. Results from the three sessions were highly consistent: Participants remembered some details from 68% of the true events in each session, whereas 29% (7 of 24) of the participants initially "recalled" something about the false event (25% of these participants recalled the false event in the two follow-up interviews).

Although these results indicate that false memories of being lost as a child are not unique to Chris, they do not address the generalizability of the phenomenon to other kinds of experiences. A series of experiments by Hyman and colleagues speaks to this issue (Hyman & Billings, 1998; Hyman, Husband, & Billings, 1995; Hyman & Pentland, 1996). They studied college undergraduates whose parents had agreed to complete a childhood events questionnaire. On the basis of parents' responses, Hyman and colleagues asked students about various childhood experiences that, according to their parents, had actually happened. In addition, however, they asked students about a false event that, parents confirmed, had never happened. For instance, Hyman and Pentland (1996) inquired about the following false event: "When you were 5 you were at the wedding reception of some friends of the family and you were running around with some other kids, when you bumped into the table and spilled the punch bowl on the parents of the bride" (p. 105).

Participants were asked about both true and false events in a series of interviews, usually separated from each other by one day. In general, participants accurately remembered 80–90% of the true events. During the initial interview, almost no participants reported any memory for the false events. However, depending on experimental conditions, approximately 20–40% of participants came to describe some memory of the false event in later interviews. For example, in an experiment by Hyman and Billings (1998), only 2 of 66 (3%) participants described any memory of the false event in an initial interview, whereas 18 of 66 (27%) did so in a second interview. Ten of these 18 participants reported "clear" false memories, which included specific details of the central event (e.g., spilling the punch), whereas eight participants reported "partial" false memories, which included some details but no specific memory of the central event.

Hyman and Billings (1998) also found that the tendency to report memories of the false events was positively correlated (.48) with scores on the Dissociative Experiences Scale (Bernstein & Putnam, 1986), which measures self-reported lapses in cognitive and memory functioning and was also positively correlated (.36) with scores on the Creative Imagination Scale (Wilson & Barber, 1978), which measures vividness of mental imagery. This latter finding is consistent with findings from Hyman and Pentland (1996), who manipulated mental imagery experimentally.

Participants who were assigned to the imagery condition were given instructions that when they failed to recall either a true or false event, they should try to form detailed images of the event. Participants in the control condition, by contrast, were instructed to sit quietly and think about the event. Participants in the imagery condition recalled more true events that they had initially failed to remember than did participants in the control condition. It is important, however, that mental imagery also produced a significant increase in memories of false events. By the third interview, 38% of participants in the imagery condition reported either a clear or partial false memory, compared with only 12% of participants in the control condition (for related evidence showing that mental imagery can contribute to false memories, see Garry et al., 1996; Goff & Roediger, 1998; Johnson et al., 1979).

Mazzoni and Loftus (1998) have recently described another kind of suggestive procedure that can produce false memories of life events—dream interpretation. Mazzoni and Loftus asked participants to indicate their confidence that various kinds of experiences had or had not ever happened to them. One group then participated in an ostensibly unrelated task 10–15 days later in which a clinical psychologist interpreted their dreams. The psychologist suggested to them that their dreams included repressed memories of events that had happened to them before the age of three—difficult experiences such as being abandoned by parents, getting lost in a public place, or being lonely and lost in an unfamiliar place. The participants had previously indicated on the life events inventory that such events had never happened to them. Nonetheless, when they completed the life events inventory again in an unrelated context 10–15 days later, the majority of these individuals now claimed to remember one or more of the three suggested experiences for which they had previously denied any memory. No such effects were observed in a control group that did not receive any suggestions regarding their dreams.

Overall, then, the studies of Loftus and Hyman and their colleagues (Hyman & Billings, 1998; Hyman et al., 1995; Hyman & Pentland, 1996; Loftus, 1993; Loftus & Pickrell, 1995; Mazzoni & Loftus, 1998) have established that it is possible to implant false memories of several different types of childhood experiences in a significant number of experimental participants. However, there may be limits to the kinds of memories that can be implanted in such studies. For example, Pezdek, Finger, and Hodge (1997) reported that whereas 15% of participants generated false recollections of being lost in a shopping mall, none generated false memories of a childhood rectal enema.

Although studies demonstrating false memories of everyday experiences are striking and important, they are characterized by a clear methodological limitation: Experimenters cannot determine definitively whether a target event actually occurred and, hence, whether and to what extent a particular memory is "true" or "false." Though not a trivial problem, this concern should not be overblown, for at least two reasons. First, reports of parents and other relatives provide reasonably convincing evidence that the kinds of highly salient target events used in these studies did or did not occur. Second, internal evidence from within an experiment, such as manipulations that increase or decrease the probability that false memories are reported, or individual-difference variables that correlate with the tendency to produce false memories, provide evidence consistent with the psychological reality of the effect.

A related domain in which suggestions contribute to the creation of false memories also has important social and legal consequences—false confessions. False confessions occur for numerous reasons (some having little to do with suggestibility and memory), but they occasionally are based on illusory recollections generated in response to highly suggestive interrogations from police (Gudjonsson, 1992; Kassin, 1997). Perhaps the best known case in recent years involved sheriff's deputy Paul Ingram, who was accused of raping his daughters and confessed to this abuse as well as to satanic rituals and murders. He later retracted the confession. No evidence for the rituals or murders was ever uncovered despite massive efforts by police, and the rape charges rested on the dubious recovered memories of his daughters (Wright, 1994).

Kassin and Kiechel (1996) have recently reported a compelling experimental analogue of false confession. Participants performed either a fast-paced or slow-paced reaction time task; all had been instructed not to press the "ALT" key because it would cause the program to crash. Although none of the participants actually hit the ALT key, the experimenter falsely accused them of doing so. After participants denied the charge, one group heard a confederate "witness" say that she saw the error; there was no witness for the other group. Overall, nearly 70% of the participants eventually signed a false confession that they had hit the ALT key. The effect was particularly pronounced in the witness–fast-paced group, where all participants signed the confession and 35% confabulated a detailed false recollection of how they made the error.

The foregoing studies clearly indicate that suggestions made at the time of memory retrieval can lead to the creation of false memories of autobiographical episodes. Perhaps it is surprising, however, that despite the theoretical and applied importance of suggestibility, cognitive neuroscience approaches have contributed little or nothing to understanding its nature and basis— or at least nothing beyond prior contributions to understanding related processes such as source misattributions. As seen in the preceding section, the cognitive neuroscience approach has begun to illuminate the neural correlates of misattributions underlying specific types of false-recall and false-recognition effects. It would therefore be desirable to carry out neuropsychological and neuroimaging studies that specifically examine forms of false-memory effects that fall under the rubric of suggestibility.

Bias

Memory encoding and retrieval are highly dependent on, and influenced by, preexisting knowledge and beliefs. Dating at least to the pioneering studies of Bartlett (1932), cognitive psychologists have known that memories can be influenced and even distorted by current knowledge, beliefs, and expectations (i.e., schemas; for a review, see Alba & Hasher, 1983). Likewise, memories of past experiences may be colored by present mood and emotional state (Bower, 1992; Ochsner & Schacter, in press). Bias refers to the distorting influences of present knowledge, beliefs, and feelings on recollection of previous experiences.

Biases of recollection have been observed in several domains (for reviews, see Dawes, 1988; M. Ross, 1989; M. Ross & Wilson, in press). A number of studies have provided evidence for the operation of a consistency bias in retrospection: People's recollections tend to exaggerate the consistency between their past and present attitudes, beliefs, and feelings. For instance, Marcus (1986) asked people in 1973 to rate their attitudes toward a variety of important social issues, including legalization of marijuana, equality of women, and aid to minorities. When asked to make the same rating again in 1982, and asked also to indicate what their attitudes had been in 1973, participants' recollections of their 1973 attitudes were more closely related to their 1982 attitudes than to what they had actually indicated in 1973. In a more recent study, Levine (1997) examined emotional reactions—hope, anger, and sadness—in supporters of candidate Ross Perot when he withdrew from the 1992 presidential campaign in July and after the election in November (following Perot's return to the campaign in early October). On this second assessment, Levine examined current feelings about Perot's candidacy and also asked the supporters to recall how they had initially felt about Perot's withdrawal in July. Although accurate in many respects, memory for past feelings was nonetheless influenced by current circumstances, show-

ing a strong consistency bias. Thus, "returning" supporters—those who initially switched their support to another candidate when Perot withdrew but later supported him again—recalled their initial reactions as less angry than they actually were. "Loyal" supporters—those who never wavered from Perot—underestimated how sad they felt when Perot withdrew. And "deserting" supporters—those who switched to another candidate and never returned—underestimated how sad and how hopeful they felt when Perot withdrew in July.

Consistency biases have also been observed in studies of memories of people involved in romantic relationships (for reviews, see Acitelli & Holmberg, 1993; Holmberg & Homes, 1994). In a study of dating couples, McFarland and Ross (1987) asked participants to evaluate themselves, their dating partner, and their relationship in an initial session and again in a second session conducted two months later. During the second session, participants were also asked to recall their earlier evaluation. McFarland and Ross found that participants whose evaluations of their partners became more negative over time recalled their initial evaluations as more negative than they actually were. In contrast, when participants reported liking or loving a partner more over time, they also tended to recall having felt more liking or loving in the past.

In a more recent study, Scharfe and Bartholomew (1998) reported similar evidence for consistency bias in a study of three kinds of couples involved in romantic relationships (i.e., dating, cohabitating, married). Each member of the couple completed a self-report attachment questionnaire in an initial session and again eight months later. During the second session, they were also asked to remember their initial attachment evaluations. Scharfe and Bartholomew (1998) found that most of the participants who inaccurately remembered their initial attachment evaluation erred by recalling their past assessment as more congruent with their present one (see also Kirkpatrick & Hazan, 1994). The consistency bias was observed in both men and women, although it was slightly more pronounced in men. Regression analyses revealed that for women, initial (past) attachment ratings accounted for about 34% of the variance in recall of those ratings, whereas present attachment ratings contributed an additional 24% of the variance. For men, past attachment ratings contributed 23% of the variance, and present attachment ratings contributed an additional 32% of the variance. Overall, then, present attachment ratings accounted for about as much of the variance in recall as did past attachment ratings.

M. Ross (1989) has argued that the specific form that retrospective bias assumes is influenced by individuals' implicit theories of whether or not they have changed over time with respect to what they are asked to remember. When individuals believe it is likely that they have been stable over time, they will tend to overestimate the consistency between past attitudes and current ones. In the foregoing examples of consistency bias, people had no particular reason to believe that their attitudes or feelings had changed over time and, hence, they relied on their current attitudes and feelings to guide reconstruction of past events. By contrast, when individuals have reason to believe that they have changed over time, they may be biased to overestimate differences between current and past attitudes. For example, Conway and Ross (1984) attempted to invoke expectancy for change by assigning a group of participants to a study-skills training group. Participants in this group diligently worked at enhancing their study skills in order to improve their grades. A second group was assigned to a waiting list control condition. When asked to remember their initial skill level, participants in the study skills group exaggerated how poor their study skills had been prior to training (compared with the assessments they had provided at the time). No such bias was observed in the control group.

In the foregoing studies, retrospective bias was observed when people attempted to recall very general features of past beliefs, attitudes, and feelings. However, similar effects have been documented when people are asked to remember specific incidents. For example, Spiro (1980) instructed participants to read a story about a man, Bob, who dearly wanted to marry his girlfriend, Margie. However, he did not want to have children and was anxious about how Margie would react to this disclosure. In one version of the story, Margie was thrilled to hear that Bob wished to remain childless because this fit well with her career plans; in another version she was horrified because she desperately wanted children. After reading the story, some participants in each condition were informed either that Bob and Margie married or that they ended their relationship. When later asked to recall the story, memory biases were observed, but only in those participants who were given poststory information that was incongruent with what they would have expected to happen, based on general knowledge of relationships. Thus, participants who read that Margie was horrified, and then learned that Bob and Margie married, incorrectly recalled various incidents that helped to explain why this would be so. For instance, one participant recalled incorrectly that "they separated but realized after discussing the matter that their love mattered more," and another misremembered that "they discussed it and decided that they could agree on a compromise: adoption." By contrast, participants who read that Margie was thrilled, and later were told that the couple split, incorrectly recalled such incidents as "there was a hassle with one or the other's parents" or that "they disagreed about having children." The fact that no such errors were made by participants who read that Margie was horrified and the couple split, or read that Margie was thrilled and that the couple married, indicates that preexisting knowledge and beliefs influenced memory retrieval only when the conclusion of the story violated schema-based expectancies.

The studies reviewed here indicate that retrospective biases have been well-established in studies by cognitive and social psychologists. Despite the pervasiveness of the phenomenon, however, it remains largely unexplored from a cognitive neuroscience perspective: I am not aware of any neuropsychological or neuro-imaging studies that have specifically examined recollective biases of the kind reviewed in this section.

Bias may also take the form of subtle influences of past experiences on current judgments about other people and groups. These kinds of biases are well-illustrated by recent studies in implicit social cognition, where various kinds of gender, racial, and related biases have been revealed by indirect or implicit tests of social judgments and beliefs (see Greenwald & Banaji, 1995). Consider, for instance, an experiment that used the previously discussed false fame paradigm (Jacoby, Kelley, Brown, et al., 1989). Banaji and Greenwald (1995) exposed participants to famous and nonfamous male and female names. On a later fame judgment task, participants were more likely to make "false fame" errors—judge incorrectly that a previously studied nonfamous name is famous—for male than for female names. Walsh, Banaji, and Greenwald (cited in Banaji & Bhaskar, in press) reported a related racial biasing effect of past experiences. Participants were shown lists of male names that were either European American (e.g., Adam Mc-Carthy) or African American (e.g., Tyrone Washington) and were asked to indicate which were the names of criminals (they were told that the names might seem familiar because they had appeared in the media). None of the individuals were in fact criminals, but across a series of experiments participants "recognized" significantly more Black than White names as those of criminals. Participants claimed that they were basing their judgments on memory and not race, but the results clearly revealed a nonconscious biasing effect of prior knowledge and experience.

As with retrospective biases, the biases revealed in studies of implicit social cognition remain unexplored from a cognitive neuroscience perspective. However, a possible model for the investigation of such biases may be provided by the numerous neuropsychological and neuro-imaging studies that have explored aspects of nonconscious or implicit memory (for recent reviews, see Schacter & Buckner, 1998; Wiggs & Martin, 1998). The wealth of data from cognitive neuroscience studies of implicit memory could provide a useful foundation for studies of bias in implicit social cognition.

Persistence

The first three of memory's sins—transience, absent-mindedness, and blocking—all entail forgetting a fact or event that one wants to remember. The final sin—persistence—involves remembering a fact or event that one would prefer to forget. Persistence is revealed by intrusive recollections of traumatic events, rumination over negative symptoms and events, and even by chronic fears and phobias.

Studies of traumatic memories reveal that failures to forget can sometimes be even more disabling than forgetting itself. Traumatic events are typically remembered repetitively and intrusively (e.g., Herman, 1992; Krystal, Southwick, & Charney, 1995). Although traumatized individuals may engage in a variety of strategies to avoid or suppress unwanted recollections, such strategies often have little or no impact on the frequency and vividness of intrusive memories (for a review, see Koutstaal & Schacter, 1997c). Relevant experimental evidence has been provided by McNally, Metzger, Lasko, Clancy, and Pitman (1998), who examined "directed forgetting" of traumatic and nontraumatic words in women with post-traumatic stress disorder (PTSD) resulting from documented sexual abuse and matched controls who had a sexual abuse history but no PTSD. In directed-forgetting procedures, individuals are instructed to try to remember some target items and to forget others. Control participants remembered fewer of the trauma-related words they had been instructed to forget than those they had been instructed to remember. However, the trauma patients showed no such directed-forgetting effect, indicating a loss of cognitive control over the encoding and retrieval of trauma-related content.

Persistence also occurs in less extreme situations than PTSD. Disturbing emotional events that are not necessarily traumatic, such as pictures that elicit negative affect, are sometimes remembered in greater detail than are positive pictures (see Ochsner & Schacter, in press). Studies by Wegner and associates have shown that instructing people not to think about a particular item or object (e.g., don't think about white bears) can produce a rebound effect. The initially suppressed item is subsequently produced at higher levels than are items for which no suppression instructions were given (e.g., Wegner & Erber, 1992).

Persistence can be influenced by aspects of current mood and emotion. Just as current feelings can distort recollections of past emotions, they can also increase the accessibility of memories whose affective tone is congruent with a current mood state (Bower, 1992; Mineka & Nugent, 1995). For example, a variety of studies have shown that depressed individuals tend to show increased memory for negative autobiographical events and experimentally presented items compared with positive events and items (for a review, see Mineka & Nugent, 1995). In the present terminology, such effects may reflect an interaction between persistence and bias. Similar considerations apply to phenomena of rumination and regret, in which individuals dwell on current and past events related to current negative mood states, generating alternative or counterfactual scenarios of what might have been (e.g., Gilovich & Medvec, 1995; Roese, 1994). Excessive rumination over depressive symptoms is associated with, and can contribute to, increased duration of depressive episodes (Nolen-Hoeksema, 1991).

Recent evidence indicates that the persistence of negative memories can be enhanced by ruminative tendencies in individuals with dysphoric moods. Lyubomirsky, Caldwell, and Nolen-Hoeksema (1998) examined recall of autobiographical memories in college students experiencing depressed and nondepressed moods. Participants engaged in a rumination task that required them to focus on self and mood (i.e., current energy level, why they turned out this way, and so forth) or they performed a distraction task that turned attention away from self and mood (e.g., thinking about the face of the Mona Lisa, clouds forming in the sky). Participants then engaged in an autobiographical memory task that required recall of specific events from their pasts. In each of four experiments using different variants of the autobiographical memory task, the rumination task resulted in increased access to negative autobiographical memories for students experiencing depressed mood, but not for students experiencing a positive mood.

Related processes occur in cases of suicidal depression. Studies by Williams and colleagues (for a review, see Williams, 1997) have shown that depressed individuals are often plagued by the persistence of "overgeneral" memories that represent the past in a nonspecific and highly negative manner. These persisting overgeneral memories can be amplified by and also contribute to depressed mood, leading to a downward spiral that may culminate in suicide.

Cognitive neuroscience analyses have increased our understanding of persistence by illuminating neurobiological factors that contribute to enduring emotional memories. A good deal of this research has followed from animal studies showing that persisting emotional memories (especially fear) depend to a large extent on a specific structure in the limbic system (the amygdala) and are promoted by a particular type of modulatory influence (stress hormones; Cahill & McGaugh, 1998; LeDoux, 1996). During the past few years, converging evidence from neuroimaging, pharmacological, and neuropsychological studies has revealed a similar picture in humans. For example, Cahill et al. (1996) carried out two PET scans: One while participants viewed emotional films and the other while participants viewed nonemotional films. Amygdala activity during viewing of the emotional films was remarkably highly correlated (.93) with subsequent recall of the emotional films three weeks later. No such correlation was observed for the nonemotional films.

Convergent with this result, studies of patients with selective damage to the amygdala have examined recall of emotional and nonemotional information about recently presented stories. Amygdala damage was associated with specific impairments in recalling emotional elements of stories, together with normal retention of nonemotional information (Cahill, Babinsky, Markowitsch, & McGaugh, 1995). Drug studies suggest that release of stress hormones that influence activity within the amygdala contribute importantly to persisting emotional memories. For example, based on prior animal studies showing that administration of beta-adrenergic antagonists ("beta blockers") interfere with the influence of stress-related hormones, Cahill, Prins, Weber, and McGaugh (1994) examined whether administration of a beta blocker (propranolol) would interfere with emotional memory. Consistent with this hypothesis, Cahill et al. (1994) found that propranolol interfered with retention of emotional but not nonemotional aspects of a story (for further review and discussion, see Cahill & McGaugh, 1998; LeDoux, 1996; Ochsner & Schacter, in press).

Conditioning studies in experimental animals have highlighted the persisting quality of certain kinds of emotional memories. For example, conditioned fear responses that depend on the amygdala, once acquired, may be resistant to erasure over time and thus are in some sense indelible (LeDoux, Romanski, & Xagoraris, 1989). In a study using brain-damaged patients, Bechara et al. (1995) reported that amygdala damage interferes with the acquisition of conditioned fear, whereas hippocampal damage does not. These kinds of persisting influences have been

implicated in the development and maintenance of powerful and sometimes disabling fears and phobias (e.g., Jacobs & Nadel, 1985). Recent PET studies of patients with PTSD have revealed activation in a variety of brain regions previously implicated in fear and anxiety, including the amygdala, when patients recall the traumatic experiences that in everyday life come to mind persistently and intrusively (e.g., Rauch et al., 1996; Shin et al., 1997).

The Seven Sins: Costs of an Adaptive System?

Considering together the seven sins of memory could easily lead one to question the wisdom of Mother Nature in building such a seemingly flawed system: It is sobering—and perhaps even depressing—to contemplate all the ways in which memory can land us in trouble. J. R. Anderson and Milson (1989) summarized the prevailing perception that memory's sins reflect poorly on its fundamental design:

Human memory is typically viewed by lay people as quite a defective system. For instance, over the years we have participated in many talks with artificial intelligence researchers about the prospects of using human models to guide the development of artificial intelligence programs. Invariably, the remark is made, "Well, of course, we would not want our system to have something so unreliable as human memory." (p. 703)

Bjork and Bjork (1988) have noted that a similar view prevails among memory researchers: "According to the modal view of human memory among today's theorists, loss of retrieval access is a central weakness of the system" (p. 283).

As tempting as such views may be, I suggest that it is a mistake to view the seven sins as flaws in system design that ought to have been corrected during the course of evolution. Instead, building on the analyses of J. R. Anderson and Bjork and their colleagues, the seven sins can be usefully viewed as by-products of otherwise adaptive features of memory. Bjork (Bjork, 1989;

Bjork & Bjork, 1988) and J. R. Anderson and colleagues (J. R. Anderson, 1990; J. R. Anderson & Milson, 1989; J. R. Anderson & Schooler, 1991; L. Schooler & Anderson, 1997) have already applied this idea to transience (i.e., forgetting over time). Thus, in their discussion of adaptive forgetting, Bjork and Bjork (1988) emphasized that it is often useful and even necessary to forget information that is no longer current, such as old phone numbers or where we parked the car yesterday. Information that is no longer needed will tend not to be retrieved and rehearsed, thereby losing out on the strengthening effects of postevent retrieval and becoming gradually less accessible over time. J. R. Anderson and Schooler (1991; L. Schooler & Anderson, 1997) have argued that forgetting over time reflects an adaptation to the structure of the environment. By their view, an adapted system retains the kind of information that is most likely to be needed in the environment in which the system operates. L. Schooler and Anderson (1997) argued that "memory's sensitivity to statistical structure in the environment allows it to optimally estimate the odds that a memory trace will be needed" (p. 219). To support this claim, they provided evidence consistent with the idea that traces of more recent and more frequently retrieved events are more likely to be needed than are traces of less recent and less frequently retrieved events. Thus, a system that exhibits gradual forgetting of the kind documented for human memory is adapted to the demands of its informational environment (for extension of this notion to animal memory, see Kraemer & Golding, 1997).

A similar analysis can be applied to blocking. As noted earlier, blocking reflects the operation of inhibitory processes in memory. Consider what might result without the operation of inhibition: A system in which all information that is potentially relevant to a retrieval cue invariably and rapidly springs to mind (Bjork, 1989). Although such a system might be free of the occasionally annoying episodes of blocking that plague hu-

man rememberers, it would likely result in mass confusion produced by an incessant coming to mind of numerous competing traces.

The third of the forgetting-related sins—absent-mindedness—involves similar considerations on the "front end" of memory. Absent-minded errors occur in part because establishment of a rich memory representation that can later be recollected voluntarily requires attentive, elaborate encoding; events that receive minimal attention have little chance of being recollected subsequently. But what if all events were registered in elaborate detail, regardless of the level or type of processing to which they were subjected? The result would be a potentially overwhelming clutter of useless details, as happened in the famous case of Shere-shevski, the mnemonist studied by Luria (1968). Shereshevski was unable to function at an abstract level because he was inundated with unimportant details of his experiences—details that are best denied entry to the system in the first place. An elaboration-dependent system ensures that only those events that are important enough to warrant extensive encoding have a high likelihood of subsequent recollection. Such a system allows us to enjoy the considerable benefits of operating on "automatic pilot," without having memory cluttered by unnecessary information about routine activities.

Similar ideas can be applied to the three sins that involve distortion of prior experiences: misattribution, suggestibility, and bias. These sins are rooted, to a large extent, in three fundamental features of memory. First, many instances of misattribution, and at least some instances of suggestibility, reflect poor memory for the source of an experience—the precise details of who told us a particular fact, where we saw a familiar face, or whether we witnessed an event ourselves or only heard about it later. When such details are not initially well-encoded, or become inaccessible over time, individuals become quite vulnerable to making the kinds of misattributions associated with false recognition or cryptomnesia, and may also be vulnerable to incorporating postevent suggestions regarding the nature of specific details that are remembered only vaguely. But what would be the consequences and costs of retaining the myriad of contextual details that define our numerous daily experiences? Consider again J. R. Anderson and Schooler's (1991) notion that memory is adapted to retain information that is most likely to be needed in the environment in which it operates. How often do we need to remember all the precise, source-specifying details of our experiences? Would an adapted system routinely record all such details as a default option, or would it record such details only when circumstances dictate?

A second and related factor that contributes to misattributions involving false recall and recognition concerns the distinction between memory for gist and verbatim or specific information (Reyna & Brainerd, 1995). False recall and recognition often occur when people remember the semantic or perceptual gist of an experience but do not recall specific details. However, memory for gist may also be fundamental to such abilities as categorization and comprehension and may facilitate the development of transfer and generalization across tasks. In a neural network analysis of memory distortions, McClelland (1995, p. 84) noted that generalization often results from gist-like, accumulated effects of prior experiences. Noting that such generalization "is central to our ability to act intelligently" and constitutes a foundation for cognitive development, McClelland further observed that "such generalization gives rise to distortions as an inherent by-product."

A third factor that is particularly relevant to many instances of bias concerns the influences of preexisting knowledge and schemas. Although they can sometimes contribute to distorted recollections of past events, schemas also perform important organizing functions in our cognitive lives (Mandler, 1979). Schemas are especially important in guiding memory retrieval, promoting memory for schema-relevant information,

and allowing us to develop accurate expectations of events that are likely to unfold in familiar settings on the basis of past experiences in those settings (Alba & Hasher, 1983). In a somewhat different vein, as discussed earlier, retrospective biases frequently involve memory distortions that exaggerate consistency or change between present and past attitudes and beliefs. M. Ross and Wilson (in press) have argued that such distortions often serve to enhance appraisals of one's current self and thus in some sense contribute to life satisfaction (see also Singer & Salovey, 1993; Strack, Schwarz, & Gschneidinger, 1985; Taylor, 1991).

Of all the seven sins, it is perhaps easiest to see the positive or adaptive side of persistence. Although intrusive recollections of trauma can be disabling, it is critically important that emotionally arousing experiences, which may occur in response to dangers that can be life threatening, persist over time and provide a basis for long-lasting memories (cf. LeDoux, 1996; McGaugh, 1995). The fact that the amygdala and related structures help to increase the persistence of such experiences by modulating memory formation may sometimes result in memories we wish we could forget. But it also provides us with a mechanism that increases the likelihood that we will retain information about arousing or traumatic events whose recollection may be crucial for survival.

The idea that the seven sins of memory are by-products of otherwise adaptive features of memory requires some cautions and clarifications. As noted recently by Buss, Haselton, Shackelford, Bleske, and Wakefield (1998), psychologists use the term "adaptation" or "adaptive features" in at least two different ways. One comes from evolutionary theory and involves a highly specific, technical definition of an adaptation as a feature of a species that came into existence through the operation of natural selection because it in some way increased reproductive fitness. The other is a more colloquial, nontechnical sense of the term that refers to a feature of an organism that has generally beneficial consequences, whether or not it arose directly in response to natural selection during the course of evolution. As discussed by Buss et al. (1998), many generally useful or "adaptive" features of humans and other animals are not, strictly speaking, adaptations. Sometimes termed "exaptations" (Gould & Vrba, 1982), these useful functions arise as a consequence of other related features that are adaptations in the technical sense. Such adaptations are sometimes co-opted to perform functions other than the one for which they were originally selected. In an evolutionary analysis of memory systems, Sherry and Schacter (1987) emphasized the possible role of exaptations in human memory:

few of the current functions that memory serves can be genuine adaptations of memory. Human memory is clearly not an adaptation for remembering telephone numbers, though it performs these functions fairly well, nor is it an adaptation for learning to drive a car, though it handles this rather different function effectively, too. The ideal of exaptation emphasizes the difference between the current functions memory systems perform and their evolutionary histories. (p. 449)

In view of these considerations, we must be cautious about making any strong claims for the evolutionary status of the adaptive features of memory considered here; they might be adaptations, exaptations, or both. As far as the seven sins go, it seems possible that some are genuine adaptations, whereas others are clearly by-products of adaptations or exaptations. For example, J. R. Anderson and colleagues' analysis of forgetting (J. R. Anderson, 1990; J. R. Anderson & Milson, 1989; J. R. Anderson & Schooler, 1991; L. Schooler & Anderson, 1997) would lead us to view transience as a genuine adaptation to the structure of the environment. By contrast, misattributions involved in source memory confusions are clearly not adaptations, but are more likely by-products of adaptations and exaptations that have yielded a memory system that does not routinely preserve all the details required to specify the exact source of an experi-

ence. Similarly, false recall and recognition may be by-products of gist-based memory processes that themselves could have arisen either as adaptations or exaptations.

These kinds of by-products resemble what Gould and Lewontin (1979) called "spandrels." A spandrel is a type of exaptation that is a side consequence of a particular function. The term spandrel is used in architecture to designate the leftover spaces between structural elements in a building. As an example, Gould and Lewontin described the four spandrels in the central dome of Venice's Cathedral of San Marco: leftover spaces between arches and walls that were subsequently decorated with four evangelists and four Biblical rivers. The spandrels were not built in order to house these paintings, although they do so very well (for further discussion of spandrels, see Buss et al., 1998; Gould, 1991). Architectural spandrels generally have benign consequences. Perhaps some of the seven sins discussed here can be thought of as spandrels gone awry—side consequences of a generally adaptive architecture that sometimes get us into trouble. Future research in psychology and cognitive neuroscience that incorporates an evolutionary perspective should help to increase our understanding of the nature and source of the seven sins of memory.

Note

Preparation of this article was supported by grants from the National Institute on Aging, National Institute of Mental Health, and Human Frontiers Science Program. I thank Wilma Koutstaal, Susan McGlynn, and Anthony Wagner for useful comments and discussion, and I thank Sara Greene and Carrie Racine for help with preparation of the article.

References

Acitelli, L. K., & Holmberg, D. (1993). Reflecting on relationships: The role of thoughts and memories. *Advances in Personal Relationships*, 4, 71–100.

Alba, J. W., & Hasher, L. (1983). Is memory schematic? *Psychological Bulletin,* 93, 203–231.

Anderson, J. R. (1990). *The adaptive character of thought.* Hillsdale, NJ: Erlbaum.

Anderson, J. R., & Milson, R. (1989). Human memory: An adaptive perspective. *Psychological Review,* 96, 703–719.

Anderson, J. R., & Schooler, L. J. (1991). Reflections of the environment in memory. *Psychological Science,* 2, 396–408.

Anderson, M. C., Bjork, R. A., & Bjork, E. L. (1994). Remembering can cause forgetting: Retrieval dynamics in long-term memory. *Journal of Experimental Psychology: Learning, Memory, and Cognition,* 20, 1063–1087.

Anderson, M. C., & Spellman, B. A. (1995). On the status of inhibitory mechanisms in cognition: Memory retrieval as a model case. *Psychological Review,* 102, 68–100.

Awh, E., & Jonides, J. (1998). Spatial working memory and spatial selective attention. In R. Parasuraman (Ed.), *The attentive brain* (pp. 353–380). Cambridge, MA: MIT Press.

Baddeley, A. D. (1986). *Working memory.* Oxford, England: Clarendon Press.

Baddeley, A. D., Gathercole, S., & Papagano, C. (1998). The phonological loop as a language learning device. *Psychological Review,* 105, 158–173.

Bailey, C. H., & Chen, M. (1989). Time course of structural changes at identified sensory neuron synapses during long-term sensitization in aplysia. *Journal of Neuroscience,* 9, 1774–1781.

Balota, D., Cortese, M. J., Duchek, J. M., Adama, D., Roediger, H. L., III, McDermott, K. B., & Yerys, B. E. (in press). Veridical and false memories in healthy older adults and in dementia of the Alzheimer's type. *Cognitive Neuropsychology.*

Banaji, M. R., & Bhaskar, R. (in press). Implicit stereotypes and memory: The bounded rationality of social beliefs. In D. L. Schacter & E. Scarry (Eds.), *Memory, brain, & belief.* Cambridge, MA: Harvard University Press.

Banaji, M. R., & Greenwald, A. G. (1995). Implicit gender stereotyping in judgments of fame. *Journal of Personality and Social Psychology,* 68, 181–198.

Bartlett, F. C. (1932). *Remembering.* Cambridge, England: Cambridge University Press.

Bechara, A., Tranel, D., Damasio, H., Adolphs, R., Rockland, C., & Damasio, A. R. (1995, November 17). Double dissociation of conditioning and declarative knowledge relative to the amygdala and hippocampus in humans. *Science,* 269, 1115–1118.

Bekerian, D. A., & Bowers, J. M. (1983). Eyewitness testimony: Were we misled? *Journal of Experimental Psychology: Human Learning and Memory,* 9, 139–145.

Belli, R. F., Windschitl, P. D., McCarthy, T. T., & Winfrey, S. E. (1992). Detecting memory impairment with a modified test procedure: Manipulating retention interval with centrally presented event items. *Journal of Experimental Psychology: Learning, Memory, & Cognition,* 18, 356–367.

Bernstein, E. M., & Putnam, F. W. (1986). Development, reliability, and validity of a dissociation scale. *Journal of Nervous and Mental Disease,* 174, 727–735.

Bjork, R. A. (1988). Retrieval practice and the maintenance of knowledge. In M. M. Gruneberg, P. E. Morris, & R. N. Sykes (Eds.), *Practical aspects of memory: Current research and issues* (Vol. 1, pp. 396–401). Chichester, England: Wiley.

Bjork, R. A. (1989). Retrieval inhibition as an adaptive mechanism in human memory. In H. L. Roediger, III, & F. I. M. Craik (Eds.), *Varieties of memory and consciousness* (pp. 309–330). Hillsdale, NJ: Erlbaum.

Bjork, R. A., & Bjork, E. L. (1988). On the adaptive aspects of retrieval failure in autobiographical memory. In M. M. Gruneberg, P. E. Morris, & R. N. Sykes (Eds.), *Practical aspects of memory: Current research and issues* (Vol. 1, pp. 283–288). Chichester, England: Wiley.

Bower, G. H. (1992). How might emotions affect learning? In S.-Å. Christianson (Ed.), *The handbook of emotion and memory: Research and theory* (pp. 3–31). Hillsdale, NJ: Erlbaum.

Brandimonte, M., Einstein, G. O., & McDaniel, M. A. (Eds.). (1996). *Prospective memory: Theory and applications.* Mahwah, NJ: Erlbaum.

Bransford, J. D., & Franks, J. J. (1971). The abstraction of linguistic ideas. *Cognitive Psychology,* 2, 331–350.

Brewer, J. B., Zhao, Z., Desmond, J. E., Glover, G. H., & Gabrieli, J. D. E. (1998, August 21). Making memories: Brain activity that predicts whether visual experiences will be remembered or forgotten. *Science,* 281, 1185–1187.

Brown, A. S. (1991). A review of the tip-of-the-tongue experience. *Psychological Bulletin,* 109, 204–223.

Brown, A. S., & Murphy, D. R. (1989). Cryptomnesia: Delineating inadvertent plagiarism. *Journal of Experimental Psychology: Learning, Memory, and Cognition,* 15, 432–442.

Brown, A. S., & Nix, L. A. (1996). Age-related changes in the tip-of-the-tongue experience. *American Journal of Psychology,* 109, 79–91.

Brown, J. (1958). Some tests of the decay theory of immediate memory. *Quarterly Journal of Experimental Psychology,* 10, 12–21.

Brown, R., & McNeill, D. (1966). The "tip-of-the-tongue" phenomenon. *Journal of Verbal Learning and Verbal Behavior,* 5, 325–337.

Buckner, R. L., & Koutstaal, W. (1998). Functional neuroimaging studies of encoding, priming, and explicit memory retrieval. *Proceedings of the National Academy of Sciences,* 95, 891–898.

Burke, D., MacKay, D. J., Worthley, J. S., & Wade, E. (1991). On the tip of the tongue: What causes word failure in young and older adults? *Journal of Memory and Language,* 30, 237–246.

Buss, D. M., Haselton, M. G., Shackelford, T. K., Bleske, A. L., & Wakefield, J. C. (1998). Adaptations, exaptations, and spandrels. *American Psychologist,* 53, 533–548.

Cabeza, R., & Nyberg, L. (1997). Imaging cognition: An empirical review of PET studies with normal subjects. *Journal of Cognitive Neuroscience,* 9, 1–26.

Cahill, L., Babinsky, R., Markowitsch, H. J., & McGaugh, J. L. (1995). The amygdala and emotional memory. *Nature,* 377, 295–296.

Cahill, L., Haier, R., Fallon, J., Alkire, M., Tang, C., Keator, D., Wu, J., & McGaugh, J. L. (1996). Amygdala activity at encoding correlated with long-term, free recall of emotional information. *Proceedings of the National Academy of Sciences,* 93, 8016–8021.

Cahill, L., & McGaugh, J. L. (1998). Mechanisms of emotional arousal and lasting declarative memory. *Trends in Neurosciences,* 21, 294–299.

Cahill, L., Prins, B., Weber, M., & McGaugh, J. L. (1994). B-Adrenergic activation and memory for emotional events. *Nature,* 371, 702–704.

Ceci, S. J. (1995). False beliefs: Some developmental and clinical considerations. In D. L. Schacter (Ed.), *Memory distortion: How minds, brains, and societies reconstruct the past* (pp. 91–128). Cambridge, MA: Harvard University Press.

Ceci, S. J., & Bruck, M. (1995). *Jeopardy in the courtroom.* Washington, DC: American Psychological Association.

Cockburn, J. (1995). Task interruption in prospective memory: A frontal lobe function? *Memory,* 31, 87–97.

Cohen, G. (1989). *Memory in the real world.* London: Erlbaum.

Cohen, G., & Burke, D. (1993). A review of memory for proper names. *Memory,* 1, 249–264.

Conway, M. A. (Ed.). (1997). *Recovered memories and false memories.* Oxford, England: Oxford University Press.

Conway, M. A., & Ross, M. (1984). Getting what you want by revising what you had. *Journal of Personality and Social Psychology,* 39, 406–415.

Cowley, G., & Underwood, A. (1998, June 15). Memory. *Newsweek,* 49–54.

Craik, F. I. M., Govoni, R., Naveh-Benjamin, M., & Anderson, N. D. (1996). The effects of divided attention on encoding and retrieval processes in human memory. *Journal of Experimental Psychology: General,* 125, 159–180.

Craik, F. I. M., & Lockhart, R. S. (1972). Levels of processing: A framework for memory research. *Journal of Verbal Learning and Verbal Behavior,* 11, 671–684.

Craik, F. I. M., & Tulving, E. (1975). Depth of processing and the retention of words in episodic memory. *Journal of Experimental Psychology: General,* 104, 268–294.

Crook, T. H., & Adderly, B. (1998). *The memory cure.* New York: Simon & Schuster.

Crowder, R. G. (1989). Modularity and dissociations in memory systems. In H. L. Roediger, III & F. I. M. Craik (Eds.), *Varieties of memory and consciousness: Essays in honor of Endel Tulving* (pp. 271–294). Hillsdale, NJ: Erlbaum.

Dale, A. M., & Buckner, R. L. (1997). Selective averaging of rapidly presented individual trials using fMRI. *Human Brain Mapping,* 5, 329–340.

Damasio, H., Grabowski, T. J., Tranel, D., Hichwa, R. D., & Damasio, A. R. (1996). A neural basis for lexical retrieval. *Nature,* 380, 499–505.

Dawes, R. (1988). *Rational choice in an uncertain world.* San Diego, CA: Harcourt, Brace, Jovanovich.

Deese, J. (1959). On the prediction of occurrence of particular verbal intrusions in immediate recall. *Journal of Experimental Psychology, 58,* 17–22.

Demb, J. B., Desmond, J. E., Wagner, A. D., Vaidya, C. J., Glover, G. H., & Gabrieli, J. D. E. (1995). Semantic encoding and retrieval in the left inferior prefrontal cortex: A functional MRI study of task difficulty and process specificity. *Journal of Neuroscience, 15,* 5870–5878.

Dywan, J., & Jacoby, L. L. (1990). Effects of aging on source monitoring: Differences in susceptibility to false fame. *Psychology and Aging, 3,* 379–387.

Ebbinghaus, H. (1885). *Über das Gedächtnis [Memory].* Leipzig, Germany: Duncker and Humblot.

Einstein, G. O., & McDaniel, M. A. (1996). Retrieval processes in prospective memory: Theoretical approaches and some new empirical findings. In M. Brandimonte, G. O. Einstein, & M. A. McDaniel (Eds.), *Prospective memory: Theory and applications* (pp. 115–142). Mahwah, NJ: Erlbaum.

Estes, W. K. (1997). Processes of memory loss, recovery, and distortion. *Psychological Review, 104,* 148–169.

Freyd, J. J. (1996). *Betrayal trauma: The logic of forgetting childhood abuse.* Cambridge, MA: Harvard University Press.

Gabrieli, J. D. E. (1998). Cognitive neuroscience of human memory. *Annual Review of Psychology, 49,* 87–115.

Gallo, D. A., Roberts, M. J., & Seamon, J. G. (1997). Remembering words not presented in lists: Can we avoid creating false memories? *Psychonomic Bulletin & Review, 4,* 271–276.

Gardiner, J. M., & Java, R. I. (1993). Recognizing and remembering. In A. F. Collins, S. E. Gathercole, M. A. Conway, & P. E. Morris (Eds.), *Theories of memory* (pp. 163–188). Hove, England: Erlbaum.

Garry, M., Manning, C., Loftus, E. F., & Sherman, S. J. (1996). Imagination inflation: Imagining a childhood event inflates confidence that it occurred. *Psychonomic Bulletin & Review, 3,* 208–214.

Gathercole, S. E., & Baddeley, A. D. (1994). *Working memory and language.* East Sussex, England: Erlbaum.

Gazzaniga, M. (Ed.). (1995). *The cognitive neurosciences.* Cambridge, MA: MIT Press.

Gilovich, T., & Medvec, V. (1995). The experience of regret: What, when, and why. *Psychological Review, 102,* 379–395.

Goff, L., & Roediger, H. L., III. (1998). Imagination inflation for action events: Repeated imaginings lead to illusory recollections. *Memory & Cognition, 26,* 20–33.

Gould, S. J. (1991). Exaptation: A crucial tool for evolutionary psychology. *Journal of Social Issues, 47,* 43–65.

Gould, S. J., & Lewontin, R. C. (1979). The spandrels of San Marco and the Panglossian paradigm: A critique of the adaptationist programme. *Proceedings of the Royal Society of London: Series B, 205,* 581–598.

Gould, S. J., & Vrba, E. S. (1982). Exaptation: A missing term in the science of form. *Paleobiology, 8,* 4–15.

Greenwald, A. G., & Banaji, M. R. (1995). Implicit social cognition: Attitudes, self-esteem, and stereotypes. *Psychological Review, 102,* 4–27.

Gudjonsson, G. H. (1992). *The psychology of interrogations, confessions and testimony.* New York: Wiley.

Hanley, J. R., & Kay, J. (1998). Proper name anomia and anomia for the names of people: Functionally dissociable impairments? *Cortex, 34,* 155–158.

Harley, T. A., & Brown, H. E. (1998). What causes the tip-of-the-tongue state? Evidence for lexical neighbourhood effects in speech production. *British Journal of Psychology, 89,* 151–174.

Herman, J. L. (1992). *Trauma and recovery.* New York: Basic Books.

Hintzman, D. L. (1988). Judgments of frequency and recognition memory in a multiple-trace memory model. *Psychological Review, 95,* 528–551.

Holmberg, D., & Homes, J. G. (1994). Reconstruction of relationship memories: A mental models approach. In N. Schwarz & S. Sudman (Eds.), *Autobiographical memory and the validity of retrospective reports* (pp. 267–288). New York: Springer-Verlag.

Hyman, I. E., & Billings, F. J. (1998). Individual differences and the creation of false childhood memories. *Memory, 6,* 1–20.

Hyman, I. E., Husband, T. H., & Billings, F. J. (1995). False memories of childhood experiences. *Applied Cognitive Psychology, 9,* 181–197.

Hyman, I. E., Jr., & Pentland, J. (1996). The role of mental imagery in the creation of false childhood memories. *Journal of Memory and Language, 35,* 101–117.

Israel, L., & Schacter, D. L. (1997). Pictorial encoding reduces false recognition of semantic associates. *Psychonomic Bulletin & Review*, 4, 577–581.

Jacobs, W. J., & Nadel, L. (1985). Stress-induced recovery of fears and phobias. *Psychological Review*, 92, 512–531.

Jacoby, L. L., Kelley, C. M., Brown, J., & Jasechko, J. (1989). Becoming famous overnight: Limits on the ability to avoid unconscious influences of the past. *Journal of Personality and Social Psychology*, 56, 326–338.

Jacoby, L. L., Kelley, C. M., & Dywan, J. (1989). Memory attributions. In H. L. Roediger, III & F. I. M. Craik (Eds.), *Varieties of memory and consciousness: Essays in honour of Endel Tulving* (pp. 391–422). Hillsdale, NJ: Erlbaum.

Janowsky, J. S., Shimamura, A. P., & Squire, L. R. (1989). Source memory impairment in patients with frontal lobe lesions. *Neuropsychologia*, 27, 1043–1056.

Johnson, M. K., Hashtroudi, S., & Lindsay, D. S. (1993). Source monitoring. *Psychological Bulletin*, 114, 3–28.

Johnson, M. K., Nolde, S. F., Mather, M., Kounios, J., Schacter, D. L., & Curran, T. (1997). The similarity of brain activity associated with true and false recognition memory depends on test format. *Psychological Science*, 8, 250–257.

Johnson, M. K., Raye, C. L., Wang, A. Y., & Taylor, T. H. (1979). Fact and fantasy: The roles of accuracy and variability in confusing imaginations with perceptual experiences. *Journal of Experimental Psychology: Human Learning and Memory*, 5, 229–240.

Jones, G. V., & Langford, S. (1987). Phonological blocking and the tip of the tongue state. *Cognition*, 26, 115–122.

Kapur, S., Craik, F. I. M., Tulving, E., Wilson, A. A., Houle, S., & Brown, G. M. (1994). Neuroanatomical correlates of encoding in episodic memory: Levels of processing effect. *Proceedings of the National Academy of Sciences*, 91, 2008–2011.

Kassin, S. (1997). The psychology of confession evidence. *American Psychologist*, 52, 221–233.

Kassin, S., & Kiechel, K. L. (1996). The social psychology of false confessions: Compliance, internalization, and confabulation. *Psychological Science*, 7, 125–128.

Kelley, W. M., Miezin, F. M., McDermott, K. B., Buckner, R. L., Raichle, M. E., Cohen, N. J., Ollinger, J. M., Akbudak, E., Conturo, T. E., Snyder, A. Z., & Petersen, S. E. (1998). Hemispheric specialization in human dorsal frontal cortex and medial temporal lobe for verbal and nonverbal memory encoding. *Neuron*, 20, 927–936.

Kensinger, E., & Schacter, D. L. (in press). When true recognition suppresses false recognition: Effects of aging. *Cognitive Neuropsychology*.

Kihlstrom, J. F. (1995). The trauma-memory argument. *Consciousness and Cognition*, 4, 63–67.

Kirkpatrick, L. A., & Hazan, C. (1994). Attachment styles and close relationships: A four year prospective study. *Personal Relationships*, 1, 123–142.

Koutstaal, W., & Schacter, D. L. (1997a). Gist-based false recognition of pictures in older and younger adults. *Journal of Memory and Language*, 37, 555–583.

Koutstaal, W., & Schacter, D. L. (1997b). Inaccuracy and inaccessibility in memory retrieval: Contributions from cognitive psychology and cognitive neuropsychology. In P. S. Appelbaum, L. Uyehara, & M. Elin (Eds.), *Trauma and memory: Clinical and legal controversies* (pp. 93–137). New York: Oxford University Press.

Koutstaal, W., & Schacter, D. L. (1997c). Intentional forgetting and voluntary thought suppression: Two potential methods for coping with childhood trauma. In L. J. Dickstein, M. B. Riba, & J. M. Oldham (Eds.), *Review of Psychiatry* (Vol. 16, pp. 79–121). Washington, DC: American Psychiatric Press.

Koutstaal, W., Schacter, D. L., Johnson, M. K., Angell, K., & Gross, M. S. (1998). Post-event review in older and younger adults: Improving memory accessibility of complex everyday events. *Psychology and Aging*, 13, 277–296.

Koutstaal, W., Schacter, D. L., Johnson, M. K., & Galluccio, L. (in press). Facilitation and impairment of event memory produced by photograph review. *Memory & Cognition*.

Koutstaal, W., Schacter, D. L., Verfaellie, M., Brenner, C. J., & Jackson, E. M. (in press). Perceptually based false recognition of novel objects in amnesia: Effects of category size and similarity to category prototypes. *Cognitive Neuropsychology*.

Kraemer, P. J., & Golding, J. M. (1997). Adaptive forgetting in animals. *Psychonomic Bulletin & Review*, 4, 480–491.

Krystal, J. H., Southwick, S. M., & Charney, D. S. (1995). Post traumatic stress disorder: Psychobiological mechanisms of traumatic remembrance. In D. L. Schacter (Ed.), *Memory distortion: How minds, brains, and societies reconstruct the past* (pp. 150–172). Cambridge, MA: Harvard University Press.

Laurence, J. R., & Perry, C. (1983, November 4). Hypnotically created memory among highly hypnotizable subjects. *Science, 222*, 523–524.

LeDoux, J. E. (1996). *The emotional brain.* New York: Simon & Schuster.

LeDoux, J. E., Romanski, L., & Xagoraris, A. (1989). Indelibility of subcortical emotional memories. *Journal of Cognitive Neuroscience, 1*, 238–243.

Lepage, M., Habib, R., & Tulving, E. (1998). Hippocampal PET activations of memory encoding and retrieval: The HIPER model. *Hippocampus, 8*, 313–322.

Levin, D. T., & Simons, D. J. (1997). Failure to detect changes to attended objects in motion pictures. *Psychonomic Bulletin & Review, 4*, 501–506.

Levine, L. J. (1997). Reconstructing memory for emotions. *Journal of Experimental Psychology: General, 126*, 165–177.

Lindsay, D. S. (1990). Misleading suggestions can impair eyewitnesses' ability to remember event details. *Journal of Experimental Psychology: Learning, Memory, and Cognition, 16*, 1077–1083.

Lindsay, D. S., & Read, J. D. (1994). Psychotherapy and memories of childhood sexual abuse: A cognitive perspective. *Applied Cognitive Psychology, 8*, 281–338.

Loftus, E. F. (1993). The reality of repressed memories. *American Psychologist, 48*, 518–537.

Loftus, E. F., Feldman, J., & Dashiell, R. (1995). The reality of illusory memories. In D. L. Schacter (Ed.), *Memory distortion: How minds, brains and societies reconstruct the past* (pp. 47–68). Cambridge, MA: Harvard University Press.

Loftus, E. F., & Ketcham, K. (1994). *The myth of repressed memory: False memories and allegations of sexual abuse.* New York: St. Martin's Press.

Loftus, E. F., & Loftus, G. R. (1980). On the permanence of stored information in the human brain. *American Psychologist, 35*, 409–420.

Loftus, E. F., Miller, D. G., & Burns, H. J. (1978). Semantic integration of verbal information into a visual memory. *Journal of Experimental Psychology: Human Learning and Memory, 4*, 19–31.

Loftus, E. F., & Pickrell, J. E. (1995). The formation of false memories. *Psychiatric Annals, 25*, 720–725.

Luria, A. R. (1968). *The mind of a mnemonist: A little book about a vast memory* (L. Solotaroff, Trans.). New York: Basic Books.

Lynn, S. J., & Nash, M. R. (1994). Truth in memory: Ramifications for psychotherapy and hypnotherapy. *American Journal of Hypnosis, 36*, 194–208.

Lyubomirsky, S., Caldwell, N. D., & Nolen-Hoeksema, S. (1998). Effects of ruminative and distracting responses to depressed mood on retrieval of autobiographical memories. *Journal of Personality and Social Psychology, 75*, 166–177.

Mandler, J. M. (1979). Categorical and schematic organization in memory. In C. R. Puff (Ed.), *Memory organization and structure* (pp. 259–299). New York: Academic Press.

Marcus, G. B. (1986). Stability and change in political attitudes: Observe, recall, and "explain." *Political Behavior, 8*, 21–44.

Marsh, R. L., & Landau, J. D. (1995). Item availability in cryptomnesia: Assessing its role in two paradigms of unconscious plagiarism. *Journal of Experimental Psychology: Learning, Memory, and Cognition, 21*, 1568–1582.

Mather, M., Henkel, L. A., & Johnson, M. K. (1997). Evaluating characteristics of false memories: Remember/know judgments and memory characteristics questionnaire compared. *Memory and Cognition, 25*, 826–837.

Mayes, A. R., & Downes, J. J. (1997). What do theories of the functional deficit(s) underlying amnesia have to explain? *Memory, 5*, 3–36.

Maylor, E. A. (1990). Recognizing and naming faces: Aging, memory retrieval and the tip of the tongue state. *Journal of Gerontology: Psychological Sciences, 46*, 207–217.

Maylor, E. A. (1996). Does prospective memory decline with age? In M. Brandimonte, G. O. Einstein, & M. A. McDaniel (Eds.), *Prospective memory: Theory and applications* (pp. 173–198). Mahwah, NJ: Erlbaum.

Maylor, E. A. (1997). Proper name retrieval in old age: Converging evidence against disproportionate impairment. *Aging, Neuropsychology, and Cognition, 4*, 211–226.

Mazzoni, G., & Loftus, E. F. (1998). Dream interpretation can change beliefs about the past. *Psychotherapy,* 35, 177–187.

McClelland, J. L. (1995). Constructive memory and memory distortions: A parallel-distributed processing approach. In D. L. Schacter (Ed.), *Memory distortion: How minds, brains, and societies reconstruct the past* (pp. 69–90). Cambridge, MA: Harvard University Press.

McCloskey, M., & Zaragoza, M. (1985). Misleading postevent information and memory for events: Arguments and evidence against memory impairment hypotheses. *Journal of Experimental Psychology: General,* 114, 1–16.

McConkey, K. M., Barnier, A. J., & Sheehan, P. W. (1998). Hypnosis and pseudomemory: Understanding the findings and their implications. In S. Lynn & K. M. McConkey (Eds.), *Truth in memory* (pp. 227–259). New York: Guilford Press.

McDaniel, M. A., & Einstein, G. O. (1993). The importance of cue familiarity and cue distinctiveness in prospective memory. *Memory,* 1, 23–41.

McDermott, K. B., & Roediger, H. L., III. (1998). Attempting to avoid illusory memories: Robust false recognition of associates persists under conditions of explicit warnings and immediate testing. *Journal of Memory & Language,* 39, 508–520.

McFarland, C., & Ross, M. (1987). The relation between current impressions and memories of self and dating partners. *Personality and Social Psychology Bulletin,* 13, 228–238.

McGaugh, J. L. (1995). Emotional activation, neuromodulatory systems and memory. In D. L. Schacter (Ed.), *Memory distortion: How minds, brains, and societies reconstruct the past* (pp. 255–273). Cambridge, MA: Harvard University Press.

McIntyre, J. S., & Craik, F. I. M. (1987). Age differences in memory for item and source information. *Canadian Journal of Psychology,* 41, 175–192.

McNally, R. J., Metzger, L. J., Lasko, N. B., Clancy, S. A., & Pitman, R. K. (1998). Directed forgetting of trauma cues in adult survivors of childhood sexual abuse with and without posttraumatic stress disorder. *Journal of Abnormal Psychology,* 107, 596–601.

Mineka, S., & Nugent, K. (1995). Mood-congruent memory biases in anxiety and depression. In D. L. Schacter (Ed.), *Memory distortion: How minds, brains,* *and societies reconstruct the past* (pp. 173–196). Cambridge, MA: Harvard University Press.

Multhaup, K. S. (1995). Aging, source, and decision criteria: When false fame errors do and do not occur. *Psychology and Aging,* 10, 492–497.

Nadel, L., & Moscovitch, M. (1997). Memory consolidation, retrograde amnesia, and the hippocampal complex. *Current Opinion in Neurobiology,* 7, 217–227.

Nolen-Hoeksema, S. (1991). Responses to depression and their effects on the duration of depressive episodes. *Journal of Abnormal Psychology,* 100, 569–582.

Norman, K. A., & Schacter, D. L. (1997). False recognition in young and older adults: Exploring the characteristics of illusory memories. *Memory & Cognition,* 25, 838–848.

Nyberg, L., McIntosh, A. R., Cabeza, R., Nilsson, L. G., Houle, S., Habib, R., & Tulving, E. (1996). Network analysis of positron emission tomography regional cerebral blood flow data: Ensemble inhibition during episodic memory retrieval. *Journal of Neuroscience,* 16, 3753–3759.

Ochsner, K. N., & Schacter, D. L. (in press). Constructing the emotional past: A social-cognitive-neuroscience approach to emotion and memory. In J. Borod (Ed.), *The neuropsychology of emotion.* New York: Oxford University Press.

Okuda, J., Fujii, T., Yamadori, A., Kawashima, R., Tsukiura, T., Fukatsu, R., Suzuki, K., Ito, M., & Fukuda, H. (1998). Participation of the prefrontal cortices in prospective memory: Evidence from a PET study in humans. *Neuroscience Letters,* 253, 127–130.

Park, D. C., & Kidder, D. P. (1996). Prospective memory and medication adherence. In M. Brandimonte, G. O. Einstein, & M. A. McDaniel (Eds.), *Prospective memory: Theory and applications* (pp. 369–390). Mahwah, NJ: Erlbaum.

Park, D. C., Puglisi, J. T., & Smith, A. D. (1986). Memory for pictures: Does an age-related decline really exist? *Psychology and Aging,* 1, 11–17.

Parkin, A. J., Bindschaedler, C., Harsent, L., & Metzler, C. (1996). Pathological false alarm rates following damage to the left frontal cortex, *Brain and Cognition,* 32, 14–27.

Parkin, A. J., & Leng, N. R. C. (1993). *Neuropsychology of the amnesic syndrome.* Hillsdale, NJ: Erlbaum.

Paulesu, E., Frith, C. D., & Frackowiak, R. S. J. (1993). The neural correlates of the verbal component of working memory. *Nature, 362,* 342–345.

Payne, D. G., Elie, C. J., Blackwell, J. M., & Neuschatz, J. S. (1996). Memory illusions: Recalling, recognizing, and recollecting events that never occurred. *Journal of Memory and Language, 35,* 261–285.

Pendergrast, M. (1995). *Victims of memory: Incest accusations and shattered lives.* Hinesburg, VT: Upper Access.

Peterson, L. R., & Peterson, M. J. (1959). Short-term retention of individual verbal items. *Journal of Experimental Psychology, 58,* 193–198.

Pezdek, K., Finger, K., & Hodge, D. (1997). Planting false childhood memories: The role of event plausibility. *Psychological Science, 8,* 437–441.

Poole, D. A., Lindsay, S. D., Memon, A., & Bull, R. (1995). Psychotherapy and the recovery of memories of childhood sexual abuse: U.S. and British practitioners' opinions, practices, and experiences. *Journal of Consulting and Clinical Psychology, 63,* 426–487.

Pope, K. S. (1996). Memory, abuse, and science: Questioning claims about the false memory syndrome epidemic. *American Psychologist, 51,* 957–974.

Posner, M. I., & Keele, S. W. (1968). On the genesis of abstract ideas. *Journal of Experimental Psychology, 77,* 353–363.

Posner, M. I., & Raichle, M. E. (1994). *Images of the mind.* New York: Scientific American Library.

Postman, L., & Underwood, B. J. (1973). Critical issues in interference theory. *Memory & Cognition, 1,* 19–40.

Rapcsak, S. Z., Reminger, S. L., Glisky, E. L., Kaszniak, A. W., & Comer, J. F. (in press). Neuropsychological mechanisms of false facial recognition following frontal lobe damage. *Cognitive Neuropsychology.*

Rauch, S. L., van der Kolk, B. A., Fisler, R. E., Alpert, N. M., Orr, S. P., Savage, C. R., Fishman, A. J., Jenike, M. A., & Pitman, R. K. (1996). A symptom provocation study of posttraumatic stress disorder using positron emission tomography and script-driven imagery. *Archives of General Psychiatry, 35,* 380–387.

Read, J. D. (1994). Understanding bystander misidentifications: The role of familiarity and contextual knowledge. In D. F. Ross, J. D. Read, & M. P. Toglia (Eds.), *Adult eyewitness testimony: Current trends and developments* (pp. 56–78). New York: Cambridge University Press.

Read, J. D., & Lindsay, D. S. (Eds.). (1997). *Recollections of trauma: Scientific research and clinical practice.* New York: Plenum Press.

Reason, J. T., & Lucas, D. (1984). Using cognitive diaries to investigate naturally occurring memory blocks. In J. E. Harris & P. E. Morris (Eds.), *Everyday memory, actions, and absentmindedness* (pp. 53–69). Orlando, FL: Academic Press.

Reason, J. T., & Mycielska, K. (1982). *Absent-minded?: The psychology of mental lapses and everyday errors.* Englewood Cliffs, NJ: Prentice-Hall.

Reyna, V. F., & Brainerd, C. J. (1995). Fuzzy-trace theory: An interim synthesis. *Learning and Individual Differences, 7,* 1–75.

Roediger, H. L., III. (1974). Inhibiting effects of recall. *Memory & Cognition, 2,* 261–269.

Roediger, H. L., III. (1996). Memory illusions. *Journal of Memory and Language, 35,* 76–100.

Roediger, H. L., III, & McDermott, K. B. (1995). Creating false memories: Remembering words not presented in lists. *Journal of Experimental Psychology: Learning, Memory, and Cognition, 21,* 803–814.

Roediger, H. L., III, McDermott, K. B., & Robinson, K. J. (1998). The role of associative processes in creating false memories. In M. Conway, S. Gathercole, & C. Cornoldi (Eds.), *Theories of memory* (Vol. 2, pp. 187–245). East Sussex, England: Psychology Press.

Roediger, H. L., III, & Neely, J. (1982). Retrieval blocks in episodic and semantic memory. *Canadian Journal of Psychology, 36,* 213–242.

Roese, N. J. (1994). The functional basis of counterfactual thinking. *Journal of Personality and Social Psychology, 66,* 805–818.

Ross, D. F., Ceci, S. J., Dunning, D., & Toglia, M. P. (1994). Unconscious transference and mistaken identity: When a witness misidentifies a familiar but innocent person. *Journal of Applied Psychology, 79,* 918–930.

Ross, M. (1989). Relation of implicit theories to the construction of personal histories. *Psychological Review, 96,* 341–357.

Ross, M., & Wilson, A. E. (in press). Constructing and appraising past selves. In D. L. Schacter & E. Scarry (Eds.), *Memory, brain, & belief.* Cambridge, MA: Harvard University Press.

Schacter, D. L. (1987). Implicit memory: History and current status. *Journal of Experimental Psychology: Learning, Memory, and Cognition, 13,* 501–518.

Schacter, D. L. (1992). Understanding implicit memory: A cognitive neuroscience approach. *American Psychologist, 47,* 559–569.

Schacter, D. L. (1996). *Searching for memory: The brain, the mind, and the past.* New York: Basic Books.

Schacter, D. L., & Buckner, R. L. (1998). Priming and the brain. *Neuron, 20,* 185–195.

Schacter, D. L., Buckner, R. L., Koutstaal, W., Dale, A. M., & Rosen, B. R. (1997). Late onset of anterior prefrontal activity during retrieval of veridical and illusory memories: An event-related fMRI study. *NeuroImage, 6,* 259–269.

Schacter, D. L., Curran, T., Galluccio, L., Milberg, W., & Bates, J. (1996). False recognition and the right frontal lobe: A case study. *Neuropsychologia, 34,* 793–808.

Schacter, D. L., Harbluk, J. L., & McLachlan, D. R. (1984). Retrieval without recollection: An experimental analysis of source amnesia. *Journal of Verbal Learning and Verbal Behavior, 23,* 593–611.

Schacter, D. L., Israel, L., & Racine, C. A. (1999). Suppressing false recognition in younger and older adults: The distinctiveness heuristic. *Journal of Memory & Language, 40,* 1–24.

Schacter, D. L., Koutstaal, W., Johnson, M. K., Gross, M. S., & Angell, K. A. (1997). False recollection induced by photographs: A comparison of older and younger adults. *Psychology and Aging, 12,* 203–215.

Schacter, D. L., Norman, K. A., & Koutstaal, W. (1997). The recovered memory debate: A cognitive neuroscience perspective. In M. A. Conway (Ed.), *False and recovered memories* (pp. 63–99). New York: Oxford University Press.

Schacter, D. L., Norman, K. A., & Koutstaal, W. (1998). The cognitive neuroscience of constructive memory. *Annual Review of Psychology, 49,* 289–318.

Schacter, D. L., Reiman, E., Curran, T., Yun, L. S., Bandy, D., McDermott, K. B., & Roediger, H. L., III. (1996). Neuroanatomical correlates of veridical and illusory recognition memory: Evidence from positron emission tomography. *Neuron, 17,* 267–274.

Schacter, D. L., Verfaellie, M., Anes, M. D., & Racine, C. A. (1998). When true recognition suppresses false recognition: Evidence from amnesic patients. *Journal of Cognitive Neuroscience, 10,* 668–679.

Schacter, D. L., Verfaellie, M., & Pradere, D. (1996). The neuropsychology of memory illusions: False recall and recognition in amnesic patients. *Journal of Memory and Language, 35,* 319–334.

Schacter, D. L., & Wagner, A. D. (1999). Medial temporal lobe activations in fMRI and PET studies of episodic encoding and retrieval. *Hippocampus, 9,* 7–24.

Schacter, D. L., Wagner, A. D., & Buckner, R. L. (in press). Memory systems of 1999. In E. Tulving & F. I. M. Craik (Eds.), *Handbook of Memory.* New York: Oxford University Press.

Scharfe, E., & Bartholomew, K. (1998). Do you remember? Recollections of adult attachment patterns. *Personal Relationships, 5,* 219–234.

Schooler, J. W. (1994). Seeking the core: The issues and evidence surrounding recovered accounts of sexual trauma. *Consciousness and Cognition, 3,* 452–469.

Schooler, L., & Anderson, J. R. (1997). The role of process in the rational analysis of memory. *Cognitive Psychology, 32,* 219–250.

Scoville, W. B., & Milner, B. (1957). Loss of recent memory after bilateral hippocampal lesions. *Journal of Neurology, Neurosurgery and Psychiatry, 20,* 11–21.

Seamon, J. G., Luo, C. R., & Gallo, D. A. (1998). Creating false memories of words with or without recognition of list items: Evidence for nonconscious processes. *Psychological Science, 9,* 20–26.

Semenza, C., Mondini, S., & Zettin, M. (1995). The anatomical basis of proper name processing: A critical review. *Neurocase, 1,* 183–188.

Shallice, T., & Burgess, P. W. (1991). Deficits in strategy application following frontal lobe damage in man. *Brain, 114,* 727–741.

Shaw, J. S., Bjork, R. A., & Handal, A. (1995). Retrieval-induced forgetting in an eyewitness memory paradigm. *Psychonomic Bulletin & Review, 2,* 249–253.

Sherry, D. F., & Schacter, D. L. (1987). The evolution of multiple memory systems. *Psychological Review, 94,* 439–454.

Shin, L. M., Kosslyn, S. M., McNally, R. J., Alpert, N. M., Thompson, W. L., Rauch, S. L., Macklin, M. L., & Pitman, R. K. (1997). Visual imagery and perception in posttraumatic stress disorder: A positron emission tomographic investigation. *Archives of General Psychiatry, 54,* 233–241.

Simons, D. J., & Levin, D. T. (1997). Change blindness. *Trends in Cognitive Sciences, 1,* 261–267.

Simons, D. J., & Levin, D. T. (1998). Failure to detect changes to people during a real-world interaction. *Psychonomic Bulletin & Review,* 4, 644–649.

Singer, J. A., & Salovey, P. (1993). *The remembered self: Emotion and memory in personality.* New York: The Free Press.

Slamecka, N. J. (1968). An examination of trace storage in free recall. *Journal of Experimental Psychology,* 76, 504–513.

Sloman, S. A., Bower, G. H., & Rohrer, D. (1991). Congruency effects in part-list cueing inhibition. *Journal of Experimental Psychology: Learning, Memory, and Cognition,* 17, 974–982.

Smith, E. E., & Jonides, J. (1997). Working memory: A view from neuroimaging. *Cognitive Psychology,* 33, 5–42.

Smith, S. M., & Tindell, D. R. (1997). Memory blocks in word fragment completion caused by involuntary retrieval of orthographically related primes. *Journal of Experimental Psychology: Learning, Memory, and Cognition,* 23, 355–370.

Spiro, R. J. (1980). Accommodative reconstruction in prose recall. *Journal of Verbal Learning and Verbal Behavior,* 19, 84–95.

Squire, L. R. (1987). *Memory and brain.* New York: Oxford University Press.

Squire, L. R., & Alvarez, P. (1995). Retrograde amnesia and memory consolidation: A neurobiological perspective. *Current Opinion in Neurobiology,* 5, 169–177.

Strack, F., Schwarz, N., & Gschneidinger, E. (1985). Happiness and reminiscing: The role of time perspective, affect, and mode of thinking. *Journal of Personality and Social Psychology,* 49, 1460–1469.

Suengas, A. G., & Johnson, M. K. (1988). Qualitative effects of rehearsal on memories for perceived and imagined complex events. *Journal of Experimental Psychology: General,* 117, 377–389.

Taylor, S. E. (1991). *Positive illusions.* New York: Basic Books.

Thomson, D. M. (1988). Context and false recognition. In G. M. Davies & D. M. Thompson (Eds.), *Memory in context: Context in memory* (pp. 285–304). Chichester, England: Wiley.

Tulving, E. (1985). Memory and consciousness. *Canadian Psychologist,* 26, 1–12.

Tulving, E., & Pearlstone, Z. (1966). Availability versus accessibility of information in memory for words. *Journal of Verbal Learning and Verbal Behavior,* 5, 381–391.

Tun, P. A., Wingfield, A., Rosen, M. J., & Blanchard, L. (1998). Response latencies for false memories: Gist-based processes in normal aging. *Psychology and Aging,* 13, 230–241.

Underwood, B. J. (1965). False recognition produced by implicit verbal responses. *Journal of Experimental Psychology,* 70, 122–129.

Ungerleider, L. G. (1995, November 3). Functional brain imaging studies of cortical mechanisms for memory. *Science,* 270, 760–775.

Vallar, G., & Baddeley, A. D. (1984). Fractionation of working memory: Neuropsychological evidence for a phonological short-term store. *Journal of Verbal Learning and Verbal Behavior,* 23, 151–161.

Vallar, G., & Shallice, T. (1990). *Neuropsychological impairments of short-term memory.* Cambridge, England: Cambridge University Press.

Vortac, O. U., Edwards, M. B., & Manning, C. A. (1995). Functions of external cues in prospective memory. *Memory,* 3, 201–219.

Wagner, A. D., Poldrack, R. A., Eldridge, L., Desmond, J. E., Glover, G. H., & Gabrieli, J. D. E. (1998). Material-specific lateralization of prefrontal activation during episodic encoding and retrieval. *NeuroReport,* 9, 3711–3713.

Wagner, A. D., Schacter, D. L., Rotte, M., Koutstaal, W., Maril, A., Dale, A. M., Rosen, B. R., & Buckner, R. L. (1998, August 21). Building memories: Remembering and forgetting of verbal experiences as predicted by brain activity. *Science,* 281, 1188–1191.

Wegner, D. M., & Erber, R. (1992). The hyperaccessibility of suppressed thoughts. *Journal of Personality and Social Psychology,* 63, 903–912.

Wells, G. L., & Bradfield, A. L. (1998). Good, you identified the suspect: Feedback to eyewitnesses distorts their reports of the witnessing experience. *Journal of Applied Psychology,* 83, 360–376.

Wells, G. L., Small, M., Penrod, S., Malpass, R. S., Fulero, S. M., & Brimacombe, C. A. E. (in press). Eyewitness identification procedures: Recommendations for lineups and photospreads. *Law and Human Behavior.*

Wheeler, M. A., Stuss, D. T., & Tulving, E. (1997). Toward a theory of episodic memory: The frontal lobes and autonoetic consciousness. *Psychological Bulletin,* 121, 331–354.

Wiggs, C. L., & Martin, A. (1998). Properties and mechanisms of perceptual priming. *Current Opinion in Neurobiology,* 8, 227–233.

Williams, M. (1997). *Cry of pain.* London: Penguin.

Wilson, S. C., & Barber, T. X. (1978). The Creative Imagination Scale as a measure of hypnotic responsiveness: Applications to experimental and clinical hypnosis. *American Journal of Clinical Hypnosis,* 20, 235–249.

Wixted, J. T., & Ebbesen, E. B. (1997). Genuine power curves in forgetting: A quantitative analysis of individual subject forgetting functions. *Memory & Cognition,* 25, 731–739.

Wright, L. (1994). *Remembering Satan: A case of recovered memory and the shattering of an American family.* New York: Knopf.

Zaragoza, M. S., & Lane, S. M. (1994). Source misattributions and the suggestibility of eyewitness memory. *Journal of Experimental Psychology: Learning, Memory, and Cognition,* 20, 934–945.

9 Double Dissociation of Conditioning and Declarative Knowledge Relative to the Amygdala and Hippocampus in Humans

Antoine Bechara, Daniel Tranel, Hanna Damasio, Ralph Adolphs, Charles Rockland, and Antonio R. Damasio

Studies in animals have established that the amygdala is critical for emotional conditioning (1), whereas several human and nonhuman primate studies have established that the hippocampus and surrounding regions are necessary for establishing declarative knowledge (2). Because of the rarity of patients with selective bilateral damage restricted to either the amygdala or hippocampus, the exact roles of these structures in emotional and declarative learning have not been established clearly for humans (3). Here, we report the relative contributions of the amygdala and hippocampus to emotional conditioning and to the establishment of declarative knowledge in humans. We studied three people with distinct brain lesions: SM046 had bilateral destruction of the amygdala, but bilaterally intact hippocampi; WC1606 had bilateral hippocampal damage, but bilaterally intact amygdalae; and RH1951 had bilateral damage to both hippocampus and amygdala (4) (Table 9.1 and Fig. 9.1). Four normal participants of comparable age and education served as controls.

Two conditioning experiments were carried out. The first, a visual-auditory conditioning experiment, used monochrome slides as the conditioned stimuli (CS) and a startlingly loud sound (a boat horn delivered at 100 dB) as the unconditioned stimulus (US). The second, an auditory-auditory conditioning experiment, used computer-generated tones as the CS (the US was the same as in the visual-auditory experiment). In both experiments, the skin conductance response (SCR) was the dependent measure of autonomic response (5). Each conditioning experiment was performed three times in SM046 and twice in WC1606 and RH1951. For each participant one visual-auditory and one auditory-auditory conditioning experiment were carried out on the same day, separated by 1 to 2 hours. Conditioning experiments were repeated on the following day (or days), about 24 hours after the first set of experiments. The order of visual-auditory (slide-sound) and auditory-auditory (tone-sound) conditioning was counterbalanced across the conditioning experiments (6).

The conditioning protocol consisted of three phases. In the habituation phase, slides of four different colors (green, blue, yellow, and red) were presented repeatedly to the participant (6 to 12 times) in an irregular order, until the SCRs to these slides approached zero (<0.05 μS). In the conditioning phase, 26 slides of the same four colors were presented in an irregular order. Six of the slides were blue and were followed immediately by a startling sound (US) of 1-s duration. There were six further presentations of a blue slide not followed by the US. Thus, only the blue slides served as the CS. The remainder of the slides (non-CS) were 14 red, green, or yellow slides never paired with the US (7). Finally, in the extinction phase, the participant was exposed to 6 to 12 repeated presentations of the CS (blue slide) without the US, and without any other colors, until the SCR activity returned to the level seen during habituation (<0.05 μS). The auditory-auditory conditioning experiment was identical to the one just described, except that four computer-generated tones were used in place of the color slides. Five minutes after completion of the conditioning experiment, the participant was asked to answer the following questions, using an oral question-and-answer format: (i) How many different colors did you see? (ii) Tell me the names of those colors. (iii) How many different colors were followed by the horn? (iv) Tell me the name (or names) of the color (or colors) that were followed by the horn (8).

Bilateral damage to the amygdala entirely blocked the ability of SM046 to acquire conditioned SCRs to the CS but did not preclude the acquisition of facts about which stimuli (CS)

Table 9.1

Demographic and neuropsychological data for experimental participants

Characteristic	Participant		
	SM046	WC1606	RH1951
Sex	Female	Male	Male
Age (years)	30	47	42
Handedness	Right	Right	Right
Years of education	12	12	16
Verbal IQ*	86	83	110
Performance IQ*	90	80	116
General memory index†	89	71	75
Delayed memory index†	88	52	53
Speech	Normal	Normal	Normal

Underlined scores are defective.
* From the Wechsler Adult Intelligence Scale—Revised (WAIS-R) (16).
† From the Wechsler Memory Scale—Revised (WMS-R) (16).

were followed by the US. Specifically, during the conditioning phase of the experiments SM046 failed to generate SCRs to the CSs in both the visual and auditory experiments but was able to provide accurate and complete factual information regarding which stimuli had been followed by the US. The opposite result was obtained with participant WC1606. His bilateral hippocampal damage did not interfere with his ability to acquire conditioned SCRs but blocked his ability to acquire new facts. During the conditioning phase, WC1606 generated normal SCRs to the CSs in both the visual and auditory experiments. However, he could not provide factual information about the nature of the CS-US pairings; for example, he was never able to report that it had been the blue slide that had been paired with the boat horn. In participant RH1951, combined bilateral hippocampal and amygdala damage halted both the acquisition of conditioned SCRs

and new facts. In the conditioning phases of the experiments, RH1951 never evidenced SCRs to the CSs and could not report factual information about which stimuli had been paired with a US or other details about the nature of the conditioning experiments (Figs. 9.2 and 9.3).

It is important to note that our results cannot be explained on the basis of a defect in electrodermal response in these participants. All three showed normal SCRs whenever the US was presented together with the CS (Fig. 9.4). This is consistent with the notion that the amygdala is not necessary for the generation of electrodermal activity per se (9, 10) but that it is indeed essential for the coupling of sensory stimuli with affect—that is, the establishment of sensory-affective associations (11). Also, the fact that the results from the visual-auditory conditioning did not differ from those of the auditory-auditory conditioning rules out any major difference in the association of a CS and a US of different sensory modalities (intermodal associations) versus a CS and a US of the same sensory modality (intramodal associations) (Figs. 9.2 and 9.3).

The neuroanatomical connectivity of the amygdala enables it to associate converging inputs from various exteroceptive sensory modalities with the comprehensive changes in somatic state that define an emotional response (12). We suggest that the amygdala is indispensable for emotional conditioning and for the coupling of exteroceptive sensory information with interoceptive information concerning somatic states (emotion and affect) (13, 14). On the other hand, the hippocampus, and the medial temporal lobe memory system of which it is a part, are essential for the learning of relations among various exteroceptive sensory stimuli. Our findings are consistent with previous studies in animals, which suggested that the amygdala is essential for the association of contextual (complex) or discrete (simple) cues with affect, whereas the hippocampus is critical for learning the relations among contextual cues (15). Our findings, however, demonstrate this double dissociation be-

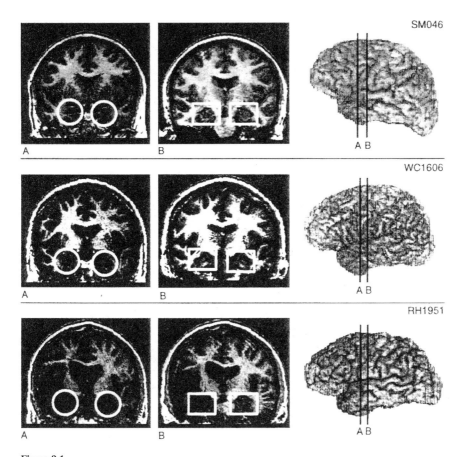

Figure 9.1

Neuroanatomical findings in the three experimental participants. (A) and (B) show coronal sections through the amygdala and hippocampus, respectively, taken from the three-dimensional reconstruction of each participant's brain. The reconstruction was based on magnetic resonance data and obtained with Brainvox (17). The region of the amygdala is highlighted by white circles and the region of the hippocampus by white rectangles. SM046 has extensive bilateral damage to the amygdala, but not to the hippocampus. Detailed anatomical analyses of her magnetic resonance imaging (MRI) scans are presented in reference 13. The damage begins in the rostral portion of the amygdala and extends throughout the caudal portion. Damage to the left amygdala is somewhat more extensive than damage to the right amygdala, but considering the connectivity and pathology of the amygdala, it is reasonable to conclude that both are severely dysfunctional as a result of the damage (13). The most anterior sector of the entorhinal cortex shows some damage, but there is no indication that this makes any contribution to her memory profile. No other areas of damage are detected. Specifically, the hippocampus is intact bilaterally. WC1606 has bilateral damage to the hippocampus proper, but not to the amygdala. We base this conclusion on several lines of evidence: (i) The mechanism of injury (ischemia-anoxia), which is known to produce damage to CA1 neurons in the hippocampus (3); (ii) the neuropsychological outcome (a declarative learning defect); and (iii) a comparison of the hippocampal volumes of WC1606 to those of two age-matched controls (one with brain damage [a stroke in the occipital lobe] and one without) with the use of chronic neuroanatomical data—that is, neuroimaging (MR) data collected several years after the onset of the lesion. The results of this analysis indicated that the left and right hippocampi of WC1606 are reduced by about 33% each, relative to the two control subjects. A similar analysis was conducted on the amygdala volumes of WC1606 and the controls. The results indicated that there is no reduction in the volumes of WC1606's amygdalae. In short, the circumstances of his injury, and the neuroimaging and neuropsychological evidence, are suggestive of hippocampal, but not amygdala, damage. RH1951 has extensive bilateral damage to the amygdala, hippocampus proper, and surrounding cortices. The amygdalae and entorhinal cortices are destroyed bilaterally. The hippocampus is destroyed on the right and severely damaged on the left.

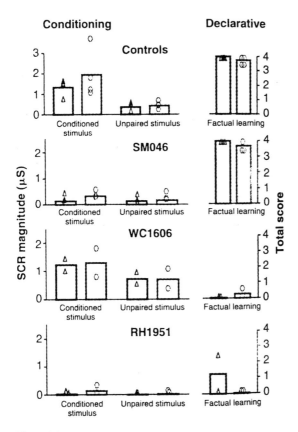

Figure 9.2
Magnitudes of SCRs and total factual learning scores (8) from the visual-auditory (blue) and auditory-auditory (red) conditioning experiments, from normal controls ($n = 4$), SM046 (three trials), WC1606 (two trials), and RH1951 (two trials). Each triangle or circle on the graph represents data from one participant (in the case of controls) or one trial (in the case of patients). Each bar represents the mean magnitude or score from all participants or trials. (Each circle or triangle on the graph represents the mean magnitude of SCRs from six presentations of the conditioned stimuli [blue slides or tones not followed by the US], 14 presentations of unpaired stimuli, or the total factual learning score from the conditioning experiment.)

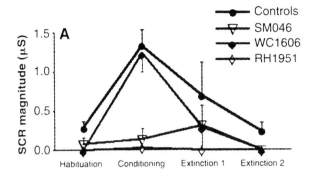

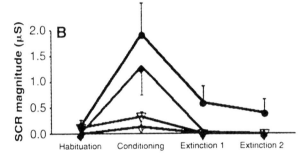

Figure 9.3
Magnitudes of SCRs in the conditioning phase as compared to the SCRs in the habituation and extinction phases. Each point on the visual-auditory conditioning (A) and auditory-auditory conditioning (B) plots represents the mean ± SEM of the magnitudes of SCRs generated by controls, SM046, WC1606, and RH1951 during each phase of the conditioning experiment. Each habituation score represents the mean (from $n = 4$ controls, three trials for SM046, two trials for WC1606, and two trials for RH1951) of the mean magnitude of SCRs generated in response to the last three slides or sounds preceding conditioning. Each conditioning score represents the mean of the mean magnitude of the SCRs generated in response to six presentations of the CS (not followed by the US). Each extinction 1 score represents the mean of the mean magnitude of SCRs generated in response to the first three repeated presentations of the CS during extinction. Each extinction 2 score represents the mean of the mean magnitude of SCRs in response to the last three repeated presentation of the CS.

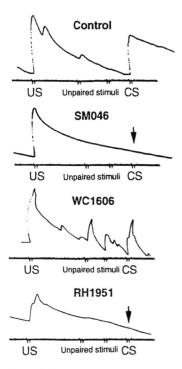

Figure 9.4
Sample copies from the original polygraph records of one control, SM046, WC1606, and RH1951. All samples are presented with the same magnitude scale (microsiemens) on the y axis and the same time scale (seconds) on the x axis (6). Each sample depicts a continuous record of electrodermal activity across the same series of slides (trials) in the conditioning phase of visual-auditory conditioning. The US corresponds to the blue slide followed by the US on the 13th trial of the conditioning phase. Unpaired stimuli correspond to the yellow and red slides on the 14th and 15th trials. CS corresponds to the blue slide not followed by the US on the 16th trial (see [7] for slide sequence). Note the complete absence of conditioned SCRs (black arrows) in SM046 and RH1951, but the preserved SCRs to the US itself. Indeed, the mean SCR magnitudes in response to the six blue slides followed by the US in the three participants were 2.4 μS (SM046), 2.6 μS (WC1606), and 1.5 μS (RH1951). These values are well within the normal range, relative to controls in our study (SCR magnitudes from the six blue-US slides were 2.0 μS (control 1) and 2.4 μS [control 2]). Both controls and patient WC1606 initially produced SCRs to the unpaired slides or tones. However, after two to three CS-US pairings, the SCRs produced by controls to the unpaired stimuli subsided, whereas those produced by the patient WC1606 did not, although the magnitudes of his SCRs to the CS were higher than those to the unpaired stimuli as shown here. Together, the combined results from SM046, WC1606, and RH1951 suggest that the amygdala is necessary for the acquisition of paired and unpaired stimuli. The observation that hippocampal damage interfered with WC1606's ability to respond differentially, at low magnitude, to a stimulus that initially was responded to at high magnitude is reminiscent of previous work in rabbits, in which hippocampal damage disrupted discrimination reversal conditioning of the rabbit nictitating membrane response (18). Hippocampal damage selectively disrupted the animals' ability to respond differentially, at a low rate, to a stimulus previously responded to at a high rate.

tween emotional and declarative learning in humans and thus offer insight on how the ensuing and different forms of knowledge may come together in the human brain.

References and Notes

1. J. E. LeDoux, in *Handbook of Physiology: The Nervous System V*, F. Plum, Ed. (American Physiological Society, Bethesda, MD, 1987), pp. 419–459; J. E. LeDoux, *Sci. Am.* 270, 50 (June 1994); M. Davis, *Annu. Rev. Neurosci.* 15, 353 (1992); *Trends Neurosci.* 17, 208 (1994).
2. M. Mishkin and E. A. Murray, *Curr. Opin. Neurobiol.* 4, 200 (1994); L. R. Squire and S. Zola-Morgan, *Science* 253, 1380 (1991).
3. S. Zola-Morgan, L. R. Squire, D. G. Amaral, *J. Neurosci.* 6, 2950 (1986).
4. Participant SM046 has bilateral amygdala damage because of Urbach-Wiethe disease. Detailed information pertaining to her neuropsychological profile, her neuroanatomical status, and facts about her daily life (especially with regard to impairments in emotional reactivity) is published [R. Adolphs, D. Tranel, H. Damasio, A. Damasio, *Nature* 372, 669 (1994); R. Adolphs, D. Tranel, H. Damasio, A. R. Damasio, *J. Neurosci.*, in press]. In brief, she has low average intellect and normal anterograde declarative memory, as measured by conventional procedures (Table 9.1). Although the exact point at which SM046 acquired her amygdala damage is not clear, the literature on Urbach-Wiethe disease and reports of SM046's childhood suggest that the neurological symptoms resulting from the disease were progressively acquired throughout late childhood and adolescence. In her daily life, SM046 has a history of inadequate decision-making and inappropriate social behavior. WC1606 has bilateral hippocampal damage. Four years before our experiments, he suffered a series of cardiac arrests and ventricular fibrillation, which produced severe ischemia-anoxia and consequent bilateral hippocampal injury (see Fig. 9.1). He was left with a severe anterograde declarative memory impairment. He has low average intellect (Table 9.1). RH1951 has bilateral damage to both the hippocampus and amygdala because of herpes simplex encephalitis, suffered 14 years before our experiments. The disease produced bilateral medial

temporal lobe lesions and a severe impairment in anterograde declarative memory. His intellectual abilities remain well above average (Table 9.1). Based on (i) review of the academic and occupational histories of the patients, (ii) multiple assessments over several years, which indicate stable intellectual functioning, and (iii) lack of significant "scatter" among the various subsets from the WAIS-R (16), there is no indication of general intellectual deterioration in these patients. The fact that SM046 and WC1606 are well-matched in intelligence quotient (IQ), but have different conditioning and declarative learning outcomes, argues against the possibility that intellectual factors could account for our findings.
5. Procedures of SCR recordings have been described in detail elsewhere [D. Tranel and H. Damasio, *Psychophysiology* 31, 427 (1994)].
6. All participants gave informed consent before participation in the experiments. After electrodes were attached, each participant was seated in a comfortable chair, 0.45 m in front of the screens of a Caramate 4000 slide projector and of a computer for generating tones. The participant was asked to relax, to remain silent, and to attend to the color of the slides appearing on the screen. No motor or verbal response was to be given. Each slide was shown for 2 s, and the interval between two consecutive slides was between 10 and 20 s. The intertrial interval was determined by the status of the electrodermal activity. A new slide was not presented if the participant was generating, or was in the steep recovery limb, of an SCR. The auditory-auditory conditioning procedure was identical to the visual-auditory procedure, except that computer-generated tones were used instead of color slides. Each tone was presented for 2 s, and the interval between two consecutive tones was 10 to 20 s.
7. In the conditioning phase, the sequence of blue slides followed by the US, blue slides not followed by the US, and unpaired slides was as follows: (B-US)-R-(B-no US)-R-(B-US)-R-R-(B-US)-R-(B-no US)-G-R-(B-US)-Y-R-(B-no US)-(B-US)-R-G-(B-no US)-G-R-(B-no US)-G-(B-US)-(B-no US) (where B, blue; G, green; R, red; and Y, yellow).
8. In auditory-auditory conditioning, the same format of questions was used, but because it was difficult to give a verbal description of the computer tones, six tones were replayed and the participant was asked to identify the familiar tones as well as the tone followed

by the horn. To quantify each participant's ability to acquire these specific facts about the experiment, we ascribed a maximum score of 4 if all answers were correct. Because the most significant fact in the conditioning experiment was to learn that the blue slide (or the one computer tone) was followed by the horn, a correct answer to this question was ascribed a score of 2.5. Any answer to this question that included more than one color (or tone), or a color other than blue (or other than the specific tone paired with the horn), resulted in a score of 0. Each of the remaining three questions was ascribed a score of 0.5 for a correct answer, and a score of 0 for an incorrect one. Participants were asked to declare their knowledge, and they were not required to guess an answer or to respond in a forced choice format. All participants answered all the questions.

9. D. Tranel and B. T. Hyman, *Arch. Neurol.* 47, 349 (1990).

10. D. Tranel and H. Damasio, *Neuropsychologia* 27, 381 (1989); G. P. Lee et al., *Neuropsychiat. Neuropsychol. Behav. Neurol.* 1, 119 (1988).

11. In follow-up experiments, we have found that some patients, though not all, with unilateral amygdala damage resulting from right or left temporal lobectomies failed to acquire conditioned SCRs. These findings are consistent with a recent report [K. S. LeBar, E. A. Phelps, J. E. LeDoux, *Soc. Neurosci. Abstr.* 20, 360 (1994); K. S. LeBar, J. E. LeDoux, D. D. Spencer, E. A. Phelps, *J. Neurosci.,* in press] that unilateral temporal lobectomies may produce impaired fear conditioning.

12. G. W. Van Hoesen, *Ann. N.Y. Acad. Sci.* 444, 97 (1985); D. G. Amaral, in *Handbook of Physiology: The Nervous System V,* F. Plum, Ed. (American Physiological Society, Bethesda, MD, 1987), pp. 211–294.

13. F. K. D. Nahm, D. Tranel, H. Damasio, A. R. Damasio, *Neuropsychologia* 31, 727 (1993).

14. A. R. Damasio, *Descartes' Error: Emotion, Reason, and the Human Brain* (Grosset/Putnam, New York, 1994).

15. R. G. Phillips and J. E. LeDoux, *Behav. Neurosci.* 106, 274 (1992); J. J. Kim and M. S. Fanselow, *Science* 256, 675 (1992); R. J. McDonald and N. M. White, *Behav. Neurosci.* 107, 3 (1993); J. J. Kim, R. A. Rison, M. S. Fanselow, *ibid.,* p. 1093.

16. D. Wechsler, *Manual for the Wechsler Adult Intelligence Scale—Revised* (New York Psychological Corporation, New York, 1991); *Manual for the Wechsler Memory Scale—Revised* (New York Psychological Corporation, New York, 1987).

17. H. Damasio and R. Frank, *Arch. Neurol.* 49, 137 (1992).

18. T. W. Berger and W. B. Orr, *Behav. Brain Res.* 8, 49 (1983).

Supported by the National Institute of Neurological Disease and Stroke (grant PO1 NS19632, the James S. McDonnell Foundation, and the Medical Research Council (Canada). R.A. is a Burroughs-Wellcome Fund Fellow of the Life Sciences Research Foundation.

10 Imaging Unconscious Semantic Priming

Stanislas Dehaene, Lionel Naccache, Gurvan Le Clec'H, Etienne Koechlin, Michael Mueller, Ghislaine Dehaene-Lambertz, Pierre-François van de Moortele, and Denis Le Bihan

Visual words that are masked and presented so briefly that they cannot be seen may nevertheless facilitate the subsequent processing of related words, a phenomenon called masked priming.[1,2] It has been debated whether masked primes can activate cognitive processes without gaining access to consciousness.[3-5] Here we use a combination of behavioural and brain-imaging techniques to estimate the depth of processing of masked numerical primes. Our results indicate that masked stimuli have a measurable influence on electrical and haemodynamic measures of brain activity. When subjects engage in an overt semantic comparison task with a clearly visible target numeral, measures of covert motor activity indicate that they also unconsciously apply the task instructions to an unseen masked numeral. A stream of perceptual, semantic and motor processes can therefore occur without awareness.

We presented a numeral between 1 and 9, the prime, to subjects for a very short duration (43 ms). The prime was masked by two nonsense letter strings, and followed by another numeral, the target (figure 10.1). Under these conditions, even when subjects focused their attention on the prime, they could neither reliably report its presence or absence nor discriminate it from a nonsense string (table 10.1). Nevertheless, we show here that the prime is processed to a high cognitive level.

We asked subjects to perform a simple semantic categorization task on the target numeral. Subjects were asked to press a response key with one hand if the target was larger than 5, and with the other hand if the target was smaller than 5. Unknown to them, each target number was preceded by a masked prime which was varied from trial to trial so it too could be larger or smaller than 5. In some trials the prime was congruent with the target (both numbers fell on the same side of 5), and in other trials it was incongruent

(one number being larger than 5, and the other being smaller; figure 10.1). We first established that prime-target congruity has a significant influence on behavioural, electrical and haemodynamic measures of brain function. We then showed that the interference between prime and target can be attributed to a covert, prime-induced activation of motor cortex, a response bias that must be overcome in incongruent trials. This indicates that the prime was unconsciously processed according to task instructions, all the way down to the motor system.

The effect of prime-target congruity on behaviour is shown in figure 10.2. Subjects responded more slowly in incongruent trials than in congruent trials ($P < 0.0001$). All 12 subjects showed a positive priming effect, ranging from 2 to 43 ms (average 24 ms, s.d. 13.5 ms). Furthermore, the entire response time distribution was shifted by ~ 24 ms in incongruent trials compared with congruent trials. Thus, there was no evidence that the effect was found in only a small proportion of subjects or a small number of trials with a distinct distribution of response times.

Two characteristics of the priming effect link it to a semantic level of analysis. First, we varied the notations used for the prime number and for the target number independently. Either number could be presented as an arabic digit (for example, 1 or 4) or as a written word (for example, ONE or FOUR). Although the target notation had a significant main effect on response times ($P < 0.0001$), the amount of priming itself was similar under all conditions of notation and did not interact with target notation, prime notation, or notation change. Priming remained significant even when the notations of the prime and target numbers differed (for example, prime 4, target ONE; $P = 0.0006$). Thus, priming occurred at a notation-independent level of numerical representation.[6] Second, priming remained significant

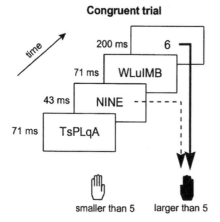

Congruent trial

time

71 ms | TsPLqA

43 ms | NINE

71 ms | WLuIMB

200 ms | 6

smaller than 5   larger than 5

Incongruent trial

TsPLqA

ONE

WLuIMB

6

smaller than 5   larger than 5

Figure 10.1
Experimental design. In each trial, the following four
visual stimuli appeared successively, centred on the
same screen location: a random-letter-string mask, a
prime number, another mask, and a target number.
Subjects were not informed of the presence of the
prime. They were simply told that a "signal" preceded
the target number that they had to classify as larger or
smaller than 5. Half of the trials were of the congruent
type (prime and target both falling on the same side of
5), and half were incongruent.

even after trials with repeated numbers (for example, prime ONE, target 1) were excluded from
the analysis ($P = 0.001$). Hence, priming did not
simply reflect a word repetition effect, but depended on the similarity of the prime and target
numbers at a semantic level (larger or smaller
than 5).

Event-related potentials (ERPs) recorded during the task also showed a prime-target congruity
effect. The central positivity, which culminated
at about the time of the subject's response and
is thought to index post-perceptual processing,[7]
was delayed by ~24 ms in incongruent trials
compared with congruent trials (figure 10.3a).
We proposed that the slower responses in incongruent trials might be due to response competition. Subjects would unconsciously apply the
task instructions to the prime, would therefore
categorize it as smaller or larger than 5, and
would even prepare a motor response appropriate to the prime (figure 10.1). In incongruent trials, this prime-induced covert motor activation
would mismatch with the overt response required
to the target, resulting in response competition
and hence slower response times relative to congruent trials.

According to this theory, we should be able to
detect an early covert motor activation on the
correct response side during congruent trials, and
on the incorrect response side during incongruent
trials. We tested this prediction using the lateralized readiness potential (LRP), an ERP measure
that indexes the activation of lateralized motor
circuits[8] (figure 10.3b). The LRP can detect low
levels of covert response activation that do not
necessarily result in an overt motor response.[8–10]
As it unfolds in time, the LRP departs from zero
as soon as task-relevant information becomes
available to bias the motor response towards the
left or right hand. Conventionally, positive deflections indicate response preparation on the correct side, whereas negative deflections indicate
a transient covert activation on the incorrect response side. Here, the LRP revealed the predicted covert prime-induced motor preparation.

Table 10.1
Experimental measures of prime awareness

	Prime duration (ms)					
	0	29	43	57	114	200
Task 1						
Hit rate (%)	4.2	10.4	12.5	25.0	85.4	97.9
False alarms (%)	4.2	7.3	7.3	3.1	5.2	1.0
d'	0.0	0.20	0.30	1.19**	2.68**	4.36**
Task 2						
Hit rate (%)	28.6	40.2	49.1	46.4	78.6	95.5
False alarms (%)	34.8	32.1	41.1	30.4	28.6	16.1
d'	−0.17	0.22	0.20	0.42*	1.36**	2.69**

In two control experiments, subjects were fully informed of the precise structure of the stimuli and were then presented with trials with numerical primes intermixed with trials in which the primes were omitted (explicit detection, task 1; six subjects, 96 trials per cell) or replaced by random strings with the same number of characters (number versus letter-string discrimination, task 2; seven subjects, 112 trials per cell). Prime duration was systematically varied. At the prime duration used in the main experiments (43 ms), subjects consistently reported not seeing the numerical primes (task 1), did not respond differently to prime-absent and prime-present trials (task 1) and were unable to discriminate numerical primes from letter strings (task 2). Discrimination performance, as measured by d', a bias-free measure of stimulus discriminability derived from signal-detection theory, began to deviate from chance only for a prime duration of 57 ms or more (χ^2 test; asterisk indicates $P < 0.05$; double asterisk indicates $P < 0.001$).

In response-locked averages, before the large positive deviation which reflected the activation of motor circuits on the correct response side, the LRP showed a significant difference in the predicted direction between congruent and incongruent trials (one-tailed $P = 0.015$). In incongruent trials, the LRP showed a significant negative deviation (one-tailed $P = 0.005$), indicating motor preparation on the incorrect side of response, whereas in congruent trials a nonsignificant positive deviation occurred (one-tailed $P = 0.22$). Hence, a period of covert prime-induced response competition preceded the overt execution of the correct response.

Covert prime processing could be observed even more directly. Because the primes and targets were varied independently in the experimental list, we could test their impact on ERP recordings separately. Primes that induced a co-

vert left-hand or right-hand bias produced a distinct pattern of brain activity over the left and right motor cortices (figure 10.4). Primes that were associated with the left hand during a given block caused a contralateral right-hemispheric negativity, and primes that were associated with the right hand caused a left-hemispheric negativity. This covert motor priming effect had a similar scalp topography to the overt motor effect that was found before the actual motor response to the target, but it was smaller and arrived earlier.

Because ERPs have a notoriously imprecise spatial resolution, we wanted to confirm that covert priming originated at least in part from motor circuits using the spatially accurate method of functional magnetic resonance imaging (fMRI). Response times recorded during fMRI recording replicated the prime-target congruity effect ($P = 0.0027$; effect size 20 ms). In fMRI, how-

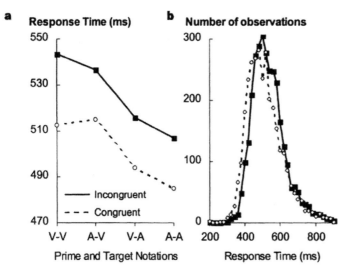

Figure 10.2
Behavioural priming effect. (a) Average correct response times recorded during the ERP experiment are plotted as a function of prime-target congruity for different prime and target notations (A, Arabic; V, verbal). (b) The distribution of correct responses showed a rightward shift in incongruent trials relative to congruent trials (bin size 20 ms).

ever, trials were now separated by 14 s, during which the rise and fall of the haemodynamic signal was measured in the whole brain every 2 s. Although this coarse haemodynamic measure cannot resolve the small activation delays associated with masked priming, we reasoned that it should be proportional to the total brain activity accumulated during a given trial, and should therefore reflect the sum of overt and covert activation in motor areas. We therefore extracted the fMRI signal profile from the left and right motor cortices, and used it to derive an index of lateralized motor activation analogous to the LRP, the lateralized bold response (LBR; figure 10.5). This measure showed a highly significant positive peak following each motor response. The LBR was smaller in incongruent trials than in congruent trials. The direction of this effect is identical to that seen in the LRP (figure 10.3b). Both effects indicate a significant prime-induced activation on the wrong response side on incongruent trials

relative to congruent trials, diminishing the overall size of the activation on the correct motor side. Electrical and haemodynamic measures of covert masked priming were complementary: fMRI localized the priming effect to motor cortex, but was insensitive to its time course, whereas ERPs pinpointed the priming effect to a small window of time before the overt target-related motor activation.

Our results resolve the issue of the depth of processing of masked primes.[3] First, the results show that the processing of masked primes is accompanied by measurable modifications of electrical brain activity and of cerebral blood flow. This concurs with the observation of a modulation of amygdala activity by masked visual faces.[11,12] As shown previously,[13,14] brain imaging now has the potential to image unconscious cerebral processing. Second, unconscious activity is not confined to brain areas involved in sensory processing. Even areas involved in motor

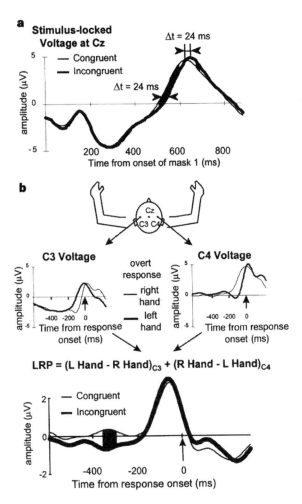

Figure 10.3
ERP measures of prime-target congruity. (a) A late positivity (P3) recorded from the vertex from electrode Cz showed a significant delay in incongruent trials relative to congruent trials (shaded areas, $P < 0.05$). (b) Derivation of the lateralized readiness potential (LRP). Individual trials were averaged in synchrony with the time of the key press, thus suppressing the effects of response delays. Electrodes C3 and C4 showed large voltage differences in opposite directions (top two graphs) before left-hand versus right-hand responses, reflecting the activation of the underlying motor circuits. The LRP (bottom) is the average of the differences at C3 and at C4, calculated according to the formula shown. In incongruent trials, before the main positive-going wave-form reflecting overt response preparation, the LRP was significantly more negative than in congruent trials (shaded areas, $P < 0.05$), reflecting covert motor priming.

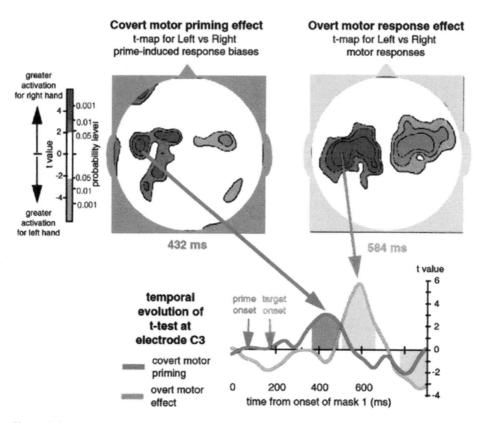

Figure 10.4

ERP measures of covert and overt motor activation. At each electrode site, two independent *t*-tests were performed on scalp voltages. The first test compared trials with overt target-induced right-hand or left-hand responses (green curve and top right map). The second test compared trials with primes inducing a covert left-hand or right-hand bias (orange curve and top left map). Statistical parameter maps in polar coordinates (top) show colour-coded *t*-test values at each site on the scalp, at the delay at which the effect was maximal. The sign and topography of the covert motor priming effect and of the overt motor response effect are similar, indicating that primes and targets were processed in a similar way according to task instructions. The bottom curve shows the temporal evolution of the two independent *t*-tests at electrode site C3, positioned over the left motor cortex (coloured areas, $P < 0.05$). The covert effect preceded the overt effect by 152 ms, a delay roughly comparable to the interval between the onsets of the prime and target (114 ms).

programming were covertly activated here, depending on the side of the motor response that subjects should have made if they had responded to the primes according to the task instructions. Because this motor parameter was determined by whether the prime was larger or smaller than 5, the prime must have been categorized at the semantic level. By showing that a large amount of cerebral processing, including perception, semantic categorization and task execution, can be performed in the absence of consciousness, our results narrow down the search for its cerebral substrates.

Methods

Procedure

All experiments were approved by the French ethical committee for biomedical research, and subjects gave informed consent. The stimulus set consisted of 64 pairs of prime and target numbers 1, 4, 6 and 9, each in either Arabic or spelled-out format. Subjects performed the number-comparison task twice in counterbalanced order. In one block, the instruction was to press the right-hand key for targets larger than 5 and the left-hand key for targets smaller than 5. In another block, the opposite instruction was used. Within each block, subjects received initial training (ERPs, 16 trials; fMRI, 25 trials) before the experimental session (ERPs, 256 trials; fMRI, 64 trials).

Event-Related Potentials

Twelve subjects were tested (six males; mean age 25; one other subject was rejected because of excessive motion). We presented a total of 512 stimuli at a 3-s rate on a standard PC-compatible SVGA screen (EGA mode, 70 Hz refresh rate). The electroencephalogram was digitized at 125 Hz from 128 scalp electrodes referenced to the vertex,[15] for a 2,048-ms period starting 400 ms before the onset of the first mask. We rejected trials with incorrect responses, voltages exceeding $\pm$ 100 μV, transients exceeding $\pm$ 50 μV, electro-oculogram activity exceeding $\pm$ 70 μV, or response times outside a 250–1,000-ms interval. The remaining trials were averaged in synchrony either with stimulus or with response onset, digitally transformed to an average reference, band-pass filtered (0.5–20 Hz), and corrected for baseline over a 400-ms window before stimulus onset (similar results were observed with the raw, unfiltered data). Experimental conditions were compared by sample-by-sample t-tests on electrodes C3, C4 and Cz, with a criterion of $P < 0.05$ for five consecutive samples. Two-dimensional maps of scalp voltage and t-values were constructed by spherical spline interpolation.[16]

Functional Magnetic Resonance Imaging

Nine new subjects were tested (seven males; mean age 26). We used an event-related design.[17] We presented a list of 128 randomly intermixed stimuli through mirror glasses and an active matrix video projector (EGA mode, 70 Hz refresh rate), with a 14-s interstimulus interval. In each trial, stimulus onset was synchronized with the acquisition of the first slice in a series of seven volumes of eighteen slices each. We used a gradient-echo echo-planar imaging sequence sensitive to brain oxygen-level-dependent contrast (18 contiguous axial slices, 6-mm thickness, repetition time/echo time = 2,000/40 ms, in-plane resolution 3×4 mm^2, 64×64 matrix) on a 3-Tesla whole-body system (Bruker). High-resolution anatomical images (three-dimensional gradient-echo inversion-recovery sequence, inversion time = 700 ms, repetition time = 1,600 ms, field of view = 192×256 mm^2, matrix = $256 \times 128 \times 256$, slice thickness = 1 mm) were also acquired.

Analysis was done with SPM96 software. Images were corrected for subject motion, normalized to Talairach coordinates using a linear

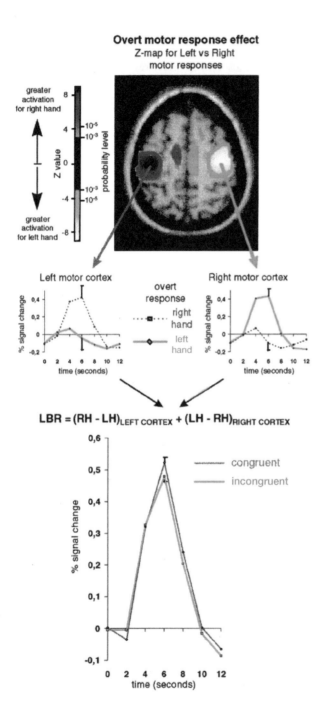

Overt motor response effect
Z-map for Left vs Right
motor responses

$$LBR = (RH - LH)_{LEFT\ CORTEX} + (LH - RH)_{RIGHT\ CORTEX}$$

Figure 10.5

fMRI measure of motor priming. (Top) Voxels that showed significant differences in bold signal intensity between overt left-hand and right-hand responses are coded using the colour scale at left. The two voxels with the most significant overt motor effects were located in the left and right precentral cortex (Talairach coordinate -39, -21, 66 and 39, -15, 63). Centre, plots of the average fMRI signal of the two voxels as a function of time show activation for contralateral movements following a haemodynamic delay of about 4–8 s (planned contrast for an increase in left-right differences from baseline (time points 0 and 2 s) to activated state (time points 4, 6, and 8 s): left motor cortex, $F(1,8) = 20.1$, $P = 0.0021$; right motor cortex, $F(1,8) = 27.0$, $P = 0.0001$). Bottom, it was therefore possible to construct an fMRI measure similar to the event-related LRP, indexing the time course of overt motor activation, which we term the lateralized bold response (LBR). The LBR was significantly larger ($+9\%$) in congruent trials than in incongruent trials (interaction of the congruity factor with the baseline-to-activated-state contrast, $F(1,8) = 6.23$, $P = 0.037$).

transform calculated on the anatomical images, smoothed (full-width at half-maximum = 15 mm), and averaged to define four types of event (congruent or incongruent × left-hand or right-hand response). Images from all nine subjects were then analysed together. We used the generalized linear model to model the intensity level of each pixel as a linear combination, for each subject and each event type, of two activation functions with haemodynamic lags 4 and 7 s, thus allowing for differences in acquisition and activation times across slices and brain regions. We used a voxelwise significance level of 0.001, corrected to $P < 0.05$ for multiple comparisons across the brain volume.

References

1. Marcel, A. J. Conscious and unconscious perception: experiments on visual masking and word recognition. *Cogn. Psychol.* 15, 197–237 (1983).

2. Forster, K. I. & Davis, C. Repetition priming and frequency attenuation in lexical access. *J. Exp. Psychol. Learn. Mem. Cogn.* 10, 680–698 (1984).

3. Holender, D. Semantic activation without conscious identification in dichotic listening, parafoveal vision and visual masking: a survey and appraisal. *Behav. Brain Sci.* 9, 1–23 (1986).

4. Cheesman, J. & Merikle, P. M. Priming with and without awareness. *Percept. Psychophys.* 36, 387–395 (1984).

5. Merikle, P. M. Perception without awareness: critical issues. *Am. Psychol.* 47, 792–796 (1992).

6. Dehaene, S. & Akhavein, R. Attention, automaticity and levels of representation in number processing. *J. Exp. Psychol. Learn. Mem. Cogn.* 21, 314–326 (1995).

7. McCarthy, G. & Donchin, E. A metric for thought: a comparison of P300 latency and reaction time. *Science* 211, 77–80 (1981).

8. Coles, M. G. H., Gratton, G. & Donchin, E. Detecting early communication: using measures of movement-related potentials to illuminate human processing. *Biol. Psychol.* 26, 69–89 (1988).

9. Miller, J. O. & Hackley, S. A. Electrophysiological evidence for temporal overlap among contingent mental processes. *J. Exp. Psychol. Gen.* 121, 195–209 (1992).

10. van Turennout, M., Hagoort, P. & Brown, C. M. Brain activity during speaking: from syntax to phonology in 40 milliseconds. *Science* 280, 572–574 (1998).

11. Whalen, P. J. et al. Masked presentations of emotional facial expressions modulate amygdala activity without explicit knowledge. *J. Neurosci.* 18, 411–418 (1998).

12. Morris, J. S., Öhman, A. & Dolan, R. J. Conscious and unconscious emotional learning in the human amygdala. *Nature* 393, 467–470 (1998).

13. Berns, G. S., Cohen, J. D. & Mintun, M. A. Brain regions responsive to novelty in the absence of awareness. *Science* 276, 1272–1275 (1997).

14. Sahraie, A. et al. Pattern of neuronal activity associated with conscious and unconscious processing

of visual signals. *Proc. Natl Acad. Sci. USA* 94, 9406–9411 (1997).

15. Tucker, D. Spatial sampling of head electrical fields: the geodesic electrode net. *Electroencephalogr. Clin. Neurophysiol.* 87, 154–163 (1993).

16. Perrin, F., Pernier, J., Bertrand, D. & Echallier, J. F. Spherical splines for scalp potential and current density mapping. *Electroencephalogr. Clin. Neurophysiol.* 72, 184–187 (1989).

17. Buckner, R. L. et al. Detection of cortical activation during averaged single trials of a cognitive task using functional magnetic resonance imaging. *Proc. Natl Acad. Sci. USA* 93, 14878–14883 (1996).

Storage and Executive Processes in the Frontal Lobes

Edward E. Smith and John Jonides

The frontal cortex comprises a third of the human brain; it is the structure that enables us to engage in higher cognitive functions such as planning and problem solving (1). What are the processes that serve as the building blocks of these higher cognitive functions, and how are these implemented in the frontal cortex?

Recent discussions of this issue have focused on working memory, a system used for temporary storage and manipulation of information. The system is divided into two general components: short-term storage and a set of "executive processes." Short-term storage involves active maintenance of a limited amount of information for a matter of seconds; it is a necessary component of many higher cognitive functions (2) and is mediated in part by the prefrontal cortex (PFC) (3). Executive processes are implemented by PFC as well (4). Although executive processes often operate on the contents of short-term storage, the two components of working memory can be dissociated: there are neurological patients who have intact short-term storage but defective executive processes and vice versa (5).

We review here neuroimaging studies of these two components of working memory. We consider experiments that have used positron emission tomography (PET) or functional magnetic resonance imaging (fMRI) to image participants while they engage in cognitive tasks that are designed to reveal processes of interest, such as tasks that isolate short-term storage of verbal material. We concentrate on studies in which participants performed an experimental and a control task while being scanned and in which the control task has typically been chosen so that it differs from the experimental task only in a process of interest; a comparison of the experimental and control tasks thus reveals activations due to the process of interest (6). These paradigms contrast with standard neuropsychological tasks that may have diagnostic value for patients with frontal cortical lesions but that do not reveal individual cognitive processes.

Storage Processes and the Frontal Lobes

Many neuroimaging studies are founded on Baddeley's (7) model of working memory. In part, it posits separate storage buffers for verbal and visual-spatial information. Baddeley further argued that verbal storage can be decomposed into a phonological buffer for short-term maintenance of phonological information and a subvocal rehearsal process that refreshes the contents of the buffer. We examine evidence about each aspect of this model as it relates to frontal cortex.

Verbal Storage

Some evidence about storage mechanisms comes from experiments with the item-recognition task (8) (figure 11.1A). In most of these studies, a small set of target letters was presented simultaneously, followed by an unfilled delay interval of several seconds, followed by a single-letter probe; the participant's task was to decide whether the probe matched any of the target letters. Compared with a control task, the item-recognition task results in activations in the left posterior parietal cortex [Brodmann's area (BA) 40] and three frontal sites [Broca's area (BA 44) and left supplementary motor and premotor areas (BA 6)]. (The latter three areas, along with other important frontal areas and divisions, are presented schematically in figure 11.2.) Given that these frontal areas are known to be involved in the preparation of speech (9) and that participants rehearse the targets silently during the delay, the frontal speech areas likely mediate subvocal rehearsal of the targets. As evidence for this claim, the activation in Broca's area closely matches that obtained in an explicitly phonological task,

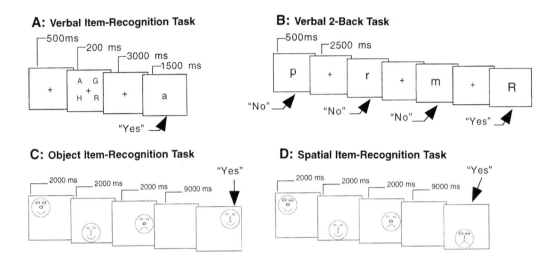

Figure 11.1
Schematic representations of four tasks used to study working memory. (A) Verbal item-recognition task, which taps mainly short-term storage for verbal information. A trial includes (i) fixation point, (ii) four uppercase letters, (iii) blank delay interval, and (iv) a lowercase probe letter. The participant's task is to decide whether the probe names one of the four target letters. (B) Verbal 2-back task, which presumably involves executive processes (temporal coding) as well as storage of verbal material. Each letter is followed by a blank delay interval, and the participant's task is to decide whether each letter has the same name as the one that occurred two back in the sequence. (C) Object item-recognition task, which taps short-term storage for object information. A trial includes (i) a sequence of three target faces, (ii) a blank delay interval, and (iii) a probe face. The participant's task is to decide whether the probe face is the same as any of the target faces. (D) Spatial item-recognition task, which taps short-term storage for spatial information. A trial includes the same events as in the object task, but the participant's task is to decide whether the probe face is in the same location as any of the target faces.

rhyme judgments (10). [Evidence from neurological patients suggests that the posterior parietal region mediates a storage buffer (11, 12).]

Further evidence for localizing rehearsal in the frontal speech areas comes from a PET study that used a "2-back" task (13) (see figure 11.1B). Participants viewed a sequence of single letters separated by 2.5 s each; for each letter they had to decide whether it was identical in name to the letter that appeared two items back in the sequence. The experiment used two different controls. In one, participants saw a sequence of letters but simply had to decide whether each letter matched a single target letter. Subtracting this control from the 2-back condition yielded many of the areas of activation that have been obtained in item-recognition tasks, including the left frontal speech regions and the parietal area. The second control required participants to rehearse each letter silently. Subtracting this rehearsal control from the 2-back task should have removed much of the rehearsal circuitry since rehearsal is needed in both tasks; indeed, in this subtraction, neither Broca's area nor the premotor area remained active. Hence, this experiment isolated a frontal rehearsal circuit.

Several other PET and fMRI studies have used 2-back and 3-back tasks. All have found activa-

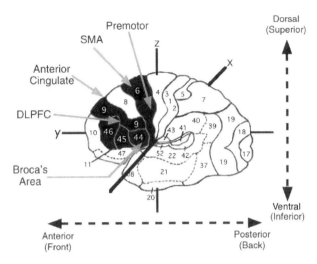

Figure 11.2
Schematic of the left lateral cortex, displaying major prefrontal areas (numbers correspond to Brodmann areas). The areas of greatest interest are shaded, and they include Broca's area, DLPFC, the anterior cingulate (not visible in the schematic, as it lies on the medial side of the cortex), SMA, and premotor. Also shown are the x, y, and z dimensions, which are used to report the coordinates of activations (where the three dimensions intersect, all coordinates are zero). In addition, anterior-posterior and dorsal-ventral directions, which are used in anatomical descriptions, are indicated.

tion in Broca's area and the premotor cortex (14, 15). In addition, two studies have used a free-recall paradigm to study short-term storage, and they also found activation in frontal speech regions (16). Thus, frontal regions that no doubt evolved for the purpose of spoken language appear to be recruited to keep verbal information active in working memory.

Figure 11.3 summarizes the relevant results; figure 11.3A shows data from item-recognition tasks, which require mainly storage, whereas figure 11.3B shows data from *n*-back tasks and free-recall tasks, which presumably require executive processes as well as storage. In figure 11.3A, in the sagittal view, the activations cluster posteriorly in the frontal lobes—running from the premotor and supplementary motor area (SMA) ventrally to Broca's area; this is the rehearsal circuit. In the coronal and axial views of figure

11.3A, the activation foci show a left lateral tendency; indeed, the mean x coordinate is significantly less than zero [$t(31) = -2.9$; $P < 0.01$], indicating a center of mass in the left hemisphere. The lateralization pattern changes when nonstorage processes are added to the task. In the axial and coronal projections of figure 11.3B, the activation foci were bilateral, not left-lateralized. Furthermore, in addition to the clusters in premotor and SMA, Broca's, and posterior parietal lobe, these tasks also produce a cluster in dorsolateral prefrontal cortex (DLPFC), as shown in the sagittal view of figure 11.3B. In fact, the mean y coordinate of frontal activations ($y > 0.25$) in figure 11.3B is significantly anterior to that in figure 11.3A [$t(79,52) = 4.18$; $P < 0.001$]. These activations therefore reflect the distinction between tasks requiring mainly storage and those requiring additional processing.

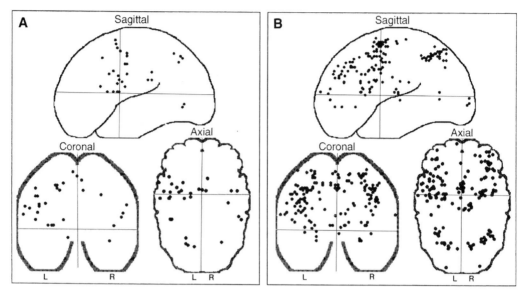

Figure 11.3
Neuroimaging results for verbal working memory are summarized by sets of three projections, with each containing points and axes conforming to standard Talairach space.[40] Each projection collapses one plane of view for each activation focus—that is, the sagittal view collapses across the x plane as though one were looking through the brain from the side; the coronal view collapses across the y plane as though one were looking through the brain from the front or back; and the axial view collapses across the z plane as though one were looking through the brain from the top. Included in the summary are published [15]O PET or fMRI studies of verbal working memory that reported coordinates of activation and had a memory load of six or fewer items. (Cerebellar activation foci, not shown, were predominantly in the right hemisphere, which is consistent with the crossed connections of cerebellum and cerebrum.) (A) Activation foci from studies that involve mainly storage. Awh et al.,[13] item recognition; Jonides et al.,[15] 0- and 1-back; Jonides et al.,[33] item recognition; Paulesu et al.,[10] item recognition. (B) Activation foci from studies that require executive processing as well as storage. Awh et al.,[13] 2-back; Braver et al.,[15] 2- and 3-back; Cohen et al.,[14] 2-back; Cohen et al.,[15] 2- and 3-back; D'Espositio et al.,[28] 2-back; Fiez et al.,[16] free recall; Jonides et al.,[15] 2- and 3-back; Jonides et al.,[16] free recall; Schumacher et al.,[15] 3-back; Smith et al.,[15] 3-back.

Spatial and Object Storage

Research on nonverbal working memory has been influenced by physiological work with non-human primates (3). Single-cell recordings made while monkeys engage in spatial-storage tasks have found "spatial memory" cells in DLPFC (which is usually taken to include BA 46 and 9). These cells selectively fire during a delay period and are position specific. Recordings made while monkeys engage in object-storage tasks have found delay-sensitive "object memory" cells in a more ventral region of PFC that are object specific (17). The implications of these findings are that (i) spatial and object working memory have different neural bases, and (ii) at least part of the circuitry for these two types of memory is in PFC, with spatial information being represented more dorsally than object information (18).

Neuroimaging evidence supports a distinction between human spatial and object working memory as well (19–21). In one paradigm used to demonstrate the distinction, three target faces were presented sequentially in three different locations, followed by a probe face in a variable location. In the object working-memory task (see figure 11.1C), participants decided whether the probe matched any of the three targets in identity; in the spatial task (see figure 11.1D), they decided whether the probe matched any of the targets in position. The object task activated regions in the right DLPFC whereas the spatial task activated a region in the right premotor cortex. Follow-up studies have shown that the region in DLPFC remains active during a delay period in the object task, whereas the premotor area remains active during a delay in the spatial task, thus strengthening the case that the two areas mediate separate kinds of storage (22, 23).

Figure 11.4 summarizes the relevant results. The sagittal and coronal projections reveal a dorsal-ventral difference between spatial and object working-memory tasks, respectively, particularly in posterior cortex. For posterior cortex ($y > -25$), the average z coordinate of the spatial-memory activation foci was significantly greater (more dorsal) than that of object-memory activation foci [$t(41,45) = 9.87$; $P < 0.001$]. The anterior cortex ($y > -25$) also shows a significant dorsal-ventral difference [$t(37,47) = 3.24$; $P < 0.004$]. Specifically, spatial working-memory activations seem to cluster primarily in the premotor area, whereas object working-memory activations spread from premotor to DLPFC.

Although the dorsal-ventral difference is in line with the results from monkeys, there are two findings from spatial tasks that differ from the results obtained with monkeys: the presence of activation in premotor cortex and the failure to consistently find activation in DLPFC. The first finding has considerable support, as spatial tasks routinely activate the right premotor area

(24). Perhaps the true functional homologue of DLPFC in monkeys is the premotor region in humans (25), or perhaps the major site of spatial working-memory in monkeys is more posterior than was originally believed (18). The issue remains unresolved.

Can the activations obtained in the spatial tasks be divided into storage and rehearsal functions, parallel to verbal working memory? One possibility is that the right premotor activation is a reflection of spatial rehearsal. By this account, spatial rehearsal involves covertly shifting attention from location to location, and doing so requires recruitment of an attentional circuit, including premotor cortex (26). Support for this account comes from the fact that neuroimaging results from studies of spatial working memory and spatial attention show overlap in activation in a right premotor site (27).

Implications

The research reviewed and the meta-analyses presented in figures 11.3 and 11.4 are relevant to two major proposals about the organization of PFC. One is that PFC is organized by the modality of the information stored; for example, spatial information is represented more dorsally than object information (17). The second proposal is that PFC is organized by process, with ventrolateral regions (BA 45 and 47) mediating operations needed to sustain storage and dorsolateral regions (BA 46 and 9) implementing the active manipulation of information held in storage [see references in (28)]. Our review provides support for both organizational principles. Relevant to the first, we have noted that verbal storage tasks activate left-hemisphere speech areas, spatial storage activates the right premotor cortex, and object storage activates more ventral regions of PFC (as shown in figure 11.4). Relevant to the second, verbal tasks that require only storage lead primarily to activations that typically do not extend into DLPFC, whereas verbal tasks that require executive processes as well as

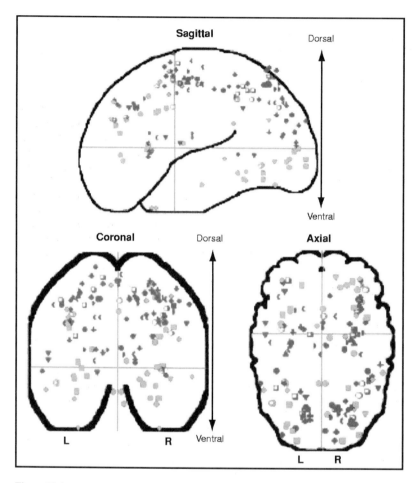

Figure 11.4

Neuroimaging results for spatial (blue) and object (red) working memory are summarized on three projections, with each containing points and axes conforming to standard Talairach space[40] (see figure 11.3 legend). Included in the summary are published ^{15}O PET or fMRI studies of spatial or object working memory that reported coordinates of activation. Courtney et al.[19] ([symbol unavailable]): item recognition (faces), item recognition (locations); Courtney et al.[22] ([symbol unavailable]): item recognition (faces); Courtney et al.[23] ([symbol unavailable]): item recognition (faces), item recognition (locations); D'Esposito et al.[28] ([symbol unavailable]): 2-back (locations); Faillenot et al.[21] ([symbol unavailable]): item recognition (objects), item recognition (orientation); Jonides et al.[24] ([symbol unavailable]): item recognition (locations); McCarthy et al.[19] ([symbol unavailable]): item recognition (locations); Owen et al.[20] ([symbol unavailable]): item recognition (locations), spatial span; Owen et al.[21] ([symbol unavailable]): n-back (locations), n-back (objects); Smith et al.[19] ([symbol unavailable]): item recognition (locations), item recognition (objects); Smith et al.[15] ([symbol unavailable]): 2-back (locations); Sweeney et al.[41] ([symbol unavailable]): memory guided saccades (locations).

storage lead to activations that include DLPFC (figure 11.3) (28).

Executive Processes and Frontal Cortex

Most researchers concur that executive processes are mediated by PFC and are involved in the regulation of processes operating on the contents of working memory. Although there is lack of consensus about a taxonomy of executive processes, there is some agreement that they include (i) focusing attention on relevant information and processes and inhibiting irrelevant ones ("attention and inhibition"); (ii) scheduling processes in complex tasks, which requires the switching of focused attention between tasks ("task management"); (iii) planning a sequence of subtasks to accomplish some goal ("planning"); (iv) updating and checking the contents of working memory to determine the next step in a sequential task ("monitoring"); and (v) coding representations in working memory for time and place of appearance ("coding"). Tasks manifesting each of these executive processes are known to be selectively impaired in patients with prefrontal damage (4). Of the five executive processes noted, the first two appear to be the most elementary and the most interrelated; for these reasons, we focus on attention and inhibition and task management.

Attention and Inhibition

A paradigmatic case of attention and inhibition is the Stroop test (29). Participants are presented a set of color names printed in different colors and asked to report the print colors; performance is poorer when the print color differs from the color name than when it is the same (it takes longer to say blue to the word red printed in blue than to the word blue printed in blue). The effect arises because two processes are in conflict: a prepotent one that automatically names the word and a weaker but task-relevant process that names the print color. Successful performance requires focusing attention on the task-relevant process and inhibiting the task-irrelevant one (30). More generally, the executive process of attention and inhibition is recruited whenever two processes are in conflict.

PET studies of the Stroop test show substantial variation in regions of activation, although one broad region is the anterior one-third of cingulate cortex (31). Activations in the anterior cingulate have been obtained in other experiments that induce a conflict between processes or response tendencies as well (32). These studies suggest that the anterior cingulate may be involved in the resolution of cognitive conflict.

If executive processes are indeed distinct from short-term storage, it should be possible to add attention and inhibition to a short-term storage task. Two recent studies have attempted to do this by introducing conflict into the verbal item-recognition task (again, see figure 11.1A) (33, 34). These studies included trials in which distractor probes—probes that were not in the memory set—were familiar, thereby putting into competition a decision based on familiarity and one based on the target items being coded as "current targets." Conflict led to activation in the left lateral prefrontal cortex, however, not the anterior cingulate.

Why are different areas of activation found in studies of attention and inhibition? One possibility is that the anterior-cingulate region mediates the inhibition of preprogrammed responses. Incorrect responses may often be preprogrammed in tasks such as Stroop's but not in the item-recognition task; hence, only the former would recruit the cingulate region. By contrast, the frontal site activated in studies of item-recognition may reflect operation of attention and inhibition earlier in the processing sequence. This interpretation is consistent with an fMRI study in which participants were led to prepare a response to an expected probe but on occasional trials had to respond differently to an unexpected probe and hence had to inhibit the prepared response (35). Statistical techniques were used to isolate trials that should have involved response inhibition; analyses of these trials revealed activations in the anterior cingulate, not in prefrontal cortex (36, 37).

Task Management

A canonical case of task management arises when participants are presented with dual tasks. For example, they might be presented a series of numbers and have to add three to the first number, subtract three from the second, and so on through successive trials (38). Both tasks require some nonautomatic or "controlled" processes, and a critical aspect of task management is switching from one controlled process to another.

An fMRI study has examined dual-task performance (39). In one task, participants had to decide whether each word presented in a series named an instance of the category Vegetable; in the other task, participants had to decide whether two visual displays differed only by a matter of rotation; in the dual-task condition, participants performed the categorization and rotation tasks concurrently. Only the dual-task condition activated frontal areas, including DLPFC (BA 46) and the anterior cingulate. The frontal areas overlap those found in attention and inhibition tasks, but in this case the anterior cingulate does not dominate the picture. The communality of results should be expected if a critical component of scheduling is management of the same attentional process that is involved in attention and inhibition tasks.

Concluding Remarks

Neuroimaging studies of humans show that storage and executive processes are major functions of the frontal cortex. The distinction between short-term storage and executive processes appears to be a major organizational principle

of PFC. With regard to storage, the PFC areas most consistently activated show modality specificity (verbal versus spatial versus object information), and generally they appear to mediate rehearsal processes, at least for verbal and spatial information. Neuroimaging analyses of executive processes are quite recent, and they have yet to lead to clear dissociations between processes. Perhaps the highest priority, then, is to turn further attention to executive processes and their implementation in frontal cortex.

References and Notes

1. A. R. Luria, *Higher Cortical Functions in Man* (Basic Books, New York, 1966).
2. P. A. Carpenter, M. A. Just, P. Shell, *Psychol. Rev.* 97, 404 (1990).
3. J. M. Fuster, *The Prefrontal Cortex: Anatomy, Physiology, and Neuropsychology of the Frontal Lobe* (Lippincott-Raven, New York, 1997); P. S. Goldman-Rakic, in *Handbook of Physiology. Nervous System,* vol. 5, Higher Functions of the Brain, F. Plum, Ed. (American Physiological Society, Bethesda, MD, 1987), pp. 373–417.
4. D. T. Stuss and D. F. Benson, *The Frontal Lobes* (Raven, New York, 1986).
5. M. D'Esposito and B. R. Postle, *Attention and Performance XVIII* (Academic Press, New York, in press).
6. M. I. Posner, S. E. Petersen, P. T. Fox, M. E. Raichle, *Science* 240, 1627 (1988).
7. A. Baddeley, *Working Memory* (Clarendon Press/Oxford Univ. Press, Oxford, 1986).
8. E. E. Smith, J. Jonides, C. Marshuetz, R. A. Koeppe, *Proc. Natl. Acad. Sci. U.S.A.* 95, 876 (1998).
9. J. M. Fuster, *Memory in the Cerebral Cortex: An Empirical Approach to Neural Networks in the Human and Nonhuman Primate* (MIT Press, Cambridge, MA, 1995).
10. E. Paulesu, C. D. Frith, R. S. Frackowiak, *Nature* 362, 342 (1993).
11. T. Shallice, *From Neuropsychology to Mental Structure* (MIT Press, Cambridge, MA, 1988).
12. None of the cited item-recognition studies found activation in DLPFC. However, a recent item-

recognition experiment found DLPFC activation with a memory load of six items compared with three items, which suggests a role for DLPFC with larger memory loads (B. Rypma, V. Prabhakaran, J. E. Desmond, *Neuroimage,* in press). Follow-up work suggests that the role of DLPFC in this task is to mediate executive processes during encoding of the larger loads (M. D'Esposito, personal communication).

13. E. Awh et al., *Psychol. Sci.* 7, 125 (1996).

14. J. D. Cohen et al., *Hum. Brain Mapp.* 1, 293 (1994).

15. E. H. Schumacher et al., *Neuroimage* 3, 79 (1996); E. E. Smith, J. Jonides, R. A. Koeppe, *Cereb. Cortex* 6, 11 (1996); T. S. Braver, J. D. Cohen, J. Jonides, E. E. Smith, D. C. Noll, *Neuroimage* 5, 49 (1997); J. D. Cohen et al., *Nature* 386, 604 (1997); J. Jonides et al., *J. Cognit. Neurosci.* 9, 462 (1997).

16. J. A. Fiez et al., *J. Neurosci.* 16, 808 (1996); J. Jonides et al., *ibid.* 18, 5026 (1998).

17. F. A. Wilson, S. P. Scalaidhe, P. S. Goldman-Rakic, *Science* 260, 1955 (1993).

18. There is currently some controversy about the degree of separation of object and spatial regions in PFC in nonhuman primates. Recent findings indicate that dorsal or ventral regions can contain neurons that process either spatial or object information or both [S. C. Rao, G. Rainer, E. K. Miller, *Science* 276, 821 (1997); G. Rainer, W. F. Asaad, E. K. Miller, *Proc. Natl. Acad. Sci. U.S.A.* 95, 15008 (1998)]. However, even these studies find some neural segregation—a sizable proportion of neurons tested by Rainer et al. are selective only for location, and these neurons predominate in posterior locations.

19. E. E. Smith et al., *J. Cogn. Neurosci.* 7, 337 (1995); G. B. McCarthy et al., *Proc. Natl. Acad. Sci. U.S.A.* 91, 8690 (1994); S. M. Courtney, L. G. Ungerleider, K. Keil, *Cereb. Cortex* 6, 39 (1996).

20. A. M. Owen, A. C. Evans, M. Petrides, *Cereb. Cortex.* 6, 31 (1996).

21. I. Faillenot, H. Sakata, N. Costes, *Neuroreport* 8, 859 (1997); A. M. Owen et al., *Proc. Natl. Acad. Sci. U.S.A.* 95, 7721 (1998).

22. M. Courtney, L. G. Ungerleider, K. Keil, J. V. Haxby, *Nature* 386, 608 (1997).

23. S. M. Courtney, L. Petit, J. M. Maisog, L. G. Ungerleider, J. V. Haxby, *Science* 279, 1347 (1998).

24. J. Jonides et al., *Nature* 363, 623 (1993); P. A. Reuter-Lorenz et al., in press; references cited in (19, 21).

25. L. G. Ungerleider, S. M. Courtney, J. V. Haxby, *Proc. Natl. Acad. Sci. U.S.A.* 95, 883 (1998).

26. E. Awh, J. Jonides, P. A. Reuter-Lorenz, *J. Exp. Psychol. Hum. Percept. Perform.* 24, 780 (1998).

27. E. Awh and J. Jonides, in *The Attentive Brain,* R. Parasurama, Ed. (MIT Press, Cambridge, MA, 1997), pp. 353–380.

28. Two other recent meta-analyses of neuroimaging studies of working memory also found evidence that PFC is organized by storage versus executive processes [M. D'Esposito et al., *Cogn. Brain Res.* 7, 1 (1998); A. M. Owen, *Eur. J. Neurosci.* 9, 1329 (1997)]. However, neither of these meta-analyses found evidence that PFC was organized by modality. There are at least two reasons for this discrepancy from the present analyses. Neither of the previous meta-analyses focused on verbal storage or included recent fMRI studies that isolate delay-period activity and that provide relatively strong evidence for a difference between spatial and object storage (22, 23).

29. J. R. Stroop, *J. Exp. Psychol.* 18, 643 (1935).

30. F. N. Dyer, *Mem. Cogn.* 1, 106 (1973); J. D. Cohen, K. Dunbar, J. L. McClelland, *Psychol. Rev.* 97, 332 (1990); C. M. Macleod, *Psychol. Bull.* 109, 163 (1991).

31. J. V. Pardo, P. J. Pardo, K. W. Janer, *Proc. Natl. Acad. Sci. U.S.A.* 87, 256 (1990); C. J. Bench et al., *Neuropsychologia* 31, 907 (1993); C. S. Carter, M. Mintun, J. D. Cohen, *Neuroimage* 2, 264 (1995); M. S. George et al., *J. Neuropsychol. Clin. Neurosci.* 9, 55 (1997); S. F. Taylor, S. Kornblum, E. J. Lauber, *Neuroimage* 6, 81 (1997); S. W. Derbyshire, B. A. Vogt, A. K. Jones, *Exp. Brain Res.* 118, 52 (1998).

32. S. F. Taylor, S. Kornblum, S. Minoshima, *Neuropsychologia* 32, 249 (1994); M. Iacoboni, R. P. Woods, J. C. Mazziotta, *J. Neurophysiol.* 76, 321 (1996); G. Bush, P. J. Whalen, B. R. Rosen, *Hum. Brain Mapp.* 6, 270 (1998).

33. J. Jonides, E. E. Smith, C. Marshuetz, R. A. Koeppe, P. A. Reuter-Lorenz, *Proc. Natl. Acad. Sci. U.S.A.* 95, 8410 (1998).

34. M. D'Esposito et al., paper presented at Cognitive Neuroscience Society Meeting, San Francisco (1998).

35. C. S. Carter et al., *Science* 280, 74 (1998).

36. The anterior cingulate is also activated in tasks that do not involve response inhibition, indicating that the cingulate serves multiple functions. [R. D. Badgaiyan and M. I. Posner, *Neuroimage* 7, 255 (1998); P. J. Whalen et al., *Biol. Psychiatry* 44, 1219 (1998).

37. Attention and inhibition may also be involved in self-ordering tasks, such as the following: on each series of trials, a set of forms is presented in random positions, and participants must point to a form they have not selected on a previous trial in that series. This task activates the anterior cingulate and DLPFC, similar to tasks that involve attention and inhibition [M. Petrides, B. Alivisatos, A. C. Evans, *Proc. Natl. Acad. Sci. U.S.A.* 90, 873 (1993)]. Some researchers have proposed that self-ordering tasks reflect the executive process of monitoring, but alternatively they may involve an appreciable working memory load and some inhibition, either of which may cause the frontal activations.

38. A. Spector and I. Biederman, *Am. J. Psychol.* 89, 669 (1976).

39. M. D'Esposito et al., *Nature* 378, 279 (1995).

40. J. Talairach and P. Tournoux, *A Co-Planar Stereotaxic Atlas of the Human Brain: An Approach to Medical Cerebral Imaging* (Thieme, New York, 1988).

41. J. A. Sweeney et al., *J. Neurophysiol.* 75, 454 (1996).

42. Supported by grants from the National Institute on Aging and the Office of Naval Research. We are indebted to the members of our laboratory for discussion of these issues and to D. Badre for his substantial contributions to the preparation of this manuscript.

12   Memory—A Century of Consolidation

James L. McGaugh

A century has passed since Müller and Pilzecker proposed the perseveration-consolidation hypothesis of memory (1). In pioneering studies with human subjects, they found that memory of newly learned information was disrupted by the learning of other information shortly after the original learning and suggested that processes underlying new memories initially persist in a fragile state and consolidate over time. At the beginning of this new millennium, the consolidation hypothesis still guides research investigating the time-dependent involvement of neural systems and cellular processes enabling lasting memory (2–4).

Retrograde Amnesia and Memory Enhancement

Clinical evidence that cerebral trauma induces loss of recent memory was reported two decades before the publication of Müller and Pilzecker's monograph, and shortly after its publication, it was noted that the consolidation hypothesis provided an explanation for such retrograde amnesia (5). Ignored for almost half a century, the consolidation hypothesis was reinvigorated in 1949, when two papers reported that electroconvulsive shock induced retrograde amnesia in rodents (6, 7), triggering a burst of studies of experimentally induced retrograde amnesia (2–4). That same year, Hebb and Gerard proposed dual-trace theories of memory, suggesting that the stabilization of reverberating neural activity underlying short-term memory produces long-term memory (7, 8). The finding that protein synthesis inhibitors did not prevent the learning of tasks but disrupted memory of the training (9) supports the view that there are (at least) two stages of memory and indicates that protein synthesis is required only for consolidation of long-term memory. The issue of whether short- and long-term memory (and, perhaps, other memory stages) (figure 12.1) are sequentially linked, as

proposed by Hebb and Gerard, or act independently in parallel (3, 10) remains central to current inquiry. The discovery that stimulant drugs administered within minutes or hours after training enhance memory consolidation further stimulated studies of memory consolidation (3, 10, 11). The use of treatments administered shortly after training to impair or enhance memory provides a highly effective and extensively used method of influencing memory consolidation without affecting either acquisition or memory retrieval (11).

Endogenous Modulation of Consolidation

Memory consolidation appears to be a useful function, because evidence of consolidation is found in a wide variety of animal species (12, 13). Why do our memories and those of other animals consolidate slowly? The answer might simply be that the molecular and cellular machinery creating memory works slowly. But that answer is clearly wrong, because "short-term" or "working" memories are created almost immediately. All our cognitive and motor skills require quickly accessible new memory. Furthermore, there is no a priori reason to assume that biological mechanisms are not capable of quickly consolidating memory. Considerable evidence suggests that the slow consolidation of memories serves an adaptive function by enabling endogenous processes activated by an experience to modulate memory strength (14). Emotionally arousing experiences are generally well remembered (15). Adrenal stress hormones, epinephrine and cortisol (corticosterone in the rat), released by emotional arousal appear to play an important role in enabling the significance of an experience to regulate the strength of memory of the experience. Epinephrine (16, 17) and corticosterone (13, 18, 19), as well as drugs that activate adrenergic receptors and glucocorticoid (type II)

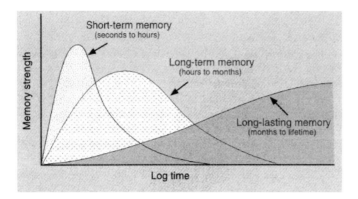

Figure 12.1
Memory consolidation phases. Studies of memory and neuroplasticity support Müller and Pilzecker's hypothesis proposing that the consolidation of new memory into long-term memory is time dependent,[1] but strongly suggest that short-term and different stages of long-term memory are not sequentially linked, as proposed by the dual-trace hypothesis.[9] Evidence that drugs can selectively block either short-term (seconds to hours) or long-term memory (hours to months) suggests that time-dependent stages of memory are based on independent processes acting in parallel. Later stages of consolidation resulting in memory lasting a lifetime likely involve interaction of brain systems in reorganizing and stabilizing distributed connections.

receptors (13, 18, 19), enhance memory for many kinds of training experiences.

Critical Involvement of the Amygdala in Memory Consolidation

Epinephrine does not freely pass the blood-brain barrier and appears to modulate memory consolidation by activating β-adrenergic receptors located peripherally on vagal afferents projecting to the nucleus of the solitary tract in the brainstem. Noradrenergic projections from this region influence neuronal activity in other brain regions, including the amygdala (20). Glucocorticoids released from the adrenal cortex readily enter the brain and activate intracellular glucocorticoid receptors (figure 12.2). Activation of the amygdala, a brain region important for emotional arousal, is critical for mediating the influences of epinephrine and glucocorticoids, because amygdala lesions block the effects of these modulators

on consolidation. Most important, activation of β-adrenergic receptors in the amygdala is essential. Infusions of β-adrenergic receptor antagonists into the amygdala after training block epinephrine effects, whereas infusions of β-adrenergic receptor agonists enhance memory (21). Lesions of the amygdala and infusions of β-adrenergic receptor antagonists into the amygdala also block the memory-modulating effects of drugs affecting systems containing γ-amino-butyric acid (GABA) and opioid peptides (20).

The basolateral nucleus of the amygdala (BLA) mediates the influences of drugs and hormones on memory consolidation. β-Adrenergic receptor agonists infused selectively into the BLA after training enhance memory, and lesions of the BLA or infusion of β-adrenergic receptor antagonists into the BLA block the memory-enhancing effects of systemically administered dexamethasone (a synthetic glucocorticoid) (22, 23). Modulatory influences on consolidation in-

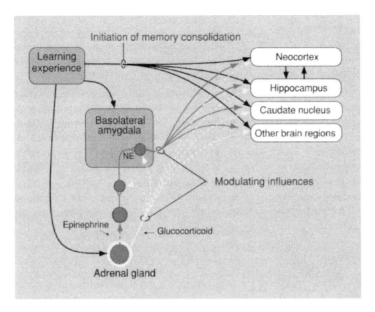

Figure 12.2
Neurobiological systems regulating memory consolidation. Experiences activate time-dependent cellular storage processes in various brain regions involved in the forms of memory represented. The experiences also initiate the release of the stress hormones from the adrenal medulla and adrenal cortex and activate the release of norepinephrine in the basolateral amygdala, an effect critical for enabling modulation of consolidation. The amygdala modulates memory consolidation by influencing neuroplasticity in other brain regions.

clude release of norepinephrine (NE) within the amygdala. For example, foot-shock stimulation induces NE release in the amygdala; administration of epinephrine or drugs that enhance consolidation (such as GABA and opioid receptor antagonists) increases NE release in the amygdala; and the use of drugs that impair memory (such as GABA and opioid receptor agonists) decreases NE release (24).

Locus of Modulation: Brain Systems and Forms of Memory

It is increasingly clear that different brain regions process different forms of memory (25). Evidence from rat studies indicates that the hippocampus and striatum process different forms of memory (26) and that the amygdala modulates consolidation by regulating processing in these brain regions. Amphetamine infused into the dorsal hippocampus after training selectively enhances memory of the spatial localization of a slightly submerged (and thus not visible to the rat) escape platform in a water-maze, whereas amphetamine infused into the striatum selectively enhances memory of a prominent visual cue located on an escape platform placed in varying locations on different training trials. Most important, amphetamine infused into the amygdala after training enhances memory of both types of training. The amygdala is clearly not the locus of the enhanced memory, because inactivation of the amygdala (with lidocaine infusions) before the retention test does not block expression of the enhanced memory for either type of training (27).

Because glucocorticoid receptors are densely located in the hippocampus, these receptors are likely involved in mediating glucocorticoid influences on consolidation (19). Evidence that infusions of a glucocorticoid agonist into the dorsal hippocampus after training enhance memory supports this view. The BLA is critically involved in enabling this glucocorticoid influence. BLA lesions or infusions of β-adrenergic receptor antagonists into the BLA block the effects of glucocorticoids either administered systemically or infused directly into the dorsal hippocampus (23, 28). These findings provide further evidence that modulating influences from the BLA regulate memory consolidation occurring within or mediated by the hippocampus. As discussed below, the molecular and cellular changes mediating the induction of long-term potentiation (LTP) in the hippocampus are widely considered to provide a basis for memory. Thus, it is of considerable interest that lesions of the BLA or infusions of a β-adrenergic receptor antagonist into BLA block the induction of LTP in the dentate gyrus of the hippocampus and that stimulation of the BLA enhances such LTP (29).

It is clear from these findings that memory consolidation involves interactions among neural systems, as well as cellular changes within specific systems, and that amygdala is critical for modulating consolidation in other brain regions. Although research has focused primarily on amygdala influences on memory related to the caudate nucleus and hippocampus, the modulation is most certainly not restricted to these brain regions.

Emotional Arousal and Memory Consolidation in Humans

Although the consolidation hypothesis was based on human memory results, most research on consolidation has studied memory in animals.

The animal memory findings have reactivated interest in human memory consolidation. Amphetamine administered to human subjects either before or after learning of word lists enhances memory of the words (30). Results of human studies, like those of animal studies, indicate that adrenergic systems and amygdala activation influence memory consolidation. Recent studies found that β-adrenergic receptor antagonists block the memory-enhancing effects of emotional arousal (31). Studies examined the effects of β-adrenergic receptor antagonists or a placebo on the memory of pictures accompanied by an emotionally arousing story. Subjects given a placebo before presentation of the pictures and story remembered best the pictures presented during the most emotional part of the story. In contrast, in subjects given a β-adrenergic receptor antagonist, memory for those pictures was not enhanced. β-Adrenergic receptor antagonists (taken as medication) also blocked arousal-induced enhancement of memory in elderly subjects. Emotional arousal also does not enhance long-term memory of the arousing material in human subjects with selective lesions of the amygdala (32). Additionally, studies using PET (positron emission tomography) scans to assess amygdala activity induced by emotionally arousing stimuli (both pleasant and unpleasant) found that long-term memory correlates with the degree of amygdala activation during the original encoding (33).

As Time Goes By: The Orchestration of Consolidation

Changes in brain activity after learning provide additional insights into the time course of consolidation processes. A study of functional brain activity in human subjects (with PET) revealed shifts in activity among different brain regions occurring over a period of several hours after the learning of a motor skill, suggesting that consolidation involves time-dependent reorganization of the brain representation underlying the motor skill (34). Studies of learning-induced changes in receptive fields in the auditory cortex provide additional evidence that neural processes activated by training continue to change for several days, after completion of training (35). Neurons in the auditory cortex of animals given a brief training session in which a specific tone was paired with foot shock subsequently responded more to that tone and less to other tones. Furthermore, the degree of selectivity in the "frequency tuning" continued to increase for several days, suggesting continuing consolidation of the memory of the tone's increased significance. It would be of considerable interest to know whether inactivation of the BLA blocks such consolidation.

Most research on memory consolidation examined the effects of treatments administered within several hours after training. It cannot be concluded from such research that consolidation is completed within hours, because the effectiveness of a treatment in modulating consolidation depends on the locus and mechanism(s) of action of the treatment, as well as the state of consolidation when the treatment is administered (14). Lesions of the hippocampus (or adjacent cortical areas) and sustained drug infusions into the hippocampus impair memory for training given days, or even weeks, earlier (36). Thus, although the hippocampus and anatomically related structures are no doubt involved in consolidation, and may well be a locus of temporary neural changes that influence the establishment of long-term memory, those brain regions are clearly not unique loci of long-term memory. This conclusion was first drawn from studies of the patient H.M. after bilateral surgical excision of his medial temporal lobes (37) The hippocampus may have a long-term or perhaps even a sustained role in consolidating memory (36, 38). Such consolidation may involve extensive interaction of the hippocampus and related cortex with the neocortex as well as other brain regions, serving to link the sites and enable regions to strengthen or reorganize connections with the others, as well as to organize and reorganize the information being consolidated (38, 39).

Cellular Machinery of Consolidation

Because of evidence suggesting that the hippocampus is active in memory consolidation (for some forms or aspects of memory), as well as the hypothesis that cellular and molecular mechanisms underlying LTP may enable memory consolidation, the relation between hippocampal LTP and memory is the focus of intense investigation (40, 41). It is important to note that because the cellular and molecular changes occur mostly within hours after LTP induction or training, they are reasonable candidates for consolidation mechanisms occurring within that time frame. Different processes occurring in other brain regions are likely involved in memory consolidation occurring over days, months, or years (36).

As discussed above, extensive evidence indicates that the BLA influences memory processes and LTP in other brain regions. Treatments known to affect memory consolidation also modulate the maintenance of hippocampal LTP in freely moving rats (42). Water given to thirsty rats within 30 min after induction of LTP enhanced the maintenance of LTP. Foot shock administered after LTP induction also enhanced LTP. A β-adrenergic receptor antagonist blocked the enhancing effects of both the water reward and foot shock on LTP. As with learning in intact animals, inhibition of protein synthesis after the induction of LTP in a hippocampal slice blocks the maintenance (that is, late phase) of LTP but does not block the induction (that is, early phase) of LTP (43).

Many recent experiments examined the effects, on memory consolidation, of drugs regulating specific molecular stages in the development and maintenance of LTP. Extensive evidence indicates the involvement of CaMKII (calcium-calmodulin–dependent protein kinase II) in both consolidation and LTP. CaMKII is known to phosphorylate the α-amino-3-hydroxy-5-methyl-4-isoxazolepropionic acid (AMPA) receptor subunit GluR1. Inhibitors of CaMKII block the induction of LTP and impair consolidation when infused into the amygdala or CA1 region of the hippocampus immediately after training (41, 44). However, CaMKII appears to have different roles in consolidation in these two brain regions (44). Infusions of any of several drugs, including 8-bromo cyclic adenosine monophosphate (8-Br-cAMP), a dopamine D1 receptor agonist, or NE into the hippocampus (CA1 region) 3 hours after training attenuate the amnesic effect of a CaMKII inhibitor infused into the amygdala immediately after training. In contrast, such treatments administered 3 hours after training do not block the amnesia induced by a CaMKII inhibitor infused into the hippocampus immediately after training. These findings provide additional evidence that the amygdala plays a modulatory role in consolidation, whereas the hippocampus is more likely a locus of memory processing or consolidation.

Inhibitors of the signal-transducing enzyme protein kinase C (PKC) are also known to block the maintenance of hippocampal LTP and to induce retrograde amnesia when infused into the hippocampus of rats after training. Similarly, inhibitors of protein kinase A (PKA) disrupt the late, protein synthesis–dependent phase of LTP and impair memory when infused into the hippocampus several hours after training (45). Additionally, PKA activity and CREB (cAMP response element–binding protein) immunoreactivity increase in the hippocampus after training. Such findings suggest that late-phase LTP and memory consolidation involve cAMP-mediated activation, by PKA phosphorylation, of the CREB transcription factor (46). Evidence that infusions of CREB antisense oligonucleotides into the hippocampus block the consolidation of water-maze learning without affecting acquisition also supports this hypothesis (47). Discovering which of the myriad of CREB-regulated genes is (or are) selectively involved in memory consolidation will be an interesting quest. Selective gene activation or inactivation after learning may regulate consolidation by modulating the stabilization of synaptic changes required for long-term memory (4, 48). Neural cell adhesion molecules also appear to play a role in memory consolidation by regulating time-dependent processes underlying synaptic stabilization (49).

Memory: The Short and the Long of It

Many treatments affect late LTP and memory consolidation without affecting early LTP or short-term or working memory. Although such findings are consistent with the hypothesis that early and later stages of memory are serially linked (9), they do not exclude the possibility that different stages of memory are based on parallel, independent processes (3, 10). Moreover, studies of memory in many species strongly support this latter view (12, 13), and studies of synaptic facilitation in *Aplysia* clearly indicate that short-term facilitation (STF) and long-term facilitation (LTF) are not serially linked (50). Drugs and other conditions that block STF do not block the expression of LTF and, as with other forms of plasticity and memory, only LTF requires protein synthesis. Additionally, evidence that some drugs infused into the hippocampus and entorhinal cortex after training block short-term memory without affecting long-term memory provides critical evidence that short- and long-term memory processes are independent (51).

Evaluation of this evidence requires several caveats. First, it remains a hypothesis that the synaptic mechanisms of LTP and LTF underlie memory, whether fleeting or lasting (or long-lasting). Second, although studies of the mechanisms of LTP and memory have focused on the involvement of the hippocampus, much evidence indicates that the hippocampus has a time-limited role in the consolidation or stabilization of lasting memory, or both. Third, there are forms of memory that do not involve the hippocampus and may not use any known mechanisms of synaptic plasticity. Third, despite theoretical conjectures, little is as yet known about system and cellular processes mediating consolidation that continues for several hours or longer after learning to create our lifelong memories. These issues remain to be addressed in this new century of research on memory consolidation.

References and Notes

1. G. E. Müller and A. Pilzecker, *Z. Psychol.* 1, 1 (1900).
2. S. E. Glickman, *Psychol. Bull.* 58, 218 (1961); J. L. McGaugh and M. J. Herz, *Memory Consolidation* (Albion, San Francisco, 1972); H. Weingartner and E. S. Parker, Eds., *Memory Consolidation* (Erlbaum, Hillsdale, NJ, 1984); H. A. Lechner, L. R. Squire, J. H. Byrne, *Learn. Mem.* 6, 77 (1999); M. R. Polster, L. Nadel, D. L. Schacter, *J. Cogn. Neurosci.* 3, 95 (1991).
3. J. L. McGaugh, *Science* 153, 1351 (1966).
4. Y. Dudai, *Neuron* 17, 367 (1996).
5. T. Ribot, *Diseases of Memory* (Appleton, New York, 1882); W. McDougall, *Mind* 10, 388 (1901); W. H. Burnham, *Am. J. Psychol.* 14, 382 (1903).
6. C. P. Duncan, *J. Comp. Physiol. Psychol.* 42, 32 (1949).
7. R. W. Gerard, *Am. J. Psychiatry* 106, 161 (1949).
8. D. O. Hebb, *The Organization of Behavior* (Wiley, New York, 1949) and (7). It is of interest that Hebb did not refer to the perseveration-consolidation hypothesis in his seminal 1949 book.
9. B. W. Agranoff, R. E. Davis, J. J. Brink, *Brain Res.* 1, 303 (1965).
10. J. L. McGaugh, in *Recent Advances in Learning and Retention,* D. Bovet, F. Bovet-Nitti, A. Oliverio, Eds. (Accademia Nazionale dei Lincei, Rome, 1968), pp. 13–24.
11. J. L. McGaugh, *Annu. Rev. Pharmacol.* 13, 229 (1973); *Brain Res. Bull.* 23, 339 (1989).
12. T. M. Alloway and A. Routtenberg, *Science* 158, 1066 (1967); T. Tully, T. Preat, S. C. Boynton, M. Del Vecchio, *Cell* 79, 35 (1994); R. Menzel and U. Müller, *Annu. Rev. Neurosci.* 19, 379 (1966); U. Müller, *Neuron* 16, 1249 (1996).
13. C. Sandi and S. P. R. Rose, *Brain Res.* 647, 106 (1994).
14. P. E. Gold and J. L. McGaugh, in *Short-Term Memory,* D. Deutsch and J. A. Deutsch, Eds. (Academic Press, New York, 1975), pp. 355–378.
15. S.-A. Christianson, Ed., *Handbook of Emotion and Memory: Current Research and Theory* (Erlbaum, Hillsdale, NJ, 1992).
16. P. E. Gold and R. van Buskirk, *Behav. Biol.* 13, 145 (1975).
17. J. L. McGaugh and P. E. Gold, in *Psychoendocrinology,* R. B. Brush and S. Levine, Eds. (Academic Press, New York, 1989), pp. 305–339.
18. E. R. de Kloet, *Front. Neuroendocrinol.* 12, 95 (1991); ———, S. Kock, V. Schild, H. D. Veldhuis, *Neuroen-docrinology* 47, 109 (1988); B. Roozendaal, L. Cahill, J. L. McGaugh in *Brain Processes and Memory,* K. Ishikawa, J. L. McGaugh, H. Sakata, Eds. (Elsevier, Amsterdam, 1996), pp. 39–54.
19. S. J. Lupien and B. S. McEwen, *Brain Res. Rev.* 24, 1 (1997).
20. M. G. Packard, C. L. Williams, L. Cahill, J. L. McGaugh, in *Neurobehavioral Plasticity: Learning, Development and Response to Brain Insults,* N. E. Spear, L. Spear, M. Woodruff, Eds. (Erlbaum, Hillsdale, NJ, 1995), pp. 149–184; J. L. McGaugh, L. Cahill, B. Roozendaal, *Proc. Natl. Acad. Sci. U.S.A.* 93, 13508 (1996). There is also evidence that epinephrine influences memory through the release of glucose, which then enters the brain; however, the effects of glucose on memory differ from those mediated by the activation of vagal afferents. P. E. Gold, in *Cellular Mechanisms of Conditioning and Behavioral Plasticity,* C. D. Woody, D. L. Alkon, J. L. McGaugh, Eds. (Plenum, New York, 1988), pp. 329–341.
21. K. C. Liang, R. G. Juler, J. L. McGaugh, *Brain Res.* 368, 125 (1986).
22. B. Roozendaal and J. L. McGaugh, *Neurobiol. Learn. Mem.* 65, 1 (1996); T. Hatfield and J. L. McGaugh, *Neurobiol. Learn. Mem.* 71, 232 (1999); B. Ferry and J. L. McGaugh, *Neurobiol. Learn. Mem.* 72, 8 (1999).
23. G. L. Quirarte, B. Roozendaal, J. L. McGaugh, *Proc. Natl. Acad. Sci. U.S.A.* 94, 14048 (1997).
24. R. Galvez, M. Mesches, J. L. McGaugh, *Neurobiol. Learn. Mem.* 66, 253 (1996); G. L. Quirarte, R. Galvez, B. Roozendaal, J. L. McGaugh, *Brain Res.*

808, 134 (1998); C. L. Williams, D. Men, E. C. Clayton and P. E. Gold, *Behav. Neurosci.* 112, 1414 (1998); T. Hatfield, C. Spanis, J. L. McGaugh, *Brain Res.* 835, 340 (1999).

25. L. R. Squire and E. R. Kandel, *Memory from Mind to Molecules* (Scientific American Library, New York, 1999).

26. For example, M. G. Packard and N. M. White, *Behav. Neurosci.* 105, 295 (1991); M. G. Packard, R. Hirsh, N. M. White, *J. Neurosci.* 9, 1465 (1989).

27. M. G. Packard, L. Cahill, J. L. McGaugh, *Proc. Natl. Acad. Sci. U.S.A.* 91, 8477 (1994); M. G. Packard and L. Teather, *Neurobiol. Learn. Mem.* 69, 163 (1998).

28. B. Roozendaal and J. L. McGaugh, *Euro. J. Neurosci.* 9, 76 (1997); B. Roozendaal, B. T. Nguyen, A. Power, J. L. McGaugh, *Proc. Natl. Acad. Sci. U.S.A.* 96, 11642 (1999).

29. Y. Ikegaya, H. Saito, K. Abe, *Brain Res.* 671, 351 (1995); *Neurosci. Res.* 22, 203 (1995); ———, K. Nakanishi, *NeuroReport* 8, 3143 (1997). BLA stimulation also induces NMDA-dependent LTP in the insular cortex, a brain region known to be important for several forms of learning [F. Bermudez-Rattoni, I. B. Introini-Collison, J. L. McGaugh, *Proc. Natl. Acad. Sci. U.S.A.* 88, 5379 (1991); M. L. Escobar, V. Chao, F. Bermudez-Rattoni, *Brain Res.* 779, 314 (1998); M. W. Jones, P. J. French, T. V. P. Bliss, K. Rosenblum, *J. Neurosci* 19, RC36 (1999)].

30. E. Soetens, S. Casaer, R. D'Hooge, J. E. Hueting, *Psychopharmacology* 119, 155 (1995).

31. L. Cahill, B. Prins, M. Weber, J. L. McGaugh, *Nature* 371, 702 (1994); A. H. van Stegeren, W. Everaerd, L. Cahill, J. L. McGaugh, L. J. G. Gooren, *Psychopharmacology* 138, 305 (1998); K. Nielson and R. Jensen, *Behav. Neural Biol.* 62, 190 (1994).

32. L. Cahill, R. Babinsky, H. J. Markowitsch, J. L. McGaugh, *Nature* 377, 295 (1995); R. Adolphs, L. Cahill, R. Schul, R. Babinsky, *Learn. Mem.* 4, 291 (1997).

33. L. Cahill et al., *Proc. Natl. Acad. Sci. U.S.A.* 93, 8016 (1996); S. Hamann, T. Ely, S. Grafton, C. Kilts, *Nature Neurosci.* 2, 289 (1999).

34. R. Shadmehr and H. H. Holcomb, *Science* 277, 821 (1997).

35. N. M. Weinberger, in *The Cognitive Neurosciences,* M. S. Gazzaniga, Ed. (MIT Press, Cambridge, MA, 1995), pp. 1071–1089; N. M. Weinberger, *Trends Cogn. Sci.* 2, 271 (1998); T. S. Bjordahl, M. A. Dimyan, N. M. Weinberger, *Behav. Neurosci.* 112, 467 (1998); V. V. Galvan, J. Chen, N. M. Weinberger, *Soc. Neurosci. Abstr.* 24, 1422 (1998).

36. G. Winocur, *Behav. Brain Res.* 38, 145 (1990); S. Zola-Morgan and L. R. Squire, *Science* 250, 288 (1990); J. J. Kim and M. S. Fanselow, *Science* 256, 675 (1992); Y. H. Cho, D. Beracochea, R. Jaffard, *J. Neurosci.* 13, 1759 (1993); J. J. Kim, R. E. Clark, R. F. Thompson, *Behav Neurosci.* 109, 195 (1995); G. Reidel et al., *Nature Neurosci.* 3, 898 (1999).

37. W. B. Scoville and B. Milner, *J. Neurol. Neurosurg. Psychiatry* 20, 11 (1957); B. Milner, in *Amnesia,* C. W. M. Whitty and O. L. Zangwill, Eds. (Butterworths, London, 1966), pp. 109–133.

38. L. R. Squire and P. Alvarez, *Curr. Opin. Neurobiol.* 5, 169 (1995).

39. T. J. Tyler and P. DiScenna, *Behav. Neurosci.* 100, 147 (1986); J. L. McClelland, B. L. McNaughton, R. C. O'Reilly, *Psychol. Rev.* 102, 419 (1995).

40. T. J. Shors and L. D. Matzel, *Behav. Brain Sci.* 20, 597 (1997).

41. R. C. Malenka and R. A. Nicoll, *Science* 285, 1870 (1999).

42. T. Seidenbacher, K. G. Reymann, D. Balschun, *Proc. Natl. Acad. Sci. U.S.A.* 94, 1494 (1997).

43. U. Frey, M. Krug, K. G. Reymann, H. Matthies, *Brain Res.* 452, 57 (1988).

44. D. M. Barros et al., *Neurobiol. Learn. Mem.* 71, 94 (1999).

45. P. A. Colley, F.-S. Sheu, A. Routtenberg, *J. Neurosci.* 10, 3353 (1990); Y.-Y. Huang, P. A. Colley, A. Routtenberg, *Neuroscience* 49, 819 (1992); D. Jerusalinsky et al., *Behav. Neural Biol.* 61, 107 (1994).

46. Y.-Y. Huang and E. R. Kandel, *Proc. Natl. Acad. Sci. U.S.A.* 92, 2446 (1995); R. Bernabeu et al., *Proc. Natl. Acad. Sci. U.S.A.* 94, 7041 (1997); G. E. Schafe, N. V. Nadel, G. M. Sullivan, A. Harris, J. E. LeDoux, *Learn. Mem.* 6, 97 (1999).

47. J. F. Guzowski and J. L. McGaugh, *Proc. Natl. Acad. Sci. U.S.A.* 94, 2693 (1997); T. Tully, *Proc. Natl. Acad. Sci. U.S.A.* 94, 4239 (1997).

48. A. Routtenberg, in *Four Decades of Memory,* P. E. Gold and W. T. Greenough, Eds. (American Psychological Association, Washington, DC, in press); T.

Abel, K. C. Martin, D. Bartsch, E. R. Kandel, *Science* 279, 338 (1998).

49. K. J. Murphy and C. M. Regan, *Neurobiol. Learn. Mem.* 70, 73 (1998); P. Roullet, R. Mileusnic, S. P. R. Rose, S. J. Sara, *NeuroReport* 8, 1907 (1997).

50. N. J. Emptage and T. J. Carew, *Science* 262, 253 (1993); J. Mauelshagen, G. R. Parker, T. J. Carew, *J. Neurosci.* 15, 7099 (1996); U. Müller and T. J. Carew, *Neuron* 21, 1423 (1996).

51. I. Izquierdo, D. M. Barros, T. Mello e Souza, M. M. de Souza, L. A. Izquierdo, *Nature* 393, 635 (1998).

52. I thank L. Cahill, I. Izquierdo, A. Routtenberg, G. Streidter, and N. M. Weinberger for their helpful comments and N. Collett for assistance in preparation of the manuscript. Supported by National Institute of Mental Health grant MH12526.

III SOCIAL COGNITION AND THE BRAIN

B. Social Applications

i. The Self

In Search of the Self: A Positron Emission Tomography Study

Fergus I. M. Craik, Tara M. Moroz, Morris Moscovitch, Donald T. Stuss, Gordon Winocur, Endel Tulving, and Shitij Kapur

It is well established that encoding and retrieval processes in episodic memory involve different regions in the frontal lobes of the cerebral cortex. Specifically, encoding processes differentially engage left prefrontal areas, whereas retrieval processes for the same materials predominantly involve right prefrontal areas. This observed difference was embodied in the hemispheric encoding/retrieval asymmetry model (HERA; Tulving, Kapur, Craik, Moscovitch, & Houle, 1994), and the empirical observations on which the model is based have since been replicated many times (for reviews, see Buckner, 1996; Nyberg, Cabeza, & Tulving, 1996; Tulving, 1998).

One question that can be asked is whether these asymmetrical cortical activations reflect the processes of memory encoding and retrieval as such, or whether they reflect the involvement of necessary constituents of encoding and retrieval, respectively. It is known, for example, that effective encoding processes typically involve deep, elaborate, semantic-processing operations (Craik & Tulving, 1975), and also that such types of processing are consistently associated with activation of the left lateral prefrontal cortex, most commonly around Brodmann's Areas (BA) 46 and 47 (Cabeza & Nyberg, 1997). It seems possible, therefore, that one major function of the left prefrontal cortex is the processing of meaning. This type of processing, in turn, is associated with good episodic memory for the processed event (Kapur et al., 1994; Petersen, Fox, Posner, Mintun, & Raichle, 1988). It should be noted that this confluence of meaningful processing, left prefrontal activation, and high levels of subsequent episodic memory performance is not restricted to verbal information; the same results have been reported for pictures (Grady, McIntosh, Rajah, & Craik, 1998).

What are the necessary constituents of memory retrieval? James (1890, Vol. I, p. 650) made

the point that for a mental event to be experienced as a personal memory, the imagined event must, first, be referred to the past and, second, be associated with feelings of self; that is, it must be dated in the rememberer's own personal past. Recent work involving positron emission tomography (PET) has shown that the retrieval of episodic memories is associated with activation of the prefrontal cortex, predominantly on the right (for reviews, see Cabeza & Nyberg, 1997; Nyberg, 1998; Nyberg et al., 1996). One interpretation of this right prefrontal activation is that it represents a set to interpret incoming stimuli as memory retrieval cues—a "retrieval mode" (Tulving, 1983) or "retrieval attempt" separable from the actual processes of successful retrieval (Kapur et al., 1995). In turn, it can be argued that the major constituents of retrieval mode are pastness and the involvement of self.

One major purpose of the present study was to examine the possibility that the association of episodic memory retrieval with activation of the right prefrontal cortex is attributable (in part at least) to the representation of self in this area of the brain. This conjecture receives some support from studies of brain-damaged patients with disturbances of self-awareness; such disorders are often associated with lesions of the right frontal cortex (Luria, 1973; Stuss, 1991; Wheeler, Stuss, & Tulving, 1997). Also, a PET study in which subjects retrieved emotional memories from their past showed activation of right prefrontal areas as well as other regions in the right hemisphere (Fink et al., 1996). We investigated this question by inducing participants to carry out self-related processing in the context of a memory encoding paradigm. If the involvement of self activates right frontal regions regardless of the nature of the cognitive operation, then self-referential encoding should also be associated with PET activations that are predominantly right lateralized. Alternatively, if self-referential encoding is associated with activations in left frontal regions, this finding would extend the generality of the HERA model, and suggest that self-referential encoding is not different in kind from other types of deeper processing.

A related purpose of the study was to gather evidence on the neural correlates of self-referential processing. It has been shown that words processed with reference to the self are very well remembered, usually even better than words processed in general semantic terms (Symons & Johnson, 1997). Thus, a person would remember the word *stubborn* better after answering the self-referential question "Does the word *stubborn* describe you?" than after answering the general semantic question "Does *stubborn* mean the same as *obstinate?*" (Rogers, Kuiper, & Kirker, 1977). This self-reference effect has been investigated extensively in the past 20 years. Its explanation is still debated, but one reasonable account is that the concept of self provides a rich schematic cognitive structure, and that new information learned with reference to self is encoded in a rich and distinctive manner. Furthermore, the organized, interdependent nature of the self-schema facilitates the formation of organizational links among the events to be remembered (Klein & Kihlstrom, 1986; Klein & Loftus, 1988), and the high accessibility of the self-schema facilitates the construction of compatible retrieval operations at the time of remembering (Wells, Hoffman, & Enzle, 1984). In the present study, we were interested in the neural correlates of self-referential encoding, as indexed by PET neuroimaging. The comparison between self-referential and general semantic encoding enabled us to determine whether these two types of encoding are associated with the same or different processes in the brain.

Participants in the PET scanner made judgments about lists of personality trait adjectives. Four types of judgments were made (only one type during any one scan); in all cases, participants rated each word on a 4-point scale by pressing one of four response keys. The four types of judgments were (a) *self* ("How well does the adjective describe you?"), (b) *other* ("How well does the adjective describe Brian Mulroney?"—a former Canadian prime minister), (c) *general* ("How socially desirable is the trait described by the adjective?"), and (d) *syllable* ("How many syllables does the adjective contain?"). Processing words in terms of the number of syllables reflects a relatively shallow type of verbal processing with little involvement of meaning; activations from these scans formed the baseline for PET measurements. The *other* condition was included to see whether personal judgments not related to self would be associated with activations different from those associated with self-referential and general semantic encoding. Behavioral studies have shown that subsequent memory for words judged with reference to another person depends on how well known the target person is to the participant. When the other in question is well known (e.g., parent, best friend), subsequent memory levels are almost as high as those associated with self judgments (Bower & Gilligan, 1979; Keenan & Baillet, 1980); but when the other is a public figure (e.g., Walter Cronkite, Jimmy Carter, John Major), memory for self-referential judgments is consistently higher than memory for other-related judgments (Bower & Gilligan, 1979; Conway & Dewhurst, 1995; Keenan & Baillet, 1980). In the present study, the other was also a public figure (Brain Mulroney), so we expected to find higher memory levels associated with self than with other judgments (see also Symons & Johnson, 1997, for recent meta-analytic support for this prediction).

Method

Participants

Eight right-handed volunteers (4 men and 4 women) were recruited for participation in the present investigation. The volunteers were between the ages of 19 and 26 years ($M = 22.8$), and had a mean education of 15.5 years. All participants were screened for a history or current evidence of any serious medical, neurological, or psychological disorder; they were also screened for recreational drug abuse. Informed consent was obtained from all volunteers before they participated, and they received a $50 reimbursement for their participation. The study was approved by the local ethics committee of the University of Toronto.

Task Design

Relative regional cerebral blood flow (rCBF) was measured while participants performed one of four encoding tasks; each task was performed twice, for a total of eight relative rCBF measurements (i.e., scans). The four tasks were presented in an ABCDDCBA design (counterbalanced across participants) to minimize order effects. Each task involved making judgments about personality trait adjectives on a 4-point scale. Sixteen similar lists of 32 personality trait adjectives were constructed using the personality trait adjectives found in Anderson (1968) and Kirby and Gardner (1972). These lists were used in the encoding tasks and in a subsequent recognition test. Each adjective occurred in only one list. Within each list, half of the words were positive and half were negative. A word was considered to be positive if it was one of the first 253 words listed by Anderson (1968; his words were ordered according to their likability ratings) or if it fell within the first five deciles of Kirby and Gardner's (1972) ratings of evaluation and social desirability; words occurring later in these lists were considered to be negative. Additionally, each list contained approximately equal numbers of two-, three-, four-, and five-syllable positive and negative adjectives. Eight additional lists of 8 personality trait adjectives were constructed for the practice trials. These practice lists were constructed using criteria similar to but less strict

than the criteria used to construct the sixteen 32-adjective lists (e.g., some of the practice adjectives were from Allport & Odbert, 1936). Eight of the 32-word lists were shown for the participants' judgments during the scans, and eight served as distractors on a recognition test at the end of scanning. Half of the participants made judgments on Lists 1 through 8; in this case, Lists 9 through 16 contributed distractors for the recognition test. The remaining participants made their initial judgments on Lists 9 through 16; in this case, Lists 1 through 8 contributed distractors for the recognition test. The lists were presented in a pseudorandom order, counterbalanced across subjects. The words within each list were randomly presented. Each word was presented in the center of a computer screen suspended a comfortable viewing distance from the participant.

In one task, representing encoding of self-referential information (*self* task), participants were requested to judge how well they thought each trait adjective described them. To indicate their judgment, they were instructed to press one of the four keys on the keypad beneath their right fingers. More specifically, they were requested to press the key beneath their index, middle, ring, or little finger if they thought that the trait adjective almost never, rarely, sometimes, or almost always described them, respectively. In a second task, representing encoding of information about another person (*other* task), participants were requested to judge how well they thought each trait adjective described Brian Mulroney by responding in the same way as in the *self* task. In a third task, representing encoding of semantic information not specific to a person (*general* task), participants were requested to judge how socially desirable the trait described by each adjective was. They judged each trait as being almost never, rarely, sometimes, or almost always socially desirable by pressing designated keys. In a fourth task, representing the encoding of nonsemantic information (*syllable* task), participants were requested to judge the number of syllables in each trait adjective. They pressed one of four keys depending on whether the adjective had two, three, four, or five syllables.

Each trial consisted of a 500-ms fixation point followed by an adjective with a maximum duration of 2,000 ms. If the participant made his or her judgment within the 2,000 ms, then the screen went blank for the duration of the 2,000 ms, and then a fixation point appeared for 1,500 ms. If the participant did not make his or her judgment within 2,000 ms, the adjective was replaced with the fixation point. The fixation point was displayed continuously for the 1,500 ms at the end of one trial and throughout the 500 ms preceding the next adjective; participants thus had a total of 4,000 ms to perceive and respond to each adjective. Participants were told that if they had not made a judgment by the time the fixation point appeared, they should do so quickly because the next trait adjective was about to appear. If a judgment had not been made within the 4,000-ms window, then the next adjective automatically appeared. This strict timing was used to ensure that each participant made the same number of judgments during each scan. The behavioral data and verbal reports from the participants confirmed that 4,000 ms was a comfortable window within which the various tasks could be performed.

Approximately 10 min after the last scan, participants were given an unexpected yes/no recognition test. The recognition test was divided into four blocks, one for each type of judgment. We made this division so that we could determine variations in the criterion participants used to recognize the adjectives from a particular judgment type. Block order was pseudorandom, counterbalanced across participants. Within each block, half of the adjectives from the two lists for a particular judgment and half of the adjectives from two distractor lists (i.e., 64 words/block) were randomly presented one at a time on a computer screen (half of the participants saw half of the adjectives, and the other half of the participants saw the remaining half of the adjec-

tives from the encoding and distractor lists). Each adjective remained on the screen until the participant pressed one of two keys to indicate whether or not he or she recognized the adjective as one that had been presented during scanning.

PET Scanning Techniques

Relative rCBF was measured by recording the regional distribution of cerebral radioactivity using a GEMS-Scanditronix PC-2048 head scanner. Full details of the method may be obtained from other PET scanning articles from the Toronto group (e.g., Kapur et al., 1994; Tulving, Kapur, Craik, Moscovitch, & Houle, 1994). Each task lasted approximately 2 min; data acquisition for each scan occurred in the middle 1 min of the task. The scans were 11 min apart to allow for adequate decay of the radioactivity. Three minutes before each scan, participants were given instructions for the next task and some practice trials.

Statistical Parametric Mapping (SPM 94) software (provided by the MRC Cyclotron Unit, Hammersmith Hospital, London, England) was used to realign, normalize, and smooth the images (using a 15-mm filter) from each participant. The data were statistically analyzed on a voxel-by-voxel basis. A given voxel was considered to be significantly activated if, in comparison with a reference task, there was an increase in relative rCBF and the corresponding z score was 4.10 or above. This z score corresponded to a p value of approximately .05 (corrected for multiple comparisons). Note, however, that we report significantly activated voxels only if they fell in a region (i.e., spatially contiguous set of voxels) that both was significantly activated ($z > 4.10$) and consisted of at least 20 voxels. Six planned comparisons (all possible pairs of conditions) were made; in all cases, the reverse comparison was also made so that both increases and decreases in relative rCBF could be assessed.

In addition to the SPM analysis, we carried out a partial least squares (PLS) analysis on

Table 13.1
Mean values of initial encoding time, recognition memory proportions (hits minus false alarms), and recognition latency

Task	Encoding reaction time (ms)	Hits—false alarms	Recognition reaction time (ms)
Self	1,454 (70)	.59 (.06)	1,349 (145)
Other	1,657 (123)	.50 (.06)	1,614 (223)
General	1,321 (79)	.51 (.06)	1,516 (198)
Syllable	1,542 (84)	.29 (.06)	1,483 (143)

Note. Standard errors are given in parentheses.

the PET data (McIntosh, Bookstein, Haxby, & Grady, 1996). This multivariate analysis operates on the covariance between brain voxels and the experimental design to identify a new set of variables (latent variables, or LVs) that optimally relate the two sets of measurements. In general, PLS is a more powerful analysis than SPM because it uses all the information from the two sets of measurements in a single step. In the present report, the PLS analysis is treated as an adjunct to the SPM analysis because it yielded an interesting result, relevant to our hypotheses; fuller details of the method are provided by McIntosh et al. (1996).

Results

Behavioral Data

Participants made a judgment about a trait adjective within the allotted 4-s window 99.5% of the time. Table 13.1 (left column) shows the mean times taken to make the judgments for each encoding condition; the *general* (social desirability) judgments were made most rapidly ($M = 1,321$ ms), and the *other* (Brian Mulroney) judgments were made most slowly ($M = 1,657$ ms). An analysis of variance (ANOVA) on these four means yielded a significant effect, $F(3, 21) = 8.78$, $p < .001$. Subsequent pair-wise comparisons (least squares means) revealed significant

differences (uncorrected $p < .05$) between the *general* and *other* tasks, *general* and *syllable* tasks, and *self* and *other* tasks.

Table 13.1 (right column) also shows the mean times taken to make correct recognition decisions in the retrieval phase. An ANOVA showed no significant differences among the four means, $F(3, 21) = 1.45$, $p > .05$, but the table shows that self-related encoding was associated with the fastest subsequent recognition reaction time (RT). Deeper encoding conditions typically lead to faster recognition latencies (Vincent, Craik, & Furedy, 1996). Recognition memory performance was indexed by the proportion of hits minus false alarms for each condition. Table 13.1 (center column) shows that the *syllable* condition yielded the lowest recognition score, and that the *self* condition was associated with the highest level of recognition performance. An ANOVA revealed a significant effect of encoding task, $F(3, 21) = 5.35$, $p < .01$, and subsequent pairwise comparisons showed that recognition was significantly higher on the *self, other,* and *general* tasks than on the *syllable* task, but that there were no reliable differences among the three semantic tasks. Thus, in the present data, the *other* and *general* tasks yielded very similar levels of recognition memory, and the *self* condition yielded a somewhat higher level. The lack of statistical significance for this latter result is likely attributable to the lack of power associated with a study involving only 8 participants.

Table 13.2
Increases in brain activity associated with encoding of self-related, other-related, general semantic, and phonological information

Task comparison and region	Side	Coordinates			z statistic
		x	*y*	*z*	
Self versus *other*					
No significant increases					
Self versus *general*					
Anterior cingulate (BA 24)	Right	6	34	4	4.47
Other versus *general*					
No significant increases					
Self versus *syllable*					
Medial frontal lobe (BA 8/9)	Left	−4	46	36	7.25
Inferior frontal gyrus (BA 47)	Left	−32	24	−8	5.77
Other versus *syllable*					
Medial frontal lobe (BA 10)	Left	−6	52	−4	6.09
Medial frontal lobe (BA 8/9)	Left	−6	44	40	7.16
Anterior cingulate (BA 32)	Left	−4	20	−8	4.50
Superior temporal gyrus (BA 38)	Left	−38	10	−16	6.44
Posterior cingulate (BA 23)	Left	−6	−54	16	4.84
Middle temporal gyrus (BA 39)	Left	−44	−68	20	5.23
General versus *syllable*					
Medial frontal lobe (BA 10)	Left	−8	52	−4	5.13
Medial frontal lobe (BA 8/9)	Left	−6	44	36	6.58
Inferior frontal gyrus (BA 47)	Left	−36	36	−4	5.60
Middle temporal gyrus (BA 39)	Left	−42	−66	20	4.97

Note. BA = Brodmann's Area, as identified in Talairach and Tournoux (1988).

SPM Analysis

Tables 13.2 and 13.3 show the increases and decreases, respectively, in brain activity associated with the planned comparisons between the different encoding conditions. With respect to the three semantic conditions (*self, other,* and *general*), table 13.3 shows that there were no significant decreases in relative rCBF between the conditions, and table 13.2 shows only one significant effect: The right anterior cingulate area was more activated in the *self* than in the *general* condition.

Self-Syllable Comparison

Table 13.2 lists two regions of relative rCBF increase in this comparison. Increases occurred in the left hemisphere only—in the medial aspect of the superior frontal gyrus (BA 8/9) and in the inferior frontal gyrus (BA 47). These regions are shown in figure 13.1a. Four regions of relative rCBF decrease were also observed (figure 13.2a).

Table 13.3
Decreases in brain activity associated with encoding of self-related, other-related, general semantic, and phonological information

Task comparison and region	Side	Coordinates			z statistic
		x	y	z	
Self versus *other*					
No significant decreases					
Self versus *general*					
No significant decreases					
Other versus *general*					
No significant decreases					
Self versus *syllable*					
Precentral gyrus (BA 6)	Right	40	6	24	4.43
Inferior parietal lobule (BA 40)	Left	−56	−38	32	5.56
Superior parietal lobule (BA 7)	Right	32	−54	36	5.50
Fusiform gyrus (BA 37)	Left	−44	−62	−12	5.46
Other versus *syllable*					
Middle frontal gyrus (BA 6)	Right	20	−2	48	5.07
Inferior parietal lobule (BA 40)	Left	−58	−38	32	4.62
Superior parietal lobule (BA 7)	Right	32	−54	36	6.07
Fusiform gyrus (BA 37)	Left	−44	−58	−12	6.39
Superior parietal lobule (BA 7)	Left	−22	−66	40	5.02
General versus *syllable*					
Anterior cingulate (BA 24)	Right	4	10	32	4.51
Inferior parietal lobule (BA 40)	Left	−54	−40	36	4.49
Inferior parietal lobule (BA 40)	Right	38	−46	36	5.53
Fusiform gyrus (BA 37)	Left	−42	−58	−12	6.34
Superior parietal lobule (BA 7)	Left	−22	−66	40	5.09

Note. BA = Brodmann's Area, as identified in Talairach and Tournoux (1988).

These regions were located in the left inferior parietal gyrus (BA 40), right superior parietal lobule (BA 7), left fusiform gyrus (BA 37), and right precentral gyrus (BA 6). The coordinates of the points of maximal activation are given in table 13.3.

Other-Syllable Comparison
Table 13.2 lists the anatomical coordinates, brain regions, and z statistics associated with relative

rCBF increases in this comparison; the six areas are illustrated in figure 13.1b. Increases occurred in the left hemisphere only—in the medial aspect of the superior frontal gyrus (BA 8/9 and 10), superior temporal gyrus (BA 38), middle temporal gyrus (BA 39), and posterior (BA 23) and anterior (BA 32) cingulate gyrus. Table 13.3 and figure 13.2b show the regions associated with relative rCBF decreases in this comparison. Decreases occurred in the right superior frontal

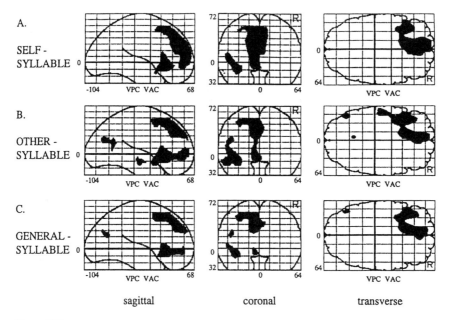

A.

SELF -
SYLLABLE

B.

OTHER -
SYLLABLE

C.

GENERAL -
SYLLABLE

sagittal   coronal   transverse

Figure 13.1
Areas of significant increase in relative regional cerebral blood flow during the encoding of self-referential information (a: *self* minus *syllable* condition), other-referential information (b: *other* minus *syllable* condition), and general semantic information (c: *general* minus *syllable* condition). The anatomical space corresponds to that of Talairach and Tournoux (1988). R, right hemisphere; VPC, vertical line through posterior commissure; VAC, vertical line through anterior commissure.

gyrus (BA 6), left inferior parietal lobule (BA 40), left and right superior parietal lobules (BA 7), and left fusiform gyrus (BA 37).

General-Syllable Comparison
Table 13.2 and figure 13.1c show the regions associated with relative rCBF increases in this comparison. These regions were all in the left hemisphere—in the medial aspect of the superior frontal gyrus (BA 8/9 and 10), the inferior frontal gyrus (BA 47), and the middle temporal gyrus (BA 39). Relative decreases in rCBF were seen in the left and the right inferior parietal lobules (BA 40), left superior parietal lobule (BA 7), right anterior cingulate gyrus (BA 24), and left fusiform gyrus (BA 37). These areas are shown in table 13.3 and figure 13.2c.

Summary
A summary of the comparisons between the semantic (*self, other, general*) and nonsemantic (*syllable*) tasks is provided in table 13.4. Given the general absence of differences among the semantic tasks, the similarity of their contrasts with the nonsemantic task is not surprising. In a sense, however, the different tasks serve as replications of semantic-nonsemantic differences, and together they yield a rather coherent picture. First, table 13.4 emphasizes the fact that all significant increases were associated with left-hemisphere activations. This finding strikingly corroborates the HERA model. Second, increases in activation tended to occur in frontal areas (8 out of 12 cases), whereas decreases in activation were concentrated in posterior areas (11 out of

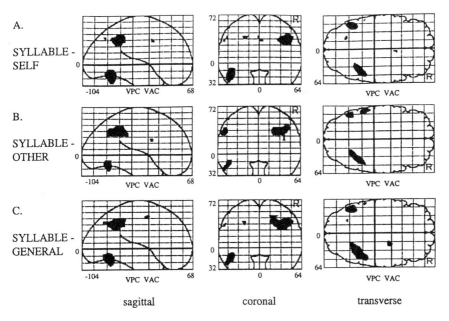

Figure 13.2
Areas of significant decrease in relative regional cerebral blood flow during the encoding of self-referential information (a: *syllable* minus *self* condition), other-referential information (b: *syllable* minus *other* condition), and general semantic information (c: *syllable* minus *general* condition). The anatomical space corresponds to that of Talairach and Tournoux (1988). R, right hemisphere; VPC, vertical line through posterior commissure; VAC, vertical line through anterior commissure.

14 cases). Third, decreases in frontal areas were all right-sided, in contrast to the frontal increases, which were all left-sided. Fourth, there was some tendency for the posterior decreases to be bilateral (BA 40 and 7), apart from the consistent activation in the left fusiform gyrus. Finally, given the present investigation's focus on activations relating to self, it is worth noting that every significant activation in the *self-syllable* contrast was also found in either the *other-syllable* contrast or the *general-syllable* contrast, or both.

PLS Analysis

Table 13.5 shows the major areas of maximum activation associated with the three LVs. In this additional analysis, we show only areas in the frontal lobes, given the present hypotheses of interest. Also, table 13.5 is restricted to clusters of 100 voxels or more, and to contrasts with positive salience. For example, the first latent variable (LV1) accounted for 66% of the variance and shows cortical areas that were relatively more active in the contrast when the combination of the *self, other,* and *general* conditions was compared with the *syllable* condition. The preceding SPM analysis and figure 13.1 would lead one to expect that this contrast should be associated with strong left frontal activation, and table 13.5 shows that this is the case. In addition, LV1 includes a smaller area in the right inferior frontal gyrus (BA 47).

Table 13.4
Regions of significant increased and decreased activation in comparisons between semantic and nonsemantic tasks

Region	Task comparison		
	Self versus *syllable*	*Other* versus *syllable*	*General* versus *syllable*
Increases			
Frontal			
Medial frontal lobe		L–10	L–10
Medial frontal lobe	L–8/9	L–8/9	L–8/9
Inferior frontal gyrus	L–47		L–47
Anterior cingulate		L–32	
Posterior			
Superior temporal gyrus		L–38	
Middle temporal gyrus		L–39	L–39
Posterior cingulate		L–23	
Decreases			
Frontal			
Frontal gyrus	R–6	R–6	
Anterior cingulate			R–24
Posterior			
Inferior parietal lobule	L–40	L–40	L–40
			R–40
Superior parietal lobule	R–7	R–7	
		L–7	L–7
Fusiform gyrus	L–37	L–37	L–37

Note. Numbers represent Brodmann's Areas. L = left hemisphere; R = right hemisphere.

The second latent variable (LV2) accounted for 18% of the variance, and table 13.5 shows frontal areas of activation associated with the contrast in which the *general* condition was greater than the combination of the *self, other,* and *syllable* conditions). These areas are both in the left frontal cortex and appear to be specifically related to general semantic encoding.

The third latent variable (LV3) accounted for 15% of the variance and contrasts the *self* condition with the other three conditions (i.e., *self >* *other, general, syllable*). The first area table 13.5 shows for this contrast is in the frontal pole; its maximum activation is slightly left of the mid-line, but the cluster spreads upward and to the right. The other two areas of activation are in right frontal areas, one in the middle frontal gyrus (BA 10) and the other in the inferior frontal gyrus (BA 45). Thus, the areas of the frontal lobes that were more activated in the *self* condition, contrasted to the other three conditions, were situated in either medial or right frontal locations.

Discussion

The behavioral results showed that adjectives judged semantically (*self, other,* and *general*

Table 13.5
Partial least squares (PLS) analysis: Areas of maximum frontal activation associated with positive saliences in three latent variables (LVs)

LV and region	Side	Coordinates			Voxel size	z statistic[a]
		x	y	z		
LV1 (*self, other, general > syllable*)						
Medial frontal lobe (BA 10)	Left	−8	52	0	5,073	8.0
Superior frontal gyrus (BA 8)	Left	−16	18	48		11.3
Frontal opercular (BA 47)	Left	−32	16	−8		10.6
Inferior frontal gyrus (BA 47)	Right	48	24	−4	157	4.3
LV2 (*general > self, other, syllable*)						
Superior frontal gyrus (BA 8)	Left	−8	24	48	158	3.2
Precentral gyrus (BA 6)	Left	−56	0	24	127	3.3
LV3 (*self > other, general, syllable*)						
Medial frontal lobe (BA 10)	Left	−6	56	8	281	4.7
Medial frontal lobe (BA 9)	Right	6	40	28		3.0
Middle frontal gyrus (BA 10)	Right	30	60	20	127	3.4
Inferior frontal gyrus (BA 45)	Right	52	26	4	110	3.7

Note. BA = Brodmann's Area, as identified in Talairach and Tournoux (1988).
a. The statistic from PLS analyses is roughly analogous to a z statistic (see McIntosh, Bookstein, Haxby & Grady, 1996).

tasks) were better recognized in a later test than adjectives judged in terms of number of syllables (table 13.1). Also, adjectives in the *self* condition were somewhat better recognized than those in the *other* and *general* conditions; that is, the present results showed a self-reference effect in memory, in line with previous work (Symons & Johnson, 1997).

The SPM analysis of the neuroimaging data is striking primarily because of the similarity among the *self, other,* and *general* conditions when compared with the *syllable* condition. As shown in table 13.4 and figure 13.1, the increases in activation in these three semantic tasks compared with the *syllable* task were restricted to the left hemisphere and were predominantly located in the left prefrontal cortex.

The common areas of relative activation in the three semantic conditions included the medial aspect of the superior frontal gyrus (BA 8/9, 10), inferior frontal gyrus (BA 47), superior temporal gyrus (BA 38), middle temporal gyrus (BA 39), and cingulate gyrus (BA 23/32). These are the areas associated with meaningful processing of individual words in a number of previous studies (Buckner, 1996; Cabeza & Nyberg, 1997; Nyberg et al., 1996; Tulving et al., 1994). The decreases in relative rCBF shown in table 13.4 may be interpreted as indicating the engagement of areas concerned with phonological analysis of visually presented words. The frontal activations (BA 6, BA 24) are associated with the motor programming of language. The posterior regions that are activated in the *syllable* task are those associated with directing attention (BA 7, BA 40) to the visual word form area (BA 37); this allocation of attention may precede and accompany processing of the printed word into syllables. The preferential activation of left frontal and temporal areas during encoding in all three semantic tasks provides additional support for the HERA model (Tulving et al., 1994).

The similarity in cortical activation patterns between the *self* condition and the *other* and *general* conditions suggests that thoughts of self may largely involve a generalized "conceptual self"—a schematic representation abstracted from many personal episodes. In this sense, then, self-related judgments may not differ substantially from other judgments requiring retrieval from semantic memory. The conclusion that the self is simply "an unusually rich and highly organized cognitive structure" (Higgins & Bargh, 1987, p. 389) abstracted from individual instances is in line with observations that brain-damaged patients with a complete absence of episodic memory can nonetheless make accurate judgments about their personality characteristics (Klein, Loftus, & Kihlstrom, 1996; Tulving, 1993).

However, the PLS analysis, while substantially corroborating the conclusions from the SPM analysis, also demonstrated frontal activations specific to the *self* condition when contrasted with the other three conditions. Moreover, these specific self-related activations were located predominantly in the right frontal lobe. There is thus good evidence for an encoding manipulation activating right prefrontal regions when encoding involves the person's self-concept. This conclusion was also reached by Velichkovsky, Klemm, Dettmar, and Volke (1996) in a study involving evoked coherence of electroencephalograms.

In a recent survey of frontal lobe functions, Grady (1998) listed activations from PET studies of episodic memory. Her survey shows that of the 39 activations reported in BA 10 and BA 9, all but one are associated with episodic retrieval.

The first two activations listed for LV3 in the present table 13.5 are in the same region as those listed by Grady in her tables 13.6 and 13.7, yet the latter activations were overwhelmingly associated with episodic retrieval whereas the present activations were associated with encoding. Our suggested conclusion is that episodic retrieval necessarily involves the concept of self, and that this involvement is signaled by neural activity in the right frontal lobe. An alternative possibility is that judgments concerning the self involve retrieval of episodic instances; this possibility is somewhat unlikely, however, given the evidence that patients with no episodic memory can make accurate self-assessments (Klein et al., 1996; Tulving, 1993).

In summary, the present study examined the neural correlates of the self-reference effect in the context of an episodic memory encoding experiment using verbal materials. The SPM analysis of the PET data showed that the *self* encoding condition was associated with left prefrontal activations similar to the activations associated with other-related and general semantic encoding. This finding suggests that part of the self-concept exists in the form of context-free schematic knowledge, similar in type to other forms of semantic knowledge (cf. Higgins & Bargh, 1987; Klein et al., 1996). In addition, however, the PLS analysis revealed some right-sided prefrontal activations related to the *self* condition in areas typically associated with episodic retrieval. We suggest that these activations signal the involvement of the self as a necessary component of episodic retrieval, much as suggested by William James more than a century ago.

Acknowledgments

We wish to thank Boris Velichkovsky for discussion of the ideas behind the present study. We also wish to thank Doug Hussey, Kevin Cheung, and Corey Jones of the Clarke Institute of Psychiatry for technical assistance, and Stefan Kohler and Randy McIntosh for advice and assistance on the PLS analysis.

The work was supported by a grant from the Natural Sciences and Engineering Research Council of Canada to the first author.

References

Allport, G. W., & Odbert, H. S. (1936). Trait-names: A psycho-lexical study. *Psychological Monographs, 47.*

Anderson, N. (1968). Likableness ratings of 555 personality-trait words. *Journal of Personality and Social Psychology,* 9, 272–279.

Bower, G. M., & Gilligan, S. G. (1979). Remembering information related to one's self. *Journal of Research in Personality,* 13, 420–432.

Buckner, R. (1996). Beyond HERA: Contributions of specific prefrontal areas to long-term memory. *Psychonomic Bulletin & Review,* 3, 149–158.

Cabeza, R., & Nyberg, L. (1997). Imaging cognition: An empirical review of PET studies with normal subjects. *Journal of Cognitive Neuroscience,* 9, 1–26.

Conway, M. A., & Dewhurst, S. A. (1995). The self and recollective experience. *Applied Cognitive Psychology,* 9, 1–19.

Craik, F. I. M., & Tulving, E. (1975). Depth of processing and the retention of words in episodic memory. *Journal of Experimental Psychology: General,* 104, 268–294.

Fink, G. R., Markowitsch, H. J., Reinkemeier, M., Bruckbauer, T., Kessler, J., & Heiss, W. (1996). Cerebral representation of one's own past: Neural networks involved in autobiographical memory. *The Journal of Neuroscience,* 16, 4275–4282.

Grady, C. L. (1998). Neuroimaging and activation of the frontal lobes. In B. L. Miller & J. L. Cummings (Eds.), *The human frontal lobes: Functions and disorders* (pp. 196–230). New York: Guilford Press.

Grady, C. L., McIntosh, A. R., Rajah, M. N., & Craik, F. I. M. (1998). Neural correlates of the episodic encoding of pictures and words. *Proceedings of the National Academy of Sciences, USA,* 95, 2703–2708.

Higgins, E. T., & Bargh, J. A. (1987). Social cognition and social perception. *Annual Review of Psychology,* 38, 369–425.

James, W. (1890). *The principles of psychology.* New York: Henry Holt.

Kapur, S., Craik, F. I. M., Jones, C., Brown, G. M., Houle, S., & Tulving, E. (1995). Functional role of the prefrontal cortex in memory retrieval: A PET study. *NeuroReport,* 6, 1880–1884.

Kapur, S., Craik, F. I. M., Tulving, E., Wilson, A. A., Houle, S., & Brown, G. M. (1994). Neuroanatomical correlates of encoding in episodic memory: Levels of processing effect. *Proceedings of the National Academy of Sciences, USA,* 91, 2008–2111.

Keenan, J. M., & Baillet, S. D. (1980). Memory for personally and socially significant events. In R. S. Nickerson (Ed.), *Attention and performance* (Vol. 8, pp. 651–669). Hillsdale, NJ: Erlbaum.

Kirby, D. M., & Gardner, R. C. (1972). Ethnic stereotypes: Norms on 208 words typically used in their assessment. *Canadian Journal of Psychology,* 26, 140–154.

Klein, S. B., & Kihlstrom, J. F. (1986). Elaboration, organization, and the self-reference effect in memory. *Journal of Experimental Psychology,* 115, 26–38.

Klein, S. B., & Loftus, J. (1988). The nature of self-referent encoding: The contributions of elaborative and organizational processes. *Journal of Personality and Social Psychology,* 55, 5–11.

Klein, S. B., Loftus, J., & Kihlstrom, J. F. (1996). Self-knowledge of an amnesic patient: Toward a neuropsychology of personality and social psychology. *Journal of Experimental Psychology: General,* 125, 250–260.

Luria, A. R. (1973). *The working brain.* New York: Basic Books.

McIntosh, A. R., Bookstein, F. L., Haxby, J. V., & Grady, C. L. (1996). Spatial pattern analysis of functional brain images using partial least squares. *Neuroimage,* 3, 143–157.

Nyberg, L. (1998). Mapping episodic memory. *Behavioural Brain Research,* 90, 107–114.

Nyberg, L., Cabeza, R., & Tulving, E. (1996). PET studies of encoding and retrieval: The HERA model. *Psychonomic Bulletin & Review,* 3, 135–148.

Petersen, S. E., Fox, P. T., Posner, M. I., Mintun, M., & Raichle, M. E. (1988). Positron emission tomographic studies of the cortical anatomy of single-word processing. *Nature,* 331, 585–589.

Rogers, T. B., Kuiper, N. A., & Kirker,W. S. (1977). Self-reference and the encoding of personal information. *Journal of Personality and Social Psychology,* 35, 677–688.

Stuss, D. T. (1991). Self awareness and the frontal lobes: A neuropsychological perspective. In J. Strauss & G. R. Goethals (Eds.), *The self: Interdisciplinary approaches* (pp. 255–278). New York: Spring-Verlag.

Symons, C. S., & Johnson, B. T. (1997). The self-reference effect in memory: A meta-analysis. *Psychological Bulletin,* 121, 371–394.

Talairach, J., & Tournoux, P. (1988). *Co-planar stereotaxic atlas of the human brain.* New York: Thieme Medical Publishers.

Tulving, E. (1983). *Elements of episodic memory.* New York: Oxford University Press.

Tulving, E. (1993). Self-knowledge of an amnesic individual is represented abstractly. In T. K. Srull & R. S. Wyer (Eds.), *Advances in social cognition* (Vol. 5, pp. 147–156). Hillsdale, NJ: Erlbaum.

Tulving, E. (1998). Brain/mind correlates of human memory. In M. Sabourin, F. I. M. Craik, & M. Robert (Eds.), *Advances in psychological science: Vol. 2. Biological and cognitive aspects* (pp. 441–460). Hove, England: Psychology Press.

Tulving, E., Kapur, S., Craik, F. I. M., Moscovitch, M., & Houle, S. (1994). Hemispheric encoding/retrieval asymmetry in episodic memory: Positron emission tomography findings. *Proceedings of the National Academy of Sciences, USA,* 91, 2016–2020.

Velichkovsky, B. M., Klemm, T., Dettmar, P., & Volke, H.-J. (1996). Evozierte koharenz des EEG II: Kommunikation der Hirnareale und Verarbeitungtiefe [Evoked coherence of EEG II: Communication of brain areas and depth of processing]. *Zeitschrift fur EEG-EMG,* 27, 111–119.

Vincent, A., Craik, F. I. M., & Furedy, J. J. (1996). Relations among memory performance, mental workload and cardiovascular responses. *International Journal of Psychophysiology,* 23, 181–198.

Wells, G. L., Hoffman, C., & Enzle, M. E. (1984). Self-versus other-referent processing at encoding and retrieval. *Personality and Social Psychology Bulletin,* 10, 574–584.

Wheeler, M. A., Stuss, D. T., & Tulving, E. (1997). Toward a theory of episodic memory: The frontal lobes and autonoetic consciousness. *Psychological Bulletin,* 121, 331–354.

14 Brain and Conscious Experience

Michael S. Gazzaniga

As we stumble forward into the next century, groping for a way to think about the problem of conscious experience, it is good to remember we do know something about the brain and psychological process. There are a set of facts, of observations that can help guide our thinking about how the brain enables the mind. I would like to outline these milestones and argue that progress on the mind-brain issue is being made (1).

We start with the simple realization that our mind is the product of natural selection. This fact has many implications for how we should think about the nature of conscious experience.

The Evolutionary Perspective

The central nervous system did not spontaneously arise in mammals. The function and structure of the extant mammalian brain is the consequence of millions of years of interaction with the environment. For a species to have survived, let alone evolve, it had to come to terms with the challenges of its niche. To cope with those challenges, it had to develop specialized neural circuitry that supports adaptations and programs for response to an environmental challenge. In short, any organism from *Escherichia coli* to a human has built-in responses that are ready to be applied to environmental challenges.

This position is part of a large issue in biology that has to do with whether information from the environment instructs biologic systems or that biologic systems select information it already has built into it. The best example of this distinction has come from immunology. For years it was thought that when a foreign substance (antigen) invaded the body, its unique structure instructed the lymphocyte cells to form an antibody. The antigen-antibody response subsequently occurred, and the foreign element would be neutralized.

For almost 30 years we have known this is not how the system works. Human beings are born with all their antibodies, and when an antigen is tied up by an antibody, it is because that antibody had been selected from the millions already present in the body. This immunologic fact was first applied to the nervous system by Niels Jerne (2), who proposed that perhaps all the nerve circuits we will ever need to perform tasks are already built into the brain. This would imply that more complex organisms, which possess more complex behaviors (language, abstract thought), must possess complex and specialized circuits. As William James noted (3), humans must have more instincts, not fewer, than lower animals.

Peter Marler reported many years ago on a fascinating aspect of bird song that directly relates to Jerne's suggestion (4). Young males learn their song from their fathers, and although there are all kinds of parameters for correct song learning, the most intriguing is that the young male can learn only a limited song. It must hear the adult males' song of its own species or only a slight dialect, but it cannot learn a related song. In short, the environment triggers the expression of a song pattern, but a pattern is selected from a small array of possibilities built into the young male; it cannot learn any random song. A related example from human research is the reduced ability to not only produce but also to perceive phonemes of different languages (5) if a child is not exposed to the language early in life.

These examples set the stage for a view of the nervous system that suggests the cerebral cortex is not a dynamic, general purpose, learn-anything, anytime, anywhere kind of device. It has built-in constraints, huge ones. Although some investigators believe that constant Darwinian competition is ongoing in the cerebral cortex (6), my view is that during learning, selection processes are at work to find the built-in circuit, the already existing adaptation, to meet the environment challenge at hand. Although all researchers studying reorganizations of cortical maps are aware of what their work may or may not mean, it is represented as showing that synapses constantly reorganize to handle new environmental circumstances (7, 8). The evolutionary view would indicate little or no recrafting of synapses; the cerebral cortex is hard wired with circuitry crafted to meet specific challenges. If the brain was not hard wired, why would the same bird be able to learn one song pattern but not another?

Timing and Automatic Actions

Timing is everything. With our brains chock full of marvelous devices, one would think they do their duties more or less automatically and before we are truly aware of the act. As reviewed by Libet, that is precisely what happens in the brain. Recent research confirms that not only are there mechanisms that seem to create this illusion, there are modern studies on the primate brain that show how cells are preparing for decisive action way before the animal is even thinking about making its decision (9).

It is also clear that, when activated, these automatic processes give rise to illusions, as in Roger Shepard's turning table illusion (10). The explanation for this striking phenomenon can be found in how the brain computes information residing on a two-dimensional structure, the retina, and transforms it into a three-dimensional reality. The cues that give perspective, the long axis lines, suggest that the table on the left is going back in depth. The long axis cues for the table on the right are at right angles to the line of sight, and now the brain reacts to these cues. The image on the retina of these two tables is exactly the same. However, the brain automatically responds to depth cues of the left table and infers (for us) that because the table is going back in depth, the image is foreshortened, and because it is foreshortened as a real table in real depth, it

must be longer. The same is true for why the horizontal table appears wider. Even though one can fully understand that the images are exactly the same and that at a level of personal consciousness one knows this to be true, it has no effect on perception. The brain automatically supplies the inference, and there is nothing one can do about it.

There are also demonstrations that our motor system, the system that makes operational any decision about the world our brains might make, works with a high degree of independence from our conscious perceptions (11). Too often our perceptions are in error, and it would be disastrous in many instances to have our lives depend on those perceptions. It would be better if our brains reacted to real sensory truths, not illusory ones.

Conscious versus Unconscious Processes

If so many processes are automatic, it would seem logical to think they could function outside the realm of conscious awareness. And yet we have come to think that the part of our brain that has grown so large, the cerebral cortex, is reserved for our conscious activities. It now seems clear that brain scientists have been wrong about this issue. The cortex is involved in all sorts of unconscious processes.

A series of reports over the past 20 years indicates that although a patient suffering damage to the primary visual system may not consciously see in a blind field of vision, the hand or even the mouth might be able to respond to stimuli presented in the blind field. Patients who exhibit this condition, which has been dubbed "blindsight," can actually respond to such stimuli without being consciously aware of the stimulus. The hope of this research was that the site of unconscious processing had been discovered and could now be examined.

Ever since the psychodynamic ideas of Freud, there has been a fascination with the unconscious.

There in that great platform for our mental life, ideas are sewn together, true relationships between information are seen, and plans are made. Although Freud never really suggested which parts of the brain might be involved in managing the unconscious, there has been a tacit assumption and sometimes an explicit claim that such things go on in the older and more primitive regions.

In the collective enthusiasm for this view, we all have missed a fundamental point. It is a fact that 98% of what the brain does, it does outside of conscious awareness. Starting with basics, no one would argue that virtually all of our sensory-motor activities are unconsciously planned and executed. As I sit here and type this sentence, I have no idea how the brain actually pulls off the task of directing my fingers to the correct keys on the keyboard. I have no idea how the bird, sitting on the outside deck, a glimpse of which I must have caught in my peripheral vision, just caught my attention, while I nonetheless continue to type these words. Furthermore, the same goes for rational behaviors. As I sit and write, I am not aware of how the neural messages arise from various parts of my brain and are programmed into something resembling a rational argument. It all just sort of happens.

Surely we are not aware of how much of anything gets done in the realm of our so-called "conscious" lives. As we use one word and find that suddenly a related word comes into our consciousness with a greater probability than another, do we really think that we have such processes under conscious control? Do we really think that we have consciously achieved an understanding of what a logarithm represents? Indeed, only a few members of our species possess such an understanding and among those who do, it just sort of happened.

It is easy to see why very clever psychologists began to wonder if formal cognitive psychology had missed the boat. Perhaps the challenge is to study that great platform of life, the unconscious. It was in this context that my colleagues and I became interested in the work of Weiskrantz and the phenomeon of blindsight (12).

The unconscious now seemed to be explorable in scientific terms. It looked as though various subcortical and parallel pathways and centers could now be studied in the human brain. A large body of subhuman primate literature on the subject also developed. Monkeys with occipital lesions were reported as being not only able to localize objects in space but were also able to perform color and object discriminations.

As the early reports on blindsight accumulated, we began to examine related issues in other types of brain patients (13, 14). Damage to the parietal lobe of the brain, for example, causes strange symptoms to appear. If it occurs on the right side of the brain, most patients experience neglect. Thus, when looking straight ahead, they deny seeing anything to the left of where they are looking, even though their primary visual system is perfectly intact. A milder symptom of damage to the right parietal lobe is extinction, which is often present when both visual fields are stimulated at the same time.

When all of these behaviors are considered, it becomes clear that the parietal lobe somehow is involved with the attentional mechanism. Something distinct is at work from the parts of the brain that simply represent visual information. Information is getting into the brain, but it operates outside the realm of conscious experience. We showed this basic fact in a number of ways. In one study, we asked patients with neglect to judge whether two lateralized visual stimuli, one appearing in each visual field, were the same or different. So, a patient might see an apple in one part of the visual field and an orange in the other. Conversely, two apples or two oranges might be presented, one in each half visual field. The patients were able to perform this task accurately. However, when questioned as to the nature of the stimuli after a trial, they could easily name the stimulus in the right visual field but denied having seen the stimulus presented in the neglected left field.

These studies were the first in a long series that have now been conducted by several laboratories. Taken together, they show that the information presented in the neglected field could be used to make decisions, even though it could not be consciously described. A decision was correctly made that two objects were different, but the patient could name only one of them.

We discovered other related phenomena while studying split-brain patients, who have had the cortical connections between the two halves of their brains severed in an attempt to control their epilepsy. In consequence of this surgery, information presented to one half of the brain can no longer consciously influence information presented to the other half of the brain (15). Thus, an apple held in one hand will not help the patient find a matching apple with the other hand, J.W., a patient we have been studying for some 15 years, was the first to provide insight into how a visual stimulus is transmitted from the visual cortex into the realm of conscious awareness. We tested J.W. during all phases of his recent medical history: before his first surgery, between the two surgeries when only the posterior half of the corpus callosum had been sectioned, and dozens of times since the callosum was completely sectioned. Before his initial surgery, J.W. performed normally on all tests of whether information presented to the right hemisphere could be named by the left. Clearly, his corpus callosum was functioning normally, and conscious unity was intact.

We were astounded by J.W.'s behavior after only the posterior half of his callosum had been sectioned, the portion of the brain that connects the primary visual areas (16). After posterior callosal sectioning, the brain messages that encode the visual images from the left visual field are no longer directly connected to the left, speech-dominant hemisphere. Thus, we expected that pictures of objects presented to J.W.'s left visual field would not be named, and that was indeed the case, but only for a couple of weeks. Unlike previous split-brain patients, who had undergone complete callosal sectioning, J.W. began to name

pictures presented solely to his right hemisphere. Somehow, information was being transferred to the left brain via the remaining callosal fibers. What proved to be most interesting was the nature of this information.

Upon careful analysis of J.W.'s spoken commentary after a picture was presented to his right hemisphere, it was clear that attributes of the original stimulus were being communicated to the left hemisphere, not the actual stimulus itself. For example, when the word "knight" was flashed to the right hemisphere, J.W. would initiate with himself a process not unlike a game of 20 questions. He would avert his eyes after the word had been presented and report, "I have a picture in mind but can't say it ... two fighters in a ring ... ancient, wearing uniforms and helmets ... on horses trying to knock each other off ... knights?"

As the partial information was being communicated from the right hemisphere to the left through the uncut part of his callosum, the left hemisphere pieced each clue together until an intelligent guess was possible. Observing this behavior, trial after trial, was a very powerful experience. These observations showed that the brain's cortical pathways handle identifiable and qualitatively different information. In this case, a communication channel in the brain was transmitting abstract information about a stimulus, not the stimulus itself. These processes are largely unconscious, and yet they go on at the level of the cortex, not among the older, subcortical parts of the brain.

In a series of studies on these same patients, we began to see that one hemisphere could influence the attentional properties of the other. Somehow, through remaining neural connections, one half of the brain was manipulating the state of the other half of the brain in an unconscious way (17). It appeared that perceptual information presented to one hemisphere subtly influenced the decision processes of the other. In light of blind-sight reports, it hardly seemed surprising that subjects could make use of visually presented information not accessible to consciousness. Subcortical networks, with their interhemispheric connections, seemed to be the anatomic structures that allowed for this transfer of information. It would be difficult to argue against the concept that perceptual decisions or cognitive activities routinely result from processes outside of conscious awareness, and it looked as if we were observing such processes in the form of subcortical, interhemispheric semantic transfer.

As our studies progressed, however, we were not able to support our original hypothesis that higher order, perceptual information interacts between the hemispheres after surgical sectioning of the corpus callosum. There were also new reports of high-level hemispheric interactions after full commissurotomy. These studies prompted us to carefully reexamine our split-brain patients, and when we did so, we could find no interhemispheric interactions of this kind. This was the case even when we used stabilized images to permit extended stimulus presentations. Moreover, we could not reproduce our original findings on semantic priming, and we have been forced to conclude that this report was in error. It also has become apparent that there are grounds for uncertainty regarding an interpretation of blindsight in terms of subcortical systems (12, 18). If the subcortex was the answer, split-brain patients should be able to show interactions of perceptual information, which they cannot. At this point, we began to suspect that the multitudinous reports of the subcortical basis of blindsight were in error.

In the early 1980s, Jeffrey Holtzman began to study blindsight in my laboratory. We were fortunate to have a piece of equipment that allowed for the very careful assessment of the position of the eye in relation to where a stimulus might appear, allowing for the precise presentation of stimuli within the scotoma.

We first studied a 34-year-old woman who had undergone surgery to clip an aneurysm in the right half of her brain (18). The surgery was expected to have the consequence of producing blindness in part of the patient's vision, because damage would occur to her right occipital lobe, the brain area with the aneurysm. Sure enough, after surgery, there was a dense, left homonymous hemianopia. Magnetic resonance imaging (MRI) showed an occipital lesion that clearly spared both extrastriate regions as well as the main midbrain candidate for residual vision, the superior colliculus. These intact areas should have been able to support many of the blindsight phenomena commonly reported.

Holtzman started out by presenting the patient with a very simple task. In each visual field, he presented a matrix of four crosses. The patient was asked to fixate a point in the middle of a visual monitor and to move her eyes to the point in the matrix that flashed. The four crosses were randomly highlighted. Of course, the patient had no problem doing the task when the matrices were flashed into her intact field of vision. What Holtzman wanted to see was good performance in her blind field. He wanted her to be able to move her eyes accurately but not be able to claim that she actually saw the lights.

The patient was shown to be blind even though she had the brain structures intact that should support the phenomenon of blindsight; he studied her for months and got nothing. Holtzman moved on to several other studies. He studied other patients who had been reported to show the phenomenon, and when he did the experiments correctly, none had it. Working with Steven Hillyard at the University of California, San Diego, he also showed that none of these patients had what are called evoked responses to light flashed into their blind fields.

We left the problem alone for a few years. It was not until a new graduate student, Mark Wessinger, came along to the laboratory that my colleague Robert Fendrich and I renewed our interest in this issue (19, 20). By this time, we had moved to Dartmouth Medical School and were calling on a different kind of patient. Our first case was a woodsman from New Hampshire who had had a stroke involving his right primary visual cortex. Nonetheless, he pursued life with vigor and was quite a marksman. Before studying what could or could not be done in the blind visual field, basic perimetry was performed to discover the exact character of the scotoma.

For these tests, we were able to use a newly acquired image stabilizer, which allowed us to keep images steady on the retina despite observer eye motions. Our woodsman's scotoma was carefully explored using high-contrast black dots on a white background. In fact, a whole matrix of dots was presented in an area of his scotoma. Hundreds of trials were presented over many testing sessions.

The efforts paid off. In the sea of blindness, we found what we called a "hot spot," an island of vision. In one small area, about 1 degree in diameter, the woodsman could detect the presence of visual information. If it were truly a 1 degree window, a 2 degree stimulus that was either a square or a diamond shape should not be detected. Even though a 2 degree stimulus is larger and under normal conditions would be easier to detect, the patient should not be able to see it because the black dot would be larger than the window the island provided. In fact, the patient could not see the larger stimulus. Follow-up testing showed that the patient could detect differences between light of different wavelengths in the "hot spot." Could it be that the island was the source of so-called blindsight?

There are many aspects of our finding that correspond directly to the original reports. First, the woodsman was not at all confident of his decisions about the lights he could detect. On a scale of 1 to 5, his confidence hovered around 1. When a spot had been presented in his good field of vision, it was closer to 5. At some level, therefore, he was responding above chance but outside of conscious awareness, which is the very definition of blindsight phenomena. But like everything else, the true answer is in the details. Our findings suggested that blindsight was not a property of subcortical systems taking over the visual function because vision was not possible in the vast majority of the blind area. Our patient

could see only in the islands of vision, whereas the original reports had maintained that patients could detect visual information throughout their visual fields.

Without an eye-tracking device of the kind we used, there are real problems with interpreting the results using standard testing procedures of the type used by Weiskrantz and colleagues. One simply cannot be sure what part of the patient's visual field one is stimulating with any kind of precision. His extensively studied patient also had a shrinking blind spot; although it started out large, by the time many studies were done, it was quite small. Overall, the smaller the blind spot, the less certain one is that discrete stimulation of the blind area, and only the blind area, is occurring. Moreover, an area approximately 10 degrees in diameter of partially preserved vision was embedded within the scotoma that remained in his patient. Many of the studies on case D.B. were conducted without any eye motion monitoring or control, so one simply must have faith that stimuli were properly placed.

There is another way of examining the issue of whether residual vision is supported by visual cortex or by subcortical structures. Through advances in modern brain imaging, one can take pictures of a patient's brain and look for spared cortex. Our woodsman had several studies done of this kind. First, using MRI, a method of taking a picture that shows the basic anatomic structure of the brain, there was the clear suggestion that part of his visual cortex was spared. Yet, MRI does not show if the remaining tissue is functional; it might be in place but damaged.

We followed up these studies on case C.L.T. with a positron emission tomography study. We tested the woodsman using that method, and discovered his spared cortex as detected with MRI was also metabolically active. We also recently confirmed and extended the finding of islands of vision in other patients who have suffered lesions to the primary visual system (21). Thus, before one can assert that blindsight occurs due to subcortical structures, one first must be extremely careful to rule out the possibility of spared visual cortex.

Finally, we have studied two patients who underwent either partial or complete functional hemispherectomy (22). Neither patient showed any evidence of residual vision even though both patients had collicular systems intact.

None of this, of course, is to suggest that unconscious processes are not of constant and primary importance to our vision. It is yet another demonstration of the truth that most of what our brain does, it does outside of the realm of conscious awareness. However, my colleagues and I do reject the proposition that because blindsight demonstrates vision outside the realm of conscious awareness, it supports the view that perception can occur in the absence of sensation, as sensations are presumed to be our experiences of impinging stimuli. Because it is the role of the primary visual cortex to process sensory inputs, advocates of this view have found it useful to attribute blindsight to alternative visual processing pathways. I submit that this formulation is unnecessary and implausible. It is commonplace to design demanding perceptual tasks where non-neurologic subjects routinely report low confidence values for tasks they are performing above chance. However, it is not necessary to proposed secondary visual systems to account for such data because the primary visual system is intact and fully functional.

As previously noted, it is also the case that patients with parietal lobe damage but spared visual cortex can perform perceptual judgments outside the realm of conscious awareness. These subjects can compare two stimuli, although they deny awareness of one of them. The failure of these patients to consciously access the information used to compare the stimuli should not be attributed to processing within a secondary visual system because the geniculostriate pathway was still intact. Many other examples of phenomena can be found where, as the MIT philosopher Ned Block has said, conscious access to brain events is impaired or nonexistent. The vast

staging for our mental activities happens largely without our monitoring, and it is to be expected that this situation can be identified by various experimental means.

The Concept of Modularity and the Role of the Interpreter

Human brains are large because of the great number of things they can do. The uniquely human skills we possess may well be produced by minute and circumscribed neuronal networks sometimes referred to as modules. And yet our highly modularized brain generates this feeling in all of us that we are integrated and unified. How does that come about, even though we are a collection of specialized modules?

The answer appears to be that there is a specialized left hemisphere system we have designated as the "interpreter," a device that seeks explanations for why events occur. The advantage of having such a system is obvious. By going beyond observing contiguous events and asking why they happened, a brain can cope with these same events more effectively, should they happen again.

We first showed the interpreter using a simultaneous concept test. The patient is shown two pictures, one exclusively to the left hemisphere and one exclusively to the right, and is asked to choose from an array of pictures placed in full view in front of him or her, the ones associated with the pictures lateralized to the left and right brain. In one example of this kind of test, a picture of a chicken claw was flashed to the left hemisphere and a picture of a snow scene to the right. Of the array of pictures placed in front of the subject, the obviously correct association is a chicken for the chicken claw and a shovel for the snow scene. Split-brain subject P.S. responded by choosing the shovel with the left hand and the chicken with the right. When asked why he chose these items, his left hemisphere replied, "Oh, that's simple. The chicken claw goes with the chicken, and you need a shovel to clean out the chicken shed." Here, the left brain, observing the left hand's response, interprets that response into a context consistent with its sphere of knowledge—one that does not include information about the right hemisphere snow scene.

There are many ways to influence the left brain interpreter. As already mentioned in the foregoing example, we wanted to know whether or not the emotional response to stimuli presented to one half of the brain would have an effect on the affective tone of the other half. Using an optical computer system that detects the slightest movement of the eyes, we were able to project an emotion-laden movie to the right hemisphere. If the patient tried to cheat and move the eye toward the movie, it was electronically shut off.

We studied patient V.P. The movie her right hemisphere saw was about a vicious man pushing another off a balcony and then throwing a fire bomb on top of him. It then showed other men trying to put the fire out. When V.P. was first tested on this problem, she could not access speech from her right hemisphere. When asked what she had seen, she said, "I don't really know what I saw. I think just a white flash." When I asked, "Were there people in it?", V.P. replied, "I don't think so. Maybe just some trees, red trees like in the fall." I asked, "Did it make you feel any emotion?", and V.P. answered, "I don't really know why, but I'm kind of scared. I feel jumpy. I think maybe I don't like this room, or maybe it's you, you're getting me nervous." Then V.P. turned to one of the research assistants and said, "I know I like Dr. Gazzaniga, but right now I'm scared of him for some reason."

The foregoing experimental evidence represents a commonly occurring event in all of us. A mental system sets up a mood that alters the general physiology of the brain. The verbal system notes the mood and immediately attributes cause to the feeling. It is a powerful mechanism, and once so clearly seen, it makes you wonder how often we are victims of spurious emotional/cognitive correlations.

There have been recent studies that examine further the properties of the interpreter and how its presence influences other mental skills. There are, for example, hemisphere-specific changes in the accuracy of memory process (23). The predilection of the left hemisphere to interpret events has an impact on the accuracy of memory. When subjects were presented with a series of pictures that represented common events (i.e., getting up in the morning or making cookies) and then asked several hours later to identify whether pictures in another series had appeared in the first, both hemispheres were equally accurate in recognizing the previously viewed pictures and rejecting the unrelated ones. Only the right hemisphere, however, correctly rejected pictures in the second set that were not previously viewed but were related or semantically congruent with pictures from the first. The left hemisphere incorrectly "recalled" significantly more of these pictures as having occurred in the first set, presumably because they fit into the schema it had constructed regarding the event. This finding is consistent with the view of a left hemisphere interpreter that constructs theories to assimilate perceived information into a comprehensible whole. In doing so, however, the elaborative processing involved has a deleterious effect on the accuracy of perceptual recognition. This result has been extended to include verbal material (24).

A more recent example of the interpreter in action comes from studies that now document the patient J.W. who can speak out of his right hemisphere as well as his left. In brief, naming of left field stimuli appears to be increasing at a rapid rate (25, 26). An interesting phenomenon that occurred during these naming tasks was J.W.'s tendency to sometimes report that he saw a stimulus in his right visual field that was actually presented to his left visual field. Although there is no convincing evidence of any genuine visual transfer between the hemispheres, on trials where he was certain of the name of the stimulus, he maintained that he saw the stimulus well. On trials where he was not certain of the name of the stimulus, he maintained that he did not see it well. This is consistent with the view that the left hemisphere's interpreter actively constructs a mental portrait of past experience, even though that experience did not directly occur in that hemisphere. We speculate that this experience was caused by the left hemisphere interpreter giving meaning to right hemisphere spoken responses, possibly by activating the left hemisphere mental imagery systems.

A related phenomenon is seen in patients with cochlear implants. Implant surgery can enable patients who have become deaf after experiencing normal development of language to regain their capacity to hear (27). The cochlear implant transduces auditory information into discrete patterns of stimulation on an eight-electrode array that is implanted on the cochlear nerve. After 3 months of practice, subjects begin to be able to decode the implant's output as speech. As they become adept at this decoding task, they report that the speech they hear sounds normal. Because the eight electrodes are unlikely to be stimulating the cochlear nerve in the way it was naturally activated before their hearing loss, the new auditory code must undergo a transformation such that the patients feel they are hearing undistorted speech. In short, a new kind of auditory input is converted to a form that resembles the patients' stored representations. Observations of this kind are consistent with our present findings concerning visual input. J.W.'s left hemisphere maintains that he sees the objects presented to the right hemisphere; because the evidence suggests that there is no actual sensory transfer, J.W.'s interpretive system appears to be constructing this reality from speech cues provided by the right hemisphere.

The left hemisphere's capacity for continual interpretation suggests that it is always looking for order and reason, even where there is none. Nowhere has this been more dramatically realized than in a recent study by George Wolford at Dartmouth College. In a simple test that requires one simply to guess if a light is going to appear on the top or bottom of a computer screen, we humans perform in an inventive way. The experiment manipulates the stimulus to appear on the top 80% of the time. Although it quickly becomes evident the top button is being illuminated more often, we keep trying to figure out the whole sequence and deeply believe we can. Yet by adopting this strategy we are rewarded only 68% of the time. If we simply always pressed the top button, we would be rewarded 80% of the time. Rats and other animals are more likely to "learn to maximize" and only press the top button. It turns out the right hemisphere behaves in the same way. It does not try to interpret its experience and find the deeper meaning but continues to live only in the thin moment of the present. And when the left is asked to explain why it is attempting to figure out the whole sequence, it always comes up with a theory, even though it is spurious.

Summary and Conclusions

There is a deep belief that we can attain not only a neuroscience of consciousness but a neuroscience of human consciousness. It is as if something terribly new and complex happens as the brain enlarges to its human form. Whatever this is, it triggers our capacity for self-reflection, for ennui, and for lingering moments.

I would like to propose a simple, three-step suggestion. First, we should focus on what we mean when we talk about conscious experience. It is merely the awareness we have of our capacities as a species, but not the capacities themselves—only the awareness or feelings we have about them. The brain is clearly not a general purpose computing device but is a collection of circuits devoted to quite specific capacities. This is true for all brains, but what is wonderful about the human brain is that we have untold numbers of these capacities. We have more than the chimp, which has more than the monkey, which has more than the cat, which runs circles around the rat. Because we have so many specialized systems and because they can frequently do things they were not designed to do, it appears our brains have a single, general computing device. But we do not. Thus, step 1 requires that we recognize we are a collection of adaptations and, furthermore, we recognize the distinction between a species' capacities and its feelings about those capacities. Now consider step 2.

Can there be any doubt that a rat at the moment of copulation is as sensorially fulfilled as a human? Of course it is. Do you think a cat does not enjoy a good piece of cod? Of course it does. Or, a monkey does not enjoy a spectacular swing? Again, it has to be true. Each species is aware of its special capacities. So, what is human consciousness? It is the very same awareness, save for the fact that we can be aware of so much more, so many wonderful things. A circuit—perhaps a single system or one duplicated over and over again—is associated with each brain capacity. The more systems a brain possesses, the greater the awareness of capacities.

Think of the variations in capacity within our own species; they are not unlike the vast differences between species. Years of split-brain research have informed us that the left hemisphere has many more mental capacities than the right one. The left is capable of logical feats that the right hemisphere cannot manage. Although the right has capacities such as facial recognition systems, it is a distant second with problem-solving skills. In short, the right hemisphere's level of awareness is limited. It knows precious little about a lot of things, but the limits to human capacity are everywhere in the population. No one need be offended to realize that just as someone with normal intelligence can understand Ohm's law, others, like yours truly, are clueless about Kepler's laws. I am ignorant about them and will remain so. I am unable to be aware about what they mean for the universe. The circuits that enable me to understand these things are not present in my brain.

By emphasizing specialized circuits that arise from natural selection, we see that the brain is not a unified neural net that supports a general problem-solving device. With this being understood, we can concentrate on the possibility that smaller, more manageable circuits produce awareness of a species' capacities. Holding fast to the notion of a unified neural net means we can understand human conscious experience only by figuring out the interactions of billions of neurons. That task is hopeless. My scheme is not.

Hence step 3. The very same split-brain research that exposed shocking differences between the two hemispheres also showed that the human left hemisphere has the interpreter. The left brain interpreter's job is to interpret our behavior and our responses, whether cognitive or emotional, to environmental challenges. It constantly establishes a running narrative of our actions, emotions, thoughts, and dreams. It is the glue that keeps our story unified and creates our sense of being a unified, rational agent. It brings to our bag of individual instincts the illusion that we are something other than what we are. It builds our theories about our own life, and these narratives of our past behavior ooze into our awareness.

The problem of consciousness, then, is tractable. We do not have to find the code of one huge, interacting neural network. Instead, we must find the common and perhaps simple neural circuit(s) that allows vertebrates to be aware of their species-specific capacities, and the problem is solved. The same enabling circuit(s) in the rat is most likely present in the human brain, and understanding that basic point makes the problem scientifically tractable. What makes us so grand is that the basic circuit has so much more to work with in the human brain.

Finally it becomes clear. The insertion of an interpreter into an otherwise functioning brain delivers all kinds of by-products. A device that begins to ask how one thing relates to another, a device that asks about an infinite number of things, and a device that can get productive answers to those questions cannot help give birth to the concept of self. Surely one of the questions the device would ask is, who is solving these problems? Let us call that me, and away it goes! The device that has its rules for solving a problem of how one thing relates to another must be reinforced for such an action, just as solving where the evening meal is for an ant reinforces the ant's food-seeking devices.

Our brains are automatic because physical tissues perform what we do. How could it be any other way? That means they do it before our conceptual self knows about it. But the conceptual self grows and grows and reaches proportions that find the biologic fact of interest but not paralyzing. The interpretation of things past has liberated us from the sense of being tied to the demands of the environment and has produced the wonderful sensation that our self is in charge of our destiny. All of our everyday success at reasoning through life's data convinces us of our centrality. Because of that we can drive our automatic brains to greater accomplishment and enjoyment of life.

Acknowledgment

This work was supported by National Institutes of Health Grants NIND S 8 R01, NS22626-09, NINDS 5 PO1, and NS1778-014, and by the James S. McDonnell Foundation. Parts of this chapter have appeared in *The Cognitive Neurosciences*, ed. by M. S. Gazzaniga, MIT Press, Cambridge, MA.

References

1. Gazzaniga MS. *Interpretations of things past*. Berkeley, CA: University of California Press, 1998.

2. Jerne N. Antibodies and learning: selection versus instruction. In: Quarton G, Melnechuck T, Schmidt FO, eds. *The neurosciences: a study program*. Vol. 1. Rockefeller University Press, 1967:200–205.

3. James W. *The principles of psychology*. Vol. I. New York: Dover, 1890.

4. Marler P. An ethological theory of the origin of vocal learning. *Ann NY Acad Sci* 1976; 280:386–395.

5. Kuhl PK. Learning and representation in speech and language. *Curr Opin Neurobiol* 1994; 4:812–822.

6. Edelman GM. *Neural Darwinism: the theory of neuronal group selection*. New York: Basic Books, 1987.

7. Merzenich MM, Kaas JH, Wall JT, Nelson RJ, Sur M, Felleman DH. Topographic reorganization of somatosensory cortical areas 3b and 1 in adult monkeys following restricted deafferentation. *Neuroscience* 1983; 10:33–55.

8. Merzenich MM, Schreiner C, Jenkins WM, Wang X. Neural mechanisms underlying temporal integration, segmentation, and input sequence representation: some implications for the origin of learning disabilities. *Ann NY Acad Sci* 1993; 682:1–22.

9. Platt (manuscript in preparation).

10. Shephar RN. *Mindsights*. San Francisco: WH Freeman, 1992.

11. Goodale MA, Milner AD. Separate visual pathways for perception and action. *Trends Neurosci* 1992; 15:20–25.

12. Weiskrantz L. *Blindsight: a case study and implications*. Oxford, England: Oxford University Press, 1986.

13. Gazzaniga MS, Ledoux JE. *The integrated mind*. New York: Plenum, 1978.

14. Volpe BT, LeDoux JE, Gazzaniga MS. Information processing of visual stimuli in an extinguished field. *Nature* 1979; 282:722–724.

15. Gazzaniga MS. Principles of human brain organization derived from split-brain studies. *Neuron* 1995; 14:217–228.

16. Sidtis JJ, Volpe BT, Holtzman JD, Wilson DH. Gazzaniga MS. Cognitive interaction after staged callosal section: evidence for a transfer of semantic activation. *Science* 1982; 212:344–346.

17. Holtzman JD, Sidtis JJ, Volpe BT, Wilson DH, Gazzaniga MS. Dissociation of spatial information for stimulus localization and the control of attention. *Brain* 1981; 104:861–872.

18. Holtzman JD. Interactions between cortical and subcortical visual areas: evidence from human commissurotomy patients. *Vision Res* 1984; 24:801–813.

19. Gazzaniga MS, Fendrich R, Wessinger, CM. Blindsight reconsidered. *Curr Directions Psychol Sci* 1994; 3:93–96.

20. Gazzaniga MS, Fendrich R, Wessinger CM. Blindsight reconsidered. *Curr Directions Psychol Sci* 1994; 3:93–96.

21. Wessinger CM, Fendrich R, Gazzaniga MS. Islands of residual vision in hemianopic patients. *J Cognitive Neurosci* 1997; 9:203–221.

22. Wessinger CM, Fendrich R, Gazzaniga MS. Residual vision with awareness in the field contralateral to a partial or complete functional hemispherectomy. *Neuropsychologia* 1996; 34:1129–1137.

23. Phelps EA, Gazzaniga MS. Hemispheric differences in mnemonic processing: the effects of left hemisphere interpretation. *Neuropsychologia* 1992; 30:293–297.

24. Metcalfe J, Funnell M, Gazzaniga MS. Right hemisphere superiority: studies of a split-brain patient. *Psychol Sci* 1995; 6:157–164.

25. Baynes K, Wessinger CM, Fendrich R, Gazzaniga MS. The emergence of the capacity of the disconnected right hemisphere to control naming: implications for functional plasticity. *Neuropsychologia* 1995; 33:1225–1242.

26. Gazzaniga MS, Eliassen JC, Nisenson L, Wessuger CM, Baynes KB. Collaboration between the hemispheres of a callosotomy patient—emerging right hemisphere speech and the left brain interpreter. *Brain* 1996; 119:1255–1262.

27. Schindler RA, Kessler DK. The UCSF Storz cochlear implant: patient performance. *Am J Otol* 1987; 8:247–255.

Attention, Self-Regulation, and Consciousness

Michael I. Posner and Mary K. Rothbart

Consider the direction of your mind at any moment you like to choose; you will find that it is occupied with what now is, but always and especially with regard to what is about to be. Attention is expectation, and there is no consciousness without a certain attention to life. The future is there; it calls up, or rather, it draws us to it.... All action is an encroachment on the future. To retain what no longer is, to anticipate what as yet is not—these are the primary functions of consciousness. Bergson (1920, p. 6)

Aspects of Consciousness

The problem of consciousness involves many difficult and overlapping issues (Block 1995; Posner 1994). Perhaps the most frequently discussed role of consciousness involves awareness of our sensory world. Another aspect of consciousness is the fact or illusion of voluntary control. In the course of development, a central issue is the awareness of one's self, and another is the form of voluntary control involved in self-regulation. These functions develop within the dyad involving the child and the care-giver as a carrier of the culture's socialization process. It is possible, even likely, that brain mechanisms subserving these various forms of consciousness may cut across definitions in ways that defy the usual logical and philosophical distinctions.

Within neuroscience, most students have followed Crick's (1994) suggestion that sensory awareness is the aspect of consciousness most amenable to scientific analysis, placing awareness at the centre of discussions of brain mechanisms of consciousness. In this chapter, however, we focus on the voluntary control of mental processes that might fit more closely with the self regulation of behaviour and thought. We believe the developmental shifts in self-regulation during the early years of life form a tractable behavioural model for studying changes in voluntary self-regulation.

In the psychology of adult cognition, systems involved in the regulation of thought, emotion and behaviour have been given the label "supervisory" or "executive attention." We note that the set of functions suggested for this system appear to be implemented by a brain network that includes the midfrontal cortical areas and underlying basal ganglia.

This system is the source of attention and operates in conjunction with other structures to carry out specific cognitive and emotional computations. While we have outlined this view previously (Posner & Rothbart 1992, 1994), new data have accumulated from our studies and the work of others to provide an enlarged perspective for the theme of this chapter.

In this chapter, we first outline how the idea of executive control developed within cognitive psychology. Next, we review links between these functions and a specific anatomy and circuitry that have arisen from neuroimaging studies of selection, conflict and error detection. We then examine evidence on how this system begins its development in early infancy with the control of distress and assumes the control and regulation of cognition in later childhood. We conclude with consideration of new directions for furthering our understanding of conscious control.

Executive Control

All normal people have a strong subjective feeling of intentional or voluntary control of their behaviour. These subjective feelings can be freely verbalized. Indeed, asking people about their goals or intentions is probably the single most predictive indicator of their behaviour during problem solving (Newell & Simon 1972). The importance of intention and goals is illustrated in observations of patients with frontal lesions (Duncan 1994) or mental disorders (Frith 1992) who show disruption in either their central control over behaviour or their subjective feelings of control. Despite these indices of central control, it has not been easy to specify exactly the functions or mechanisms of central control. Norman & Shallice (1986) argued that a supervisory system would be necessary for situations in which routine or automatic processes are inadequate. These functions include selection among competing inputs, resolution of conflict among responses, and monitoring and correcting errors.

The idea of executive control was made more concrete in cognitive studies of the 1970s and 1980s (see Posner (1978) for a review). In this research, it was possible to separate conscious control of mental events from automatic activation of the same events. The research approach involved semantic priming of a target word by a related (prime) word. If the prime was masked so that subjects were unaware of its identity, priming could still take place. However, the effects of priming were somewhat different from trials in which the prime had been carefully attended. When masked, ambiguous primes (e.g., palm referring to tree or hand) improved performance on targets related to both of its meanings (e.g. tree and hand). However, when presented in context and unmasked, only the relevant meaning was primed (Marcel 1983).

If a word from one category (e.g. animal) was presented as a prime and subjects were instructed they should associate animal primes with the category "building," target words in the associated category (e.g. window) were faster in comparison with those in a category unrelated to the instructed category (e.g. tin). The subject had voluntarily activated the instructed category. If an animal target (e.g. dog) was presented before subjects could switch from the prime category "animal" to the instructed category "building," fast reaction times were shown to the word "dog," but if dog was delayed until after subjects had a chance to execute the switch to the instructed category, the target "dog" would have

a slow reaction time since subjects were now attending to the wrong category (Neeley 1977).

These findings gave a concrete reality to the difference between the voluntary control of mental events and the same event when driven by input. Priming could be produced by an automatic activation of a pathway without attention, facilitating reaction times for primed items. Imaging studies have shown that automatic priming of this sort is produced by a reduction of blood flow within the brain area related to the form of priming. For semantic priming, this reduction would be within areas of the brain related to the meaning of the word (Demb et al. 1995). A second form of priming could be produced by attention. Within one second, subjects could voluntarily choose an associated category and the consequence of that selection was faster processing of related targets and retarded processing of unrelated targets. When a category was attended, items within the category were facilitated in reaction time, but items in other categories were retarded over what they would be if unprimed. Imaging studies have suggested that attention to a computation increases blood flow within the attended area. Thus, priming may be produced by different brain mechanisms and have quite different consequences for performance.

Brain Mechanisms

When studies were begun using neuroimaging with PET, it was possible to discover brain areas that might reflect the various functions of attention (Posner & Petersen 1990). These include orienting to sensory stimuli and maintenance of the alert state as well as higher level executive attention. The executive network was found to be active in tasks involving selection, conflict and error detection, the very functions outlined in the earlier cognitive models (Shallice & Burgess 1996). In all of these cases, there was evidence of activity within the frontal midline, most often within the anterior cingulate gyrus.

Selection

One task that has been analysed in great detail involves reading individual words. In a typical task, subjects are shown a series of 40 simple nouns (e.g., hammer). In the experimental condition they indicate the use of each noun (for example, hammer → pound). In the control condition, they read the word aloud. The difference in activation between the two tasks illustrates what happens in the brain when subjects are required to develop a very simple thought, in this case how to use a hammer. Brain activity obtained during reading words aloud is then subtracted from the activity found in the generate condition. Results illustrate the surprising fact that the anatomy of this high-level cognitive activity is similar enough among individuals to produce focal average activations that are both statistically significant and reproducible.

There are four focal but well separated areas of increases in brain activity during the simple thought needed to find the use of the word. The first is activity in the midline of the frontal lobe in the anterior cingulate gyrus. This area is involved in higher level aspects of attention, regardless of whether the task involves language, spatial location or object processing. We believe it relates to what we called above executive attention (Posner & DiGirolamo 1998). Two additional activations are in the left lateral frontal and posterior cortex in areas involved with processing the meaning of words or sentences. Finally, there is activation in the right cerebellum, which is closely connected to the left frontal areas.

We have been able to find the scalp signatures of three of these activations in our high density electrical recording studies and to trace the time-course of this activation (Abdullaev & Posner 1997, 1998; Snyder et al. 1995). When subjects obtain the use of a noun, there is an area of positive electrical activity over frontal electrodes starting about 150 ms after the word appears. This early electrical activity is most likely to be generated by the large area of activation in the anterior cingulate shown by the PET studies.

Two other areas active during generating word meanings occur in the left frontal and left posterior cortex. The left frontal area (anterior to and overlapping classical Broca's area) begins to show activity about 220 ms after the word occurs. During this interval, both the cingulate and the left frontal semantic area are active. We assume that the left frontal activation is related to the meaning of the individual word presented on that trial. The time-course of the left frontal area during processing the meaning of words is further supported by results obtained from cellular recording in patients with depth electrodes implanted for neurosurgery (Abdullaev & Bechtereva 1993). This area is active early enough to influence motor and eye movement responses, typically occurring by 200–300 ms, that can be influenced by the meaning of a word.

On the other hand, the left posterior brain area found to be more active during the processing of the meaning of visual words does not show up in the electrical maps until about 600 ms after input. This activity is near the classical Wernicke's area and lesions of this area are known to produce a loss of understanding of meaningful speech. We think this area is important in the storage and integration of words into larger meaningful units. Damage to this area makes it difficult to understand speech or written material. These results demonstrate how one can approach both the anatomy and circuitry of higher mental processes. By observing the brain areas activated in PET studies and relating them to scalp electrical activity, we have a picture of the temporal dynamics in creating a simple thought.

Recent fMRI studies have confirmed the presence of the semantic areas shown by PET and have provided more information on individual differences. For example, an fMRI study has shown that within the anterior and posterior semantic areas, different portions are active when processing different semantic categories (Spitzer et al. 1996). In Spitzer's data, the exact organization of individual categories within the general anterior and posterior semantic brain areas appears to differ from one subject to another. Nevertheless, the presence of category specific semantic areas indicates that the brain uses the same general mapping strategy to handle semantic relations as it does to handle sensory processing.

This form of semantic mapping by word category helps explain the automatic effect of semantic priming described above. If a category is activated by input, it simply makes more available words related to the same category. Automatic priming in the brain seems to be produced by a reduction in blood flow by neurons in the primed area (Demb et al. 1995; Raichle et al. 1994). However, priming can also occur as the result of attending to items. Attention appears to involve the midline frontal activity described above, and has the effect of boosting activity within the attended area. Cognitive studies argue that attended activation produces both an improvement in the processing of related items and

also a reduction in the efficiency of processing unrelated items. It is as though the increase in neuronal activity in one area induced by attending to that area actually inhibits other items far outside of the attended category. By bringing together methods for examining anatomy and circuitry of brain activity with analysis of the cognitive consequences it is now possible to see much of what is involved when carrying out the conscious or voluntary act of selecting a thought.

Conflict

The next step was to test whether these midfrontal activations were generally involved when elements of the task were in conflict, requiring executive control to perform the selected function. The most frequently studied conflict task is the Stroop effect in which subjects are instructed to name the colour of ink of a word which may be either the same as the ink colour (congruent), a different colour word (incongruent), or a noncolour word (neutral) (Pardo et al. 1990).

Figure 15.1 shows the results of six studies using variants of this task. All of them have activation in the frontal midline, but at a variety

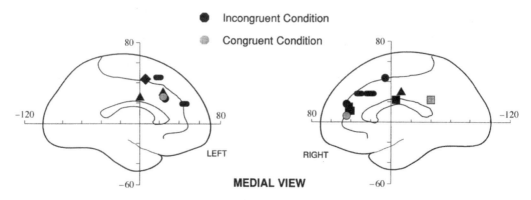

Figure 15.1
Activations in various Stroop and Stroop-like experiments in areas of the frontal midline. Activations in congruent and incongruent blocks are plotted as dark and light figures. The data are from the following studies: circle, Carter et al. (1995); diamond, Taylor et al. (1994); triangle, George et al. (1994); oval, Bench et al. (1990).

of locations. Although the colour word task is effective for eliciting conflict, it is by no means required. Conflict between word and location (e.g. the word right on the left of the screen), or between the number of items present and their names (e.g. reporting that there are four items present when the items are the word two), are other examples of conflict. A recent fMRI study of word–number conflict, for example, found strong activation of the anterior cingulate and also some motor areas (Bush et al. 1998).

The studies summarized in figure 15.1 show quite a spread over areas of the cingulate. Since the studies shown in figure 15.1 differ in subjects, methods and experimental procedure, this is not surprising. However, somewhat more disturbing, some studies showed the same degree of activation in the cingulate whether the trials were congruent or incongruent, although both differed from neutral trials. Since these trials give very different reaction times, and quite different subjective impressions of conflict, it appeared as though the frontal midline activation might not relate to conflict after all.

However, the PET method provides little evidence on how the frontal activation relates to the overall task. Because trials of a given type have to be blocked together, it is hard to know for all congruent trials whether subjects are responding based on reading the name or whether they really inhibit the name to respond based on the ink colour, since the output would be the same in both cases. To discover exactly what the internal processing is like, it is important to ask when conflict is occurring and for what range of trials.

We have recently completed two studies using high-density electrical study to address these issues (DiGirolamo et al. 1998). Both experiments demonstrated similar temporal and spatial patterns of data for the congruent (e.g. the word "BLUE" in blue ink) and incongruent (e.g. the word "RED" in blue ink) Stroop conditions. These two conditions first diverged from a neutral

condition (a non-colour word; e.g. "KNIFE" in blue ink) at 268 ms over midline and lateral posterior electrode sites (see figure 15.2).

Dipole models of the congruent and incongruent conditions produced matching neural solutions accordant with a cingulate gyrus generator, suggesting the activity of an anterior attentional system during both conditions. These results support an analysis of the Stroop effect postulating comparable selective attentional processes to resolve conflict in both the congruent and incongruent conditions. These occur at multiple levels of processing, from stimulus selection through response choice. The data help to resolve some of the controversies in this literature.

The instruction to select by ink colour is implemented by amplifying computations in prestriate colour areas when there is simultaneous activity in colour name areas, as occurs on both congruent and incongruent trials. It appears that at the time of selection, the subject does not know if the activation in the colour name area matches or mismatches the ink colour. Thus the same cingulate activity is found on both trial types. Presumably both the ink colour and the colour name activate response tendencies. The congruent trials activate only the correct response, while incongruent trials activate conflicting responses, which accounts for the difference in RT and errors. However, the attention network is apparently dominated by the more fundamental conflict involved in executing the instruction to respond based on the ink colour.

The Stroop effect is compelling because it produces such a profound feeling of effort on trials in which the word and ink colour conflict. However, according to our result the selection process is the same as long as the stimulus is a coloured word. This finding supports the idea that the midline frontal areas are involved in resolving conflict, but perhaps are not involved in the feelings of conflict and effort, which must arise more from the conflicting response tendencies and errors produced by incongruent trials.

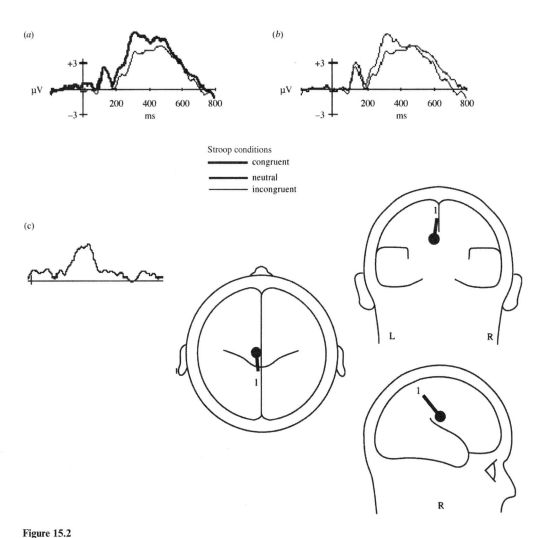

Figure 15.2
Scalp electrical activity from a study of the Stroop effect. Event-related potentials for congruent trials (a), and in-congruent trials (b). Each is compared to neutral trials. Data are from midline electrodes. Best fitting single dipole solutions to 64 channel difference waves between incongruent-neutral trials (c) (DiGirolamo et al. 1998).

Error Detection

One of the functions of the supervisory attention system (Norman & Shallice 1986) was error detection. Error detection has been studied extensively in reaction time tasks within cognitive psychology (Rabbitt 1967) and neuropsychology (Bechtereva 1997). Usually it is thought of as part of a conscious strategy that seeks to adjust the speed of performance to an adequate level of accuracy.

A negative component of the scalp recorded electrical activity (error-related negativity) is recorded following the subject's detection of an error (Gehring et al. 1993). This error negativity occurs about 80 ms after the key press and appears to be localized in the anterior cingulate gyrus (Dehaene et al. 1994; Luu et al. 1998); see figure 15.3.

Error negativity does not occur if the error is undetected by the subject. However, if the subject receives feedback from the experimenter concerning a prior error, negativity can also be recorded (Miltner et al. 1998). The error detection process may also relate to the emotion of making an error, since errors are frequently accompanied by negative vocalization and negative facial expression. Recently, it has been shown that the amplitude of error-related negativity is correlated with self reports of negative emotionality, one of the temperament and personality dimensions most frequently found in psychological self-report scales (Luu et al. 1998). Since the cingulate is anatomically an important part of the limbic system involved in the coding of emotions, its relationship to negative emotionality seems appropriate.

Thus, cognitive tasks involving different operations, all related to executive control, have been shown to activate areas of the anterior cingulate. These observations seem unified only by their involvement in higher level attentional activity related to focal aspects of voluntary control. It is not clear if the same group of cingulate neurons is involved in these various cognitive operations.

To explore this question, an experiment was run in which two tasks known to activate the cingulate gyrus were studied in the same trials with the same subjects (Badgaiyan & Posner 1998). The subject was instructed to generate the use of a visually presented noun and do so within a pre-specified window of time. The window was constructed so that about half the time, subjects' responses fell within the selected window, and half the time they were outside of it. When subjects were outside the window, they received error feedback.

There was evidence of midfrontal activity in the generate use task in comparison to reading aloud. This activity was quite far forward, at about the same location reported previously (Abdullaev & Posner 1997, 1998). However, it occurred somewhat later in time, perhaps reflecting the level of practice or the dual nature of the task in generating the word within an appropriate temporal window. When error feedback trials were compared with correct trials, another activation of the anterior cingulate was found. This activation was much more posterior and clearly different than that obtained for the generate task. Since the two tasks involved the same subjects and trials, it appears that different tasks activate distinct sets of cingulate and that the cingulate does not act as a single unit for processing complex cognitive tasks.

The finding that areas of activation of the cingulate differ according to task demands helps to explain the failure to find common activation in the cingulate during a meta-analysis of nine tasks (Shulman et al. 1997a,b). When passive presentation of the stimuli and responses was subtracted from active performance of the tasks there was activity in the supplementary motor area but not in the cingulate (Shulman et al. 1997a,b). However, a common cingulate focus of activation was found when merely presenting the stimuli was compared with passive presentation of fixation. This finding could suggest that there is an area of the cingulate related to awareness involved in the passive reception of verbal or non-verbal stimuli.

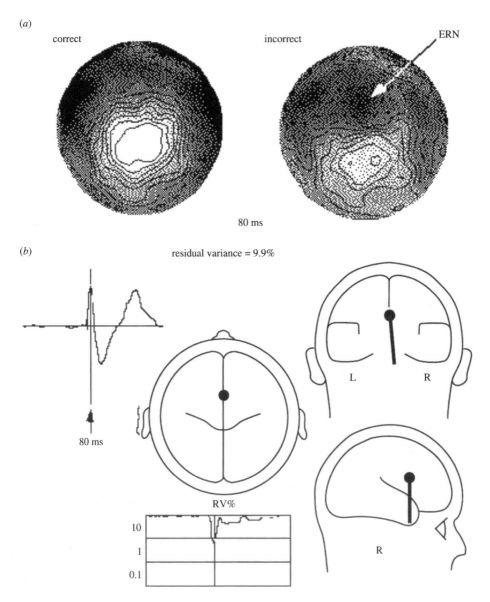

Figure 15.3
Scalp electrical activity at 80 ms following correct and incorrect (error) trials (a) in a speeded reaction time task with distractors. (b) Shows best fitting dipole solutions. (Luu et al. 1998.)

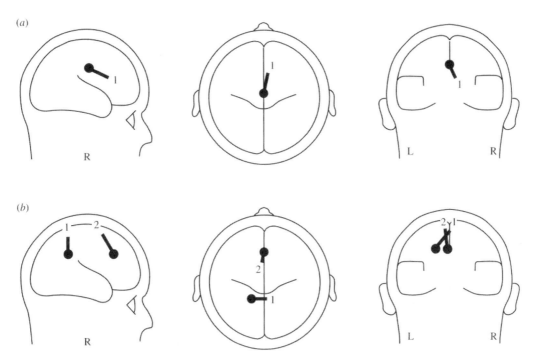

Figure 15.4
Best fitting dipole solutions to 128 channels of ERP following error feedback (a), and use generation (b). (After Badgaiyan & Posner 1998.)

However, each task demand may require processing from different areas of the cingulate.

We have reviewed evidence that areas of the anterior cingulate are involved in many of the features of executive control over mental processing in a wide variety of task domains. It appears that a common area of the cingulate may be involved in the reception of the input, perhaps related to awareness, but that very different areas are involved with different task demands. This data may seem surprising since the anterior cingulate does not appear at first to be likely to be involved in non-emotional responding as in the many cognitive tasks we have examined. We turn now to the question of how this form of brain organization may have arisen in development.

Development

The human infant has the longest period of dependence upon care-givers of any mammal. During this period, infants must gain control of their behaviour and mental state. As we have seen in the last section, it appears that adults exercise a degree of central control over their thoughts and action, and this control involves specific areas within the frontal midline. We ask now how this form of control develops.

Luria (1973) distinguished between an early developing, largely involuntary biological attention system and a later developing, more voluntary social attention system. A major theme emerging from our work shows that Luria (1973) was roughly correct in making a distinction between voluntary and involuntary attention systems, but that contrary to his original belief, both are shaped by a complex interaction between biology and socialization that together determine their regulatory properties.

Soothing

There is clear evidence that anterior cingulate activity is a part of the brain's system for evaluating pain (Rainville et al. 1997) and for distress vocalization (Devinsky et al. 1995). The pain studies have shown cingulate activity when heat stimuli were judged as painful in comparison to merely warm. Moreover, the cingulate appears more involved in the distress caused by the pain rather than merely in the sensory stimuli involved (Rainville 1997). When an effort was made to control the distress produced by a given stimulus using hypnotic suggestion, the amount of cingulate activation reflected felt distress while the somatosensory cortex reflected stimulus intensity rather than perceived pain. A PET study using both pain and Stroop trials with the same subjects (Derbyshire et al. 1998) found that both types of trials activated anterior cingulate sites, but there appeared to be different loci when individual subjects were examined.

How does the cingulate become involved in the control of both pain and in cognitive tasks? In our view this may arise from the experience of early life. The early life of the infant is concerned with the regulation of state, including distress. During the first year of life, attention appears important in developing this form of control. Care-givers provide a hint of how attention is used to regulate the state of the infant. Earlier than three months, care-givers usually report holding and rocking as the main means of quieting their infant. However, at about three months, many care-givers, particularly in western cultures, attempt to distract their infants by bring-

ing their attention to other stimuli. As infants attend, they are often quieted and their distress appears to diminish.

We have conducted a systematic study of attention and soothing in three- to six-month-old infants (Harman et al. 1997). Infants first become distressed to over-stimulation from lights and sounds, but then strongly orientate to interesting visual and auditory events when these are presented. While they orientate, facial and vocal signs of distress disappear. However, as soon as the orienting stops, for example, when the new object is removed, we found that the infant distress returned to almost exactly the levels shown prior to presentation of the object. Apparently the loss of overt signs of distress is not always accompanied by a genuine loss of distress. Instead, some internal system which we termed "the distress keeper" appears to hold the initial level of distress and it returns if the infant's orientation to the novel event is lost. In our later studies, we quieted infants by distraction for as long as one minute without changing the eventual level of distress reached once orienting is ended. The effectiveness of a novel stimulus in achieving sustained orienting in the infant also appeared to be reduced at six months over its influence at 3–4 months.

There are possibly related phenomena present in the adult. Adults who report themselves as having good ability to focus and shift attention, also say they experience less negative affect (Derryberry & Rothbart 1988). Attention may serve to control levels of distress in adults in a somewhat similar way to that found early in infancy. Indeed, many of the ideas of modern cognitive therapy are based upon links between attention and negative ideation.

We do not yet know very much about how orienting serves to control distress either in infancy or for adults. However, as we have noted in the control of pain, a system in which distress and attention are closely coordinated lies in the anterior cingulate gyrus. Of course pain has a

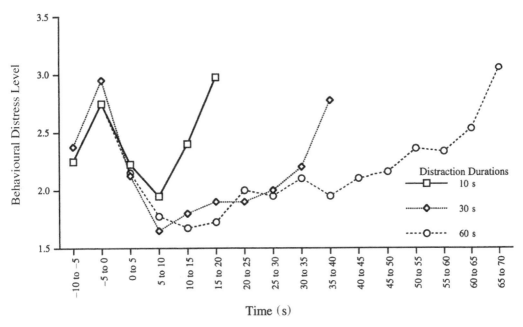

Figure 15.5
Pattern of distress ratings before, during and after presentation of an orienting stimulus to 4- and 6-month-old infants for 10, 30, or 60 s. (Harman et al. 1993.)

very intrusive character and this could be related to its close physical proximity to the anterior attention network.

Recent studies of negative emotion in the adult suggest that distress is related to activity in the amygdala (Irwin et al. 1996). When pictures depicting frightening or horrible scenes are shown to subjects, there is a strong area of amygdala activation. Evidence now exists that activation of the amygdala is modulated by left prefrontal cortical activity. These findings suggest a negative correlation between left prefrontal and amygdala activation in both non-depressed and depressed subjects. One effort to move beyond correlations has been made in studies of rats in which lesions of the medial frontal areas were shown to interfere with extinction of a classically conditioned fear response, suggesting an inhibitory control

of the amygdala by midfrontal regions (Morgan et al. 1993).

One way of measuring emotional awareness of individuals (called the level of emotional awareness) has them describe how they feel about situations, coding their use of emotional terms and descriptors in their written responses (Lane & Schwartz 1992). In a recent study, 12 subjects were shown each of three highly emotional movies and three neutral movies during a PET scan (Lane et al. 1998). Differences in anterior cingulate blood flow between the emotional and neutral movies were correlated with the person's level of emotional awareness score. These data suggest that something about the subjects' awareness of their emotions during sad or happy events is related to changes in the anterior cingulate.

We have no direct evidence that the exquisite control of negative affect by attention in our infant experiments is mediated by midfrontal control systems as might be suggested by the literature above. However, if it were, we might be able to explain why it is that midfrontal areas are so frequently seen as a control system involved in the self-regulation of behaviour.

It is not so much the stimulus of pain or distress that activates cingulate, but the feelings of distress related to the pain or efforts to cope with or control these feelings. Thus amygdala-cingulate interaction might be a reasonable candidate for the earliest form of self-regulation in the infant. In the infant, control of orienting is partly in the hands of care-givers' presentation of relevant information. However, the infant is clearly also involved in soliciting attention from the adults (Stern 1985). During the first years of life, more direct control of attention passes from care-givers to infant. It seems likely that the same mechanisms used to cope with self-regulation of emotion are then transferred to issues of control of cognition during later infancy and childhood.

Executive Control

Many psychologists agree with Denckla (1996) that "the difference between the child and adult resides in the unfolding of executive functions" (p. 264). Luria (1973) referred to the development of a higher level more voluntary attentional mechanism during the second year of life. Individual differences in executive attention have important implications for the early development of behavioural and emotional control (Rothbart & Bates 1998).

The central issue of this chapter is to describe an approach to examining executive function as a developmental process in early childhood. Our goal is to provide an experimental means to link individual differences in self-regulatory behaviours developing in early childhood to the maturation of underlying neural systems. According

to the Norman & Shallice (1986) model discussed above, executive attention comes into play in adults in resolving conflict, correcting errors, and planning new actions. There appears to be excellent data that the ability to resolve conflict undergoes development in early childhood.

For example, Diamond (1991) showed the stages from 9–12 months through which the child passes in resolving conflict between reaching and the line of sight in order to retrieve an object in a box. At nine months, the line of sight dominates completely. Even if the child's hand should touch the toy through the open side of the box, if it is not in line with the side they are looking, infants will withdraw their hand and reach along the line of sight, striking the closed side. Three months later, they are able to look at a closed side but reach through the open end to retrieve the toy.

However, being able to reach for a target away from the line of sight is only a very limited form of conflict resolution, and Gerstadt et al. (1994) extended a verbal conflict modelled on the Stroop paradigm to children as young as 3.5 years. Two cards were prepared to suggest day and night to the children: one depicted a line-drawing of the sun, the other a picture of the moon surrounded by stars. Cards for the control condition were intended to suggest neither day nor night. Children in the conflict condition were instructed to reply "day" to the moon card and "night" to the sun card. Children in the control condition were divided into two groups and instructed to say "day" to either a checkerboard or ribbon card and "night" to the other. At every age, accuracy scores were significantly lower for conflict relative to control trials. Although all children performed at 80% accuracy or better for the first four trials of the session, by the last four trials, performance of the youngest declined to chance. Older children were able to maintain above-chance performance throughout the 16-trial session. Latency scores for conflict relative to control trials were also significantly longer for 3.5- and 4-year-old groups, suggesting that younger children needed more time to formulate their responses when faced with conflict. Other efforts have been made with Stroop-like tasks (Jerger et al. 1988), and with the Wisconsin card sort task (Zelazo et al. 1995), to study children as young as 31 months; little evidence of successful inhibitory control below three years has been found.

However, we believed that children as young as 18 months might be undergoing a development in frontal midline areas that would allow the limited conflict resolution related to eye position to become more general. We have found that children at 18 months can show context sensitive learning of sequences (Clohessy 1993; Posner et al. 1999). This is a form of learning which in adults appears to require access to the kind of higher level attention needed to resolve conflict. Adults can learn sequences of spatial locations implicitly when each location is invariably associated with another location (e.g. 13241324). This occurs even when the adult is distracted with a secondary task known to occupy focal attention (Curran & Keele 1993). The implicit form of skill learning seems to rely mainly upon subcortical structures. However, when distraction is present, adults are not able to learn context sensitive sequences (e.g. 123213) in which each association is ambiguous.

We found that infants as young as four months could learn the unambiguous associations, but not until 18 months did they show the ability to learn ambiguous or context sensitive associations (e.g. 1213). Individual children showed wide differences in their learning abilities, and in our study the ability to learn context sensitive cues was correlated with the care-givers report of the child's vocabulary development.

According to the analysis of the last section, a more direct measure of the development of executive attention might be reflected in the ability to resolve conflict between simultaneous stimulus events as in the Stroop effect. Since children of this age do not read we reasoned that the use of basic visual dimensions of location and identity might be the most appropriate way to study the early resolution of conflict.

The variant of the Stroop effect we designed to be appropriate for ages 2–3 years involved presenting a simple visual object on one side of a screen in front of the child and requiring the child to respond with a button that matched the stimulus they were shown (Gerardi 1996). The child had been trained to "pat" the button that matched the stimulus they were shown. The appropriate button could be either on the side of the stimulus (congruent trial) or on the side opposite the stimulus (incongruent trial). The prepotent response was to press the button on the side of the target irrespective of its identity. However, the task required the child to inhibit that prepotent response and to act instead based on identity. The ability to resolve this conflict is measured by the accuracy and speed of their key press responses.

Results of the study strongly suggested that executive attention undergoes dramatic change during the third year of life. Performance by toddlers at the very beginning of this period was dominated by a tendency to repeat the previous response. Perseverance is associated with frontal dysfunction and this finding is consistent with the idea that executive attention is still very immature at 24 months. Even at this young age, however, toddlers were already showing a significant accuracy difference between compatible and incompatible trials (63% versus 53%). Children at the end of the third and beginning of the fourth year showed a strikingly different pattern of responses. Children who were 36–38 months old performed with high accuracy for both compatible and incompatible conditions (92% and 85%, respectively), showing the expected slowing for incompatible relative to compatible trials (30% longer reaction times).

The transition between these two extremes appears to take place at about 30 months. Cluster analysis divided 30-month-olds into three groups: one group (50%) performed similarly to 24-month-olds, one group (37%) approximated 36–

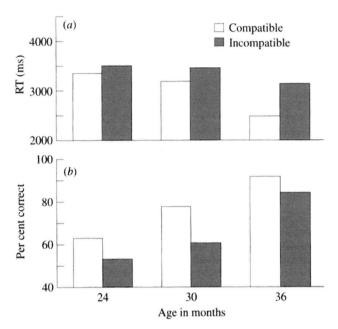

Figure 15.6
RT and per cent correct for compatible (open columns) and incompatible (closed columns) trials of a conflict task in which responses must be made based on identity, but location also varies as a function of age between two and three years. (Gerardi 1996.)

38-month-olds' performance, and a very small group (13%) responded almost exclusively to the location of the stimulus rather than to its identity. In other words, if the picture appeared on the left, these toddlers responded on the left and vice versa, regardless of picture identity.

It was also possible to examine the relationship of our laboratory measures of conflict resolution to a battery of tasks requiring the young child to exercise inhibitory control over their behaviour. We found substantial correlations between these two measures. Even more impressive, elements of the laboratory task were significantly correlated with aspects of effortful control and negative affect in parental reports of infant behaviour in their normal environment. Cingulate activity relates to the control of distress and the cognitive measure of conflict resolution also relates to aspects of infant self control in daily life as reported by their parents.

In the Stroop effect, conflict is introduced between two elements of a single stimulus. We reasoned that an even more difficult conflict might be introduced by the task of executing instructions from one source while inhibiting those from another (L. Jones and M. K. Rothbart, unpublished data). This conflict task is the basis of the "Simon says" game. Previous studies had suggested that the ability to perform this task emerged at about four years of age (Reed et al. 1984). In a recent study we asked children of 40–48 months of age to execute a response when they were given the command by a bear toy but to inhibit it when given by a toy elephant. Children up to 42 months were unable to carry out the instruction at better than a chance level.

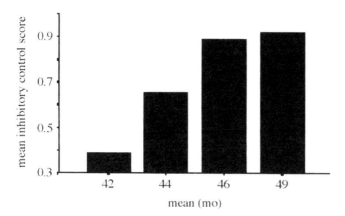

Figure 15.7
Ability to withhold a response to one animal while executing the instruction of another animal (inhibitory control score) as a function of age between 3.5 and 4 years. (L. Jones and M. K. Rothbart, unpublished studies.)

However, just two months later they were virtually perfect. The older children tend to use physical control to inhibit themselves from executing the commands given by the elephant. It is quite amazing to observe the lengths they go to control their own behaviour (see figure 15.7).

One remarkable aspect of this study was that children whose performance was at chance showed by their behaviour that they also had some recognition they were not supposed to respond to the elephant. This was demonstrated by the pattern of slowing down on trials following an error that is characteristic of error detection (A. Revutchi, L. Jones and M. K. Rothbart, unpublished data). This and the fact that they responded more slowly to the elephant than to the bear suggested they somehow were experiencing the conflict when receiving the instruction from the elephant. As shown in figure 15.8, the pattern of slowed response following an error emerged well before children were able to do the task, suggesting that error monitoring is in place well before inhibitory control is shown.

There is also some direct evidence that the anterior cingulate is developing during this part of childhood in a way that might support the data on conflict and error correction. In children aged 5.3–16 years there is a significant correlation between the volume of the area of the right anterior cingulate and the ability to perform tasks relying upon focal attentional control (Casey et al. 1997a). Moreover, in a recent fMRI study, performance of children aged 7–12 years and adults was studied when performing a go–no-go task in which they were required to withhold pressing to an X while responding to non-Xs. This condition was compared to control tasks where subjects responded to all stimuli and thus never had to withhold a response. Both children and adults showed strong activity in prefrontal cortex when required to withhold responses. Moreover, the number of false alarms made in the task was significantly correlated with the extent of cingulate activity (Casey et al. 1997b).

Volition and Awareness

The problem of consciousness includes both awareness and volition. In this chapter, we have concentrated chiefly upon evidence linking activation of specific brain areas to voluntary

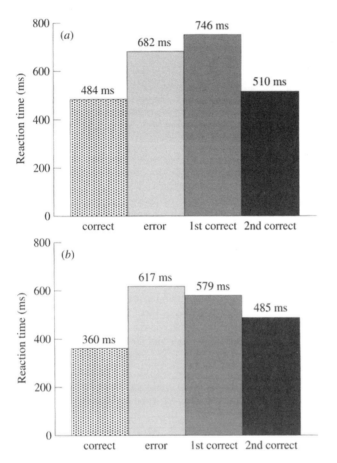

Figure 15.8
Reaction time for correct trials, error trials and correct trials following an error trial for children of 40–42 months who cannot inhibit (a) and 43–50 months who almost always successfully inhibit (b). (A. Revutchi, L. Jones and M. K. Rothbart, unpublished studies.)

control of behaviour. In part our choice reflects the importance of self-regulation to the individual and to collective human interest in the socialization of children. This perhaps is not the most usual concern of neuroscientists striving to develop a model of consciousness, but it does fit with classical issues raised about consciousness by philosophers concerned with the relation of the individual human to society.

As we have seen, Luria (1973) remarked on the social construction of consciousness. The infant development data we have reviewed provides concrete reality to the importance of a slow progression of self control in early life. This development allows society to influence the child's own control mechanisms through socialization. However, we believe that Luria (1973) stressed too strongly the social nature of this higher form of attention, because our review shows it to be woven out of specific biological tissue. If our story is accurate, control begins with the regulation of distress and most likely involves the specific interaction of midfrontal (cingulate) systems with the amygdala. The effort to develop ways of controlling distress provides a locus of control in the cingulate which may, step-by-step, generalize to other situations where conflicting demands must be resolved. Many years are devoted to development of systems of self-regulation. Indeed it seems likely that this development continues into adolescence and may be open to change in adult life, providing a basis for what is attempted in therapy.

Self regulation is a key to a successful society, as the philosopher Bergson has pointed out:

Society, which is the community of individual energies, benefits from the efforts of all its members and renders effort easier to all. It can only subsist by subordinating the individual, it can only progress by leaving the individual free: contradictory requirements, which have to be reconciled. Human societies ... bring about that individual wills should insert themselves in the social will without losing their individual form.... here too, across innumerable obstacles, life is working both by individualization and integration to obtain the greatest

quantity, the richest variety, the highest qualities, of invention and effort. Bergson (1920, p. 33)

How does the issue of self-regulation relate to the other major aspect of consciousness that involves our awareness of the sensory world? We have found that the development of visual orientating precedes the major events we have described for cingulate development by at least a year (Posner & Rothbart 1992). Infants seem to function well visually at a time when their volitional self-regulation has not yet undergone the development we have described above. This suggests that Crick may be right in his idea that visual awareness is a simpler function of consciousness and perhaps the one easiest to study.

On the other hand, the meta-analysis of cortical activity conducted by Shulman et al. (1997a,b) suggests that specific areas of cingulate activity accompany the presentation of almost any stimulus to a subject, even when the instruction is to make no effort to process it. While it is unclear exactly what subjects do with this instruction, it is likely that they are aware of the stimulus, but do little else with it. This result suggests a possible connection between cingulate activity and awareness of the stimulus.

It is also clear from studies of complex scenes that the presentation of a stimulus does not lead very automatically to awareness of its presence (Schneider 1995). Even though subjects report themselves as aware of the whole scene, only when their attention is drawn to a change in the scene do they become aware of that change. Attention may be summoned to the location of the change as the result of energy transients, or as the result of voluntary search. Focal attention is therefore a necessary condition for awareness of detail within a scene as well as a mechanism of voluntary control. Perhaps the distinction between focal attention to limited aspects of the external world and a more general ambient awareness of the scene as a whole (Iwasaki 1993) will prove important in understanding the parts of the brain related to consciousness of sensory events.

Certain conditions of the organism lead to dissociations between awareness and volition. We have discussed in previous papers the conditions of vigilance in which subjects suspend thought while awaiting an infrequent near-threshold signal (Posner & Rothbart 1992, 1994). Several studies have shown that the clearing of the mind of conscious content necessary to avoid missing the signal is accompanied by a reduction in activity within the anterior cingulate.

One condition in which voluntary control is lost but awareness, at least in the form of dream content, can remain high is during REM sleep. Most people would regard the dream as consciousness that is imposed without regard to volition. One PET study of the REM state (Maquet et al. 1996) showed activation of the anterior cingulate together with the amygdala and other parts of the subcortical arousal systems and portions of the parietal lobe. Another study (Braun et al. 1997) compared waking, slow wave and REM sleep and again found increased activity in the cingulate during REM which was accompanied by other arousal and sensory brain areas. Thus, we find substantial reason to suppose that cingulate activation is a part of systems related to awareness as well as to cognitive control.

There is no reason to suppose that the distinctions between awareness and volition made in scientific and philosophical speculations will prove to neatly divide anatomical or developmental systems. Nonetheless, we believe progress has been made in understanding mechanisms of self-regulation, and that it will be important to continue to study aspects of the anatomy, circuitry and development of mechanisms that provide the basis for our voluntary control of thought, emotion and action.

References

Abdullaev, Y. G. & Bechtereva, N. P. 1993 Neuronal correlates of the higher-order semantic code in human prefrontal cortex in language tasks. *Int. J. Psychophysiol.* 14, 167–177.

Abdullaev, Y. G. & Posner, M. I. 1997 Time course of activating brain areas in generating verbal associations. *Psychol. Sci.* 8, 56–59.

Abdullaev, Y. G. & Posner, M. I. 1998 Event-related brain potential imaging of semantic encoding during processing single words. *Neuroimage* 7, 1–13.

Badgaiyan, R. & Posner, M. I. 1998 Mapping the cingulate cortex in response selection and monitoring. *Neuroimage* 7, 255–260.

Bechtereva, A. 1997 *On the human brain.* St. Petersburg: Notabene.

Bench, C. J., Frith, C. D., Grasby, P. M., Friston, K. J., Paulesu, E., Frackowiak, R. S. J. & Dolan, R. J. 1993 Investigations of the functional anatomy of attention using the Stroop test. *Neuropsychologia* 31, 907–922.

Bergson, H. 1920 *Mind-energy: lectures and essays.* New York: Holt Co.

Block, N. 1995 On a confusion about a function of consciousness. *Behav. Brain Sci.* 18, 227–287.

Braun, A. R., Balkin, T. J., Wesensten, N. J., Carson, R. E., Varga, M., Baldwin, P., Selbie, S., Belenky, G. & Herscovitch, P. 1997 Regional cerebral blood flow throughout the sleep–wake cycle: an $H_2{}^{15}O$ PET study. *Brain* 120, 1173–1197.

Bush, G., Whalen, P. J., Rose, B. R., Jenike, M. A., McInerney, S. C. & Rauch, S. L. 1998 The counting Stroop: an interference task specialized for functional neuroimaging—validation study with functional MRI. *Hum. Brain Mapp.* 6, 270–282.

Carter, C. S., Mintun, M. & Cohen, J. D. 1995 Interference and facilitation effects during selective attention: an $H_2{}^{15}O$ PET study of Stroop task performance. *Neuroimage* 2, 264–272.

Casey, B. J., Trainor, R., Giedd, J., Vauss, Y., Vaituzis, C. K., Hamburger, S., Kozuch, P. & Rapoport, J. L. 1997a The role of the anterior cingulate in automatic and controlled processes: a developmental neuroanatomical study. *Devl. Psychobiol.* 3, 61–69.

Casey, B. J. (and 12 others) 1997b A developmental function MRI study of prefrontal activation during performance of a go-no-go task. *J. Cog. Neurosci.* 9, 835–847.

Clohessy, A. B. 1993 Anticipatory eye movement learning in infants and adults: using visual cues to predict event locations. Unpublished PhD thesis, University of Oregon.

Crick, F. 1994 *The astonishing hypothesis*. New York: Basic Books.

Curran, T. & Keele, S. W. 1993 Attentional and non-attentional forms of sequence learning. *J. Exp. Psychol.: Learn. Mem. & Cogn.* 19, 189–202.

Dehaene, S., Posner, M. I. & Tucker, D. M. 1994 Localization of a neural system for error detection and compensation. *Psychol. Sci.* 5, 303–305.

Demb, J. B., Desmond, J. E., Wagner, A. D., Vaidya, C. J., Glover, G. H. & Gabrieli, J. D. E. 1995 Semantic encoding and retrieval in the left inferior prefrontal cortex: a functional MRI study of task difficulty and process specificity. *J. Neurosci.* 15, 5870–5878.

Denckla, M. B. 1996 A theory and model of executive function: a neuropsychological perspective. In *Attention, memory and executive function* (ed. G. R. Lyon & N. A. Krasnegor), pp. 263–278. Baltimore, MD: Paul H. Brookes.

Derbyshire, S. W. G., Vogt, B. A. & Jones, A. K. P. 1998 Pain and Stroop interference tasks activate separate processing modules in anterior cingulate cortex. *Exp. Brain Res.* 11, 52–60.

Derryberry, D. & Rothbart, M. K. 1988 Arousal, affect, and attention as components of temperament. *J. Personality Social Psychol.* 55, 958–966.

Devinsky, O., Morrell, M. J. & Vogt, B. A. 1995 Contributions of anterior cingulate to behaviour. *Brain* 118, 279–306.

Diamond, A. 1991 Neuropsychological insights into the meaning of object concept development. In *The epigenesis of mind: essays on biology and cognition* (ed. S. Carey & R. Gelman), pp. 67–110. Hillsdale, NJ: Lawrence Erlbaum.

DiGirolamo, G., Heidrich, A. & Posner, M. I. 1998 Similar time course and neural circuitry across congruent and incongruent Stroop condition. Cognitive Neuroscience Society Poster, April, San Francisco.

Duncan, J. 1986 Disorganization of behaviour after frontal lobe damage. *J. Cog. Neuropsychol.* 3, 271–290.

Frith, C. D. 1992 *The cognitive neuropsychology of schizophrenia*. Hove, UK: Lawrence Erlbaum.

Gehring, W. J., Gross, B., Coles, M. G. H., Meyer, D. E. & Donchin, E. 1993 A neural system for error detection and compensation. *Psychol. Sci.* 4, 385–390.

George, M. S., Ketter, T. A., Parekh, P. I., Rosinsky, N., Ring, H., Casey, B. J., Trimble, M. R., Horwitz, B., Herscovitch, P. & Post, R. M. 1994 Regional brain activity when selecting response despite interference: an $H_2^{15}O$ PET study of the Stroop and an emotional Stroop. *Hum. Brain Mapp.* 1, 194–209.

Gerardi, G. 1996 Early development of attention and self regulation. Unpublished PhD thesis, University of Oregon.

Gerstadt, C. L., Hong, Y. J. & Diamond, A. 1994 The relationship between cognition and action: performance of children 3.5–7 years old on a Stroop-like day–night test. *Cognition* 53, 129–153.

Harman, C., Rothbart, M. K. & Posner, M. I. 1997 Distress and attention interactions in early infancy. *Motivation & Emotion* 21, 27–43.

Iwasaki, S. 1993 Spatial attention and two modes of visual consciousness. *Cognition* 49, 211–233.

Jerger, S., Martin, R. C. & Pirozzolo, F. J. 1988 A developmental study of the auditory Stroop effect. *Brain Lang.* 35, 86–104.

Lane, R. D. & Schwartz, G. E. 1992 Levels of emotional awareness: implications for psychotherapeutic integration. *J. Psychother. Integration* 2, 1–18.

Lane, R. D., Reiman, E. M., Axelrod, B., Yun, L.-S., Holmes, A. & Schwartz, G. E. 1998 Neural correlates of levels of emotional awareness: evidence of an interaction between emotion and attention in the anterior cingulate cortex. *J. Cog. Neurosci.* 10, 525–535.

Luria, A. R. 1973 *The working brain*. New York: Basic Books.

Luu, P., Collins, P. & Tucker, D. M. 1998 Mood personality and self-monitoring: negative affect and emotionality in related to frontal lobe mechanisms of error detection. *J. Exp. Psychol. Gen.* (Submitted.)

Maquet, P., Peters, J.-M., Aerts, J., Delfiore, G., Deguelldre, C., Luxen, A. & Franck, G. 1996 Functional neuroanatomy of human rapid-eye-movement sleep and dreaming. *Nature* 164, 163–166.

Marcel, A. J. 1983 Conscious and unconscious perception: experiments on visual masking. *Cogn. Psychol.* 15, 197–237.

Miltner, W. H. R., Braun, C. H. & Coles, M. G. H. 1998 Event related potentials following incorrect feedback I a time-estimation task: evidence for a 'generic' neural system for error detection. *J. Cog. Neurosci.* 9, 788–798.

Morgan, A. H., Romanski, L. M. & LeDoux, J. E. 1993 Extinction of emotional learning: contributions of medial prefrontal cortex. *Neurosci. Lett.* 163, 109–113.

Neeley, J. H. 1977 Semantic priming and retrieval from lexical memory. The role of inhibitionless spreading activity and limited capacity attention. *J. Exp. Psychol. Gen.* 106, 1–66.

Newell, A. & Simon, H. A. 1972 *Human problem solving.* Englewood Cliffs, NJ: Prentice-Hall.

Norman, D. A. & Shallice, T. 1986 Attention to action: willed and automatic control of behaviour. In *Consciousness and self regulation* (ed. R. J. Davidson, G. E. Schwartz & D. Shapiro), pp. 1–18. New York: Plenum Press.

Pardo, J. V., Pardo, P. J., Janer, K. W. & Raichle, M. E. 1990 The anterior cingulate cortex mediates processing selection in the Stroop attentional conflict paradigm. *Proc. Natn. Acad. Sci. USA* 87, 256–259.

Posner, M. I. 1978 *Chronometric explorations of mind.* Hillsdale, NJ: Lawrence Erlbaum.

Posner, M. I. 1994 Attention: the mechanism of consciousness. *Proc. Natn. Acad. Sci. USA* 91, 7398–7402.

Posner, M. I. & DiGirolamo, G. J. 1998 Executive attention: conflict, target detection, and cognitive control. In *The attentive brain* (ed. R. Parasuraman), pp. 401–423. Cambridge, MA: MIT Press.

Posner, M. I. & Petersen, S. E. 1990 The attention system of the human brain. *A. Rev. Neurosci.* 13, 25–42.

Posner, M. I. & Rothbart, M. K. 1992 Attention and conscious experience. In *The neuropsychology of consciousness* (ed. A. D. Milner & M. D. Rugg), pp. 91–112. London: Academic Press.

Posner, M. I. & Rothbart, M. K. 1994 Constructing neuronal theories of mind. In *High level neuronal theories of the brain* (ed. C. Koch & J. Davis), pp. 183–199. Cambridge, MA: MIT Press.

Posner, M. I., Clohessy, A. B. & Rothbart, M. K. 1999 Development of the functional visual field. *Acta Psychol.* (Submitted.)

Rabbitt, P. M. A. 1967 Time to detect errors as a function of factors affecting choice-response time. *Acta Psychologia* 27, 131–142.

Raichle, M. E., Fiez, J. A., Videen, T. O., MacLeod, A.-M. K., Pardo, J. V., Fox, P. T. & Petersen, S. E. 1994 Practice-related changes in human brain functional anatomy during nonmotor learning. *Cerebr. Cortex* 4, 8–26.

Rainville, P., Duncan, G. H., Price, D. D., Carrier, B. & Bushness, M. C. 1997 Pain affect encoded in human anterior cingulate but not somatosensory cortex. *Science* 277, 968–970.

Reed, M., Pien, D. L. & Rothbart, M. K. 1984 Inhibitory self-control in preschool children. *Merrill-Palmer Quart.* 30, 131–147.

Rothbart, M. K. & Bates, J. E. 1998 Temperament. In *Handbook of child psychology. 3. Social, emotional and personality development* (ed. W. Damon & N. Eisenberg), pp. 105–176. New York: Wiley.

Schneider, W. X. 1995 VAM: a neurocognitive model for visual attention control of segmentation, object recognition and space based motor action. *Visual Cogn.* 2, 331–375.

Shallice, T. & Burgess, P. 1996 The domain of supervisory processes and temporal organization of behaviour. *Phil. Trans. R. Soc. Lond.* B 351, 1405–1412.

Shulman, G. L., Corbetta, M., Buckner, R. L., Fiez, J. A., Miezin, F. M., Raichle, M. E. & Petersen, S. E. 1997a Common blood flow changes across visual tasks. I. Increases in subcortical structures and cerebellum but not in nonvisual cortex. *J. Cog. Neurosci.* 9, 624–647.

Shulman, G. L., Fiez, J. A., Corbetta, M., Buckner, R. L., Miezin, F. M., Raichle, M. E. & Petersen, S. E. 1997b Common blood flow changes across visual tasks. II. Decreases in cerebral cortex. *J. Cog. Neurosci.* 9, 648–663.

Snyder, A. Z., Abdullaev, Y., Posner, M. I. & Raichle, M. E. 1995 Scalp electrical potentials reflect regional cerebral blood flow responses during processing of written words. *Proc. Natn. Acad. Sci. USA* 92, 1689–1693.

Spitzer, M., Bellemann, M. E., Kammer, T., Friedemann, G., Kichka, U., Maier, S., Schwaartz, A. & Brix, G. 1996 Functional MR imaging of semantic information processing and learning-related effects using psychometrically controlled stimulation paradigms. *Cog. Brain Res.* 4, 149–161.

Stern, D. N. 1985 *The interpersonal world of the infant.* New York: Basic Books.

Taylor, S. F., Kornblum, S., Minoshima, S., Oliver, L. M. & Koeppe, R. A. 1994 Changes in medial cortical blood flow with a stimulus-response compatibility task. *Neuropsychologia* 32, 249–255.

Zelazo, P. D., Resnick, J. S. & Pinon, D. E. 1995 Response control and the execution of verbal rules. *Devl. Psychol.* 31, 508–517.

16 Neural Correlates of Theory-of-Mind Reasoning: An Event-Related Potential Study

Mark A. Sabbagh and Marjorie Taylor

Many philosophers, psychologists, and anthropologists support the view that everyday understanding of human behavior rests on a theory of mind—an appreciation of how people's behaviors relate to their internal mental states, such as beliefs (Wellman, 1990). An important cognitive prerequisite to having a theory of mind is the ability to think about mental states as representations of reality (Perner, 1991). Recent research suggests that thinking about mental representations of reality (e.g., beliefs) may be computationally dissociated from thinking about other kinds of representations of reality (e.g., photographs). For instance, autistic children typically fail the standard false-belief task in which participants are asked to reason about a person's mental representation of a particular scene that has become outdated, or false, because that scene has changed in his or her absence. Yet, they show strong performance on similarly structured false-photograph tasks in which participants are asked to recognize that a photograph can be outdated if the scene changes after the photograph has been taken (Leekam & Perner, 1991; Leslie & Thaiss, 1992). For young preschoolers, performance on these two tasks is typically not correlated (Slaughter, 1998). These dissociations are striking given that the false-belief and false-photograph tasks are similar in inferential structure, memory load, and story content; they differ only in the nature of the representation.

To account for these dissociations, a number of researchers have suggested that there may be a distinct neural system that supports reasoning about mental states and is impaired in the case of autism (Baron-Cohen, 1994). A handful of studies have attempted to investigate this question directly (e.g., Fletcher et al., 1995; Goel, Grafman, Sadato, & Hallett, 1995). However, none have used tasks as well matched as the false-belief and false-photograph tasks, thereby leaving unanswered a number of questions regarding

their interpretation. The present study capitalized on the matched nature of the false-belief and false-photograph tasks to investigate the brain electrophysiological activity associated with reasoning about mental versus nonmental representations in adults.

Identifying a brain electrophysiological marker for theory-of-mind reasoning is important for two reasons. First, there is presently a wide range of theories regarding the cognitive mechanisms and rate-limiting factors underlying theory-of-mind reasoning in young children (see Carruthers & Smith, 1996). Gaining a cognitive neuroscience perspective on this question could be an important step in constraining theorizing and guiding research in this interesting area. Second, identifying such a marker has the potential to provide insight into the neurophysiological bases of autism. Although the search for a common neurological substrate in autism has been elusive (Minshew & Rattan, 1992), several researchers have identified a number of brain electrophysiological abnormalities that seem to be common in individuals with autism, such as electroencephalographic (EEG) abnormalities at left frontal locations (e.g., Dawson, Klinger, Panagiotides, & Lewy, 1995) and abnormal cognitive event-related potential (ERP) characteristics (i.e., P300; e.g., Lincoln, Courchesne, Harms, & Allen, 1993). Convergence between the electrophysiological correlates of theory-of-mind reasoning in normal adults and the known cognitive and electrophysiological characteristics of autism would give insight into the neuropathology of this developmental disorder.

Method

Participants

Twenty-three right-handed college students participated in this study for pay. Participants were between the ages of 18 and 42 years (median = 21). There were 12 females and 11 males. All participants reported that they were native English speakers without history of significant psychiatric or neurological illness.

ERP Collection

Electrophysiological data were recorded from the scalp using a 128-channel Geodesic Sensor Net (Tucker, 1993), a network of 128 Ag/AgCl sponge sensors knitted into an elastic geodesic tension structure. The Sensor Net has an even interelectrode distance of 2.7 cm, and electrode impedances between 10 and 20 kΩ. The EEG was amplified (band-pass filtered at 0.1 Hz–100 Hz), digitized at 250 Hz for 1,256 ms starting 256 ms prior to the onset of the test stimulus. Single-trial data were edited with algorithmic artifact-rejection software that combed the data for evidence of lateral eye movements, eyeblinks, and muscle artifacts. All participants had at least 25 artifact-free trials per condition. These artifact-free trials were averaged, transformed using the average-reference method (Hjorth, 1982), corrected to baseline, and digitally filtered (low-pass filter with 20-Hz cutoff) to reduce environmental noise.

Participants were tested in a sound-attenuated booth approximately 50 cm from a computer screen. An adjustable chin rest ensured that this distance remained constant and minimized head movement. A closed-circuit video system allowed monitoring of participants' position, eye movements, eyeblinks, and correct placement of the Sensor Net throughout each 1.5-hr session.

Experimental Task and Procedure

Participants were presented with 80 short (six-line) narratives, 40 describing a character's belief regarding the location of two objects and 40 describing a character who took a photograph of two objects. In both types of stories, the representations were subsequently outdated when one

Table 16.1
Examples of belief and photo stories

Belief Story

Ben put a folder and a clipboard on his desk.

His friend, Maggie, noticed that he had lots of work to do.

Then, Maggie went out for a coffee.

While Maggie was gone, Ben moved the clipboard.

Ben put the clipboard on the bookshelf.

He left the folder on his desk.

Photo Story

Ben put a folder and a clipboard on his desk.

His friend, Maggie, took a picture of these things.

Then, Maggie put the camera away.

After a little while, Ben moved the clipboard.

Ben put the clipboard on the bookshelf.

He left the folder on his desk.

of the two objects was displaced during the character's absence. To ensure that the narratives differed only on the relevant dimension (beliefs vs. photos), each story had both a belief and a photo variant (see table 16.1). Both variants of each story were presented to all participants. The 80 stories were presented in one of two random orders.

Narratives were presented line by line and read at the participants' own pace. Participants were asked to ensure that they comprehended each line fully before they moved on to the next. To facilitate good comprehension and ensure that they were completing the task by making reference to the representations in question, we told participants to "make a mental picture" of the events depicted in each line.

At the end of each narrative, participants were asked control questions designed to assess their attention to story details and a test question about the location of one of the objects according to the character's belief or photograph. Questions were presented word by word at a 512-ms interstimulus interval. Participants did not know which object (displaced or not displaced) they were going to be asked about until the final word of the question (e.g., "According to [Mary/the photo], where is the [object]?"), which served as the stimulus onset for the ERP analysis. ERP data were collected for a 1,500-ms time period, during which participants were asked to mentally generate the answer while remaining fixated on the screen. The computer then displayed a possible answer to the question, and the participants' task was to press the appropriate key to indicate, after a 1,000-ms delay, whether the computer's answer was correct (yes/no). The computer's answer was correct 50% of the time.

Results

There were no significant differences in the participants' accuracy for belief versus photo questions ($Ms = 94\%$ and 95% correct, respectively), paired $t(22) = 1.04$, $p > .10$. Further, there were no significant differences in the time it took participants to read the belief stories versus the photo stories ($Ms = 18.79$ s and 18.35 s, respectively), paired $t(22) = 1.54$, $p > .10$. These findings suggest that the two types of stories were equivalent in reading and comprehension difficulty.

Nonparametric Wilcoxon signed-ranks tests and factorial analyses of variance (ANOVAs) were used in concert to characterize differences in the ERPs associated with beliefs versus photos. The Wilcoxon signed-ranks tests were performed for all time points on all 128 channels ($p < .05$, two-tailed). To avoid false positives, we adopted strict criteria whereby differences were considered significant only if they were (a) maintained on a single channel for eight continuous samples (32 ms) and (b) neighbored by at least two other channels that showed a similar pattern of activity. Assuming independence, this procedure is associated with a very stringent alpha level ($p < 3.9 \times 10^{-11}$). Starting at 300 ms poststimulus, ERPs for the belief condition were more positive

than ERPs for the photograph condition at a cluster of four left frontal sensors and less positive than ERPs for the photograph condition at a cluster of four left parietal sensors (see figure 16.1). These differences were maintained intermittently throughout the ERP epoch, and were most clearly recapitulated at 820 ms poststimulus. No differences meeting the significance criteria were present at right-hemisphere sites.

A series of follow-up 2 (condition) × 2 (hemisphere) repeated measures ANOVAs were carried out to further characterize both the frontal and the parietal effects. Voltages from representative channels (sites corresponding to 10–20 sites) identified in the nonparametric analyses and from their right-hemisphere analogues (frontal: FP1, FP2; parietal: P3, P4) were averaged across two different time windows: 300–400 ms (25 samples) and 600–840 ms (60 samples). The ANOVAs for the frontal sites revealed a significant Condition × Hemisphere interaction in both time windows, $F(1, 22) = 13.60$, $p < .005$, for 300–400 ms and $F(1, 22) = 9.93$, $p < .005$, for 600–840 ms (see figure 16.2). Planned means comparisons indicated that the interactions were due to a focal increase in the positivity associated with beliefs at FP1 (left frontal) relative to FP2 (right frontal) in both time windows, $F(1, 22) = 11.22$, $p < .005$, for 300–400 ms and $F(1, 22) = 10.01$, $p < .005$, for 600–840 ms. There was also a hemispheric asymmetry (more positive at FP1 than FP2) for the belief condition in both time windows, $F(1, 22) = 15.14$, $p < .005$, for 300–400 ms and $F(1, 22) = 13.91$, $p < .005$, for 600–840 ms. Contrary to the nonparametric findings, the ANOVAs for the parietal sites did not reveal significant main effects or interactions.

To confirm the replicability of these findings, we randomly split the subject sample into two groups (Group 1: $n = 12$, Group 2: $n = 11$) and conducted the same analyses. The analyses for both groups revealed a pattern of differences congruent with that of the full-sample analysis.

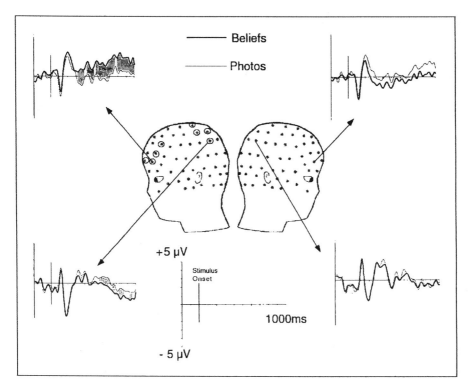

Figure 16.1
Event-related potentials in the photograph (thin lines) and belief (thick lines) conditions, recorded from selected frontal and parietal sites. Gray-shaded regions indicate time windows in which the condition differences met criteria for statistical significance. Circled sites showed condition differences at 300–400 ms and at 600–840 ms.

Discussion

The purpose of this study was to characterize the brain electrophysiology of theory-of-mind reasoning in adults using the false-belief and false-photograph tasks in an ERP paradigm. In doing so, we have provided an important link between theory-of-mind abilities and their neural underpinnings, a link that can play an important role in constraining research and theorizing about theory-of-mind development and disorders (Klein & Kihlstrom, 1998). Results indicated that ERPs elicited by these two tasks differed beginning at 300 ms post-stimulus: Beliefs were associated with an enhanced positivity over left frontal sites and a stronger negativity over left parietal sites. Given the close structural match between these two tasks, and the control analyses indicating that the two kinds of stories were of equal reading difficulty, we can be confident that this dissociation indexes activity that can be attributed to theory-of-mind reasoning.

Both the time course and the spatial distribution of the dissociations are noteworthy. With respect to time course, the dissociations we ob-

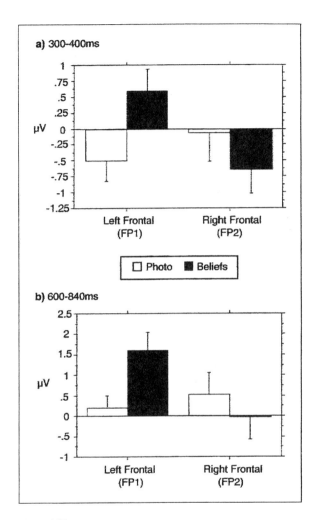

Figure 16.2
Mean amplitude of evoked potentials recorded from selected frontal sites in the photograph and belief conditions. Results are shown separately for two time windows: 300–400 ms poststimulus (a) and 600–840 ms poststimulus (b).

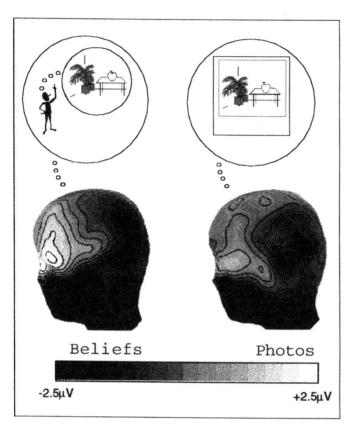

Figure 16.3
Three-dimensional interpolations of the scalp electrical activity recorded at 820 ms poststimulus. The interpolations were created using the spherical splines method (Perrin, Pernier, Bertrand, & Eschallier, 1989).

served in the 300- to 400-ms window and in the 600- to 840-ms window are thought to index the point at which contextual variables appear in the ERP record (e.g., Chung et al., 1996). It is possible that the dissociations we observed reflect the processes associated with integrating mental versus nonmental representations within a given context. With respect to spatial distribution, the focal nature of the increased positivity for beliefs (see figure 16.3) suggests the possibility of a radially oriented generator within the left frontal lobe. Though this idea is speculative, the possibility of a left frontal generator is consistent with two positron emission tomography studies that found increased activation of the left medial frontal gyrus during tasks that required social cognitive reasoning (Fletcher et al., 1995; Goel et al., 1995).

Implications for Theories of Theory of Mind

Executive Function and Inhibitory Control
Recent studies have suggested that performance on false-belief tasks hinges on having adequate

inhibitory control (Carlson, Moses, & Hix, 1998; Ozonoff, Pennington, & Rogers, 1991). We doubt that inhibitory-control differences alone can account for the observed differences between false-belief and false-photograph tasks because the two tasks are well matched for inhibitory demands. In addition, the extended time course over which the ERP differences were maintained is inconsistent with the time course of brain activation shown in previous ERP studies designed to investigate inhibitory control more directly (Keifer, Marzinzik, Weisbrod, Scherg, & Spitzer, 1998).

Subtle Task Differences

Despite the fact that the belief and photograph tasks were structurally well matched, it is possible that they imposed different cognitive demands. For example, beliefs differ from photographs in the explicitness of their origins. A photograph is an explicitly made representation: The photograph is taken and the scene is represented. In contrast, understanding that a person's perception of a scene results in a belief about that scene requires an inference (Wimmer, Hogrefe, & Perner, 1988). A second difference between beliefs and photographs is that only beliefs require integrating propositional contents with propositional attitudes (Perner, 1991). That is, a belief involves a commitment to a representation (i.e., thinking that a situation is true), and not just a representation itself (i.e., photograph of a past situation). Both of these observations suggest that reasoning about beliefs requires an additional inferential or integrative step that is not required when thinking about photos. It is possible that the left frontal differences reflect this cognitive disparity (Grafman, Holyoak, & Boller, 1995).

Theory-of-Mind "Module"

A number of researchers have suggested that the mental operations required for thinking about mental representations may be carried out in an automatic and modularized fashion (Baron-Cohen, 1994; Brothers & Ring, 1992). However,

the late onset and extended time course of the ERP differentiations cast doubt on the idea that reasoning about mental representations is automatic. Nevertheless, it remains possible that there is a specialized region of cortex responsible for thinking about mental representations. This localization proposal is not necessarily inconsistent with the suggestion that the difference can be attributed to more general mental operations (Karmiloff-Smith, 1992).

Implications for Autism

Identifying a neurophysiological marker for theory-of-mind reasoning has potentially important implications for considering the neurobiological bases of autism. Lincoln et al. (1993) have found that individuals with autism have a greatly reduced P300 (or P3) component in response to novel stimuli in the standard oddball paradigm. Although it is difficult to identify strong cognitive similarities between the oddball paradigm and the methods used in the present study, it is interesting to note that cognitive processes engaging at 300 ms poststimulus seem to be especially important for considering specifically mental representations, and are known to be impaired in autism.

A second aspect of our findings that can be linked with known neurological deficits in autism concerns the location of the main effects. In standard neuropsychiatric tests, autistic individuals show greater impairment on items designed to tap left- as opposed to right-hemisphere dysfunction (Dawson, 1983). In addition, autistic individuals have demonstrated reduced EEG power over frontal electrode sites, and this effect is more pronounced over the left hemisphere (Dawson et al., 1995). The present findings linking theory-of-mind reasoning with regions in the left frontal lobe suggest that these characteristic neurophysiological abnormalities seen in autistic individuals may be related to their social cognitive deficits.

Acknowledgments

This research was supported by a National Science Foundation Graduate Fellowship to Mark Sabbagh, and by a McDonnell-Pew Investigator-Initiated Cognitive Neuroscience Award to Marjorie Taylor.

Special thanks go to Brandon Pol for his assistance in data collection, and to Dare Baldwin, Ben Clegg, Gregg DiGirolamo, Bill Gehring, Louis Moses, Helen Neville, and Don Tucker for their assistance at various stages of study design and manuscript preparation.

References

Baron-Cohen, S. (1994). How to build a baby that can read minds: Cognitive mechanisms in mind reading. *Cahiers de Psychologie Cognitive, 13*, 513–552.

Brothers, L., & Ring, B. (1992). A neuroethological framework for the representation of minds. *Journal of Cognitive Neuroscience, 4*, 107–118.

Carlson, S. M., Moses, L. J., & Hix, H. (1998). The role of inhibitory processes in young children's difficulties with deception and false belief. *Child Development, 69*, 672–691.

Carruthers, P., & Smith, P. K. (1996). *Theories of theories of mind.* Cambridge, England: Cambridge University Press.

Chung, G., Tucker, D. M., West, P., Potts, G. F., Liotti, M., Luu, P., & Hartry, A. L. (1996). Emotional expectancy: Brain electrical activity associated with an emotional bias in interpreting life events. *Psychophysiology, 33*, 218–233.

Dawson, G. (1983). Lateralized brain dysfunction in autism: Evidence from the Halstead-Reitan neuropsychological battery. *Journal of Autism and Developmental Disorders, 13*, 269–286.

Dawson, G., Klinger, L. G., Panagiotides, H., & Lewy, A. (1995). Subgroups of autistic children based on social behavior display distinct patterns of brain activity. *Journal of Abnormal Child Psychology, 23*, 569–583.

Fletcher, P. C., Happé, F., Frith, U., Baker, S. C., Dolan, R. J., Frackowiak, R. S. J., & Frith, C. D.

(1995). Other minds in the brain: A functional imaging study of "theory of mind" in story comprehension. *Cognition, 57*, 109–128.

Goel, V., Grafman, J., Sadato, N., & Hallett, M. (1995). Modeling other minds. *NeuroReport, 6*, 1741–1746.

Grafman, J., Holyoak, K. J., & Boller, F. (1995). *Structure and functions of the human prefrontal cortex.* New York: New York Academy of Sciences.

Hjorth, B. (1982). An adaptive EEG derivation technique. *Electroencephalography and Clinical Neurophysiology, 54*, 654–661.

Karmiloff-Smith, A. (1992). *Beyond modularity: A developmental perspective on cognitive science.* Cambridge, MA: MIT Press.

Keifer, M., Marzinzik, F., Weisbrod, M., Scherg, M., & Spitzer, M. (1998). The time course of brain activations during response inhibition: Evidence from event-related potentials in a go/no go task. *NeuroReport, 9*, 765–770.

Klein, S. B., & Kihlstrom, J. F. (1998). On bridging the gap between social-personality psychology and neuropsychology. *Personality and Social Psychology Review, 2*, 228–242.

Leekam, S. R., & Perner, J. (1991). Does the autistic child have a metarepresentational deficit? *Cognition, 40*, 203–218.

Leslie, A. M., & Thaiss, L. (1992). Domain specificity in conceptual development: Neuropsychological evidence from autism. *Cognition, 43*, 225–251.

Lincoln, A. J., Courchesne, E., Harms, L., & Allen, M. (1993). Contextual probability evaluation in autistic, receptive developmental language disorder and control children: Event-related brain potential evidence. *Journal of Autism and Developmental Disorders, 23*, 37–58.

Minshew, N. M., & Rattan, A. I. (1992). The clinical syndrome of autism. In F. Boller (Series Ed.) & S. J. Segalowitz & I. Rapin (Vol. Eds.), *Handbook of neuropsychology: Vol. 7. Child neuropsychology* (pp. 401–441). Amsterdam: Elsevier.

Ozonoff, S., Pennington, B. F., & Rogers, S. J. (1991). Executive function deficits in high-functioning autistic individuals: Relationship to theory of mind. *Journal of Child Psychology and Psychiatry, 32*, 1081–1105.

Perner, J. (1991). *Understanding the representational mind.* Cambridge, MA: MIT Press.

Perrin, F., Pernier, J., Bertrand, O., & Echallier, J. F. (1989). Spherical splines for scalp potential and current density source mapping. *Electroencephalography and Clinical Neurophysiology, 72*, 184–187.

Slaughter, V. (1998). Children's understanding of pictorial and mental representations. *Child Development, 69*, 321–332.

Tucker, D. M. (1993). Spatial sampling of head electrical fields: The geodesic sensor net. *Electroencephalography and Clinical Neurophysiology, 87*, 154–163.

Wellman, H. M. (1990). *The child's theory of mind.* Cambridge, MA: MIT Press.

Wimmer, H., Hogrefe, G., & Perner, J. (1988). Children's understanding of informational access as source of knowledge. *Child Development, 59*, 386–396.

III SOCIAL COGNITION AND THE BRAIN

B. Social Applications

ii. Perceiving Others

17 Language within Our Grasp

Giacomo Rizzolatti and Michael A. Arbib

In all communication, sender and receiver must be bound by a common understanding about what counts; what counts for the sender must count for the receiver, else communication does not occur. Moreover the processes of production and perception must somehow be linked; their representation must, at some point, be the same.

What is said here by Alvin Liberman[1] for speech where individuals have an explicit intent to communicate, must apply also for "communications" in which such an overt intention is absent. We understand when one individual is attacking another or when someone is peacefully eating an apple. How do we do it? What is shared by the (involuntary) sender and by the receiver? Is this mechanism the precursor of willed communications? The present review addresses these questions.

The Mirror System

Neurons located in the rostral part of monkey inferior area 6 (area F5) discharge during active movements of the hand or mouth, or both.[2-4] Some years ago we found that in most F5 neurons, the discharge correlates with an action, rather than with the individual movements that form it.[3] Accordingly, we classified F5 neurons into various categories corresponding to the action associated with their discharge. The most common are: "grasping with the hand" neurons, "holding" neurons and "tearing" neurons.[3,5] Further study revealed something unexpected: a class of F5 neurons that discharge not only when the monkey grasped or manipulated the objects, but also when the monkey observed the experimenter making a similar gesture.[6-8] We called the neurons endowed with this property "mirror neurons" (Fig. 17.1).

The response properties of mirror neurons to visual stimuli can be summarized as follows: mirror neurons do not discharge in response to object presentation; in order to be triggered they require a specific observed action. The majority of them respond selectively when the monkey observes one type of action (such as grasping). Some are highly specific, coding not only the action aim, but also how that action is executed. They fire, for example, during observation of grasping movements, but only when the object is grasped with the index finger and the thumb.

All mirror neurons show visual generalization: they discharge when the agent of the observed action (typically a hand) is far away from or close to the monkey. A few neurons respond even when the object is grasped by the mouth. The actions most represented are: grasp, manipulate, tear, and put an object on a plate. Mirror neurons also have motor properties that are indistinguishable from those of F5 neurons that do not respond to action observation. In this review, they will be referred to collectively and regardless of their other properties, as "canonical neurons." Typically, mirror neurons show congruence between the observed and executed action. This congruence can be extremely strict, that is, the effective motor action (for example, precision grip) corresponds with the action that, when seen, triggers the neuron (that is, precision grip). For other neurons the congruence is broader: the motor requirements (for example, precision grip) are usually stricter than the visual ones (for example, any type of hand grasping). An example of a highly congruent mirror neuron is shown in figure 17.2. What is the function of mirror neurons? The proposal that we[7,8] and others[9] have advanced is that their activity "represents" actions. This representation can be used for imitating actions and for understanding them. By "understanding" we mean the capacity that individuals have to recognize that another individual is performing an action, to differentiate the observed action from other actions, and to use this

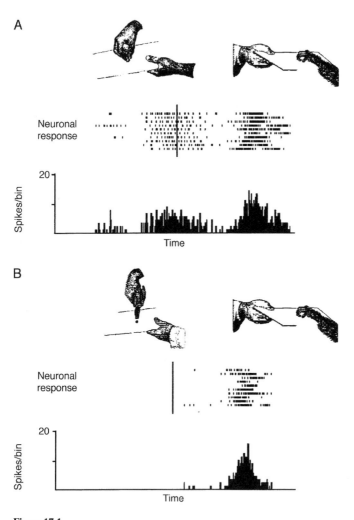

Figure 17.1
An example of a mirror neuron. The behavioral situation is schematically represented in the upper part of each panel. The responses of the neuron are shown in the middle and lower parts of each panel. The responses are shown as discharges using ten individual behavioral trials (each short vertical line corresponds to an action potential) and expressed as relative-response histograms. (A) The experimenter grasps a piece of food with his hand then moves it toward the monkey, who, at the end of the trial, grasps it. The neuron discharges during observation of the grip, ceases to fire when the food is given to the monkey and discharges again when the monkey grasps it. (B) The experimenter grasps the food with a tool. The subsequent sequence of events is as in (A). Note the lack of response of the neuron when the food is grasped with the tool. (C) The monkey grasps food in darkness. In (A) and (B) the rasters are aligned with the moment when the food is grasped by the experimenter (vertical line). In (C) the alignment is with the approximate beginning of the grasping movement. Each small vertical line in the rasters corresponds to a spike. Histogram bin width: 20 ms. (Reproduced with permission from Ref. 7.)

C

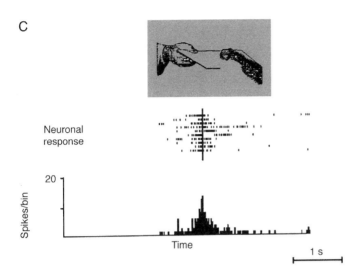

Neuronal
response

Spikes/bin

20

Time   1 s

Figure 17.1 (continued)

information to act appropriately. According to this view, mirror neurons represent the link between sender and receiver that Liberman postulated in his motor theory of speech perception as the necessary prerequisite for any type of communication.[1,10,11]

What Is Area F5?

Although doubts have been expressed,[12] most authors share the view that the rostral part of the monkey ventral premotor cortex (area F5) is the monkey homologue of Broca's area in the human brain. The reasons for this view are: that both F5 and Broca's area are parts of inferior area 6 (Refs. 13–15) and their location within the agranular frontal cortex is similar (Box 17.1); and cytoarchitectonically, there are strong similarities between area 44 (the caudal part of Broca's area) and F5 (Refs. 14,16,17).

Functionally, a difference between Broca's area and F5 is that Broca's area is most commonly thought of as an area for speech, whereas

F5 is often considered as an area for hand movements. F5 is somatotopically organized—its dorsal part contains a representation of hand movements[2,3,18] and its large ventral part contains a representation of mouth and larynx movement;[19,20] a similar organization is present in the ventral premotor cortex of other primates.[21] Similarly, the motor properties of human Broca's area do not relate only to speech: recent PET data indicate that Broca's area might also become active during the execution of hand or arm movements,[22,23] during mental imagery of hand grasping movement (mostly area 44),[24,25] and during tasks involving hand–mental rotations (areas 44 and 45).[26] Finally, Broca's area becomes active in patients who have recovered from subcortical infarctions when they are asked to use their paralyzed hand.[27]

It is intriguing that the area, which in the monkey contains a system that links action recognition and action production, is precisely that area that, for completely different reasons, has been proposed as the homologue of Broca's area. Is this a mere coincidence? Or, on the contrary,

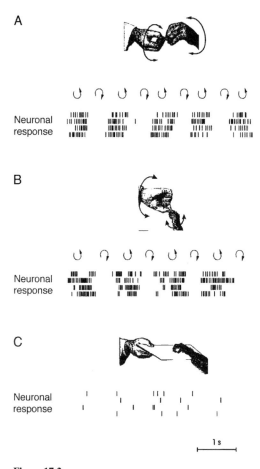

Figure 17.2
An example of a highly congruent mirror neuron. The behavioural situation is schematically represented in the upper part of each panel. The responses of the neuron are shown in the middle and lower parts of each panel; four sketches of continuous recordings are shown in each panel, with each vertical line corresponding to an action potential. (A) The monkey observes the experimenter who rotates his hand around an object in opposite directions to break it. The neuronal response is present in one rotation direction only. (B) The monkey rotates a piece of food held by the experimenter who opposes the monkey movement making a rotation in the opposite direction. (C) The monkey grasps food using the same finger as during rotation. Small arrows above the records (A and B) indicate the directions of rotations. (Reproduced with permission from ref. 7.)

has the mirror system been fundamental for the development of speech and, before speech, of other forms of intentional communication? Before discussing these points, we examine the evidence for a mirror system in humans.

The Mirror System in Humans

The first demonstration of a mirror system in humans was provided by Fadiga et al.[28] The rationale of their experiment was the following: if the observation of an action activates the premotor cortex in humans as it does in monkeys, then magnetic transcranial stimulation should induce, during action observation, an enhancement of motor-evoked potentials recorded from those muscles that are active when the observed action is executed. Their results confirmed the hypothesis: during the observation of various actions, a selective increase of motor evoked potentials occurred in the muscles that the subjects usually use for producing them.

Although these data indicate that an action production and action observation matching system exists in humans, they do not give information on the circuits that underlie it. Data on this issue were provided by two PET experiments.[25,29] The two experiments differed in many aspects, but both had a condition in which subjects observed the experimenter grasping a 3-dimensional object; object observation was used as a control situation. Grasp observation significantly activated the superior temporal sulcus (STS), the inferior parietal lobule and the inferior frontal gyrus (area 45); all activations were in the left hemisphere.

Hemispheric differences aside, the cortical areas active during action observation in humans match well with those active in the monkey under the same conditions. Neurons that become selectively active in the STS during the sight of hand actions were described by Perrett and his co-workers.[30,31] There is evidence, although limited, that mirror neurons might be present in area

Box 17.1

Cytoarchitectonic map of the caudal part of the monkey frontal lobe and possible homologies with human frontal cortex

Figure 17.3A shows parcellation of prearcuate cortex[a] and agranular frontal cortex[b] of the macaque monkey and figure 17.3B shows parcellation of the region of the human frontal cortex defined as "intermediate precentral cortex" by Campbell.[c] The terminology of Foerster[d] and Vogt and Vogt[e] has been adopted for the human cortex. Similar colors in 17.3A and 17.3B indicate areas with anatomical and functional homologies. Brain regions colored yellow are areas with anatomical and functional homologies, mostly related to orienting behavior; areas colored red also share anatomical and functional homologies and are mostly related to interactions with the external world.[e–h] The homology is based on cytoarchitectonics, electrical stimulation[i] and sulci embryology.[j]

The superior frontal sulcus (SF) and the superior precentral sulcus (SP) of human brain are drawn in dark green as the superior limb of the monkey arcuate sulcus (AS). The inferior frontal sulcus (IF) and the ascending branch of the inferior precentral sulcus (IPa) of human brain are drawn in blue as the inferior limb of the monkey arcuate sulcus (AI). The descending branch of the inferior precentral sulcus (IPd) of human brain is drawn in pale green and is labeled as the inferior precentral dimple (ipd) of the monkey brain figure 17.3A. The reasons for these homologies are the following. The precentral sulcus develops from two separate primordia. Both of them have, during development, a horizontal branch representing the primordia of SF and IF, respectively. Typically, in the adult brain, the precentral sulcus[j] is formed by two separate segments. Thus, we suggest that the human homologue of the monkey arcuate sulcus is formed by SF plus SP (dark green) and by the IF plus IPa (blue). The descending branch of inferior precentral sulcus (IPd, pale green) corresponds, in this view, to the inferior precentral dimple of the monkey. In humans it abuts IF. The proposed sulcal equivalence fits well the available data on the anatomical and functional organization of the premotor cortices in the two species. The equivalence between human IPd and monkey ipd is well supported by the fact that this sulcus marks the border between F4 and

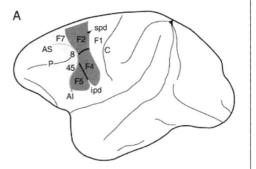

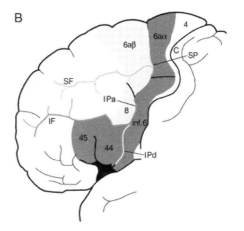

Figure 17.3

F5 in monkey and the border between inferior area 6 (inf. 6) and area 44 in humans. Abbreviations: 4, cortical area 4; C, central sulcus; F1, cortical area F1; P, principal sulcus; spd, superior precentral dimple.

References

a. Walker, A. E. (1940) *J. Comp. Neurol.* 262, 256–270.

Box 17.1 (continued)

b. Matelli, M., Luppino, G. and Rizzolatti, G. (1985) *Behav. Brain Res.* 18, 125–137.

c. Campbell, A. W. (1905) *Histological Studies on the Localisation of Cerebral Function,* Cambridge University Press.

d. Foerster, O. (1936) *Brain* 59, 135–159

e. Vogt, C. and Vogt, O. (1926) *Naturwissenschaften* 14, 1190–1194.

f. Bruce, C. J. (1988) In *Neurobiology of Neocortex* (Rakic, P. and Singer, W., eds), pp. 297–329, Wiley

g. Suzuki, H. and Azuma, M. (1983) *Exp. Brain Res.* 53, 47–58.

h. Matelli, M. and Luppino, G. (1992) *Exp. Brain Res.* (Suppl.) 22, 85–102.

i. Preuss, T. M., Stepniewska, I. and Kaas, J. H. (1996) *J. Comp. Neurol.* 371, 649–676.

j. Ono, M., Kubik, S. and Abernathey, C. D. (1990) *Atlas of the Cerebral Sulci,* Thieme.

7b in monkeys (Ref. 32). Finally, as discussed earlier, it is likely that F5 is the monkey homologue of Broca's area.

Taken together, human and monkey data indicate that, in primates, there is a fundamental mechanism for action recognition. We argue that individuals recognize actions made by others because the neural pattern elicited in their premotor areas during action observation is similar to that internally generated to produce that action. This mechanism in humans is circumscribed to the left hemisphere. In the next section we will posit that this action–recognition mechanism has been the basis for language development.

Action Recognition and Communication

Animals' calls and human speech are undoubtedly different phenomena. Among the many aspects that differentiate them is a marked difference in the anatomical structures underlying the two behaviors. Animals' calls are mediated primarily by the cingulate cortex plus some diencephalic and brain stem structures.[33,34] Speech is mediated essentially by a circuit whose main nodes are the classical Broca's and Wernicke's areas, both located on the lateral cortical surface.

Our proposal is that the development of the human lateral speech circuit is a consequence of the fact that the precursor of Broca's area was endowed, before speech appearance, with a mechanism for recognizing actions made by others. This mechanism was the neural prerequisite for the development of interindividual communication and finally of speech. We thus view language in a more general setting than one that sees speech as its complete basis.

There is obviously an enormous gap between recognizing actions and sending messages with communicative intent. We offer now a hypothesis (for an earlier version, see Ref. 35) on how this gap might have been bridged. Whether an individual is about to perform an action or observes another individual performing an action, premotor areas are activated. Normally, a series of mechanisms prevents the observer from emitting a motor behaviour that mimics the observed one, and the "actor" from initiating the action prematurely. In the case of action observation, for example, there is a strong spinal cord inhibition that selectively blocks the motoneurons involved in the observed action execution (L. Fadiga, pers. commun.). Sometimes, however, for example when the observed action is of particular interest, the premotor system will allow a brief prefix of the movement to be exhibited. This prefix will be recognized by the other individual. This fact will affect both the actor and the observer. The actor will recognize an intention in the observer, and the observer will notice that its involuntary response affects the behaviour of the actor. The development of the capacity of the observer to control his or her mirror system is crucial in order to emit (voluntarily) a signal. When this occurs, a primitive dialogue between observer and actor is established. This dialogue forms the core of language. The capacity to notice that one has emitted a signal and associating it with changes of the behavior of others might or might not have developed simultaneously. However, there is no doubt that, once established, this new association should have yielded enormous benefits of adaptive value for the group of individuals that started to make use of it, providing the selective pressure for the extension of communicative capacities to larger groups.

This new use of the mirror system, at both individual and species levels, marks the beginning of intentional communication. What actions were used for this new function in primates? Hand gestures or oro-facial movements? Before examining this issue, it is necessary to examine whether or not a "prelinguistic grammar" can be assigned to the control and observation of actions. If this is so, the notion that evolution could yield a language system "atop" of the action system becomes much more plausible.

A Pre-Linguistic "Grammar" of Action in the Monkey Brain

In order to provide abstract expression of the "meanings" of neural activity in premotor cortex (monkey area F5), we have chosen "case grammar" as a representation of sentence structure. Case grammar organizes sentences around action frames with slots for different roles. The key paper for case structure is "The Case for Case" by Fillmore,[36] although many of the ideas about case have now been absorbed in the thematic structure of the lexicon that is an integral component of the Chomskian approach to syntax known as "government and binding theory."[37]

In a case analysis, the sentence "John hit Mary with his hand" is viewed as the "surface structure" for a case structure "hit" (John, Mary, John's hand), which is an instance of the case frame "hit" (agent, recipient, instrument), which makes explicit the roles of "John," "Mary" and "John's hand." Clearly, many different sentences can express the underlying case structure. Our analysis will deal with the two main types of F5 neurons: the mirror neurons and the "canonical" F5 neurons.

(1) Imperative structure for "canonical" F5 neurons. We view the activity of "canonical" F5 neurons as part of the code for an imperative case structure, for example,

Command: grasp-A (raisin)

as an instance of grasp-A (object), where grasp-A is a specific kind of grasp, to be applied to the raisin. Note that this case structure is an "action description," not a linguistic representation. "Raisin" denotes the specific object towards which the grasp is directed, whereas grasp-A is a specific command directed towards an object with well-specified physical properties, but whose semantic properties are unspecified. The idea is that grasp type generalizes across similar grasps of varied objects has been postulated in opposition space theory.[38] Note that the slots in a case frame come with restrictions on what can fill those slots, for example, any x in grasp-A (x) must be a small object. As actions become more refined and as the transition to language occurs, the constraints on slot fillers might become more rigorous. From this, it follows that if the same principle holds for linguistic commands as for motor commands, Broca's area would code "verb phrases" and constraints on the noun phrases that can fill the slots, but not details of the noun phrases themselves. This knowledge (objects or noun phrases) could be completely outside F5 or Broca's area; for example, in the temporal lobe.

(2) Declarative structure for mirror neurons. Having viewed the activity of canonical F5

neurons as coding a command (compared with an imperative sentence), we might say that the firing of "mirror" F5 neurons is part of the code for a declarative case structure, for example,

Declaration: grasp-A (Luigi, raisin)

which is a special case of grasp-A (agent, object), where grasp-A is a specific kind of grasp, applied to the raisin (the object) by Luigi (the agent). Again, this is an "action description," not a linguistic representation. If attention is focused on the agent's hand, then the appropriate case structure would be grasp-A (hand, object) as a special case of grasp-A (instrument, object). Thus, the same act can be perceived in different ways: "who" grasps versus "what" grasps. An interesting aspect of mirror-neuron properties is that they do not fire when the monkey observes the experimenter grasping the raisin with pliers, rather than his hand (Fig. 17.1B). However, after repetitive observation, a response to the tool may appear (G. Rizzolatti, unpublished). We thus see the ability to learn new constraints on a case slot: in this case the observed generalization of the "instrument" role from hands alone to include pliers.

(3) Declarative structure for non-mirror "canonical" F5 neurons. In the case of grasp-A (object), once the grasp is initiated, can it be asserted that the activity in F5 now becomes part of the declarative "grasp-A (self, object)"? This is not an easy question. The neuronal discharge observed after hand-shaping onset might have command functions. It might, for example, reinforce the initial command to open the hand, or command the hand closure. Some "canonical" F5 neurons, however, when tested passively, show proprioceptive responses.[3,4] For these neurons, the discharge that accompanies the hand movement might have a specific declarative function concerning the agent of the action. The sentence in this case would be "grasp-A (self, object)."

From Action to Speech

Returning to our previous query as to which was the initial communicative gestural system in primates, we now distinguish between systems that are closed in the sense that they have a small, fixed repertoire and systems whose elements can be combined to yield an open repertoire of meaning. We argue that: (1) the mimetic capacity inherent to F5 and Broca's area had the potential to produce various types of closed systems related to the different types of motor fields present in that area (hand, mouth and larynx); (2) the first open system to evolve en route to human speech was a manual gestural system that exploited the observation and execution matching system described earlier; and (3) that this paved the way for the evolution of the open vocalization system we know as speech.

As far as the first point is concerned, both F5 and Broca's areas have the neural structures for controlling oro-laryngeal, oro-facial and brachio-manual movements. Furthermore, they are both endowed with mechanisms that link action perception and action production. This is true for brachio-manual gestures (as discussed in this review) as well as, in the case of human Broca's area, for linguistic tasks, including those not requiring speech production.[39–41] It is likely that the human capacity to communicate beyond that of other primates depended on the progressive evolution of the mirror system in its globality. Congruent with this view is the observation by Donald[42] that mimetic capacity, a natural extension of action recognition, is central to human culture (such as dances, games and tribal rituals), and that the evolution of this capacity was a necessary precursor to the evolution of language.

Even so, it is interesting to speculate on the sequence of events that led from gestural communication to speech. The gestures of primates that were most likely to be first used for person-to-person communication (as distinct from signals that are directed to "everybody," rather than to a specific receiver) are the oro-facial ones. In favor of this view are the following facts: oro-facial movements are used for communication by monkeys, apes and humans, and neither monkeys nor humans use manuo-brachial gestures as their main natural way to communicate. Exceptions are deaf people who naturally use sign language,[43] some Indian populations in North America and some Aboriginal Australian tribes.[44] The open–close alternation of the mandible that is typical of oro-facial communication of monkeys ("lipsmacks," "tonguesmacks"[45]) appears to persist in humans where it forms the syllabic "frame" in speech production.[46,47]

Was speech, therefore, a direct evolution of oro-facial gestures, after which followed an expansion stage during which an open vocalization system appeared? A first reason for doubting this scenario is that by using oro-facial communication, the exchange of communication is essentially limited to two actors. The possibility of introducing a third element in this one-to-one communication is very limited. By contrast, if manual gestures are associated with oro-facial communication, the sender's possibilities dramatically increase. The sender might indicate to the receiver the position of a third person or of an object, or even give a certain description of their characteristics. A second reason lies in the fact that the combinatorial properties for the openness of speech are virtually absent in the basic primate form of oro-facial communication. By contrast, they are inherent to the brachio-manual system, both when it is used for transitive actions (actions directed towards objects) and when it is employed for intransitive gestures (as in the case of American Sign Language).

These considerations suggest that, at a certain stage, a brachio-manual communication system evolved complementing the oro-facial one. This development greatly modified the importance of vocalization and its control. Whereas during the closed oro-facial stage, sounds could add very little to the gestural message (for example, oro-

facial gesture "be scared"; oro-facial gesture plus vocalization "be more scared"), their association with gestures allowed them to assume the more open, referential character that brachio-manual gestures had already achieved.[48,49] An object or event described gesturally (such as, large object—large gesture of the arms, and small object—tiny opening of the fingers) could now be accompanied by vocalization. If identical sounds were constantly used to indicate identical elements (such as, large object—large opening of the mouth, vowel "a," and small object—tiny opening of the mouth, vowel "i"), a primitive vocabulary of meaningful sounds could start to develop.[50,51]

An important consequence of this new functional use of vocalization was the necessity of its skillful control. In the oro-facial communication system, the addition of a sound had only an emotional valence that simply reinforced the meaning conveyed by the facial expression; its precise execution had a relative importance. Therefore, vocalization could remain under the control of the old system located in the brain medial areas. The situation changed radically when sounds acquired a descriptive value and thus had to remain the same in identical situations and, in addition, had to be imitated when emitted by other individuals. These new requirements could not be fulfilled by the ancient emotional vocalization centers. This new situation was most likely to be the cause of the emergence of human Broca's area from an F5-like precursor that already had mirror properties, a control of oro-laryngeal movements and, in addition, a tight link with the adjacent primary motor cortex. The evolutionary pressure for more complex (combinatorial) sound emission, and the anatomical possibility for it, were thus the elements that moved language from its manuo-brachial origins to sound emission. Manual gestures progressively lost their importance, whereas, by contrast, vocalization acquired autonomy, until the relation between gestural and vocal communication inverted and gesture became purely an accessory factor to sound communication. At this point speech took off.

A Historical Coda

The debate on the origin of language has a long history. Clearly we side with those authors who see a common origin for human speech and some forms of communications in primates, with gestural communication playing an important role in human language genesis.[52-56] Chomsky has long argued that language is determined by innate, biologically determined abilities in conjunction with exposure to the language in the environment[57]; to learn a grammar the child must simply use a few fragments of a particular language to "set" parameters in the Universal Grammar, a genetically determined, biological endowment relevant to language (for a critique of this view see Ref. 58).

Chomsky also downplays the role of natural selection in language evolution. Pinker and Bloom[59] offer convincing arguments against this view, but their approach to language evolution differs from ours on one major point. They see what has evolved for language as Universal Grammar. Our suggestion, by contrast, is that natural selection yielded a set of generic structures for matching action observation and execution. These structures, coupled with appropriate learning mechanisms, proved great enough to support cultural evolution of human languages in all their richness. We hold that human language (as well as some dyadic forms of primate communication) evolved from a basic mechanism that was not originally related to communication: the capacity to recognize actions.

Imprints in fossil cranial cavities indicate that "speech areas" were already present in early hominids such as *Homo habilis* (Ref. 60), but there is debate over whether or not such areas were already present[61] or not[62] in australopithecines. A plausible hypothesis is that the transition from the australopithecines to the first forms

of "*Homo*" coincided with the transition from a mirror system, enlarged, but used only for action recognition, to a human-like mirror system used for intentional communication. Our view on the subsequent scenario is close to that of Corballis.[53] The "proto-speech" areas of early hominids mediated oro-facial and brachio-manual communication, but not speech. The long period from the appearance of these areas to the appearance of speech[63,64] coincided with an increased capacity to communicate with gesture and the progressive association of gesture with vocalization.

In conclusion, the discovery of the mirror system suggests a strong link between speech and action representation. "One sees a distinctly linguistic way of doing things down among the nuts and bolts of action and perception, for it is there, not in the remote recesses of cognitive machinery, that the specifically linguistic constituents make their first appearance."[1]

Acknowledgements

We thank Massimo Matelli for his help with the anatomical figure. The work was supported by HFSP and BIOMED 2.

Selected References

1. Liberman, A. M. (1993) *Haskins Laboratories Status Report on Speech Research* 113, 1–32.
2. Kurata, K. and Tanji, J. (1986) *J. Neurosci.* 6, 403–411.
3. Rizzolatti, G. et al. (1988) *Exp. Brain Res.* 71, 491–507.
4. Hepp-Reymond, M.-C. et al. (1994) *Can. J. Physiol. Pharmacol.* 72, 571–579.
5. Jeannerod, M. et al. (1995) *Trends Neurosci.* 18, 314–320.
6. Di Pellegrino, G. et al. (1992) *Exp. Brain Res.* 91, 176–180.
7. Rizzolatti, G. et al. (1996) *Cogn. Brain Res.* 3, 131–141.
8. Gallese, V. et al. (1996) *Brain* 119, 593–609.

9. Jeannerod, M. (1994) *Behav. Brain Sci.* 17, 187–245.

10. Liberman, A. M. and Mattingly, I. G. (1985) *Cognition* 21, 1–36.

11. Liberman, A. M. and Mattingly, I. G. (1989) *Science* 243, 489–494.

12. Passingham, R. (1981) *Philos. Trans. R. Soc. London Ser. B* 292, 167–175.

13. Campbell, A. W. (1905) *Histological Studies on the Localisation of Cerebral Function,* Cambridge University Press.

14. Von Bonin, G. and Bailey, P. (1947) *The Neocortex of* Macaca Mulatta, University of Illinois Press.

15. Passingham, R. (1993) *The Frontal Lobes and Voluntary Action,* Oxford University Press.

16. Galaburda, A. M. and Pandya, D. N. (1982) in *Primate Brain Evolution* (Armstrong, E. and Falk, D., eds.), pp. 203–216, Plenum Press.

17. Petrides, M. and Pandya, D. N. (1994) in *Handbook of Neuropsychology* (Vol. IX) (Boller, F. and Grafman, J., eds.), pp. 17–58, Elsevier.

18. Rizzolatti, G. et al. (1981) *Behav. Brain Res.* 2, 147–163.

19. Hast, M. H. et al. (1974) *Brain Res.* 73, 229–240.

20. Gentilucci, M. et al. (1988) *Exp. Brain Res.* 71, 475–490.

21. Preuss, T. M. (1995) in *The Cognitive Neurosciences* (Gazzaniga, M. S., ed.), pp. 1227–1241, MIT Press.

22. Bonda, E. et al. (1994) *Soc. Neurosci. Abstr.* 20, 353.

23. Schlaug, G., Knorr, U. and Seitz, R. J. (1994) *Exp. Brain Res.* 98, 523–534.

24. Decety, J. et al. (1994) *Nature* 371, 600–602.

25. Grafton, S. T. et al. (1996) *Exp. Brain Res.* 112, 103–111.

26. Parsons, L. M. et al. (1995) *Nature* 375, 54–58.

27. Chollet, F. et al. (1991) *Ann. Neurol.* 29, 63–71.

28. Fadiga, L. et al. (1995) *J. Neurophysiol.* 73, 2608–2611.

29. Rizzolatti, G. et al. (1996) *Exp. Brain Res.* 111, 246–252.

30. Perrett, D. I. et al. (1989) *J. Exp. Biol.* 146, 87–113.

31. Perrett, D. I. et al. (1990) in *Vision and Action: The Control of Grasping* (Goodale, M. A., ed.), pp. 163–180, Ablex.

32. Leinonen, L. and Nyman, G. (1979) *Exp. Brain Res.* 34, 321–333.

33. Jurgens, U. (1995) in *Current Topics in Primate Vocal Communication* (Zimmerman, E., Newman, J. D. and Jurgens, U., eds.), pp. 199–206, Plenum Press.

34. MacLean, P. D. (1993) in *Neurobiology of Cingulate Cortex and Limbic Thalamus: A Comprehensive Handbook* (Vogt, B. A. and Gabriel, M., eds.), pp. 1–15, Birkhäuser.

35. Arbib, M. A. and Rizzolatti, G. (1997) *Commun. Cogn.* 29, 393–424.

36. Fillmore, C. J. (1966) in *Universals in Linguistic Theory* (Bach, E. and Harms, R. T., eds.), pp. 1–88, Rinehart and Winston.

37. van Riemsdijk, H. and Williams, E. (1986) *Introduction to the Theory of Grammar,* MIT Press.

38. Iberall, T. et al. (1986) *Exp. Brain Res.* 15, 158–173.

39. Demonet, J.-F. et al. (1992) *Brain* 115, 1753–1768.

40. Zatorre, R. J. et al. (1992) *Science* 256, 846–849.

41. Demonet, J.-F., Wise, R. and Frackowiak, R. S. J. (1993) *Hum. Brain Mapp.* 1, 39–47.

42. Donald, M. (1991) *Origins of the Modern Mind: Three Stages in the Evolution of Culture and Cognition,* Harvard University Press.

43. Klima, E. S. and Bellugi, U. (1979) *The Signs of the Language,* Harvard University Press.

44. Kendon, A. (1988) *Sign Languages of Aboriginal Australians,* Cambridge University Press.

45. Redican, W. K. (1975) in *Primate Behavior: Developments in Field and Laboratory Research* (Vol. 4) (Rosenblum, L. A., ed.), pp. 104–194, Academic Press.

46. MacNeilage, P. F. (1997) in *Approaches to the Evolution of Language* (Hurford, J. R., Knight, C. and Studdert-Kennedy, M. G., eds.), pp. 234–252, Cambridge University Press.

47. MacNeilage, P. F. *Behav. Brain Sci.* (in press).

48. Paget, R. A. S. (1963) *Human Speech: Some Observations, Experiments and Conclusions as to the Nature, Origin, Purpose and Possible Improvement of Human Speech,* Routledge and Kegan Paul.

49. Johanesson, A. (1950) *Nature* 166, 60–61.

50. Holland, M. and Wertheimer, M. (1964) *Percept. Motor Skill* 19, 111–117.

51. Weiss, J. H. (1964) *Psychol. Bull.* 61, 454–458.

52. Hewes, G. W. (1973) *Curr. Anthropol.* 14, 5–24.

53. Corballis, M. C. (1992) *Cognition* 44, 197–226.

54. Corballis, M. C. (1991) *The Lopsided Ape: Evolution of the Generative Mind,* Oxford University Press.

55. Kimura, D. (1993) *Neuromotor Mechanisms in Human Communication,* Oxford University Press.

56. Armstrong, D. F., Stokoe, W. C. and Wilcox, S. E. (1995) *Gesture and the Nature of Language,* Cambridge University Press.

57. Chomsky, N. (1986) *Knowledge of Language: Its Nature, Origin and Use,* Praeger.

58. Arbib, M. A. and Hill J. C. (1988) in *Explaining Language Universals* (Hawkins, J. A., ed.), pp. 56–72, Blackwell.

59. Pinker, S. and Bloom, P. (1990) *Behav. Brain Sci.* 12, 707–784.

60. Tobias, P. V. (1987) *J. Hum. Evol.* 16, 741–761.

61. Holloway, R. L. (1981) *Am. J. Phys. Anthropol.* 56, 43–58.

62. Falk, D. (1983) *Science* 222, 1072–1074.

63. Lieberman, P., Crelin, E. S. and Klatt, D. H. (1972) *Am. Anthropol.* 74, 287–307.

64. Lieberman, P. (1984) *The Biology and Evolution of Language,* Harvard University Press.

18

The Fusiform Face Area: A Module in Human Extrastriate Cortex Specialized for Face Perception

Nancy Kanwisher, Josh McDermott, and Marvin M. Chun

Evidence from cognitive psychology (Yin, 1969; Bruce et al., 1991; Tanaka and Farah, 1993), computational vision (Turk and Pentland, 1991), neuropsychology (Damasio et al., 1990; Behrmann et al., 1992), and neurophysiology (Desimone, 1991; Perrett et al., 1992) suggests that face and object recognition involve qualitatively different processes that may occur in distinct brain areas. Single-unit recordings from the superior temporal sulcus (STS) in macaques have demonstrated neurons that respond selectively to faces (Gross et al., 1972; Desimone, 1991; Perrett et al., 1991). Evidence for a similar cortical specialization in humans has come from epilepsy patients with implanted subdural electrodes. In discrete portions of the fusiform and inferotemporal gyri, large N200 potentials have been elicited by faces but not by scrambled faces, cars, or butterflies (Ojemann et al., 1992; Allison et al., 1994; Nobre et al., 1994). Furthermore, many reports have described patients with damage in the occipitotemporal region of the right hemisphere who have selectively lost the ability to recognize faces (De Renzi, 1997). Thus, several sources of evidence support the existence of specialized neural "modules" for face perception in extrastriate cortex.

The evidence from neurological patients is powerful but limited in anatomical specificity; however, functional brain imaging allows us to study cortical specialization in the normal human brain with relatively high spatial resolution and large sampling area. Past imaging studies have reported regions of the fusiform gyrus and other areas that were more active during face than object viewing (Sergent et al., 1992), during face matching than location matching (Haxby et al., 1991, 1994; Courtney et al., 1997), and during the viewing of faces than of scrambled faces (Puce et al., 1995; Clark et al., 1996), consonant strings (Puce et al., 1996), or textures (Malach et al., 1995; Puce et al., 1996). Although these studies are an important beginning, they do not establish that these cortical regions are *selectively* involved in face perception, because each of these findings is consistent with several alternative interpretations of the mental processes underlying the observed activations, such as (1) low-level feature extraction (given the differences between the face and various control stimuli), (2) visual attention, which may be recruited more strongly by faces, (3) "subordinate-level" visual recognition (Damasio et al., 1990; Gauthier et al., 1996) of particular exemplars of a basic-level category (Rosch et al., 1976), and (4) recognition of any animate (or human) objects (Farah et al., 1996).

Such ambiguity of interpretation is almost inevitable in imaging studies in which only two or three conditions are compared. We attempted to overcome this problem by using functional magnetic resonance imaging (fMRI) to run multiple tests applied to the same cortical region within individual subjects to search for discrete regions of cortex *specialized* for face perception. (For present purposes, we define face perception broadly to include any higher-level visual processing of faces from the detection of a face as a face to the extraction from a face of any information about the individual's identity, gaze direction, mood, sex, etc.). Our strategy was to ask first whether any regions of occipitotemporal cortex were significantly more active during face than object viewing; only one such area (in the fusiform gyrus) was found consistently across most subjects. To test the hypothesis that this fusiform region was specialized for face perception, we then measured the activity in this same functionally defined area in individual subjects during four subsequent comparisons, each testing one or more of the alternative accounts listed in the previous paragraph.

Materials and Methods

General Design

This study had three main parts. In Part I, we searched for any occipitotemporal areas that might be specialized for face perception by looking within each subject for regions in the ventral (occipitotemporal) pathway that responded significantly more strongly during passive viewing of photographs of faces than photographs of assorted common objects. This comparison served as a scout, allowing us to (1) anatomically localize candidate "face areas" within individual subjects, (2) determine which if any regions are activated consistently across subjects, and (3) specify precisely the voxels in each subject's brain that would be used as that subject's previously defined region of interest (ROI) for the subsequent tests in Parts II and III.

We used a stimulus manipulation with a passive viewing task (rather than a task manipulation on identical stimuli) because the perception of foveally presented faces is a highly automatic process that is difficult to bring under volitional control (Farah et al., 1995). Imagine, for example, being told that a face will be flashed at fixation for 500 msec and that you must analyze its low-level visual features but not recognize the face. If the face is familiar it will be virtually impossible to avoid recognizing it. Thus when faces are presented foveally, all processes associated with face recognition are likely to occur no matter what the task is, and the most effective way to generate a control condition in which those processes do not occur is to present a nonface stimulus (Kanwisher et al., 1996).

The results of Part I showed only one region that was activated consistently across subjects for the faces versus objects comparison; this area was in the right fusiform gyrus (and/or adjacent sulci). We hypothesized that this region was specialized for some aspect of face perception, and we tested alternatives to this hypothesis with several different stimulus comparisons in Parts II

and III. In Part II, each of five subjects who had revealed a clear fusiform face activation in Part I was tested on two new stimulus comparisons. In each, the methodological details were identical to those of the faces versus objects runs, and only the stimulus sets differed. Our first new stimulus comparison in Part II was between intact two-tone faces (created by thresholding the photographs used in Part I) and scrambled two-tone faces in which the component black regions were rearranged to create a stimulus unrecognizable as a face (see Fig. 18.3b). This manipulation preserved the mean luminance and some low-level features of the two-tone face stimuli and avoided producing the "cut-and-paste" marks that have been a problem in the scrambling procedures of some earlier studies; this contrast therefore served as a crude test of whether the "face areas" were simply responding to the low-level visual features present in face but not nonface stimuli. Our second stimulus contrast—front view photographs of faces versus front view photographs of houses (see Fig. 18.3c)—was designed to test whether the "face area" was involved not in face perception per se but rather in processing and/or distinguishing between any different exemplars of a single class of objects.

In Part III, a new but overlapping set of five subjects who had revealed clear candidate face areas in Part I were tested on two new comparisons. (Subjects S1 and S2 participated in both Parts II and III.) In the first new comparison, subjects passively viewed three-quarter-view photographs of faces (all were of people whose hair was tucked inside a black knit ski hat) versus photographs of human hands (all shot from the same angle and in roughly the same position). This comparison (see Fig. 18.4b) was designed to test several different questions. First, would the response of the candidate face area generalize to different viewpoints? Second, is this area involved in recognizing the face on the basis of the hair and other external features of the head (Sinha and Poggio, 1996) or on the basis of its internal features? Because the external features were largely hidden (and highly similar across exemplars) in the ski hat faces, a response of this area to these stimuli would suggest that it is primarily involved in processing the internal rather than external features of the face. Third, the use of human hands as a control condition also provided a test of whether the face area would respond to any animate or human body part. In the second new comparison, the same stimuli (three-quarter-view faces vs hands) were presented while subjects performed a "1-back" task searching for consecutive repetitions of identical stimuli (pressing a button whenever they detected a repetition). For this task, a 250 msec blank gray field was sandwiched between each successive 500 msec presentation of a face. The gray field produced sensory transients over the whole stimulus and thereby required subjects to rely on higher-level visual information to perform the task (Rensink et al., 1997). Because the 1-back task was, if anything, more difficult for hand than face stimuli, the former should engage general attentional mechanisms at least as strongly as the latter, ruling out any account of greater face activation for faces in terms of general attentional mechanisms.

Tests of each subject in Parts II and III were run on the basic face versus object comparison from Part I in the same session, so that the results of Part I could be used to generate the precise ROIs for that subject for the comparisons in Parts II and III. For the passive viewing conditions, subjects were instructed to maintain fixation on the dot when it was present, and otherwise to simply look at the stimuli attentively without carrying out other mental games at the same time.

Subjects

Tests of 20 normal subjects under the age of 40 were run, and all of the subjects reported normal or corrected-to-normal vision and no previous neurological history. The data from five of them were omitted because of excessive head motion or other artifacts. Of the remaining 15 subjects (9 women and 6 men), 13 participants described themselves as right-handed and two as left-handed. All 15 subjects participated in Part I. (Subject S1 was run on Part I many times in different scanning sessions spread over a 6 month period both to measure test–retest reliability within a subject across sessions and to compare the results from Part I with a number of other pilot studies conducted over this period.) Subjects S1, S2, S5, S7, and S8 from Figure 18.2 were run in Part II, and subjects S1, S5, S9, S10, and S11 from Figure 18.2 were run in Part III. Subjects S1–S10 described themselves as right-handed, whereas subjects S11 and S12 described themselves as left-handed. The experimental procedures were approved by both the Harvard University Committee on the Use of Human Subjects in Research and the Massachusetts General Hospital Subcommittee on Human Studies; informed consent was obtained from each participant.

Stimuli

Samples of the stimuli used in these experiments are shown in Figures 18.3 and 18.4. All stimuli were $\sim 300 \times 300$ pixels in size and were grayscale photographs (or photograph-like images), except for the intact and scrambled two-tone faces used in Part II. The face photographs in Parts I and II were 90 freshmen ID photographs obtained with consent from members of the Harvard class of 1999. The three-quarter-view face photos used in Part II were members of or volunteers at the Harvard Vision Sciences Lab. (For most subjects none of the faces were familiar.) The 90 assorted object photos (and photo-like pictures) were obtained from various sources and included canonical views of familiar objects such as a spoon, lion, or car. The 90 house photographs were scanned from an architecture book and were unfamiliar to the subjects.

Each scan lasted 5 min and 20 sec and consisted of six 30 sec stimulus epochs interleaved with seven 20 sec epochs of fixation. During

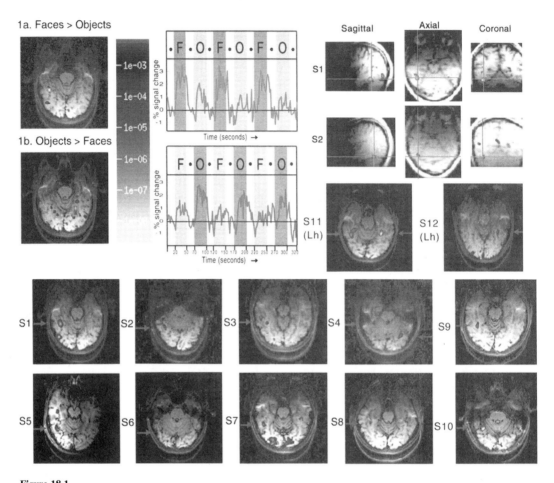

Figure 18.1
Results from subject S1 on Part I. The right hemisphere appears on the left for these and all brain images in this chapter (except the resliced images labeled "Axial" in Figure 18.2). The brain images at the left show in color the voxels that produced a significantly higher MR signal intensity (based on smoothed data) during the epochs containing faces than during those containing objects (1a) and vice versa (1b) for 1 of the 12 slices scanned. These significance images (see color key at right for this and all figures in this chapter) are overlaid on a T1-weighted anatomical image of the same slice. Most of the other 11 slices showed no voxels that reached significance at the $P < 10^{-3}$ level or better in either direction of the comparison. In each image, and ROI is shown outlined in green, and the time course of raw percentage signal change over the 5 min 20 sec scan (based on unsmoothed data and averaged across the voxels in this ROI) is shown at the right. Epochs in which faces were presented are indicated by the vertical gray bars marked with an F; gray bars with an O indicate epochs during which assorted objects were presented; white bars indicate fixation epochs.

each stimulus epoch in Parts I and II, 45 different photographs were presented foveally at a rate of one every 670 msec (with the stimulus on for 500 msec and off for 170 msec). Stimulus epochs alternated between the two different conditions being compared, as shown in Figures 18.1, 18.3, and 18.4. The 45 different stimuli used in the first stimulus epoch were the same as those used in the fifth stimulus epoch; the stimuli used in the second stimulus epoch were the same as those used in the sixth. The stimuli in Part III were the same in structure and timing, except that (1) a total of 22 face stimuli and 22 hand stimuli were used (with most stimuli occurring twice in each epoch), and (2) the interval between face or hand stimuli was 250 msec.

Stimulus sequences were generated using Mac-Probe software (Hunt, 1994) and recorded onto videotape for presentation via a video projector during the scans. Stimuli were back-projected onto a ground-glass screen and viewed in a mirror over the subject's forehead (visual angle of the stimuli was ~15 × 15°).

MRI Acquisition
Scans were conducted using the 1.5 T MRI scanner (General Electric Signa, Milwaukee, WI) at the Massachusetts General Hospital NMR Center (Charlestown, MA), using echo-planar imaging (Instascan, ANMR Systems, Wilmington, MA) and a bilateral quadrature receive-only surface coil (made by Patrick Ledden, Massachusetts General Hospital NMR Center). Functional data were obtained using an asymmetric spin echo sequence (TR = 2 sec, TE = 70 msec, flip angle = 90°, 180° offset = 25 msec). Our 12 6 mm slices were oriented parallel to the inferior edge of the occipital and temporal lobes and covered the entire occipital and most of the temporal lobe (see Fig. 18.5). Head motion was minimized with a bite bar. Voxel size was 3.25 × 3.25 × 6 mm. Details of our procedure are as described in Tootell et al. (1995), except as noted here.

Data Analysis
Five subjects of the 20 scanned had excessive head motion and/or reported falling asleep during one or more runs; the data from these subjects were omitted from further analysis. Motion was assessed within a run by looking for (1) a visible shift in the functional image from a given slice between the first and last functional image in one run, (2) activated regions that curved around the edge of the brain and/or shifted sides when the sign of the statistical comparison was reversed, and/or (3) ramps in the time course of signal intensity from a single voxel or set of voxels. Motion across runs was assessed by visually inspecting the raw functional images for any change in the shape of a brain slice across runs.

For the remaining 15 subjects no motion correction was carried out. Pilot data had indicated that the significance from a single run was sometimes weak, but became much stronger when we averaged across two identical runs within a subject (i.e., when the two corresponding values for each voxel, one from each scan, were averaged together for each of the 160 images × 12 slices collected during a single 5 min 20 sec scan). We therefore ran each test twice on each subject, and averaged over the two runs of each test. The

Figure 18.2
Anatomical images overlaid with color-coded statistical maps from the 10 right-handed subjects in Part I who showed regions that produced a significantly stronger MR signal during face than object viewing. For each of the right-handed subjects (S1–S10), the slice containing the right fusiform face activation is shown; for left-handed subjects S11 and S12 (in Figure 18.1), all the fusiform face activations are visible in the slices shown. Data from subjects S1 and S2 resliced into sagittal, coronal, and axial slices (top right). Data from the three subjects who showed no regions that responded significantly more strongly for faces than objects are not shown.

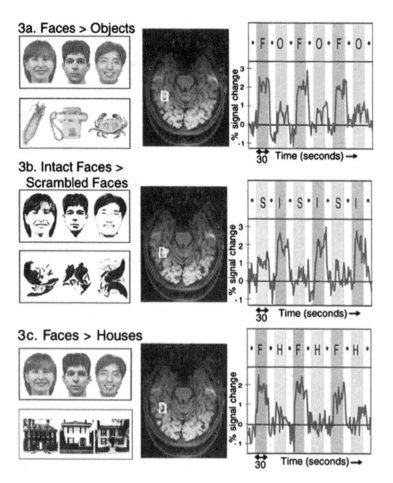

Figure 18.3
Results of Part II. (Left column) Sample stimuli used for the faces versus objects comparison as well as the two subsequent tests. (Center column) Areas that produced significantly greater activation for faces than control stimuli for subject S1. (a) The faces versus objects comparison was used to define a single ROI (shown in green outline for S1), separately for each subject. The time courses in the right column were produced by (1) averaging the percentage signal change across all voxels in a given subject's ROI (using the original unsmoothed data), and then (2) averaging these ROI-averages across the five subjects. F and O in (a) indicate face and object epochs; I and S in (b) indicate intact and scrambled face epochs; and F and H in (c) indicate face and hand epochs.

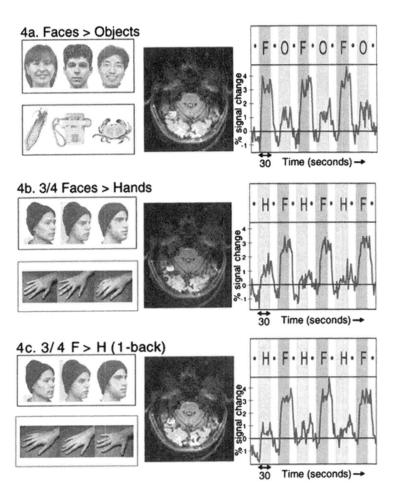

Figure 18.4
Results of Part III. Stimulus contrasts for each test are shown in the left column. (a) Face ROIs were defined separately for each subject using the average of two face versus object scans as described for Figure 18.3a. The resulting brain slice with statistical overlay for one subject (S10) is shown in the center column, and the time course of signal intensity averaged over the five subjects' ROIs is shown at the right. As described for Figure 18.3a (Part II), the ROI specified on the basis of the faces versus objects comparison was used for the two subsequent comparisons of passive viewing of three-quarter faces versus hands (b), and the consecutive matching task on three-quarter faces versus hands (c).

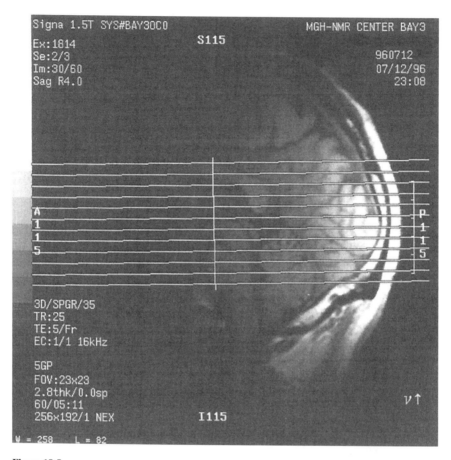

Signa 1.5T SYS#BAY30C0   S115   MGH-NMR CENTER BAY3
Ex:1814
Se:2/3   960712
Im:30/60   07/12/96
Sag R4.0   23:08

3D/SPGR/35
TR:25
TE:5/Fr
EC:1/1 16kHz

5GP
FOV:23x23
2.8thk/0.0sp
60/05:11
256x192/1 NEX   I115

W = 258   L = 82

Figure 18.5
Midsagittal anatomical image from subject S1 showing the typical placing of the 12 slices used in this study. Slices were selected so as to include the entire ventral surface of the occipital and temporal lobes.

data were then analyzed statistically using a Kolmogorov–Smirnov test, after smoothing with a Hanning kernel over a 3×3 voxel area to produce an approximate functional resolution of 6 mm. This analysis was run on each voxel (after incorporating a 6 sec lag for estimated hemodynamic delay), testing whether the MR signal intensity in that voxel was significantly greater during epochs containing one class of stimuli (e.g., faces) than epochs containing the other

(e.g., objects). Areas of activation were displayed in color representations of significance level, overlaid on high-resolution anatomical images of the same slice. Voxels of significant activation were also inspected visually by plotting the time course of raw (unsmoothed) signal intensity over the 5 min 20 sec of the scan.

To identify all regions within our chosen slices and coil range that responded more strongly to faces than objects in Part I, as well as their

Talairach coordinates, each subject's anatomical and functional data were first fitted into their own Talairach space and then analyzed (using the program Tal-EZ by Bush et al., 1996) to find all the regions that produced a stronger signal for faces than objects at the $p < 10^{-4}$ level of significance (uncorrected for multiple comparisons). This analysis was intended as a scout for candidate face areas and revealed that the only region in which most of our subjects showed a significantly greater activation for faces than objects was in the right fusiform gyrus. This region therefore became the focus of our more detailed investigations in Parts II and III.

For each subject in Parts II and III, a face ROI was identified that was composed of all contiguous voxels in the right fusiform region in which (1) the MR signal intensity was significantly stronger during face than object epochs at the $p < 10^{-4}$ level, and (2) a visual inspection of the raw time course data from that voxel did not reveal any obvious ramps, spikes, or other artifacts. For subject S11, who was left-handed and had very large and highly significant activations in both left and right fusiform gyri, the ROI used in Part III included both of these regions.

For each of the comparisons in Parts II and III we first averaged over the two runs from each subject and then averaged across the voxels in that subject's predefined face ROI (from Part I) to derive the time course of raw signal intensity in that subject's ROI. Two further analyses were then carried out. First, the average MR signal intensity in each subjects' ROI for each epoch was calculated (by averaging within a subject across all the voxels in their ROI and across all the images collected in each epoch). The average MR signal intensities for each subject and stimulus epoch were then entered into a three-way ANOVA across subjects (epoch number × face/ control × test) separately for Parts II and III. The factor of epoch number had three levels corresponding to the first, second, and third epochs for each condition; the test factor had three levels for the three different stimulus compar-

isons (faces vs objects/scrambled vs intact faces/ faces vs houses for Part II and faces vs objects/ passive faces vs hands/1-back faces vs hands for Part III). These ANOVAs allowed us to test for the significance of the differences in signal intensity between the various face and control conditions and also to test whether this difference interacted with epoch number and/or comparison type.

Second, for each subject we converted the raw time course of MR signal intensity from that subject's face ROI into a time course of percent signal change, using that subject's average signal across all the fixation epochs in the same runs (in the face ROI) as a baseline. These time courses of percent signal change for each subject's face ROI could then be averaged across the five subjects who were run on the same test, for all the tests in Parts I through III. By averaging across each subject's ROI and across all the data collected during each epoch type, we derived an average percentage signal change for the face and control conditions for each test. The ratio of the percentage signal change for the faces versus control condition for each test provides a measure of the selectivity of the face ROI to the stimulus contrast used in that test.

Results

Part I

In Part I we asked whether any brain areas were significantly more active during face viewing than object viewing. Figure 18.1a shows the results from a single subject (S1), revealing a region in the right fusiform gyrus that produced a significantly higher signal intensity during epochs in which faces were presented than during epochs in which objects were presented (in five adjacent voxels at the $p < 10^{-4}$ level based on an analysis of smoothed data). This pattern is clearly visible in the raw (unsmoothed) data for this single subject shown in Figure 18.1a (*right*), where the percentage signal change is plotted over the 5 min 20 sec of the scan, averaged over the five voxels outlined in green (Fig. 18.1a, *left*). The opposite effect, a significantly higher MR signal (each significant at the $p < 10^{-4}$ level) during the viewing of objects than during face viewing, was seen in a different, bilateral and more medial area including two adjacent voxels in the right hemisphere and eight in the left in the same slice of the same data set (Fig. 18.1b). A similar bilateral activation in the parahippocampal region for objects compared with faces was seen in most of the subjects run in this study; this result is described briefly in Kanwisher et al. (1996), where images of this activation are shown for three different subjects. The two opposite activations for faces and objects constitute a double dissociation and indicate that the face activation cannot merely be an artifact of an overall tendency for the faces to be processed more extensively than the objects or vice versa.

To scout for any regions of the brain that might be specialized for face perception consistently across subjects, we tabulated (in Table 18.1) the Talairach coordinates of all the regions in each subject that produced a stronger signal for faces than objects at the $p < 10^{-4}$ level of significance (uncorrected for multiple comparisons). The only region in which most of our subjects showed a significantly greater activation for faces than objects was in the right fusiform gyrus. This region therefore became the focus of our more detailed investigations in Parts II and III.

Fusiform activations for faces compared with objects were observed in the fusiform region in 12 of the 15 subjects analyzed; for the other three subjects no brain areas produced a significantly stronger MR signal intensity during face than object epochs at the $p < 10^{-4}$ level or better. [Null results are difficult to interpret in functional imaging data: the failure to see face activations in these subjects could reflect either the absence of a face area in these subjects or the failure to detect a face module that was actu-

ally present because of (1) insufficient statistical power, (2) susceptibility artifact, or (3) any of numerous other technical limitations.] The slice showing the right fusiform face activation for each of the 12 subjects is shown in Figure 18.2. An inspection of flow-compensated anatomical images did not reveal any large vessels in the vicinity of the activations. Despite some variability, the locus of this fusiform face activation is quite consistent across subjects both in terms of gyral/sulcal landmarks and in terms of Talairach coordinates (see Table 18.1). Half of the 10 right-handed subjects showed this fusiform activation only in the right hemisphere; the other half showed bilateral activations. For the right-handed subjects, the right hemisphere fusiform area averaged 1 cm^3 in size and was located at Talairach coordinates 40x, -55y, -10z (mean across subjects of the coordinates of the most significant voxel). The left hemisphere fusiform area was found in only five of the right-handed subjects, and in these it averaged 0.5 cm^3 in size and was located at -35x, -63y, -10z. (As shown in Table 18.1, the significance level was also typically higher for right hemisphere than left hemisphere face activations.) For cortical parcellation, the data for individual subjects were resliced into sagittal, coronal, and axial slices (as shown for S1 and S2 in Fig. 18.2). This allowed localization of these activated areas to the fusiform gyrus at the level of the occipitotemporal junction (parcellation unit TOF in the system of Rademacher et al., 1993), although in several cases we cannot rule out the possibility that the activation is in the adjacent collateral and/or occipitotemporal sulci.

Subject S1 was run on the basic faces versus objects comparison in Part I in many different testing sessions spread over a period of 6 months. A striking demonstration of the test–retest reliability of this comparison can be seen by inspecting the activation images for this subject from four different sessions in which this same faces versus objects comparison was run; these are shown in Figure 18.1a, the two different axial

Table 18.1
Talairach coordinates of brain regions with stronger responses to faces than objects in individual subjects

Subject	Fusiform face area	MT gyrus/ST sulcus	Other activation loci	Other activation loci
A. Right-handed subjects				
S1	(40, −48, −12), 2.1, −10		(43, −75, −6), 2.1, −10	
S2	(37, −57, −9), 0.4, −7	(50, −54, 15), 0.3, −6	(−37, −57, 21), 0.6, −5 (0, −54, 28), 6.1, −8	(−43, −72, 25), 0.7, −5
S3	(43, −54, −18), 1.8, −9	(65, −51, 9), 3.6, −6 (56, −60, 3), 1.6, −5	(37, −78, −15), 0.6, −8 (56, −27, 18), 1.1, −5	(40, −69, 40), 2.8, −5
S4	(31, −62, −6), 0.9, −10 (−31, −62, −15), 1.3, −6	(56, −57, 6), 0.9, 2e−7	(34, −42, −21), 0.3, −4	
S5	(50, −63, −9), 2.1, −10		(34, −81, 6), 0.6, −6	(40, −30, −9), 0.2, −6
S6	(37, −69, −3), 0.1, −4 (−34, −69, 0), 0.1, −4	(46, −48, 12), 0.7, −4	(−34, −69, 0), 0.2, −4	
S7	(46, −54, −12), 0.8, −6 (−40, −69, −12), 0.5, −5		(43, −69, −3), 0.4, −5 (0, −75, 6), 1.9, −9 (−6, −75, 34), 4.2, −8	(−12, −87, 0), 3.1, −5 (21, −90, −3), 3.7, −6 (40, 54, 34), 2.8, −5 (12, −81, 46), 1.7, −6
S8	(40, −39, −6), 0.06, −6 (−34, −75, −3), 0.06, −8		(3, −72, 31), 2.7, −6	
S9	(40, −51, −12), 0.7, −1.10			
S10	(34, −57, −15), 1.4, −13 (−37, −41, −12), 0.4, −6	(56, −60, 6), 0.2, −5		
B. Left-handed subjects				
S11	(−37, −42, −12), 1.9, −12 (40, −48, −12), 1.1, −8	(46, −69, 0), 0.4, −5 (−53, −54, 0), 1.4, −5	(−62, −30, 12), 0.4, −5	
S12	(−34, −48, −6), 0.4, −8	(56, −42, 21), 0.5, −5	(3, −60, 12), 0.3, −5 (6, −60, 31), 3.5, −5	(34, −90, 6), 0.3, −4

Regions that responded significantly (at the $p < 10^{-4}$ level) more strongly during face than object epochs (Part I) for each activated region is given (1) the Talairach coordinates (M-Lx, A-Py, S-Iz), (2) size (in cm^3), and (3) exponent (base 10) of the p level of the most significant voxel (based on an analysis of unsmoothed data) in that region (in italics). This table was generated using a program (Tal-EZ) supplied by G. Bush et al. (1996). Subject S5 was run with a surface coil placed over the right hemisphere, so only right hemisphere activations could be detected.

Table 18.2A
Part I

Faces	Objects	Ratio	Intact	Scrambled	Ratio	Face	House	Ratio
1.9%	0.7%	2.8	1.9%	0.6%	3.2	1.6%	0.2%	6.6

Table 18.2B
Part II

			Passive			1-Back repetition detection		
Faces	Objects	Ratio	3/4 Faces	Hands	Ratio	3/4 Faces	Hands	Ratio
3.3%	1.2%	2.7	2.7%	0.7%	4.0	3.2%	0.7%	4.5

Mean percent signal change (from average fixation baseline) across all five subjects for face epochs versus control epochs for each of the comparisons in Parts II and III. The ratio of percent signal change for faces to the percent signal change for the control condition is a measure of face selectivity.

images for subject S1 in Figure 18.2 (*bottom left* and *top right*), and Figure 18.3a. The high degree of consistency in the locus of activation suggests that the complete lateralization of the face activation to the right hemisphere in this subject is not an artifact of partial voluming (i.e., a chance positioning of the slice plane so as to divide a functional region over two adjacent slices, thereby reducing the signal in each slice compared with the case in which the entire region falls in a single slice). Although our sample size is too small to permit confident generalizations about the effects of handedness, it is worth noting that our 10 right-handed subjects showed either unilateral right-hemisphere or bilateral activations in the fusiform region, whereas one left-handed subject (S11) showed a unilateral left-hemisphere and the other (S12) showed a bilateral activation.

In addition to the activation in the fusiform region, seven subjects also showed an activation for faces compared with objects in the region of the middle temporal gyrus/superior temporal (ST) sulcus of the right hemisphere. Talairach coordinates for these activations are provided in the second column of Table 18.1. Most subjects also showed additional face (compared with object) activations in other regions (Table 18.2, third and fourth columns), but none of these appeared to be systematic across subjects.

Part II

Part II tested whether the activation for faces compared with objects described in Part I was attributable to (1) differences in luminance between the face and object stimuli and/or (2) the fact that the face stimuli but not the object stimuli were all different exemplars of the same category. Five subjects who had also been run in Part I were run on Part II in the same scanning session, allowing us to use the results from Part I to derive previous face ROIs for the analysis of the data in Part II.

First we defined a "face" ROI in the right fusiform region separately for each of the five subjects, as described above, and then averaged the response across all the voxels in that subject's own face ROI during the new tests. The pattern of higher activation for face than nonface stimuli was clearly visible in the raw data from each subject's face ROI for each of the tests in Part II. To test this quantitatively, we averaged the mean MR signal intensity across each subject's ROI and across all the images collected within a given stimulus epoch and entered these data into a three-way ANOVA across subjects (face/control × epoch number × test). This analysis revealed a main effect of higher signal intensity during face epochs than during control stimulus epochs ($F_{(1,4)} = 27.1$; $p < 0.01$). No other main effects or interactions reached significance. In particular, there was no interaction of face/control × test ($F < 1$), indicating that the effect of higher signal intensity during face than control stimuli did not differ significantly across the three tests. As a further check, separate pairwise comparisons between the face and control stimuli were run for each of the three tests, revealing that each reached significance independently ($p < 0.001$ for faces vs objects, $p < 0.05$ for intact vs scrambled faces, and $p < 0.01$ for faces vs houses). Note that because the ROI and exact hypothesis were specified in advance for the latter two tests (and because we averaged over all the voxels in a given subject's ROI to produce a single averaged number for each ROI), only a single comparison was carried out for each subject in each test, and no correction for multiple comparisons is necessary for the intact versus scrambled faces and faces versus houses comparisons.

For each subject the ROI-averaged time course data were then converted into percentage signal change (using the average MR signal intensity across the fixation epochs in that subject's face ROI as a baseline). The average across the five subjects' time courses of percentage signal change are plotted in Figure 18.3, where the data clearly show higher peaks during face epochs than during nonface epochs. An index of selectivity of the face ROI was then derived by calculating the average percentage signal change across all subjects' face ROIs during face epochs to the average percentage signal change during nonface epochs. This ratio (see Table 18.2) varies from 2.8 (the faces vs objects test) to 6.6 (faces vs houses), indicating a high degree of stimulus se-

lectivity in the face ROIs. For comparison purposes, note that Tootell et al. (1995) reported analogous selectivity ratios from 2.2 to 16.1 for the response of visual area MT to moving versus stationary displays.

In sum, these data indicate that the region in each subject's fusiform gyrus that responds more strongly to faces than objects also responds more strongly to intact than scrambled two-tone faces and more strongly to faces than houses.

The selectivity of the MT gyrus/ST sulcus activation could not be adequately addressed with the current data set because only one of the five subjects run in Part II showed a greater response for faces than objects in this region. (For this subject, S2, the ST/MT gyrus region activated for faces vs objects was activated only weakly if at all in the comparisons of intact vs scrambled faces and faces vs houses.)

Part III

Part III tested whether the activation for faces compared with objects described in Part I was attributable to (1) a differential response to animate (or human) and inanimate objects, (2) greater visual attentional recruitment by faces than objects, or (3) subordinate-level classification. Five subjects (including two who were run on Part II in a different session) were run on Parts I and III in the same session. The data were analyzed in the same way as the data from Part II: fusiform face ROIs were defined on the basis of the faces versus objects data from Part I, and these ROIs were used for the analysis of the two new tests. Each subjects' individual raw data clearly showed higher signal intensities in the face ROI during the two new face compared with nonface tests (passive three-quarter faces vs hands and 1-back faces vs hands). The 3-way ANOVA across subjects on the mean signal intensity in each subject's face ROI for each of the stimulus epochs (face/control × epoch number × test) revealed a significant main effect of higher signal intensity for face than nonface stimuli

$(F_{(1,4)} = 35.2; \; p < 0.005)$; no other main effects or interactions reached significance. Separate analyses of the mean signal intensity during face versus control stimulus epochs confirmed that each of the three tests independently reached significance ($p < 0.001$ for faces vs objects, $p < 0.02$ for faces vs hands passive, and $p < 0.005$ for faces 1-back vs hands 1-back).

As in Part II, we also calculated the percentage signal change in each subject's prespecified face ROI. The averages across the five subjects' time courses of percentage signal change are plotted in Figure 18.4, where the data clearly show higher peaks during face than nonface epochs. The face selectivity ratios (derived in the same way described in Part II) varied from 2.7 for faces versus objects to 4.5 for faces versus hands 1-back (Table 18.2), once again indicating a high degree of selectivity for faces. Thus, the data from Part III indicate that the same region in the fusiform gyrus that responds more strongly to faces than objects also responds more strongly during passive viewing of three-quarter views of faces than hands, and more strongly during the 1-back matching task on faces than hands.

We have only partial information about the selectivity of the MT gyrus/ST sulcus activation in the two comparisons of Part III, because only two of the five subjects run in Part III contained activations in the MT/ST region for faces versus objects (S10 and S11). Both of these subjects showed significantly greater signal intensities in this region for faces versus hands, suggesting that it is at least partially selective for faces; however, this result will have to be replicated in future subjects to be considered solid.

Although a technical limitation prevented recording of the behavioral responses collected from subjects in the scanner during the 1-back task, the experimenters were able to verify that the subject was performing the task by monitoring both the subject's responses and the stimulus on-line during the scan. All subjects performed both tasks well above chance. Subsequent behavioral measurements on different subjects ($n = 12$)

in similar viewing conditions in the lab found similar performance in the two tasks (86% correct for hands and 92% correct for faces, corrected for guessing), although all subjects reported greater difficulty with the hands task than the faces task. Thus the hands task was at least as difficult as the faces task, and general attentional mechanisms should be at least as actively engaged by the hands task as the faces task.

Discussion

This study found a region in the fusiform gyrus in 12 of 15 subjects that responded significantly more strongly during passive viewing of face than object stimuli. This region was identified within individual subjects and used as a specific ROI within which further tests of face selectivity were conducted. One test showed that the face ROIs in each of five subjects responded more strongly during passive viewing of intact two-tone faces than scrambled versions of the same faces, ruling out luminance differences as accounting for the face activation. In a second test, the average percentage signal increase (from the fixation baseline) across the five subjects' face ROIs was more than six times greater during passive viewing of faces than during passive viewing of houses, indicating a high degree of stimulus selectivity and demonstrating that the face ROI does not simply respond whenever any set of different exemplars of the same category are presented. In a third test, the face ROIs in a new set of five subjects responded more strongly during passive viewing of three-quarter-view faces with hair concealed than during viewing of photographs of human hands, indicating that (1) this region does not simply respond to any animal or human images or body parts and (2) it generalizes to respond to images of faces taken from a different viewpoint that differed considerably in their low-level visual features from the original set of face images. Finally, in a fourth test, each of the five subjects' face ROIs were shown to respond more strongly during a consecutive matching task carried out on the three-quarter-view faces than during the same matching task on the hand stimuli. Because both tasks required subordinate-level categorization, and the hand task was at least as difficult as the face task, the greater activation of the face ROIs during the face task indicates that the activity of this region does not reflect general processes associated either with visual attention or with subordinate-level classification of any class of stimuli (contrary to suggestions by Gauthier et al., 1996). The elimination of these main alternative hypotheses provides compelling evidence that the fusiform face area described in this study, which we will call area "FF," is specifically involved in the perception of faces.

Area FF responds to a wide variety of face stimuli, including front-view gray-scale photographs of faces, two-tone versions of the same faces, and three-quarter-view gray-scale faces with hair concealed. Although it is possible that some low-level visual feature present in each of these stimuli can account for the activation observed, this seems unlikely given the diversity of faces and nonface control stimuli used in the present study. Furthermore, another study in our lab (E. Wojciulik, N. Kanwisher, and J. Driver, unpublished observations) has shown that area FF also responds more strongly during attention to faces than during attention to houses, even when the retinal stimulation is identical in the two cases. (The faces in that study were also smaller and were presented to the side of fixation, indicating further that area FF generalizes across the size and retinal position of the face stimuli.) We therefore conclude that area FF responds to faces in general rather than to some particular low-level feature that happens to be present in all the face but not nonface stimuli that have been tested so far. In addition, the fact that area FF responds as strongly to faces in which the external features (e.g., hair) are largely concealed under a hat suggests that area FF is more involved in face recognition proper than in "head recognition" (Sinha and Poggio, 1996).

Our use of a functional definition of area FF allowed us to assess the variability in the locus of the "same" cortical area across different individual subjects. Before considering the variability across individuals, it is important to note that our face-specific patterns of activation were highly consistent across testing sessions within a single subject. The remarkable degree of test–retest reliability can be seen in the results from four different testing sessions in subject S1 (see the brain images in Fig. 18.1a, S1 in the bottom left of Fig. 18.2, S1 in the top right of Fig. 18.2, and in Fig. 18.3a). Given the consistency of our within-subject results, it is reasonable to suppose that the variation observed across individuals primarily reflects actual individual differences.

Area FF was found in the fusiform gyrus or the immediately adjacent cortical areas in most right-handed subjects (Fig. 18.2, Table 18.1). This activation locus is near those reported in previous imaging studies using face stimuli, and virtually identical in Talairach coordinates to the locus reported in one (40x, -55y, -10z for the mean of our right-hemisphere activations; 37x, -55y, -10z in Clark et al., 1996). We found a greater activation in the right than left fusiform, a finding that is in agreement with earlier imaging studies (Sergent et al., 1992; Puce et al., 1996). We suspect that our face activation is somewhat more lateralized to the right hemisphere than that seen in Courtney et al. (1997) and Puce et al. (1995, 1996), because our use of objects as comparison stimuli allowed us to effectively subtract out the contribution of general object processing to isolate face-specific processing. In contrast, if scrambled faces are used as comparison stimuli (Puce et al., 1995; Courtney et al., 1997), then regions associated with both face-specific processing and general shape analysis are revealed and a more bilateral activation is produced. (See the image in Fig. 18.3b for a bilateral activation in our own intact vs scrambled faces run.) Our results showing complete lateralization of face-specific processing in some subjects (e.g., S1) but not in others (e.g., S4) are consistent with the developing consensus from the neuropsychology literature that damage restricted to the posterior right hemisphere is often, although not always, sufficient to produce prosopagnosia (De Renzi, 1997).

In addition to the fusiform face area described above, seven subjects in the present study also showed a greater activation for faces than objects in a more superior and lateral location in the right hemisphere in the region of the middle temporal gyrus/STS (Table 18.1). Although other areas were observed to be activated by faces compared with objects in individual subjects (Table 18.1), they were not consistent across subjects.

Physiological studies in macaques have shown that neurons that respond selectively to faces (Gross et al., 1972; Desimone, 1991; Perrett et al., 1991) are located in both the inferior temporal gyrus and on the banks of the STS. Cells in inferotemporal cortex tend to be selective for individual identity, whereas cells in STS tend to be selective for facial expression (Hasselmo et al., 1989) or direction of gaze or head orientation (Perrett et al., 1991). Lesion studies have reinforced this view, with bilateral STS lesions leaving face-identity matching tasks unimpaired but producing deficits in gaze discrimination (Heywood and Cowey, 1993). Similarly, studies of human neurological patients have demonstrated double dissociations between the abilities to extract individual identity and emotional expression from faces, and between individual identity and gaze direction discrimination, suggesting that there may be two or three distinct brain areas involved in these different computations (Kurucz and Feldmar, 1979; Bruyer et al., 1983; Adolphs et al., 1996). A reasonable hypothesis is that the fusiform face area reported here for humans is the homolog of the inferotemporal region in macaques, whereas the face-selective regions in the STS of humans and macaques are homologs of each other. If so, then we would expect future studies to demonstrate that the human fusiform face area is specifically involved in the discrimination of individual identity, whereas the MT gyrus/STS area is involved in the extraction of emotional expression and/or gaze direction.

The import of our study is threefold. First, it demonstrates the existence of a region in the fusiform gyrus that is not only responsive to face stimuli (Haxby et al., 1991; Sergent et al., 1992; Puce et al., 1995, 1996) but is *selectively* activated by faces compared with various control stimuli. Second, we show how strong evidence for cortical specialization can be obtained by testing the responsiveness of the same region of cortex on many different stimulus comparisons (also see Tootell et al., 1995). Finally, the fact that special-purpose cortical machinery exists for face perception suggests that a single general and overarching theory of visual recognition may be less successful than a theory that proposes qualitatively different kinds of computations for the recognition of faces compared with other kinds of objects.

Recent behavioral and neuropsychological research has suggested that face recognition may be more "holistic" (Behrmann et al., 1992; Tanaka and Farah, 1993) or "global" (Rentschler et al., 1994) than the recognition of other classes of objects. Future functional imaging studies may clarify and test this claim, for example, by asking (1) whether area FF can be activated by inducing similarly holistic or global processing on nonface stimuli, and (2) whether the response of area FF to faces is attenuated if subjects are induced to process the faces in a more local or part-based fashion. Future studies can also evaluate whether extensive visual experience with any novel class of visual stimuli is sufficient for the development of a local region of cortex specialized for the analysis of that stimulus class, or whether cortical modules like area FF must be innately specified (Fodor, 1983).

Acknowledgments

We thank the many people who helped with this project, especially Oren Weinrib, Roy Hamilton,

Mike Vevea, Kathy O'Craven, Bruce Rosen, Roger Tootell, Ken Kwong, Lia Delgado, Ken Nakayama, Susan Bookheimer, Roger Woods, Daphne Bavelier, Janine Mendola, Patrick Ledden, Mary Foley, Jody Culham, Ewa Wojciulik, Patrick Cavanagh, Nikos Makris, Chris Moore, Bruno Laeng, Raynald Comtois, and Terry Campbell.

References

Adolphs R, Damasio H, Tranel D, Damasio AR (1996) Cortical systems for the recognition of emotion in facial expressions. J Neurosci 16:7678–7687.

Allison T, Ginter H, McCarthy G, Nobre AC, Puce A, Belger A (1994) Face recognition in human extrastriate cortex. J Neurophysiol 71:821–825.

Behrmann M, Winocur G, Moscovitch M (1992) Dissociation between mental imagery and object recognition in a brain-damaged patient. Nature 359:636–637.

Breiter HC, Etcoff NL, Whalen PJ, Kennedy WA, Rauch SL, Buckner RL, Strauss MM, Hyman SE, Rosen BR (1996) Response and habituation of the human amygdala during visual processing of facial expression. Neuron 17:875–887.

Bruce V, Doyle T, Dench N, Burton M (1991) Remembering facial configurations. Cognition 38:109–144.

Bruyer R, Laterre C, Seron X, Feyereisen P, Strypstein E, Pierrand E, Rectem D (1983) A case of prosopagnosia with some preserved covert remembrance of familiar faces. Brain Cogn 2:257–284.

Bush G, Jiang A, Talavage T, Kennedy D (1996) An automated system for localization and characterization of functional MRI activations in four dimensions. NeuroImage 3:S55.

Clark VP, Keil K, Maisog JM, Courtney S, Ungerleider LG, Haxby JV (1996) Functional magnetic resonance imaging of human visual cortex during face matching: a comparison with positron emission tomography. NeuroImage 4:1–15.

Courtney SM, Ungerleider LG, Keil K, Haxby JV (1997) Transient and sustained activity in a distributed neural system for human working memory. Nature, in press.

Damasio AR, Tranel D, Damasio H (1990) Face agnosia and the neural substrates of memory. Annu Rev Neurosci 13:89–109.

De Renzi E (1997) Prosopagnosia. In: Behavioral neurology and neuropsychology (Feinberg TE, Farah MJ, eds), pp 245–255. New York: McGraw-Hill.

Desimone R (1991) Face-selective cells in the temporal cortex of monkeys. Special issue: face perception. J Cognit Neurosci 3:1–8.

Farah MJ, Wilson KD, Drain WH, Tanaka JR (1995) The inverted face inversion effect in prosopagnosia: evidence for mandatory, face-specific perceptual mechanisms. Vision Res 35:2089–2093.

Farah MJ, Meyer MM, McMullen PA (1996) The living/nonliving dissociation is not an artifact: giving an a priori implausible hypothesis a strong test. Cognit Neuropsychol 13:137–154.

Fodor J (1983) Modularity of mind. Cambridge, MA: MIT.

Gauthier I, Behrmann M, Tarr MJ, Anderson AW, Gore J, McClelland JL (1996) Subordinate-level categorization in human inferior temporal cortex: converging evidence from neuropsychology and brain imaging. Soc Neurosci Abstr 10:11.

Gross CG, Roche-Miranda GE, Bender DB (1972) Visual properties of neurons in the inferotemporal cortex of the macaque. J Neurophysiol 35:96–111.

Hasselmo ME, Rolls ET, Baylis GC (1989) The role of expression and identity in the face-selective responses of neurons in the temporal visual cortex of the monkey. Behav Brain Res 32:203–218.

Haxby JV, Grady CL, Horwitz B, Ungerleider LG, Mishkin M, Carson RE, Herscovitch P, Schapiro MB, Rapoport SI (1991) Dissociation of spatial and object visual processing pathways in human extrastriate cortex. Proc Natl Acad Sci USA 88:1621–1625.

Haxby JV, Horwitz B, Ungerleider LG, Maisog JM, Pietrini P, Grady CL (1994) The functional organization of human extrastriate cortex: a PET-rCBF study of selective attention to faces and locations. J Neurosci 14:6336–6353.

Heywood CA, Cowey A (1993) Colour and face perception in man and monkey: the missing link. In: Functional organisation of human visual cortex (Gulyas B, Ottoson D, Roland PE, eds), pp 195–210. Oxford: Pergamon Press.

Hunt SMJ (1994) MacProbe: A Macintosh-based experimenter's work station for the cognitive sciences. Behav Res Methods Instrum Comput 26:345–351.

Kanwisher N, Chun MM, McDermott J, Ledden P (1996) Functional imaging of human visual recognition. Cognit Brain Res 5:55–67.

Kurucz J, Feldmar G (1979) Prosop-affective agnosia as a symptom of cerebral organic disease. J Am Geriatr Soc 27:91–95.

Malach R, Reppas JB, Benson RB, Kwong KK, Jiang H, Kennedy WA, Ledden PJ, Brady TJ, Rosen BR, Tootell RBH (1995) Object-related activity revealed by functional magnetic resonance imaging in human occipital cortex. Proc Nat Acad Sci USA 92:8135–8138.

Nobre AC, Allison T, McCarthy G (1994) Word recognition in the human inferior temporal lobe. Nature 372:260–263.

Ojemann JG, Ojemann GA, Lettich E (1992) Neuronal activity related to faces and matching in human right nondominant temporal cortex. Brain 115:1–13.

Perrett DI, Oram MW, Harries MH, Bevan R, Hietanen JK, Benson PJ, Thomas S (1991) Viewer-centered and object-centered coding of heads in the macaque temporal cortex. Exp Brain Res 86:159–173.

Perrett DI, Hietanen JK, Oram MW, Benson PJ (1992) Organisation and functions of cells responsive to faces in the temporal cortex. Philos Trans R Soc Lond [Biol] 335:23–30.

Puce A, Allison T, Gore JC, McCarthy G (1995) Face-sensitive regions in human extrastriate cortex studied by functional MRI. J Neurophysiol 74:1192–1199.

Puce A, Allison T, Asgari M, Gore JC, McCarthy G (1996) Differential sensitivity of human visual cortex to faces, letterstrings, and textures: a functional magnetic resonance imaging study. J Neurosci 16:5205–5215.

Rademacher J, Caviness Jr VS, Steinmetz H, Galaburda AM (1993) Topographical variation of the human primary cortices: implications for neuroimaging, brain mapping, and neurobiology. Cereb Cortex 3:313–329.

Rensink RA, O'Regan JK, Clark JJ (1997) To see or not to see: the need for attention to perceive changes in scenes. Psychol Sci, in press.

Rentschler I, Treurwein B, Landis T (1994) Dissociation of local and global processing in visual agnosia. Vision Res 34:963–971.

Rosch E, Mervis CB, Gray WD, Johnson DM, Boyes-Braem P (1976) Basic objects in natural categories. Cognit Psychol 8:382–439.

Sergent J, Ohta S, MacDonald B (1992) Functional neuroanatomy of face and object processing: a positron emission tomography study. Brain 115:15–36.

Sinha P, Poggio T (1996) I think I know that face. Nature 384:404.

Tanaka JW, Farah MJ (1993) Parts and wholes in face recognition. Q J Exp Psychol [A] 46A:225–245.

Tootell RBH, Reppas JB, Kwong KK, Malach R, Born RT, Brady TJ, Rosen BR, Belliveau JW (1995) Functional analysis of human MT and related visual cortical areas using magnetic resonance imaging. J Neurosci 15:3215–3230.

Turk M, Pentland A (1991) Eigenfaces for recognition. Special issue: face perception. J Cognit Neurosci 3:71–86.

Yin RK (1969) Looking at upside-down faces. J Exp Psychol 81:141–145.

19 Expertise for Cars and Birds Recruits Brain Areas Involved in Face Recognition

Isabel Gauthier, Pawel Skudlarski, John C. Gore, and Adam W. Anderson

Face and object recognition differ in at least two ways. First, faces are recognized at a more specific level of categorization (for example, "Adam") than most objects (for example, "chair" or "car"). Second, although we are experts with faces, we have much less experience discriminating among members of other categories. Level of categorization and expertise are relevant even for unfamiliar faces and objects. A person passed on the street may be encoded at the individual level and recognized the next day, whereas a mug may be replaced by another mug without our noticing. Processing biases for different categories depend on our experience with levels of categorization and our expertise in extracting diagnostic features.[1]

Viewing faces activates a small extrastriate region called the fusiform face area (FFA).[2–10] Neuropsychological studies suggest that the brain areas responsible for face and object processing can be dissociated.[11–14] According to one view, extrastriate cortex contains a map of visual features,[15–16] suggesting that the same region should not be recruited for processing different object categories when the relevant features differ.

On the other hand, prosopagnosia is often associated with deficits discriminating among nonface objects within categories. For example, a bird watcher became unable to identify birds,[17] whereas another patient could no longer identify car makes.[18] Thus, one hypothesis holds that prosopagnosia is a deficit in evoking a specific context from a stimulus belonging to a class of visually similar objects.[19] At least some prosopagnosic patients have difficulty with classes in which objects are both visually and semantically homogeneous.[20,21] Evidence from brain-lesion studies is still under debate;[13,22] however, additional data from brain imaging may help resolve these questions.

Several lines of research converge to suggest that level of categorization and expertise account for a large part of the activation difference between faces and objects. First, behavioral effects[23–25] once thought unique to faces have been obtained with objects, often with expert subjects.[26–29] Second, nonface objects elicit more activation in the FFA when matched to specific labels as compared to more categorical ones (for example, "ketchup bottle" versus "bottle").[3,30] Third, expertise with animal-like unfamiliar objects ("greebles") recruits the right FFA.[4] However, it remains unclear whether expertise with any homogeneous category is capable of recruiting the neural substrate of face recognition.

This experiment had three purposes. First, we tested whether long-term expertise with birds and cars would recruit face-selective areas. Second, the interaction between level of categorization and expertise was investigated. Third, we tested how these two factors depend on attention to stimulus identity. The FFA typically activates more for faces than objects, even during passive viewing.[7] This suggests that faces are processed automatically at the subordinate level. Here we asked whether this is also true for other expertise domains.

Results

We tested 11 car experts and 8 bird experts with many years of experience recognizing car models or bird species (Table 19.1). The right and left FFA and right occipital face area (OFA) were defined in passive-viewing localizer scans (see Methods). The OFA is also face selective[31] and active in greeble experts.[4] A right FFA was found in all subjects (median size, 6 voxels), a left FFA was found in 13 subjects (4 bird experts, 9 car experts; median size, 5 voxels) and a right OFA in 15 subjects (7 bird experts, 8 car experts; median size, 7 voxels).

Subjects also underwent identity and location scans. Stimulus presentation was identical in

Table 19.1
Subject information and behavioral results

	Bird experts	Car experts
Mean age $\pm$ SE	34.4 $\pm$ 2.0	31 $\pm$ 2.5
Mean years experience $\pm$ SE	18 $\pm$ 3.3	20.6 $\pm$ 3.8
Behavioral data during fMRI (% correct identity $\pm$ SE; location $\pm$ SE)		
Objects	86 $\pm$ 3; 81 $\pm$ 4	93 $\pm$ 3; 88 $\pm$ 3
Faces	85 $\pm$ 3; 82 $\pm$ 3	92 $\pm$ 3; 91 $\pm$ 3
Cars	84 $\pm$ 3; 81 $\pm$ 3	92 $\pm$ 2; 91 $\pm$ 2
Birds	87 $\pm$ 3; 81 $\pm$ 4	92 $\pm$ 3; 89 $\pm$ 3
Behavioral data pre-test (d$'$ $\pm$ SE)		
Birds upright	2.53 $\pm$ 0.10	1.06 $\pm$ 0.07
Cars upright	1.41 $\pm$ 0.12	2.42 $\pm$ 0.14
Birds inverted	2.23 $\pm$ 0.20	1.01 $\pm$ 0.09
Cars inverted	0.84 $\pm$ 0.13	1.58 $\pm$ 0.20

both conditions, and subjects detected immediate (1-back) repetitions in either the identity of the picture or its location while ignoring the other dimension. Blocks of 16 grayscale faces, objects, cars or birds shown sequentially were alternated with periods of fixation (Fig. 19.1). Pilot experiments indicated that the absence of color cues did not eliminate the advantage of experts over novices. Behavioral data in the scanner was available for 16 of the 19 subjects. Performance was better in the identity than the location runs (identity performance $\pm$ s.e., 89.4 $\pm$ 2.1; location, 86.0 $\pm$ 2.3; $F_{1,14} = 9.98$, $p < 0.01$) and this effect was larger for birds and objects than for cars and faces (task $\times$ category interaction, $F_{1,14} = 5.86$, $p < 0.01$). These categories varied more in shape, making location judgments more difficult.

The percent signal changes in the three regions of interest (ROIs) were assessed using a fixation baseline. First, we describe all significant effects pooled across task, coming back to this factor later. The level of categorization effect was measured by comparing activation in novices to cars or birds versus objects. The effect of level of categorization was significant in the right FFA ($F_{1,17} = 14.36$, $p < 0.02$) and in the left FFA ($F_{1,11} = 8.76$, $p = 0.02$). This effect was marginal in the right OFA ($F_{1,13} = 3.67$, $p < 0.08$). The interaction between level and group was significant in both the right FFA ($F_{1,17} = 6.61$, $p < 0.02$) and the left FFA ($F_{1,11} = 6.47$, $p < 0.05$). Post-hoc tests ($p < 0.05$) indicated that the level effect was only significant for car experts viewing birds. It may be tempting to believe that birds activate the FFA because of their faces.[10] However, the difference between birds and cars for novices was not significant in either area ($p > 0.5$ for both), and the group effect arises from a difference in activity for common objects (larger in birders).

Inspection of Fig. 19.2 suggests baseline differences between categories and between groups. First, responses to birds were larger than to cars in FFAs of both hemispheres (right, $F_{1,17} = 11.13$, $p < 0.05$; left, $F_{1,11} = 5.47$, $p < 0.05$). Again, although animal faces may activate this area more than objects,[10] here we found no difference between cars and birds in novices. Bird experts showed more activation for any object category than car experts, although not significantly in any ROI. Given these baseline trends, it was crucial to measure the effect of expertise by comparing activation for cars and birds in the two groups. The predicted expertise effect was significant (a group $\times$ category interaction) in the right FFA (Figs. 19.2 and 19.3; $F_{1,17} = 19.22$, $p < 0.0005$) and in the right OFA ($F_{1,13} = 4.86$, $p < 0.05$). There was no expertise effect in the left FFA ($F < 1$).

One important question is whether this expertise effect arises from the same area as face expertise. To test this, we used a set of criteria (see Methods) based on a definition of face cells in neurophysiology.[32] This defines a smaller FFA

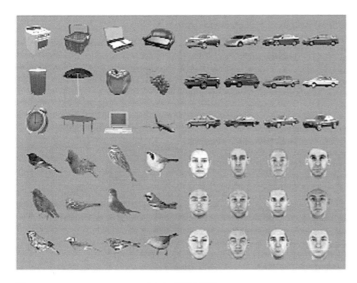

a

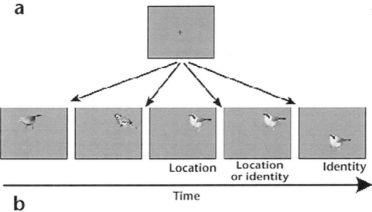

b

Figure 19.1
Examples of stimuli and tasks for the fMRI protocol. (a) Images (256 × 256 pixels in size, 256 grays) from each of four categories (Caucasian faces without hair, passerine birds from New England, car models for the years 1995 and 1998, and various familiar objects) were used in the fMRI study. (b) Example of stimulus presentation during the fMRI runs. Subjects made 1-back repetition judgments regarding either location or identity (an identity repeat would show identical images, although sometimes in different locations—see Methods for details).

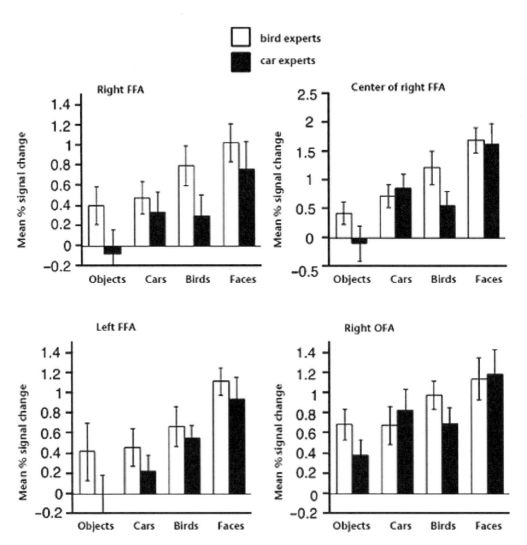

Figure 19.2
Mean percent signal change for each object category in the two expert groups in three face-specific ROIs and in the center of the right FFA. The average percent signal increase from fixation for each object category in the different ROIs was averaged across subjects in each ROI for each expert group. Error bars indicate standard error of the mean. The Talairach coordinates for the center of each ROI $\pm$ standard error were right FFA, $x = 38 \pm 2$, $y = -50 \pm 1$, $z = -7 \pm 1$; left FFA, $x = -38 \pm 2$, $y = -56 \pm 4$, $z = -6 \pm 2$; right OFA, $x = 40 \pm 2$, $y = -75 \pm 3$, $z = -3 \pm 1$.

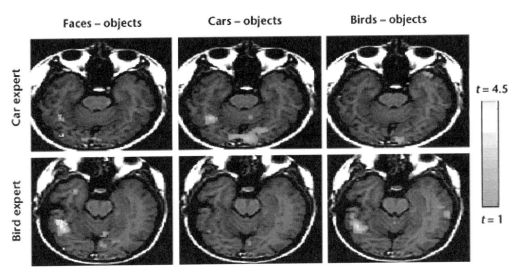

Figure 19.3
The right FFA shows an expertise effect for birds and cars. One axial oblique slice through the FFA for one expert for each category shows the *t*-maps obtained when comparing the activation for faces, cars and birds with the activation elicited by objects during the location 1-back runs. The voxels marked by white crosses indicate the right FFA and OFA as defined in the passive viewing runs for these two subjects. (In this car expert, the OFA was actually in the slice immediately below and is shown on the same slice as the FFA only to illustrate its in-plane location.) Note that the center of the right FFA may be slightly different depending on the task (here passive viewing versus 1-back location) and that its size varies between subjects.

than any other definition to our knowledge (also eliminating the majority of OFA and left FFA ROIs, which were not analyzed further). We call this ROI the center of the FFA (median = 3 voxels), in which each voxel is highly face selective. Even in this ROI, both the level of categorization effect in novices ($F_{1,17} = 6.37$, $p < 0.02$) and the expertise effect were present ($F_{1,17} = 10.25$, $p < 0.006$; Fig. 19.3). These effects also held when analyzed in a subset of subjects whose FFA could be defined using described criteria[6,10] (see supplemental material at http://neurosci. nature.com/web_specials/). To assess the magnitude of the expertise effect, we plotted the main effects and interaction separately for the center of the right FFA[33] (Fig. 19.4). The statistically significant expertise effect contributed a differ-

ence of about 0.4% signal change between groups, whereas the group and category main effects contributed about 0.3% and 0.1% signal change, respectively, and were not significant ($F < 1$ for both). Corresponding values in the larger right FFA ROI were 0.2, 0.1 and 0.3, respectively. The expertise effect alone accounted for 32% of the difference between faces and objects in the right FFA defined at $t = 2$ and for 36% in the center of the right FFA.

We measured the center of mass of the signal change for activated voxels for birds, cars and faces (relative to objects). This was done in a ROI of 25×25 voxels (each 1.3 mm by 1.7 mm, $y \times x$ over 3 slices in Talairach space, centered on the right and left FFA from the localizer). The only significant differences for cars or birds

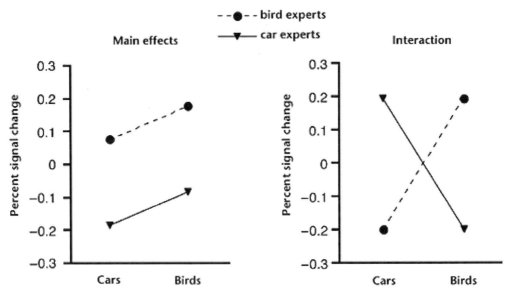

Figure 19.4
Main effects with grand mean and interaction partialed out and interaction effect with the grand mean and main effects partialed out, in the center of the right FFA. Each observed condition mean can be constructed by adding the value for the main effects and the interaction effect to the grand mean (in this case, 0.845).

relative to faces were obtained in novice subjects (see Table 19.2). Center of mass for expert categories was indistinguishable from that obtained for faces (even using a lenient statistical test). We also compared the activation distribution in the right FFA for the three categories by averaging nonspatially smoothed individual maps, centered on the most face-selective voxel in the localizer. This is shown in a 5×5 voxel (each $3.125 \times 3.125 \times 7$ mm^3) window in Fig. 19.5. Experts (and to some extent birders viewing cars) showed a distribution of activation for birds and cars that was relatively limited to the localizer peak of the FFA. The mean percent signal change in the center voxel was compared to that in the 8 voxels surrounding it, and to the surrounding "outside" 16 voxels. An ANOVA (3 regions × 3 categories × 2 groups) revealed a main effect of region ($F_{2,22} = 7.18$, $p < 0.004$) with more activ-

ity in the center than in both outer regions. Because of greater activity for faces than birds and cars only in the center, the category × region interaction was marginal ($F_{4,44} = 2.18$, $p < 0.09$), consistent with our other analyses. Crucially, there was no significant difference among the three categories in activity for each of the two surrounding regions, suggesting that activation is as focused for objects as for faces.

As a more direct way of assessing the expertise effect, we measured the correlation between behavioral performance outside the scanner with the signal change in the three ROIs during the location and identity tasks. In the behavioral test, subjects judged whether sequentially presented pairs of birds and cars (upright or inverted) belonged to the same species or car model. The expertise effect was significant (group × category interaction; Table 19.1), bird experts being more

Table 19.2
Center of mass coordinates in the middle temporal lobe for category-selective areas, given in Talairach coordinates

	Left hemisphere			Right hemisphere		
	x	y	z	x	y	z
Bird experts						
Faces	−31.3	−49.8	−7.6	40.8	−48.2	−8.5
Cars	−29.3*	−47.3*	−7.8	39.9	−47.5	−9.0
Birds	−30.8	−49.6	−7.9	40.3	−48.1	−8.3
Car experts						
Faces	−29.0	−48.7	−9.1	38.6	−48.1	−9.1
Cars	−28.9	−49.2	−8.1	38.3	−47.2	−8.5
Birds	−30.5*	−49.8	−7.0	41.2*	−47.8	−8.9

*Value significantly different from the coordinate for faces in the same expert group according to a least significant difference test; $p < 0.05$.

sensitive for birds than cars and *vice versa* for car experts ($F_{1,17} = 59.40$, $p < 0.0001$). The effect of orientation and interaction of category with orientation were significant, with the inversion effect stronger for cars than for birds ($F_{1,17} = 14.27$, $p < 0.002$). Both groups were poorer with inverted than upright cars, whereas the inversion effect for birds only approached statistical significance in birders ($p = 0.068$).

A group analysis was performed on the fMRI data during all 1-back tasks with cars and birds (see Methods). This less precise analysis allowed us to seek other regions showing an expertise effect regardless of the category, beyond the ones we could define functionally. This showed an area in right ventral temporal cortex that was more activated in experts than novices (Fig. 19.6). In addition to this stream of activation, going from the right OFA toward the right FFA, a bilateral region in the parahippocampal gyrus was also more active in experts. This area overlaps with the parahippocampal place area (PPA),[34] functionally defined as the region responding more to scenes than objects. (It also responds more to objects than faces.) Further work will be required to identify the role of this area in perceptual expertise. The only region more activated in nov-

ices than experts was a small bilateral area of the lateral occipital gyrus, superior to the OFA. This area has been found to activate more for letter strings than faces,[35] and its selective activation for novices could reflect a switch from a featural to a more configural strategy.

In each ROI, we correlated the percent signal change for birds minus cars with relative expertise, the difference in sensitivity (d') for upright birds minus upright cars. As the 2 groups combined would produce a bimodal distribution, the correlation coefficients were calculated for each group separately using our largest homogeneous sample (the 12 subjects scanned with axial slices). For both groups, relative expertise was positively correlated with relative percent signal change for birds versus cars in the right FFA and only for the location task (car experts, $r = 0.75$; bird experts, $r = 0.82$; $p < 0.05$ for both; Fig. 19.7).

We also considered task effects beyond that found in the correlation analyses. The only ROI showing a significant influence of task was the right FFA, where this factor interacted with level of categorization ($F_{1,17} = 6.58$, $p < 0.02$): the subordinate-level advantage was larger when novices attended to the identity than to the location of the stimuli. In prior studies,[6,10] the effect

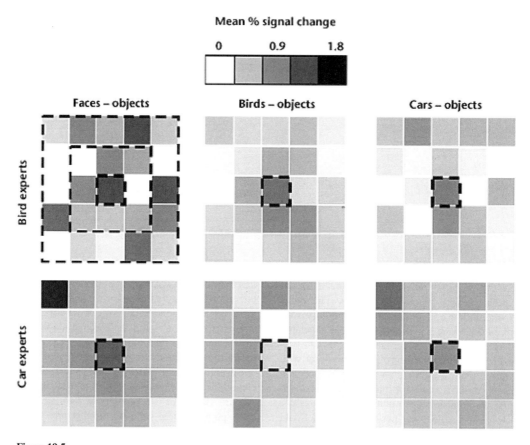

Figure 19.5
Spatial distribution of percent signal change for faces, birds and cars (relative to an objects baseline) in a 5 × 5 voxel window in the right FFA, centered on the most strongly activated voxel in the localizer. Dashed lines indicate the three regions within which activation was averaged for analyses. Note that the highest activation during experimental runs for faces may not be identical to the highest peak in the localizer (consider car experts in the faces—objects condition).

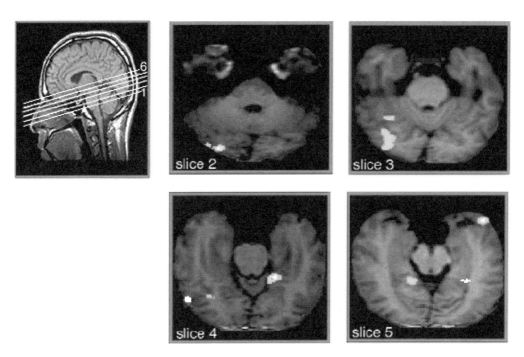

Figure 19.6
Expertise effect in the temporal cortex. The *t*-maps for all subjects with axial slices (14) were transformed into a common standard space. Voxels showing a significant expertise effect across subjects (*P* < 0.01) are displayed on the transformed anatomical images for slices 2–5 for a single subject. The red to yellow voxels were more active for experts than novices across the identity and location tasks, whereas the blue voxels were more active for novices. The right hemisphere is shown on the left. The FFA is typically found in slice three.

of task in the FFA was small (1-back identity versus passive viewing; but see ref. 36). We also found no effect of task on the advantage of faces over objects in the right FFA (*p* > 0.28), nor on the expertise effect. Expertise may influence how objects are automatically processed, an idea that we come back to in our discussion.

Discussion

Previous studies suggest that level of categorization and expertise contribute to the specialization of the FFA. The present results show how their contributions add up to account for a con-

siderable part of the difference typically found between objects and faces.

In our experiment, experts would know more names for the birds or cars than novices would. However, naming is not likely to account for the effects in the FFA because unfamiliar faces activated this area the most, whereas common objects that are easily named elicited the least activation. In addition, expertise effects for novel objects can be obtained in the FFA for unfamiliar exemplars of a trained category.[4]

Why would faces recruit the FFA more than expert recognition of objects? There are many possibilities. First, the FFA may be dedicated to

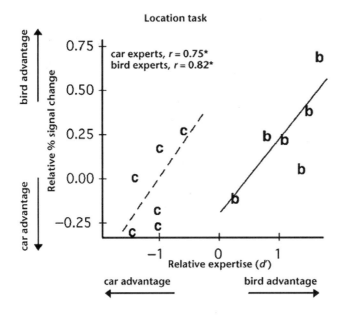

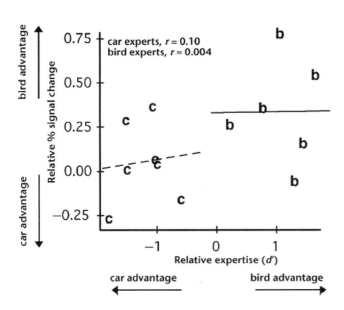

face recognition (innately or through experience), although it may mediate the processing of other objects to some extent. At the least, our study demonstrates that an innate bias is unnecessary for objects to recruit this area with expertise. Second, we cannot claim to have equated objects with faces on level of categorization and expertise.[22] The faces may constitute a more visually homogeneous set than our bird or car images. Faces are recognized as individual exemplars, whereas even experts mainly recognize cars and birds at the model/species level. Although our subjects had years of experience with cars or birds, they still had been practicing face recognition for many more years. Thus, face recognition being in a sense "more subordinate" and relying on "greater expertise" may be what make it seem "special," leaving little contribution for a component of object category *per se*. Additionally, categorization level and expertise may be only two of several factors that determine the specialization of this area. (Other factors may include symmetry, properties of associated semantic knowledge, number of exemplars, value to the perceiver.)[37]

The effect obtained in the right OFA suggests that expertise may be responsible for specialization of a large part of the face recognition system (at least in the right hemisphere). In the left FFA, we found an effect of level of categorization, with no detectable contribution of expertise. Whereas subordinate-level processing may recruit both hemispheres, here visual expert recognition of homogeneous categories seems to be mainly a right hemisphere process.

Our most striking result may be a very strong correlation between a behavioral test of object expertise and the relative activation in the right FFA for birds and cars. It is remarkable that the

expertise of a subject was so accurately predicted from the activation in a small part (six voxels) of the brain, especially as the behavioral and fMRI experiments shared neither a common task nor stimulus set. In addition, this analysis suggests that activation of the right FFA was more directly correlated with expert performance than the right OFA.

There seems to be an important interaction between automaticity of processing at the subordinate level and expertise. It is argued that the preference of the FFA for faces does not depend on the task[6,10] (but see ref. 35), a claim also supported by our results. However, we found an interaction between level of categorization and task for novices, indicating that, for most people, simply seeing an object among similar exemplars may not prompt complete subordinate-level processing. Automatic subordinate-level processing for experts could also explain a surprising finding: the correlation between behavior and activation in the right FFA was significant only when subjects attended to the location of the objects. During the identity task, subjects had to perform subordinate-level recognition with both categories, regardless of expertise. Novices may then use a featural strategy, whereas experts may use a more configural strategy.[26–28] Perhaps only configural processing is a good predictor of behavioral expertise. In contrast, during the location task novices may not access the subordinate level, whereas experts did so automatically.

Birds and cars differ in many aspects. (Birds are small animals with movable parts, covered with feathers that have specific markings; cars are large man-made objects made of metal and typically uniform in texture.) Combined with a previous study showing an expertise effect in the FFA with "greebles,"[4] our results suggest very

Figure 19.7
Relationship between a behavioral measure of expertise and activation in the right FFA. Relative expertise is the sensitivity (d') for bird minus car matching. The dashed and full lines respectively indicate the best linear fits for car and bird experts. Significant correlation coefficients are marked with an asterisk ($p < 0.05$).

few constraints on the structure of the objects for which expertise can recruit this small area. This is important for any theory of visual representation in the ventral pathway, because it suggests that responses of neurons in extrastriate cortex may not be organized according to the visual features that they detect;[15,16] rather, their functional organization may depend on the different processes important for object recognition. For instance, some areas may be more suited for featural processing, whereas other areas may support configural and holistic processing, hallmarks of subordinate-level expertise. Our results suggest that expert subordinate-level recognition for any category may be mediated in the same regions, either by virtue of activating common cells or through selectively activating different populations that are intermingled. Other techniques, such as single-cell recording, will be necessary to distinguish between these two alternatives.

Methods

Subjects

Subjects, all male, included 11 car experts and 8 bird experts. Informed consent was obtained from each subject, and the study was approved by the Human Investigation Committee at the School of Medicine, Yale University. Eight subjects were left handed. Handedness did not correlate with any effect reported here.

Stimuli

One hundred and seventy six images each of passerine birds and cars were obtained from public sources on the World Wide Web. Images were converted to 8-bit grayscale 256×256-pixel format, and objects were isolated and placed on a 50% gray background. Objects were selected to be familiar to our expert population. For each category, 112 images were used in the behavioral

test, whereas the remaining 64 objects from each category were used for experimental scans. Faces without hair ($n = 64$, scanned in a 3-D laser scanner, courtesy of Niko Troje and Heinrich Bülthoff, Max Planck Institute, Tübingen, Germany) and 64 images of non-living familiar objects were prepared in the same way as the cars and birds and also used in experimental scans. Localizer scans used 90 grayscale photographs of faces and 90 pictures of familiar objects.

Behavioral Task

Each subject performed 10 blocks of 56 sequential matching trials, alternating between blocks showing birds or cars. There were four conditions (upright and inverted cars and birds). Each trial showed two images from the same category and orientation. Upright and inverted trials were randomly intermixed. On each trial, a fixation cross appeared for 500 ms, followed by stimulus 1 for 1000 ms and a pattern mask for 500 ms before stimulus 2 appeared and remained on the screen until a response was made. Subjects judged whether the two images showed birds from the same species or whether cars were from the same model but different years (mostly 1995 versus 1998). No difference was found in mean sensitivity between categories for novices. However, responses to cars were slower than responses to birds for all subjects (RTs for hits with cars, 1138 ms; birds, 1046 ms; $p < 0.05$, suggesting that the cars were more difficult).

fMRI Task

Experimental scans consisted of three runs of a one-back location task alternated with three runs of a one-back identity task. The only difference between identity and location runs was instructions to detect immediate repetitions in either location or identity (Fig. 19.1). Each run lasted 5 min, 36 s and consisted of 16 epochs (16 s each) with 5 fixation periods (16 s each) interleaved at regular intervals. During each epoch, 16 objects appeared, each shown for 725 ms followed by a 275 ms blank. Objects (each $12° \times 12°$) appeared in one of 8 locations within an overall area subtending $18° \times 18°$ of visual angle. The order of the four categories was counterbalanced across runs.

ROI Selection

Regions of interests were functionally defined using two localizer scans, which included 16 epochs (16 s each) of passive viewing of faces or common objects centered on the screen (25 pictures per epoch). Each run began with 16 s of fixation, and an 8-s fixation period was included after every 2 passive viewing epochs. The right and left FFA and right OFA were defined as contiguous voxels activated at an arbitrary threshold of $t = 2$ in the middle fusiform gyri (c–d, F–G, 9–10 in Talairach space), and the same threshold was applied in the right ventral occipital lobe (c–d, H–I, 9–10) for the right OFA. The raw data were noisier than when using a higher field scanner and a surface coil[6,10] so the same level of significance for ROI definitions could not be applied. However, the magnitude and spatial extent of the effect for a given functional area should be similar regardless of statistical power, and we used a criterion leading to ROIs comparable in size to those in published studies.[6,10] Our FFAs show at least twice as much percent signal change for faces as for objects (each compared to fixation). To eliminate the influence of less face-selective voxels, we defined the "center of the right FFA" using criteria more stringent than in any published study. The only voxels selected were found within the cluster of contiguous voxels selected using the less stringent criterion, showed twofold greater percentage signal change for faces as objects (compared with fixation) and, in each subject, did not have less than half the percentage signal change for faces of the voxel showing the maximum signal change for faces.

fMRI Imaging Parameters and Analyses

Most (16) subjects were scanned at the Yale School of Medicine on a 1.5 T GE Signa scanner equipped with resonant gradients (Advanced NMR, Wilmington, Massachusetts) using echo-planar imaging (gradient echo single shot sequence, 168 images per slice, FOV = 40×20 cm, matrix = 128×64, NEX = 1, TR = 2000 ms, TE = 60 ms, flip angle = 60 ms). Six contiguous 7-mm-thick axial-oblique slices aligned along the longitudinal extent of the fusiform gyrus covered most of the temporal lobe. Some subjects (two car experts and one bird expert) were scanned using coronal-oblique slices. Three more subjects (two car experts and 1 bird expert, I. G. et al., *Soc. Neurosci. Abstr.* 25, 212.9, 1999) were scanned using coronal slices on the 3 T GE scanner at the MGH-NMR Center in Charlestown, Massachusetts. In this case, a custom bilateral surface coil was used to collect 168 images per slice in 12 near-coronal slices, 6 mm-thick. The imaging parameters were TR = 2000 ms, TE = 70 ms, flip angle = 90°, 180 degrees and offset = 25 ms.

Before statistical analysis, images from the 1.5 T scanner were motion corrected for three translation directions and the three possible rotations using SPM-96 software (Wellcome Department of Cognitive Neurology, London, UK). On the 3 T scanner, a bite bar was used to minimize head motion. Maps of t-values and percent signal change, both corrected for a linear drift in the signal,[38] were created. Maps were spatially smoothed using a Gaussian filter with a full-width half-maximum value of two voxels, except for analyses in the center of the right FFA, where regions of interests were very small and no smoothing was performed.

In group composite maps, the percent signal change relative to fixation baseline for both birds and cars was multiplied with contrast weights for each subject (1 and −1 for bird experts and −1 and 1 for car experts). Under the null hypothesis of no expertise effect, the expected value for this contrast was equal to zero. We used a randomization test to asses the statistical significance of percent signal changes. A population distribution for each voxel was generated by calculating randomized mean values (1000 times) of the contrast in which randomly chosen subsets of half the subjects got reversed weights. The observed contrast, calculated without sign reversal, was assigned a p value or proportion of times that the observed contrast was more extreme than the randomized contrast. To show the anatomy clearly, the p values were overlaid on the normalized anatomical images for a single subject (threshold at $p < 0.01$; Fig. 19.6).

Acknowledgements

We thank Nancy Kanwisher and René Marois for discussions and Jill Moylan, Terry Hickey and Hedy Sarofin for technical assistance. This work was supported by NINDS grant NS33332 to J.C.G. and NIMH grant 56037 to N. Kanwisher. I.G. was supported by NSERC.

References

1. Archambault, A., O'Donnell, C. & Schyns, P. G. Blind to object changes: When learning the same object at different levels of categorization modifies its perception. *Psychol. Sci.* 10, 249–255 (1999).

2. Allison, T. et al. Face recognition in human extrastriate cortex. *J. Neurophysiol.* 71, 821–825 (1994).

3. Gauthier, I., Tarr, M. J., Moylan, J., Anderson, A. W. & Gore, J. C. The functionally-defined "face area" is engaged by subordinate-level recognition. *Cognit. Neuropsychol.* (in press).

4. Gauthier, I., Tarr, M. J., Anderson, A. W., Skudlarski, P. & Gore, J. C. Activation of the middle fusiform "face area" increases with expertise in recognizing novel objects. *Nat. Neurosci.* 2, 568–573 (1999).

5. Haxby, J. V. et al. The functional organization of human extrastriate cortex: A PET-RCBF study of selective attention to faces and locations. *J. Neurosci.* 14, 6336–6353 (1994).

6. Kanwisher, N., McDermott, J. & Chun, M. M. The fusiform face area: A module in human extrastriate cortex specialized for face perception. *J. Neurosci.* 17, 4302–4311 (1997).

7. McCarthy, G., Puce, A., Gore, J. C. & Allison, T. Face-specific processing in the human fusiform gyrus. *J. Cogn. Neurosci.* 9, 605–610 (1997).

8. Puce, A., Allison, T., Asgari, M., Gore, J. C. & McCarthy, G. Face-sensitive regions in extrastriate cortex studied by functional MRI. *Neurophysiology* 74, 1192–1199 (1996).

9. Sergent, J., Otha, S. & MacDonald, B. Functional neuroanatomy of face and object processing. *Brain,* 115, 15–36 (1992).

10. Kanwisher, N., Stanley, D. & Harris, A. The fusiform face area is selective for faces not animals. *Neuroreport* 10, 183–187 (1999).

11. Sergent, J. & Signoret, J. L. Varieties of functional deficits in prosopagnosia. *Cereb. Cortex* 2, 375–388 (1992).

12. McNeil, J. E. & Warrington, E. K. Prosopagnosia: A face-specific disorder. *Q. J. Exp. Psychol. A* 46, 1–10 (1993).

13. Moscovitch, M., Winocur, G. & Behrmann, M. What is special in face recognition? Nineteen experiments on a person with visual object agnosia and dyslexia but normal face recognition. *J. Cogn. Neurosci.* 9, 555–604 (1997).

14. Assal, G., Favre, C. & Anderes, J. P. Non-reconnaissance d'animaux familiers chez un paysan. *Rev. Neurol.* 140, 580–584 (1984).

15. Ishai, A., Ungerleider, L. G., Martin, A., Schouten, J. L. & Haxby, J. Distributed representation of objects in the human ventral visual pathway. *Proc. Natl. Acad. Sci. USA* 96, 9379–9384 (1999).

16. Tanaka, K. Inferotemporal cortex and object vision. *Annu. Rev. Neurosci.* 19, 109–139 (1996).

17. Bornstein, B. in *Problems of Dynamic Neurology* (ed. Halpern, L.) 283–318 (Hadassah Medical Organization, Jerusalem, 1963).

18. Lhermitte, J., Chain, F., Escouroole, R. Ducarne, B. & Pillon, B. Étude anatomo-clinique d'un cas de prosopagnosie. *Rev. Neurol.* (*Paris*) 126, 329–346 (1972).

19. Damasio, A. R. & Damasio, H. & Van Hoesen, G. W. Prosopagnosia: anatomic basis and behavioral mechanisms. *Neurology* 32, 331–341 (1982).

20. Dixon, M. J., Bub, D. N. & Arguin, M. Semantic and visual determinants of face recognition in a prosopagnosic patient. *J. Cogn. Neurosci.* 10, 362–376 (1998).

21. Riddoch, J. M. & Humphreys, G. W. Visual processing in optic aphasia: A case of semantic access agnosia. *Cognit. Neuropsychol.* 4, 131–186 (1987).

22. Gauthier, I., Behrmann, M. & Tarr, M. J. Can face recognition really be dissociated from object recognition? *J. Cogn. Neurosci.* 11, 349–370 (1999).

23. Yin, R. K. Looking at upside-down faces. *J. Exp. Psychol.* 81, 141–145 (1969).

24. Tanaka, J. W. & Farah, M. J. Parts and wholes in face recognition. *Q. J. Exp. Psychol. A* 46, 225–245 (1993).

25. Farah, M. J., Wilson, K. D., Drain, H. M. & Tanaka, J. W. The inverted face inversion effect in prosopagnosia: Evidence for mandatory, face-specific perceptual mechanisms. *Neuropsychologia* 33, 661–674 (1995).

26. Diamond, R. & Carey, S. Why faces are and are not special: An effect of expertise. *J. Exp. Psychol. Gen.* 115, 107–117 (1986).

27. Gauthier, I. & Tarr, M. J. Becoming a "Greeble" expert: Exploring the face recognition mechanisms. *Vision Res.* 37, 1673–1682 (1997).

28. Gauthier, I., Williams, P., Tarr, M. J. & Tanaka, J. W. Training "Greeble" experts: A framework for studying expert object recognition processes. *Vision Res.* 38, 2401–2428 (1998).

29. deGelder, B., Bachoud-Lévi, A.-C. & Degos, J.-D. Inversion superiority in visual agnosia may be common to a variety of orientation-polarised objects besides faces. *Vision Res.* 38, 2855–2861 (1998).

30. Gauthier, I., Anderson, A. W., Tarr, M. J., Skudlarski, P. & Gore, J. C. Levels of categorization in visual object recognition studied with functional MRI. *Curr. Biol.* 7, 645–651 (1997).

31. Halgren, E., Dale, A. M., Sereno, M. I., Tootell, R. B., Marinkovic, K. & Rosen, B. R. Location of human face-selective cortex with respect to retinotopic areas. *Hum. Brain Mapp.* 7, 29–37 (1999).

32. Rolls, E. T. & Baylis, G. C. Size and contrast have only small effects on the response to faces of neurons in the cortex of the superior temporal sulcus of the monkey. *Exp. Brain Res.* 65, 38–48 (1986).

33. Rosnow, R. L. & Rosenthal, R. "Some things you learn aren't so": Cohen's paradox, Asch's Paradigm, and the interpretation of interaction. *Psychol. Sci.* 6, 3–9 (1995).

34. Epstein, R., Harris, A., Stanley, D. & Kanwisher, N. The parahippocampal place area: Recognition, navigation, or encoding? *Neuron* 23, 115–125 (1999).

35. Puce, A., Allison, T., Asgari, M., Gore, J. C. & McCarthy, G. Differential sensitivity of human visual cortex to faces, letterstrings, and textures: A functional magnetic resonance imaging study, *J. Neurosci.* 16, 5205–5215 (1996).

36. Wojciulik, E., Kanwisher, N. & Driver, J. Modulation of activity in the fusiform face area by covert attention: an fMRI study. *J. Neurophysiol.* 79, 1574–1578 (1998).

37. Tranel, D., Logan, C. G., Frank, R. J. & Damasio, A. R. Explaining category-related effects in the retrieval of conceptual and lexical knowledge for concrete entities: operationalization and analysis of factors. *Neuropsychologia* 35, 1329–1339 (1997).

38. Skudlarski, P., Constable, R. T. & Gore, J. C. ROC analysis of statistical methods used in functional MRI: Individual subjects. *Neuroimage* 9, 311–329 (1999).

Voice-Selective Areas in Human Auditory Cortex

Pascal Belin, Robert J. Zatorre, Philippe Lafaille, Pierre Ahad, and Bruce Pike

The human voice contains in its acoustic structure a wealth of information on the speaker's identity and emotional state which we perceive with remarkable ease and accuracy.[1-3] Although the perception of speaker-related features of voice plays a major role in human communication, little is known about its neural basis.[4-7] Here we show, using functional magnetic resonance imaging in human volunteers, that voice-selective regions can be found bilaterally along the upper bank of the superior temporal sulcus (STS). These regions showed greater neuronal activity when subjects listened passively to vocal sounds, whether speech or non-speech, than to non-vocal environmental sounds. Central STS regions also displayed a high degree of selectivity by responding significantly more to vocal sounds than to matched control stimuli, including scrambled voices and amplitude-modulated noise. Moreover, their response to stimuli degraded by frequency filtering paralleled the subjects' behavioural performance in voice-perception tasks that used these stimuli. The voice-selective areas in the STS may represent the counterpart of the face-selective areas in human visual cortex;[8,9] their existence sheds new light on the functional architecture of the human auditory cortex.

Experiment 1 sought to identify brain regions showing higher neuronal activity during auditory stimulation with voices than with non-vocal sounds, using a functional magnetic resonance imaging (fMRI) paradigm adapted for auditory presentation (see Methods). Eight right-handed adults were scanned during silence and while they listened passively to stimuli from two categories (Fig. 20.1a): (1) vocal sounds produced by several speakers of different gender and age, either speech (for example, isolated words, connected speech in several languages) or non-speech (such as laughs, sighs and coughs); and (2) energy-matched, non-vocal sounds (for example, natural sounds, animal cries, mechanical sounds) from a variety of environmental sources. In all eight subjects, vocal sounds elicited significantly ($t > 5.7$, $P < 0.001$, t-test) greater activation than non-vocal sounds bilaterally in several regions of non-primary auditory cortex. The maximum of voice-sensitive activation was located along the upper bank of the central part of the STS in seven out of the eight subjects (Fig. 20.1b). Averaged in the group of subjects, voice-sensitive activity appeared stronger in the right hemisphere, and was distributed in three bilateral clusters along the STS (Fig. 20.1c): one in the anterior portion close to the temporal pole; one in the central portion approximately at the level of the anterior extension of Heschl's gyrus; and one in the STS portion posterior to Heschl's gyrus, extending dorsally and caudally to the planum temporale in the superior temporal gyrus (Table 20.1). Importantly, there were no regions of significantly greater activation for non-vocal than for vocal stimuli ($t < 4.9$, $P > 0.05$).

Experiment 1 thus demonstrated that the brain contains several regions that are sensitive to voices; yet there is no clear evidence that they are selectively activated by voices. Vocal and non-vocal stimuli in expt 1 differed in a number of low-level acoustic features, and the areas activated might have simply been responding to some acoustic component more strongly present in the vocal stimuli. We therefore performed a second experiment in the same group of subjects to determine whether we would find a selective activation pattern when comparing vocal stimuli with more carefully matched control sounds. In expt 2, vocal stimuli were contrasted to four classes of control stimuli: (1) recordings of various bells, to assess whether the same regions would be activated by presentation of exemplars of a single category, rather than voices;[8] (2) human non-vocal sounds (for example, finger snaps, handclaps), to examine the possibility that the

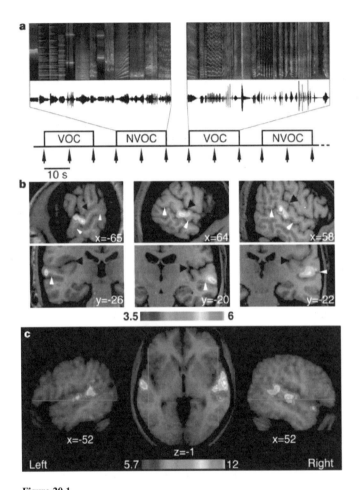

Figure 20.1

Experiment 1. (a) Experimental paradigm. Spectrograms (0–4 kHz) and amplitude waveforms of examples of auditory stimuli. Vocal (VOC) and non-vocal (NVOC) stimuli are presented in 20-s blocks with 10-s silent interblock intervals, while scanning (arrows) occurs at regular 10-s intervals. (b) Individual voice-sensitive activations. Maxima of vocal and non-vocal activation maps from three subjects are indicated in colour scale (t-value) on anatomical images in sagittal (upper panel) and coronal (lower panel) orientations (x and y: Talairach coordinates). Arrows indicate relative positions of the Sylvian fissure (black arrows) and of the superior temporal sulcus (white arrows). (c) Voice-sensitive activation in the group average. Regions with significantly ($P < 0.001$) higher response to human voices than to energy-matched non-vocal stimuli are shown in colour scale (t-value) on an axial slice of the group-average MR image (centre, Talairach coordinate $z = -1$) and on sagittal slices of each hemisphere (sides; Talairach coordinates $x = -52$ and $x = 52$). See Table 20.1 and Methods for details.

Table 20.1
Voice-sensitivity maxima

Anatomical location	Talairach coordinates			t-value		
	x	y	z	Expt 1	Expt 2	Expt 3
Right hemisphere						
STS, anterior	58	6	−10	9.2		
STS, anterior	60	−1	−4	9.6	7.9	
STS, middle	63	−13	−1	12.0	11.0	6.7
Middle temporal gyrus	52	−19	−1	9.9	7.8	9.6
STS, posterior	56	−30	6	8.0	7.2	9.7
STS, posterior	46	−44	6	9.2		
Precuneus	4	−52	30	6.0		
Left hemisphere						
Middle temporal gyrus, anterior	−60	−2	−9	6.3		
STS, middle	−62	−14	0	10.1	7.9	8.7
Planum temporale	−40	−37	13	7.1	5.9	7.2
STS, posterior	−62	−40	10	9.7		10.5

Coordinates in standard stereotaxic space[25] (mm) and approximate anatomical location are given for voice-sensitivity maxima of expt 1, as well as corresponding t-values above 5.7 ($P < 0.001$), for expts 1, 2 and 3. STS, superior temporal sulcus; x, lateral distances to anterior commissure–posterior commissure (AC–PC) line (positive = right); y, anterior–posterior distance to the anterior commissure (positive = in front of AC); z, distance above–below AC–PC line (positive = above).

above areas would respond to any sound of human origin; (3) white noise modulated with the same amplitude envelope as the vocal sounds; and (4) scrambled voices, which preserve the amplitude envelope of vocal sounds, but sound nothing like voices (see Methods and Fig. 20.2a–c). In addition, we separated vocal speech from vocal non-speech sounds. As expected, regions of significantly greater ($t > 5.7$; $P < 0.001$) response to the vocal than to the control stimuli were again distributed along the central STS and with maxima (right: $x = 62$, $y = −14$, $z = 0$; left: $x = −58$, $y = −18$, $z = −24$; see Table 20.1 for description of coordinates) located close (2–7 mm) to those from expt 1. Analysis of variance shows that neuronal response in these two nearly symmetrical locations was significantly affected by stimulus class (right: $F(4, 28) = 6.63$, $P <$

0.001; left: $F(4, 28) = 6.49$, $P < 0.001$; Fig. 20.2). Interestingly, response to both speech and non-speech vocal stimuli was significantly greater than to the pooled control stimuli (right: speech $F(1, 28) = 31$, $P < 0.001$; non-speech $F(1, 28) = 6.8$, $P < 0.02$; left: speech $F(1, 28) = 24.6$, $P < 0.001$; non-speech $F(1, 28) = 4.1$, $P = 0.05$), indicating that the voice-sensitive response was not entirely due to the presence of speech in the vocal stimuli. Experiment 2 also shows that the voice-sensitive areas do not simply respond to the presentation of various sound exemplars of a same category such as bells, or to sounds of human origin, since response to voices was stronger than to these two categories, particularly in the right hemisphere (Fig. 20.2d, e). Moreover, expt 2 suggests that frequency structure plays a more prominent role in voice-sensitive activation than does amplitude

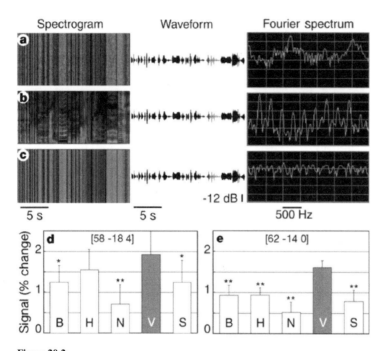

Figure 20.2
Experiment 2. (a–c) Control stimuli. Scrambled vocal sounds (a) and amplitude-modulated white noise (c) have the same amplitude waveforms as the vocal stimuli (b), but not its characteristic spectral shape. (d, e) Activation at voice-sensitivity maxima in expt 2. Bars (mean ± SE) indicate signal change for the five classes of stimuli at peak of voice selectivity in the left (d) and right (e) hemispheres. B, bells; H, human non-vocal sounds; N, amplitude-modulated noise; V, vocal sounds; S, scrambled voices; numbers in brackets: coordinates in standard stereotaxic space.[25] Difference with vocal stimuli: asterisk, $P < 0.05$; two asterisks, $P < 0.01$. Signal changes (in per cent) are measured from the signal mean during silence.

envelope: both the amplitude-modulated noise and the scrambled voice stimuli, which elicited significantly lower responses than the vocal stimuli (left, $P < 0.015$; right, $P < 0.001$), were similar to voices in amplitude envelope but not in spectral structure (Fig. 20.2a–c).

A third experiment was conducted in a different group of subjects with two goals: first, to control the spectral distribution of the vocal and non-vocal stimuli, to verify that the results of expts 1 and 2 were not attributable to any difference in this variable; second, to examine how activity of the voice-sensitive areas, as well as the

subjects' performance on voice-perception tasks, would be affected by modifying the spectral structure of the stimuli. Sets of vocal and non-vocal sounds were presented during scanning, both in their original form and after spectral filtering that removed either high or low frequencies, and equating vocal and non-vocal stimuli in spectral distribution (Fig. 20.3a). After scanning, subjects performed a vocal/non-vocal decision task and a speaker's gender-identification task that used the same filtered and unfiltered stimuli. The images corresponding to the unfiltered vocal and non-vocal sounds, averaged

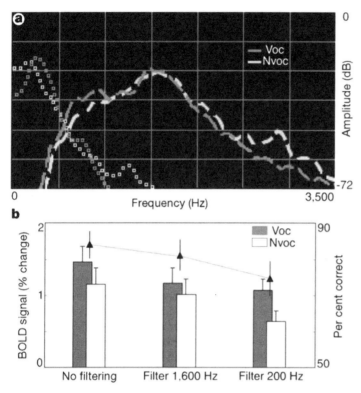

Figure 20.3
Experiment 3. (a) Frequency distribution of frequency-filtered stimuli. Dashed lines, bandpass filter centred at 1,600 Hz (400-Hz bandwidth). Open squares, bandpass filter centred at 200 Hz (50-Hz bandwidth). (b) Activation at voice-sensitivity maxima in expt 3. Bars: signal change (mean ± SE) for vocal stimuli is greater than for non-vocal stimuli even after their frequency distribution has been nearly equated by filtering. Behavioral performance: triangles show combined performance (mean ± SE in per cent correct) on the vocal/non-vocal decision task and the speaker's gender-identification task, showing a decrease with filtering that parallels that of signal change in that area.

in the group, were very similar to those from expts 1 and 2, with voice-sensitive activity concentrated along the STS (Table 20.1). Maxima of voice sensitivity were located at approximately 1 cm behind and above those of expts 1 and 2 (right: $x = 54$, $y = -13$, $z = 4$; left: $x = -60$, $y = -23$, $z = 6$). Figure 20.3 shows that the mean activity in these regions was always greater for vocal than for non-vocal stimuli ($F(1, 7) = 27.8$, $P < 0.001$), and was significantly decreased by filtering ($P > 0.05$), with no hemisphere difference ($F(1, 7) = 1.46$, $P > 0.25$). Interestingly, the signal decrease was paralleled by subjects' performances on the two voice-perception tasks (Fig. 20.3b). Experiment 3 thus replicates the findings of expts 1 and 2, and shows that the identified regions are indeed sensitive to voice: their response to the vocal sounds was greater than to the non-vocal sounds even after their frequency distribution had been equated by filtering (Fig. 20.3a). Moreover, expt 3 suggests that the voice-sensitive areas might respond selectively to combination of both the high- and low-frequency components characteristic of voices,[10] since excluding one or the other by filtering significantly reduced both neuronal activity and subjects' accuracy on the voice-perception tasks (Fig. 20.3b).

In all three experiments, peaks of voice selectivity could be found in most subjects along the upper bank of the STS, a deep, long sulcus (> 8 cm) running along the whole temporal lobe that is also found in many non-human primates. Activations along the STS are often reported in neuroimaging studies of human speech-processing,[11,12] but their exact functional role remains unclear.[13] Anatomical studies in the macaque brain have shown that the STS is composed of several distinct uni- or multimodal areas, in particular, one homogeneous region lying entirely in the upper bank of the STS (area TAa),[14] in a location homologous to those identified in the present study, receives its input exclusively from the auditory-related areas of the superior temporal gyrus. This area forms part of a hierarchically organized system extending

anteriorly and ventrally beyond the lateral belt of the auditory cortex,[15] in a cortical stream that may be specialized for extracting auditory object features.[16–18] This region is well situated to be involved in high-level analysis of complex acoustic information, such as extraction of speaker-related cues, and transmission of this information to other areas for multimodal integration and long-term memory storage.[19] Here, voice-selective regions were found in the STS on both sides, but voice selectivity was stronger in the right hemisphere in the first two experiments, in good agreement with the available clinical and psychological literature.[4–7,20] However, the same pattern was not found in expt 3, suggesting that the neural substrate of voice perception might be less clearly lateralized than in the case of speech perception.

In conclusion, these experiments provide strong evidence that the human brain contains regions that are not only sensitive to, but also strongly selective to, human voices. This finding is important for several reasons. First, it draws a strong parallel with the architecture of the visual cortex, where face-selective regions have been observed following similar experimental paradigms.[8,9] It strengthens the view that the different sensory cortices could share common principles of functional organization. Second, it could lead to new comparisons between species, by suggesting that areas sensitive to species-typical vocalizations could be found in the homologous regions in other primates. Indeed, language is probably unique to humans, and its possible evolutionary precursors are hard to define and study in other animals. In contrast, we share the ability to reliably extract affective- and identity-related cues from the species-specific vocalizations with many other species, at least of primates.[21,22] Finally, these data extend the current knowledge on the organization of the human auditory cortex, by identifying regions of the brain involved in the analysis of human voices, a class of auditory objects of high occurrence and ecological interest.

Methods

Subjects

Fourteen adult subjects (age 22–47 yr), six males and eight females, participated in this study. Six subjects performed expts 1 and 2, six subjects performed expt 3, and two subjects performed all three experiments. They were all right-handed and had normal audition.

Task and Stimuli

In all three experiments, subjects were instructed to simply close their eyes and listen to the sounds that would be presented. Auditory stimuli were delivered binaurally at a mean 88–90-dB sound-pressure level, using foam insert earplugs (Etymotic Research) and an MR-compatible pneumatic sound transmission in expts 1 and 2, and electrostatic, MR-compatible headphones (KOSS) in expt 3. Auditory stimuli consisted of sounds from a variety of sources arranged in 20-s blocks of similar overall energy (RMS) using Mitsyn (WLH) and CoolEdit Pro (Syntrillium Software Corporation). In each experiment, all blocks were composed of sounds from the same number of speakers/sources (12 in expts 1 and 3, 10 in expt 2). Vocal stimuli were obtained from 47 speakers: 7 babies, 12 adults, 23 children and 5 elderly people. In expt 1, stimuli were divided into 21 blocks of vocal sounds only, and 21 of non-vocal sounds only; vocal stimuli within the same block could be either speech (33%: words, non-words, foreign language) or non-speech (67%: laughs, sighs, various onomatopoeia). Sounds that did not involve vocal-fold vibration were excluded (for example, whistling, whispered speech). Non-vocal stimuli consisted of sounds from nature (14%: for example, wind, streams), animals (29%: cries, gallops), the modern human environment (37%: cars, telephones, aeroplanes) or musical instruments (20%: bells, harp, instru-mental orchestra). In expt 2, stimuli consisted of 40 blocks divided into 8 blocks for each of 5 classes: bells; human non-vocal sounds (snaps, footsteps); amplitude-modulated white-noise shaped by the same amplitude envelope as the vocal sounds; vocal sounds, divided in 4 blocks of speech sounds, and 4 of non-speech sounds; and scrambled vocal sounds, obtained by randomly intermixing the magnitude and phase of each Fourier component of the vocal stimuli (Fig. 20.3c). In expt 3, stimuli consisted of 80 500-ms samples of vocal and non-vocal sounds selected among stimuli from expt 1, and either presented in their original form or frequency-filtered through bandpass filters with peaks at 200 Hz (50 Hz bandwidth) or 1,600 Hz (400 Hz bandwidth). After scanning, subjects performed a two-alternative forced-choice task on pairs of stimuli, one vocal and one non-vocal but with the same filtering, where they had to decide which of the two sounds was the vocal sound, and what was the gender of the speaker who produced that sound.

MRI Acquisition

Scanning was performed on a 1.5-T Siemens Vision imager. After obtaining a high-resolution T1 anatomical scan, one series of 128 gradient-echo images (TE = 50 ms, head coil, matrix size: 64×64; voxel size: $4 \times 4 \times 5$ mm^3; 10 slices acquired in the orientation of the Sylvian fissure) of blood-oxygenation-level-dependent (BOLD) signal—an indirect index of neuronal activity—was acquired for each experiment at a 10-s interacquisition interval (21 min 40 s scanning time). The long interacquisition interval ensures low signal contamination by noise artefacts of image acquisition.[23,24] In all experiments, the 20-s auditory-stimulation blocks were presented in a randomized order with a 10-s silence inter-block interval using Media Control Function (Digivox); the beginning of each block was synchronized with scanning (see Fig. 20.1a).

Data Analysis

BOLD signal images were smoothed (6-mm Gaussian kernel), corrected for motion artefact and transformed into standard stereotaxic space[25] using in-house software.[26] Statistical maps were obtained in each individual by computing for each voxel the t-value of the Spearman correlation of the voxel's value time-series with an ideal curve representing the desired contrast.[27] Group-average statistical images were obtained by computing an omnibus test on individual t-maps using a pooled estimate of standard deviation,[28] and a threshold established at $t = 5.7$ ($P < 0.001$), based on the number of resolution elements in the acquisition volume (2,880 resels).

Acknowledgements

We thank S. Milot, P. Bermudez, M. Bouffard, C. Hurst, A. Cormier, G. Leroux, V. Petre and J. Fiedsend for assistance in data acquisition and analysis, T. Paus, A. Evans, M.-H. Grosbras, I. Lussier, J. Hillenbrand, R. Hoge, G. Legoualher, M.-C. Masure, P. Neelin, K. Worsley and Y. Samson for advice, and N. Kanwisher for seminal discussion. This work was supported by France-Télécom, MRC (Canada), McDonnel-Pew, INSERM-FRSQ and NSERC.

References

1. Doehring, D. G. & Bartholomeus, B. N. Laterality effect in voice recognition. Neuropsychologia 9, 425–430 (1971).
2. Papcun, G., Kreiman, J. & Davis, A. Long-term memory for unfamiliar voices. J. Acoust. Soc. Am. 85, 913–925 (1989).
3. Van Dommelen, W. A. Acoustic parameters in human speaker recognition. Lang. Speech 33(3), 259–272 (1990).
4. Assal, G., Aubert, C. & Buttet, J. Asymétrie cérébrale et reconnaissance de la voix. Rev. Neurol. 137, 255–268 (1981).
5. Van Lancker, D. R. & Canter, G. J. Impairment of voice and face recognition in patients with hemispheric damage. Brain Cogn. 1, 185–195 (1982).
6. Van Lancker, D. R., Kreiman, J. & Cummings, J. Voice perception deficits: Neuroanatomic correlates of phonagnosia. J. Clin. Exp. Neuropsychol. 11, 665–674 (1989).
7. Imaizumi, S. Vocal identification of speaker and emotion activates different brain regions. NeuroReport 8, 2809–2812 (1997).
8. Kanwisher, N., McDermott, J. & Chun, M. M. The fusiform face area: a module in human extrastriate cortex specialized for face perception. J. Neurosci. 17, 4302–4311 (1997).
9. McCarthy, G., Puce, A., Gore, J. C. & Allison, T. Face-specific processing in the human fusiform gyrus. J. Cogn. Neurosci. 9, 605–610 (1997).
10. Klatt, D. H. & Klatt, L. C. Analysis, synthesis, and perception of voice quality variations among female and male talkers. J. Acoust. Soc. Am. 87, 820–857 (1990).
11. Zatorre, R. J., Evans, A. C., Meyer, E. & Gjedde, A. Lateralization of phonetic and pitch discrimination in speech processing. Science 256, 846–849 (1992).
12. Dehaene, S. et al. Anatomical variability in the cortical representation of first and second language. NeuroReport 8, 3809–3815 (1997).
13. Binder, J. R., Frost, J. A. & Bellgowan, P. S. F. Superior temporal sulcus (STS) responses to speech and nonspeech auditory stimuli. J. Cogn. Neurosci. 11 (Suppl. 1), 99 (1999).
14. Seltzer, B. & Pandya, D. N. Afferent connections and architectonics of the superior temporal sulcus and surrounding cortex in the rhesus monkey. Brain Res. 149, 1–24 (1978).
15. Pandya, D. N. Anatomy of the auditory cortex. Rev. Neurol. 151, 486–494 (1995).
16. Jones, E. G., Dell'Anna, M. E., Molinari, M., Rausell, E. & Hashikawa, T. Subdivisions of macaque monkey auditory cortex revealed by calcium-binding protein immunoreactivity. J. Comp. Neurol. 362, 153–170 (1995).
17. Rauschecker, J. P. Parallel processing in the auditory cortex of primates. Audiol. Neuro-Otol. 3, 86–103 (1998).

18. Kaas, J. H., Hackett, T. A. & Tramo, M. J. Auditory processing in primate cerebral cortex. *Curr. Opin. Neurobiol.* 9, 154–170 (1999).

19. Mesulam, M. M. From sensation to cognition. *Brain* 121, 1013–1052 (1998).

20. Ellis, A. W. in *Handbook of Research on Face Processing* (eds Young, A. W. & Ellis, H. D.) 207–215 (Elsevier, Amsterdam, 1989).

21. Watzlawick, P., Beavin, J. H. & Jackson, D. D. in *A Study of Interactional Patterns, Pathologies and Paradoxes* (Norton, New York, 1967).

22. Rendall, D., Owren, M. J. & Rodman, P. S. The role of vocal trace filtering in identity cueing in rhesus monkey (Macaca mulatta) vocalizations. *J. Acoust. Soc. Am.* 103, 602–614 (1998).

23. Belin, P., Zatorre, R. J., Hoge, R., Pike, B. & Evans, A. C. Event-related fMRI of the auditory cortex. *NeuroImage* 10, 417–429 (1999).

24. Hall, D. et al. "Sparse" temporal sampling in auditory fMRI. *Hum. Brain Map* 7, 213–223 (1999).

25. Talairach, J. & Tournoux, P. *Co-Planar Stereotaxic Atlas of the Human Brain* (Thieme, New York, 1988).

26. Collins, D. L., Neelin, P., Peters, T. M. & Evans, A. C. Automatic 3D intersubject registration of MR volumetric data in standardized Talairach space. *J. Comput. Assist. Tomogr.* 18, 192–205 (1994).

27. Turner, R. & Jezzard, P. in *Functional Neuroimaging Technical Foundations* (eds Thatcher, R. W., Hallett, M., Zeffiro, T., John, E. R. & Huerta, M.) 69–78 (Academic, San Diego, 1994).

28. Worsley, K. J., Evans, A. C., Marrett, S. & Neelin, P. A three-dimensional statistical analysis for CBF activation studies in human brain. *J. Cereb. Blood Flow Metab.* 12, 900–918 (1992).

21 Evidence from Turner's Syndrome of an Imprinted X-Linked Locus Affecting Cognitive Function

D. H. Skuse, R. S. James, D. V. M. Bishop, B. Coppin, P. Dalton, G. Aamodt-Leeper, M. Bacarese-Hamilton, C. Creswell, R. McGurk, and P. A. Jacobs

Turner's syndrome is a sporadic disorder of human females in which all or part of one X chromosome is deleted.[1] Intelligence is usually normal[2] but social adjustment problems are common.[3] Here we report a study of 80 females with Turner's syndrome and a single X chromosome, in 55 of which the X was maternally derived (45,X^m) and in 25 it was of paternal origin (45,X^P). Members of the 45,X^P group were significantly better adjusted, with superior verbal and higher-order executive function skills, which mediate social interactions.[4] Our observations suggest that there is a genetic locus for social cognition, which is imprinted[5] and is not expressed from the maternally derived X chromosome. Neuropsychological and molecular investigations of eight females with partial deletions of the short arm of the X chromosome[6] indicate that the putative imprinted locus escapes X-inactivation,[7] and probably lies on Xq or close to the centromere on Xp. If expressed only from the X chromosome of paternal origin, the existence of this locus could explain why 46,XY males (whose single X chromosome is maternal) are more vulnerable to developmental disorders of language and social cognition, such as autism, than are 46,XX females.[8]

An increasing number of mammalian genes are known to be subject to genomic imprinting, defined as parental origin-specific differential gene expression.[5] No imprinted gene has yet been described on the X chromosome in humans,[9] although the *Xist* gene has been shown to be imprinted in the mouse.[10] We considered that it should be possible to identify the effects of an X-linked imprinted locus by comparing classes of females with Turner's syndrome. In this chromosomal disorder all, or a substantial part, of one X chromosome is missing as a result of non-disjunction (chromosome loss during gametogenesis or early cleavage of the zygote). In 70%

of monosomic (45,X) Turner-syndrome females, the single X chromosome is maternal in origin;[1] in the remainder it is paternal. Normal females (46,XX) possess both a maternally derived X chromosome (X^m) and a paternally derived X chromosome (X^P), one of which is randomly inactivated in any given somatic cell.[7] In monosomy X, the single chromosome is never inactivated. Differences in physical or behavioural phenotype between 45,X^P and 45,X^m Turner-syndrome subjects might therefore indicate the existence of an imprinted genetic locus.

Impaired social competence and adjustment are frequent in Turner's syndrome,[3] but a minority have good social skills.[11] Intelligence is usually normal in monosomic (45,X) cases.[2] We wished to test the hypothesis that 45,X^P females would be distinguishable from 45,X^m females by their social behaviour.

We karyotyped 80 monosomic (45,X) females and eight with deletions of the short arm of one X chromosome (46,XXp-). The parental origin of the normal X chromosome was determined by comparing proband and parental DNA polymorphisms located on distal Xp, in a region that was deleted in both 45,X and 46,XXp-patients. Of the 80 45,X females, 25 were 45,X^P and 55 were 45,X^m, with ages from 6 to 25 years. Clinical records did not reveal any significant group differences in terms of physical phenotype or in the provision of hormone-replacement therapy.[12] From a first-stage screening survey[13] of parents and teachers, using standardized instruments,[14–16] we discovered that 40% of 45,X^m girls of school age had received a statement of special educational needs, indicating academic failure, compared with 16% of 45,X^P subjects ($P < 0.05$); the figure in the general population is just 2%. We also found that clinically significant social difficulties affected 72.4% of the 45,X^m subjects over 11 years of age (21 of 29), compared with 28.6% of $45,X^p$ females (4 of 14) ($P < 0.02$).

Such phenotypic variability between the two classes of monosomy X subjects could indicate the existence of an imprinted genetic locus, at which gene(s) that influence social adjustment are expressed only from the paternally derived X chromosome. On the maternally derived X chromosome, the corresponding locus would be silenced. This could account for the excess of social and learning difficulties among $45,X^m$ females compared with the $45,X^p$ variant. Pilot interviews and observations showed that $45,X^m$ females in particular lacked flexibility and responsiveness in social interactions. We therefore devised a questionnaire relevant to social cognition to summarize the main features of their behaviour (Box 21.1). Parents of our sample of Turner's syndrome females and the parents of age-matched normal male and female comparisons completed the questionnaire. The results for subjects aged from 6 to 18 years of age confirm there are significant differences between $45,X^m$ and $45,X^p$ females in the predicted direction (Fig. 21.1). We found that $45,X^m$ subjects obtained significantly higher scores than $45,X^p$ females on our measure of social-cognitive dysfunction. Normal boys also obtained significantly higher scores on the questionnaire than did normal girls, indicating poorer social cognition (Fig. 21.1). The magnitude and direction of this difference are compatible with the hypothesis that there is an imprinted locus on the X chromosome that influences the development of social cognitive skills (although the finding is of course also compatible with other explanations of gender differences in behaviour[17]). If the putative locus only expressed a gene (or genes) from the X chromosome of paternal origin (X^p), we would expect a tendency for normal females to have superior social cognitive skills than males. Because males (46,XY) invariably inherit their single X chromosome from their mothers, the genetic locus would be silenced. In contrast, the gene(s) would be expressed from X^p in approxi-

Box 21.1
Scale measuring social cognition

> Complete the following section by circling 0 if the statement is not at all true of your child, 1 if it is quite or sometimes true of your child, and 2 if it is very or often true of your child:
>
> • lacking an awareness of other people's feelings
> • does not realise when others are upset or angry
> • is oblivious to the effect of his/her behaviour on other members of the family
> • behaviour often disrupts normal family life
> • very demanding of people's time
> • difficult to reason with when upset
> • does not seem to understand social skills: e.g., interrupts conversation
> • does not pick up on body language
> • unaware of acceptable social behaviour
> • unknowingly offends people with behaviour
> • does not respond to commands
> • has difficulty following commands unless they are carefully worded
>
> Internal consistency for set of 12 questions: Standardised item alpha 0.94.
>
> *Source:* Skuse, *Nature*, 387 (6634) June 12, 1997:705–708.

mately half of the cells of normal females if it were inactivated, and from all cells if it escaped X-inactivation.[7]

We hypothesized that an imprinted X-linked locus, either without a Y-linked homologue or with a Y homologue showing a lower level of expression, could also explain why males are markedly more vulnerable than females to pervasive developmental disorders affecting social adjustment and language, such as autism.[8] Accordingly, $45,X^m$ Turner females should be exceptionally vulnerable to disorders of language and social adjustment that are usually more

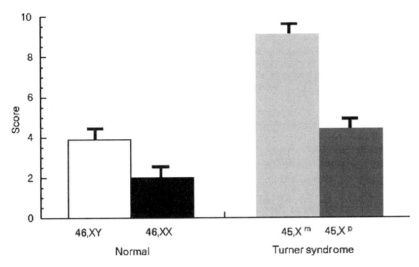

Figure 21.1
Subscale scores (mean ± SE) of questionnaire on social-cognitive impairment (Box 21.1). Higher scores indicate poorer social cognitive skills. The $45,X^m$ Turner-syndrome females score higher than $45,X^p$ females and both normal groups ($P < 0.0001$). Normal males score higher than normal females ($P < 0.001$); the effect size of this difference is 0.58, implying that the upper 50% of females score higher than approximately 72% of males. The ratios of mean social-dysfunction scores male:female and $45,X^m$:$45,X^p$ are very similar, 2.2:1 and 2.1:1, respectively). The overall higher scores for Turner-syndrome subjects, compared with normal females, may reflect the contribution made by visuospatial abilities to social cognition.[11] These abilities are impaired equally in both monosomic groups. No information regarding parental origin of the normal X chromosome was made available to parents, their consultants, or members of the research team gathering these or other data.

common in males. Consistent with this hypothesis, we identified three Turner-syndrome females with autism (meeting ICD-10 criteria),[18] out of the total unbiased sample assessed personally in the course of this investigation (3.75%). All three females had retained a normal maternal X chromosome. The population prevalence of autism is less than 1 per 10,000 females.[8]

We then sought corresponding differences in the results of neuropsychological testing of both normal and Turner-syndrome subjects. We found that $45,X^p$ females were significantly superior in verbal intelligence to $45,X^m$ females (Table 21.1). Verbal IQ was negatively correlated with the social dysfunction score in the sample as a whole ($r = -0.41$, $P < 0.002$). Both monosomic

Turner subgroups were equivalently impaired in non-verbal (including visuospatial) abilities.

We subsequently performed several more focused neuropsychological assessments. First, although we had found that verbal abilities were moderately good predictors of social cognition, we hypothesized that higher-order cognitive skills would be better predictors. These are not measured directly by conventional intelligence tests. The executive functions of the prefrontal cortex[4] exert an important influence on social interactions, and include skills that allow for the development of strategies of action and the inhibition of distracting impulses when striving towards a goal. Developmental disorders of social adjustment and language are associated with im-

Table 21.1
Neuropsychological test results

	Turner's syndrome		Normal	
	45,X^m (mean ± s.d.)	45,X^p (mean ± s.d.)	46,XX (mean ± s.d.)	46,XY (mean ± s.d.)
IQ				
Verbal	96.2 ± 15.9	106.4 ± 14.4	100.1 ± 16.7	98.6 ± 17.1
Non-verbal	79.5 ± 18.8	82.1 ± 15.9	—	—
Executive function tasks				
Behavioural inhibition	8.7 ± 7.1	5.7 ± 4.8	5.3 ± 4.1	6.8 ± 3.4
Planning ability	6.1 ± 1.7	7.4 ± 1.7	6.6 ± 1.6	7.2 ± 1.4

The 45,X^p females have significantly higher verbal IQ than 45,X^m subjects ($P < 0.02$), but neither Turner group differs significantly from the normal female comparisons. Non-verbal IQ was measured only in Turner-syndrome subjects and does not significantly distinguish the subgroups; it incorporates tests of visuospatial abilities, which are known to be specifically impaired in this condition.[2,29] In all analyses using the executive function measures, age has been covaried because, unlike conventional IQ measures, these tests are not yet standardized for age. Behavioural inhibition scores (Same–Opposite World) are measured in seconds, higher scores indicating more difficulty completing the task accurately. The 45,X^m females are less competent than either 45,X^p subjects ($P < 0.02$) or normal females ($P < 0.03$). Males are less competent than normal females ($P < 0.03$). On the planning task (Tower of Hanoi), neither the two Turner subgroups nor normal males and females are significantly distinguished from one another by the mean highest level achieved.

pairment in measures of executive function.[19] Many monosomic Turner-syndrome subjects have executive-function deficits.[2] We also predicted that 45,X^p females would perform better than 45,X^m females in tests of executive function skills. Finally, we predicted that abilities in which 45,X^p subjects were superior to 45,X^m subjects would also distinguish normal females from males, and in the same direction.

We chose tests of both planning ability (Tower of Hanoi) and behavioural inhibition (Same–Opposite World). The results were consistent with the initial hypothesis. Although the social-cognitive impairment score correlated independently with verbal IQ and with both measures of executive function, only planning ability ($r = -0.4$; $P < 0.006$) and behavioural inhibition ($r = -0.37$; $P < 0.015$) retained significance when the three variables were forced into a multiple regression analysis. The second prediction was partly confirmed: there were significant differences between 45,X^p and 45,X^m subjects

in terms of the behavioural inhibition task, although not on the test of planning ability. The third prediction was fully confirmed (Table 21.1): there was no significant difference in the highest level achieved on the planning task between normal males and females. However, on the behavioural-inhibition task, normal females were superior to males and their mean scores were very similar to those of the 45,X^p subjects. Previous reports have noted gender differences on inhibition tasks, and they have been conceptually linked to corresponding differences in social behaviour.[20]

We then attempted to map the putative imprinted locus, provisionally, by studying eight females, ascertained as part of the Turner-syndrome project, who had large terminal deletions of the short arm of the paternally derived X chromosome (a 46,X^m X^p p-karyotype). These deletions all extended to a point proximal to the *MLS* gene at Xp22.3 (Table 21.2); the paternal X chromosome was consequently preferentially

Table 21.2
Cytogenetic and molecular information

Patient	Karyotype	Breakpoints between	
		proximal	distal
85/5142	46,X,del(X)(qter → p22:)	DXS8036	DXS1053
95/4894	46,X,del(X)(qter → p21.2:)	DXS1036	DXS985
95/4247	45,X[33]/46,X,del(X)(qter → p21.2:)[17]	DXS1036	DXS985
95/3557	45,X[32]/46,del(X)(qter → p22.11:)[68]	DXS8039	DXS8049
91/219	46,X,del(X)(qter → p11:)	DXS1208	DXS1055
96/863	46,X,del(X)(qter → 11.2:)	DXS8062	DXS1003
96/8266	46,X,del(X)(qter → p11.23:)	DXS423E	*UBE1*
96/5509	45,X[9]/46,X,der(X)del(X)(p21.2 → pter)inv(X)(p21.2 q22.1)[166]	DXS1067	DXS8039

Cytogenetic analysis was performed by standard techniques and the chromosomes were examined in a minimum of 100 cells. To map the position of the breakpoints in the deleted X chromosomes, DNA from probands and parents was tested using PCR amplification of polymorphic microsatellite repeat sequences located along the length of Xp. For DXS423E and UBE1, the status of the locus in the proband was determined by fluorescence in situ hybridization (FISH) using metaphase chromosome spreads. The breakpoints lie between the most distal non-deleted marker and the most proximal deleted marker.

inactivated.[6] On examination, no one in this series was found to have any significant learning difficulties. The mean verbal intelligence score for the group was 103.4 (s.d., 13.7), and their mean non-verbal IQ was 93 (s.d., 11.2). Their mean social dysfunction score was 3.75 (s.d., 3.1), a value very similar to that of the $45,X^p$ subjects (Fig. 21.1). We drew the following conclusions from these data. First, the imprinted locus had not been deleted on the structurally abnormal paternal X chromosome, and so it must lie on Xq or on Xp closer to the centromere than, *UBE1* at Xp11.23. Second, the imprinted locus was not subject to X-inactivation, or the preferentially inactivated, partly deleted chromosome would not have expressed it. We already know of several genes that escape X-inactivation.[21]

We expected that isochromosomes of the long arm of the X chromosome [i(Xq)] would help in the mapping of the putative imprinted locus. However, virtually all i(Xq) chromosomes have been shown to contain proximal Xp sequences.[22] Duplication and consequent trisomy of the long arm of the X chromosome further complicate the

interpretation of correlations between phenotype and genotype. Accordingly, this approach did not provide unambiguous evidence to assist in the deletion mapping of the locus.

An imprinted locus is not the only possible explanation for our findings. Among the $45,X^p$ females, there may have been a greater degree of cryptic mosaicism (with a normal 46,XX cell line) than among those who were $45,X^m$. Some degree of mosaicism in apparently monosomic females may be essential for the fetus to avoid spontaneous abortion.[23] We examined both blood and cheek cells, tissues of mesodermal and ectodermal origin, respectively, and found two cryptic mosaics, but both were from the $45,X^m$ group.

Males are substantially more vulnerable to a variety of developmental disorders of speech, language impairment and reading disability, as well as more severe conditions such as autism.[8] Our findings are consistent with the hypothesis that the locus described, which we propose to be silent both in males and $45,X^m$ females, acts synergistically with susceptibility loci elsewhere on the genome to increase the male-to-female prevalence ratio of such disorders. Our data on normally developing children suggest it may also exert an effect on social and cognitive abilities in the normal range. These preliminary findings could thus provide evidence for the evolution of an imprinted X-linked locus that underlies the development of sexual dimorphism in social behaviour.[17]

Method

Subjects

This study, which was approved by the local hospital ethics committee, involved 88 females with Turner's syndrome (80 monosomic and 8 partial X-chromosome deletions; age range, 6–25 years). They were selected from a national survey of Turner's syndrome and from records of the Wessex Regional Laboratory. The mean age of the 45,X^m females was 162.3 months (s.d., 57.6), that of the 45,X^p females was 164.5 months (s.d., 57.7), and that of the Xp- females was 185.8 months (s.d., 74.9). All subjects were healthy, with no significant neurological disease. Females with an Xp- chromosome were all referred for investigation because of short stature in middle childhood, with one exception who was karyotyped at birth. Neuropsychological test results are presented for subjects with verbal IQs $\geqq 65$ (three 45,X^m subjects and one 45,X^p subject had verbal IQs that fell out of range). Parents rated 70 normal males and 71 normal females (age range, 6–18 years) on the social-cognition scale. The neuropsychological test battery was used to assess 68 normal males and 91 normal females (age range, 6–25 years). Verbal IQs were in the range 65–151. All normal comparison subjects were recruited from urban and suburban schools (6–18 years) and from hospital staff (18–25 years).

Behavioural and Cognitive Measures

Initial screening was conducted by postal questionnaires using a well-standardized set of instruments.[14–16] These were completed by parents, teachers and the Turner-syndrome subjects themselves (11 years and over). The social cognition questionnaire (Box 21.1) was completed by parents only. In a survey of 175 Turner-syndrome subjects for whom we obtained parental ratings on two occasions, a mean of 2.7 years apart, the intraclass correlation coefficient was 0.81 ($P < 0.01$). Scores correlate with the self-rated social problem subscale of the YSR[16] 0.58 ($P < 0.002$), with the teacher rating on the TRF[15] 0.54 ($P < 0.001$), and with the parent-rated CBCL[14] 0.69 ($P < 0.001$). The range of scores was 0–23 in the Turner-syndrome sample and 0–21 in the normal sample (maximum score of 24). The CBCL[14] was completed by 70 parents, the YSR[16] was completed by 40 subjects over 11 years of age, and the TRF[15] was completed by 45 teachers. Clinical significance of social problems was estimated according to clinical T scores.[14–16] Measures of cognition included the Wechsler Intelligence Scales for Children (WISC III-UK)[24] and the Wechsler Adult Intelligence Scales–Revised (WAIS-R).[25] The behavioural inhibition task was the Same–Opposite World subtest from the Test of Everyday Attention for Children.[26] This yields a time measure that ascertains the difference in latency for a subject responding to a series of stimuli on a task of sequential responses, which are named both as they appear and then opposite to their appearance. The subject reads a random series of numbers (1 and 2) saying "one" to 1, and "two" to 2. The subjects then repeat the task on a new series, but this time they have to inhibit the prepotent response and instead say "two" to 1, and "one" to 2, correcting any errors before proceeding. Test–retest reliability on a sample of 70 normal children gave an intraclass correlation coefficient of 0.62 ($P <$ 0.001). The Tower of Hanoi task was based on the procedure described previously.[27] It was scored according to the most complex level of the problem the child could solve reliably. Test–retest reliability gave an intraclass correlation coefficient for the highest level achieved of 0.45 ($P < 0.001$), which is in line with expectations for a test that makes novel demands of this nature.[28]

Acknowledgements

We thank E. Percy, S. Cave, A. O'Herlihy, R. South, J. Smith, M. Power and D. Robinson for assistance; M. Pembrey for comments and discussion; many paediatric consultants for assisting with the recruitment of patients, the schools who participated, and all of the subjects of our investigation and their families for their time. This research was supported by the Wellcome Trust and the Child Growth Foundation. Compilation of the national register of Turner syndrome was supported by the British Society for Paediatric Endocrinology and by Pharmacia.

References

1. Jacobs, P. A. et al. A cytogenetic and molecular reappraisal of a series of patients with Turner's syndrome. *Ann. Hum. Genet.* 54, 209–223 (1990).

2. Pennington, B. F. et al. The neuropsychological phenotype in Turner syndrome. *Cortex* 21, 391–404 (1985).

3. McCauley, E., Ito, J. & Kay, T. Psychosocial functioning in girls with the Turner syndrome and short stature. *J. Am. Acad. Child Psychiat.* 25, 105–112 (1986).

4. Damasio, A. R. On some functions of the human prefrontal cortex. *Proc. N. Y. Acad. Sci.* 769, 241–251 (1995).

5. Barlow, D. P. Gametic imprinting in mammals. *Science* 270, 1610–1613 (1995).

6. Ballabio, A. & Andria, G. Deletions and translocations involving the distal short arm of the human X chromosome: review and hypotheses. *Hum. Mol. Genet.* 1, 221–227 (1995).

7. Lyon, M. F. Gene action in the X-chromosome of the mouse (*Mus musculus* L). *Nature* 190, 372–373 (1961).

8. Bailey, A., Philips, W. & Rutter, M. Autism: towards an integration of clinical, genetic, neuropsychological and neurobiological perspectives. *J. Child Psychol. Psychiat.* 37, 89–126 (1996).

9. Ledbetter, D. H. & Engel, E. Uniparental disomy in humans: development of an imprinting map and its implications for prenatal diagnosis. *Hum. Mol. Genet.* 4, 1757–1764 (1995).

10. Zuccotti, M. & Monk, M. Methylation of the mouse *Xist* gene in sperm and eggs correlates with imprinted *Xist* expression and paternal X-inactivation. *Nature Genet.* 9, 316–320 (1995).

11. McCauley, E., Kay, T., Ito, J. & Trader, R. The Turner syndrome: cognitive deficits, affective discrimination and behaviour problems. *Child Dev.* 58, 464–473 (1987).

12. Saenger, P. Clinical Review 48: The current status of diagnosis and therapeutic intervention in Turner's syndrome. *J. Clin. Endocrinol. Metabol.* 77, 297–301 (1993).

13. Skuse, D., Percy, E. L. & Stevenson, J. in *Growth, Stature, and Adaptation. Behavioral, Social, and Cognitive Aspects of Growth Delay* (eds Stabler, B. & Underwood, L.) 151–164 (UCP, Chapel Hill, 1994).

14. Achenbach, T. M. *Manual for the Child Behavior Checklist/4-18 and 1991 Profile* (Department of Psychiatry, University of Vermont, Burlington, VT, 1991).

15. Achenbach, T. M. *Manual for the Teacher's Report Form and 1991 Profile* (Department of Psychiatry, University of Vermont, Burlington, VT, 1991).

16. Achenbach, T. M. *Manual for the Youth Self-Report Form and 1991 Profile* (Department of Psychiatry, University of Vermont, Burlington, VT, 1991).

17. Eagley, A. H. The science and politics of comparing men and women. *Am. Psychol.* 50, 145–158 (1995).

18. World Health Organization *The ICD-10 Classification of Mental and Behavioural Disorders: Clinical Descriptions and Diagnostic Guidelines* (World Health Organization, Geneva, 1992).

19. Pennington, B. F. & Ozonoff, S. Executive functions and developmental psychopathology. *J. Child Psychol. Psychiat.* 37, 51–87 (1996).

20. Bjorklund, D. F. & Kipp, K. Parental investment theory and gender differences in the evolution of inhibition mechanisms. *Psychol. Bull.* 120, 163–188 (1996).

21. Disteche, C. M. Escape from X inactivation in human and mouse. *Trends Genet.* 11, 17–22 (1995).

22. Wolff, D. J., Miller, A. P., Van Dyke, D. L., Schwartz, S. & Willard, H. F. Molecular definition of breakpoints associated with human Xq isochromosomes: implications for mechanism of formation. *Am. J. Hum. Genet.* 58, 154–160 (1996).

23. Hassold, T., Pettay, D., Robinson, A. & Uchida, I. Molecular studies of parental origin and mosaicism in 45,X conceptuses. *Hum. Genet.* 89, 647–652 (1992).

24. Wechsler, D. *Wechsler Intelligence Scale for Children* 3rd UK edn (Psychological Corporation, London, 1992).

25. Wechsler, D. *Wechsler Adult Intelligence Scales-Revised* (Psychological Corporation, New York, 1986).

26. Borys, S. V., Spitz, H. H. & Dorans, B. A. Tower of Hanoi performance of retarded young adults and nonretarded children as a function of solution length and goal state. *J. Exp. Child Psychol.* 33, 87–110 (1982).

27. Manly, T., Robertson, I. H. & Anderson, V. *The Test of Everyday Attention for Children (TEACh)* (Thames Valley Test Company, Bury St Edmunds, in press).

28. Rabbitt, P. M. A. in *Methodologies of Frontal and Executive Function* (ed. Rabbitt, P. M. A.) (Psychology Press, Hove, in press).

29. Temple, C. M. & Carney, R. A. Patterns of spatial functioning in Turner's syndrome. *Cortex* 31, 109–118 (1995).

III SOCIAL COGNITION AND THE BRAIN

B. Social Applications

iii. Social Information Processing

22 Social Cognition and the Human Brain

Ralph Adolphs

Social cognition refers to the processes that subserve behavior in response to conspecifics (other individuals of the same species), and, in particular, to those higher cognitive processes subserving the extremely diverse and flexible social behaviors that are seen in primates. Its evolution arose out of a complex and dynamic interplay between two opposing factors: on the one hand, groups can provide better security from predators, better mate choice, and more reliable food; on the other hand, mates and food are available also to competitors from within the group. An evolutionary approach to social cognition therefore predicts mechanisms for cooperativity, altruism, and other aspects of prosocial behavior, as well as mechanisms for coercion, deception and manipulation of conspecifics. The former are exemplified in the smallest groups, in the bond between mother and infant; the latter in the largest groups by the creation of complex dominance hierarchies.

It is clear that primates are exceedingly adept at negotiating the social environment. This ability is most striking in the most social primate, *Homo sapiens*, suggesting the hypothesis that our exceptional cognitive skills may be traced back to evolution in an environment in which there was a premium on social skills. In support of this idea, there is a correlation between mean group size among various primate species and their neocortex volume (specifically, the ratio of neocortex volume to the rest of the brain).[1] Such a correlation has been found also for several other mammals that all feature a complex social structure (e.g. bats, carnivores and toothed whales)—the larger the social groups, the larger the brains (relative to body size). Although it has been proposed that brain size correlates with a number of other factors, including dietary foraging strategy, tool use and longevity,[2,3] it might be that large brain size is at least a partial consequence of the fact that primates have a complex ecological

niche with respect to social structure (including its effect on food and mate availability). This hypothesis, variously dubbed the "Machiavellian Intelligence Hypothesis"[4] or the "Social Brain Hypothesis,"[1] depending on what theorists take to be its most salient features, suggests that the complexity of primate social structure, together with certain of its unique features, such as cooperativity and deception, led to an advantage for larger brains.

Aside from sheer brain volume, one would of course like to know more about the specific neural systems that subserve various aspects of social cognition. A seminal review[5] argued for the importance of the following set of structures: amygdala, temporal cortex, anterior cingulate cortex, and orbitofrontal cortex.[6] The neurobiological underpinnings of social cognition in humans, the topic of this review, are being investigated using various methods, including lesion studies and functional imaging, and can be situated in the context of what we know about social cognition from anthropological, comparative and developmental studies.

An Overview of the Neurobiology of Social Cognition in Primates

Non-human Primates

Two sets of findings, one at a macroscopic level, the other at a microscopic level, first suggested that the primate brain might contain neural systems specialized for processing socially relevant information. In the 1930s, Kluver and Bucy made large bilateral lesions in monkey brains, encompassing amygdala, temporal neocortex, and surrounding structures.[7] The animals subsequently appeared able to perceive and respond to objects in their environment, but they behaved inappropriately with respect to the emotional significance that objects would normally signal. This included a compulsive examination of objects, especially with the mouth, hypersexual behavior, unusual tameness, and a complete lack of awareness of the emotional significance of stimuli ("psychic blindness"; e.g. handling of snakes). Selective neurotoxic lesions of the monkey amygdala result in more subtle impairments; however they do still appear to impair disproportionately those behaviors normally elicited by social cues.[8–10] Although the amygdala is a heterogeneous collection of nuclei that participate in several different functional systems,[11] at least some of its components thus appear to contribute disproportionately to social behavior.

The other set of findings that first sparked interest in the neural basis of social cognition pertains to the level of single neurons. Neurophysiological studies in non-human primates have shown that single neurons in the monkey inferotemporal cortex respond relatively selectively to the sight of faces.[12] Moreover, specific neurons modulate their response preferentially with specific information about faces, such as their identity, social status or emotional expression.[13–15] There are also neurons whose responses are modulated by viewing complex scenes of social interaction,[16,17] as well as by specific features of faces that can signal social information, such as gaze direction.[18] A neural code in which the responses of individual neurons are tuned relatively selectively to highly specific feature conjunctions may permit a neuronal ensemble to distinguish among complex, similar members of a large class of stimuli, such as the faces of conspecifics. Current information-theoretical approaches are providing more detail on how such socially relevant information might be encoded in a neuronal population.[19]

Humans

Human social cognition has received extensive attention from cognitive, developmental and social psychologists. Some important current issues that might be informed by findings from cognitive neuroscience concern how social cognitive abilities develop in infants, and to what extent genetic factors might influence such abilities. Clearly, the emotional and social development of humans is extraordinarily complex, involving a multi-factorial interplay between genes, parental behavior, and the influence of culture.

There have been two major sets of studies that first argued for neural systems critical to social cognition in humans: social impairments following damage to the frontal lobe, and, more recently, social impairments in subjects with autism. The observation that the frontal lobes can contribute relatively specifically to behavior in the social domain was first made on the basis of a rather horrible accident: the injury of the railroad worker Phineas Gage.[20] Gage received a large bilateral lesion of his frontal lobe, including the ventromedial prefrontal cortex, from an accidental explosion that shot a metal rod through his head (see Fig. 22.1 for neuroanatomical structures highlighted in this review). Whereas Gage had been a diligent, reliable, polite and socially adept person before his accident, he subsequently became uncaring, profane, and socially inappropriate in his conduct. This change in his personality remained a mystery until it could be interpreted in the light of similar patients in modern times: like Gage, other subjects with bilateral damage to the ventromedial frontal lobes show a severely impaired ability to function in society, despite an entirely normal profile on standard neuropsychological measures, such as IQ, language, perception and memory. Recent theoretical explanations propose that the ventromedial frontal cortices play an important role in associating emotional experience with decision making in complex situations, especially perhaps situations in the social domain (see below).

A second line of evidence that has been used to argue for the functional modularity of social cognition (see Box 22.1) comes from a developmental disorder, childhood autism. Interest in the social cognitive abilities of subjects with autism was fueled by the argument that autism features a disproportionate impairment in one specific aspect of social cognition: the ability

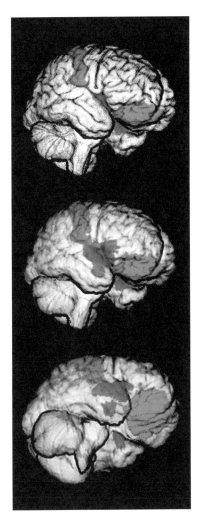

to attribute mental states, such as beliefs, to others.[21,22] While there is debate on the basic hypothesis, and while the link between autism and brain systems is also not well understood, the data point towards neural components that appear to have a high degree of domain-specific function. This idea is strengthened by comparison with another psychiatric disorder, entirely genetic in etiology: Williams syndrome. Subjects with Williams syndrome exhibit social behavior that comes close to being the opposite of that seen in autism—they are hypersocial, and their unusual social skills in the face of impairments in non-social domains have been taken as further evidence for the modularity of social cognition.[23] Of particular interest will be comparisons among subjects with Williams syndrome, autism, and focal brain lesions, some of which are now underway. For example, a recent study found that subjects with Williams syndrome showed selective sparing in their ability to recognize other people's mental states from photographs of their eyes,[24] a task that high-functioning subjects with autism fail,[25] and which in normal individuals, but not in subjects with autism, has been shown to activate the amygdala in functional imaging studies.[26] Subjects with Williams syndrome also show abnormally positive judgments of approachability when shown unfamiliar people's faces, one component of impaired social judgment that might share commonalities with im-

Figure 22.1
Summary of neuroanatomical structures involved in social cognition. These renderings of a normal human brain, reconstructed from serial magnetic resonance (MR) images, show the neuroanatomical structures highlighted in this review. The same brain is shown in different views and with differing amounts of transparency, to permit visualization of interior structures. The images were generated by first tracing the structures on 2-D MR images, and then co-rendering these regions of interest in various colors together with the rest of the brain. Highlighted are ventromedial prefrontal cortex (green), amygdala (red), right somatosensory cortex (blue) and insula (purple), all of which play key roles in various aspects of social cognition discussed here. Additionally, other structures (not colored), such as the cingulate cortices, visual association cortices in temporal lobe, and structures in hypothalamus, thalamus, and brainstem contribute to social function. All of these structures also play varied roles in regulating emotion. (Figure kindly provided by Deema Fattal and Hanna Damasio, Human Neuroanatomy and Neuroimaging Laboratory, Department of Neurology, University of Iowa.)

Box 22.1
Social cognition, modularity and innateness

Focal brain damage can result in impaired processing that is limited to highly specific categories. For instance, patients have been reported who are specifically unable to recognize, or to name, tools, animals, people, or a variety of other selective categories. There is thus very strong evidence that categories are, in some sense, mapped in the brain (but in a way that differs from aspects of objects that are a direct consequence of topography at the sensory epithelium). While initially surprising, the finding is in fact predicted from the assumption of a few, very simple, local rules that specify how brains represent stimuli (Ref. a). In essence, local rules for organizing neural tissue as a function of activity suffice to generate topographic representations of abstract stimulus categories. The categories that are abstracted emerge naturally out of the covariances of our interactions with certain classes of stimuli in the environment. Thus, we typically interact with members of the class of animals in a similar way; that is, the similarity is greater among animals than it is to how we typically interact with members of the class of tools, or members of the class of people. Similarity in sensorimotor interaction can thus translate into functional and anatomical similarity in the brain (Refs. b,c).

The above view suggests a strong component of experience and learning in such self-organized topographic maps. A different explanation comes from the view that there are innately specified modules in the brain for processing specific categories of knowledge. The evidence for this latter view is strongest from domains such as language, and it is the view that has historically been associated with the notion of "modularity" (Ref. d).

As with many dichotomies, it is likely that both the above views are right, in the proper context, and recent interpretations suggest a softer version of "modularity" that does not require a rigid set of criteria (Ref. e). It may well be that there are domain-specific modules for processing certain kinds of information that are ecologically highly relevant and that would benefit from a particular, idiosyncratic processing strategy that does not apply to other kinds of information. That is, one would expect the brain to provide problem-specific structures for processing information from those domains in which there is a premium on speed and survival. Within, and beyond, such a module there might also be topographic mapping of the same domain. It is likely that domain-specific processing draws upon innately specified modules, as well as upon self-organized maps that emerged as a consequence of experience with the world.

Is social cognition modular? And if so, is it innate, or is it a consequence of learning? It is likely that both are true, and that whether or not social cognition is modular will depend both on one's notion of modularity and on the aspects of social cognition under consideration. Some rather basic attributes of stimuli, such as self-directed motion, bilateral symmetry, presence of eyes, and so forth, might be processed similarly by different primate species, by mechanisms that are largely innately specified. But there also seems little doubt that the class of social stimuli needs to be explored during development in order to be able to make more fine-grained distinctions—a developmental process that is likely to include parental behavior and pretend play as critical aspects. The most plausible scenario, then, would view social cognition as relying on a neural architecture in which there is interaction between components that are innately specified and others whose operation emerges through experience in the context of a specific culture.

A similar answer would presumably obtain in regard to the broader question of cognition, not only with respect to the social world, but the animate world in general (see Ref. f for more extensive discussions of this topic). Future goals will be to provide a more detailed account of the relative contributions that innate and culturally acquired components make to social cognition, and to explore how such functional components might be subserved by specific neuroanatomical structures.

References

a. Kohonen, T. and Hari, R. (1999) Where the abstract feature maps of the brain might come from *Trends Neurosci.* 22, 135–139

Box 22.1
(continued)

b. Solomon, K. O., Medin, D. L. and Lynch, E. (1999) Concepts do more than categorize *Trends Cognit. Sci.* 3, 99–104

c. Tranel, D., Damasio, A. R. and Damasio, H. (1997) A neural basis for the retrieval of conceptual knowledge *Neuropsychologia* 35, 1319–1327

d. Fodor, J. A. (1983) *The Modularity of Mind,* MIT Press

e. Coltheart, M. (1999) Modularity and cognition *Trends Cognit. Sci.* 3, 115–119

f. Medin, D. L. and Atran, S., eds (1999) *Folkbiology,* MIT Press

paired social judgment seen in patients with bilateral amygdala damage.[27]

The Amygdala: Social Judgment of Faces

We glean considerable social information from faces, and there is evidence to suggest that faces are processed in a relatively domain-specific fashion by neocortical sectors of the temporal lobe. For instance, visual processing in regions of the human fusiform gyrus appears to contribute disproportionately to the perception of faces,[28] and viewing dynamic information from faces that convey socially relevant information (such as eye or mouth movements) activates regions in the superior temporal sulcus.[29] Recent data suggest that it is a particular property of how we interact with faces that leads to the specific neuroanatomical processing seen, namely, that we need to become expert at distinguishing many exemplars that are visually extremely similar and yet socially highly distinctive.[30]

High-level visual cortices in the temporal lobe project to the amygdala,[31] which has also received historical and recent interest in regard to its role in processing emotionally and socially salient information from faces. A small proportion of neurons within the amygdala show responses that are relatively selectively modulated by the sight of faces, compared with other visual stimuli.[32,33] Studies that have used functional neuroimaging in normal subjects,[34,35] and studies that have examined patients with damage

to the amygdala,[36–38] have provided evidence that the amygdala is critical to recognize emotions from facial expressions, specifically certain negative emotions, such as fear. The findings have been broadly consonant with the amygdala's contribution to social behavior that was suggested by earlier lesion studies in animals, as well as with the large number of animal studies that have investigated the amygdala's role in fear conditioning.[39,40] While these threads of research have pointed to a disproportionately important role for the amygdala in processing stimuli related to danger and threat, there are also findings, primarily from studies in animals, that suggest a more general role for the amygdala in processing emotionally arousing stimuli that are either pleasant or aversive. One recent theoretical view suggests that the amygdala, in both humans and animals, might subserve a more general role in allocating processing resources to biologically salient stimuli that are ambiguous, and about which additional information needs to be acquired, regardless of the valence of those stimuli.[41]

Given the above findings, one might expect that the amygdala would make important contributions also to higher-level social cognition, especially to those aspects of it that rely on recognizing social information from faces. This prediction is indeed borne out by recent studies. One important cue, direction of eye gaze in a face, has been shown to be processed by the amygdala in both some lesion[36] and functional imaging studies.[42] Other studies have examined the amygdala's role in more global social judgments. We investigated subjects' ability to judge how trustworthy or how approachable other people looked, from perceiving their faces. Such an ability would be expected to draw on aspects of social recognition, as well as on social decision making. In our study, we found that three subjects who had bilateral amygdala damage all shared the same pattern of impairment: they judged to be abnormally trustworthy and approachable the faces of those people who are normally judged to look the most untrustworthy or most unapproachable[43] (Fig. 22.2A). While the subjects with amygdala damage showed a general positive bias in judging all faces, they showed a disproportionate impairment when judging those faces normally given the most negative ratings (Fig. 22.2B). The amygdala's role in processing stimuli related to potential threat or danger thus appears to extend to the complex judgments on the basis of which we regulate our social behavior. Clearly, the cues that we normally use to make such judgments will be complex, and there will be multiple strategies available to utilize them, a topic deserving further study.

There are two issues of additional interest: the specificity of the above impairment to faces, and its consequences for social behavior in the real world. In regard to specificity, follow-up studies revealed that bilateral amygdala damage also impaired judgments for the preferences of nonsocial visual stimuli, such as color patterns or landscapes, although the effect was not as large. In one such study, subjects with amygdala damage liked pictures of non-social stimuli more than did controls.[44] Thus, the amygdala's contribution does not appear to be entirely restricted to processing stimuli in the social domain, but may encompass a more general function which is of disproportionate importance to social cognition. A further experiment assessed social judgments that were made about other people on the basis of written descriptions of them. Judgments

about people from such lexical stimuli were not impaired by amygdala damage,[43] perhaps because the stimuli provided sufficient explicit information such that normal task performance could result from reasoning strategies that did not necessarily require the amygdala. However, two other recent studies have suggested that the amygdala is involved in processing lexical stimuli, when such stimuli signal potential threat or danger.[45,46]

The second question, concerning the social impairments following amygdala damage in real life, is more difficult to investigate. However, observation of patients with complete bilateral amygdala damage suggests a common aspect to their social behavior: they tend to be unusually friendly towards others, consistent with the idea that they lack the normal mechanisms for detecting individuals that should be avoided. Similar changes in behavior are seen in non-human primates with selective bilateral amygdala damage.[8,9] On the other hand, the human patients do not appear to be as severely impaired in their social behavior as do monkeys with similar brain damage. It may be that humans with amygdala damage, unlike other animals, possess additional mechanisms for social reasoning and decision making, and are able also to draw substantially on declarative knowledge encoded in language, resulting in partial compensation for their impairment.[47]

One would also like to extend the above line of investigations to additional types of stimuli, and to additional types of social information that can be gleaned from such stimuli. We have begun such an investigation, using visual motion cues to provide information about biological and psychological categories. In one experiment, subjects were shown a short video that depicts three geometric shapes moving on a plain, white background.[48] Although visual motion is the only available cue in this experiment, normal subjects have no difficulty interpreting the motion of the shapes in terms of social categories: the shapes are attributed psychological states, such as goals,

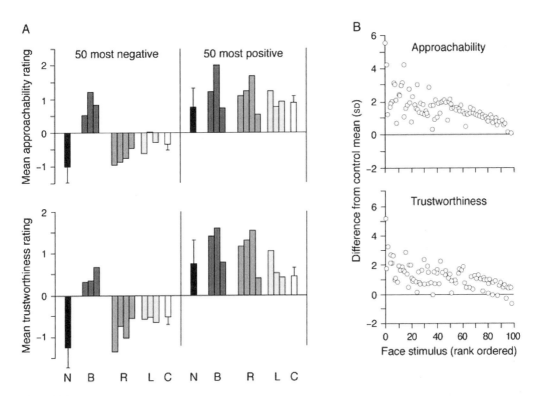

Figure 22.2
Mean judgments of approachability and trustworthiness of 100 unfamiliar faces. (A) Means and SD for data from 46 normal controls are given at the left of each panel ("N"). Individual means are shown for each of three subjects with bilateral amygdala damage ("B"), four subjects with unilateral right ("R") and three with unilateral left ("L") amygdala damage. Group means and SEM are shown for seven brain-damaged controls with no damage to amygdala ("C"). The data, broken down into those obtained from the 50 faces that received the most negative mean ratings from normal controls (left) and the most positive (right) on each attribute, show that subjects with bilateral amygdala damage gave abnormally positive ratings to the half of the stimuli that normally receive the most negative ratings. (B) Standard deviations from the control mean are shown for one of the three subjects with bilateral amygdala damage (subject SM). Each face was judged on a scale of −3 (very unapproachable or untrustworthy) to +3 (very approachable or trustworthy). The data show that SM rated nearly all faces as positive. (Data redrawn from Ref. 43.)

beliefs, desires and emotions, on the basis of their relative motion. By contrast, a subject with selective bilateral amygdala damage did not spontaneously make such attributions.[49] When shown the same stimulus, she described it in purely geometric terms, lacking the normal, automatic social interpretation (Box 22.2).

A final important consideration concerns the amygdala's role beyond recognition and judgment, to encompass such processes as attention and memory. It is clear from studies in animals that the amygdala contributes importantly to these processes,[50] and that its role extends well beyond a function restricted to recognizing potential threat or danger; but such a possible role in humans is just beginning to be explored. For instance, emotionally[51] or socially[52] salient stimuli are remembered better by normal individuals, an effect that correlates with activation of the amygdala in functional imaging studies[53,54] and one whose function is impaired in patients with amygdala lesions.[55]

Taken together, all the above findings argue that the amygdala is one component of the neural systems by which stimuli trigger emotional reactions, broadly construed. Such emotional reactions would include autonomic, endocrine and somatomotor changes in the body, as well as neurophysiological and neuromodulatory changes in brain function. Such multidimensional emotional responses would serve to modulate and to bias cognition and behavior in important ways, as a function of the emotional and social significance of the stimulus that is perceived. This role for the amygdala may be of special importance for relatively fast, automatic evaluation of biologically important stimuli, and will no doubt function in parallel with other systems.

An active program of research has explored why it might be adaptive to make certain social judgments about faces with certain properties. For instance, average faces are perceived to be highly attractive,[56] but very slight deviations from the average may be considered even more attractive.[57] A possible evolutionary explanation of this effect proposes that averageness, symmetry, or slight deviations from it, are correlated with fitness; consequently, one would predict that such features could have signal value, and one would predict the evolution of perceptual mechanisms for their detection. However, these interpretations are very contentious (see Ref. 58 for a review). Contrary to prediction, some recent data suggest that people with attractive faces are not more healthy,[59] and that at least some aspects of attractiveness also do not correlate with social dominance,[60] but may be a more complex function of weighing multiple short-term versus long-term benefits.[61] Notwithstanding the current debates, it will be essential in future studies to attempt to link specific physical features that plausibly index fitness, with specific neurobiological adaptations for their detection, hopefully subserved by neuroanatomically and neurofunctionally identifiable structures.

While the studies reviewed above strongly implicate the amygdala in several of the processes that are important for normal social cognition, they are problematic from an anatomical point of view: they are both too macroscopic and too microscopic. They are too macroscopic because it is clear that different nuclei within the amygdala subserve different functions,[11] an issue that is addressed in animal studies by lesioning specific nuclei rather than the entire amygdala. Functional imaging studies using fMRI with high field strengths, as well as rare studies of human patients with chronically implanted depth electrodes for monitoring seizures,[62,63] will provide some further neuroanatomical resolution in this regard.

Of equal importance, lesion studies of the amygdala are too microscopic in that it is important to consider the amygdala as one component of a distributed neural system for social cognition. In particular, amygdala and prefrontal cortex appear to function together in processing the rewarding contingencies of emotionally salient stimuli,[64,65] and it is likely that they function as

Box 22.2
Attribution of social meaning from visual motion

Subjects were shown a short movie of simple geometric shapes in motion (a still from the movie is
shown in Fig. 22.3). After seeing the movie, they
were asked to describe what they saw. While normal subjects immediately ascribe social meaning
to what they see, a subject with developmental
amygdala damage (subject SM) failed to do so,
interpreting the stimulus in purely geometric terms.
The findings suggest that the amygdala may be
critical in order to acquire the social knowledge by
which normal individuals automatically assign social meaning to stimuli.

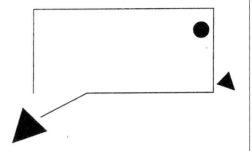

Figure 22.3
A still from the movie of simple geometric shapes in
motion that was shown to the subjects (see text for
description). (Redrawn from Ref. a.)

Normal Control Subject

"I saw a box, like a room, that had an opening to it.
There was a large triangle chasing around a smaller
triangle, and a circle ... got into the box, or the
room, and hid. And then the big triangle chased the
little triangle around. Finally he went in, got inside
the box to go after the circle, and the circle was
scared of him ... but manoeuvred its way around
and was able to get out the opening, and they shut
it on him. And the little circle and the little triangle
were happy that they got that, the big one, caught.
And they went off on their way, and the big triangle
got upset and started breaking the box open."

Subject SM

"OK, so, a rectangle, two triangles, and a small circle. Let's see, the triangle and the circle went inside

the rectangle, and then the other triangle went in,
and then the triangle and the circle went out and
took off, left one triangle there. And then the two
parts of the rectangle made like an upside-down V,
and that was it."

Reference

a. Heberlein, A. S. et al. (1998) Impaired attribution of social meanings to abstract dynamic visual
patterns following damage to the amygdala *Soc.
Neurosci. Abstr.* 24, 1176

two components of a system also in social cognition, a topic I address next.

The Ventromedial (VM) Prefrontal Cortex: Social Reasoning and Decision Making

Decision Making: The Somatic Marker Hypothesis

The frontal lobes have a long history in social behavior, going back to the story of Phineas Gage discussed above. More recently, it has become clear that the frontal lobes, specifically their ventromedial sectors, are critical in linking perceptual representations of stimuli with representations of their emotional and social significance.[66] This function bears some resemblance to that of the amygdala outlined above, but with two important differences. First, it is clear that the ventromedial frontal cortices play an equally important role in processing stimuli with either rewarding or aversive contingencies; whereas the amygdala's role, at least in humans, is clearest for aversive contingencies. Second, reward-related representations in the ventromedial frontal cortex are less stimulus-driven than in the amygdala, and can be the substrate of more flexible computations, playing a general monitoring role in regard to both punishing and rewarding contingencies.[67]

The impaired social behavior in humans with ventromedial frontal lobe injury is notable for an inability to organize and plan future activity, a diminished capacity to respond to punishment, stereotyped and sometimes inappropriate social manners, and an apparent lack of concern for other individuals, all in the face of otherwise normal intellectual functioning.[66,68,69] Particularly striking are the patients' often gross lack of concern for the well-being of others and remarkable lack of empathy. While the details of impaired emotional and social function following damage to the ventromedial frontal lobes can be complex, and can vary from case to case, the impairments share a core dysfunctional mechanism that no longer permits cognitive processes to incorporate certain types of emotional knowledge.

The role of the human ventromedial prefrontal cortex in decision making has been explored in a series of studies that used a task in which subjects had to gamble in order to win money. As with gambling in real life, the task involved probabilistic contingencies that required subjects to make choices based on incomplete information. Normal subjects learn to maximize their profits on the task by building a representation of the statistical contingencies gleaned from prior experiences: certain choices tend to pay off better than others, in the long run. The key ingredient that distinguishes this task from other tasks of probabilistic reasoning is that subjects discriminate choices by feeling; they develop hunches that certain choices are better than others, and these hunches can be measured both by asking subjects verbally, and by measuring autonomic correlates of emotional arousal, such as skin conductance response. Subjects with damage to the ventromedial frontal cortex fail this task,[70] and they fail it precisely because they are unable to represent choice bias in the form of an emotional hunch.[71] Not only do subjects with VM frontal damage make poor choices on the task, they also acquire neither any subjective feeling regarding their choices,[71] nor any anticipatory autonomic changes.[72]

These findings are consonant with prior reports that subjects with VM frontal lobe damage do not trigger a normal emotional response to stimuli, including socially relevant stimuli,[73] and support a specific hypothesis that has been put forth to explain the data: the somatic marker hypothesis.[66,74] According to this hypothesis, the VM frontal cortex participates in implementing a particular mechanism by which we acquire, represent, and retrieve the values of our actions. This mechanism relies on generating somatic states, or representations of somatic states, that correspond to the anticipated future outcome of decisions. The function of these somatic states is to steer the decision making process toward those outcomes that are advantageous for the individual, based on the individual's past experience with similar situations. Such a mechanism may be of special importance in the social domain, where the enormous complexity of the decision space precludes an exhaustive analysis.

Reasoning: The Wason Selection Task

The ventromedial frontal cortex appears to play a key role in a second domain of high relevance to social cognition: social reasoning. Human reasoning strategies have been intensively investigated using the Wason selection task, the most popular experimental design for probing deductive reasoning.[75] The Wason selection task consists of a conditional statement ("if P then Q"), often presented in some context (e.g. "If you are drinking beer, then you must be over the age of 18"), and subjects must use deductive reasoning in order to decide its truth. Typically, the proportion of logically correct choices made by normal subjects on this task is facilitated by conditionals about social rules, threats, and promises (see Ref. 76 for a review). Cosmides and her colleagues have argued that these data provide evidence for evolved mechanisms for reasoning about social exchange. Specifically, the findings from the Wason selection task support the hypothesis of an evolved skill to detect deception in the context of social contracts (cheating), because an ability to rapidly and reliably detect such deception would have been adaptive[77] (although there is considerable debate regarding the interpretation of the data, and alternative models have been proposed).

We investigated the role of the VM frontal cortex in such deductive reasoning, using three groups of subjects: patients with damage centered on the VM frontal cortex, patients with damage centered on the dorsolateral frontal cortex (specifically excluding the VM frontal cortex), and

patients with damage outside the frontal cortex. Subjects with bilateral damage to the VM frontal cortex were disproportionately impaired in normal reasoning about social and familiar scenarios, whereas they showed no abnormality when reasoning about more abstract material[78] (Fig. 22.4). These findings are consonant with those presented above, and support a role for the VM frontal cortex in guiding reasoning and decision making by the elicitation of emotional states that serve to bias cognition. While the ventromedial frontal cortices, together with the amygdala, would participate in a more general function of linking stimuli to emotionally valued responses, they may be notably indispensable when reasoning and making decisions about social matters. Additional future studies that attempt to dissect the broad collection of processes that comprise social cognition will help to shed light on the question of the specificity and modularity of ventromedial frontal cortex function. The evolutionary implications that can be drawn from such a disproportionate importance to social cognition remain a difficult and open question (Box 22.1).

The above findings from humans can be related to a large number of studies from non-human primates,[79-81] which have shown abnormal social behavior, especially social isolation and avoidance[82] following damage to the orbital frontal cortices. The role of the orbitofrontal cortex in social affiliative behaviors is also of interest from a pharmacological point of view: the density of certain subtypes of serotonin receptors in the orbitofrontal cortex of monkeys correlates with the animal's social status. Pharmacological manipulation of serotonergic neurotransmission targeted at these receptors influences social affiliative behavior, and results in changes in social status.[83] These findings from monkeys may offer some explanation of the changes in social behaviors that can also be observed in humans following serotonergic manipulation [e.g. with drugs such as Prozac (fluoxetine) or ecstasy (MDMA)]. A further specification of neurotransmitter and

A

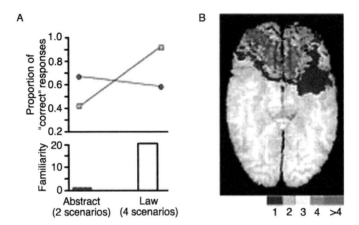

B

Figure 22.4

Reasoning on the Wason Selection Task. (A) Subjects with ventromedial (VM) frontal lesions (circles) gave the logically correct answer more often than did control subjects (squares) when reasoning about scenarios where the subject matter was logical and abstract (e.g. If a student got an "A" grade, then his card must be marked with the numeral "3"); however, they gave the logically correct answer less often than controls when the subject matter concerned familiar social situations, specifically social laws (e.g. "If you are drinking beer, then you must be over the age of 18") (result significant at $p = 0.001$ level). These findings support the idea that, in normal subjects, the VM frontal cortices may be part of a system that facilitates correct reasoning about social matters. The results were especially striking, as the scenarios on which subjects with VM frontal damage failed are in fact the ones that are normally the easiest, and the most familiar, to reason about. When subjects were asked to indicate how familiar they found each of the scenarios, both VM frontal and normal control subjects judged the social laws to be much more familiar than the abstract scenarios (bottom, grouped data). (B) Volumetric overlap image of the lesions of all subjects with VM frontal lobe damage. Color encodes the number of subjects (indicated below) who have a lesion at a given anatomical location, rendered onto a ventral view of the human brain. The anatomical sites shared in common by all subjects in the group were the ventromedial frontal cortex, bilaterally. (Data redrawn from Refs. 78, 92.)

neuromodulator systems will clearly be important in our understanding of the neural basis of social cognition; a more detailed discussion of this topic falls outside the scope of this review. Of special interest is the neurotransmitter serotonin (acting on specific subtypes of serotonin receptor), and the neuropeptide oxytocin, both of which appear to play a role in neurochemical systems relatively specialized for social behaviors (see Ref. 84 for a review).

Ultimately, one would like to see comparative investigations that examine frontal lobe structure and function in humans and other primates, but such studies are exceedingly difficult. While it

is clear that primate species vary tremendously in terms of their social behaviors, it is not at all clear to what extent this variation might result from innate or from acquired factors,[85] and it is also far from clear that there is any correlation between aspects of social behavior and comparative anatomy of the frontal lobes.[86]

Somatosensory Cortices: Empathy and Simulation

I have mentioned several examples of processes that all appear to operate in a relatively domain-specific fashion on socially relevant information. The examples range from specialized perceptual processing of eyes and faces to reasoning about social exchange. To qualify truly as high-level cognition, social cognition must rely on particular types of representations. Specifically, a social organism must be able to represent not only its own body states in response to conspecific stimuli, but must also possess mechanisms for constructing detailed representations of the conspecific stimuli themselves. Social cognition should permit the construction of a mental model, a comprehensive representation, of other individuals, and of what it is about those individuals that is important to know about them as social agents who have the possibility of interacting with us.

In order to answer the question of how we represent other individuals, it is useful to consider how we represent ourselves. In fact, one line of thinking has argued that we represent the minds of others by attempting to simulate another person's state in our own brain (see Box 22.3). Our ability to judge other people's emotions, behavioral dispositions, beliefs and desires might draw substantially on our ability to empathize with them: that is, to create a model in our own minds of what the other person is feeling. It would seem that such an ability would be essential in order to adopt another person's point of view in a comprehensive manner, and that it would aid in the ability to predict other people's behavior.

This idea might help to explain why emotion and social cognition are closely related, not only in terms of shared processing strategies, but in fact in terms of their neural substrates: most structures important to social cognition are also important to normal emotional functioning. The common ingredient may be what we commonly call "feeling": the representation of emotional body states, either in regard to one's own emotional reaction, or in regard to the empathy for, or simulation of, another person's internal state.

In addition to the amygdala and ventromedial frontal cortices, which can trigger emotional responses to socially relevant stimuli, there is evidence for a third important structure that contributes directly to our ability to construct representations of other individuals. In a study of subjects with focal brain lesions, we found that recognition of emotions from other people's facial expressions critically relied on the integrity of somatosensory-related cortices in the right hemisphere (including S-I, S-II, and insula[87,88]). In our study, somatosensory structures were particularly important in order to judge complex blends of multiple emotions in a single face. The finding may be explained as follows. When asked to judge the emotion shown in a face, there are at least two different strategies that could conceivably contribute to performance. Subjects might reason about the other person's emotion from knowledge regarding the facial configurations normally associated with certain emotions (e.g. reasoning that a smile signals happiness). A second strategy would be to generate somatosensory images that correspond to the way one would feel if one were making the facial expression shown in the stimulus; such a procedure might work best in cases where no prior factual knowledge is readily available (e.g. asking difficult questions concerning how much anger there is in a sad face, or an afraid face, as we did in our task). This second idea proposes that subjects judge another person's emotional state from the facial expression by reconstructing in their own brains a simulation of what the other person might be feeling. That is, subjects who are looking at pictures of facial expressions ask themselves how they would feel if they were making the facial expression shown in the stimulus (either overtly or covertly). The finding from our study is consistent with many other studies that have found social and emotional impairments following right hemisphere damage,[89,90] including an impaired ability to attribute higher-order mental states to other people in theory-of-mind tasks[91] (Box 22.3).

Box 22.3
How do we represent the minds of others?

Primates appear to be highly skilled at predicting other individuals' behavior, but there is vigorous debate about how to interpret such an ability. The mechanisms by which we represent and predict other people's behavior have been viewed from two different theoretical perspectives. The two main camps argue either for a "theory of mind," or for a set of processes that permits "simulation" of other minds. The "theory"-theory has been floated for some time in philosophy of mind as a possible explanation of what is commonly called "folk psychology": our commonsense understanding of other people's behavior in terms of intervening mental states, such as beliefs, desires and intentions, on the basis of which people act. The other camp, however, views our ability to recognize and reason about other people's states of mind as an example of experience projection; in essence, we know other minds by empathy, or by simulation. It is likely that both these views have some truth to them, depending on the circumstances (see Ref. a for examples of both sides of the debate). The theory-view might afford greater economy and generalizability of prediction, or might be particularly suited to information that can be lexically encoded; but simulation may be the only option in cases that are sufficiently idiosyncratic, or in cases where the information is not easily encoded into language. In the latter situation, it could be that the only way to predict what another person will do is to run in one's own brain the processes that the other person is running in theirs. If this possibility is taken seriously, it suggests a role for conscious experience in social cognition: to obtain information about another person's internal mental state, it may be necessary to imagine what it would be like to be the other person via direct simulation. Simulation might find its developmental origins in infants' ability to mimic facial expressions spontaneously (Ref. b), and it has found some recent neurophysiological support from the finding of so-called "mirror neurons," which appear to participate in simulating the actions of other individuals (Ref. c).

Research into how we represent other minds began with a question about whether or not chimpanzees might possess a theory of mind (Ref. d), a question that is still unanswered (Ref. e). In humans, the theory-of-mind question was posed concretely in terms of the ability to attribute beliefs, specifically false beliefs, to other individuals. It has been shown that this ability begins to emerge around age four or possibly earlier (Refs. f,g). The abilities that constitute a theory of mind have been fractionated into several distinct components, such as the ability to attribute desires, to recognize objects of shared attention, and to monitor others' direction of gaze. All these different components appear at distinct developmental stages in humans, and there is evidence that some of them may be selectively impaired in subjects with autism, a disorder that exhibits marked difficulties in social behavior (Ref. h).

Several lesion and functional imaging studies have investigated the neural structures by which subjects generate knowledge about other people's mental states. In addition to a large literature demonstrating the involvement of amygdala, orbitofrontal cortices, and right hemisphere cortices in more general processing of emotion, including recognition of emotion in others, some studies have explicitly investigated attribution of higher-order mental states, such as beliefs and intentions. A recent study by Stone et al. found that subjects with bilateral damage to the orbitofrontal cortex were specifically impaired in their ability to attribute higher-order mental states to other people from stories (Ref. i). In particular, they were unable to detect a *faux pas*, something that subjects with high-functioning autism (Asperger syndrome) also fail. A functional imaging study that compared brain activation during theory-of-mind tasks between normal and high-functioning autistic subjects found evidence that sectors of left medial prefrontal cortex were also important to reason about other people's mental states (Ref. j), a finding consistent with earlier studies that showed that processing words for mental states (Ref. k), or reasoning about the beliefs and intentions of others (Ref. l), normally activates regions in medial prefrontal cortex. In regard to the amygdala, an fMRI study

Box 22.3
(continued)

demonstrated amygdala activation when normal subjects had to attribute mental states and intentions to other people from looking at pictures of their eyes (Ref. m). Interestingly, this is a task that high-functioning subjects with autism fail behaviorally (Ref. n), and also in which, unlike normal individuals, the amygdala does not appear to be activated (Ref. m). As far as right hemisphere somatosensory-related cortex is concerned, in addition to a large literature implicating this region in more general emotional processing, a recent lesion study showed that damage to this area can impair the ability to attribute mental states, such as false beliefs, to other individuals (Ref. o).

References

a. Carruthers, P. and Smith, P. K., eds (1996) *Theories of Theories of Mind,* Cambridge University Press

b. Meltzoff, A. N. and Moore, M. K. (1977) Imitation of facial and manual gestures by human neonates *Science* 198, 74–78

c. Gallese, V. and Goldman, A. (1999) Mirror neurons and the simulation theory of mind-reading *Trends Cognit. Sci.* 2, 493–500

d. Premack, D. and Woodruff, G. (1978) Does the chimpanzee have a theory of mind? *Behav. Brain Sci.* 1, 515–526

e. Povinelli, D. J. and Preuss, T. M. (1995) Theory of mind: evolutionary history of a cognitive specialization *Trends Neurosci.* 18, 418–424

f. Wimmer, H. and Perner, J. (1983) Beliefs about beliefs: representation and constraining function of wrong beliefs in young children's understanding of deception *Cognition* 13, 103–128

g. Perner, J. and Lang, B. (1999) Development of theory of mind and executive control *Trends Cognit. Sci.* 3, 337–344

h. Baron-Cohen, S. (1995) *Mindblindness: an Essay on Autism and Theory of Mind,* MIT Press

i. Stone, V. E., Baron-Cohen, S. and Knight, R. T. (1998) Frontal lobe contributions to theory of mind *J. Cogn. Neurosci.* 10, 640–656

j. Happe, F. et al. (1996) "Theory of mind" in the brain. Evidence from a PET scan study of Asperger syndrome *NeuroReport* 8, 197–201

k. Baron-Cohen, S. et al. (1994) Recognition of mental state terms *Br. J. Psychiatry* 165, 640–649

l. Goel, V. et al. (1995) Modeling other minds *NeuroReport* 6, 1741–1746

m. Baron-Cohen, S. et al. (1999) Social intelligence in the normal and autistic brain: an fMRI study *Eur. J. Neurosci.* 11, 1891–1898

n. Baron-Cohen, S., Wheelwright, S. and Jolliffe, T. (1997) Is there a "language of the eyes"? Evidence from normal adults and adults with autism or Asperger Syndrome *Visual Cognit.* 4, 311–332

o. Happe, F., Brownell, H. and Winner, E. (1999) Acquired "theory of mind" impairments following stroke *Cognition* 70, 211–240

Conclusions

Social cognition draws upon a vast set of abilities. Some of these are quite specific to the social domain, and others may be more general in their application. Some classes of emotions, such as guilt, shame, embarrassment and jealousy, only make sense in a social context and may have evolved to subserve very specific roles in social communication. Other social signals, and other types of social judgments, draw upon systems that subserve emotional processing in general, systems that permit us to build models of other individuals through simulation, and a vast network of structures that contribute to reasoning, inference and language.

Three structures have been highlighted in this review: amygdala, ventromedial frontal cortex, and right somatosensory-related cortex. Normally, in a typical, complex, emotionally salient situation in real life, all three component structures will operate in parallel: the amygdala will provide a quick and automatic bias with respect to those aspects of the response that pertain to evaluating the potentially threatening nature of the situation, or with respect to allocating processing resources to those stimuli that are potentially important but ambiguous; ventromedial frontal cortex will associate elements of the situation with elements of previously encountered situations, and trigger a re-enactment of the corresponding emotional state; and right somatosensory-related cortices will be called upon to the extent that a detailed, comprehensive representation of the body state associated with emotional or social behavior needs to be made available. All of these components would be important to guide social behavior in a typical situation in real life, and all of them emphasize the close link between emotion and social cognition.

There is no doubt that humans differ from other animals in their social skills, in that they are able to form higher-order representations of the social environment, and to manipulate those representations in reasoning that can be quite flexible. On the other hand, there is also good evidence that our reasoning is biased in domain-specific ways, and that our judgment of other individuals, and our behavioral responses towards them, are strongly influenced by mechanisms that we share in common with other animals. The challenge for the future will be to offer a more precise account of the interplay between all these different processes as a function of the detailed specification of the performance demands required by a given experimental task, or by a given situation in real life.

Acknowledgements

I thank my colleagues for their support of, and participation in, several of the studies reviewed here: Antonio Damasio, Hanna Damasio, Daniel Tranel, Antoine Bechara and Andrea Heberlein. Thanks also go to Leslie Brothers, Andrea Heberlein and the anonymous reviewers in providing helpful critiques of earlier drafts. Supported by NINDS Program Project Grant NS19632 to Antonio R. Damasio; and by NIMH Grant MH57905-02, and grants from the EJLB Foundation and the Alfred P. Sloan Foundation to R.A.

References

1. Dunbar, R. (1998) The social brain hypothesis *Evol. Anthropol.* 6, 178–190.

2. Allman, J. M. (1999) *Evolving Brains,* Scientific American Library.

3. Potts, R. (1998) Environmental hypotheses of hominin evolution *Yearbook Phys. Anthropol.* 41, 93–136.

4. Whiten, A. and Byrne, R. W. (1997) *Machiavellian Intelligence II: Extensions and Evaluations,* Cambridge University Press.

5. Brothers, L. (1990) The social brain: a project for integrating primate behavior and neurophysiology in a new domain *Concepts Neurosci.* 1, 27–51.

6. Brothers, L. (1997) *Friday's Footprint,* Oxford University Press.

7. Kluver, H. and Bucy, P. C. (1939) Preliminary analysis of functions of the temporal lobes in monkeys *Arch. Neurol. Psychiatry* 42, 979–997.

8. Emery, N. J. et al. (1998) Role of the amygdala in dyadic social interactions and the stress response in monkeys *Soc. Neurosci. Abstr.* 24, 780.

9. Meunier, M. et al. (1996) Effects of aspiration vs neurotoxic lesions of the amygdala on emotional reactivity in rhesus monkeys *Soc. Neurosci. Abstr.* 22, 1867.

10. Zola-Morgan, S. et al. (1991) Independence of memory functions and emotional behavior: separate contributions of the hippocampal formation and the amygdala *Hippocampus* 1, 207–220.

11. Swanson, L. W. and Petrovich, G. D. (1998) What is the amygdala? *Trends Neurosci.* 21, 323–331.

12. Perrett, D. I., Rolls, E. T. and Caan, W. (1982) Visual neurons responsive to faces in the monkey temporal cortex *Exp. Brain Res.* 47, 329–342.

13. Hasselmo, M. E., Rolls, E. T. and Baylis, G. C. (1989) The role of expression and identity in the face-selective responses of neurons in the temporal visual cortex of the monkey *Behav. Brain Res.* 32, 203–218.

14. Nakamura, K., Mikami, A. and Kubota, K. (1992) Activity of single neurons in the monkey amygdala during performance of a visual discrimination task *J. Neurophysiol.* 67, 1447–1463.

15. Young, M. P. and Yamane, S. (1992) Sparse population coding of faces in the inferotemporal cortex *Science* 256, 1327–1330.

16. Brothers, L., Ring, B. and Kling, A. (1990) Response of neurons in the macaque amygdala to complex social stimuli *Behav. Brain Res.* 41, 199–213.

17. Brothers, L. and Ring, B. (1993) Mesial temporal neurons in the macaque monkey with responses selective for aspects of social stimuli *Behav. Brain Res.* 57, 53–61.

18. Perrett, D. I. et al. (1985) Visual cells in the temporal cortex sensitive to face view and gaze direction *Proc. R. Soc. London Ser. B* 223, 293–317.

19. Oram, M. W. et al. (1998) The "ideal homunculus": decoding neural population signals *Trends Neurosci.* 21, 259–265.

20. Damasio, H. et al. (1994) The return of Phineas Gage: clues about the brain from the skull of a famous patient *Science* 264, 1102–1104.

21. Leslie, A. (1987) Pretense and representation: the origins of "theory of mind" *Psychol. Rev.* 94, 412–426.

22. Baron-Cohen, S. (1995) *Mindblindness: an Essay on Autism and Theory of Mind,* MIT Press.

23. Karmiloff-Smith, A. et al. (1995) Is there a social module? Language, face processing, and theory of mind in individuals with Williams Syndrome *J. Cogn. Neurosci.* 7, 196–208.

24. Tager-Flusberg, H., Boshart, J. and Baron-Cohen, S. (1998) Reading the windows to the soul: evidence of domain-specific sparing in Williams Syndrome *J. Cogn. Neurosci.* 10, 631–640.

25. Baron-Cohen, S., Wheelwright, S. and Jolliffe, T. (1997) Is there a "language of the eyes"? Evidence from normal adults and adults with autism or Asperger Syndrome *Visual Cognit.* 4, 311–332.

26. Baron-Cohen, S. et al. (1999) Social intelligence in the normal and autistic brain: an fMRI study *Eur. J. Neurosci.* 11, 1891–1898.

27. Bellugi, U. et al. (1999) Towards the neural basis for hypersociability in a genetic syndrome *NeuroReport* 10, 1653–1659.

28. Kanwisher, N., McDermott, J. and Chun, M. M. (1997) The fusiform face area: a module in human extrastriate cortex specialized for face perception *J. Neurosci.* 17, 4302–4311.

29. Puce, A. et al. (1998) Temporal cortex activation in humans viewing eye and mouth movements *J. Neurosci.* 18, 2188–2199.

30. Gauthier, I. et al. (1999) Activation of the middle fusiform "face area" increases with expertise in recognizing novel objects *Nat. Neurosci.* 2, 568–573.

31. Amaral, D. G. et al. (1992) Anatomical Organization of the Primate Amygdaloid Complex, in *The Amygdala: Neurobiological Aspects of Emotion, Memory, and Mental Dysfunction* (Aggleton, J. P., ed.), pp. 1–66, John Wiley & Sons.

32. Leonard, C. M. et al. (1985) Neurons in the amygdala of the monkey with responses selective for faces *Behav. Brain Res.* 15, 159–176.

33. Rolls, E. T. (1992) Neurophysiology and Functions of the Primate Amygdala, in *The Amygdala: Neurobiological Aspects of Emotion, Memory, and Mental Dysfunction* (Aggleton, J. P., ed.), pp. 143–167, John Wiley & Sons.

34. Morris, J. S. et al. (1996) A differential neural response in the human amygdala to fearful and happy facial expressions *Nature* 383, 812–815.

35. Breiter, H. C. et al. (1996) Response and habituation of the human amygdala during visual processing of facial expression *Neuron* 17, 875–887.

36. Adolphs, R. et al. (1994) Impaired recognition of emotion in facial expressions following bilateral damage to the human amygdala *Nature* 372, 669–672.

37. Young, A. W. et al. (1995) Face processing impairments after amygdalotomy *Brain* 118, 15–24.

38. Adolphs, R. et al. (1999) Recognition of facial emotion in nine subjects with bilateral amygdala damage *Neuropsychologia* 37, 1111–1117.

39. Le Doux, J. (1996) *The Emotional Brain,* Simon & Schuster.

40. Davis, M. (1992) The role of the amygdala in conditioned fear, in *The Amygdala: Neurobiological Aspects of Emotion, Memory, and Mental Dysfunction* (Aggleton, J. P., ed.), pp. 255–306, John Wiley & Sons.

41. Whalen, P. (1999) Fear, vigilance, and ambiguity: initial neuroimaging studies of the human amygdala *Curr. Dir. Psychol. Sci.* 7, 177–187.

42. Kawashima, R. et al. (1999) The human amygdala plays an important role in gaze monitoring *Brain* 122, 779–783.

43. Adolphs, R., Tranel, D. and Damasio, A. R. (1998) The human amygdala in social judgment *Nature* 393, 470–474.

44. Adolphs, R. and Tranel, D. (1999) Preferences for visual stimuli following amygdala damage *J. Cogn. Neurosci.* 11, 610–616.

45. Isenberg, N. et al. (1999) Linguistic threat activates the human amygdala *Proc. Natl. Acad. Sci. U. S. A.* 96, 10456–10459.

46. Adolphs, R., Russell, J. A. and Tranel, D. (1999) A role for the human amygdala in recognizing emotional arousal from unpleasant stimuli *Psychol. Sci.* 10, 167–171.

47. Adolphs, R. et al. (1995) Fear and the human amygdala *J. Neurosci.* 15, 5879–5892.

48. Heider, F. and Simmel, M. (1944) An experimental study of apparent behavior *Am. J. Psychol.* 57, 243–259.

49. Heberlein, A. S. et al. (1998) Impaired attribution of social meanings to abstract dynamic visual patterns following damage to the amygdala *Soc. Neurosci. Abstr.* 24, 1176.

50. Holland, P. C. and Gallagher, M. (1999) Amygdala circuitry in attentional and representational processes *Trends Cognit. Sci.* 3, 65–73.

51. Bradley, M. M. et al. (1992) Remembering pictures: pleasure and arousal in memory *J. Exp. Psychol. Learn. Mem. Cognit.* 18, 379–390.

52. Mealey, L., Daood, C. and Krage, M. (1996) Enhanced memory for faces of cheaters *Ethol. Sociobiol.* 17, 119–128.

53. Cahill, L. et al. (1996) Amygdala activity at encoding correlated with long-term, free recall of emotional information *Proc. Natl. Acad. Sci. U. S. A.* 93, 8016–8021.

54. Hamann, S. B. et al. (1999) Amygdala activity related to enhanced memory for pleasant and aversive stimuli *Nat. Neurosci.* 2, 289–293.

55. Adolphs, R. et al. (1997) Impaired declarative memory for emotional material following bilateral amygdala damage in humans *Learn. Mem.* 4, 291–300.

56. Langlois, J. H. and Roggman, L. A. (1990) Attractive faces are only average *Psychol. Sci.* 1, 115–121.

57. Perrett, D. I., May, K. A. and Yoshikawa, S. (1994) Facial shape and judgments of female attractiveness *Nature* 368, 239–242.

58. Miller, G. F. and Todd, P. M. (1998) Mate choice turns cognitive *Trends Cognit. Sci.* 2, 190–198.

59. Kalick, S. M. et al. (1998) Does human facial attractiveness honestly advertise health? Longitudinal data on an evolutionary question *Psychol. Sci.* 9, 8–13.

60. Perrett, D. I. et al. (1998) Effects of sexual dimorphism on facial attractiveness *Nature* 394, 884–887.

61. Penton-Voak, I. S. et al. (1999) Menstrual cycle alters face preference *Nature* 399, 741–742.

62. Mirsky, R. et al. (1997) Single-unit neuronal activity in human amygdala and ventral frontal cortex recorded during emotional experience *Soc. Neurosci. Abstr.* 23, 1318.

63. Fried, I., MacDonald, K. A. and Wilson, C. L. (1997) Single neuron activity in human hippocampus and amygdala during recognition of faces and objects *Neuron* 18, 753–765.

64. Gaffan, D., Murray, E. A. and Fabre-Thorpe, M. (1993) Interaction of the amygdala with the frontal lobe in reward memory *Eur. J. Neurosci.* 5, 968–975.

65. Rolls, E. T. (1999) *The Brain and Emotion,* Oxford University Press.

66. Damasio, A. R. (1994) *Descartes' Error: Emotion, Reason, and the Human Brain,* Grosset/Putnam.

67. Schoenbaum, G., Chiba, A. A. and Gallagher, M. (1998) Orbitofrontal cortex and basolateral amygdala encode expected outcomes during learning *Nat. Neurosci.* 1, 155–159.

68. Ackerly, S. S. and Benton, A. L. (1948) Report of a case of bilateral frontal lobe defect *Res. Publ. Assoc. Res. Nerv. Ment. Disord.* 27, 479–504.

69. Brickner, R. M. (1932) An interpretation of frontal lobe function based upon the study of a case of partial bilateral frontal lobectomy: localization of function in the cerebral cortex *Proc. Assoc. Res. Nerv. Ment. Dis.* 13, 259.

70. Bechara, A. et al. (1994) Insensitivity to future consequences following damage to human prefrontal cortex *Cognition* 50, 7–15.

71. Bechara, A. et al. (1997) Deciding advantageously before knowing the advantageous strategy *Science* 275, 1293–1295.

72. Bechara, A. et al. (1996) Failure to respond autonomically to anticipated future outcomes following damage to prefrontal cortex *Cereb. Cortex* 6, 215–225.

73. Damasio, A. R., Tranel, D. and Damasio, H. (1990) Individuals with sociopathic behavior caused by frontal damage fail to respond autonomically to social stimuli *Behav. Brain Res.* 41, 81–94.

74. Damasio, A. R. (1996) The somatic marker hypothesis and the possible functions of the prefrontal cortex *Phil. Trans. R. Soc. London Ser. B* 351, 1413–1420.

75. Wason, P. C. and Johnson-Laird, P. N. (1972) *Psychology of Reasoning: Structure and Content,* Batsford.

76. Wharton, C. M. and Grafman, J. (1998) Deductive reasoning and the brain *Trends Cognit. Sci.* 2, 54–59.

77. Cosmides, L. and Tooby, J. (1992) Cognitive adaptations for social exchange, in *The Adapted Mind: Evolutionary Psychology and the Generation of Culture* (Barkow, J. H., Cosmides, L. and Tooby, J., eds), pp. 163–228, Oxford University Press.

78. Adolphs, R. et al. (1995) Neuropsychological approaches to reasoning and decision-making, in *Neurobiology of Decision Making* (Christen, Y., Damasio, A. and Damasio, H., eds), pp. 157–179, Springer-Verlag.

79. Fuster, J. M. (1989) *The Prefrontal Cortex. Anatomy, Physiology, and Neuropsychology of the Frontal Lobe,* Raven Press.

80. Kolb, B. and Taylor, L. (1990) Neocortical substrates of emotional behavior. In: *Psychological and Biological Approaches to Emotion* (Stein, N. L., Leventhal, B. and Trabasso, T., eds), pp. 115–144, Erlbaum.

81. Butter, C. M. and Snyder, D. R. (1972) Alternations in aversive and aggressive behaviors following orbital frontal lesions in rhesus monkeys *Acta Neurobiol. Exp.* 32, 525–565.

82. Butter, C. M., Mishkin, M. and Mirsky, A. F. (1968) Emotional responses toward humans in monkeys with selective frontal lesions *Physiol. Behav.* 3, 213–215.

83. Raleigh, M. J. et al. (1996) Neural mechanisms supporting successful social decisions in simians, in *Neurobiology of Decision Making* (Christen, Y., Damasio, A. and Damasio, H., eds), pp. 63–82, Springer-Verlag.

84. Panksepp, J. (1998) *Affective Neuroscience,* Oxford University Press.

85. Whiten, A. et al. (1999) Cultures in chimpanzees *Nature* 399, 682–685.

86. Semendeferi, K. et al. (1997) The evolution of the frontal lobes: a volumetric analysis based on three-dimensional reconstructions of magnetic resonance scans of human and ape brains *J. Hum. Evol.* 32, 375–388.

87. Adolphs, R. et al. (1996) Cortical systems for the recognition of emotion in facial expressions *J. Neurosci.* 16, 7678–7687.

88. Adolphs, R. et al. (1996) The right second somatosensory cortex (S-II) is required to recognize emotional facial expressions in humans *Soc. Neurosci. Abstr.* 22, 1854.

89. Bowers, D. et al. (1985) Processing of faces by patients with unilateral hemisphere lesions *Brain Cognit.* 4, 258–272.

90. Borod, J. C. et al. (1998) Right hemisphere emotional perception: evidence across multiple channels *Neuropsychology* 12, 446–458.

91. Happe, F., Brownell, H. and Winner, E. (1999) Acquired "theory of mind" impairments following stroke *Cognition* 70, 211–240.

92. Adolphs, R. and Damasio, A. R. (1995) Human reasoning and the frontal cortex *Soc. Neurosci. Abstr.* 21, 1213.

23 Impairment of Social and Moral Behavior Related to Early Damage in Human Prefrontal Cortex

Steven W. Anderson, Antoine Bechara, Hanna Damasio, Daniel Tranel, and Antonio R. Damasio

It is well established that in adults who have had normal development of social behavior, damage to certain sectors of prefrontal cortex produces a severe impairment of decision-making and disrupts social behavior, although the patients so affected preserve intellectual abilities and maintain factual knowledge of social conventions and moral rules.[1-6] Little is known for certain, however, about the consequences of comparable damage occurring before the maturation of the relevant neural and cognitive systems, namely in infancy, because such cases are exceedingly rare. Information about the early onset condition is vital to the elucidation of how social and moral competencies develop from a neurobiological standpoint. A number of questions have arisen in this regard. First, would early-onset lesions lead to the appearance of persistent defects comparable to those seen in adult-onset lesions, or would further development and brain plasticity reduce or cancel the effects of the lesions and prevent the appearance of the defects? Second, assuming early-onset lesions cause a comparable defect, would there be a dissociation between disrupted social behavior and preserved factual social knowledge, as seen in the adult-onset condition, or would the acquisition of social knowledge at factual level be compromised as well? We addressed these questions by investigating two young adults who received focal nonprogressive prefrontal damage before 16 months of age.

Results

The evidence presented here is based on detailed histories obtained from medical and school records, as well as legal documents, extensive interviews with the patients' parents, clinical and experimental cognitive tasks and neuroimaging studies.

Clinical Evidence

The first patient (subject A) was 20 years old at the time of these studies and was ambidextrous. She had been run over by a vehicle at age 15 months. At the time of the accident, she appeared to recover fully within days. No behavioral abnormalities were observed until the age of three years, when she was first noted to be largely unresponsive to verbal or physical punishment. Her behavior became progressively disruptive, so much so that, by age 14, she required placement in the first of several treatment facilities. Her teachers considered her to be intelligent and academically capable, but she routinely failed to complete assigned tasks. Her adolescence was marked by disruptive behavior in school and at home (for example, failure to comply with rules, frequent loud confrontations with peers and adults). She stole from her family and from other children and shoplifted frequently, leading to multiple arrests. She was verbally and physically abusive to others. She lied chronically. Her lack of friends was conspicuous. She ran away from home and from treatment facilities. She exhibited early and risky sexual behavior leading to a pregnancy at age 18. Contingency management in residential treatment facilities and the use of psychotropic medication were of no help. After repeatedly putting herself at physical and financial risk, she became entirely dependent on her parents and on social agencies for financial support and oversight of her personal affairs. She did not formulate any plans for her future and she sought no employment. Whenever employment was arranged, she was unable to hold the job due to lack of dependability and gross infractions of rules. Affect was labile and often poorly matched to the situation, but superficial social behavior was unremarkable. She never expressed guilt or remorse for her misbehavior. There was little or no evidence that she experienced empathy, and her maternal behavior was marked by dangerous insensitivity to the infant's needs. She blamed her misdeeds and social difficulties on other people, and she denied any difficulties with cognition or behavior.

When first seen by us, the second patient (subject B) was 23 years old. He had undergone resection of a right frontal tumor at age three months. He had an excellent recovery and there were no signs of recurrence. Developmental milestones were normal and he was left handed. In early grade school, mild difficulties were noted with behavior control and peer interactions, but he was not especially disruptive in school or at home. By age nine, however, he showed a general lack of motivation, had limited social interactions, usually exhibited a neutral affect and suffered from occasional brief and explosive outbursts of anger. His work habits were poor, and tutoring was recommended. He was able to graduate from high school, but perhaps because of the loss of structure for daily activities, his behavioral problems escalated after graduation. Left to himself, he limited his activities to viewing television and listening to music. His personal hygiene was poor and his living quarters were filthy. He consumed large quantities of foods with high fat and sugar content, and became progressively more obese. He also displayed abnormal food choices, for instance, eating uncooked frozen foods. Given his frequent absences, tardiness and general lack of dependability, he could not hold a job. He showed reckless financial behavior which resulted in large debts, and engaged in poorly planned petty thievery. He frequently threatened others and occasionally engaged in physical assault. He lied frequently, often without apparent motive. He had no lasting friendships and displayed little empathy. His sexual behavior was irresponsible. He fathered a child in a casual relationship, and did not fulfill his paternal obligations. He was dependent on his parents for financial support and legal guardianship. He showed no guilt or remorse for his

behavior and could not formulate any realistic plans for his future.

Both patients were raised in stable, middle-class homes by college-educated parents who devoted considerable time and resources to their children. In neither case was there a family history of neurologic or psychiatric disease, and both patients had socially well-adapted siblings whose behavior was normal. The neurological evaluation was normal in both patients, except for their behavioral defects.

Neuropsychological Evidence

Comprehensive neuropsychological evaluations (Table 23.1) revealed normal performances on measures of intellectual ability (for example, fund of general information, ability to repeat and reverse random sequence of digits, mental arithmetic, verbal reasoning, nonverbal problem solving, verbal and visual anterograde memory, speech and language, visuospatial perception, visuomotor abilities and academic achievement). As in the case of patients with adult-onset lesions, the behavioral inadequacy of the two patients with early-onset lesions cannot be explained by a failure in basic mental abilities.

The patients were asked to perform several cognitive tasks designed to assess their ability to plan and execute multistep procedures, use contingencies to guide behavior, reason through social dilemmas and generate appropriate responses to social situations. Both patients had significant impairments on these tasks. They failed to show normal learning of rules and strategies from repeated experience and feedback (Wisconsin Card Sorting Test, Subject A; Tower of Hanoi, both subjects). They also had significant impairments of social-moral reasoning and verbal generation of responses to social situations (Fig. 23.1). Moral reasoning was conducted at a very early ("preconventional") stage, in which moral dilemmas were approached largely from the egocentric perspective of avoiding punishment.[7] This stage of moral reasoning is characteristic of

Table 23.1
Standardized neuropsychological test data

		Subject A	Subject B
WAIS-R			
	Information	37	63
	Digit span	25	37
	Arithmetic	37	63
	Similarities	37	25
	Block design	75	75
	Digit symbol	25	25
RAVLT			
	Trial 5	78	11
	30 min. recall	99	68
JLO		40	57
Complex figure test			
	Copy	21	39
	30 min. recall	32	66
WRAT-R			
	Reading	86	63
	Spelling	81	63
	Arithmetic	32	58
COWA		43	15
WCST			
	Categories	>16	>16
	Persev. errors	1*	88
TOH			
	Trial 1	7*	7*
	Trial 2	1*	51
	Trial 3	1*	1*
	Trial 4	1*	1*
	Trial 5	1*	1*

WAIS-R, Wechsler Adult Intelligence Scale-Revised; RAVLT, Rey Auditory Verbal Learning Test; JLO, Judgment of Line Orientation; WRAT-R, Wide Range Achievement Test-Revised; COWA, Controlled Oral Word Association; WCST, Wisconsin Card Sorting Test; TOH, Tower of Hanoi. All tests were administered according to standardized procedures.[27,28,29] Test performances are represented as percentile scores and impairment is indicated by an asterisk.

10-year-olds, and is surpassed by most young adolescents. The patients demonstrated limited consideration of the social and emotional implications of decisions, failed to identify the primary issues involved in social dilemmas and generated few response options for interpersonal conflicts. Their performance was in stark contrast to that of patients with adult-onset prefrontal damage, who can access the "facts" of social knowledge in the format used in the laboratory (verbally packaged, outside of real life and real time[8]).

To explore the decision-making process further, the patients participated in a computerized version of the Gambling Task.[9,10] This task simulates real-life decision-making in the way it factors uncertainty of rewards and punishments associated with various response options. Unlike normal controls, but precisely as patients with adult-onset prefrontal lesions, both patients failed to develop a preference for the advantageous response options. They failed to choose options with low immediate reward but positive long-term gains; rather, they persisted in choosing response options which provided high immediate reward but higher long-term loss (Fig. 23.2).

The electrodermal skin conductance response (SCR) was used as a dependent measure of somatic-state activation, according to methods described elsewhere.[11] After repeated trials, normal controls begin to generate anticipatory SCRs when pondering the selection of a risky response (a response which may lead to long-term punishment). However, both patients failed to acquire these anticipatory SCRs, although they did show normal SCRs to a variety of unconditioned stimuli. Again, these findings were similar to those from patients with adult-onset prefrontal damage.[11]

Neuroimaging Evidence

The patients were studied with research-protocol magnetic resonance imaging, which permitted reconstruction of their brains in three dimensions

Level 3: Postconventional Stage 6: Personal commitment to universal moral principles. Stage 5: Recognition that moral perspective may conflict with law. Consider rights and welfare of all.	Achieved by a minority of adults. One of 6 adult-onset patients at this level.
Level 2: Conventional Stage 4: Recognition of obligations to society. The individual is viewed within the system. Stage 3: Reliance on the Golden Rule. Be a good person in your own eyes and those of others.	Characteristic of most adults and adolescents. Five of 6 adult-onset patients at this level.
Level 1: Preconventional Stage 2: Concrete reasoning that, to serve one's own needs, you must recognize others' rights. Stage 1: Egocentric perspective with decisions based on avoidance of punishment.	Characteristic of most children under age 9. Both early-onset patients at this level.

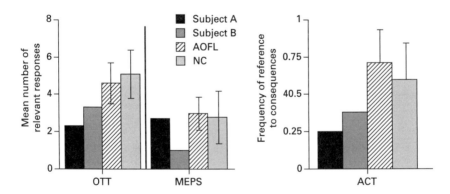

Figure 23.1
Social and moral reasoning. (Top) Kohlberg Moral Judgment Task. (Bottom) Social fluency; OTT, optional thinking test; MEPS, means-ends problem solving; ACT, awareness of consequences.

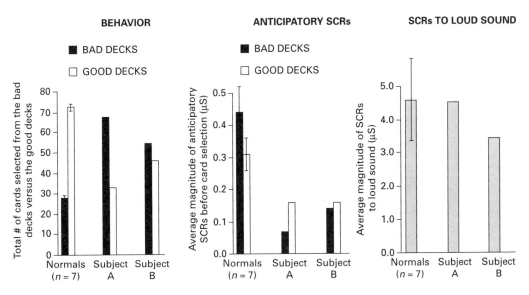

Figure 23.2
Experimental decision-making and psychophysiology. (Left) Responses on the gambling task. (Middle) Anticipatory skin conductance responses (SCRs). (Right) SCRs to an unconditioned stimulus (sudden onset of 110-dB noise).

using the Brainvox technique and subsequent analysis of their anatomical defects. Both patients had focal damage to prefrontal regions, and had no evidence of damage in other brain areas (Fig. 23.3). The lesion in subject A was bilateral and involved the polar and ventromedial prefrontal sectors. The lesion in subject B was unilateral, located in the right prefrontal region, and involved the polar sector, both medially and dorsally. The lesions of both patients were located in sites whose damage in adults is known to produce the emotional and decision-making defects discussed above.[2,3,12] Most frequently, these defects are caused by ventromedial and bilateral lesions, but the condition also has been noted with exclusively right, medial or lateral prefrontal lesions. The critical issue seems to be dysfunction in the medial prefrontal cortices (which can be caused either by direct cortical damage or white matter undercutting) and the sparing of at least one dorsolateral prefrontal sector.

Discussion

We begin by acknowledging that our sample was small, but our findings accord with the only two other recorded instances of patients with early-onset frontal lobe damage,[13,14] both with life-long behavior dysfunction, although in neither case is there precise neuroanatomical information. (One case, from 1947, predates modern neuropsychological and neuroimaging techniques, and lesions of the other are not described satisfactorily and may not be confined to the prefrontal region.) The sample is valuable, nonetheless, because of its rarity, and the evidence is offered in the hope that it calls attention to other existing cases and facilitates their study and the extension of the preliminary investigation noted here.

In answer to the first question we posed, the evidence presented above suggests that patients

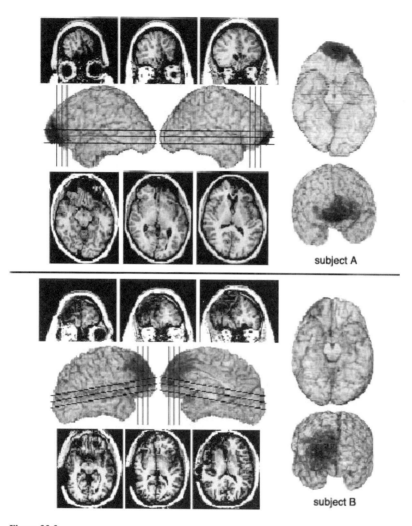

Figure 23.3
Neuroanatomical analysis. (a) 3-D reconstructed brain of patient 1 (Subject A). There was a cystic formation occupying the polar region of both frontal lobes. This cyst displaced and compressed prefrontal regions, especially in the anterior orbital sector, more so on the left than on the right. Brodmann areas 11, 10, and 9 bilaterally, and 46 and 47 on the left, were involved. Additionally, there was structural damage in the right mesial orbital sector and the left polar cortices (Brodmann areas 11, 47, and 10). (b) 3-D reconstructed brain of patient 2 (Subject B). There was extensive damage to the right frontal lobe, encompassing prefrontal cortices in mesial, polar and lateral sectors (Brodmann areas 10, 9, 46, and 8). Both the lateral half of the orbital gyri and the anterior sector of the cingulate gyrus were damaged (Brodmann areas 12, 24, and 32). The cortex of the inferior frontal gyrus was intact (Brodmann areas 44, 45, and 47), but the underlying white matter was damaged, especially in the anterior sector.

with early-onset prefrontal lesions in bilateral ventromedial or right sectors resembled patients with comparable adult-onset lesions in a number of ways. In early-onset patients, emotional responses to social situations and behavior in situations that require knowledge of complex social conventions and moral rules were inadequate. But whereas the early-onset patients were comparable, at first glance, to patients with adult-onset prefrontal lesions, a comprehensive analysis reveals several distinctive features. First, the inadequate social behaviors were present throughout development and into adulthood; second, those behavioral defects were more severe in early-onset patients; third, the patients could not retrieve complex, socially relevant knowledge at the factual level.

The greater severity of impairment in these two subjects was especially notable. The adult-onset prefrontal-lesion patients we studied ($n > 25$) generally do not show the sort of antisocial behavior noted in the early-onset patients, for example, stealing, violence against persons or property. Beyond the acute period, the disruptive behavior of adult-onset patients tends to be more constrained, although impulsiveness and susceptibility to immediately present environmental cues leave them at risk of violating the rights of others. More often than not, the victims are the adult-onset patients themselves, not others, and their social and moral ineptitude can hardly be described as antisocial.

Patients with impairments of social behavior caused by adult-onset lesions of the prefrontal cortex acquire varied aspects of socially relevant knowledge during normal development, and usually have had decades of appropriate application of such knowledge to social situations before incurring brain damage. As shown here and previously, following lesion onset in adulthood, they can continue to access socially relevant knowledge at the level of declarative facts,[5] and they can even solve social problems when presented in a laboratory setting, that is, in a verbal format, outside of real time. This distinction might ex-

plain why the two patients described here seemed to show less of a sense of guilt and remorse relative to their conduct than do adult-onset patients. Admittedly, however, this is a clinical impression, and we have no controlled measurement yet to substantiate it.

The mechanisms whereby adult-onset patients fail in social behaviors are still under investigation, but we have suggested that an important mechanism of the defect is the disruption of the systems that hold covert, emotionally related knowledge of social situations.[2,9] Emotionally related knowledge is presumed to bias the reasoning process covertly, namely, by enhancing attention and working memory related to options for action and future consequences of choices, as well as to bias the process overtly, by qualifying options for action or outcomes of actions in emotional terms. When emotionally related knowledge, covert or overt, is no longer available or cannot be retrieved, as shown in experiments involving failure of anticipatory psychophysiological responses,[10,11] the declarative recall of socially relevant facts either does not occur or is insufficient to ensure adequate social behavior in real-life and real-time circumstances. Given that early-onset patients failed in both emotionally-related and factual modes of retrieval, it is possible that they never acquired socially relevant knowledge, either in emotional or factual modes, and that their profound behavioral inadequacy is explained by an absence of the diverse knowledge base necessary for social and moral behavior.

The cognitive and behavioral defects present in these patients arose in the context of stable social environments that led to normal and well-adapted social behavior in their siblings. In spite of extensive exposure to appropriate social behavior in their home and school environments, and in spite of the relevant instruction, the patients failed to acquire complex social knowledge during the regular development period. Moreover, they failed to respond to programs aimed at correcting their inappropriate behavior during adolescence and young adulthood. This is an intriguing finding. Although comparison of different complex functions should be cautious, it is noteworthy that patients with early damage to language cortices, including those who undergo ablations of the entire left cerebral cortex at ages comparable to those at which our patients acquired their lesions, emerge into adolescence and adulthood with language defects whose magnitude seems smaller than the defects we encounter in the prefrontal patients described here. That the magnitude of compensation seemed smaller in our patients suggests that neural systems impaired by their lesions were critical for the acquisition of social knowledge, at least in the manner in which that acquisition traditionally occurs. It is possible, for instance, that by destroying a critical cortical control for the punishment and reward system, the acquisition of knowledge that depends on the coordinated contributions of punishment and reward situations becomes severely compromised. Should this be the case, it is possible that other neural systems might be recruited for the learning and processing of social knowledge, provided appropriate behavioral or pharmacological interventions could be developed. For example, cognitive-behavioral strategies that rely on a different balance of punishment and reward contributions might prove successful, and administration of neuromodulators such as serotonin and dopamine might conceivably help those interventions.

The cognitive and behavioral profiles resulting from early prefrontal damage resembled, in several respects, the profiles resulting from adult-onset damage. Unlike adult-onset patients, however, early-onset patients could not retrieve complex social knowledge at the factual level, and may never have acquired such knowledge. Overall, the profiles of early-onset patients bore considerable similarity to those of patients with psychopathy or sociopathy ("Conduct Disorder" or "Antisocial Personality Disorder," according to DSM-IV nosology),[15] another early onset disorder characterized by a pervasive disregard for

social and moral standards, consistent irresponsibility and a lack of remorse. Psychopathy may be associated with dysfunction in prefrontal regions,[16-18] especially in persons without predisposing psychosocial risk factors.[18] Also of note, children with antisocial tendencies have deficiencies of moral reasoning relative to age-matched controls,[19,20] and abnormal psychophysiological arousal and reactivity are found in adults with antisocial behavior.[21] The behavior of our patients differed from the typical profile of psychopathy in that our patients' patterns of aggression seemed impulsive rather than goal-directed, and also in the highly transparent, almost child-like nature of their transgressions and their attempts to cover them.

In conclusion, early dysfunction in certain sectors of prefrontal cortex seems to cause abnormal development of social and moral behavior, independently of social and psychological factors, which do not seem to have played a role in the condition of our subjects. This suggests that antisocial behavior may depend, at least in part, on the abnormal operation of a multi-component neural system which includes, but is not limited to, sectors of the prefrontal cortex. The causes of that abnormal operation would range from primarily biological (for instance, genetic, acting at the molecular and cellular levels) to environmental. Further clarification of these questions requires not only additional studies in humans, relying on both lesions and functional neuroimaging, but also experimental studies in developing animals, such as those demonstrating defects in social interactions of neonate monkeys with lesions of the amygdala and inferotemporal cortex.[22]

Methods

The behavioral histories were based on evidence obtained from medical and school records and legal documents, as well as extensive interviews with the patients' parents. Participants in this research provided informed consent in accord with the policies of the Institutional Review Board of the University of Iowa College of Medicine. Neuroimaging analysis was conducted by an investigator blind to neuropsychological information, on the basis of thin-cut T1 weighted magnetic resonance (MR) images using Brainvox.[23,24]

Comprehensive clinical neuropsychological evaluations were conducted according to standardized procedures (Table 23.1). Assessment of social knowledge and moral reasoning was based on four measures, Standard Issue Moral Judgement (SIMJ),[7] the Optional Thinking Test (OTT),[25] the Awareness of Consequences Test (ACT)[25] and the Means-Ends Problem Solving Procedure (MEPS).[26] All of these procedures involve standardized verbal presentation to the subject of moral dilemmas or social situations, and require verbal responses.

In the SIMJ task, a subject is presented with a conflict between two moral imperatives (a man must steal a drug in order to save his wife's life). The subject is asked to describe the protagonist's proper actions and their rationale through a series of standard questions (for example, "Should he steal the drug?" "Is it right or wrong for him to steal it?" or "Why do you think that?"). Responses were scored according to explicit criteria to allow staging of specific levels of moral development. The OTT is designed to measure the ability to generate alternative solutions to hypothetical social dilemmas (for instance, two people disagree on what TV channel to watch). A series of probes are used to elicit as many potential solutions as the subject could produce. The number of discrete relevant alternative solutions is scored. The ACT is intended to sample a subject's spontaneous consideration of the consequences of actions. Hypothetical predicaments involving temptation to transgress ordinary rules of social conduct are presented (for instance, receiving too much money in a business transaction through a mistake), and the subject must describe how the scenario evolves, including the

protagonist's thoughts prior to the action and the subsequent events. Scoring reflects the frequency with which the likely consequences of response options are considered. The MEPS is intended to measure a subject's ability to conceptualize effective means of achieving social goals. Scoring is based on the number of effective instrumental acts described as methods of achieving goals in hypothetical scenarios (for example, how to meet people in a new neighborhood).

In the Gambling Task, subjects are presented with four decks of cards (named A, B, C and D) and instructed to select cards from the decks in a manner to win as much play money as possible. After each card selection, they are awarded some money, but certain selections are also followed by a loss of money. The magnitude of the yield of each deck and the magnitude and frequency of punishment associated with each deck are controlled such that choosing from the decks with low initial reward turns out to be the most advantageous strategy over a long series of selections.[9] Subjects are required to make a series of 100 card selections, but they are not told in advance how many card selections they will be allowed to make. Cards can be selected one at a time from any deck, and subjects are free to switch from any deck to another at any time and as often as they wish. The decision to select from one deck or another is largely influenced by schedules of rewards and punishment. These schedules are pre-programmed and known to the examiner, but not to the subject. They are arranged in such a way that every time a card is selected from deck A or B, the subject gets $100, and every time a card deck is selected from C or D, the subject gets $50. However, in each of the four decks, subjects encounter unpredictable money loss (punishment). The punishment is set to be higher in the high-paying decks, A and B, and lower in the low-paying decks, C and D. In decks A and B, the subject encounters a total loss of $1,250 in every 10 cards. In decks C and D, the subject encounters a total loss of $250 in every 10 cards. In the longer term, decks A and

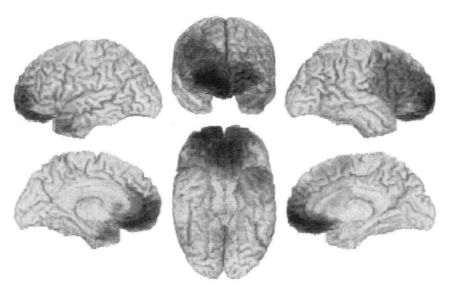

Figure 23.4
Control subjects with adult-onset prefrontal damage. The overlap of lesions in the 6 patients with adult-onset lesions is depicted on a normal reference brain. Lesions of individual subjects were transferred onto the reference brain using MAP-3 (ref. 24). Darker shade indicates a higher number of overlapping subjects. The areas involved include all sectors damaged in the target subjects.

B are disadvantageous because they cost more (a loss of $250 in every 10 cards). Decks C and D are advantageous because they result in an overall gain in the end (a gain of $250 in every 10 cards).[6]

The methods for the psychophysiological recordings (Fig. 23.2) are described.[11] Response selection in the gambling task was temporally linked by computer to ongoing SCR recordings, and SCRs generated in the four seconds before behavioral response selection were considered to be anticipatory responses. The normal control subjects (three male, four female) were matched to the target subjects for age and education. The control subjects with adult onset prefrontal damage (three male, three female) were selected from our database on the basis of lesion location, in order to provide representation of adult-onset damage to prefrontal areas including, and more

extensive than, the areas of damage in the early-onset cases (Fig. 23.4). Lesions were due to a vascular event ($n = 3$) or resection of a meningioma ($n = 3$). Age of lesion onset ranged from 26 to 51 years, and subjects were studied at least one year following onset.

Acknowledgements

Supported by the National Institute of Neurological Diseases and Stroke Grant PO1 NS19632 and the Mathers Foundation.

References

1. Damasio, A. R., Tranel, D. & Damasio, H. in *Frontal Lobe Function and Dysfunction* (eds. Levin, H. S., Eisenberg, H. M. & Benton, A. L.) 217–229 (Oxford Univ. Press, New York, 1991).

2. Damasio, A. R. *Descartes' Error* (Grosset/Putnam, New York, 1994).

3. Damasio, A. R. The somatic marker hypothesis and the possible functions of the prefrontal cortex. *Philos. Trans. R. Soc. Lond. B Biol. Sci.* 351, 1413–1420 (1996).

4. Grafman, J. in *Structure and Functions of the Human Prefrontal Cortex* (eds. Grafman, J., Holyoak, K. J. & Boller, F.) 337–368 (1995).

5. Shallice T. & Burgess, P. W. Deficits in strategy application following frontal lobe damage in man. *Brain* 114, 727–741 (1991).

6. Stuss, D. T. & Benson, D. F. *The Frontal Lobes* (Raven, New York, 1986).

7. Colby, A. & Kohlberg, L. *The Measurement of Moral Judgment* (Cambridge Univ. Press, New York, 1987).

8. Saver, J. & Damasio, A. R. Preserved access and processing of social knowledge in a patient with acquired sociopathy due to ventromedial frontal damage. *Neuropsychologia* 29, 1241–1249 (1991).

9. Bechara, A., Damasio, A. R., Damasio, H. & Anderson, S. W. Insensitivity to future consequences following damage to human prefrontal cortex. *Cognition* 50, 7–15 (1994).

10. Bechara, A., Damasio, H., Tranel, D. & Damasio, A. R. Deciding advantageously before knowing the advantageous strategy. *Science* 275, 1293–1295 (1997).

11. Bechara, A., Tranel, D., Damasio, H. & Damasio, A. R. Failure to respond autonomically to anticipated future outcomes following damage to prefrontal cortex. *Cereb. Cortex* 6, 215–225 (1996).

12. Damasio, A. R. & Anderson, S. W. in *Clinical Neuropsychology,* 3rd edn. (eds. Heilman, K. M. & Valenstein, E.) 409–460 (Oxford Univ. Press, New York, 1993).

13. Ackerly, S. S. & Benton, A. L. Report of a case of bilateral frontal lobe defect. *Assoc. Res. Nerv. Ment. Dis.* 27, 479–504 (1947).

14. Price, B. H., Daffner, K. R., Stowe, R. M. & Mesulam, M. M. The comportmental learning disabilities of early frontal lobe damage. *Brain,* 113, 1383–1393 (1990).

15. American Psychiatric Association. *Diagnostic and Statistical Manual of Mental Disorders* 4th edn. (APA, Washington, District of Columbia, 1994).

16. Deckel, A. W., Hesselbrock, V. & Bauer, L. Antisocial personality disorder, childhood delinquency, and frontal brain functioning: EEG and neuropsychological findings. *J. Clin. Psychol.* 52, 639–650 (1996).

17. Kuruoglu, A. C. et al. Single photon emission computerised tomography in chronic alcoholism. *Br. J. Psychiatry* 169, 348–354 (1996).

18. Raine, A., Stoddard, J., Bihrle, S. & Buchsbaum, M. Prefrontal glucose deficits in murderers lacking psychosocial deprivation. *Neuropsychiatry Neuropsychol. Behav. Neurol.* 11, 1–7 (1998).

19. Campagna, A. F. & Harter, S. Moral judgment in sociopathic and normal children. *J. Pers. Soc. Psychol.* 31, 199–205 (1975).

20. Blair, R. J. R. Moral reasoning and the child with psychopathic tendencies. *Pers. Individ. Diff.* 22, 731–739 (1997).

21. Scarpa, A. & Raine, A. Psychophysiology of anger and violent behavior. *Psychiatr. Clin. North Am.* 20, 375–394 (1997).

22. Newman, J. D. & Bachevalier, J. Neonatal ablations of the amygdala and inferior temporal cortex alter the vocal response to social separation in rhesus macaques. *Brain Res.* 758, 180–186 (1997).

23. Damasio, H. & Frank, R. J. Three-dimensional in vivo mapping of brain lesions in humans. *Arch. Neurol.* 49, 137–143 (1992).

24. Frank, R. J., Damasio, H. & Grabowski, T. J. Brainvox: An interactive, multimodal visualization and analysis system for neuroanatomical imaging. *Neuroimage* 5, 13–30 (1997).

25. Platt, J. J. & Spivack, G. *Measures of Interpersonal Problem-Solving for Adults and Adolescents* (Department of Mental Health Sciences, Hahnemann Medical College, Philadelphia, 1977).

26. Platt, J. J. & Spivack, G. *Manual for the Means-Ends Problem Solving Procedure* (Widener University Institute for Graduate Psychology, Chester, Pennsylvania, 1975).

27. Lezak, M. *Neuropsychological Assessment* 3rd edn. (Oxford Univ. Press, New York, 1995).

28. Davis, H. P., Bajsjar, G. M. & Squire, L. R. *Tower of Hanoi Test—Colorado Neuropsychology Tests Version 2.0* (Western Psychological Services, Los Angeles, 1995).

29. Heaton, R. K. et al. *Wisconsin Card Sorting Test Manual* (Psychological Assessment Resources, Odessa, Florida, 1993).

24   The Human Amygdala in Social Judgment

Ralph Adolphs, Daniel Tranel, and Antonio R. Damasio

Studies in animals have implicated the amygdala in emotional[1-3] and social[4-6] behaviours, especially those related to fear and aggression. Although lesion[7-10] and functional imaging[11-13] studies in humans have demonstrated the amygdala's participation in recognizing emotional facial expressions, its role in human social behaviour has remained unclear. We report here our investigation into the hypothesis that the human amygdala is required for accurate social judgments of other individuals on the basis of their facial appearance. We asked three subjects with complete bilateral amygdala damage to judge faces of unfamiliar people with respect to two attributes important in real-life social encounters: approachability and trustworthiness. All three subjects judged unfamiliar individuals to be more approachable and more trustworthy than did control subjects. The impairment was most striking for faces to which normal subjects assign the most negative ratings: unapproachable and untrustworthy looking individuals. Additional investigations revealed that the impairment does not extend to judging verbal descriptions of people. The amygdala appears to be an important component of the neural systems that help retrieve socially relevant knowledge on the basis of facial appearance.

Data from three subjects with complete bilateral amygdala damage (subjects SM, JM and RH) and seven with unilateral amygdala damage were compared to those from normal and from brain-damaged control subjects (see Table 24.1 and Methods). Ratings of approachability and of trustworthiness were analysed separately for the 50 faces to which normal controls assigned the most negative ratings, and for the 50 most positive faces. Subjects with bilateral amygdala damage rated the 50 most negative faces more positively than did either normal controls ($P < 0.01$) or brain-damaged controls ($P < 0.05$; Mann–Whitney U-tests on subjects' mean rat-

ings, Bonferroni corrected) (Fig. 24.1). Groups with unilateral amygdala lesions did not differ from controls on either rating. All subject groups gave similar ratings to the 50 most positive faces. Subject SM spontaneously commented during the experiment that, in real life, she would not know how to judge if a person were trustworthy, consistent with her tendency to approach and engage in physical contact with other people rather indiscriminately.[7,14] All subjects with bilateral amygdala damage had normal ability to discriminate faces (Table 24.1), clear evidence that there were no visuoperceptual impairments that might account for the above findings.

Data from subjects with bilateral amygdala damage showed two effects: the subjects tended to rate all faces more positively than did controls, and they also showed the largest deviation from control ratings specifically when rating the most negative faces (Fig. 24.2). This suggests an overall positive bias, as well as a disproportionate impairment in rating the most negative faces. To establish the independence of these two effects, we carried out a detailed two-alternative forced-choice task with JM, RH and SM, using the same 100 face stimuli. We asked JM and RH to choose the more approachable face in pairwise comparisons between an anchor face that received a mean normal rating of 0.0 and each of the remaining 99 faces. We compared subjects' choices on this task to the choices that would be expected from the mean approachability ratings given to the faces in each pair by normal controls. JM and RH consistently made more incorrect choices when making comparisons to very negative faces, than when making comparisons to very positive faces (Fig. 24.3a). By contrast, the small number of errors made by normal controls occurred in the opposite direction, with positive rather than with negative faces (Fig. 24.3a), indicating that the impairments seen in amygdala subjects cannot be explained by stimulus difficulty.

Table 24.1
Neuropsychology background data

Subject	SM	JM	RH	Left	Right	BD Ctrl	N Ctrl
N				3	4	10	46
Age	31	67	42	29 ± 5	31 ± 5	66 ± 10	19 ± 1
PIQ	90	95	108	104 ± 24	103 ± 24	98 ± 11	—
Benton (percentile)	71st	12th	20th	32nd	50th	48th	—
Expression discrimination	70 (40)	45 (20)	59 (15)	—	—	—	—
Gender discrimination	75th	65th	65th	—	—	—	—
Gaze discrimination	64th	86th	86th	—	—	—	—

SM, JM, RH, bilateral amygdala damage; Left, Right, unilateral amygdala damage; BD Ctrl and N Ctrl, brain-damaged and normal controls. PIQ, performance IQ from the Wechsler Adult Intelligence Scale-revised. Benton, percentile score on the Benton Facial Recognition Test, a measure of ability to discriminate among unfamiliar faces.[18] Expression, gender, gaze discrimination, percentile score on two-alternative forced-choice discrimination tasks of emotional facial expressions (average and minimum (in parentheses) for the 6 basic emotions), gender, and direction of gaze. See Methods for details.

In subject SM, we carried out forced-choice tasks with a total of five anchor faces, including faces normally rated very negatively and very positively. Each anchor face was paired with the remaining 99 faces, for a total of $5 \times 99 = 495$ pairwise comparisons. SM made the largest number of incorrect choices in comparisons involving those of the five anchor faces that normally receive the most negative ratings, a performance that was highly abnormal compared to control subjects' forced-choices in the same task (Fig. 24.3b). The findings from the forced-choice tasks cannot be explained solely on the basis of a general positive bias, and confirm that judgments given by subjects with bilateral amygdala damage are disproportionately impaired relative to individuals who are normally classified as unapproachable.

Might the impairment seen in subjects with bilateral amygdala damage extend to judging people from word descriptions rather than from faces? We asked subjects to rate the likeability of different individuals based on short verbal biographies or on single words (adjectives describing people). All three subjects with bilateral amygdala damage made entirely normal judgments

when the stimuli were verbal (Fig. 24.4). This critical dissociation supports the following interpretation. The amygdala appears necessary to trigger the retrieval of information on the basis of prior social experience or innate bias in regard to certain classes of faces.[15] The retrieved information might be either covert or overt, or both (compare with ref. 16). The failure due to amygdala damage thus occurs after basic visual processing has taken place, by blocking the retrieval of information normally linked either to negative past experiences with similar stimuli, or to innately specified feature configurations. By contrast, sentences and words evoke a broad sweep of information directly, without the need for the amygdala's assistance, thus providing a sufficient basis for performing judgments normally.

A further question concerns the specific facial cues that would normally engage the amygdala in social judgment. Might amygdala lesions impair judgments based only on certain facial features? This does not seem to be the case, as subjects with bilateral amygdala lesions gave idiosyncratic ratings to specific negative faces (Fig. 24.2; intersubject Spearman rank correlations of ratings given by subjects with bilateral

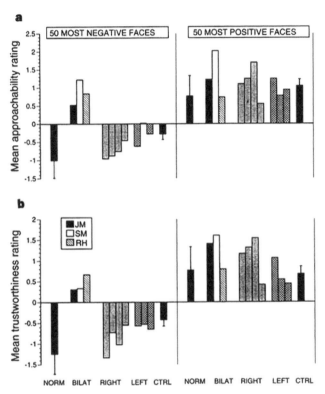

Figure 24.1
Mean judgments. (a) Approachability; (b) trustworthiness of the faces of 100 unfamiliar people, shown for the 50 faces that received the most negative (left) and most positive (right) mean ratings from normal controls. Data are shown from 46 normal controls (NORM; means and s.d.), 3 subjects with bilateral amygdala damage (BILAT; individual means), 4 subjects with unilateral right (RIGHT) and 3 with unilateral left (LEFT) amygdala damage, and 10 brain-damaged controls with no damage to amygdala (CTRL; means and SEM).

amygdala lesions for the 50 most negative faces: $-0.23 < r < 0.31$). We further explored this complex issue by choosing the 10 faces to which SM had given the most abnormal ratings of approachability (all rated very negatively by controls), and systematically manipulating individual features in each face. We showed subjects 109 pairs of faces in which each pair showed the same individual differing by only one single feature. We manipulated direction of gaze (45 stimuli), expression of the eyes (27 stimuli), ex-

pression of the mouth (14 stimuli), or visibility of the eyes (for example, with glasses of different tint; 23 stimuli), all features that might conceivably contribute to the subjects' judgments. In a two-alternative forced-choice task, SM and 16 normal controls were asked to choose the face they would prefer to approach. SM performed entirely normally on this task. Logistic linear analysis, with subjects' binary choices as the dependent variable and the manipulated features as factors, showed that SM did not differ from

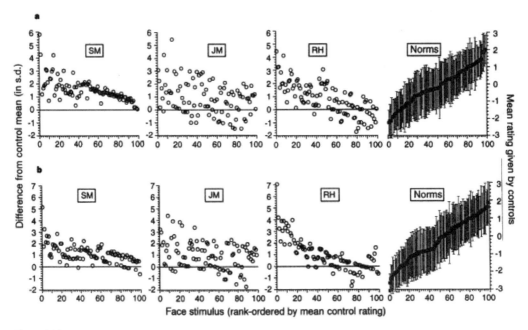

Figure 24.2
Deviations from normal judgments. (a) Approachability; (b) trustworthiness given by subjects with bilateral amygdala damage (circles; left y-axis). Units are standard deviations of the normal control ratings. Stimuli are rank-ordered on the x-axis according to the ratings normal controls gave them (squares; far right y-axis; means and SD).

controls in her choices with respect to any of the above features that we had manipulated. Insensitivity to particular features, in isolation, is thus unlikely to account for the impairment in judging approachability or trustworthiness in faces.

The findings suggest that the human amygdala triggers socially and emotionally relevant information in response to visual stimuli. The amygdala's role appears to be of special importance for social judgment of faces that are normally classified as unapproachable and untrustworthy, consistent with the amygdala's demonstrated role in processing threatening and aversive stimuli. An intriguing question that remains to be addressed is the amygdala's relative participation in triggering information that is innate, versus information that is acquired through individual experience in a cultural setting.[17]

Methods

Subjects

All subjects had given informed consent to participate in these studies. Brain-damaged subjects were selected from the Patient Registry of the Department of Neurology at the University of Iowa, and had been fully characterized neuropsychologically[18] and neuroanatomically.[19,20]

Amygdala Damage

Subject SM has complete lesions of both amygdalae, as well as minimal damage to anterior entorhinal cortex, resulting from Urbach-Wiethe disease.[7,14,21,22] Subjects RH and JM had en-

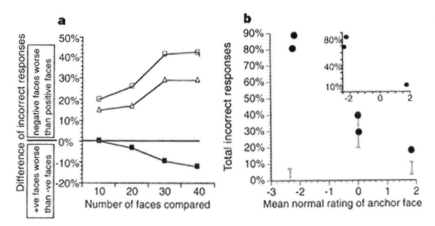

Figure 24.3
Disproportionate impairment in choosing the most unapproachable faces. (a) JM's (empty squares), RH's (triangles) and normal controls' (filled squares) judgments of approachability from two-alternative forced-choice tasks. We calculated the percent incorrect choices made for pairings involving faces at either extreme of the normal rating scale (that is, faces that were normally rated as either very approachable or very unapproachable). The x-axis shows the number of faces at either extreme of the normal rating scale over which the percent incorrect choices was calculated. The y-axis shows the difference in the errors made (unapproachable–approachable). (b) SM's judgments of approachability from two-alternative forced-choice tasks. The mean normal rating of approachability given to each of 5 anchor faces is shown on the x-axis, and the proportion of incorrect forced choices (out of 99) made by SM (circles) and by normal controls (grey bars show range) are shown on the y-axis. Inset, analysis of SM's data from this task for only those pairs of faces whose mean control rating differed by more than 2 rating points. Data from comparisons involving the two faces with mean control ratings of 0 were not analysed, as very few faces with ratings < −2 or > 2 could be paired with them. No normal control made any incorrect choices in this analysis.

cephalitis at ages 28 and 62, respectively, resulting in complete bilateral destruction of the amygdala and substantial damage to surrounding structures. Both patients are severely amnesic. Seven subjects with unilateral amygdala lesions (4 right, 3 left) had surgical temporal lobectomy for the treatment of epilepsy, and also had damage to hippocampus and surrounding temporal cortices.

Control Subjects

We examined 10 brain-damaged controls with lesions that did not include the amygdala. Four of the subjects had bilateral lesions. Three of the subjects were amnesic consequent to anoxia and

hippocampal damage. We also examined 46 normal controls (16M/30F) who were undergraduates at the University of Iowa.

Stimuli and Tasks

In all tasks, stimuli within each session were presented in randomized order, and without time limit.

Approachability and Trustworthiness Ratings of Faces

We selected from a larger set of photographs 100 final stimuli whose ratings had low variance and were evenly distributed (Fig. 24.2). There was no

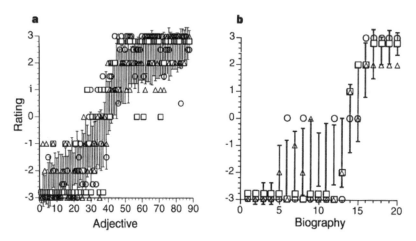

Figure 24.4
Likeability ratings of lexical stimuli. (a) Ratings given by SM (2 experiments; circles), JM (squares), RH (triangles) and 20 normal controls (s.d. shown as bars) to 88 adjectives describing personality. (b) Ratings given by SM, JM, RH and 20 normal controls to biographical descriptions of people.

effect of subject gender on rating the faces ($P >$ 0.7, ANOVA on normal data). Stimuli were black-and-white photographs of unfamiliar male ($N = 55$) and female ($N = 45$) faces in natural poses.

Subjects were asked to rate the stimuli, shown one at a time on a slide projector, on a 7-point scale (-3 to $+3$) with respect to either approachability or trustworthiness. For approachability, subjects were asked to imagine meeting the person on the street, and to indicate how much they would want to walk up to that person and strike up a conversation. For trustworthiness, subjects imagined trusting that person with all their money, or with their life. Each of the two attributes was rated in two independent sessions in counterbalanced order; there were no order effects.

Approachability and trustworthiness were chosen because (1) they are clear measures of real-life social judgment; (2) they are easy to understand; and (3) pilot data indicated that ratings of these specific attributes had lower variance than those obtained with other words, such

as "nice" or "good." Although approachability and trustworthiness ratings in normals were somewhat correlated (mean $r = 0.52$), there were many stimuli that received discrepant ratings on the two attributes, indicating that they were non-redundant measures of social judgment.

Forced-Choice Tasks

Direct pairwise comparisons of approachability were made between an anchor face, and each of the remaining 99 faces, all drawn from the same 100 face stimuli used in other tasks. We calculated the proportion of subjects' choices that differed from the choices that would be expected on the basis of the mean normal control ratings given to each of the two faces in a pair.

In one experiment (Fig. 24.3a), each of two anchor faces with a mean normal approachability rating of 0.0 was compared to other faces that were either very approachable or very unapproachable; data obtained with both anchor faces were very similar and were pooled. In a second experiment (Fig. 24.3b), each of 5 anchor faces (which included faces with a range of ratings) was compared to all other 99 faces (a total of 495 pairwise comparisons).

Lexical Stimuli

We chose 88 adjectives that described personality attributes from a large standardized set[23] so as to span the range from very likeable to very dislikeable, and to exhibit maximal reliability and common usage. Twenty short biographies described people by giving information about the person's lifestyles and activities. Subjects rated how much they liked individuals described by the stimuli, on a scale of -3 to $+3$. Words were presented visually on a sheet of paper; biographical descriptions were read to subjects.

Control Tasks

For each of the control tasks, we calculated thresholds at which subjects were just able to discriminate stimuli. Data were converted to percentiles compared to performances given by normal subjects ($N = 28$ for expression, 20 for gender, 28 for gaze).

Expression Discrimination

Two-alternative forced-choice discriminations were made between 80 images of a neutral face, and 80 images that were linear morphs between the neutral face and facial expressions of emotion[24] (happiness, surprise, fear, anger, disgust, sadness). Subjects were asked to choose the image that showed more of a stated emotion.

Gender Discrimination

Two-alternative forced-choice discriminations were made between 84 pairs of images that were morphs between an average composite of a neutral male face, and an average composite of a neutral female face, of equal age.

Gaze Discrimination

Two-alternative forced-choice discriminations were made between 16 pairs of images showing the same, neutral, male face in which only direction of gaze had been varied by manipulating the digital image on a computer.

Acknowledgements

We thank J. Suhr and J. Nath for technical assistance in testing subjects, D. Krutzfeldt for help in scheduling subjects and H. Damasio for comments on the manuscript. This study was supported by a grant from the National Institute for Neurological Diseases and Stroke.

References

1. Weiskrantz, L. Behavioral changes associated with ablation of the amygdaloid complex in monkeys. *J. Comp. Physiol. Psychol.* 49, 381–391 (1956).

2. Blanchard, D. C. & Blanchard, R. J. Innate and conditioned reactions to threat in rats with amygdaloid lesions. *J. Comp. Physiol. Psychol.* 81, 281–290 (1972).

3. Le Doux, J. *The Emotional Brain* (Simon and Schuster, New York, 1996).

4. Rosvold, H. E., Mirsky, A. F. & Pribram, K. Influence of amygdalectomy on social behavior in monkeys. *J. Comp. Physiol. Psychol.* 47, 173–178 (1954).

5. Kling, A., Steklis, H. D. & Deutsch, S. Radiotelemetered activity from the amygdala during social interactions in the monkey. *Exp. Neurol.* 66, 88–96 (1979).

6. Kling, A. S. & Brothers, L. A. in *The Amygdala: Neurobiological Aspects of Emotion, Memory, and Mental Dysfunction* (ed. Aggleton, J. P.) 353–378 (Wiley-Liss, New York, 1992).

7. Adolphs, R., Tranel, D., Damasio, H. & Damasio, A. Impaired recognition of emotion in facial expressions following bilateral damage to the human amygdala. *Nature* 372, 669–672 (1994).

8. Young, A. W. et al. Face processing impairments after amygdalotomy. *Brain* 118, 15–24 (1995).

9. Calder, A. J. et al. Facial emotion recognition after bilateral amygdala damage: differentially severe impairment of fear. *Cogn. Neuropsychol.* 13, 699–745 (1996).

10. Broks, P. et al. Face processing impairments after encephalitis: amygdala damage and recognition of fear. *Neuropsychologia* 39, 59–70 (1998).

11. Morris, J. S. et al. A differential neural response in the human amygdala to fearful and happy facial expressions. *Nature* 383, 812–815 (1996).

12. Breiter, H. C. et al. Response and habituation of the human amygdala during visual processing of facial expression. *Neuron* 17, 875–887 (1996).

13. Morris, J. S. et al. A neuromodulatory role for the human amygdala in processing emotional facial expressions. *Brain* 121, 47–57 (1998).

14. Tranel, D. & Hyman, B. T. Neuropsychological correlates of bilateral amygdala damage. *Arch. Neurol.* 47, 349–355 (1990).

15. Damasio, A. R. Toward a neurobiology of emotion and feeling: operational concepts and hypotheses. *Neuroscientist* 1, 19–25 (1995).

16. Lewicki, P., Hill, T. & Czyzewska, M. Nonconscious acquisition of information. *Am. Psychol.* 47, 796–801 (1992).

17. Saarni, C., Mumme, D. L. & Campos, J. J. in *Handbook of Child Psychology, Vol. 3: Social, Emotional, and Personality Development* (ed. Damon, W.) 237–309 (Wiley, New York, 1997).

18. Tranel, D. in *Neuropsychological Assessment of Neuropsychiatric Disorders* (eds Grant, I. & Adams, K. M.) 81–101 (Oxford Univ. Press, New York, 1996).

19. Damasio, H. & Frank, R. Three-dimensional *in vivo* mapping of brain lesions in humans. *Arch. Neurol.* 49, 137–143 (1992).

20. Frank, R. J., Damasio, H. & Grabowski, T. J. Brainvox: an interactive, multi-modal visualization and analysis system for neuroanatomical imaging. *NeuroImage* 5, 13–30 (1997).

21. Adolphs, R., Tranel, D., Damasio, H. & Damasio, A. R. Fear and the human amygdala. *J. Neurosci.* 15, 5879–5892 (1995).

22. Nahm, F. K. D., Tranel, D., Damasio, H. & Damasio, A. R. Cross-modal associations and the human amygdala. *Neuropsychologia* 31, 727–744 (1993).

23. Anderson, N. H. Likableness ratings of 555 personality-trait words. *J. Person. Social Psychol.* 9, 272–279 (1968).

24. Ekman, P. & Friesen, W. *Pictures of Facial Affect* (Consulting Psychologists, Palo Alto, CA, 1976).

Social Intelligence in the Normal and Autistic Brain: An fMRI Study

Simon Baron-Cohen, Howard A. Ring, Sally Wheelwright, Edward T. Bullmore, Mick J. Brammer, Andrew Simmons, and Steve C. R. Williams

Introduction

Social intelligence encompasses our abilities to interpret others' behaviour in terms of mental states (thoughts, intentions, desires and beliefs), to interact both in complex social groups and in close relationships, to empathize with others' states of mind, and to predict how others will feel, think and behave. The idea that social intelligence might be independent, or dissociable from, general intelligence comes from several sources. First, individuals exist who are capable of considerable understanding of the non-social world (e.g. physics, math, engineering) yet who readily admit to finding the social world confusing (Baron-Cohen et al., in press; Sacks, 1994). The opposite type of individual also exists: people who have no difficulty interacting with the social world but who find non-social problem-solving confusing (Karmiloff-Smith et al., 1995). Second, certain kinds of brain damage can cause selective impairment in social judgement (Damasio et al., 1990) without any necessary loss to general problem-solving ability. Loss of social judgement can co-occur with memory and executive dysfunction, following amygdala damage (Tranel & Hyman, 1990), but the functional double dissociation between social and non-social intelligence implies their neural independence. Finally, many primatologists now believe that social problem-solving was a key driving force behind the evolution of primate intelligence, rather than tool-use or other non-social problem solving (Whiten, 1991).

A neural basis of social intelligence was first proposed by Brothers (1990). She suggested from both animal lesion studies (Kling & Brothers, 1992), single-cell recording studies (Brothers et al., 1990) and neurological studies (cited above) that this involves the amygdala, orbito-frontal cortex (OFC) and superior temporal gyrus (STG). Together, she postulated that these comprise the "social brain." Damage to the amygdala impairs judgement of emotion (Calder et al., 1996), damage to the OFC impairs judgement of what is socially appropriate (Eslinger & Damasio, 1985), and damage to the STG impairs face-perception (Campbell et al., 1990). Single-cell recording studies in non-human primates also confirm the role of the STG in detection of gaze (Perrett et al., 1985). Recent PET and SPECT studies of "theory of mind" (or the ability to impute mental states) also implicate areas of prefrontal cortex, specifically the medial frontal cortex (MFC, Fletcher et al., 1995; Goel et al., 1995) and the OFC (Baron-Cohen et al., 1994).

The present fMRI study had two main aims. (i) To test Brothers' social brain theory that these neural regions, identified independently from several different studies and methods of investigation, are jointly activated in a group of normal subjects performing a novel social intelligence test. (ii) To test the validity of this neural model of social intelligence by comparing normal cerebral blood oxygenation changes induced by performance of this task with hypothetically abnormal changes in a group of patients with high-functioning autism or Asperger syndrome (AS), known to have social impairment (Baron-Cohen & Ring, 1994). In particular, we predicted abnormal amygdala activation in the autism group,[1] on the basis of five lines of evidence. (i) A neuroanatomical study of autism at postmortem found microscopic pathology (in the form of increased cell density) in the amygdala, in the presence of normal amygdala volume (Bauman & Kemper, 1994; Rapin & Katzman, 1998). (ii) The only animal model of autism involves ablation of the amygdala (in rhesus monkeys) (Bachevalier, 1991). Whilst there is some dispute as to whether one can have an animal model of autism when the syndrome involves deficits in higher order cognition, this is at least consistent with the amygdala theory. (iii) Patients with amygdala lesions show impairments in social judgement (Adolphs et al., 1994; Young et al., 1996). (iv) Using SPECT, patients with autism spectrum conditions show significant reductions in temporal lobe blood flow, regardless of whether they have temporal lobe epilepsy (Gillberg et al., 1993). (v) In cases of tuberous sclerosis, autistic co-morbidity is determined by hamartomata in the temporal lobe (Bolton & Griffiths, 1997). For all these reasons, a basic impairment of amygdala function in autism seems very plausible.[2]

Materials and Methods

Subjects

Six subjects with autism (four male, two female) were matched for mean age, handedness, IQ, socioeconomic status and educational level, with 12 subjects in the normal group (six male, six female). IQ was assessed with the full Wechsler Adult Intelligence Scale (WAIS-R). Subjects were only included if their IQ was in the normal range (i.e. above 85 both in terms of full-scale IQ, and in terms of performance and verbal IQ). These variables are shown in Table 25.1. There were no significant differences in any of these dimensions. Individuals in the clinical group all had a diagnosis of autism or AS, using DSM-IV (APA, 1994) and ICD-10 (1994) criteria.

Experimental Design

We used a blocked periodic ABA ... design. Each epoch (A or B) was presented for 30 s, and there were five cycles of AB alternation in total. Images were acquired from each subject during visual presentation of two tasks, both of which involved deriving socially relevant information

Table 25.1
Mean age and IQ ($\pm$ SD), and handedness of subjects in the experiment

	Autism	Controls
Age (years)	26.3 ± 2.1	25.5 ± 2.8
IQ	108.5 ± 10.5	110 ± 8.5
Handedness (R:L)	6:0	12:0

from facial stimuli. This periodically designed (ABA ...) experiment was expected to induce a periodic MR signal change with maximum signal during task A in brain regions relatively specialized for gender recognition from facial stimuli; and periodic MR signal change with maximum signal during task B in brain regions relatively specialized for mental state recognition from facial stimuli. The response involved a forced choice between the two words offered (pressing one of two buttons with the right hand to select the right or left word). Correct words were counterbalanced to left and right side. Because both tasks were social, either may have resulted in anomalous activation in the autism group, though we predicted abnormalities would only arise in task B.

Method

Task A
Subjects were visually presented with a series of photographs of eyes and asked to indicate by right-handed button press whether each stimulus was a man or a woman. In this first task (A: gender recognition), instructions to subjects were to decide for each stimulus which of two simultaneously presented words ("male" or "female") best described the face. Each stimulus was presented for 5 s and was followed by a 0.75-s interval in which the screen was blank. Stimuli were drawn from 30 faces of women or men. Stimuli were presented 3.5 m from the subject, subtending visual angles of 10° horizontally and 8° vertically.

Task B

Subjects were presented with exactly the same stimuli but were asked to indicate by button press which of two simultaneously presented words best described the mental state of the photographed person. Thus, the key difference between the two tasks was the type of judgement the subject had to make when viewing the eyes.[3] Subjects were presented with an example of the stimuli before scanning. For this second task (B: theory of mind), instructions to subjects were to decide for each stimulus which of two simultaneously presented words best described what the person in the photograph was feeling or thinking. Task B is an "advanced" theory of mind test, in that it is used with adults, and involves mind-reading.

Adults with high-functioning autism or AS, with intelligence in the normal range, show deficits on this task (Baron-Cohen et al., 1997), as do parents of children with autism/AS (Baron-Cohen & Hammer, 1997). Children with William's syndrome are not impaired on this test, despite their general retardation (Tager-Flusberg et al., 1998). Examples of the eyes used in the experimental condition, together with the forced choice words that appeared underneath each face, are shown in Fig. 25.1. Finally, as a control pretest outside the scanner, subjects were given the opportunity to pick out any words in a list of mental state words that would appear in task B that they did not recognize or understand, in which case a glossary definition was provided by the experimenter. Neither group made use of this, reflecting that the words used were relatively common, and that the adult subjects in both groups were of normal intelligence.

Image Acquisition and Analysis

Single-shot gradient echo, echoplanar images were acquired using a 1.5 Tesla GE Signa system (General Electric, Milwaukee, WI, USA) fitted with Advanced NMR hardware and software (ANMR, Woburn, MA, USA) using a standard head coil. One hundred T_2*-weighted images depicting bold contrast (Ogawa et al., 1990) were acquired over 5 min at each of 14 near-axial non-contiguous 7-mm-thick planes parallel to the intercommissural (AC-PC) line, providing whole-brain coverage: TE, 40 ms; TR, 3 s; in-plane resolution, 3 mm; interslice gap, 0.7 mm. At the same session, an inversion recovery EPI dataset was also acquired from 43 near-axial 3-mm-thick slices parallel to the AC-PC line: TE, 80 ms; TI, 180 ms; TR, 16 s; in plane resolution 1.5 mm; number of signal averages = 8.

Periodic change in T_2*-weighted signal intensity at the (fundamental) experimentally determined frequency of alternation between A and B conditions (= 1/60 Hz) was modelled by the sum of a sine wave and cosine wave at that frequency. The amplitudes of the sine and cosine waves, γ and δ, respectively, were estimated by pseudo-generalized least-squares fit to the movement-corrected time functional magnetic resonance imaging (fMRI) series at each voxel. The sum of squared amplitudes, γ^2 and δ^2, divided by its SE, provided a standardized estimate of experimentally determined power, the fundamental power quotient (FPQ, Bullmore et al., 1996). The sign of γ indicated the phase of the periodic signal change with respect to the input function. Maps were constructed to represent FPQ and γ at each voxel of each observed dataset. Each observed time series was randomly permuted 10 times, and FPQ estimated as above in each randomized time series, to generate 10 randomized parametric maps of FPQ for each subject in each anatomical plane.

To construct generic brain activation maps, observed and randomized FPQ maps derived from each subject were transformed into the standard space of Talairach and Tournoux and smoothed by a two-dimensional Gaussian filter (SD = 4.5 mm) (Talairach & Tournoux, 1988). The median value of FPQ at each intracerebral voxel in standard space was then tested against a critical value of the randomization distribution for median FPQ ascertained from the random-

1

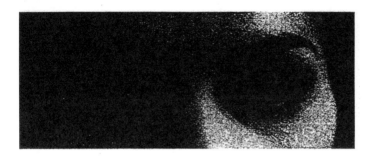

UNCONCERNED   **CONCERNED**

24

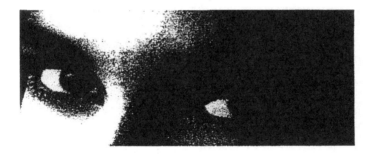

SYMPATHETIC   **UNSYMPATHETIC**

Figure 25.1
Examples of the stimuli used. During task B, photographs of eyes were presented with a choice of mental state words (examples as shown); during task A the eyes were presented with a choice of the words "male" and "female." (Top example: correct word in task B is "concerned"; correct word in task A is "female." Bottom example: correct word in task B is "sympathetic"; correct word in task A is "female.")

ized FPQ maps. For a one-tailed test of size $\alpha = 0.0008$, the critical value was the $100 \times (1 - \alpha)$th percentile value of the randomization distribution. Maps of γ observed in each individual were likewise transformed into standard space and smoothed. The median value of γ was computed for each generically activated voxel. If median $\gamma > 0$, that voxel was considered to be generically activated by the gender recognition task (A); if median $\gamma < 0$, that voxel was considered to be generically activated by the theory of mind task (B).

To estimate the difference between control and autism groups in the mean power of response to task B, we fitted the following ANOVA model at each of 1658 voxels generically activated by the ToM task in one or both of the groups:

$$FPQ_{i,j} = \mu + \beta_1 \text{Group}_j + \varepsilon_{i,j}$$

Here, $FPQ_{i,j}$ denotes the standardized power of response at the ith individual in the jth group. Group denotes a factor coding the main effects of diagnostic status. The null hypothesis of zero between-group difference in mean FPQ was tested by comparing the observed coefficient β_1 with critical values of its non-parametrically ascertained null distribution. To do this, the elements of Group were randomly permuted 10 times at each voxel; β_1 was estimated at each voxel after each permutation; and these estimates were pooled over all intracerebral voxels in standard space to sample the randomization distribution of β_1 (Brammer et al., 1997). Critical values for a two-tailed test of size $\alpha = 0.01$ were the $100^*(\alpha/2)$th and $100^*(1 - \alpha/2)$th percentiles of this distribution (Edgington, 1980). For this size of test ($\alpha = 0.01$) and search volume (1658 voxels), we expect no more than 16 voxels to be type I (false positive) errors.[4]

An analysis of variance in this context assumes that it is meaningful to characterize pathological differences in functional activation in terms of a quantitative difference in mean power of response at each voxel. This assumption has been widely adopted in previous functional imaging

studies of neuropsychiatric disorder, most notably it is central to characterization of schizophrenic abnormalities of functional anatomy in terms of hypofrontality (Weinberger & Berman, 1998). There is also evidence from previous imaging studies of normal subjects that the magnitude of functional response in a given region may be proportional to the cognitive processing load imposed by experimental design (e.g. Price et al., 1996; Price & Friston, 1997). It therefore seems reasonable to interpret differences in power of functional response between control and patient groups as a proxy measure of differences in local neural processing which reflect differences in cognitive strategy imposed by disease.

Results

Considering task performance, both the autism and normal control groups performed both tasks significantly better than chance during scanning. The control group was more accurate in both gender recognition ($x = 86\%$, SD = 3.0) and theory of mind ($x = 83\%$, SD = 7.3) than the autism group ($x = 82\%$, SD = 7.5 and $x = 74\%$, SD = 1.8 correct, respectively). For both tasks, there was a significant effect of Group, with the normal controls performing better than the subjects with autism or AS (ANOVA, theory of mind: $F_{1,16} = 6.1$, $P = 0.02$; gender recognition: $F_{1,16} = 15.6$, $P = 0.001$). Note that in larger sample studies, gender recognition on the eyes test is intact, whilst theory of mind is impaired, in adults with high-functioning autism or AS (Baron-Cohen et al., 1997).

Functional MRI data were analysed in two stages. First, generic brain activation maps were constructed separately for the control and autism groups. These maps identified voxels demonstrating significant power of periodic signal change over all subjects in each group; they also represented differences between generically activated voxels in terms of phase of response to the experimental input function. Thus it was possible to determine which voxels were activated in each group by each of the two tasks. Second, we used ANOVA to identify voxels that demonstrated a significant difference between groups in mean power of response to each task (see Materials and Methods).

Figure 25.2 shows the functional system activated by presentation of the theory of mind task in the control and autism groups. This system can be anatomically subdivided into two main components. (i) A set of fronto-temporal neocortical regions, comprising left dorsolateral prefrontal cortex (DLPFC), approximately Brodmann area (BA) 44, 45, 46; the left MFC (BA 9); supplementary motor area (SMA, medial BA 6); and bilateral temporo-parietal regions, including middle and superior temporal, angular and supramarginal gyri (BA 21, 22, 39 and 40). (ii) A number of non-neocortical areas, including the left amygdala, the left hippocampal gyrus (BA 27 and 30), bilateral insulae and left striatum.

The autism group activated the frontal components less extensively than the control group; and did not activate the amygdala at all. As shown in Table 25.2, the control group demonstrated significantly greater power of response in the left amygdala, right insula and left inferior frontal gyrus. The autism group demonstrated significantly greater power of response in bilateral superior temporal gyrus (STG). For completeness, the main brain regions significantly activated by the theory of mind task are shown in Table 25.3 (control group) and Table 25.4 (autism group).

Discussion

These results are a striking confirmation of Brothers' theory that extracting socially relevant information from visual stimuli is normally associated with activation of the STG, areas of prefrontal cortex,[5] and the amygdala. We next discuss each of these neural regions in turn, both in relation to normal functioning and to autism.

Regarding the left amygdala, this area may be critically involved in identifying mental state/ emotional information from complex visual stimuli, e.g. the eye region. This laterality effect is consistent with previous studies: the left amygdala appears to be specifically activated in emotion processing (Ketter et al., 1996; Morris et al., 1996, but also see Breiter et al., 1996; Phillips et al., 1997). The autism group appears not to perform the task using the amygdala, but instead places a greater processing load on temporal lobe structures, specialized for verbally labelling complex visual stimuli and processing faces and eyes. We interpret this as showing that people with autism may be solving the task using both language and facial memory functions, perhaps in compensation for an amygdala abnormality. Although it is known that the amygdala plays a role in the recognition of fear (Adolphs et al., 1994; Calder et al., 1996; Young et al., 1996; Scott et al., 1997), here we have also shown that it is involved in inference of a broader range of mental states, from the face and especially the eyes. We consider it unlikely that these results simply reflect emotion-processing or arousal, as the stimuli in the present study involve judging expressions of a broad range of mental states, many of which are not primarily emotional (e.g. interest, reflective, ignoring). Furthermore, whereas previous studies showing amygdala activation have involved passive perception of powerful emotional stimuli, our task involved an active judgement of a different kind: attribution of a mental state. This suggests that mental state concepts are processed in this region, both when the task involves inferring these from eyes, or other animate actions (Bonda et al., 1996).

Regarding the left prefrontal regions, these may subserve the verbal working memory/central executive function (Frith et al., 1991; D'Esposito et al., 1995; Salmon et al., 1996), entailed in matching words whilst observing the eyes. A previous study of autism suggested attenuated activation of MFC (Happe et al., 1996). In the present study we also found that MFC was acti-

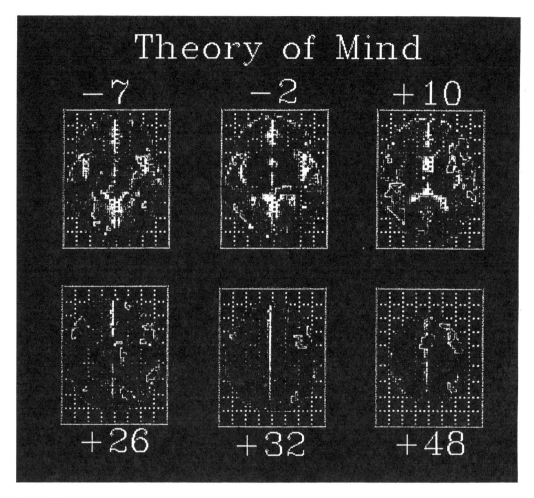

Figure 25.2
Generic brain activation maps separately computed from the control and autistic group data are superimposed in standard space. Only those voxels with maximum signal during the theory of mind task are shown. Voxel-wise probability of type I error alpha = 0.008 for both maps. Voxels activated in the control group only are coloured yellow; voxels activated in the autism group only are coloured red; voxels activated coincidentally in both groups are coloured blue. The right side of each map represents the left side of the brain. The z coordinates (mm) of each slice relative to the intercommissural line in the standard space (Talairach & Tournoux, 1988) are shown above or below each slice. At −7 mm, the control group activated regions including bilateral insulae and left amygdala: at −2 mm, the main focus of activation in the control group is located in the left parahippocampal gyrus; at +10 mm, the control group demonstrates activation of the bilateral STG and left prefrontal cortex, while the autism group demonstrates less extensive activation of predominantly left sided STG; at +26 and +32 mm, both groups activate the left prefrontal cortex.

Table 25.2
Main brain regions differentially activated by theory of mind task in control (C) and autism (A) groups

Cerebral region	BA	Side	Voxels (n)	x	y	z	Difference	P-value
Superior temporal gyrus*	22	L	12	−55	−28	15	A > C	0.004
Superior temporal gyrus	22	R	8	40	−28	15	A > C	0.002
Inferior frontal gyrus†	44/45	L	5	−46	22	9	C > A	0.001
Insula		R	5	40	11	−7	C > A	0.001
Amygdala		L	4	−23	−11	−7	C > A	0.001

BA, Brodmann area. * Or Wernicke's area. † Or Broca's area.

vated less extensively by the autism group, but this was not statistically significant.

Regarding the temporal regions, these may be involved in the processing of words and serve as a word store (Wise et al., 1991), and in the processing of eyes (Perrett et al., 1990). We consider that the STG activation seen in the theory of mind condition here is likely to reflect the processing of eyes and faces as it involved bilateral activity, whereas the processing of words would be more likely to have only activated STG lateralized to the left side.

The fundamental premise of this study is that social intelligence is modular or dissociable from general intelligence. More specifically, we have assumed that it will be possible to design a periodic contrast between two experimental conditions which differ exclusively in terms of social cognition, and that the experimental response to this design will be specific to elements of the "social brain." The validity of this set of assumptions is supported by the correspondence between our results in normal subjects and a prior model of the social brain (Brothers & Ring, 1992). But it may be instructive also to note some limitations and ambiguities inherent in our design.

The two contrasting conditions, although closely matched for stimulus frequency and motor response, may not have differed exclusively in terms of social cognition. For example, subjects may have attempted to solve the experimental problem of mental state assignment by retrieval

from long-term memory, or by inducing in themselves the emotional states represented by the stimuli. The theory of mind task involved presentation of novel word pairs with each set of visual stimuli, whereas the same pair of short, high-frequency words ("male" and "female") was repeatedly presented with each set of stimuli during the gender assignment task. It is thus possible that the experimental contrast could have caused periodic signal change in areas specialized for novelty detection, or differential engagement of language systems. Finally, the simultaneous presentation of visual and verbal stimuli, although necessary so that response during scanning could be monitored by forced choice button press, allows an important ambiguity. Do subjects match the eyes to associations or memories primarily induced by the words, or vice versa? In short, the design does not allow us to implicate a particular modality of stimulation (visual or verbal) in experimental activation of the social brain. Several of these problems are typical of periodic or subtraction designs generally, and it will be important in future work to consider so-called parametric experimental designs, in which a single task is presented at continuously variable levels of difficulty during fMRI data acquisition.

Abnormalities of functional activation by patient groups have often been attributed simply to failure of the patients to perform the task. This seems an inadequate explanation of our

Table 25.3
Main brain regions differentially activated by theory of mind task in the control group

Voxels (n)	x	y	z	Side	BA	Cerebral region
9	−26	−11	−7	L		Amygdala
1	20	−8	−7	R		Amygdala
8	−26	−67	31	L	19	Angular gyrus
14	23	−56	−13	R		Cerebellum
4	−14	−78	−13	L		Cerebellum
25	6	3	42	R	24	Cingulate gyrus
7	−3	36	−2	L	24	Cingulate gyrus
29	−3	−44	37	L	31	Cingulate gyrus
23	0	−33	31	R	31	Cingulate gyrus
50	0	44	15	R	32	Cingulate gyrus
17	29	−58	−7	R	19	Fusiform gyrus
8	−38	−44	−7	L	36	Fusiform gyrus
66	−49	11	20	L	6	Inferior frontal gyrus
26	58	8	15	R	6	Inferior frontal gyrus
101	−46	14	31	L	44	Inferior frontal gyrus
42	49	14	26	R	44	Inferior frontal gyrus
169	−43	25	4	L	45	Inferior frontal gyrus
10	52	19	20	R	45	Inferior frontal gyrus
26	−32	−56	42	L	19	Inferior parietal lobule
15	49	−53	−2	R	37	Inferior temporal gyrus
15	32	−17	4	R	72	Insula
4	−35	−17	9	L	72	Insula
14	12	−72	−2	R	18	Lingual gyrus
10	−3	−86	4	L	18	Lingual gyrus
7	20	−53	−2	R	19	Lingual gyrus
33	−14	−31	−2	L	27	Lingual gyrus
163	6	6	53	R	6	Medial frontal gyrus
13	0	47	9	R	32	Medial frontal gyrus
111	−43	3	42	L	6	Middle frontal gyrus
37	38	6	37	R	6	Middle frontal gyrus
60	−46	14	37	L	9	Middle frontal gyrus
73	32	−72	4	R	19	Middle occipital gyrus
142	43	−33	4	R	21	Middle temporal gyrus
16	−46	−22	37	L	1	Postcentral gyrus
4	−23	−44	59	L	7	Postcentral gyrus
8	35	−22	53	R	4	Precentral gyrus
82	−23	−6	59	L	6	Precentral gyrus
6	52	6	9	R	6	Precentral gyrus

Table 25.3
(continued)

Voxels (n)	x	y	z	Side	BA	Cerebral region
63	−3	−44	53	L	7	Precuneus
32	0	−47	59	R	7	Precuneus
122	−17	3	−2	L		Putamen
8	29	−22	−2	R		Putamen
13	−29	39	20	L	10	Superior frontal gyrus
7	−32	−56	48	L	7	Superior parietal lobule
75	−55	−39	9	L	22	Superior temporal gyrus
42	52	−50	15	R	22	Superior temporal gyrus
12	46	11	−7	R	38	Superior temporal gyrus
22	40	−58	20	R	39	Superior temporal gyrus
5	−49	−56	15	L	39	Superior temporal gyrus
8	−35	−25	15	L	42	Superior temporal gyrus
21	−46	−44	26	L	40	Supramarginal gyrus
22	−14	−11	15	L		Thalamus
6	0	−31	4	R		Thalamus

findings as the patients performed both tasks better than chance during scanning and had no difficulty in comprehending examples of mental state adjectives presented to them before scanning. However, a number of possible interpretations remain open. It could be that patients with autism have a general deficit in emotional processing, rather than specifically emotional processing to inform mental state assignation. Such a possibility is attractive simply because it is known that the amygdala responds to fearful faces (Breiter et al., 1996; Morris et al., 1996), and that such amygdala activity occurs regardless of whether the subjects are aware of the face (Whalen et al., 1998) or aware that different facial expressions were critical to the study (Morris et al., 1996). However, because we regard emotional processing as part of social intelligence, this interpretation is a refinement rather than a contradiction of our preferred interpretation that autistic patients fail to activate the social brain. Furthermore, whilst this might be part of the explanation, it cannot be sufficient, as some of the expressions were of non-affective mental states (e.g. "reflective").

A more problematic alternative is that the patients with autism may in fact activate the social brain, but under both experimental conditions. This pattern of response would not engender periodic signal change and cannot be excluded on the basis of these data. However, even if it were true that the subjects with autism promiscuously activated the social brain under both conditions, this would still constitute interesting evidence for abnormal modularity or modularization (Karmiloff-Smith, 1992) of social intelligence in autism. Here we use the term modularity not in the strong Fodorian (Fodor, 1983) sense, but in a weaker sense (Baron-Cohen, 1994; in press). Against this, however, analysis of the individual subject scans in each condition shows little if any evidence of amygdala activity in the volunteers with autism, which renders the amygdala theory of autism quite plausible.

A further alternative account of the present results might be that people with autism have simply had less experience of the relevant mental states or attitudes being expressed towards them.

Table 25.4
Main brain regions differentially activated by theory of mind task in the autism group

Voxels (n)	x	y	z	Side	BA	Cerebral region
28	14	−72	−13	R	71	Cerebellum
8	17	−53	9	R	23	Cingulate gyrus
7	3	−33	31	R	31	Cingulate gyrus
15	3	19	31	R	32	Cingulate gyrus
30	20	−81	9	R	18	Cuneus
9	26	−42	−13	R	36	Fusiform gyrus
65	−46	3	26	L	6	Inferior frontal gyrus
8	−43	14	20	L	45	Inferior frontal gyrus
16	−38	28	20	L	46	Inferior frontal gyrus
5	−49	−17	−2	L	21	Insula
8	−23	−75	−2	L	18	Lingual gyrus
23	−9	50	20	L	9	Medial frontal gyrus
37	−43	8	37	L	6	Middle frontal gyrus
24	−40	6	42	L	9	Middle frontal gyrus
16	−38	28	26	L	46	Middle frontal gyrus
6	−23	−75	4	L	18	Middle occipital gyrus
16	−49	−42	9	L	21	Middle temporal gyrus
8	−43	−58	26	L	39	Middle temporal gyrus
8	40	−31	59	R	1	Postcentral gyrus
4	−43	−11	42	L	4	Precentral gyrus
8	−35	−11	59	L	6	Precentral gyrus
9	−14	−44	53	L	7	Precuneus
63	6	−53	59	R	7	Precuneus
43	−46	−39	15	L	22	Superior temporal gyrus
9	43	−31	15	R	22	Superior temporal gyrus
19	−49	−17	9	L	42	Superior temporal gyrus
6	55	−11	9	R	42	Superior temporal gyrus
4	−52	−47	26	L	40	Supramarginal gyrus
5	55	−39	26	R	40	Supramarginal gyrus

(i) For brevity here, we refer to the autism group, this includes patients with high functioning autism. (ii) We emphasize the amygdala theory of autism, and it might be thought that this is too narrow, because some of the lines of evidence cited here implicate temporal lobe structures more widely, which include the amygdala but also include other adjacent mesiotemporal areas. To the extent that the results reported later support the amygdala theory, it remains for future work to establish the specificity of this finding. (iii) A secondary difference between tasks A and B is that in A the same words (male, female) always appear, whilst in B different words (describing a range of mental states) appear. This is inevitable if one uses the same pictorial stimuli in both tasks, whilst varying the social judgement required. However, we cannot see any reason why this factor should explain the results. (iv) In fact, 51 voxels were found to have significantly greater power of response to the theory of mind task in controls compared with autistics; and seven voxels had significantly greater power of response in autistics compared with controls. (v) We have no strong evidence for OFC activation in these data. This may reflect magnetic susceptibility artefacts induced by the proximity of frontal bone and air spaces.

This also seems unlikely, in relation to states, e.g. "sympathy," "reflective," "sad thought" and "friendly." These are not rare sorts of expressions, and there is no reason to expect that others would not have shown such attitudes towards the subjects in both groups equally. Of course, none of these alternative explanations rules out that the subjects with autism might not understand such concepts and expressions less well than controls, but that is precisely the hypothesis that was tested.

Three final alternative accounts might be that eye-movements made by subjects with autism during task B might have differed significantly in comparison with task A. We cannot see why the stimuli in tasks A and B might have provoked different patterns of eye-movement/visual scanning, as the stimuli were identical in both conditions. However, this remains a small possibility as it may be that when one understands a visual scene less well, one scans it less. This should be checked in future studies. A vague and untestable account might be that the autistic group simply expends less "effort" in attempting to solve such tasks. We do not consider this further as this could never be determined, and in any case would not necessarily be independent of a comprehension deficit.

Future studies are also needed as a task like this could be dismantled into multiple, simpler mental elements. First, patients with autism should be presented with the eyes and no words, and vice versa, to establish which neural activations are due to these two separate factors. Second, it will be important to attempt to activate the amygdala in these patients, using a range of cognitive paradigms, to test if the present results reflect a general hypofunctioning of this structure, or whether this is specific to tasks involving inferring mental state. Converging evidence from another social intelligence task will also be important, as the above study employs just one such task. But the present study provides strong evidence of the role of the amygdala in normal social intelligence, and abnormality of the amygdala in autism.

Acknowledgements

This work was funded by a grant to S.B.C., H.R. and S.C.W. from the Wellcome Trust, and by a grant to the first author from the Gatsby Foundation. E.B. is also supported by the Wellcome Trust. We are grateful to Barry Everitt for comments on the first draft of this paper, and Chris Andrew for technical support.

Abbreviations

AS, Asperger syndrome; BA, Brodmann area; DLPFC, dorsolateral prefrontal cortex; fMRI, functional magnetic resonance imaging; FPQ, fundamental power quotient; MFC, medial frontal cortex; OFC, orbito-frontal cortex; SMA, supplementary motor area; STG, superior temporal gyrus.

References

Adolphs, R., Tranel, D., Damasio, H. & Damasio, A. (1994) Impaired recognition of emotion in facial expressions following bilateral damage to the human amygdala. *Nature*, 372, 669–672.

APA. (1994) *DSM-IV Diagnostic and Statistical Manual of Mental Disorders,* 4th edn. American Psychiatric Association, Washington DC.

Bachevalier, J. (1991) An animal model for childhood autism: memory loss and socioemotional disturbances following neonatal damage to the limbic system in monkeys. In Tamminga, C. & Schulz, S. (eds), *Advances in Neuropsychiatry and Psychopharmacology: Vol. 1. Schizophrenia Research.* Raven Press, New York.

Baron-Cohen, S. (1994) How to build a baby that can read minds: Cognitive mechanisms in mindreading. *Cahiers Psychologie Cognitive/Current Psychol. Cognition,* 13, 513–552.

Baron-Cohen, S. (1999) Does the study of autism justify minimalist innate modularity? *Learning and Individual Differences,* (in press).

Baron-Cohen, S. & Hammer, J. (1997) Parents of children with Asperger Syndrome: what is the cognitive phenotype? *J. Cogn. Neurosci.,* 9, 548–554.

Baron-Cohen, S., Jolliffe, T., Mortimore, C. & Robertson, M. (1997) Another advanced test of theory of mind: evidence from very high functioning adults with autism or Asperger Syndrome. *J. Child Psychol. Psychiatry,* 38, 813–822.

Baron-Cohen, S. & Ring, H. (1994) A model of the mindreading system: neuropsychological and neurobiological perspectives. In Mitchell, P. & Lewis, C. (eds), *Origins of an Understanding of Mind.* Lawrence Erlbaum Associates.

Baron-Cohen, S., Ring, H., Moriarty, J., Shmitz, P., Costa, D. & Ell, P. (1994) Recognition of mental state terms: a clinical study of autism, and a functional neuroimaging study of normal adults. *Br. J. Psychiatry,* 165, 640–649.

Baron-Cohen, S., Wheelwright, S., Stone, V. & Rutherford, M. A mathematician, a physicist, and a computer scientist with Asperger Syndrome: performance on folk psychology and folk physics test. *Neurocase,* (in press).

Bauman, M. & Kemper, T. (1988) Limbic and cerebellar abnormalities: consistent findings in infantile autism. *J. Neuropathol. Exp. Neurol.,* 47, 369.

Bauman, M. & Kemper, T. (1994) *The Neurobiology of Autism.* Johns Hopkins, Baltimore.

Bolton, P. & Griffiths, P. (1997) Association of tuberous sclerosis of temporal lobes with autism and atypical autism. *Lancet,* 349, 392–395.

Bonda, E., Petrides, M., Ostry, D. & Evans, A. (1996) Specific involvement of human parietal systems and the amygdala in the perception of biological motion. *J. Neurosci.,* 15, 3737–3744.

Brammer, M., Bullmore, E., Simmons, A., Williams, S., Grasby, P., Howard, R., Woodruff, P. & Rabe-Hesketh, S. (1997) Generic brain activation mapping in fMRI: a non-parametric approach. *Magn. Reson. Imaging.,* 15, 763–770.

Breiter, H. C., Etcoff, N. L., Whalem, P. J., Kennedy, W. A., Rauch, S. L., Buckner, R. L., Strauss, M. M., Hyman, S. E. & Rosen, B. R. (1996) Response and habituation of the human amygdala during visual processing of facial expression. *Neuron,* 17, 875–887.

Brothers, L. (1990) The social brain: a project for integrating primate behaviour and neurophysiology in a new domain. *Concepts Neurosci.,* 1, 27–51.

Brothers, L. & Ring, B. (1992) A neuroethological framework for the representation of minds. *J. Cognit. Neurosci.,* 4, 107–118.

Brothers, L., Ring, B. & King, A. (1990) Responses of neurons in the macaque amygdala to complex social stimuli. *Behav. Brain Res.,* 41, 199–213.

Bullmore, E., Brammer, M., Williams, S., Rabe-Hesketh, S., Janot, N., David, A., Mellers, J., Howard, R. & Sham, P. (1996) Statistical methods of estimation and inference for functional MR image analysis. *Magn. Reson. Med.,* 35, 261–277.

Calder, A. J., Young, A. W., Rowland, D., Perrett, D. I., Hodges, J. R. & Etcoff, N. L. (1996) Facial emotion recognition after bilateral amygdala damage: Differentially severe impairment of fear. *Cognit. Neuropsychol.,* 13, 699–745.

Campbell, R., Heywood, C., Cowey, A., Regard, M. & Landis, T. (1990) Sensitivity to eye gaze in prosopagnosic patients and monkeys with superior temporal sulcus ablation. *Neuropsychologia,* 28, 1123–1142.

D'Esposito, M., Detre, J. A., Alsop, D. C., Shin, R. K., Atlas, S. & Grossman, M. (1995) The neural basis of the central executive system of working memory. *Nature,* 378, 279–281.

Damasio, A., Tranel, D. & Damasio, H. (1990) Individuals with sociopathic behaviour caused by frontal lobe damage fail to respond autonomically to socially charged stimuli. *Behav. Brain Res.,* 14, 81–94.

Edgington, E. S. (1980) *Randomisation Tests.* Marcel Dekker, New York.

Eslinger, P. & Damasio, A. (1985) Severe disturbance of higher cognition after bilateral frontal lobe ablation: Patient EVR. *Neurology,* 35, 1731–1741.

Fletcher, P. C., Happe, F., Frith, U., Baker, S. C., Dolan, R. J., Frackowiak, R. S. J. & Frith, C. D. (1995) Other minds in the brain: a functional imaging study of "theory of mind" in story comprehension. *Cognition,* 57, 109–128.

Fodor, J. (1983) *The Modularity of Mind.* MIT/Bradford Books.

Frith, C., Friston, K., Liddle, P. & Frackowiak, R. (1991) A PET study of word finding. *Neuropsychologia,* 29, 1137–1148.

Gillberg, I., Bjure, J., Uvebrant, P., Vestergren, E. & Gillberg, C. (1993) SPECT in 31 children and adolescents with autism and autistic like syndromes. *Eur. Child Adolescent Psychiatry,* 2, 50–59.

Goel, V., Grafman, J., Sadato, N. & Hallett, M. (1995) Modeling other minds. *Neuroreport,* 6, 1741–1746.

Happé, F., Ehlers, S., Fletcher, P., Frith, U., Johansson, M., Gillberg, C., Dolan, R., Frackowiak, R. & Frith, C. (1996) "Theory of mind" in the brain. Evidence from a PET scan study of Asperger Syndrome. *Neuroreport*, 8, 197–201.

Humphrey, N. (1984) The social function of the intellect. In Humphrey, N. (ed.), *Consciousness Regained*. Oxford University Press, Oxford, pp. 14–28.

Karmiloff-Smith, A. (1992) *Beyond Modularity*. MIT Press/Bradford Books, Cambridge, MA, USA.

Karmiloff-Smith, A., Grant, J., Bellugi, U. & Baron-Cohen, S. (1995) Is there a social module? Language, face-processing and theory of mind in William's Syndrome and autism, in press. *J. Cognit. Neurosci.*, 7, 196–208.

Ketter, T., Andreason, P., George, M., Lee, C., Gill, D., Parekh, P., Willis, M., Herscovitch, P. & Post, R. (1996) Anterior paralimbic mediation of procaine induced emotional and psychosensory experience. *Arch. Gen. Psychiatry*, 53, 59–69.

Kling, A. & Brothers, L. (1992) The amygdala and social behavior. In Aggleton, J. (ed.), *Neurobiological Aspects of Emotion, Memory, and Mental Dysfunction*. Wiley-Liss, New York.

Morris, J., Frith, C., Perrett, D., Rowland, D., Young, A., Calder, A. & Dolan, R. (1996) A differential neural response in the human amygdala to fearful and happy facial expressions. *Nature*, 383, 812–815.

Ogawa, S., Lee, T., Kay, A. & Tank, D. (1990) Brain magnetic resonance imaging with contrast dependent blood oxygenation. *Proc. Natl Acad. Sci. USA*, 3, 9868–9872.

Perrett, D., Harries, M., Mistlin, A., Hietanen, J., Benson, P., Bevan, R., Thomas, S., Oram, M., Ortega, J. & Brierley, K. (1990) Social signals analyzed at the single cell level: someone is looking at me, something touched me, something moved! *Int J. Comp. Psychol.*, 4, 25–55.

Perrett, D., Smith, P., Potter, D., Mistlin, A., Head, A., Milner, A. & Jeeves, M. (1985) Visual cells in the temporal cortex sensitive to face view and gaze direction. *Proc. R. Soc. Lond. B Biol. Sci.*, B223, 293–317.

Phillips, M., Young, A., Senior, C., Brammer, M., Andrew, C., Calder, A., Bullmore, E., Perrett, D., Rowland, D., Williams, S., Gray, J. & David, A. (1997) A specific neural substrate for perceiving facial expressions of disgust. *Nature*, 389, 495–498.

Price, C. & Friston, K. (1997) The temporal dynamics of reading: a PET study. *Proc. R. Soc. Lond. B Biol. Sci.*, 264, 1785–1791.

Price, C., Moore, C. & Frackowiak, R. (1996) The effect of varying stimulus rate and duration on brain activity during reading. *Neuroimage*, 3, 40–52.

Rapin, I. & Katzman, R. (1998) Neurobiology of autism. *Ann. Neurol.*, 43, 7–14.

Sacks, O. (1994) *An Anthropologist on Mars*. Picador, London.

Salmon, E., Van der Linden, M., Collette, F., Maquet, P., Degueldre, C., Luxen, A. & Franck, G. (1996) Regional brain activity during working memory tasks. *Brain*, 119, 1617–1625.

Scott, S., Young, A., Calder, A., Hellawell, D., Aggleton, J. & Johnson, M. (1997) Impaired auditory recognition of fear and anger following bilateral amygdala lesions. *Nature*, 385, 254–257.

Tager-Flusberg, H., Boshart, J. & Baron-Cohen, S. (1998) Reading the windows of the soul: evidence of domain specificity sparing in Williams syndrome. *J. Cognit. Neurosci.*, 10, 631–639.

Talairach, J. & Tournoux, P. (1988) *Coplanar Stereotaxic Atlas of the Human Brain*. Thieme Medical Publishers, New York.

Tranel, D. & Hyman, B. T. (1990) Neuropsycholocial correlates of bilateral amygdala damage. *Arch. Neurol.*, 47, 349–355.

Weinberger, D. & Berman, K. (1998) Prefrontal function in schizophrenia: confounds and controversies. In Roberts, A., Robbins, T. & Weiskrantz, L. (eds), *The Prefrontal Cortex: Executive and Cognitive Functions*. Oxford University Press, Oxford.

Whalen, P. J., Rauch, S. L., Etcoff, N. L., McInerney, S. C., Lee, M. B. & Janike, M. A. (1998) Masked presentations of emotional facial expressions modulate amygdala activity without explicit knowledge. *J. Neurosci.*, 18, 411–418.

Whiten, A. (1991) *Natural Theories of Mind*. Basil Blackwell, Oxford.

Wise, R., Chollet, F., Hadar, U., Friston, K., Hoffner, E. & Frackowiak, R. (1991) Distribution of cortical neural networks involved in word comprehension and retrieval. *Brain*, 114, 1803–1817.

Young, A., Hellawell, D., De Wal, C. & Johnson, M. (1996) Facial expression processing after amygdalectomy. *Neuropsychologia*, 34, 31–39.

26 The Social Brain: A Project for Integrating Primate Behavior and Neurophysiology in a New Domain

Leslie Brothers

1 Introduction

Understanding how the central nervous system codes behaviorally relevant information is the central goal of brain research. Since neural processing carried out by organisms operating in the natural world is complex, it is critical for the study of nervous system functions to tease out particular cognitive operations underlying an organism's behavior and to relate these in meaningful ways to sets of facts about its brain.

As a first step, we may categorize an organism's activities into cognitive subsystems such as learning, memory (especially as it is currently being refined into discrete categories), attention, perception of visual form, perception of odor, perception of the subject's own body surface, and so forth. Moving to a less general level, it has been extraordinarily productive to attend simultaneously to the behavioral specializations of particular species for certain kinds of cognition and to the corresponding neural structures underlying the specialization. Such an approach is exemplified by the comparative anatomical and neurophysiological studies, informed by ecological knowledge, which have been carried out on the primate visual system by Allman [1–3] and on avian audition by Konishi [4]. The neuroethological approach has proven fruitful because each particular instantiation of a brain-behavior relation reveals new principles in the coding of information by the nervous system.

It is the primate brain which concerns us in this essay. To take an informed approach to primate brain function, we begin by asking, "What are the relative behavioral specializations of primates?" The use of language by human primates appears to be one. Another example is reliance on activity involving the forelimbs, which has prompted the use of non-human primates for studies of hand and arm motor control. A high degree of development of central vision, while not unique to primates, is a relative specialization: its study has led to a meaningful interpretation of an anatomical arrangement which is unique to primates, namely, the separate representation of the visual hemifields in the optic tectum [2, 5].

A primate specialization which has now been amply documented by behavioral scientists, but ignored for the most part by neuroscientists, is the specialization for social cognition. What I mean by the term "social cognition" is the following: *Social cognition is the processing of any information which culminates in the accurate perception of the dispositions and intentions of other individuals.* While many non-primates (for example, ants) can interact in highly specific ways with others of their kind, it appears that primates, especially those most closely related to ourselves, have developed a unique capacity to perceive psychological facts (dispositions and intentions) about other individuals. This capacity appears to distinguish primate social behavior from that of other orders (although whether some cetaceans possess a similar sophistication is being studied). The perception of such entities as disposition and intention in others arises from the processing of the following kinds of information about other individuals: identity, direction of movement, category of posture, facial expression, quality of vocalization, knowledge of which other individuals are present and what their mutual relations are, etc. While I intend to subsume all this processing under the category "social cognition," my central assertion is that these subprocesses have come to be organized so as to produce perception of the dispositions and intentions of others.

It is reasonable to believe that this specialization is in some way stamped upon brain function and therefore accessible to investigation at the neural level: in effect, the attempt to relate growing knowledge about primate social cognition to neural activity opens up a new area for brain research. In Section 2, I present evidence for the status of social cognition in primates as a separate domain of cognition and I provide material supporting my particular definition of it. Understanding the nature of the social cognitive domain paves the way for Section 3, which is a re-evaluation of the significance of socially-responsive neurons ("face cells" and their congeners) that have been described in macaque temporal lobe structures. In Section 3, I also indicate the nature of the studies which will be needed in the future to strengthen our understanding of the link between neural activity and social cognition in non-human primates.

2 Social Cognition Is a Special Domain: The Evidence

Although the idea has been debated [6], an evolutionary viewpoint suggests that the brain's operations are specialized for solving problems of adaptive significance [7]. General criteria for cognitive modules have been proposed, for example, by Fodor. One of these is domain-specificity of input systems ("if you have a stimulus domain ... in which perceptual analysis requires a body of information whose character and content is specific to that domain, then it is plausible that psychological processes defined over that domain may be carried out by relatively special purpose computational systems" [8]). Gardner considers the following to be among the "signs" of what he terms an "intelligence": an evolutionary history and evolutionary plausibility, a distinctive developmental history, the existence of prodigies (or, conversely, of persons with selective absence of an intelligence), potential isolation by brain damage, and identifiable core operations [9].

In what follows, we will subject primate social cognition to scrutiny along the dimensions proposed by Gardner.

2.1 Evolutionary History and Plausibility

2.1.1 An Example: The Evolution of Facial Expression

Darwin [10] wrote:

The community of certain expressions in distinct though allied species, as in the movements of the same facial muscles during laughter by man and by various monkeys, is rendered somewhat more intelligible, if we believe in their descent from a common progenitor. He who admits on general grounds that the structure and habits of all animals have been gradually evolved, will look at the whole subject of Expression in a new and interesting light.

The phylogeny of facial expression in primates illustrates the evolution of one channel of social communication. Using comparative data, it appears that nocturnal primates were the earliest forms [3]. These animals lived in rather simple social groups and communicated primarily by olfaction (spraying of scent from special-purpose glands) rather than by vision—as would be expected given their nocturnal lifestyles. The switch to diurnal activity patterns was probably accompanied by two developments, one, a greater reliance on visual social communication, and two, more complex social structures [3]. That these two developments should go together is not surprising, given that vision permits a high degree of temporal sequencing and brevity of signals compared to olfaction. Lemurs are a particularly interesting group in regard to the transition from olfaction to vision, as they use both modalities. They are able to use facial expression to a limited degree but are restricted by the anatomical fact that their upper lips are attached to their gums in the middle (as are dogs' upper lips, to use a familiar example). Primates which use their visual systems extensively for social communication, such as ourselves, have non-attached, mobile upper lips. This permits the mouth region to be used for a very rich variety of facial expressions—and indeed, those muscles innervated by the seventh cranial nerve (which also include the muscles around the eyes) are sometimes referred to as "the muscles of expression."

The face and its expressions are but one channel over which information concerning an animal's internal state might be conveyed: others are vocalization, body posture and gestures. It is logical to assume that, together with the development of ever more differentiated signalling devices such as the expressive primate face, a cognitive apparatus for correct perception and response evolved as well. Evidence for sophisticated cognitive processing of social signals by non-human primates is reviewed next.

2.1.2 The Perception of Social Signals in Non-human Primates

Cheney et al. [11] have written:

As information on primate social behavior continues to accumulate, the complex and multi-faceted social relationships of non-human primates become increasingly apparent.... They employ a variety of mechanisms for sustaining relationships that combine competitive and affiliative elements, and they seem to be able to adjust their behavior to particular individuals and circumstances. These features of primate behavior raise intriguing questions about the cognitive capacities that underlie social interactions.

Examples of the sophistication of social cognition in monkeys and apes include these: baboon males engage in "psychological contests," rather than physical ones, with other males when attempting to appropriate their female consorts [12]; female chimpanzees create situations which cause reconciliations between previously antagonistic males [13]; bonobos "fix" situations which they perceive as distressing to their playmates [13]. The following is an example of a chimpanzee interaction, together with an interpretation, as described by De Waal [14].

On a hot day two mothers, Jimmie and Tepel, are sitting in the shadow of an oak tree while their two children play in the sand at their feet (playfaces, wrestling, throwing sand). Between the two mothers the oldest female, Mama, lies asleep. Suddenly the children start screaming, hitting and pulling each other's hair. Jimmie admonishes them with a soft, threatening grunt and Tepel anxiously shifts her position. The children go on quarrelling and eventually Tepel wakes Mama by poking her in the ribs several times. As Mama gets up, Tepel points to the two quarrelling children. As soon as Mama takes one threatening step forward, waves her arm in the air and barks loudly, the children stop quarrelling. Mama then lies down again and continues her siesta.

Interpretation: In order to understand this interpretation fully, it is important to know two things: first, that Mama is the highest-ranking female and is greatly respected; and second, that conflicts between children regularly engender such tension between their mothers that they too come to blows. This tension is probably caused by the fact that each mother wishes to prevent the other from interfering in the children's quarrel. In the case of the example above, when the children's game turned to fighting, both mothers found themselves in a painful situation. Tepel solved the problem by activating a dominant third party, Mama, and pointing out the problem to her. Mama obviously realized at a glance that she was expected to act as arbitrator.

De Waal [14] states:

The result (of chimpanzees' combining past experiences to achieve a goal) is considered rational behavior. In their *social* application of reason and thought, chimpanzees are truly remarkable. Technically their inventiveness is clearly inferior to that of human beings but socially, I would hesitate to make such a claim.

The behavior of the chimpanzee Mama in the anecdote above indicates that she perceived the situation and the desires of her neighbors. Terms which imply an approach to human mentality, such as "deception," "altruism" and "reason" must however be used with care. For example, there is no evidence that propositional thought invoking separate selves ("if I do such-and-such, he will likely do such-and-such") is involved. Rather, as suggested by Langer [15], sophisticated empathic and cooperative behaviors of animals may represent "a supreme development of non-human capacities, rather than an approach to human intellect." It is the nature of these non-human capacities which we wish in the first instance to understand. Accounts of chimpanzee behavior which seem to demonstrate that the animals "have ideas about" another individual's knowledge or intent may imply a stronger theory of other minds than the animals actually possess; for example, while there is agreement that chimpanzees do attribute seeing, wanting and expecting to others, which is a sort of theory of other minds, it has not been proven to everyone's satisfaction that they can maintain one set of desires themselves and simultaneously attribute a different set to another individual [16].

We are on firm ground in stating that human beings possess the capacity to perceive the inner states of others, and to a more sophisticated degree than do chimpanzees if only because of the presumed greater complexity of our mental lives. The appropriate word for such cognition in humans is "empathy," defined as "a mode of cognition which is specifically attuned to the perception of complex psychological configurations" [17]. The term should not be confused with "sympathy"; nor does it imply benevolent intentions, as knowledge of another's feelings gained by empathic perception can be used in hostile or exploitive ways equally as well as in helpful ones. The extent to which human beings have retained, and the routes along which we have developed, the social cognitive capacities of our ancestors are topics of profound interest inviting further study.

2.1.3 Social Knowledge is Operationally Distinct from other Knowledge

Having shown that non-human primates are indeed able to attribute—in some form—intentions and motivations to others, we return to the issue of the distinction between social and other domains of cognition. Investigators studying non-human primates have suggested that what at first might appear to be general-purpose cognitive operations (association, reasoning by analogy, making transitive inferences) appear to operate most strongly, indeed practically exclusively, in

the manipulation of social representations. That is, logical operations carried out by monkeys in a social setting, with other individuals as the "terms," do not seem able to be executed with inanimate objects in the laboratory [11]. There appears to be, then, a "social intelligence" distinguishable in primate evolution from general intelligence. This finding of a specialized social cognition has given rise to the suggestion that human intelligence arose secondarily from social cognitive operations in our primate ancestors, operations which developed to solve complex social problems [18]. This idea will help us to understand some neurological syndromes discussed below, in which social deficits are accompanied by analogous deficits in the processing of non-social stimuli.

Finally, we might consider the pressures favoring evolution of social skills. Increasing complexity of social groups is one which has been mentioned. Another, pointed out by Humphrey [19], is the fact that increasing competence among members of a group for deceiving and manipulating each other (that is, for masking intentions or for being ambiguous) is itself a source of ever more intense pressure to develop acute perception of subtle configurations of expression and behavior. Increasingly acute perception in turn increases the pressure to develop more ambiguity and concealment, etc. For people, it has become a form of amusement to exercise these capacities in games like poker.

2.2 A Distinctive Developmental History

The story of an evolved specialization for social interaction can also be read in the behavior of primate infants. We shall confine ourselves to human infants here.

According to classical psychoanalytic views, infants perceive the world in terms of "only the crudest representations of pleasure and unpleasure" [20]. Experimental observation has revealed however that human neonates are equipped with basic mechanisms of face and voice perception [21]. They are able to imitate facial gestures (opening and closing mouth, protruding tongue or lips) at two weeks of age [22], to imitate facial expression at 36 hours of age [23], and possess at one day of age a remarkable tendency to cry upon hearing the crying of other infants but not synthetic cries of the same loudness and duration [24]. (There is reason to believe that this innate tendency to imitate is a phylogenetically primitive substrate for perception of the emotional states of others [25].) Two-month-olds display organized expressions of affect which are systematically related to changes in the mother's behavior [26]. Beyond these sophisticated social perceptual capacities, infants have in addition a host of innate behaviors which serve to maintain dyadic (two-person) exchanges. These include the social smile, present even in blind infants [27]; patterns of cyclic gazing at the caretaker's face, accompanied by complex facial movements, established by three to four weeks of age [28]; and extremely sensitive temporal participation in the rhythm of kinesic and vocal dialogues that occur between infant and caregiver [29]. The fairly stereotyped ontogenetic development of all these repertoires is evidence of an innate neural specialization for social behavior. Their behavioral content expresses an innate disposition on the part of human infants to establish and maintain rapport.

To understand the significance of this rapport we turn to innate behaviors of parents. Adult caretakers appear instinctively to engage in expressive matching behavior with their infants when the latter are between eight and twelve months of age. In such matching, the temporal contour of an expressive movement on the part of the infant is matched in a different modality, for example by the prosodic contour of the mother's vocal expression [30]. In this way, a state of rapport is created with the infant's *feeling* and not just with its overt physical activity. The innate tendency of mother and infant to orchestrate this psychological attunement provides the basis for a remarkable achievement:

Infants gradually come upon the momentous realization that inner subjective experiences, the "subject matter" of the mind, are potentially shareable with someone else.... This discovery amounts to the acquisition of a "theory" of separate minds.

For such an experience to occur, there must be some shared framework of meaning and means of communication such as gesture, posture, or facial expression [30].

Thus under normal circumstances children perceive by one year of age that others, like themselves, have feelings and intentions.

In sum, what we can reconstruct of primate evolution from study of non-human primates and of human infants suggests the development of a specialization for perceiving and responding to social signals. The central characteristic of this trend is a capacity to detect features of the mental lives—not just the overt behaviors—of others. In the case of apes, psychological features such as seeing, wanting and expecting are able to be detected in others; in human infants, there is a developmental sequence culminating in the potential to perceive these psychological features, and many more.

2.3   Inborn Selective Absence of Social Cognition

There exist individuals with selective absence of social knowledge.

Autism is a spectrum of relatively rare disorders (4–15 per 10,000, depending on diagnostic criteria) which in its broadest manifestations may include echolalia (parroting of heard words or phrases); repetitive speech; concrete, literal interpretation of language; lack of social interest and empathy; a narrow range of activities and acute distress and anger when these are interrupted; and others. Significantly, the varying sets of diagnostic criteria for autism overlap in the emphasis on social impairments. It is clear that the disorder may result from a variety of brain diseases, either genetic or due to intrauterine factors: since other diseases affecting development do not give rise to social impairment (for example, cerebral palsy and Downs syndrome), it is hypothesized that particular brain regions or functions must be affected in autistic children in order for social impairment to result [31].

The social impairments of autism have been described in general terms as aloofness, indifference, or a tendency to use odd social approaches. A variety of deficits in dyadic behavior emerge in infancy, such as markedly reduced eye contact compared to normal infants and failure of the infant to raise its arms in anticipation of being picked up [32], a behavior which is normally well-established by four months of age. The fundamental deficit begins to be understood, however, by considering studies of slightly older autistic children.

For one thing, there appears to be a particular form of inability to share information with another person about a third object through verbal or non-verbal means. Compared to mentally retarded and normal children, autistic children fail to point, show or make eye contact with others while holding an object or watching an object in motion. In one study, for example, although they watched mechanical toys with interest, they infrequently demonstrated the joint attention behavior of looking between the toy and an adult. They were, however, able to combine eye contact with the acts of reaching to an object or handing it to an adult [33]. Interpreting these findings, Mundy [33] states:

Presumably one goal of these behaviors is to coordinate one's own focus of attention to an object or event with the attention of a social partner. (However) an important distinction is that (the latter behaviors, i.e., reaching toward or giving an object while using eye contact) involved object goals and an appreciation of other as an agent of action capable of assisting with the object goals. Alternatively, indicating behaviors (pointing, showing or making eye contact while watching or holding an object) appear to involve object goals to a lesser extent. Instead these behaviors appear to focus on the interpersonal goal of monitoring or acknowledging shared interest in an object or event.

Deficits in indicating skills mark the young autistic child's failure to develop an adequate concept of others as possessing independent psychological states, such as interest in objects.

In addition, compared to IQ-matched controls, autistic children have difficulty understanding the emotional content of facial expression and vocalizations, while their manipulation and understanding of objects is normal [34]. They are able to use gestures such as pointing with finger, upraised hand to signal "stop," finger on lips to signal "quiet"; but in contrast to control subjects they fail to use expressive gestures such as arm around shoulder in consolation or hand over mouth, signalling embarrassment, that is, gestures which express understanding of the internal state of another or which communicate one's own internal state [35]. Finally, the use of language by autistic children shows deficits in pragmatics (social aspects such as turn-taking, inter-weaving of a person's utterances into an ongoing conversation, tailoring one's utterances to the situation) and in prosody (the intonation or melody of speech), while competence is preserved in other aspects of language such as articulation, syntax and semantics [36].

It appears then that there exists a group of individuals with deficits which are selectively social. While the central quality of these deficits is a lack of ability to perceive the inner world of other persons, or to convey one's own state to others, there are also disturbances in component processes such as understanding voice intonation or establishing eye contact. This suggests that the cognitive module whose processes culminate in the perception of the dispositions and intentions of others, subsumes related and more peripheral processes as well.

2.4 Neurological Syndromes

In this section, I consider neurological syndromes under two headings: those which give rise to deficits in the peripheral operations of social cognition, and those which give rise to deficits in proposed core processes.

2.4.1 Syndromes Affecting Components of Social Perception

Prosopagnosia, the inability to identify a familiar face, may arise as a symptom of localized brain damage. Evidence suggesting face recognition shares a common substrate with identification of objects all belonging to a class of similar appearance [37] does not disqualify prosopagnosia as a defect of social cognition: neural machinery which is particularly well-adapted for one task will not be expected to be reserved only for that task (see Section 3.1 below for an extended treatment of this point). Also, as set out in Section 2.1 above, it has been hypothesized that neural mechanisms for social cognition have provided the framework for similar processing of non-social objects. Following this line of thought, it would not be unreasonable to find processing which is logically similar to face identification affected by lesions which damage face-recognition structures.

There are several reasons to consider face recognition as a lower-level subprocess of social cognition. First, it is possible to carry on complex social exchanges with people whose faces are not familiar from previous exposure and to assess their motivations and intentions. Second, identifying facial expression and recognizing faces are abilities which appear to reside in different anatomical structures [38, 39]. However, I propose that face recognition is a process with the special quality of being rapidly "pulled into" a social cognition module. In this respect, it obeys Jackendoff's [40] description of modular processes as mandatory. As an example, in the language module, "one cannot hear a speech stream as mere sound, especially in a language one understands," that is—following Jackendoff's construction—lower-level representations are obligatorily pulled up into intermediate ones, and it is the latter that become conscious. Evidence from patients who have undergone surgical disconnection of the cerebral hemispheres indicates that face-processing tasks activate a specialized circuit in the right hemisphere [41]. I suggest that the visual appearance of a face in social cognition is analogous to a stream of speech in linguistic processing: the face stimulus is immediately and obligatorily transformed into the representation of a person (with dispositions and intentions) before having access to consciousness. My evidence for this comes from an anecdote told by a colleague:

My colleague was provided with a large set of rather poor quality photographs of a class of graduate students from another university, to use as a stimulus set in an experiment. While carrying out the experiment, she saw the photographs many times. Subsequently, from time to time at scientific meetings she would find herself near someone whom she felt she knew but couldn't place ("I know that I know you but I can't quite place you ..."), which person would turn out to be one of the photographed students [42].

What is significant is that the sight of the familiar face gave rise to a conviction that *she knew the person*, rather than to the only memory which was in fact relevant, namely, that the face belonged to the photographed set. Would the same illusory familiarity be created by prior exposure to pictures of non-social stimuli? Another somewhat amusing anecdote suggests not:

A late-night television fan was being driven through Paris while on a European trip. Catching sight of one of the landmarks, he stated, "That looks just like the one in 'The Hunchback of Notre Dame.'" (It was Notre Dame.)

Notice that the sight of the building did not create the illusion "I have personally seen this actual building before," unlike the conviction inspired by the familiar face in the preceding anecdote. Rather, it called up the relevant memory, that a building with the same appearance had been seen in a movie.

In addition to prosopagnosia, there are several other neurological syndromes which affect peripheral aspects of social cognition. Right temporoparietal lesions may produce auditory affective agnosia, that is, the inability to understand emotion in voice quality [43]. There appears to be a right hemisphere specialization for producing and comprehending the affective components of language, analogous to the specialization of the left hemisphere for propositional components [44]. The aprosodic-agestural syndrome is an inability to express felt emotions through prosody (voice intonation) or spontaneous gesture, and occurs in some individuals with right hemisphere lesions [45].

2.4.2 Syndromes Affecting Core Social Cognitive Processes

2.4.2.1 Patient EVR Eslinger and Damasio [46] have reported the case of a patient who underwent resection of an orbitofrontal meningioma at age 35, with consequent loss of all of right orbital cortex, part of left orbital cortex, destruction of subjacent white matter, and some damage to right dorsolateral cortex and white matter subjacent to the premotor area. Premorbidly, the patient had superior social functioning as judged by his success in a variety of groups (vocational, church and family) and by accounts of his premorbid personality. Since his surgery, however, the patient has presented a remarkable dissociation between his fund of abstract knowledge about social situations, which is fully intact as elicited by verbal testing, and his capacity to evaluate real-life social situations. Although there were no impairments on any neuropsychological tests and his intelligence is above average, his inability to draw correct conclusions about the motivations of those around him has led him into associations with people of doubtful character, resulting in his bankruptcy (he had formerly worked as an accountant). The clinical presentation ends with a telling description:

EVR is now 44 years old. He is currently considering a third marriage to a person he described as a "spoiled 58-year-old woman," a "semi-prominent socialite." He is trying to persuade her to finance a "luxury travel business" to drive "wealthy people" on vacation around the country in a motor home.

Patient EVR has lost the ability to respond appropriately to social situations, apparently as a result of having lost access to the internal cues which the behavior of others should generate. Nor does he seem to form an accurate appraisal of the motivations and attitudes others are likely to have in the imagined future. The inability in real life situations to generate internal signals, which normally serve as guides to appropriate action, plagues EVR in other spheres as well. Trivial decisions such as what to throw away or which restaurant to select for a meal are carried on for hours without conclusion.

Orbital frontal cortex, the primary site of the patient's lesions, has extensive limbic connections [47]—EVR's deficits should be kept in mind as we consider other limbic structures in Section 2.5. Lesions of orbital frontal cortex and amygdala in monkeys, as well as kindling of the amygdala, are also known to create deficits in social behavior [48].

2.4.2.2 Capgras Syndrome A fascinating syndrome in which the link between recognition of an individual and feelings of familiarity with the person becomes broken, is Capgras syndrome. This syndrome may occur in isolation as a result of a single brain insult [49, 50] or more commonly as a feature of an evolving or full-blown psychosis. It consists of preserved ability to identify another individual by appearance, usually a close familiar such as spouse or parent, joined with an absolute conviction that the individual actually is *not* that person. The confusing percept is usually resolved by the patient concluding that a diabolically clever masquerade is taking place (e.g. "There's a man living in my house—I think the Mafia have put him there, I don't know why—he looks exactly like my husband but I just know he's not. They've switched him for my real husband.") Notice that the primary element of the syndrome is a failed feeling of rapport or familiarity with the other person's mental life (analogous to the prosopagnosic's failed feeling of familiarity with the appearance of the person's face). We cannot distinguish whether the patients actually are suffering a failure of perception of the other person's mental life, or a failure of the affect of familiarity pertaining to this perception. In either case, the syndrome circumscribes *the felt link with the mental life of another individual*. The syndrome is an uncommon, but not rare [51], occurrence in the general psychiatric population. As in prosopagnosia, careful study reveals that similar cognitive dysfunction may occur in appraisal of inanimate objects, for example, a woman with Capgras syndrome also felt her glasses case was a clever substitute which looked just like her real glasses case [52].

While many case reports of Capgras syndrome emphasize the role of organic brain lesions, the majority either involve widespread damage, or, when the lesion is discrete, show it to be superimposed on previous diffuse dysfunction. However, a few case studies document fairly localized lesions. In one patient, extensive examination revealed no focal or diffuse abnormalities, except for a CT scan finding of bilateral temporal lobe atrophy [53]. In another, symptoms began upon treatment of a left temporal cysticercum (an encapsulated parasitic infection of the brain): it was measured on CT scan at about 6×8 mm in size, and was located near the external capsule [50].

2.4.2.3 Paranoid Psychoses
Finally, distortion of the perception of other people's intentions and motivations—particularly as these are directed toward one's self—is virtually pathognomonic of the paranoid psychoses. The distortion is often an exaggerated sense of emotional or psychological relatedness between one's inner life and that of others ("people are reading my mind";

"famous Actress X is in love with me"); or it can take the form of a conviction about the intentions of unidentified agents ("it feels like people I don't know are trying to trip me up, stop me from getting what I want"; or, "there are powerful people out there who are keeping a watch on me, they have something really good in store for me and they're guiding my steps"). In effect, the paranoid person is beset by "intentions"—benevolent, hostile, erotic—in almost disembodied form. The following excerpt is typical of the exaggerated sense of being the object of others' intentions and actions [54]:

"On the streetcar there were two women talking. I did not know them at all. They were looking in my direction and one woman said to the other, 'She is always looking for a fight.' ... One of the women followed me into the grocery store."

Paranoid psychoses are also accompanied by other disturbances of mentation; the neural basis of paranoia is unknown. Although both paranoia and Capgras syndrome are somewhat unsatisfactory in providing little hard anatomical data, a description of the clinical phenomena in the terms I have provided above seems quite worthwhile—traditional psychodynamic formulations invoking ambivalence (in the case of Capgras) and attribution of one's own disavowed aggressive or erotic feelings to others (as in paranoia) have dominated explanations of the phenomena. Accounts invoking disturbances in central cognitive processes involving perception of others' intentions and motivations in my view provide a more satisfactory framework for understanding the symptoms of these illnesses.

2.5 Core Operations?

Jackendoff states, "... it is clear that intuition about how people work is quite distinct from intuition about how machines or deductive systems work; and it is equally clear that talent in one domain often does not carry over into another," however, "what representations this intelligence engages is an open question" [40]. I have suggested in the preceding section that the subject matter of social cognition is the dispositions and intentions of others. In Section 3 below, I shall describe what is known of the neural basis of this module in non-human primates. However, before proceeding to those findings, it seems worthwhile to explore the implications of some additional clinical data which bear directly upon the social cognitive module. These data are comprised in part of something subjective, namely, affect. I will suggest that what may be unique to social cognition does not concern representations *per se,* but is rather an especially intimate tie of core representations—that is, the representations of others' dispositions and intentions—to affect. Since affects strain our notions of what "cognition" is, this section may appear to lie outside the conceptual scheme I have outlined so far. A brief discussion of "affect" precedes the clinical material.

2.5.1 Human Beings have the Innate Capacity to Experience Very Many Diverse Affects
I mean to keep my discussion of affect (which can be read as "feeling") on a very common-sense plane. The idea which I wish to convey in this section is that affects in human experience are an extremely numerous and diverse kind of innate mental phenomenon.

By affects, I emphatically do not mean "basic" affects as set out in typologies ("joy–sadness–anger–surprise–disgust–fear"). These typologies tend to suggest that other affects are derived from combinations of these basic elements, much as purple pigment is derived from mixing blue and red. However, the sensation "purple" is not derivable in any way from the sensations "red" and "blue." While observation suggests that innate facial expressions fall into basic categories [55], there is actually no reason to think that feelings themselves do. In fact, it is the irreducible richness of the spectrum of affects which should attract our attention.

A second difficulty which typologies create is the idea that we have ready labels for affect experiences. In fact, feelings and the names for them are worlds apart, with the result that our general reliance on verbally expressed concepts leaves many important nuances of feeling unarticulated.

A man began to realize the significance for him of his relationship with a helpful mentor: he felt moved and his eyes became wet. Unable at first to articulate his feeling, he declared, "I must be sad—I'm crying."

Because of the limitation of conceptual terms in conveying affects, and the small number of common-currency names such as "sad" and "happy" that we have at our disposal, feeling states often are communicated from one person to another by a different means, namely, by reference to a situation (e.g. "you know, the way you feel in dreams when you find yourself in public with no clothes on and you're trying to hide," or "the way you feel at a cocktail party if you don't know anyone and everyone else is talking to someone," or "feeling like you sank the winning basket at the buzzer and you're everyone's hero"). As we turn to clinical evidence below, we will see that in order to describe certain affective experiences, people resort to the format, "as if I were in such-and-such a situation."

2.5.2 The Special Link between Affect and Social Representations
While there is no doubt that behavior indicative of fear and rage can be elicited in a non-human primate threatened by a predator, it must be hundreds of times more frequent—at least—that more modulated versions of these affects are evoked in everyday social interactions. It is to be expected that the full range of affective life in the non-human primate is experienced virtually exclusively in its social dealings.

The proposal that social cognition and affect have a special tie receives strong support from the studies of Gloor [56, 57], involving patients' reports of their subjective experiences upon stimulation of temporal lobe structures. (See [58] for the reason that experiences stimulated under these conditions should be considered as samples of the normal function of these structures rather than aberrant or artifactual.) It is worthwhile to quote at length from a few of these reports:

In a twenty-year-old man, right amygdaloid stimulation at 2 mA elicited an elaborate experience encompassing the complex visual hallucination of standing at noontime on a cliff by the seaside with a friend. This experience was associated with fear and represented an evocation of the memory of a past event. This was a fully integrated experience consisting of perceptual, mnemonic, and affective components, as is the case in real life.
... Amygdaloid stimulation at a lower intensity of 1 mA ... had elicited another experiential response ...: he reported that he had reexperienced a frightening event from his childhood which happened while he was at a picnic in Brewer Park in Ottowa. He described it as follows: "A kid was coming up to me to push me in the water. It was a certain time, a special day during the summer holidays and the boy was going to push me into the water. I was pushed down by somebody stronger than me. I have experienced that same feeling when I had 'petit mals' before."
... Upon stimulating his left amygdala at 1 mA, he had a feeling "as if I were not belonging here," which he likened to being at a party and not being welcome.... Right hippocampal stimulation at 3 mA induced anxiety and guilt, "... like you are demanding to hand in a report that was due 2 weeks ago ... as if I were guilty of some form of tardiness."
Another 32-year-old patient upon stimulation in the left amygdala at 1.5 mA reported that it felt "like someone talking to a child." It was a female voice and he thought it could have been that of his wife, but he could not understand what was being said. He believed this was an evocation of an old memory.
Upon stimulation of the right amygdala (in a forty-year-old woman) the patient looked perplexed and was reluctant to talk about what she felt. She had an abdominal feeling like nausea, but in addition she experienced a pleasant feeling in her vulva and on the inner surface of her thighs, as if she were having sexual intercourse. She did not see her partner, but knew it was "X," the boyfriend with whom she had had her first sexual intercourse at age 16, and subsequently many

times more. She affirmed that the experience was an evocation of an old memory, and although she subsequently had had intercourse with other men, she was positive that the feeling evoked by amygdaloid stimulation was the feeling of having sexual relations with her old boyfriend "X." ... She volunteered that she had the same sexual experience at the onset of her spontaneous seizures.

Gloor points out that a characteristic of these phenomena "is that they most often are set in what might be called a 'social context' in the broadest sense of the term, or better perhaps in an 'ethological' context.... They frequently bear some relationship with familiar situations or situations with an affective meaning. They frequently touch on some aspect of (the patient's) relationship with other people, either known specifically to him, or not" [57].

I would add this emphasis: the experiences tend to involve actions, attitudes or intentions of others, perceived by the subjects to be directed at themselves. These mental or behavioral attitudes on the part of others evoked feelings which sometimes were able to be named (sexual arousal, fear). When they were not able to be named, they were still quite definite in quality and able to be indicated to the investigators by reference to a situation ("like being at a party and not being welcome"; "like you are demanding and I am guilty"). I propose that these are innate social affects and that they are the experiential core of the representations of the dispositions and intentions of others.

The account of the 40-year-old female patient gives an excellent insight into the social nature of affects: her physical sensations, combined with pleasurable feelings, were fused with the idea of a particular partner. As in some of the previous examples, the feelings created by the other person's actions or intentions, be they pleasurable or scary, were intimately linked to the representation of the interaction and the person. In other examples, by contrast, the feelings brought on by others' intentions or attitudes (scolding, being talked to as a child) were virtually in isolation from specific images of other individuals or their overt behaviors. In a sense, in these experiences the intention of another was perceived, in the form of an affect, without an agent of the intention being represented. We might consider these as the experiences of core fragments, in effect, affective signals which are potentially ready to become linked with a social representation—either in current experience or in a mnemonic record. We are indebted to Gloor for his acumen in noting the significance of these patients' accounts.

The common identification of limbic structures, such as the amygdala, with affects related to "basic drives," such as fear and hunger, probably misses those structures' most remarkable role in primate phylogeny. The affective coloration of social experience, experienced as lived feeling, is a powerful signal to its possessor. Shame is a social affect, as are triumph, jealousy, parental tenderness, romantic love, and all the hard-to-name affects to which we have referred above by describing situations. Complex social life calls for subtle, differentiated and varied feelings, useful as internal signals in environments consisting of mates, offspring, allies, rivals, leaders, in-groups, bullies, and friends. I propose that the human possession of a huge "dictionary" of innate feelings has as its evolutionary origin the demands of social existence. If limbic structures such as the amygdala and orbital frontal cortex are responsible in some way for generating this vast array of discrete affective experience—as seems likely—then they are remarkable structures indeed.

Finally, although I have argued for the origin of affect diversity in primate social experience, I readily acknowledge that people experience powerful feelings in non-social contexts. The pleasure of mastering a problem or of forging an idea or aesthetic object seems to inhere in the interaction with the materials; likewise, the feelings brought on by contemplation of huge scales—existential feelings regarding one's self in relation to the ocean, the heavens, or history—are certainly

non-social and often quite strong. Their place in evolution and neurobiology would be an interesting topic of inquiry.

To summarize Section 2 briefly, we have examined social cognition, defined as cognition culminating in the perception of the dispositions and intentions of others, in light of various criteria for a separate module. The social abilities of non-human primates, evolved in the context of an increasingly complex social environment, were found to be on a continuum with the sophisticated abilities of humans to perceive others' mental states. A stereotyped development in human infants of the ability to perceive the existence of other minds, and the innate lack of it in autistic children, provided further support for the module. Next, neurologic syndromes affecting both subprocesses and core processes were presented. Finally, a special link between the perception of others' intentions and the wide array of innate affects which human beings possess, was offered as evidence for the proposal that our affective life has evolved to provide differentiated internal signals in response to the social environment.

3 Understanding Socially-Responsive Cells in the Macaque Brain: Current Findings and Future Directions

3.1 The "Face Cell" Debate

Neurons with responses which appear to be selective for the sight of faces have been described in the inferotemporal cortex and superior temporal sulcus [59–61], and in the amygdala [62]. In Section 3, I intend to show that these and other socially-responsive cells are elements of the neural machinery underlying social cognition as defined in Section 2.

A central logical issue must be made clear from the outset in discussing "face cells." It is impossible in principle to meet the requirement that all other possible non-face stimuli be tested for efficacy and excluded before concluding that certain cells respond preferentially to faces. Furthermore, such a requirement contains a false premise, namely, that a biological element may be uniquely dedicated to one function. Exclusive dedication of an element or part to only one function occurs in man-made systems, but not in biological ones.

In nature, individual elements tend to be used in multiple ways; therefore, there can only be relative, not absolute, dedication of function. Latent multi-potentiality of function exists in single neurons [63]; in whole organs it may be unmasked under pathological conditions, as when ectopic atrial pacemakers emerge as a result of reduced automaticity of the sinoatrial node [15]. Similarly, a neural system which is well-adapted for a particular purpose may under some circumstances process stimuli in other domains, without weakening the claim for a particular primary adaptation. Such shifts in function appear to take place when there is damage to lateralized structures early in life [64]. Another possible illustration of this general principle occurs in the unusual cognitive capacities displayed in about 10% of autistic individuals, the so-called "savant syndrome" [65]; some neural abnormality, one may speculate, makes the presumed social cognitive system no longer able to process social stimuli, but creates conditions for unusually enhanced processing of other material, such as music or mathematical problems.

For these reasons, instead of trying to prove that a system is strictly dedicated, we need to ask a more biologically-framed question, which is, does its design appear well-adapted to a particular important function? In discussing "face cells" and other neurons which appear to be specialized for processing social information, I do not wish to claim that there are positively no other influences on these cells. What I propose is that *these neurons are components of a system whose design has evolved to meet a very important environmental demand, namely, to enable its possessor to interpret information about other individuals.*

I am making claims, then, regarding a system which is hidden away from direct view and with which we are unable to interfere in very precise ways (compare the crudeness of correlating brain lesions with altered behavior against, for example, the precision of correlating progressive constriction of the inferior vena cava with pressure in the hepatic vein). Nevertheless, I am under an obligation either to provide evidence for my assertion, or to show how evidence could be provided. What forms would that evidence take?

Plausibility, the weakest form of evidence, has been demonstrated in Section 2 in the arguments for the existence of a separate module of cognition—a separate module implies a relatively dedicated neural subsystem. A second line of evidence would be the absence of strongly positive results from earnest attempts to demonstrate a non-social function for candidate specialized neural structures; the arguments for multi-potentiality I offered above would become moot should large numbers of putative "face cells" also turn out to be strongly responsive, under normal conditions, to views of complex inanimate objects or patterns. Such a line of evidence is developed by efforts to demonstrate that the cells are responding to incidental visual features. Procedures such as presenting a vast array of visual objects in addition to faces [59–61]; and demonstrating that responses to faces are maintained across varying viewing conditions, including changes in retinal size and orientation of the stimulus [61, 66, 67], belong to this line of experimental demonstration. The results of these experiments have been negative, that is, there does appear to exist a class of neurons which responds to faces but not to incidental features of face stimuli. Attempts to demonstrate non-social function can never be exhaustive on logical grounds but should continually be made.

Let us now turn to a different sort of evidence. A neurophysiological approach to the presumed neural system, using social stimuli, should yield data which suggest underlying operations conforming to or illuminating behavioral observations. In building a case based on underlying operations, we are in a situation logically analogous to that of Darwin attempting to demonstrate the process of speciation. It was first necessary for him to examine the morphology and behavior of many individual organisms. These observations provided indirect evidence for the interaction of two underlying operations, isolation and gradual modification [68]. Combined, these provided an elegant and sufficient mechanism to begin to explain the origin of species diversity.

By studying the response properties of many neurons, we may begin to discern underlying operations which accord interestingly with our knowledge of primate social behavior. We would further anticipate that such underlying operations, inferred from the properties of neural activity in various regions in response to a range of social stimuli, should have unanticipated properties of coherence and elegance—the signature of newly-understood biological systems. In fact, there are examples of such processes which have emerged from analysis of unit data, and we turn to them now.

3.2   A Framework for the Data

There are neurons which appear to participate in coding for elements of faces—the elements may be spatial relations of particular dimensions of a face [69]; or parts such as hairline, eyes or mouth [61]. Other cells appear tuned to head position (e.g. facing left, facing right, back of head, etc.) [59, 70]. We may understand such coding as essential building blocks for another class of neurons which codes for identity of a pictured subject; this class responds maximally to all views of that subject, regardless of facial expression, while showing diminished responses to pictures of other individuals [66, 71]. In the characteristics of these building blocks of perception, we see the operation of a "who is it?" processing of the face. *The operation of such a process is in agreement with the remarkable ability of our spe-*

cies to ascertain individual identity from among the huge class of visually similar faces, under conditions where each may be seen from a variety of perspectives.

Some neurons participate in the coding of facial expression [66, 39]. Perrett [66] has shown that such cells generalize across different faces of both humans and monkeys for one expression, and that cells responsive to threat faces, which involve opening of the mouth, do not respond to mouth opening made during chewing or other expressions [72]. Furthermore, such cells appear to respond to several attributes which are characteristic of the same expression. Of special significance is a response to both frontal and profile views of one expression but not to other facial expressions in both views [66]. These findings strongly indicate that some neurons code for the content rather than merely the visual features of the pictured facial expressions. They also imply that there is a code for facial expression regardless of orientation with respect to the viewer, that is, an object-centered description of the expression [72, 73]. Such activity is essential for coding another individual's state in absolute terms, independent of his direct relation to the viewer. *Object-centered knowledge of expression is essential for developing a scheme of another individual's motivations and disposition.*

In addition, there are neurons which code for motion of "biological objects," such as direction of rotation of a head, or direction of motion of a body—but not of an inanimate object—in space [60, 74]. There are also neurons which appear to code for direction of gaze of another animal [70]. In both monkeys and apes, direction of gaze is a potent signal—staring often presages hostile intent in macaques, for example. Bertrand [75] observes:

Stumptails, like gorillas and most other primates, are extremely "eye-conscious." They have developed specific eye signals which may be reinforced by eyebrow lifting, ear flattening, and facial mimics. They control the direction of their looking in a way that a person finds difficult to emulate. They can interact with a conspecific or human dominant and watch him without meeting his eyes, whereas a human observer requires a great deal of training to do the same. Thus the way a stumptail looks at its surroundings and uses eyesignals conveys much information about its rank, character, mood and intentions.

Consistent with the importance of the signal is the fact that behavioral response to gaze direction has a defined ontogeny in juvenile macaques [76]. *The finding of cells sensitive to direction of gaze accords well with the social importance of this information.*

A sensitivity to hands as a visual stimulus also appears in these regions [59, 77]. While Perrett's studies emphasize sensitivity to hand-object interactions, it is also worth observing that hands are used socially in a variety of ways. In chimpanzees, they are presented outstretched to solicit reconciliation, as in the "come here" gesture described by De Waal ("then Vernon would make the typical 'come here' gesture—open hand and rapid finger movements toward himself" [13]), or to enlist the aid of a third animal during a confrontation between two others. Pats, slaps and cuffs are described as part of the threat sequence in stumptail macaques; grabbing, pinching and plucking of the fur are also part of the stumptail repertoire and are used in serious and play fighting as well as in play invitations [75].

Where an animal is going, what it is looking at, and what it is doing with its hands, even if there is no immediate social contact involved, are all important bits of information to an observer trying to construct its fellow's intentions and purposes. Based on his observations, Perrett [74] has proposed a classification into viewer-centered, object-centered and goal-centered categories of socially-responsive cells. Goal-centered cells in Perrett's interpretation respond to the relation between an agent and the object it acts upon; such neurons may fire, for example, at any view of a hand plucking an object, but fail to respond when the same motions are carried out with the hand and object in slightly different

planes such that there is no contact between them. *Such responses are what would be expected in neural activity coding "action-with-purpose" on the part of another individual.*

To summarize, another animal's intentions, as expressed in its purposeful actions and gaze direction; its disposition as revealed by expressive behavior; and its identity, which is the mnemonic record of its past interactions with the observing subject, together constitute critical information which must be rapidly integrated by an observer in order to construct a representation of its mental state. The underlying processes which appear to be emerging from these single-unit studies, then, are sufficient for coding the aspects of primate social perception which I have emphasized in Section 2.

3.3 Future Directions

The above studies have employed still photos or drawings of animal and human faces; three-dimensional inanimate models; live human faces, bodies and heads; moving figures; and to a more limited extent, videotapes of monkey faces. We may imagine that the most potent and interesting stimuli to monkey subjects are the sights and sounds of other monkeys performing their natural behavioral repertoires. These stimuli were difficult to obtain and present under controlled conditions before the availability of laser disk players. Facial expressions in particular involve dynamic elements in the movement of features, and of accompanying postures. Expressive behaviors, of particular interest in the formulation I have offered, are only just beginning to be presented in a controlled fashion.

It should by now be apparent that in order to probe this neural system, a broad array of realistic, socially relevant stimuli must be imaginatively employed. At the least, these should include moving pictures and vocalizations of conspecifics. Regions which should be explored using such stimuli include the inferotemporal cortex and superior temporal sulcus, and, based

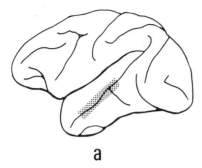

a

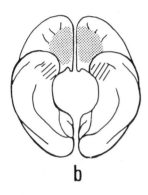

b

Figure 26.1
Macaque brain. (a) Lateral view. The stippled area of
the superior temporal sulcus indicates general location
of socially-responsive cells found in various investigations. (b) Basal view. Orbital frontal cortex, shown
by lesion studies to be important in primate social behavior, is shown stippled. The hatched regions overlie
medial portions of the amygdala, a collection of nuclei
found within the anterior temporal lobes. The amygdala contributes to emotion, is also a site for socially-
responsive cells, and is interconnected with the superior
temporal sulcus and orbital frontal cortex.

on anatomical evidence [78] as well as on the
clinical and lesion evidence cited above, orbital
frontal cortex, cingulate gyrus, temporal pole and
amygdala. Two strategies would be suitable for
controlling for the rich array of visual features
which any single stimulus picture would contain.
One is to show the same behavior (for example, a dominance bounce display) executed by
a number of individuals and from a number of
different angles. A neuron which responds regardless of identity or view can also be tested
with other samples of the same individuals performing different behaviors, and with samples of
similar body views and movements lacking the
particular behavioral content. The profile of the
cell's response across these dimensions will indicate whether its selectivity is to an individual,
a feature such as direction of motion, or to expressive content. The second strategy is to show
an action in reverse: a scene of an animal grabbing and biting another has all the same features
if shown in reverse, but the meaning is eliminated. A cell responsive to the content of the
motivation should fail to respond to the reversed
sequence.

We are in need of a large body of neural data
generated under the conditions I have suggested
and perhaps under others as well. Analysis of
such data will begin to tell us of response properties and underlying processes which may be
unanticipated at present. It will confirm and
amplify—or perhaps fail to confirm!—the picture of social information processing which
appears to be emerging. Most important at this
early stage is an open attitude toward the possibility of unexpected findings.

---

4   Summary

In this essay I have proposed that an understanding of brain function depends upon expli-
cating the relation between neural structures and
selected aspects of cognition. Behavioral observations in monkeys and apes have suggested that

sophisticated social behavior is a primate specialization. The essential characteristic of the underlying social cognition, I have suggested, is that it is organized to culminate in the perception of the dispositions and intentions of other individuals.

Using this definition of social cognition, and including related processes which contribute to it, several criteria for a cognitive module were considered. Evolutionary evidence was gathered from comparative primatological studies, showing that social cognition appears to operate separately from other domains of knowledge, and that non-human primates are indeed able to attribute qualities such as seeing, wanting and expecting to conspecifics. The ontogeny of social perception in human infants was next examined and found to be relatively stereotyped in its course; furthermore, an innate interactive sequence with caregivers contributes to the infant establishing an awareness of the existence of other minds, thus of the feelings and desires of others. The selective inborn absence of such knowledge in autism was described, as were neurological syndromes affecting both subprocesses of social cognition and the proposed central perception of others' dispositions and intentions.

In the final sub-section of Section 2, two theories were offered regarding a core cognitive process. One is that human beings are endowed with a vast spectrum of innate feelings, many of which are not conceptually labeled—clinical evidence shows these to be intimately tied to representations of the attitudes and actions of others. The second is that the richness of human affective life has evolved in response to a need for a large array of internal signals in order to respond appropriately in a complex social environment.

The evidence for considering social cognition as a separate module implies that a discrete neural system subserves it. Single neurons responsive to the sights of faces, hands and body motions have been described in macaque temporal lobe structures. The rationale for accepting these as components of a neural system which has evolved for the purpose of social perception was advanced

in Section 3. The definitive test for whether this neural system is responsible for social cognition is the extent to which cell firing characteristics reveal the presence of underlying processes that can be meaningfully related to observed behavior. Such data is beginning to emerge. Strategies are described for further probing the brain structures of interest using social stimuli.

Acknowledgments

I thank John Allman for comments on the manuscript. My research is supported by a Veterans Administration Career Development Award.

References

[1] J. Allman, F. Miezin and E. McGuinness, *Annu. Rev. Neurosci.* 8, 407 (1985); J. Allman, in *Neurobiology of Neocortex,* ed. by P. Rakic and W. Singer (Wiley, New York, 1988).

[2] J. Allman, *Prog. Physiol. Psychol.* 7, 1 (1977).

[3] J. Allman, in *Primate Brain Evolution: Methods and Concepts,* ed. by E. Armstrong and D. Falk (Plenum, New York, 1982).

[4] E. I. Knudsen and M. Konishi, *Science* 200, 745 (1978); M. Konishi, T. Takehashi, H. Wagner, W. Sullivan and C. E. Carr, in *Auditory Function: Neurobiological Bases of Hearing,* ed. by G. M. Edelman, W. E. Gall and W. M. Cowan (Wiley, New York, 1988).

[5] J. D. Pettigrew, *Science* 231, 1304 (1986).

[6] A. M. Liberman and I. G. Mattingly, *Science* 243, 489 (1989); K. R. Kluender and S. Greenberg (letter); A. M. Liberman and I. G. Mattingly (response), *Science* 244, 1530 (1989).

[7] L. Cosmides, *Cognition* 31, 187 (1989).

[8] J. A. Fodor, *The Modularity of Mind: An Essay on Faculty Psychology* (MIT Press, Cambridge, Massachusetts, 1983); *ibid.,* p. 47.

[9] H. Gardner, *Frames of Mind: The Theory of Multiple Intelligences* (Basic Books, New York, 1983); *ibid.,* p. 63.

[10] C. Darwin, *The Expression of the Emotions in Man and Animals* (D. Appleton, New York, 1873).

[11] D. Cheney, R. Seyfarth and B. Smuts, *Science* 234, 1361 (1986).

[12] B. Smuts, *Sex and Friendship in Baboons* (Aldine, Hawthorne, New York, 1985) p. 154.

[13] F. De Waal, *Peacemaking Among Primates* (Harvard University Press, Cambridge, Massachusetts, 1989) p. 42; *ibid.*, p. 195; *ibid.*, pp. 21, 215.

[14] F. De Waal, *Chimpanzee Politics: Power and Sex Among Apes* (Harper & Row, New York, 1982) p. 47; *ibid.*, p. 51.

[15] S. K. Langer, *Mind: An Essay on Human Feeling* (abridged) (Johns Hopkins University Press, Baltimore, 1988) p. 229; *ibid.*, p. 144.

[16] D. Premack, in *Machiavellian Intelligence: Social Expertise and the Evolution of Intellect in Monkeys, Apes and Humans*, ed. by R. Byrne and A. Whiten (Clarendon Press, Oxford, 1988) p. 160.

[17] H. Kohut, *The Analysis of the Self: A Systematic Approach to the Psychoanalytic Treatment of Narcissistic Personality Disorders* (International Universities Press, New York, 1971) p. 300.

[18] R. Byrne and A. Whiten (eds.), *Machiavellian Intelligence: Social Expertise and the Evolution of Intellect in Monkeys, Apes and Humans* (Clarendon Press, Oxford, 1988).

[19] N. Humphrey, *Consciousness Regained* (Oxford University Press, Oxford, 1983).

[20] J. Sandler and B. Rosenblatt, *Psychoanal. Study Child* 17, 128 (1962).

[21] R. L. Fantz, *Science* 140, 296 (1963); J. Mehler, J. Bertoncini and M. Barriere, *Perception* 7, 491 (1978).

[22] A. N. Meltzoff and M. K. Moore, *Science* 198, 75 (1977).

[23] T. M. Field, R. Woodson, R. Greenberg, et al., *Science* 218, 179 (1982).

[24] A. Sagi and M. L. Hoffman, *Dev. Psychol.* 12, 175 (1976).

[25] L. Brothers, *Am. J. Psychiatry* 146, 10 (1989).

[26] L. Murray and C. Trevarthen, in *Social Perception in Infants*, ed. by T. M. Field and N. A. Fox (Ablex, Norwood, New Jersey, 1985).

[27] I. Eibl-Eibesfeldt, *Ethology: The Biology of Behavior* (Holt, Rinehart and Winston, New York, 1970) p. 404; D. G. Freedman, *J. Child Psychol. Psychiatry* 5, 171 (1964).

[28] H. Oster, in *The Development of Affect,* ed. by M. Lewis and L. Rosenblum (Plenum, New York, 1978).

[29] B. Beebe, D. Alson, J. Jaffe, S. Feldstein and C. Crown, *J. Psycholinguist. Res.* 17, 245 (1988); B. Beebe, D. Stern and J. Jaffe, in *Of Speech and Time: Temporal Speech Patterns in Interpersonal Contexts,* ed. by A. W. Siegman and S. Feldstein (Lawrence Erlbaum, Hillsdale, New Jersey, 1979).

[30] D. Stern, *The Interpersonal World of the Infant: A View from Psychoanalysis and Developmental Psychology* (Basic Books, New York, 1985) p. 140; *ibid.,* p. 124.

[31] L. Wing (ed.), *Aspects of Autism: Biological Research* (Alden Press, Oxford, 1988).

[32] L. Kanner, *J. Pediatr.* 25, 211 (1944).

[33] P. Mundy, M. Sigman, J. Ungerer and T. Sherman, *J. Child Psychol. Psychiatry* 27, 657 (1986).

[34] R. P. Hobson, *J. Child Psychol. Psychiatry* 27, 321 (1986).

[35] A. Attwood, U. Frith and B. Hermelin, *J. Autism Dev. Disord.* 18, 241 (1988).

[36] M. Prior, *J. Ment. Defic. Res.* 21, 37 (1977).

[37] A. R. Damasio, H. Damasio and G. W. Van Hoesen, *Neurology* 32, 331 (1982).

[38] D. Tranel, A. R. Damasio and H. Damasio, *Neurology* 38, 690 (1988).

[39] M. E. Hasselmo, E. T. Rolls and G. C. Baylis, *Behav. Brain Res.* 32, 203 (1989).

[40] R. Jackendoff, *Consciousness and the Computational Mind* (MIT Press, Cambridge, Massachusetts, 1987) p. 261; *ibid.,* p. 267.

[41] M. S. Gazzaniga, *Science* 245, 947 (1989).

[42] B. A. Vermeire, personal communication.

[43] K. M. Heilman, R. Scholes and R. T. Watson, *J. Neurol. Neurosurg. Psychiatry* 38, 69 (1975).

[44] E. D. Ross, *Arch. Neurol.* 38, 561 (1981).

[45] E. D. Ross and M.-M. Mesulam, *Arch. Neurol.* 36, 144 (1979).

[46] P. J. Eslinger and A. R. Damasio, *Neurology* 35, 1731 (1985).

[47] W. J. H. Nauta, *Brain* 85, 505 (1962); J. L. Price, F. T. Russchen and D. G. Amaral, in *Handbook of Chemical Neuroanatomy,* Vol. 5, *Integrated Systems,* Part 1, ed. by L. W. Swanson, A. Bjorklund and T. Hokfelt (Elsevier, New York, 1987).

[48] C. M. Butter and D. R. Snyder, *Acta Neurobiol. Exp.* 32, 525 (1972); A. Kling and H. D. Steklis, *Brain Behav. Evol.* 13, 216 (1976); R. L. Lloyd, A. S. Kling and O. Ricci, *Neurosci. Res. Commun.* 5, 53 (1989).

[49] A. Bouckoms, R. Martuza and M. Henderson, *J. Nerv. Ment. Dis.* 174, 484 (1986); D. A. Fishbain and H. Rosomoff, *Int. J. Psychiat. Med.* 16, 131 (1986–7).

[50] A. Ardila and M. Rosseli, *Int. J. Neurosci.* 43, 219 (1988).

[51] S. F. Signer, *J. Clin. Psychiatry* 48, 147 (1987).

[52] J. Todd, in *Historical Aspects of the Neurosciences,* ed. by F. C. Rose and W. F. Bynum (Raven, New York, 1980).

[53] A. B. Joseph, *Am. J. Psychiatry* 142, 146 (1985).

[54] H. E. Lehmann, in *Comprehensive Textbook of Psychiatry* II, ed. by A. M. Freedman, H. I. Kaplan and B. J. Sadock (Williams and Wilkins Co., Baltimore, 1975).

[55] P. Ekman, E. R. Sorenson and W. V. Friesen, *Science* 164, 86 (1969).

[56] P. Gloor, in *The Neurobiology of the Amygdala,* ed. by B. E. Eleftheriou (Plenum, New York, 1972).

[57] P. Gloor, in *The Limbic System: Functional Organization and Clinical Disorders,* ed. by B. K. Doane and K. E. Livingston (Raven Press, New York, 1986); *ibid.,* p. 165.

[58] P. Gloor, A. Olivier, L. F. Quesney, F. Andermann and S. Horowitz, *Ann. Neurol.* 12, 129 (1982).

[59] R. Desimone, T. D. Albright, C. G. Gross and C. Bruce, *J. Neurosci.* 4, 2051 (1984).

[60] C. Bruce, R. Desimone and C. G. Gross, *J. Neurophysiol.* 46, 369 (1981).

[61] D. I. Perrett, E. T. Rolls and W. Caan, *Exp. Brain Res.* 47, 329 (1982).

[62] C. M. Leonard, E. T. Rolls, F. A. W. Wilson and G. C. Baylis, *Behav. Brain Res.* 15, 159 (1985).

[63] S. L. Hooper and M. Moulins, *Science* 244, 1587 (1989).

[64] R. D. Adams and M. Victor, *Principles of Neurology* (McGraw-Hill, New York, 1979) p. 321.

[65] D. A. Treffert, *Am. J. Psychiatry* 145, 563 (1988).

[66] D. I. Perrett, P. A. J. Smith, D. D. Potter, A. J. Mistlin, A. S. Head, A. D. Milner and M. A. Jeeves, *Hum. Neurobiol.* 3, 197 (1984).

[67] E. T. Rolls and G. C. Baylis, *Exp. Brain Res.* 65, 38 (1986).

[68] E. Mayr, *The Growth of Biological Thought: Diversity, Evolution, and Inheritance* (Harvard University Press, Cambridge, Massachusetts, 1982) p. 409.

[69] S. Yamane, S. Kaji and K. Kawano, *Exp. Brain Res.* 73, 209 (1988).

[70] D. I. Perrett, P. A. J. Smith, D. D. Potter, A. J. Mistlin, A. S. Head, A. D. Milner and M. A. Jeeves, *Proc. R. Soc. Lond.* Ser. B 223, 293 (1985).

[71] G. Baylis, E. T. Rolls and C. M. Leonard, *Brain Res.* 342, 91 (1985).

[72] D. I. Perrett and A. J. Mistlin, in *Comparative Perception,* ed. by M. Berkeley and W. Stebbins (Wiley and Sons, New York) in press.

[73] M. E. Hasselmo, E. T. Rolls, G. C. Baylis and V. Nalwa, *Exp. Brain Res.* 75, 417 (1989).

[74] D. I. Perrett, M. H. Harries, A. J. Chitty and A. J. Mistlin, in *Images and Understanding,* ed. by H. B. Barlow, C. Blakemore and M. Weston-Smith (Cambridge University Press, Cambridge) in press.

[75] M. Bertrand, *Bibl. Primatol.* 11, 69 (1969); *ibid.,* 82.

[76] M. J. Mendelson, M. M. Haith and P. Goldman-Rakic, *Dev. Psychol.* 2, 222 (1982).

[77] D. I. Perrett, A. J. Mistlin, M. H. Harries and A. J. Chitty, in *Vision and Action: The Control of Grasping,* ed. by M. A. Goodale (Ablex, New Jersey) in press.

[78] J. L. Price, F. T. Russchen and D. G. Amaral, in *Handbook of Chemical Neuroanatomy,* Vol. 5, *Integrated Systems,* Part 1, ed. by L. W. Swanson, A. Bjorklund and T. Hokfelt (Elsevier, New York, 1987); A. G. Herzog and G. W. Van Hoesen, *Brain Res.* 115, 57 (1976); J. P. Aggleton, M. J. Burton and R. E. Passingham, *Brain Res.* 190, 347 (1980).

IV SOCIAL NEUROSCIENCE OF MOTIVATION, EMOTION, AND ATTITUDES

A. Basic Processes

27   Emotion: Clues from the Brain

Joseph E. LeDoux

Introduction

Despite the obvious importance of emotion to human existence, scientists concerned with human nature have not been able to reach a consensus about what emotion is and what place emotion should have in a theory of mind and behavior. Controversy abounds over the definition of emotion, the number of emotions that exist, whether some emotions are more basic than others, the commonality of certain emotional response patterns across cultures and across species, whether different emotions have different physiological signatures, the extent to which emotional responses contribute to emotional experiences, the role of nature and nurture in emotion, the influence of emotion on cognitive processes, the dependence of emotion on cognition, the importance of conscious versus unconscious processes in emotion, and on and on (see Ekman & Davidson 1994).

Although there has been no shortage of psychological research on these topics, the findings have not resolved many of the issues in a compelling manner. But psychological research is not the only source of information about the nature of emotion. Information about the representation of emotion in the brain may shed light on the nature of emotional processes. First, information about how emotion is represented in the brain can provide constraints that could help us choose between alternative hypotheses about the nature of some emotional process. Second, findings about the neural basis of emotion might also suggest new insights into the functional organization of emotion that were not apparent from psychological findings alone. The brain, in other words, can constrain and inform our ideas about the nature of emotion.

This review examines the neural basis of emotion and considers how research on brain mech-

anisms can potentially help us to understand emotion as a psychological process.

Neural Basis of Emotion

Studies of the neural basis of emotion have a long history within neuroscience (see LeDoux 1987, 1991). This research culminated around mid-century in the limbic system theory of emotion (MacLean 1949, 1952), which claimed to have identified the limbic system as the mediator of emotion. However, in recent years both the limbic system concept (Brodal 1982, Swanson 1983, Kotter & Meyer 1992) and the limbic system theory of emotion (LeDoux 1991) have been questioned. Despite problems with the conceptualization of the brain system that mediates emotion in general, there has been a great deal of systematic and productive research on the neural basis of specific emotions. It is not known whether there is a general purpose system of emotion in the brain, but if there is it will be identified readily by synthesizing across studies of specific emotions. This review focuses on the neural basis of fear, an emotion that has been studied extensively at the neural level.

Neural Basis of Fear

Fear is an especially good emotion to use as a model. It is a common part of life, almost from the beginning. The expression of fear is conserved to a large extent across human cultures and at least to some extent across human and nonhuman mammalian species, and possibly across other vertebrates as well. There are well-defined experimental procedures for eliciting and measuring fear, and many of these can be used in more or less identical ways in humans and experimental animals. Further, disorders of fear regulation are at the heart of many psychopatho-

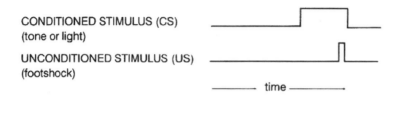

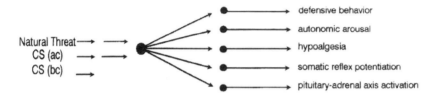

Figure 27.1
Fear conditioning involves the temporal association of an innocuous conditioned stimulus (CS), such as a light or tone, with a noxious unconditioned stimulus (US), such as footshock. After conditioning (ac), but not before conditioning (bc), the CS acquires the capacity to activate a variety of brain systems involved in the control of defensive responses. These same responses are elicited by natural or unlearned threatening stimuli. Fear conditioning is stimulus learning, not response learning, and it allows new stimuli to gain control over hard-wired, evolutionarily perfected, defensive response control networks.

logic conditions, including anxiety, panic, phobic, and posttraumatic stress disorders. It would be an important achievement if, by focusing on fear, we were able to generate an adequate theory of fear, even if it applied to no other emotion.

The following survey of the neural basis of fear concentrates on studies of fear conditioning. This approach has been particularly successful in identifying the neural system that mediates learned fear and in uncovering some of the cellular mechanisms that might be involved.

Fear conditioning is a form of Pavlovian (classical) conditioning. Pavlov is best remembered for his studies of alimentary conditioning, in which he elicited salivation in dogs by presenting stimuli that had been associated with the delivery of food (Pavlov 1927). He also determined that animals will exhibit conditioned reflexes that allow them to protect themselves against harmful

stimuli by responding to warning signals. Pavlov referred to the latter as defense conditioning. Today, Pavlovian defense conditioning is usually referred to as fear conditioning (Brown et al. 1951; Kamin 1965; McAllister & McAllister 1971; Millenson & de Villiers 1972; Bouton & Bolles 1980; Davis 1992; Kapp et al. 1992; Fanselow 1980; LeDoux 1993a).

In a typical fear conditioning experiment, the subject is exposed to a tone or light (the conditioned stimulus, CS) that is followed by a brief shock (the unconditioned stimulus, US; see Figure 27.1). Conditioning occurs after only a few pairings (one pairing is enough if the US is sufficiently intense) (Fanselow & Bolles 1979). The effects of conditioning can be assessed directly by measuring defense responses elicited by the CS, including freezing responses (Blanchard & Blanchard 1972, Bouton & Bolles 1980, Fanselow

1980, LeDoux et al. 1984) or changes in autonomic (Smith et al. 1980, Cohen & Randall 1984,
LeDoux et al. 1984) and endocrine (Mason
1968, van de Kar et al. 1991) activity. These are
hard-wired or innate reactions to threat that
come to be coupled to the CS through the conditioning process. The effects of fear conditioning can also be assessed indirectly by measuring
the potentiation of reflexes, such as the eyeblink
or startle reflex (e.g. Brown et al. 1951, Davis
et al. 1987, Weisz et al. 1992), in the presence of
the CS, by measuring the inhibition of pain by
the CS (e.g. Watkins & Mayer 1982, Fanselow &
Helmstetter 1988), or by measuring the degree to
which the animal's ongoing behavior is interfered with or suppressed by the CS (e.g. Estes &
Skinner 1941, Hunt & Brady 1955, Bouton &
Bolles 1980, Leaf & Muller 1965).

Neural Pathways Mediating Fear Conditioning

The logic underlying the search for the neural
pathways in fear conditioning is straightforward.
Conditioning is believed to involve the intersection in the brain of pathways transmitting information about the CS and the US (Pavlov 1927,
Konorski 1967, Hebb 1949). Because the US
must intersect a variety of CS pathways originating in different sensory systems, it seems that the
crucial changes that underlie conditioning should
involve modifications in the network that is involved in the processing of the specific CS used.
Thus, if one were able to follow the processing of
the CS through its sensory system and beyond to
the motor system controlling the conditioned
responses (CRs), the circuitry within which conditioning occurs would presumably be known.

How, then, should one attempt to follow the
processing of the CS? The strategy that has
worked best uses the classical lesion method in
conjunction with modern neuroanatomical tracing techniques. For example, if the CS is an
acoustic stimulus, then the CS pathway must
begin in the auditory system and should continue as an efferent projection out of the auditory

system. Since the auditory system is a linearly
organized system involving relays from lower to
higher centers, it is possible to determine, with
the lesion method, whether the auditory CS has
to rise through the entire pathway for conditioning to occur. By using neuroanatomical tracing techniques it is then possible to examine the
connections of the highest auditory station required and, thereby, define the next possible
links in the pathway, which can each in turn be
lesioned to determine which one constitutes the
key link.

Research in the early 1980s showed that lesions
of the midbrain and thalamic stations of the auditory pathway prevented conditioning but that
lesions of the auditory cortex had no effect
(LeDoux et al. 1984). This suggested that the CS
must exit the auditory system at the level of the
thalamus. Anatomical tracing techniques were
then used to show that the auditory thalamus
projects not only to the auditory cortex but also
to the amygdala (LeDoux et al. 1985). Additional studies showed that interruption of the
connections between the auditory thalamus and
the amygdala interferes with conditioning (Le-
Doux et al. 1986, Iwata et al. 1986) and that the
lateral nucleus of the amygdala is the crucial region for the reception of the auditory stimulus
(LeDoux et al. 1990a,b; Clugnet et al. 1990).

Although the auditory cortex is not necessary
for conditioning, projections from the auditory
thalamus through the auditory cortex and to the
amygdala (Romanski & LeDoux 1993a,b) are
sufficient to mediate simple acoustic fear conditioning (conditioning with a single auditory
CS paired with the US) (Romanski & LeDoux
1992). This suggests that the thalamo-amygdala
and thalamo-cortico-amygdala pathways are
equipotential in mediating simple conditioning
(Romanski & LeDoux 1992). However, auditory
cortical areas, and presumably cortico-amygdala
connections, are required for differential conditioning (in which two auditory stimuli are presented, one paired with the US and the other
not) (Jarrell et al. 1987).

The direct thalamic pathway to the amygdala is shorter and thus faster, but its capacity to represent the auditory stimulus is more limited (Bordi & LeDoux 1994a,b). The thalamo-cortico-amygdala pathway, which involves several cortico-cortical links before reaching the amygdala (Romanski & LeDoux 1993a,b), is longer and slower, but its capacity to represent the auditory stimulus is considerably greater. The thalamic pathway is sufficient for the rapid triggering of emotion by simple stimulus features (as in simple conditioning), whereas the cortical pathway appears to be needed for emotional reactions coupled to perceptually complex stimulus objects (as in differential conditioning). Within the amygdala, the quick-and-dirty thalamic inputs and the slower but more accurate cortical inputs converge in the lateral nucleus (LeDoux et al. 1991). The lateral nucleus is the sensory interface of the amygdala and possibly a crucial site of integration of information from parallel auditory projections during fear conditioning (LeDoux et al. 1990b, LeDoux 1992).

Whenever a CS is paired with a US, some conditioning accrues to the background or to contextual stimuli that are also present in the environment (e.g. Rescorla & Wagner 1972). Recent studies have shown that contextual conditioning, like conditioning to a CS, is dependent on the amygdala, but unlike CS conditioning, it is also dependent upon the hippocampus (Phillips & LeDoux 1992b, Kim & Fanselow 1992, Selden et al. 1991). Although the exact direction of information flow between these structures is not known, the hippocampus (by way of the subiculum) projects to the lateral nucleus (and several other amygdala nuclei) (Ottersen 1982, Phillips & LeDoux 1992a). As a result, the hippocampus, long believed to be involved in complex information processing functions, including spatial, contextual, and relational processing (O'Keefe & Nadel 1978, Eichenbaum 1992, McNaughton & Barnes 1990, Nadel & Willner 1980, Rudy & Sutherland 1992), may be a kind of higher-order sensory structure in

fear conditioning. That is, the hippocampus may relay environmental inputs pertaining to the conditioning context to the amygdala, where emotional meaning is added to context just as it is added to thalamic or cortical sensory information. Once learned, this kind of contextual fear conditioning might allow the organism to distinguish between those situations in which it is appropriate to defend oneself against a stimulus vs situations in which it is not necessary (e.g. a bear in the woods vs in the zoo).

Just as the lateral nucleus is the input system of the amygdala, the central nucleus is the output system (LeDoux 1993a, Davis 1992, Kapp et al. 1984, 1990). Lesions of the central nucleus interfere with the expression of conditioned responses expressed through a variety of motor modalities, including freezing behavior, sympathetic and parasympathetic autonomic responses, neuroendocrine responses, the potentiation of startle and eyeblink reflexes, and the suppression of pain. Most interestingly, lesions of areas to which the central nucleus projects interfere separately with individual responses. For example, projections to the central gray are involved in freezing responses (Iwata et al. 1987, LeDoux et al. 1988, Wilson & Kapp 1994); projections to the lateral hypothalamus are involved in sympathetic autonomic responses (Smith et al. 1980, Iwata et al. 1987, LeDoux et al. 1988); projections to the bed nucleus of the stria terminalis are involved in neuroendocrine responses (van de Kar et al. 1991); and projections to the nucleus reticularis caudalis pontis are involved in the potentiation of startle responses (Rosen et al. 1991).

The amygdala is involved in both the acquisition and the expression of fear conditioning (e.g. LeDoux 1987, 1990, 1992; Davis et al. 1987; Davis 1992; Kapp et al. 1984, 1990, 1992; Gentile et al. 1986). Even with extensive overtraining, posttraining lesions of the amygdala interfere with fear conditioning (Kim & Davis 1993).

Although much of the work on fear conditioning has used auditory CSs, some studies have used visual stimuli (e.g. Davis et al. 1987; Davis

1992; LeDoux et al. 1989). In general, the circuitry involved appears to be quite similar. However, because the visual connections with the amygdala in the rat are poorly understood, the input circuitry is not as clear as it is for auditory conditioning.

In summary, the neural pathways through which defense responses are conditioned and expressed to auditory stimuli have been well defined (see Figure 27.2). The amygdala appears to play a central role in this circuitry. It is located between the sensory system that processes the CS and the motor systems that control the conditioned responses. Although some learning may occur in the sensory and motor systems (see below), important aspects of fear conditioning probably occur in the amygdala because it is the only part of the circuitry that is involved independent of the CS and CR modalities. Studies of cellular mechanisms have thus focused on the amygdala.

Cellular Mechanisms Involved in Fear Conditioning

A main reason for wanting to understand the neural circuit underlying conditioning is that such information isolates from the vast numbers of neurons and their connections the particular neurons and connections that must be modified during learning and within which the changes might be stored either temporarily or permanently. The neural systems level of analysis thus guides the cellular level analysis, and findings at the cellular level reveal mechanisms about how the brain actually works. Although the search for the cellular basis of fear conditioning is in its infancy, important discoveries have begun to shed light on the underlying mechanisms.

CS–US Convergence
The neural basis of classical conditioning involves convergence of the CS and US pathways in the brain (Pavlov 1927, Hebb 1949, Konorski 1967). If, as the systems level of analysis suggests, the

amygdala is a crucial site of conditioning, then cells in the amygdala should respond to both the CS and the US. Recent studies have mapped the responses of amygdala neurons to auditory stimuli similar to those used in conditioning experiments (Bordi et al. 1992, 1993; Romanski et al. 1993). This work has shown that neurons in the lateral nucleus of the amygdala are particularly responsive to auditory CS-like stimulation. Responses in other areas tend to be weaker and to have longer latencies. This reinforces the conclusion that the lateral nucleus is the sensory interface of the amygdala. Romanski et al. (1993) found that essentially every cell that responded to auditory stimuli also responded to noxious somatosensory stimulation similar to that used as a US. The lateral nucleus of the amygdala is thus a site of CS–US convergence and may be a crucial site of the cellular changes that underlie learning. However, one of the key missing pieces of information about the neural basis of fear conditioning is the origin of the US inputs to the amygdala.

Physiological Plasticity Induced by CS–US Pairing
Neurons in a number of brain regions undergo physiological changes during aversive classical conditioning (see Thompson et al. 1983). This fact discourages the use of unit recording techniques to find the critical locus of learning. An alternative strategy is to first identify the essential neural circuit underlying a particular learned response through lesion studies and then examine the plastic properties of the neurons in the circuit. These are the neurons that are most likely to undergo changes in physiological responsivity that are essential to the learning task.

With key aspects of the fear learning circuitry now identified (see above), it is useful to consider the extent of physiological plasticity that has been observed in these areas. Studies of the physiology of learning have suggested that many brain regions exhibit physiological changes during learning. Thus, it is perhaps not surprising

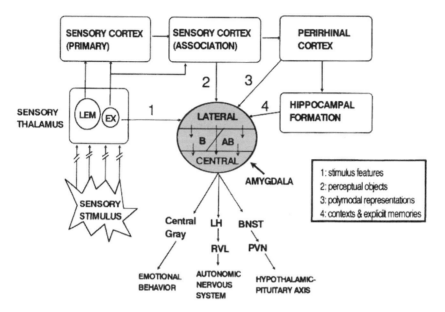

Figure 27.2

Neural circuits of fear conditioning. The neural pathways by which a sensory CS elicits emotional responses involve the relay of sensory inputs to the thalamus. While the lemniscal nuclei (LEM) transmit only to the primary sensory cortex, the extralemniscal areas (EX) transmit to primary sensory and association regions of the cortex, as well as to the lateral nucleus of the amygdala. This region of the amygdala also receives inputs from sensory association areas of the neocortex, as well as from polymodal areas such as the perirhinal cortex and the hippocampal formation. The thalamo-amygdala sensory projection (1) has been implicated in simple fear conditioning (one conditioned stimulus [CS] paired with an unconditioned stimulus [US]); the cortico-amygdala sensory projection (2) in differential fear conditioning (one CS paired with US, another not paired); and the hippocampo-amygdala projection (4) in contextural conditioning (conditioning to situational cues other than the CS). The hippocampal projection may also be involved in conditioning of fear to explicit or declarative memories that occur in the presence of an US, but this has not been studied. The role of the perirhinal projection to amygdala (3) is not known, but it may have something to do with the elicitation of fear by complex polymodal stimulus representations. The central nucleus of the amygdala is the interface with motor systems, as it connects with various brain stem areas involved in the regulation of specific defense response networks. Projections to the central gray control freezing and other defensive behaviors; projections to the lateral hypothalamus (LH) and from there to the rostral ventral lateral medulla (RVL) control sympathetic autonomic nervous system responses; and projections to the bed nucleus of the stria terminalis (BNST) and paraventricular hypothalamus control stress reactions involving the pituitary-adrenal axis. The amygdala nuclei are the sensory- and motor-independent parts of the circuitry and are likely to play important integrative roles in fear conditioning.

that plasticity has been found throughout the fear conditioning circuitry: in the auditory thalamic areas that project to the amygdala (Gabriel et al. 1976, Ryugo & Weinberger 1978, Edeline & Weinberger 1992); in the auditory cortex (Weinberger & Diamond 1987, Edeline & Weinberger 1993); in the lateral, basolateral, and central nuclei of the amygdala (LeGal LaSalle & Ben-Ari 1981, Muramoto et al. 1993, Pascoe & Kapp 1985); and in the lateral hypothalamus (Ono et al. 1988). This ubiquitous plasticity in the conditioning circuitry would be trivial if plasticity in all levels of the pathway reflects learning by some early station (such as the auditory thalamus). On the other hand, it would be significant if it means that each link in the pathway is plastic and that plasticity in different locations serves different functions. Plasticity in the sensory structures could make stimulus processing more efficient; plasticity in motor systems could make the execution of the responses more efficient; and plasticity in the amygdala could represent the integrative (stimulus- and response-independent) aspects of learning.

LTP and the Amygdala

Learning at the cellular level is generally believed to involve changes in synaptic transmission (Hebb 1949, Kandel & Spencer 1968, Squire 1987). A great deal of work has thus sought to identify the mechanisms by which experience modifies the efficiency of synaptic transmission. Most of this work has involved long-term potentiation (LTP). In an LTP experiment, a pathway is stimulated at a high frequency, and as a result, the response to a low-frequency test stimulus is amplified. LTP has been studied most extensively in the hippocampus (Lynch 1986, Cotman et al. 1988, Brown et al. 1988, Malenka & Nicoll 1993, Madison et al. 1991, Bliss & Collingridge 1993) but has also been demonstrated in other brain regions, including the lateral and basal nuclei of the amygdala (Clugnet & LeDoux 1990, Chapman et al. 1990).

Several properties of LTP make it attractive as a memory mechanism (Lynch 1986, Brown et al. 1988). LTP is experience dependent and synapse specific: Cells receive many inputs, but the response is only amplified for those inputs that were stimulated. LTP exhibits cooperativity: The induction of LTP depends on the simultaneous activation of many afferents. LTP exhibits associativity: It can be produced by simultaneous stimulation of two pathways using stimuli that are not effective individually. LTP is stable and long lasting. Although the relationship between LTP and behavioral learning and memory is still unclear and controversial (Teyler & DiScenna 1987, Morris 1992, McNaughton & Barnes 1990, O'Keefe 1993), an LTP-like phenomenon might underlie some aspects of learning, including fear conditioning mediated by the amygdala.

Pharmacological Similarity of LTP and Fear Conditioning

One way to link LTP to learning and memory is to determine whether similar pharmacological manipulations are involved (Lynch et al. 1991, Staubli 1994). The pharmacology of the classic form of LTP has been well characterized (e.g. Lynch et al. 1991, Madison et al. 1991, Malenka & Nicoll 1993). It involves the binding of the excitatory amino acid transmitter, L-glutamate, to two classes of postsynaptic excitatory amino acid receptors, NMDA and non-NMDA receptors. The NMDA receptor channel is normally opened only when the cell membrane is depolarized by the prior binding of Glu to non-NMDA receptors. The opening of the NMDA channel is a crucial step in LTP. LTP does not occur if the channel is blocked by an antagonist. In contrast, the expression of established LTP is not affected by NMDA blockade.

In 1949 Hebb postulated that learning at the cellular level involved the simultaneous activity of pre- and postsynaptic neurons. That is, if the postsynaptic neuron is depolarized when the presynaptic input arrives, the connection will be strengthened. The NMDA receptor appears to be a neural instantiation of the Hebb rule. It requires that presynaptically released Glu bind to postsynaptic NMDA receptors while the postsynaptic cell is active or depolarized.

If the classic form of LTP is a mediator of fear conditioning, then blockade of NMDA receptors in the amygdala should have two consequences: 1. The establishment but not the expression of LTP in the amygdala should be disrupted, and 2. The acquisition but not the expression of fear conditioning should be disrupted. Existing data are, for the most part, consistent with this line of reasoning. Recent studies have shown that LTP induced in the amygdala by stimulation of the endopyriform nucleus is dependent on NMDA receptors (Gean et al. 1993). However, induction of LTP in the same regions by stimulation of the external capsule does not exhibit the same dependence (Chapman & Bellavance 1992). Regardless, these studies have focused on the basal nucleus, which is not necessarily the only or even the main site of plasticity in fear conditioning (recall that the cells receiving CS–US convergent inputs are in the lateral nucleus). Further, these studies have not stimulated known CS or US pathways in their LTP paradigms. Although LTP has been demonstrated in a CS pathway to the lateral amygdala, the thalamo-amygdala auditory pathway (Clugnet & LeDoux 1990), the pharmacology of LTP in this pathway has yet to be determined. Blockade of NMDA receptors in the lateral/basal amygdala interferes with the acquisition but not the expression of Pavlovian fear conditioning to a CS (e.g. Miserendino et al. 1990) or to contextual stimuli (Fanselow & Kim 1994). Because of the small size of these brain areas it is not possible to conclude whether the site of action is in the lateral or basal nucleus. Nevertheless, NMDA receptors in this region seem to be involved.

Summary

Important steps have been taken toward understanding the cellular basis of fear conditioning.

While much work remains, this is a young research area and it holds great promise for elucidating mechanisms through which an important aspect of emotional learning occurs. Findings to date are consistent with the view that an NMDA-dependent, LTP-like phenomenon in the amygdala might mediate fear conditioning, but this remains unproved.

Extinction of Conditioned Fear

Extinction is the process through which the strength of a conditioned response is weakened by repeated exposure to the CS in the absence of the US. Considerable evidence suggests that extinction of conditioned fear does not occur passively (i.e. the memory persists in the absence of explicit extinction training), and when extinction occurs it is not passive forgetting but instead is an active process, quite possibly involving new learning (Bouton & Swartzentruber 1991). Further, conditioned fear reactions are notoriously difficult to extinguish and once extinguished they can recur spontaneously or can be reinstated by stressful experiences (e.g. Rescorla & Heth 1975, Jacobs & Nadel 1985, Campbell & Jaynes 1966). Because fear conditioning processes may contribute to such disorders as phobia, excessive fear, anxiety, posttraumatic stress, and panic, understanding how the effects of fear conditioning are modulated by extinction is of great clinical interest.

The neural basis of extinction has been studied much less extensively than has the neural basis of acquisition, but some key discoveries have been made. Although cortical areas are not required for the acquisition of conditioned defense (see above), cortical lesions can interfere with extinction. For example, lesions of auditory (Teich et al. 1989) or visual (LeDoux et al. 1989) cortex have no effect on simple conditioning involving an auditory or visual CS. However, with such lesions extinction is greatly prolonged if not prevented. This suggests that the subcortical sensory projections to the amygdala mediate learning in this situation (since the relevant cortical areas have been removed) and that subcortical learning of this type is relatively indelible (LeDoux et al. 1989). The cortical lesions, in other words, may have unmasked the existence of relatively permanent memories. Extinction, by this account, might be a process by which the cortex regulates the expression of these indelible memories. A recent study failed to replicate these effects (Falls et al. 1992), but a number of procedural differences between the studies might be responsible for the failure to replicate.

Additional studies have shown that extinction is prolonged by damage to the medial prefrontal cortex (Morgan et al. 1993), which may be the link between sensory cortex and the amygdala in behavioral extinction. That is, the medial prefrontal cortex may modulate the expression of defense responses at the level of the amygdala. A related conclusion was reached on the basis of studies recording unit activity in the prefrontal cortex and the amygdala during appetitive conditioning (e.g. Thorpe et al. 1983, Rolls 1992).

Blockade of NMDA receptors in the amygdala interferes with the extinction of conditioned fear (Falls et al. 1992). This reinforces the view that extinction is not passive forgetting but an active form of learning and suggests that NMDA-dependent synaptic plasticity may be involved. The synapses between the frontal cortex and the amygdala might be the plastic synapses in this case. Although extinction plasticity may involve modifications in the strength of the existing associations, extinction plasticity may also involve changes in the propensity with which existing memories are expressed.

Conditioned Fear and Instrumental Action (Coping)

A stimulus that warns of impending danger elicits defense responses, such as those discussed above, but it also has other consequences. Once the organism is acted on by the CS, it then prepares to act back on the environment, figuring out how to escape and/or avoid danger and the stimuli that are associated with danger. These instrumental emotional responses, which might be thought of as coping responses (Lazarus 1966, 1991), have been studied experimentally using avoidance conditioning procedures. Fear conditioning is generally assumed to be the first step in the learning of avoidance (e.g. Mowrer 1960, Mackintosh 1983). That is, the state of conditioned fear is assumed to be unpleasant or undesirable, and in the effort to reduce fear, the organism learns to escape from and ultimately avoid situations or stimuli that lead to the arousal of fear. It might therefore be expected that damage to the amygdala, which will prevent fear conditioning, would interfere with avoidance conditioning.

The literature on the effects of brain lesions on avoidance conditioning is large and fairly confusing, and is not reviewed in detail here. Several features of this literature are highlighted below.

First, many studies of active and passive avoidance demonstrate that lesions of the amygdala interfere with the acquisition of avoidance responses (Panksepp et al. 1991, Sarter & Markowitsch 1985). It is not clear why some studies fail to find this effect, but an analysis of the underlying task demands might be revealing. Even for those tasks in which the amygdala is involved, the input and output connections and intra-amygdala circuitry are not very well understood, possibly because of the variability in the eliciting stimulus conditions and in the emitted instrumental responses. At the same time, the simplicity of the eliciting stimuli and elicited responses in fear conditioning probably contribute to the greater success achieved in uncovering brain mechanisms with this procedure.

Second, most studies of passive avoidance find that the septo-hippocampal system is important. This observation provides part of the conceptual foundation for Gray's septo-hippocampal theory of fear and anxiety (Gray 1982, 1987). Although the theory is based on an impressive survey of the literature, it is unclear to what extent the septo-hippocampal system is involved in the fear part or in the stimulus processing (e.g. contextual processing) aspect of many passive avoidance tasks. As noted above, the hippocampus is involved in fear conditioning if the CS is the context in which the US occurs rather than a discrete signal. The same may be true of passive avoidance, in which diffuse contextual cues usually serve as the Pavlovian CS. Other aspects of the septo-hippocampal model of anxiety have been discussed elsewhere (see commentaries in Gray 1982, LeDoux 1992, Panksepp 1990).

Third, although the amygdala is often required for the acquisition of avoidance, it is less important and probably unnecessary for the long-term maintenance of well-trained avoidance responses. Thus, after learning is established, the defense system involving the amygdala is no longer a necessary part of the avoidance circuitry. It is thus important to keep the phase of training in mind when asking questions about brain involvement in avoidance.

Fourth, the instrumental aspects of avoidance, unlike the Pavlovian elicited responses, may require connections between the amygdala and the ventral striatum for their acquisition and/or expression (Everitt & Robbins 1992). In particular, the nucleus accumbens of the ventral striatum may be a crucial area for the initiation and control of instrumental responses motivated by either appetitive or aversive processes, possibly resulting from its innervation by dopaminergic pathways.

In summary, although the literature on avoidance is somewhat confusing, studies of avoidance conditioning, like studies of fear conditioning, point to the amygdala as probably playing some role. This should not be surprising since avoidance conditioning is believed to involve Pavlovian fear conditioning (which requires the amygdala) followed by the learning of the instrumental avoidance response. The amygdala almost certainly contributes to the Pavlovian part of avoidance learning but its role in the instrumental part is less clear.

Fear Conditioning: Conclusions

Studies of fear conditioning have successfully identified the neural system that underlies this important form of learning and memory process. Part of the reason that researchers have been so successful is that in fear conditioning, simple, well-defined stimuli can be used to elicit stereotyped or at least repeatable responses that require little training. It is always much easier to trace neural pathways when the stimulus and the response can both be precisely identified and quantified. This probably accounts for the greater success of studies of fear conditioning than of studies of avoidance conditioning in mapping the pathways of fear. At the same time, we have to be aware that the brain mechanisms of fear conditioning may not generalize to all aspects of fear. Whether fear of failure or fear of authority or fear of being afraid are mediated by the same basic system, with some cognitive baggage added on, remains to be determined.

Relation of the Neural Basis of Fear to Other Emotions

As noted above, the neural basis of fear conditioning has been studied so extensively and successfully because there are good techniques available for eliciting and quantifying conditioned fear responses. For the same reason, there has been a relative paucity of research on the neural basis of most other emotions, especially positive emotions.

Some studies have examined the neural basis of positive affective reactions and approach behavior. Unlike studies of defensive behavior, which are relevant to the emotion of fear, these studies are less specifically related to a well-defined emotion, except possibly pleasure. Most of this work has involved three paradigms: brain stimulation reward (Rolls 1975, Olds 1977, Gallistel et al. 1981), stimulus-reward association learning procedures (see Aggleton & Mishkin 1986, Gaffan 1992, Everitt & Robbins 1992, Rolls 1992, Ono

& Nishijo 1992), and appetitive classical conditioning (Gallagher & Holland 1992). The neural network underlying these tasks overlaps somewhat with the fear system in that the amygdala is involved to some extent in each of these tasks [but see Cahill & McGaugh (1990) for a comparison of the relative contribution of the amygdala to appetitive and aversive learning]. Unfortunately, the neural system is poorly understood for these positive emotional phenomena and much more work is needed. The creation of new models of positive affect is also important.

Given that the amygdala is involved to some extent in both positive and negative emotional reactions, one might be tempted to conclude that the amygdala is the centerpiece of an emotional system of the brain. However, this would be a mistake. We know far too little about the neural system–mediating emotions other than fear and far too little about variants of fear other than simple forms of conditioned fear. The amygdala is a sufficiently complex brain region that it could be involved in fear and reward processes in completely different ways and for different reasons. Other attempts at identifying emotion with a single system of the brain (e.g. the limbic system) have fared poorly (see LeDoux 1991), and we should be cautious not to overinterpret the role of the amygdala.

Implications of the Neural Basis of Fear for Understanding Emotion

Examining emotion from the point of view of the nervous system allows us to see questions about this complex process from a unique angle. Several issues have been raised about the nature of emotion in light of the neural systems analysis of emotion just presented.

Cognitive-Emotional Interactions

The nature of cognitive-emotional interactions is one of the most debated topics in the psychol-

ogy of emotion (e.g. Zajonc 1980, 1984; Lazarus 1982, 1984, 1991; Mandler 1984; Leventhal & Scherer 1987; Frijda 1986; LeDoux 1987, 1993b; Parrott & Schulkin 1993a,b; Izard 1992; Oatley & Johnson-Laird 1987; Ortony et al. 1988; Ekman 1992). Knowledge of the neural system underlying emotion can help constrain our thinking on this topic. As we have seen, the system that mediates the emotion fear is well characterized. We can thus examine how cognitive processes participate in and interact with the neural system of fear.

Dependence of Emotional Processing (Appraisal) on Cognition

By most accounts, the amygdala plays a crucial role in deciding whether a stimulus is dangerous or not. Functions mediated by the amygdala are likely to be the neural instantiation of the emotional process known as appraisal (Arnold 1960; Lazarus 1966, 1991; Ekman 1977, 1992; Leventhal & Scherer 1987; Ellsworth 1991; Scherer 1991), at least for the appraisal of danger. The anatomical inputs to the amygdala from systems involved in stimulus processing define the kinds of events that can be appraised by the amygdala and the kinds of cognitive factors that might be important in this evaluation.

For example, the amygdala receives inputs from sensory processing areas in the thalamus and cortex (summarized in Figure 27.1; see LeDoux 1992 for review). The former provide course representations, but reach the amygdala quickly, while the latter provide detailed stimulus information, but reach the amygdala more slowly because of the additional processing stations involved at the cortical level. The thalamic inputs thus may be useful for producing rapid responses on the basis of limited stimulus information, whereas cortical inputs are required to distinguish between stimuli. Rapid response to danger has obvious survival value (Ohman 1986, 1992; Ekman 1992; LeDoux 1986, 1990), suggesting the possible significance of a quick-and-dirty subcortical pathway. The amygdala also receives inputs from the hippocampal formation (Ottersen 1982, Amaral et al. 1992). These set the context in which an emotional stimulus is to be evaluated (Phillips & LeDoux 1992b, Kim & Fanselow 1992, Selden et al. 1991, Penick & Solomon 1991, Good & Honey 1991), possibly allowing the amygdala to respond to a stimulus as threatening in one situation and not in another. In addition, given the role of the hippocampus in declarative or explicit memory (Squire 1992, Eichenbaum 1992), the hippocampal inputs may also allow fear responses to be activated by explicit or conscious memories of past experiences. When the functions of the other cortical areas that project to the amygdala have been elucidated we will be able to make additional predictions about the kinds of inputs that the amygdala appraises.

The anatomical organization of the fear system thus tells us that emotional responses can be elicited by processing in a wide range of systems. This issue of whether emotional processing is dependent on prior cognitive processing is reduced to a question of how we define cognition. If cognition is defined broadly to include sensory information processing, such as that occurring in the sensory thalamus and/or sensory cortex, as well as the processing that occurs in complex association areas of cortex in the frontal lobes or hippocampus, then emotional processing by the amygdala is highly dependent on cognitive processing. If cognitive processing is defined narrowly to include only the higher mental functions most likely mediated by complex association cortex, then emotion is not necessarily dependent on prior cognitive processing.

Emotional responses also might occur in the absence of inputs from cognitive systems. On the one hand, the amygdala receives inputs about the state of various internal organs of the body (e.g. Cechetto & Calaresu 1984) and these subcortical sensory inputs, like other exteroceptive sensory inputs, might be capable of triggering emotional responses. It is known that internal

signals can precipitate emotional reactions, as in panic attacks (Klein 1993), but it is not known whether the coding of the signal by the amygdala is involved. On the other hand, in some situations spontaneous discharges of the amygdala might generate emotional responses, but little evidence supports this possibility.

In the past, cognitive-emotional interactions have often been discussed without much consideration of what the terms cognition and emotion mean. I have limited this discussion to the emotion of fear and have examined how specific cognitive processes (such as sensory processing in the thalamus, perceptual processing in the neocortex, spatial and contextual processing in the hippocampus, or mnemonic processing in the hippocampus) can influence the amygdala and thereby elicit fear responses. This perspective forces us to abandon discussions of cognitive-emotional interactions in terms of vague monolithic cognitive processes and instead consider exactly which cognitive processes are involved in fear reactions. This is a more practical and tractable problem than the problem of how cognition and emotion, in the broader sense of the terms, interact. All we have to do is to determine how a particular cognitive process is organized in the brain and then determine how that brain region interacts with the amygdala. We can then hypothesize the nature of that particular cognitive-emotional interaction, at least within the fear domain.

Emotional Influences on Cognition
A similar situation holds for the other side of the cognitive-emotional dyad. That is, we can examine projections from the amygdala to areas involved in cognitive processing and make predictions about how the appraisal of danger by the amygdala might affect these processes (see Figure 27.3). The role of these projections in information processing has not been studied empirically, but the anatomical observations are suggestive of the functions served. For example,

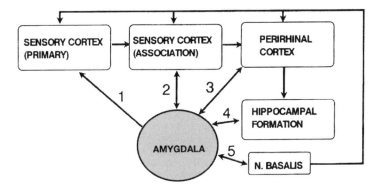

Figure 27.3
Amygdala influences on cortical cognitive processing. Once an emotional stimulus activates the amygdala, the amygdala can in turn impact cognitive processes organized in the neocortex. The amygdala receives inputs from sensory association areas but not primary sensory cortex (see figure 27.2). However, it appears to project back to primary sensory cortex (1) and to association areas (2). These projections allow the amygdala and its coding of emotional significance to control the ongoing flow of sensory information and may represent channels by which emotional processing can influence perception. The amygdala receives inputs from and projects to the perirhinal cortex and hippocampal formation (3, 4). These structures have been implicated in explicit or declarative memory processing and the interconnections may account for emotional influences on memory processing. The hippocampus is also important in adding context to emotional situations, and the interconnections between the amygdala and the hippocampus may play a role in making context an emotional stimulus. The nucleus basalis (N. Basalis) is the source of cholinergic inputs to widespread areas of the cortex (5) and plays an important role in cortical arousal and attention. Projections from the amygdala to this region may be important in attention and arousal processes.

the amygdala projects back to the cortical sensory processing systems that send projections to the amygdala (Price et al. 1987, Amaral et al. 1992). Although the amygdala receives inputs from only the later stages of sensory processing, its back projections innervate the earlier stages as well. These projections from the amygdala to sensory processing areas may allow the amygdala's appraisals of danger to influence ongoing perceptions of the environment (Rolls 1992, LeDoux 1992). The amygdala does not project back to the thalamus, but the cortical areas that receive amygdala inputs do, allowing for an indirect modulation of thalamic processing. Additionally, the amygdala projects to the nucleus basalis (Price et al. 1987, deOlmos et al. 1985), which provides widespread cholinergic modulation of cortical arousal. These projections may allow the amygdala to participate in selective attention (Weinberger 1993, Kapp et al. 1992, Gallagher & Holland 1992). The amygdala also projects to the hippocampus (Amaral et al. 1992, Price et al. 1987), allowing the appraisal of danger to modulate hippocampal functions, including spatial behavior (O'Keefe & Nadel 1978, O'Keefe 1993, McNaughton & Barnes 1990, Muller et al. 1991), contextual processing (Phillips & LeDoux 1992b, Kim & Fanselow 1992, Selden et al. 1991, Nadel & Willner 1980, Good & Honey 1991, Penick & Solomon 1991), and explicit or declarative memory storage or retrieval (Squire 1992, Eichenbaum 1992). Many other examples could be given, but these illustrate the usefulness of a neuroanatomical perspective in suggesting predictions about the nature of cognitive-emotional interactions.

Is Emotional Processing Cognitive Processing?

It has been argued that appraisal involves information processing; therefore, emotion is cognition (Lazarus 1982, 1984). However, as Zajonc (1984) and Izard (1992) have noted, cognitive processing is but one example of information processing. Noncognitive biological information processing systems include the immune system and the genome. Just because emotion involves information processing does not mean that emotion is cognition.

The issue, again, depends on how cognition is defined. It can be defined to include emotion, motivation, and similar processes, but this would seem to defeat the purpose of having a designation of cognition as opposed to the more general term mind. Hilgard (1980) has reminded psychology that cognition historically has been thought of as part of a trilogy of mind that also includes emotion and will (motivation) rather than as an all-encompassing description of mind. Certainly, early pioneers of cognitive science did not view emotion as a cognitive process. According to Neisser (1967), emotion was one of the many aspects of psychology not included in the cognitive approach.

Studies of the processing rules and transformations in areas of the brain that are involved in cognition and areas involved in emotion might be able to address the question of whether emotional and cognitive processing are fundamentally different. Studies of the brain mechanisms of emotion have pointed to the amygdala as an important part of an aversive emotional memory system, and to the hippocampus as part of the system involved in cognitive or declarative form of memory (for a discussion of emotional and cognitive memory systems, see LeDoux 1993a). This does not prove that the systems operate by different information processing rules, but it certainly leaves open the possibility. For example, given that cells in the amygdala and hippocampus both "learn" during conditioning, one might ask whether comparable representations are encoded. Although a lot has been learned about the nature of hippocampal information processing from studies of the physiology of hippocampal neurons (for review, see O'Keefe 1993), we know very little about how amygdala neurons process information. If and when physiological studies of the amygdala catch up with studies of the hippocampus, it may be possible to determine whether these systems use different processing rules or whether they simply do different things on the basis of similar processing functions.

Conscious versus Unconscious Processes in Emotion

The issue of what is conscious or unconscious in emotion was around even before James (1884) popularized it with his famous question about whether we run from a bear out of fear (conscious or subjective emotion) or whether fear comes from running away. However, all animals, invertebrates as well as vertebrates, must have a way of defending themselves from danger. When a fruitfly is conditioned to avoid shock by flying out of the chamber where the shock occurred (Tully 1991), it is unlikely that a conscious state of fear intervenes between the reception of the stimulus and the production of the response. Comparative psychologists long ago learned the importance of parsimony in explaining findings across species. If we do not need subjective fear to explain defensive responses in lower species, then we should not explain defensive responses in higher species in this way either. At least amongst vertebrates, the neural system involved in detecting danger and producing defense responses is similarly organized in all species studied. This suggests that evolution long ago figured out how to organize the defense system and has continued to use this organizational blueprint. Subjective fear, in this view, is what occurs when the evolutionary old defense system is activated, but only in a species that also has the capacity for subjective conscious states.

This view highlights the value of studies of experimental animals in understanding emotional systems. Because the system that generates emotional responses is strongly conserved in evolution (the amygdala and its connections are involved in all vertebrates studied), we can learn about human defense or fear reactions by studying other creatures. And if fear responses and conscious emotional states of fear are the result of activation of an evolutionarily conserved system that detects danger, then studying how the neural system produces fear responses in animals will also shed light on mechanisms that contribute to conscious states of fear in humans.

Volitional Control of Emotion

Whether emotional responses are under voluntary control is an important issue with a great deal of practical application to legal issues. What seems clear from the neural systems perspective is that there are both involuntary and voluntary responses, each mediated by different neural networks emanating out of the amygdala.

Many defense responses are respondents rather than operants. That is, the responses are controlled by their antecedents rather than by their consequences (Bouton & Bolles 1980). Borrowing a term from ethology, these responses are released by the presence of stimuli that have their releasing capacity either as a result of genetic programming or associative learning processes. These responses are, in the language of cognitive psychology, effortless and automatic, and probably are controlled by unconscious appraisal processes. These involuntary emotional responses include behavioral (e.g. freezing and flight reactions, facial expressions) as well as visceral (e.g. autonomic and endocrine) responses.

Emotional respondents are only part of the story of emotional responsivity. Once emotional respondents are expressed, emotional operants begin to occur. These are instrumental responses. A rat exposed to a cat will automatically freeze in order to minimize the possibility of an attack. During the freezing episode, the rat begins planning strategies that might lead to successful

escape, using information stored from past experience and expectations about possible outcomes. These kinds of processes are related to what has been called risk-assessment behavior (Blanchard et al. 1993). This may be the point at which Gray's (1982, 1987) septo-hippocampal system (which may be involved in the instrumental and cognitive phase of fear and anxiety) meets the amygdala-based system (which is probably more involved in the automatic, elicited aspects of fear and anxiety).

Respondents are not learned. They are hardwired into the nervous system, and are subject to Pavlovian conditioning. But conditioning does not modify the responses; it allows new stimuli to activate the responses. In contrast, emotional operants are learned through instrumental (operant) conditioning procedures. Although the respondents are controlled by outputs of the amygdala to brainstem motor systems, the instrumental actions (such as escape and avoidance) appear to be mediated by projections from the amygdala to a forebrain region known as the ventral striatum (Everitt & Robbins 1992), an important link to the extrapyramidal motor system. The emotional respondent system has been examined in detail, but less is known about emotional operants, which are much more difficult to study because they are considerably more complex. However, this is an important area for future research because it may help shed light on emotional coping responses (Lazarus 1991).

Psychopathological Issues

Disorders of fear regulation make up an important set of psychopathologic conditions. To the extent that we understand the anatomy of these systems, we will be in a better position to develop more selective drug therapies that are targeted for the specific brain networks involved in fear regulation. In addition, knowledge of the anatomy of fear may help us understand some other aspects of pathological fear, and perhaps other emotions, as well.

The anatomy of the fear processing system tells us that fear can be triggered by many different kinds of information processing functions that lead to the amygdala. If, for genetic or experiential reasons, the lower-order pathways are more efficient at triggering the amygdala than are the higher-order pathways in some individuals, we would expect those individuals to have rather limited insight into the nature of their emotional reactions. People have different degrees of insight into their emotions and the anatomical findings suggest a possible explanation.

Another point to consider is that emotional memories mediated by the amygdala system are indelible. That is, the memories persist even after emotional behavior is extinguished. This has been demonstrated in behavioral studies (e.g. Bouton & Swartzentruber 1991), but is also illustrated dramatically by studies showing that with cortical lesions, extinction can be prolonged or eliminated (Teich et al. 1989, LeDoux et al. 1989, Morgan et al. 1993). Extinction thus appears to involve cortical inhibition of indelible, amygdala-mediated memories. It is not a process of emotional memory erasure. The role of therapy may be to allow the cortex to establish more effective and efficient synaptic links with the amygdala.

Finally, consider the issues of infantile amnesia and the inaccessibility of memory for early trauma. Jacobs & Nadel (1985) made the intriguing suggestion that our inability to remember early experiences may be because the hippocampus is not sufficiently mature to allow us to form declarative or conscious memories until around the second or third year of life. They suggest that early trauma might not be accessible consciously because the system that encodes conscious memories is not fully functional. At the same time, we know that early trauma can have long lasting influences on behavioral and mental states, which suggests that the system that encodes these unconscious traumatic memories is present and functional. We know that the amygdala is crucial for at least some forms of aversive

or traumatic learning and memory, but little definitive work has been done on the maturational time course of the amygdala that would allow us to clearly state whether it develops before the hippocampus. However, a recent study showed that rats can be conditioned to an auditory CS at an earlier age than they can to contextual stimuli (Rudy 1993). This finding implies strongly that the amygdala matures earlier than does the hippocampus.

There are several implications of these observations. First, early memories may be emotional memories (and not explicit, declarative conscious memories) because the emotional memory system (and not the declarative system) is functional at the time. Second, early emotional memories, including traumatic as well as nontraumatic memories, may be inaccessible to consciousness not because of active repression but because of the time course of brain maturation. Third, the extent to which one can gain conscious access to these early memories, which were encoded in the absence of the conscious or declarative memory system, may be limited.

Conclusions

Progress in understanding the neural basis of fear has been rapid in the last decade. We now understand the anatomy of this system in great detail. This information can help us see emotions in a different light and suggests some insights and constraints concerning important issues about the nature of emotion. Although much remains to be done, especially in terms of determining the generality of the findings, we are well on the way to understanding how one important aspect of emotional life is represented in the brain.

Literature Cited

Aggleton JP. 1992. *The Amygdala: Neurobiological Aspects of Emotion, Memory, and Mental Dysfunction.* New York: Wiley-Liss.

Aggleton JP, Mishkin M. 1986. The amygdala: sensory gateway to the emotions. In *Emotion: Theory, Research and Experience,* ed. R Plutchik, H Kellerman, 3:281–99. Orlando: Academic.

Amaral DG, Price JL, Pitkänen A, Carmichael ST. 1992. Anatomical organization of the primate amygdaloid complex. See Aggleton 1992, pp. 1–66.

Arnold MB. 1960. *Emotion and Personality.* New York: Columbia Univ. Press.

Blanchard DC, Blanchard RJ. 1972. Innate and conditioned reactions to threat in rats with amygdaloid lesions. *J. Comp. Physiol. Psychol.* 81(2):281–90.

Blanchard RJ, Yudko EB, Rodgers RJ, Blanchard DC. 1993. Defense system psychopharmacology: an ethological approach to the pharmacology of fear and anxiety. *Behav. Brain Res.* 58:155–66.

Bliss TVP, Collingridge GL. 1993. A synaptic model of memory: long-term potentiation in the hippocampus. *Nature* 361:31–39.

Bordi F, LeDoux J. 1992. Sensory tuning beyond the sensory system: an initial analysis of auditory properties of neurons in the lateral amygdaloid nucleus and overlying areas of the striatum. *J. Neurosci.* 12(7): 2493–2503.

Bordi F, LeDoux JE. 1994a. Response properties of single units in areas of rat auditory thalamus that project to the amygdala. I: Acoustic discharge patterns and frequency receptive fields. *Exp. Brain Res.* 98:261–74.

Bordi F, LeDoux JE. 1994b. Response properties of single units in areas of rat auditory thalamus that project to the amygdala. II: Cells receiving convergent auditory and somatosensory inputs and cells antidromically activated by amygdala stimulation. *Exp. Brain Res.* 98:275–86.

Bordi F, LeDoux JE, Clugnet MC, Pavlides C. 1993. Single unit activity in the lateral nucleus of the amygdala and overlying areas of the striatum in freely-behaving rats: rates, discharge patterns, and responses to acoustic stimuli. *Behav. Neurosci.* 107:757–69.

Bouton ME, Bolles RC. 1980. Conditioned fear assessed by freezing and by the suppression of three different baselines. *Anim. Learn. Behav.* 8:429–34.

Bouton ME, Swartzentruber D. 1991. Sources of relapse after extinction in Pavlovian and instrumental learning. *Clin. Psychol. Rev.* 11:123–40.

Brodal A. 1982. *Neurological Anatomy.* New York: Oxford Univ. Press.

Brown JS, Kalish IH, Farber IE. 1951. Conditioned fear as revealed by magnitude of startle response to an auditory stimulus. *J. Exp. Psychol.* 41:317–28.

Brown TH, Chapman PF, Kairiss EW, Keenan CL. 1988. Long-term synaptic potentiation. *Science* 242:724–28.

Cahill L, McGaugh JL. 1990. Amygdaloid complex lesions differentially affect retention of tasks using appetitive and aversive reinforcement. *Behav. Neurosci.* 104:532–43.

Campbell BA, Jaynes J. 1966. Reinstatement. *Psychol. Rev.* 73:478–80.

Cechetto DF, Calaresu FR. 1984. Units in the amygdala responding to activation of carotid baro- and chemoreceptors. *Am. J. Physiol.* 246:R832–36.

Chapman PF, Bellavance LL. 1992. NMDA receptor-independent LTP in the amygdala. *Synapse.*

Chapman PF, Kairiss EW, Keenan CL, Brown TH. 1990. Long-term synaptic potentiation in the amygdala. *Synapse* 6:271–78.

Clugnet MC, LeDoux JE. 1990. Synaptic plasticity in fear conditioning circuits: induction of LTP in the lateral nucleus of the amygdala by stimulation of the medial geniculate body. *J. Neurosci.* 10:2818–24.

Clugnet MC, LeDoux JE, Morrison SF. 1990. Unit responses evoked in the amygdala and striatum by electrical stimulation of the medial geniculate body. *J. Neurosci.* 10:1055–61.

Cohen DH, Randall DC. 1984. Classical conditioning of cardiovascular responses. *Annu. Rev. Physiol.* 46:187–97.

Cotman CW, Monaghan DT, Ganong AH. 1988. Excitatory amino acid neurotransmission: NMDA receptors and Hebb-type synaptic plasticity. *Annu. Rev. Neurosci.* 11:61–80.

Davis M. 1992. The role of the amygdala in conditioned fear. See Aggleton 1992, pp. 255–306.

Davis M, Hitchcock JM, Rosen JB. 1987. Anxiety and the amygdala: pharmacological and anatomical analysis of the fear-potentiated startle paradigm. In *The Psychology of Learning and Motivation,* ed. GH Bower, 21:263–305. San Diego: Academic.

deOlmos J, Alheid G, Beltramino C. 1985. Amygdala. In *The Rat Nervous System,* ed. G Paxinos, pp. 223–334. Orlando: Academic.

Edeline J-M, Weinberger NM. 1992. Associative retuning in the thalamic source of input to the amygdala and auditory cortex: receptive field plasticity in the medial division of the medial geniculate body. *Behav. Neurosci.* 106:81–105.

Edeline J-M, Weinberger NM. 1993. Receptive field plasticity in the auditory cortex during frequency discrimination training: selective retuning independent of task difficulty. *Behav. Neurosci.* 107:82–103.

Eichenbaum H. 1992. The hippocampal system and declarative memory in animals. *J. Cogn. Neurosci.* 4(3):217–31.

Ekman P. 1977. Biological and cultural contributions to body and facial movement. In *Anthropology of the Body,* ed. J Blacking, pp. 39–84. London: Academic.

Ekman P. 1992. An argument for basic emotions. *Cogn. Emot.* 6:169–200.

Ekman P, Davidson R. 1994. *The Nature of Emotion: Fundamental Questions.* New York: Oxford Univ. Press.

Ellsworth P. 1991. Some implications of cognitive appraisal theories of emotion. In *International Review of Studies on Emotion,* ed. KT Strongman, pp. 143–61. Chichester, UK: Wiley.

Estes WK, Skinner BF. 1941. Some quantitative properties of anxiety. *J. Exp. Psychol.* 129:390–400.

Everitt BJ, Robbins TW. 1992. Amygdala-ventral striatal interactions and reward-related processes. See Aggleton 1992, pp. 401–29.

Falls WA, Miserendino MJD, Davis M. 1992. Extinction of fear-potentiated startle: blockade by infusion of an NMDA antagonist into the amygdala. *J. Neurosci.* 12(3):854–63.

Fanselow MS. 1980. Conditional and unconditional components of postshock freezing. *Pavlovian J. Biol. Sci.* 15:177–82.

Fanselow MS, Bolles RC. 1979. Naloxone and shock-elicited freezing in the rat. *J. Comp. Physiol. Psychol.* 93(4):736–44.

Fanselow MS, Helmstetter FJ. 1988. Conditional analgesia, defensive freezing, and benzodiazepines. *Behav. Neurosci.* 102(2):233–43.

Fanselow MS, Kim JJ. 1994. Acquisition of contextual Pavlovian fear conditioning is blocked by application of an NMDA receptor antagonist D,L-2-amino-5-phosphonovaleric acid to the basolateral amygdala. *Behav. Neurosci.* 108:210–12.

Frijda N. 1986. *The Emotions.* Cambridge: Cambridge Univ. Press.

Gabriel M, Slatwick SE, Miller JD. 1976. Multiple unit activity of the rabbit medial geniculate nucleus in conditioning, extinction, and reversal. *Physiol. Psychol.* 4:124–34.

Gaffan D. 1992. Amygdala and the memory of reward. See Aggleton 1992, pp. 471–483.

Gallagher M, Holland PC. 1992. Understanding the function of the central nucleus: Is simple conditioning enough? See Aggleton 1992, pp. 307–21.

Gallistel CR, Shizgal P, Yeomans JS. 1981. A portrait of the substrate for self-stimulation. *Psychol. Rev.* 88:228–73.

Gean P-W, Chang F-C, Huang C-C, Lin J-H, Way L-J. 1993. Long-term enhancement of EPSP and NMDA receptor-mediated synaptic transmission in the amygdala. *Brain Res. Bull.* 31:7–11.

Gentile CG, Jarrell TW, Teich A, McCabe PM, Schneiderman N. 1986. The role of amygdaloid central nucleus in the retention of differential Pavlovian conditioning of bradycardia in rabbits. *Behav. Brain Res.* 20:263–73.

Good M, Honey RC. 1991. Conditioning and contextual retrieval in hippocampal rats. *Behav. Neurosci.* 105:499–509.

Gray JA. 1982. *The Neuropsychology of Anxiety.* New York: Oxford Univ. Press.

Gray JA. 1987. *The Psychology of Fear and Stress.* New York: Cambridge Univ. Press.

Hebb DO. 1949. *The Organization of Behavior.* New York: Wiley.

Hilgard ER. 1980. The trilogy of mind: cognition, affection, and conation. *J. Hist. Behav. Sci.* 16:107–17.

Hunt HF, Brady JV. 1955. Some effects of punishment and intercurrent "anxiety" on a simple operant. *J. Comp. Physiol. Psychol.* 48:305–10.

Iwata J, Chida K, LeDoux JE. 1987. Cardiovascular responses elicited by stimulation of neurons in the central amygdaloid nucleus in awake but not anesthetized rats resemble conditioned emotional responses. *Brain Res.* 418:183–88.

Iwata J, LeDoux JE, Meeley MP, Arneric S, Reis DJ. 1986. Intrinsic neurons in the amygdaloid field projected to by the medial geniculate body mediate emotional responses conditioned to acoustic stimuli. *Brain Res.* 383:195–214.

Izard CE. 1992. Four systems for emotion activation: cognitive and noncognitive. *Psychol. Rev.* 99:561–65.

Jacobs WJ, Nadel L. 1985. Stress-induced recovery of fears and phobias. *Psychol. Rev.* 92:512–31.

James W. 1884. What is emotion? *Mind* 9:188–205.

Jarrell TW, Gentile CG, Romanski LM, McCabe PM, Schneiderman N. 1987. Involvement of cortical and thalamic auditory regions in retention of differential bradycardia conditioning to acoustic conditioned stimuli in rabbits. *Brain Res.* 412:285–94.

Kamin LJ. 1965. Temporal and intensity characteristics of the conditioned stimulus. In *Classical Conditioning*, ed. WF Prokasy, pp. 118–47. New York: Appleton-Century-Crofts.

Kandel ER, Spencer WA. 1968. Cellular neurophysiological approaches to the study of learning. *Physiol. Rev.* 48:65–134.

Kapp BS, Pascoe JP, Bixler MA. 1984. The amygdala: a neuroanatomical systems approach to its contributions to aversive conditioning. In *Neuropsychology of Memory*, ed. N Buttlers, LR Squire, pp. 473–88. New York: Guilford.

Kapp BS, Whalen PJ, Supple WF, Pascoe JP. 1992. Amygdaloid contributions to conditioned arousal and sensory information processing. See Aggleton 1992, pp. 229–54.

Kapp BS, Wilson A, Pascoe J, Supple W, Whalen PJ. 1990. A neuroanatomical systems analysis of conditioned bradycardia in the rabbit. In *Learning and Computational Neuroscience: Foundations of Adaptive Networks*, ed. M Gabriel, J Moore, pp. 53–90. Cambridge, MA: MIT Press.

Kim JJ, Fanselow MS. 1992. Modality-specific retrograde amnesia of fear. *Science* 256:675–77.

Kim M, Davis M. 1993. Lack of a temporal gradient of retrograde amnesia in rats with amygdala lesions assessed with the fear-potentiated startle paradigm. *Behav. Neurosci.* 107:1088–92.

Klein DF. 1993. False suffocation alarms and spontaneous panics: subsuming the CO_2 hypersensitivity theory. *Arch. Gen. Psychiatry* 50:306–17.

Konorski J. 1967. Transient (or dynamic) memory. In *Integrative Activity of the Brain*, ed. Anonymous, pp. 490–505. Chicago: Univ. Chicago Press.

Kotter R, Meyer N. 1992. The limbic system: a review of its empirical foundation. *Behav. Brain Res.* 52:105–27.

Lazarus RS. 1966. *Psychological Stress and the Coping Process.* New York: McGraw Hill.

Lazarus RS. 1982. Thoughts on the relations between emotion and cognition. *Am. Psychol.* 37:1019–24.

Lazarus RS. 1984. On the primacy of cognition. *Am. Psychol.* 39:124–29.

Lazarus RS. 1991. Cognition and motivation in emotion. *Am. Psychol.* 46(4):352–67.

Leaf RC, Muller SA. 1965. Simple method for CER conditioning and measurement. *Psychol. Rep.* 17:211–15.

LeDoux JE. 1986. Sensory systems and emotion. *Integr. Psychiatry* 4:237–48.

LeDoux JE. 1987. Emotion. In *Handbook of Physiology. 1: The Nervous System*, ed. F Plum, 5:419–60. Bethesda, MD: Am. Physiol. Soc.

LeDoux JE. 1990. Information flow from sensation to emotion: plasticity in the neural computation of stimulus value. See Kapp et al. 1990, pp. 3–52.

LeDoux JE. 1991. Emotion and the limbic system concept. *Concepts Neurosci.* 2:169–99.

LeDoux JE. 1992. Brain mechanisms of emotion and emotional learning. *Curr. Opin. Neurobiol.* 2:191–98.

LeDoux JE. 1993a. Emotional memory systems in the brain. *Behav. Brain Res.* 58:69–79.

LeDoux JE. 1993b. Cognition versus emotion, again—this time in the brain: a response to Parrott and Schulkin. *Cogn. Emot.* 7:61–64.

LeDoux JE, Cicchetti P, Xagoraris A, Romanski LM. 1990a. The lateral amygdaloid nucleus: sensory interface of the amygdala in fear conditioning. *J. Neurosci.* 10:1062–69.

LeDoux JE, Farb C, Ruggiero DA. 1990b. Topographic organization of neurons in the acoustic thalamus that project to the amygdala. *J. Neurosci.* 10:1043–54.

LeDoux JE, Farb CR, Romanski L. 1991. Overlapping projections to the amygdala and striatum from auditory processing areas of the thalamus and cortex. *Neurosci. Lett.* 134:139–44.

LeDoux JE, Iwata J, Cicchetti P, Reis DJ. 1988. Different projections of the central amygdaloid nucleus mediate autonomic and behavioral correlates of conditioned fear. *J. Neurosci.* 8:2517–29.

LeDoux JE, Romanski LM, Xagoraris AE. 1989. Indelibility of subcortical emotional memories. *J. Cogn. Neurosci.* 1:238–43.

LeDoux JE, Ruggiero DA, Reis DJ. 1985. Projections to the subcortical forebrain from anatomically defined regions of the medial geniculate body in the rat. *J. Comp. Neurol.* 242:182–213.

LeDoux JE, Sakaguchi A, Iwata J, Reis DJ. 1986. Interruption of projections from the medial geniculate body to an archi-neostriatal field disrupts the classical conditioning of emotional responses to acoustic stimuli in the rat. *Neuroscience* 17:615–27.

LeDoux JE, Sakaguchi A, Reis DJ. 1984. Subcortical efferent projections of the medial geniculate nucleus mediate emotional responses conditioned by acoustic stimuli. *J. Neurosci.* 4(3):683–98.

LeGal La Salle G, Ben-Ari Y. 1981. Unit activity in the amygdaloid complex: a review. In *The Amygdaloid Complex*, ed. Y Ben-Ari, pp. 227–237. New York: Elsevier/North-Holland Biomed. Press.

Leventhal H, Scherer K. 1987. The relationship of emotion to cognition: a functional approach to a semantic controversy. *Cogn. Emot.* 1:3–28.

Lynch G. 1986. *Synapses, Circuits, and the Beginnings of Memory*. Cambridge, MA: MIT Press.

Lynch G, Larson J, Staubli U, Granger R. 1991. Variants of synaptic potentiation and different types of memory operations in hippocampus and related structures. In *Memory: Organization and Locus of Change*, ed. LR Squire, NM Weinberger, G Lynch, JL McGaugh, pp. 330–63. New York: Oxford Univ. Press.

Mackintosh NJ. 1983. *Conditioning and Associative Learning*. New York: Oxford Univ. Press.

MacLean PD. 1949. Psychosomatic disease and the "visceral brain": recent developments bearing on the Papez theory of emotion. *Psychosom. Med.* 11:338–53.

MacLean PD. 1952. Some psychiatric implications of physiological studies on frontotemporal portion of limbic system (visceral brain). *Electroencephalogr. Clin. Neurophysiol.* 4:407–18.

Madison DV, Malenka RC, Nicoll RA. 1991. Mechanisms underlying long-term potentiation of synaptic transmission. *Annu. Rev. Neurosci.* 14:379–97.

Malenka RC, Nicoll RA. 1993. NMDA-receptor-dependent synaptic plasticity: multiple forms and mechanisms. *Trends Neurosci.* 16:521–27.

Mandler G. 1984. *Mind and Body: The Psychology of Emotion and Stress*. New York: Norton.

Mason JW. 1968. A review of psychoendocrine research on the sympathetic-adrenal medullary system. *Psychosom. Med.* 30:631–53.

McAllister WR, McAllister DE. 1971. Behavioral measurement of conditioned fear. In *Aversive Conditioning and Learning*, ed. FR Brush, pp. 105–79. New York: Academic.

McNaughton BL, Barnes CA. 1990. From cooperative synaptic enhancement to associative memory: bridging the abyss. *Sem. Neurosci.* 2:403–16.

Millenson JR, de Villiers PA. 1972. Motivational properties of conditioned anxiety. In *Reinforcement: Behavioral Analyses*, ed. RM Gilbert, JR Millenson, pp. 98–128. New York: Academic.

Miserendino MJD, Sananes CB, Melia KR, Davis M. 1990. Blocking of acquisition but not expression of conditioned fear-potentiated startle by NMDA antagonists in the amygdala. *Nature* 345:716–18.

Morgan MA, Romanski LM, LeDoux JE. 1993. Extinction of emotional learning: contribution of medial prefrontal cortex. *Neurosci. Lett.* 163:109–13.

Morris RGM. 1992. Is there overlap between the characteristics of learning and the physiological properties of LTP? In *Encyclopedia of Learning and Memory*, ed. LR Squire, pp. 369–72. New York: Macmillan.

Mowrer OH. 1960. *Learning Theory and Behavior*. New York: Wiley.

Muller RU, Kubie JL, Saypoff R. 1991. The hippocampus as a cognitive graph (abridged version). *Hippocampus* 1(3):243–46.

Muramoto K, Ono T, Nishijo H, Fukuda M. 1993. Rat amygdaloid neuron responses during auditory discrimination. *Neuroscience* 52:621–36.

Nadel L, Willner J. 1980. Context and conditioning: a place for space. *Physiol. Psychol.* 8:218–28.

Neisser U. 1967. *Cognitive Psychology*. New York: Appleton-Century-Crofts.

Oatley K, Johnson-Laird P. 1987. Towards a cognitive theory of emotion. *Cogn. Emot.* 1:29–50.

Öhman A. 1986. Face the beast and fear the face: animal and social fears as prototypes for evolutionary analyses of emotion. *Psychophysiology* 23:123–45.

Öhman A. 1992. Fear and anxiety as emotional phenomena: clinical, phenomenological, evolutionary perspectives, and information-processing mechanisms. In *Handbook of the Emotions*, ed. M Lewis, JM Haviland, pp. 511–36. New York: Guilford.

O'Keefe J. 1993. Hippocampus, theta, and spatial memory. *Curr. Opin. Neurobiol.* 3:917–24.

O'Keefe J, Nadel L. 1978. *The Hippocampus as a Cognitive Map.* Oxford: Clarendon.

Olds J. 1977. *Drives and Reinforcement.* New York: Raven.

Ono T, Nakamura K, Nishijo H, Tamura R, Tabuchi E. 1988. Lateral hypothalamus and amygdala involvement in rat learning behavior. *Adv. Biosci.* 70:123–26.

Ono T, Nishijo H. 1992. Neurophysiological basis of the Kluver-Bucy Syndrome: responses of monkey amygdaloid neurons to biologically significant objects. See Aggleton 1992, pp. 167–90.

Ortony A, Clore GL, Collins A. 1988. *The Cognitive Structure of Emotions.* Cambridge: Cambridge Univ. Press.

Ottersen OP. 1982. Connections of the amygdala of the rat. IV: Corticoamygdaloid and intraamygdaloid connections as studied with axonal transport of horseradish peroxidase. *J. Comp. Neurol.* 205:30–48.

Panksepp J. 1990. Gray zones at the emotion/cognition interface: a commentary. *Cogn. Emot.* 4:289–302.

Panksepp J, Sacks DS, Crepau LJ, Abbot BB. 1991. The psycho- and neurobiology of fear systems in the brain. In *Fear, Avoidance, and Phobias,* ed. MR Denny, pp. 7–59. Hillsdale, NJ: Erlbaum.

Parrott WG, Schulkin J. 1993a. What sort of system could an affective system be? A reply to LeDoux. *Cogn. Emot.* 7:65–69.

Parrott WG, Schulkin J. 1993b. Neuropsychology and the cognitive nature of the emotions. *Cogn. Emot.* 7:43–59.

Pascoe JP, Kapp BS. 1985. Electrophysiological characteristics of amygdaloid central nucleus neurons during Pavlovian fear conditioning in the rabbit. *Behav. Brain Res.* 16:117–33.

Pavlov IP. 1927. *Conditioned Reflexes.* New York: Dover.

Penick S, Solomon PR. 1991. Hippocampus, context, and conditioning. *Behav. Neurosci.* 105:611–17.

Phillips RG, LeDoux JE. 1992a. Overlapping and divergent projections of CAI and the ventral subiculum to the amygdala. *Soc. Neurosci. Abstr.* 18:518.

Phillips RG, LeDoux JE. 1992b. Differential contribution of amygdala and hippocampus to cued and contextual fear conditioning. *Behav. Neurosci.* 106:274–85.

Price JL, Russchen FT, Amaral DG. 1987. The limbic region. II: The amygdaloid complex. In *Handbook of Chemical Neuroanatomy.* Vol. 5: *Integrated Systems of the CNS,* ed. A Bjorklund, T Hokfelt, LW Swanson, pp. 279–388. Amsterdam: Elsevier.

Rescorla RA, Heth CD. 1975. Reinstatement of fear to an extinguished conditioned stimulus. *J. Exp. Psychol. Anim. Behav.* 104:88–96.

Rescorla RA, Wagner AR. 1972. A theory of Pavlovian conditioning: variations in the effectiveness of reinforcement and nonreinforcement. In *Classical Conditioning II: Current Research and Theory,* ed. AA Black, WF Prokasy, pp. 64–99. New York: Appleton-Century-Crofts.

Rolls ET. 1975. *The Brain and Reward.* Oxford: Pergamon.

Rolls ET. 1992. Neurophysiology and functions of the primate amygdala. See Aggleton 1992, pp. 143–65.

Romanski LM, Clugnet MC, Bordi F, LeDoux JE. 1993. Somatosensory and auditory convergence in the lateral nucleus of the amygdala. *Behav. Neurosci.* 107:444–50.

Romanski LM, LeDoux JE. 1992. Equipotentiality of thalamo-amygdala and thalamo-cortico-amygdala projections as auditory conditioned stimulus pathways. *J. Neurosci.* 12:4501–9.

Romanski LM, LeDoux JE. 1993a. Information cascade from primary auditory cortex to the amygdala: corticocortical and corticoamygdaloid projections of temporal cortex in the rat. *Cerebr. Cortex* 3:515–32.

Romanski LM, LeDoux JE. 1993b. Organization of rodent auditory cortex: anterograde transport of PHA-L from MGv to temporal neocortex. *Cerebr. Cortex* 3:499–514.

Rosen JB, Hitchcock JM, Sananes CB, Miserendino MJD, Davis M. 1991. A direct projection from the central nucleus of the amygdala to the acoustic startle pathway: anterograde and retrograde tracing studies. *Behav. Neurosci.* 105:817–25.

Rudy JW. 1993. Contextual conditioning and auditory cue conditioning dissociate during development. *Behav. Neurosci.* 107:887–91.

Rudy JW, Sutherland RJ. 1992. Configural and elemental associations and the memory coherence problem. *J. Cogn. Neurosci.* 4(3):208–16.

Ryugo DK, Weinberger NM. 1978. Differential plasticity of morphologically distinct neuron populations in the medial geniculate body of the cat during classical conditioning. *Behav. Biol.* 22:275–301.

Sarter M, Markowitsch HJ. 1985. Involvement of the amygdala in learning and memory: a critical review, with emphasis on anatomical relations. *Behav. Neurosci.* 99:342–80.

Scherer KR. 1991. Criteria for emotion-antecedent appraisal: a review. In *Cognitive Perspectives on Motivation and Emotion,* ed. V Hamilton, GH Bower, NH Fridja, pp. 89–126. Dordrecht: Kluwer.

Selden NRW, Everitt BJ, Jarrard LE, Robbins TW. 1991. Complementary roles for the amygdala and hippocampus in aversive conditioning to explicit and contextual cues. *Neuroscience* 42(2):335–50.

Smith OA, Astley CA, Devito JL, Stein JM, Walsh RE. 1980. Functional analysis of hypothalamic control of the cardiovascular responses accompanying emotional behavior. *Fed. Proc.* 39(8):2487–94.

Squire LR. 1987. Memory: neural organization and behavior. In *Handbook of Physiology.* 1: *The Nervous System,* ed. F Plum, 5:295–371. Bethesda, MD: Am. Physiol. Soc.

Squire LR. 1992. Memory and the hippocampus: a synthesis from findings with rats, monkeys, and humans. *Psychol. Rev.* 99:195–231.

Staubli U. 1994. Parallel properties of LTP and memory. In *Brain and Memory: Modulation and Mediation of Neuroplasticity,* ed. JL McGaugh. New York: Oxford Univ. Press. In press.

Swanson LW. 1983. The hippocampus and the concept of the limbic system. In *Neurobiology of the Hippocampus,* ed. W Seifert, pp. 3–19. London: Academic.

Teich AH, McCabe PM, Gentile CC, Schneiderman LS, Winters RW, et al. 1989. Auditory cortex lesions prevent the extinction of Pavlovian differential heart rate conditioning to tonal stimuli in rabbits. *Brain Res.* 480:210–18.

Teyler TJ, DiScenna P. 1987. Long-term potentiation. *Annu. Rev. Neurosci.* 10:131–61.

Thompson RF, Berger TW, Madden J IV. 1983. Cellular processes of learning and memory in the mammalian CNS. *Annu. Rev. Neurosci.* 6:447–91.

Thorpe SJ, Rolls ET, Meddison S. 1983. The orbitofrontal cortex: neuronal activity in the behaving monkey. *Exp. Brain Res.* 49:93–115.

Tully T. 1991. Genetic dissection of learning and memory in *Drosophila melanogaster.* In *Neurobiology of Learning, Emotion and Affect,* ed. JI Madden, pp. 29–66. New York: Raven.

van de Kar LD, Piechowski RA, Rittenhouse PA, Gray TS. 1991. Amygdaloid lesions: differential effect on conditioned stress and immobilization-induced increases in corticosterone and renin secretion. *Neuroendocrinology* 54:89–95.

Watkins LR, Mayer DJ. 1982. Organization of endogenous opiate and nonopiate pain control systems. *Science* 216:1185–92.

Weinberger NM. 1993. Learning-induced changes of auditory receptive fields. *Curr. Opin. Neurobiol.* 3:570–77.

Weinberger NM, Diamond DM. 1987. Physiological plasticity in auditory cortex: rapid induction by learning. *Prog. Neurobiol.* 29:1–55.

Weisz DJ, Harden DG, Xiang Z. 1992. Effects of amygdala lesions on reflex facilitation and conditioned response acquisition during nictitating membrane response conditioning in rabbit. *Behav. Neurosci.* 106:262–73.

Wilson A, Kapp BS. 1994. The effect of lesions of the ventrolateral periequiductal gray on the Pavlovian conditioned heart response in the rabbit. *Behav. Neural Biol.* In press.

Zajonc R. 1980. Feeling and thinking: preferences need no inferences. *Am. Psychol.* 35:151–75.

Zajonc RB. 1984. On the primacy of affect. *Am. Psychol.* 39:117–23.

28 Fear and the Brain: Where Have We Been, and Where Are We Going?

Joseph E. LeDoux

Introduction

Twenty years ago, emotion was hardly talked about in neuroscience circles. Today, it is one of the hot topics in the field. The transformation has come because research on one emotion, "fear," has been enormously successful in mapping the pathways and even in explaining some of the cellular mechanisms involved.

The key to the fear pathways in the brain is a small region called the amygdala. Damage to this area greatly changes the way animals, including people, act in the face of danger. Monkeys, for example, lose their fear of snakes, and rats their fear of cats, as a result of amygdala damage. Damage to the amygdala prevents rats and people from learning about stimuli that warn of danger.

The amygdala has in fact become quite popular as a research topic. A quick scan through various journals in the field reveals more and more papers on the structure and function of the amygdala each year. It is perhaps a sign of the times that the amygdala and its contribution to emotional behavior have even penetrated deep into popular culture. My two sons were watching Batman on The Cartoon Network the other day when I fell victim to the "cocktail party phenomenon," where your attention is grabbed by something significant that you were not paying attention to. All of a sudden, I heard the words, "the amygdala," which was described as "an almond-shaped mass of nerves in the brain that controls feelings of rage." I turned to the screen. In the story, the amygdala of Aaron Helzinger had been removed in an attempt to calm him, but instead he was transformed into a creature of perennial rage called "Amygdala." Actually, I did not remember all these details, but a quick trip to the Worldwide Web led to a site that had all the facts, and even guided me to the issue of the printed version of Batman that the show was

based on. The search also revealed a site that promised to show you how to "click your amygdala" by exposing yourself to certain kinds of stimuli.

Given all this interest in the amygdala, it seems like a good time to take stock of where we are in this field. Below, I will review the basic facts, consider some controversies, and preview some new directions.

Fear, Anxiety, and Fear Conditioning

Fear is a normal reaction to threatening situations and is a common occurrence in daily life. When fear becomes greater than that warranted by the situation, or begins to occur in inappropriate situations, a fear or anxiety disorder exists (e.g., Marks 1987; Öhman, 1992). Excluding substance abuse problems, anxiety disorders account for about half of all the conditions that people see psychiatrists for each year (Manderscheid and Sonnenschein 1994). It seems likely that the fear system of the brain is involved in at least some anxiety disorders (LeDoux 1996; Öhman 1992), and it is thus important that we understand in as much detail as possible how the fear system works. This information may lead to a better understanding of how anxiety disorders arise and how they might be prevented or controlled. If studies of the fear system shed light only on fear and no other emotion, that alone would be an important achievement.

There are a number of experimental tools for studying fear and anxiety; however, one of the simplest and most straightforward is classical fear conditioning. In fear conditioning, a relatively neutral stimulus (the conditioned stimulus, CS) is paired with an aversive event. In a typical study, an innocuous tone is paired with a mild foot shock. After very few pairings (as few as one under certain conditions) long-lasting changes are established in the brain, such that the CS

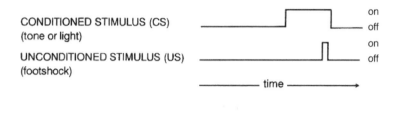

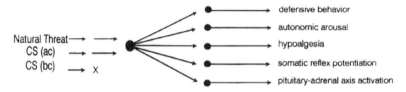

Figure 28.1
Fear conditioning involves the temporal pairing of an innocuous conditioned stimulus (CS), such as a light or tone, with a noxious unconditioned stimulus, typically a footshock (above). After conditioning (ac), but not before (bc), the CS enters fear networks and activates defense systems typically activated by a natural threat, such as a predator (below).

comes to elicit behavioral, autonomic, and endocrine responses that are characteristically expressed in the presence of danger (Figure 28.1). The responses tend to be hard-wired, species-typical expressions of fear, and are not learned or conditioned. Fear conditioning, in other words, does not involve response learning, but instead involves the coupling of new stimuli to preexisting responses. Fear conditioning occurs throughout the phyla, and within the vertebrates, it appears that very similar neural mechanisms are involved across species. Much of the relevant background information about fear conditioning is summarized in LeDoux (1996).

Fear conditioning may not tell us all we need to know about all aspects of fear, or all aspects of fear or anxiety disorders, but it is an excellent starting point. Furthermore, many of the other fear assessment procedures, such as the various forms of avoidance conditioning, crucially involve an initial phase of fear conditioning that

then provides motivational impetus for the later stages of instrumental avoidance learning (e.g., Mowrer 1939; Dollard and Miller 1950). Other fear assessment procedures do not require learning (e.g., the open field, the elevated maze, or light avoidance), but these are somewhat less amenable to a neural systems analysis than fear conditioning, due mainly to the fact that the fear-eliciting stimulus is often poorly defined in these procedures. Also, since many of the things that people fear are learned about through experience, an understanding of how fear learning occurs is an important part of an understanding of the fear system.

What Are the Brain Pathways Involved in Fear Conditioning?

Simply stated, the pathways underlying fear conditioning involve the transmission of CS information to the amygdala, and transmission from the amygdala to various conditioned response (CR) control networks in the brain stem. Several different CS modalities have been used (e.g., auditory, visual, olfactory), but I concentrate below on studies using the auditory modality, since the pathways to the amygdala are best understood for these (Figure 28.2).

An acoustic CS is transmitted through the auditory system to the level of the auditory thalamus, the medial geniculate body (MGB), and is then transmitted to two disparate targets. One is the amygdala and the other is the auditory cortex. Auditory cortical areas in turn project to the amygdala (Price et al. 1987; Amaral et al. 1992; LeDoux et al. 1990a, 1990b; Turner and Herkenham 1991; Romanski and LeDoux 1993a, 1993b; Mascagni et al. 1993). The auditory thalamus is believed to provide rapid but imprecise information, whereas the auditory cortex provides a somewhat delayed (relative to the thalamus) but more detailed representation to the amygdala (e.g., LeDoux 1986, 1996). Although damage to the auditory cortex before conditioning does not prevent conditioning to a single tone (e.g., Romanski and LeDoux 1992a, 1992b; Campeau and Davis 1995b), the auditory cortex appears to be required for some aspects of conditioned responding to more complex stimulus situations (e.g., Jarrell et al. 1987), though the exact conditions requiring the auditory cortex are poorly understood (see Armony et al. 1997).

Anatomical and physiological studies suggest that the lateral nucleus of the amygdala (LA) is a major site of termination of both thalamic and cortical auditory inputs (LeDoux et al. 1990a, 1991; Clugnet et al. 1990; Turner and Herkenham 1991; Bordi and LeDoux 1992; Romanski et al. 1993; Romanski and LeDoux 1993a; Mascagni et al. 1993; Amaral et al. 1992; Price et al. 1987). In fact, single cells in LA receive convergent inputs from the auditory thalamus and cortex (Li et al. 1996). The central nucleus (CE), on the other hand, appears to be the interface with motor systems involved in controlling conditioned responses (LeDoux 1992; Kapp et al.

1992; Davis 1994). Thus, whereas lesions of CE interfere with the expression of fear responses of all types, lesions of areas to which CE projects interfere with select responses. For example, lesions of the lateral hypothalamus interfere with sympathetic nervous system mediated responses (like changes in blood pressure), whereas lesions of the central gray interfere with behavioral conditioned responses (like freezing).

Information flows from LA to CE over well-defined intra-amygdala circuits (e.g., Price et al. 1987; Amaral et al. 1992; de Olmos et al. 1985; Pitkänen et al. 1997; Smith and Paré 1994). For example, inputs arriving in LA are distributed to the basal (B), accessory basal (AB), and CE nuclei, and to a lesser extent to several other areas (Pitkänen et al. 1995). The B and AB nuclei also project to CE (Savander et al. 1995, 1996a; Paré et al. 1995). Figure 28.2 illustrates some of the key pathways. Damage to LA and CE (but not other amygdala nuclei) disrupts fear conditioning to a tone CS (LeDoux et al. 1990b; Majidishad et al. 1996), suggesting that the direct projection from LA to CE is sufficient to mediate conditioning.

The identification of the amygdala as a key site of fear processing and fear learning has obvious implications for understanding anxiety disorders. It is conceivable that alterations in the way the amygdala processes information underlie at least some of these conditions. In addition, some cortical regions that project to the amygdala have been implicated in aspects of fear conditioning, and these findings also have implications for understanding anxiety disorders. Two of these areas include the hippocampus and its role in contexual conditioning and the medial prefrontal cortex and its role in extinction. When rats are conditioned to a tone paired with a shock, they also develop fear responses to the chamber in which the tone–shock pairings occur. The chamber cues are part of what is referred to as the conditioning context. Damage to the hippocampus interferes with conditioning to the chamber or contextual cues (Phillips and LeDoux

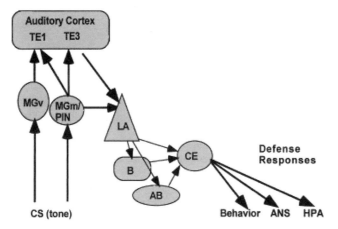

Figure 28.2
The basic neural pathways underlying fear conditioning involve transmission of sensory stimuli about a conditioned stimulus (CS) to the amygdala from the thalamus and cortex and the control of emotional responses by outputs of the amygdala. The illustration shows auditory signals from the thalamic nuclei (MGm/PIN) and auditory cortex (TE3) reaching the lateral nucleus of the amygdala (LA). LA then projects to the central nucleus (CE) directly and by way of intra-amygdala pathways involving the basal (B) and accessory basal (AB) nuclei. CE, in turn, controls the expression of defense responses, including behavioral, autonomic nervous system (ANS), and hormonal (HPA, hypothalamic-pituitary-adrenal axis) responses.

1992; Kim and Fanselow 1992; Selden et al. 1991; Blanchard et al. 1970). It is possible that the generalization of fear that occurs in some anxiety disorders is due to weakening of contextual constraints on fear. The fact that stress, a concomitant of anxiety disorders, impairs the anatomy, physiology, and behavioral functions of the hippocampus (Sapolsky 1996; McEwen and Sapolsky 1995) is consistent with this. Extinction refers to loss of the ability of the conditioned stimulus to elicit fear responses after repeated presentations in the absence of the shock. Damage to the medial prefrontal cortex results in a prolongation of extinction (Morgan et al. 1993; Morgan and LeDoux 1995). This is important, since it seems to produce something akin to clinical fears—that is, fears that, once established, are difficult to get rid of. Stress also affects functions of the prefrontal cortex (Diorio et al. 1993), suggesting that the alterations in this area may contribute to the irrational fears of patients with some anxiety disorders.

Some Controversies about the Circuitry

In spite of the general agreement about the neural circuitry of fear and fear learning (see LeDoux 1996; Davis 1994; Maren and Fanselow 1996; Kapp et al. 1992), several controversies have arisen. A brief discussion of these is in order.

Recent studies have questioned the importance of LA as the site of CS reception in the amygdala (Killcross et al. 1997); however, these studies employed a complex behavioral paradigm requiring hundreds of training trials, and the results are not directly relevant to our studies involving rapid acquisition over a few (1–5) trials. These issues are discussed in more detail in Nader and LeDoux (1997) and Killcross et al. (1997).

Another controversial point is the sufficiency of the thalamoamygdala pathway in mediating learning (see Campeau and Davis 1995b). Studies involving lesions made after training and before testing question whether the thalamic pathway alone can sustain conditioning; however, several lines of evidence support the importance of the thalamic pathway. First, unit recording studies show that physiological changes occur in LA prior to the auditory cortex both within and across trials (Quirk et al. 1995, 1997). Thus, plasticity clearly exists in the amygdala that cannot be explained by cortical transmission. Further, several functional imaging studies in humans have shown evidence for subcortical processing of masked visual emotional stimuli by the amygdala, including conditioned emotional stimuli (Whalen et al. 1998; Buchel et al. 1998).

A third controversy involves the question of whether the amygdala is a site of plasticity and storage or just a modulator of plasticity elsewhere. McGaugh and colleagues have argued that the amygdala just modulates plasticity in other areas (e.g., McGaugh et al. 1995). That the amygdala modulates storage in other brain systems seems clear from numerous studies (reviewed by McGaugh et al. 1995; Packard et al. 1995; Gold 1995); however, the stronger conclusion—that plasticity and storage do not occur in the amygdala during aversive learning—is more problematic. This conclusion is based, in part, on the finding that lesions of the amygdala made within a few days of conditioning interfere with the expression of inhibitory avoidance learning, but lesions made 10–14 days later do not (see McGaugh et al. 1995 for a discussion of this and other lines of evidence); however, inhibitory avoidance and fear conditioning differ procedurally and could also have different neural bases (see LeDoux 1996). Also, several studies (see above) have shown that plasticity occurs in the amygdala during fear conditioning (Quirk et al. 1995, 1997; Armony et al. 1998). An obvious question is whether the effects of amygdala lesions on fear conditioning are time-dependent.

It turns out that they are not (Maren 1998); however, this may not be very interesting. Given that conditioned fear responses require the amygdala for their expression (Davis 1994; LeDoux 1992; Kapp et al. 1992), it is not possible to distinguish effects of lesions on learning/memory processes as opposed to response expression (McGaugh et al. 1995). To resolve this issue we used reversible inactivation of the amygdala during acquisition (Muller et al. 1997). Infusion of the gamma-aminobutyric acid agonist muscimol into the lateral/basal amygdala during learning prevented learning from taking place. This was true for both the tone CS and for contextual stimuli. Further, the same animals, when retrained after the first test, learned just fine, showing the reversibility of the effects. For other studies related to this point, see Helmstetter (1992), Helmstetter and Bellgowan (1994). Why then might inhibitory avoidance and fear conditioning differ with respect to the role of the amygdala? There is an old literature suggesting that once avoidance is learned, the situation loses its emotional impact and the amygdala, although needed for initial learning, is not required to maintain avoidance performance (see LeDoux 1996). This sounds very similar to what goes on in inhibitory avoidance (amygdala is needed initially but not later). Conclusions based on inhibitory avoidance should not be freely generalized to fear conditioning.

Fourth, the role of the hippocampus in contextual conditioning has been questioned on two grounds. Hippocampal damage does not always impair context conditioning (Gisquet-Verrier and Doyere 1997; Phillips and LeDoux 1995; Maren et al. 1997); however, this most likely is due to the use of conditions that bias the animal toward being conditioned to specific cues in the environment rather than to the context per se, thus allowing conditioning to proceed in ways that are independent of the hippocampus (see Phillips and LeDoux 1995). If lesions are made before training, animals are more likely to become conditioned to elemental cues, since they are unable to become conditioned to the context it-self (Frankland et al. in press). The inconsistency resulting from pretraining lesions may be due to inconsistency in the degree to which individual animals become conditioned to elemental cues in the context or background when the hippocampus is damaged before learning. The second point of contention comes from studies suggesting that hippocampal effects on context conditioning, as measured by freezing behavior, are secondary to changes in activity levels produced by the lesions—more activity competes with freezing and drives down the scores, leading to a false result with respect to context (Good and Honey 1997; McNish et al. 1997); however, there are a number of problems with this interpretation (for a discussion, see Maren et al. 1998; McNish et al. 1998). One problem is that hippocampal lesions have no effect on freezing to a tone CS measured by freezing. McNish et al. argued that tone conditioning is stronger, and therefore resistant to competition by activity; however, during the early phase of training, when tone conditioning is weak, hippocampal lesions are still ineffective. Another problem is that for individual animals, the amount of general activity in a novel environment does not correlate inversely with the amount of freezing. In other words, although hippocampal lesions can lead to an increase in activity, the degree of increased activity does not predict the amount of freezing and cannot be the explanation for the freezing deficit.

Fifth, the effects of medial prefrontal cortex lesions on extinction, though replicated several times in our lab (Morgan et al. 1993; Morgan and LeDoux 1995), have not been found in another study (Gerwitz et al. 1997). Although the procedures used differed in the studies from the two labs, one would hope that the findings are sufficiently general to extend beyond a limited paradigm. That the findings may be more general is suggested by unit recordings in primates, which have indicated that the medial prefrontal cortex is crucially involved in breaking associa-

tions during reversal learning, which is similar to the process involved in extinction (Thorpe et al. 1983). More work is needed to fully understand the contribution of the prefrontal cortex to extinction, which is important given the implications of such studies for elucidating the nature of clinically debilitating fears that resist extinction.

Where Is Research on Fear and the Amygdala Going?

Best Level of Analysis of the Amygdala

Our recent studies of the connections of the amygdala suggest that the organization of this brain region is determined not at the level of nuclei but at the level of subnuclei. For example, anatomical and physiological studies suggest that auditory information is received mainly by the dorsal subnucleus of the lateral nucleus (LeDoux et al. 1990a; Bordi and LeDoux 1992), and that the medial subnucleus, which receives information from the dorsal subnucleus, gives rise to most of the intra-amygdala connections of the lateral nucleus (Pitkänen et al. 1997). A similar condition holds for the other nuclei as well. Thus if we want to understand how the amygdala processes information, we will need to work at the level of the subnuclei rather than nuclei. This means that the traditional methods of placing lesions or injections of drugs that influence one nucleus at best, but typically several nuclei, are going to be of limited value. Other techniques, though, such as unit recordings, have sufficient resolving power to be useful at this level of analysis.

Contribution of Unit Recordings

The validity of the subnuclear organization of the amygdala, revealed by anatomical tracing studies, is verified by unit recordings. Short-latency auditory responses are only found in the dorsal subregion of the lateral nucleus, and

many of these cells are responsive to both auditory (CS-like) and somatosensory (unconditioned
stimulus-like) stimuli (Bordi and LeDoux 1992;
Romanski et al. 1993). Further, during conditioning, the shortest latency conditioned unit
responses occur in the dorsal subnucleus, and
somewhat longer latency conditioned responses
in the more ventral areas, including the medial
subnucleus (Quirk et al. 1995). Response latencies are longer in the central nucleus than in both
of these areas (Pascoe and Kapp 1985). Detailed
information about how the amygdala learns and
stores information will require that the subnuclear organization be attended to.

But physiological recording studies are important for reasons other than their ability to pinpoint small areas of the amygdala. They are also
crucial for understanding how the amygdala encodes experiences. Although the focus to date
has been at the level of single units, it is clear
that, as in other brain regions, information about
how populations or ensembles encode information is going to be important. This level of analysis works in two ways. On the one hand, we
need to understand how specific regions (like the
dorsal subnucleus of the lateral nucleus) encode
stimuli. On the other, we need to understand how
pools of neurons in different regions interact
during information processing (such as between
areas of the auditory thalamus and subregions of
the lateral nucleus, between subareas of the lateral nucleus, or between subareas of the lateral
nucleus and subareas of other amygdala nuclei).
The computing power for such analyses is now
readily available and affordable. Analytic tools,
though, need to be developed further to make the
most use of the information that will be available
with these techniques.

Mechanisms of Plasticity

Long-term potentiation (LTP) of synaptic transmission is high on many people's list as an
explanation of how the brain learns and stores
information (e.g., Bliss and Collingridge 1993;

Nicoll and Malenka 1995). LTP has been studied
most extensively in the hippocampus, but it
has been very difficult to show that hippocampal
LTP has anything to do with learning (Barnes
1995; Eichenbaum 1995). Over the past several
years, we have taken a different approach. We
started with the fact that thalamoamygdala pathways are involved in fear learning, and have
asked whether LTP occurs in these pathways.
After finding evidence for LTP there (Clugnet
and LeDoux 1990), we asked whether induction
of LTP would affect the processing of a CS-like
sound stimulus in this conditioning pathway
(Rogan and LeDoux 1995). After finding that
the processing of a sound by the amygdala was
amplified by induction of LTP, we showed that
fear conditioning did the same thing to the sound
as LTP induction (Rogan et al. 1997). This latter
study and another one published at the same
time (McKernan and Shinnick-Gallagher 1997)
constitute the best evidence to date that LTP
has anything to do with learning (Malenka and
Nicoll 1997; Stevens 1998).

Because LTP is understood in such detail in
the hippocampus, all the way to the level of molecules, it may be possible to apply some of this
knowledge in the effort to understand the mechanisms of fear learning. In the best studied form
of hippocampal LTP, the induction of plasticity
involves the entry of calcium into the postsynaptic cell and activation of the N-methyl-D-
aspartate (NMDA) class of glutamate receptors
(see Bliss and Collingridge 1993; Nicoll and Malenka 1995). The maintenance of the plasticity
then requires a cascade of intracellular events
that include the cyclic adenosine monophosphate
signaling system, protein and RNA synthesis, and
gene action (see Huang et al. 1996). The specific
genes involved, though, are not known. That
some of these mechanisms may apply to fear
conditioning is suggested by studies that have
manipulated NMDA receptors in the amygdala
during learning (see Miserendino et al. 1990;
Maren and Fanselow 1996; Rogan and LeDoux
1996; Rogan et al. 1997), and that have examined

genetically altered mice that lack various components of intracellular cascades (Bourtchuladze et al. 1994; Mayford et al. 1996). Relatively little is known at this point about the molecular machinery of fear learning, and this is likely to be an important area for future research, especially given that it may open up new opportunities for drug therapy for fear and anxiety.

Role of the Human Amygdala

It has been known for some time that the primate temporal lobe (Kluver and Bucy 1937) and especially the amgydala (Weiskrantz 1956) is involved in fear and perhaps other emotional processes (Mishkin and Aggleton 1981; Aggleton 1992; Ono and Nishijo 1992; Rolls 1992); however, recent studies of humans with temporal lobe lesions that include (LaBar et al. 1995) or are restricted mainly to the amygdala (Bechara 1995) have shown deficits in fear conditioning. The perception of fear in facial expressions (Young et al. 1995; Adolphs et al. 1994; but see Hamann et al. 1996) and voices (Scott et al. 1997) is also impaired. In addition, functional imaging studies have now shown activation of the amygdala during fear conditioning (LaBar et al. 1998; Buchel et al. 1998) and while processing faces and other emotional stimuli (Breiter et al. 1996; Morris et al. 1996). It thus seems clear that the animal data apply to the human brain. Future studies of the human amygdala will be required to determine how, if at all, the amygdala contributes to the subjective experience of emotions such as fear. Speculations on this topic can be found in LeDoux (1996) and Damasio (1994).

From Reaction to Action and Feeling

Essentially all of the recent work on the amygdala and fear has concentrated on the reactions that are automatically elicited in threatening situations. But clearly there is more to understand. Automatic, evolutionarily programmed responses to danger are typically followed by willful actions. We startle and freeze, and then decide to run away or stay put. Little is known about the manner in which the transition from emotional reaction to emotional action occurs, but some evidence suggests that interactions between the amygdala and corticostriatal motor systems are important (Everitt and Robbins 1992; LeDoux 1996). As little as we know about voluntary emotional actions, we know even less about conscious emotional feelings. It seems to me, though, that to the extent that working memory is a staging area for consciousness (Baars 1988; Kosslyn and Koenig 1992; Kihlstrom 1987), then feelings may result from the representation in working memory that an emotion system, like the fear system, is active. At a minimum, this suggestion provides a research strategy for studying feelings.

What about Other Emotions?

The neural basis of emotions other than fear is not clearly understood. Part of the difficulty is that there are not, at this point, good tasks for studying other emotions. Evidence that amygdala damage produces some deficit on some task that has some emotional relevance needs to be cautiously interpreted. The reason we can say so much about fear and fear disorders from studies of the neural basis of fear is because we have a great deal of information about how fear is organized in the brain. Until that level of information is available about other emotions, it will not be easy to extrapolate from isolated findings about the effects of lesions to an understanding of how this or that emotion is mediated by the brain.

Conclusions

We have come a long way in our understanding of the amygdala and its contribution to fear and fear learning. As a result, fear is the emotion that is best understood in terms of brain mechanisms.

Although some controversies have arisen, these reflect the normal checks and balances of the scientific enterprise, and in no way detract from the fundamental fact that the amygdala is the heart and soul of the fear system. New findings, pouring in all the time, are adding to this powerful database and will hopefully set the stage for a neurobiological understanding not only of the way the fear system normally works, but also of how it breaks down in anxiety disorders.

References

Adolphs R, Tranel D, Damasio H, Damasio AR (1994): Impaired recognition of emotion in facial expressions following bilateral damage to the human amygdala. *Nature* 372:669–672.

Aggleton JP (1992): *The Amygdala: Neurobiological Aspects of Emotion, Memory, and Mental Dysfunction.* New York: Wiley-Liss.

Amaral DG, Price JL, Pitkänen A, Carmichael ST (1992): Anatomical organization of the primate amygdaloid complex. In: Aggleton JP, editor. *The Amygdala: Neurobiological Aspects of Emotion, Memory, and Mental Dysfunction.* New York: Wiley-Liss, pp 1–66.

Armony JL, Servan-Schreiber D, Cohen JD, LeDoux JE (1997): Computational modeling of emotion: Explorations through the anatomy and physiology of fear conditioning. *Trends Cogn Sci* 1:28–34.

Armony JL, Quirk GJ, LeDoux JE (1998): Differential effects of amygdala lesions on early and late plastic components of auditory cortex spike trains during fear conditioning. *J Neurosci* 18:2592–2601.

Baars BJ (1988): *A Cognitive Theory of Consciousness.* New York: Cambridge University Press.

Barnes CA (1995): Involvement of LTP in memory: Are we "searching under the streetlight"? *Neuron* 15:751–754.

Bechara A, Tranel D, Damasio H, Adolphs R, Rockland C, Damasio AR (1995): Double dissociation of conditioning and declarative knowledge relative to the amygdala and hippocampus in humans. *Science* 269:1115–1118.

Blanchard RJ, Blanchard DC, Fial RA (1970): Hippocampal lesions in rats and their effect on activity, avoidance, and aggression. *J Comp Physiol Psychol* 71:92–102.

Bliss TVP, Collingridge GL (1993): A synaptic model of memory: Long-term potentiation in the hippocampus. *Nature* 361:31–39.

Bordi F, LeDoux J (1992): Sensory tuning beyond the sensory system: An initial analysis of auditory properties of neurons in the lateral amygdaloid nucleus and overlying areas of the striatum. *J Neurosci* 12: 2493–2503.

Bourtchuladze R, Frenguelli B, Blendy J, Cioffi D, Shutz G, Silva AJ (1994): Deficient long-term memory in mice with a targeted mutation of the cAMP-responsive element binding protein. *Cell* 79:59–68.

Breiter HC, Etcoff NL, Whalen PJ, Kennedy WA, Rauch SL, Buchner RL, et al. (1996): Response and habituation of the human amygdala during visual processing of facial expression. *Neuron* 17:875–887.

Campeau S, Davis M (1995a): Involvement of the central nucleus and basolateral complex of the amygdala in fear conditioning measured with fear-potentiated startle in rats trained concurrently with auditory and visual conditioned stimuli. *J Neurosci* 15:2301–2311.

Campeau S, Davis M (1995b): Involvement of subcortical and cortical afferents to the lateral nucleus of the amygdala in fear conditioning measured with fear-potentiated startle in rats trained concurrently with auditory and visual conditioned stimuli. *J Neurosci* 15:2312–2327.

Clugnet MC, LeDoux JE (1990): Synaptic plasticity in fear conditioning circuits: Induction of LTP in the lateral nucleus of the amygdala by stimulation of the medial geniculate body. *J Neurosci* 10:2818–2824.

Clugnet MC, LeDoux JE, Morrison SF (1990): Unit responses evoked in the amygdala and striatum by electrical stimulation of the medial geniculate body. *J Neurosci* 10:1055–1061.

Damasio A (1994): *Descarte's Error: Emotion, Reason, and the Human Brain.* New York: Gosset/Putnam.

Davis M (1994): The role of the amygdala in emotional learning. *Int Rev Neurobiol* 36:225–266.

de Olmos J, Alheid G, Beltramino C (1985): Amygdala. In: Paxinos G, editor. *The Rat Nervous System.* Orlando, FL: Academic Press, pp 223–334.

Diorio D, Viau V, Meaney MJ (1993): The role of the medial prefrontal cortex (cingulate gyrus) in the regulation of hypothalamic-pituitary-adrenal responses to stress. *J Neurosci* 13:3839–3847.

Dollard JC, Miller NE (1950): *Personality and Psychotherapy.* New York: McGraw-Hill.

Eichenbaum H (1995): The LTP-memory connection. *Nature* 378:131–132.

Everitt BJ, Robbins TW (1992): Amygdala-ventral striatal interactions and reward-related processes. In: Aggleton JP, editor. *The Amygdala: Neurobiological Aspects of Emotion, Memory, and Mental Dysfunction.* New York: Wiley-Liss, pp 401–429.

Frankland PW, Cestari V, Filipkowski RK, McDonald RJ, Silva A (1998): The dorsal hippocampus is essential for context discrimination, but not for contextual conditioning. *Behav Neurosci* 112:863–874.

Gerwitz JC, Falls WA, Davis M (1997): Normal conditioned inhibition and extinction of freezing and fear potentiated startle following electrolytic lesions of medial prefrontal cortex in rats. *Behav Neurosci* 111:1–15.

Gisquet-Verrier P, Doyere V (1997): Lesions of the hippocampus in rats do not affect conditioning to context cues in classical fear conditioning. *Soc Neurosci Abstr* 23:1609.

Gold PE (1995): Modulation of emotional and non-emotional memories: Same pharmacological systems, different neuroanatomical systems. In: McGaugh JL, Weinberger NM, Lynch G, editors. *Brain and Memory.* New York: Oxford University Press, pp 41–74.

Good M, Honey RC (1997): Dissociable effects of selective lesions to hippocampal subsystems on exploratory behavior, contextual learning, and spatial learning. *Behav Neurosci* 111:487–493.

Hamann SB, Stefanacci L, Squire L, Adolphs R, Tranel D, Damasio H, et al. (1996): Recognizing facial emotion. *Nature* 379:497.

Helmstetter FJ (1992): Contribution of the amygdala to learning and performance of conditional fear. *Physiol Behav* 51:1271–1276.

Helmstetter FJ, Bellgowan PS (1994): Effects of muscimol applied to the basolateral amygdala on acquisition and expression of contextual fear conditioning in rats. *Behavior Neurosci* 108:1005–1009.

Huang YY, Nguyen PV, Abel T, Kandel ER (1996): Long-lasting forms of synaptic potentiation in the mammalian hippocampus. *Learning Memory* 3:74–85.

Jarrell TW, Gentile CG, Romanski LM, McCabe PM, Schneiderman N (1987): Involvement of cortical and thalamic auditory regions in retention of differential bradycardia conditioning to acoustic conditioned stimuli in rabbits. *Brain Res* 412:285–294.

Kapp BS, Whalen PJ, Supple WF, Pascoe JP (1992): Amygdaloid contributions to conditioned arousal and sensory information processing. In: Aggleton, editor. *The Amygdala: Neurobiological Aspects of Emotion, Memory, and Mental Dysfunction.* New York: Wiley-Liss, pp 229–254.

Kihlstrom JF (1987): The cognitive unconscious. *Science* 237:1445–1452.

Killcross S, Robbins TW, Everitt BJ (1997): Different types of fear-conditioned behavior mediated by separate nuclei within amygdala. *Nature* 388:377–380.

Kim JJ, Fanselow MS (1992): Modality-specific retrograde amnesia of fear. *Science* 256:675–677.

Kluver H, Bucy PC (1937): "Psychic blindness" and other symptoms following bilateral temporal lobectomy in rhesus monkeys. *Am J Physiol* 119:352–353.

Kosslyn SM, Koenig O (1992): *Wet Mind: The New Cognitive Neuroscience.* New York: Macmillan.

LaBar KS, LeDoux JE, Spencer DD, Phelps EA (1995): Impaired fear conditioning following unilateral temporal lobectomy in humans. *J Neurosci* 15:6846–6855.

LeDoux JE (1986): Sensory systems and emotion. *Integr Psychiatry* 4:237–248.

LeDoux JE (1992): Emotion and the amygdala. In: Aggleton JP, editor. *The Amygdala: Neurobiological Aspects of Emotion, Memory, and Mental Dysfunction.* New York: Wiley-Liss, pp 339–351.

LeDoux JE (1996): *The Emotional Brain.* New York: Simon and Schuster.

LeDoux JE, Farb CF, Ruggiero DA (1990a): Topographic organization of neurons in the acoustic thalamus that project to the amygdala. *J Neurosci* 10:1043–1054.

LeDoux JE, Cicchetti P, Xagoraris A, Romanski LM (1990b): The lateral amygdaloid nucleus: Sensory interface of the amygdala in fear conditioning. *J Neurosci* 10:1062–1069.

LeDoux JE, Farb CR, Milner TA (1991): Ultrastructure and synaptic associations of auditory thalamo-amygdala projections in the rat. *Exp Brain Res* 85:577–586.

Li XF, Stutzmann GE, LeDoux JE (1996): Convergent but temporally separated inputs to lateral amygdala neurons from the auditory thalamus and auditory cortex use different postsynaptic receptors: *In vivo* intracellular and extracellular recordings in fear conditioning pathways. *Learning Memory* 3:229–242.

Majidishad P, Pelli DG, LeDoux JE (1996): Disruption of fear conditioning to contextual stimuli but not to a tone by lesions of the accessory basal nucleus of the amygdala. *Soc Neurosci Abstr* 22:1116.

Malenka RC, Nicoll RA (1997): Learning and memory: Never fear, LTP is here. *Nature* 390:552.

Manderscheid RW, Sonnenschein MA (1994): *Mental Health, United States* 1994. Rockville, MD: U.S. Department of Public Health and Human Services.

Maren S, Fanselow MS (1996): The amygdala and fear conditioning: Has the nut been cracked? *Neuron* 16:237–240.

Maren S, Aharonov G, Fanselow MS (1997): Neurotoxic lesions of the dorsal hippocampus and Pavlovian fear conditioning in rats. *Behav Brain Res* 88:261–274.

Maren S, Anagnostaras SG, Fanselow MS (1998): The startled seahorse: Is the hippocampus necessary for contextual fear conditioning? *Trends Cogn Sci* 2:39–41.

Marks I (1987): *Fears, Phobias, and Rituals: Panic, Anxiety and Their Disorders.* New York: Oxford University Press.

Mascagni F, McDonald AJ, Coleman JR (1993): Corticoamygdaloid and corticocortical projections of the rat temporal cortex: A phaseolus vulgaris leucoagglutinin study. *Neuroscience* 57:697–715.

Mayford M, Bach ME, Huang Y-Y, Wang L, Hawkins RD (1996): Control of memory formation through regulated expression of a CaMKII transgene. *Science* 274:1678–1683.

McEwen B, Sapolsky R (1995): Stress and cognitive functioning. *Curr Opin Neurobiol* 5:205–216.

McGaugh JL, Mesches MH, Cahill L, Parent MB, Coleman-Mesches K, Salinas JA (1995): Involvement of the amygdala in the regulation of memory storage. In: McGaugh JL, Bermudez-Rattoni F, Prado-Alcala RA, editors. *Plasticity in the Central Nervous System.* Hillsdale, NJ: Lawrence Erlbaum Associates, pp 18–39.

McKernan MG, Shinnick-Gallagher P (1997): Fear conditioning induces a lasting potentiation of synaptic currents in vitro. *Nature* 390:607–611.

McNish KA, Gewirtz JC, Davis M (1997): Evidence of contextual fear after lesions of the hippocampus: A disruption of freezing but not fear-potentiated startle. *J Neurosci* 17:9353–9360.

McNish KA, Gewirtz JC, Davis M (1998): Response from McNish, Gewirtz and Davis. *Trends Cogn Sci* 2:42–43.

Miserendino MJD, Sananes CB, Melia KR, Davis M (1990): Blocking of acquisition but not expression of conditioned fear-potentiated startle by NMDA antagonists in the amygdala. *Nature* 345:716–718.

Mishkin M, Aggleton J (1981): Multiple functional contributions of the amygdala in the monkey. In: Ben-Ari Y, editor. *The Amygdaloid Complex.* Amsterdam: Elsevier/North-Holland Biomedical Press, pp 409–420.

Morgan M, LeDoux JE (1995): Differential contribution of dorsal and ventral medial prefrontal cortex to the acquisition and extinction of conditioned fear. *Behav Neurosci* 109:681–688.

Morgan MA, Romanski LM, LeDoux JE (1993): Extinction of emotional learning: Contribution of medial prefrontal cortex. *Neurosci Lett* 163:109–113.

Morris JS, Frith CD, Perret DI, Rowland D, Young AW, Calder AJ, et al. (1996): A differential neural response in the human amygdala to fearful and happy facial expressions. *Nature* 383:812–815.

Mowrer OH (1939): A stimulus-response analysis of anxiety and its role as a reinforcing agent. *Psychol Rev* 46:553–565.

Nader K, LeDoux JE (1997): Is it time to invoke multiple fear learning systems? *Trends Cogn Sci* 1:241–244.

Nicoll RA, Malenka RC (1995): Contrasting properties of two forms of long-term potentiation in the hippocampus. *Nature* 377:115–118.

Öhman A (1992): Fear and anxiety as emotional phenomena: Clinical, phenomenological, evolutionary perspectives, and information-processing mechanisms. In: Lewis M, Haviland JM, editors. *Handbook of the Emotions.* New York: Guilford, pp 511–536.

Ono T, Nishijo H (1992): Neurophysiological basis of the Kluver-Bucy syndrome: Responses of monkey amygdaloid neurons to biologically significant objects. In: Aggleton JP, editor. *The Amygdala: Neurobiological Aspects of Emotion, Memory, and Mental Dysfunction.* New York: Wiley-Liss, pp 167–190.

Packard MG, Williams CL, Cahill L, McGaugh JL (1995): The anatomy of a memory modulatory system:

From periphery to brain. In: Spear NE, Spear LP, Woodruff ML, editors. *Neurobehavioral Plasticity: Learning, Development, and Reponse to Brain Insults.* Hillsdale, NJ: Lawrence Erlbaum Associates, pp 149–150.

Paré D, Smith Y, Paré JF (1995): Intra-amygdaloid projections of the basolateral and basomedial nuclei in the cat: Phaseolus vulgaris-leucoagglutinin anterograde tracing at the light and electron microscopic level. *Neuroscience* 69:567–583.

Pascoe JP, Kapp BS (1985): Electrophysiological characteristics of amygdaloid central nucleus neurons during Pavlovian fear conditioning in the rabbit. *Behav Brain Res* 16:117–133.

Phillips RG, LeDoux JE (1992): Differential contribution of amygdala and hippocampus to cued and contextual fear conditioning. *Behav Neurosci* 106:274–285.

Phillips RG, LeDoux JE (1995): Lesions of the fornix but not the entorhinal or perirhinal cortex interfere with contextual fear conditioning. *J Neurosci* 15:5308–5315.

Pitkänen A, Stefanacci L, Farb CR, Go C-G, LeDoux JE, Amaral DG (1995): Intrinsic connections of the rat amygdaloid complex: Projections originating in the lateral nucleus. *J Comp Neurol* 356:288–310.

Pitkänen A, Savander V, LeDoux JE (1997): Organization of intra-amygdaloid circuitries: An emerging framework for understanding functions of the amygdala. *Trends Neurosci* 20:517–523.

Price JL, Russchen FT, Amaral DG (1987): The limbic region. II: The amygdaloid complex. In: Bjorklund A, Hokfelt T, Swanson LW, editors. *Handbook of Chemical Neuroanatomy. Vol. 5: Integrated Systems of the CNS, pt. 1.* Amsterdam: Elsevier, pp 279–388.

Quirk GJ, Repa JC, LeDoux JE (1995): Fear conditioning enhances short-latency auditory responses of lateral amygdala neurons: Parallel recordings in the freely behaving rat. *Neuron* 15:1029–1039.

Quirk GJ, Armony JL, LeDoux JE (1997): Fear conditioning enhances different temporal components of toned-evoked spike trains in auditory cortex and lateral amygdala. *Neuron* 19:613–624.

Rogan MT, LeDoux JE (1995): LTP is accompanied by commensurate enhancement of auditory-evoked responses in a fear conditioning circuit. *Neuron* 15:127–136.

Rogan MT, LeDoux JE (1996): Emotion: Systems, cells, synaptic plasticity. *Cell* 85:469–475.

Rogan M, Staubli U, LeDoux J (1997): Fear conditioning induces associative long-term potentiation in the amygdala. *Nature* 390:604–607.

Rogan M, Staubli U, LeDoux JE (1997): AMPA-receptor facilitation accelerates fear learning without altering the level of conditioned fear aquired. *J Neurosci* 17:5928–5935.

Rolls ET (1992): Neurophysiology and functions of the primate amygdala. In: Aggleton JP, editor. *The Amygdala: Neurobiological Aspects of Emotion, Memory, and Mental Dysfunction.* New York: Wiley-Liss, pp 143–165.

Romanski LM, LeDoux JE (1992a): Equipotentiality of thalamo-amygdala and thalamo-cortico-amygdala projections as auditory conditioned stimulus pathways. *J Neurosci* 12:4501–4509.

Romanski LM, LeDoux JE (1992b): Bilateral destruction of neocortical and perirhinal projection targets of the acoustic thalamus does not disrupt auditory fear conditioning. *Neurosci Lett* 142:228–232.

Romanski LM, LeDoux JE (1993a): Organization of rodent auditory cortex: Anterograde transport of PHA-L from MGv to temporal neocortex. *Cereb Cortex* 3:499–514.

Romanski LM, LeDoux JE (1993b): Information cascade from primary auditory cortex to the amygdala: Corticocortical and corticoamygdaloid projections of temporal cortex in the rat. *Cereb Cortex* 3:515–532.

Romanski LM, LeDoux JE, Clugnet MC, Bordi F (1993): Somatosensory and auditory convergence in the lateral nucleus of the amygdala. *Behav Neurosci* 107:444–450.

Sapolsky RM (1996): Why stress is bad for your brain. *Science* 273:749–750.

Savander V, Go CG, LeDoux JE, Pitkänen A (1995): Intrinsic connections of the rat amygdaloid complex: Projections originating in the basal nucleus. *J Comp Neurol* 361:345–368.

Savander V, Go C-G, LeDoux JE, Pitkänen A (1996a): Intrinsic connections of the rat amygdaloid complex: Projections originating in the accessory basal nucleus. *J Comp Neurol* 374:291–313.

Scott SK, Young AW, Calder AJ, Hellawell DJ, Aggleton JP, Johnson M (1997): Impaired auditory recognition of fear and anger following bilateral amygdala lesions. *Nature* 385:254–257.

Selden NRW, Everitt BJ, Jarrard LE, Robbins TW (1991): Complementary roles for the amygdala and hippocampus in aversive conditioning to explicit and contextual cues. *Neuroscience* 42:335–350.

Smith Y, Paré D (1994): Intra-amygdaloid projections of the lateral nucleus in the cat: PHA-L anterograde labeling combined with postembedding GABA and glutamate immunocytochemistry. *J Comp Neurol* 342:232–248.

Stevens CF (1998): A million dollar question: Does LTP = memory? *Neuron* 20:1–2.

Thorpe SJ, Rolls ET, Maddison S (1983): The orbitofrontal cortex: Neuronal activity in the behaving monkey. *Exp Brain Res* 49:93–115.

Turner B, Herkenham M (1991): Thalamoamygdaloid projections in the rat: A test of the amygdala's role in sensory processing. *J Comp Neurol* 313:295–325.

Weiskrantz L (1956): Behavioral changes associated with ablation of the amygdaloid complex in monkeys. *J Comp Physiol Psychol* 49:381–391.

Whalen PJ, Rauch SL, Etcoff NL, McInerney SC, Lee MB, Jenike MA (1998): Masked presentations of emotional facial expressions modulate amygdala activity without explicit knowledge. *J Neurosci* 18:411–418.

Young AW, Aggleton JP, Hellawell DJ, Johnson M, Broks P, Hanley JR (1995): Face processing impairments after amygdalotomy. *Brain* 118:15–24.

29

Anxiety and Cardiovascular Reactivity: The Basal Forebrain Cholinergic Link

Gary G. Berntson, Martin Sarter, and John T. Cacioppo

1 Introduction

Anxiogenic or fear-eliciting contexts are associated with robust autonomic responses in both humans and animals, and the DSM-IV recognizes exaggerated visceral reactivity as a common feature of anxiety disorders [3].[1] The empirical research on the autonomic features and correlates of anxiety and anxiety disorders has yielded mixed results, however, and the behavioral significance of autonomic accompaniments of fear and anxiety remain uncertain. These are important issues, not only because anxiety disorders represent a clear risk factor for cardiovascular disease and sudden cardiac death [96, 126], but because they bear on the fundamental nature of anxiety and the underlying neural mechanisms that link behavioral processes and autonomic functions. Some insight into the behavioral features and neural mechanisms of anxiety may be offered by the prototypic anxiolytic actions of the benzodiazepine receptor (BZR) agonists, and the putative anxiogenic effects of BZR inverse agonists. In the present chapter, the literature on autonomic functions in anxiety disorders is briefly reviewed, along with the relevance of these findings for neurobehavioral models of anxiety states. From this starting point, this chapter considers the research on BZR agonists and inverse agonists, and the implications of these studies for the cognitive and neural bases of anxiety. It is proposed that the basal forebrain cholinergic system may constitute an important component of the central mechanisms underlying both the cognitive and autonomic features of anxiety states. Specifically, it is suggested that this cholinergic system serves as a crucial link between cortical processing substrates, likely involved in the cognitive aspects of anxiety, and subcortical systems involved in anxiety and autonomic regulation. Finally, the relationships of this basal forebrain cholinergic mechanism to neural systems that have previously been implicated in anxiety are discussed, and a more comprehensive neurobiological model that may serve as a conceptual framework for future studies is proposed.

2 Autonomic Regulation and Its Relation to Neurobehavioral Processes

The autonomic nervous system is often considered to be a homeostatic regulatory system, serving to maintain visceral function within adaptive limits. This view had its historical origins in the early focus on peripheral anatomy, and in conceptions of the autonomic nervous system as an "involuntary" or "vegetative" system. The early works of Langley and Cannon recognized the importance of the central components of the autonomic nervous system, but this control for the most part was considered to comprise a set of interoceptive reflexes [36, 37, 140]. Cannon [37] viewed the autonomic system, including its central components, as a homeostatic system that responded to perturbations in the fluid matrix.

There is ample basis for such a view. Baroreceptor reflexes are prototypic homeostatic processes that exert powerful regulatory control over the cardiovascular system. With an increase in blood pressure, for example, enhanced activity of baroreceptor afferents to the nucleus tractus solitarius (NTS) leads to reflexive changes in autonomic outflows that oppose the perturbation [66, 243]. Baroreceptor reflexes potently inhibit sympathetic outflow, and exert an excitatory drive on vagal motor neurons. In response to the pressor disturbance, the reflexive decrease in sympathetic outflow yields vasodilation, a slowing of the heart, and a decrease in myocardial contractility. The parallel increase in vagal traffic further decreases heart rate and cardiac output. Collectively, these responses oppose the blood pressure disturbance and promote the restoration of basal levels. In direct opposition to the baroreflex, however, psychological stressors can yield both an increase in blood pressure and heart rate. It is now clear that stressors, even as mild as mental arithmetic, can lead to a reduction in the sensitivity and/or a shift in set point of the baroreceptor–heart rate reflex [56, 141, 245, 246].[2] Consistent with these perspectives, manipulations of limbic and forebrain areas implicated in behavioral processes have been shown to be capable of facilitating or inhibiting basic brainstem autonomic reflexes, and potently modulating autonomic outflow [113, 114, 133, 146, 179, 182, 187, 192]. The specific descending projections and neurochemical mechanisms that underlie the links between rostral systems and brainstem mechanisms for cardiovascular control are beginning to be clarified [25, 26, 39, 48, 109, 179, 196, 231, 237, 265].

Of additional relevance for emerging neurobehavioral models of stress and anxiety is the fact that rostral-caudal interactions are bidirectional. Ascending projections from brainstem autonomic substrates project directly to the amygdala and other forebrain and diencephalic areas that have been implicated in neurobehavioral regulation, and have been shown to potently modulate the activity of these rostral brain systems [5, 178, 237, 279]. This chapter will further consider the interactions between rostral and caudal neural systems that have been implicated in anxiety and autonomic regulation. First, however, a brief review is given of the literature on autonomic function in anxiety disorders.

3 Anxiety and Cardiovascular Regulation

3.1 Historical Literature

Early studies often reported that patients with anxiety disorders are characterized by higher autonomic arousal, as evidenced by basal heart rate, skin conductance or other autonomic indices [128, 137]. Anxious patients were also variously reported in early studies to show exag-

gerated or prolonged responses to typical laboratory stressors [151]; to evidence a slower rate of habituation of autonomic responses over trials [137, 202]; and/or to be more likely to display defensive-like tachycardia, in contrast to a typical orienting-like bradycardia to innocuous stimuli [94]. In the aggregate, these and other findings led to suggestions that anxiety disorders are associated with: (a) a shift in "autonomic balance" toward sympathetic dominance [271]; (b) an over reactivity of the sympathetic system [63]; or (c) a generalized hyperattention to environmental stimuli [264].

Results of early studies, however, were not uniform. Baseline differences between anxious and control subjects were not always observed, at least on many autonomic measures [94, 160]. In fact, autonomic responses to laboratory stressors were sometimes reported to be smaller in anxious subjects [127, 128, 137]. Although this attenuated autonomic reactivity of anxiety patients was considered by some researchers to be a ceiling effect secondary to higher baseline levels [127, 151], other studies reported neither baseline differences nor grossly exaggerated autonomic responses in anxiety disorders [94]. To some extent, these variable findings likely reflected differences in the specific test stimuli and experimental contexts, categories of anxiety disorders tested, as well as the specific measures employed. It is apparent, however, that early studies do not offer a clear and consistent picture of autonomic control, nor permit a simple characterization of potential autonomic dysfunction in anxiety disorders.

3.2 Contemporary Findings

Within the past two decades, a substantial literature has accrued on autonomic function in anxiety. Although these studies have by no means simplified the relations between anxiety states and autonomic regulation, the recent literature does offer important clarifications and insights. Recent studies provide a much broader sampling of autonomic function across a range of anxiety disorders and experimental contexts, and are more cognizant of possible differences among categories of anxiety disorders. The literature remains complex, but this is not surprising given the heterogeneity of the cognitive, affective, and physiological processes that likely interact in anxiety states. Further, studies frequently employ different or only partially overlapping subsets of autonomic measures that do not always covary. Moreover, conditions under which "baseline" autonomic measures are obtained can vary widely across studies and an important question arises as to what constitutes an appropriate context to assess basal autonomic state. Experimental contexts, stimuli and challenges also differ substantially across studies. This is an especially important issue because behavioral and autonomic responses can vary among categories of anxiety disorder, and individual differences are apparent even within a given category. Additional complexity arises as anxiety conditions often show considerable comorbidity with other psychological disorders [129, 148].

Some preliminary generalizations can be derived from the existing literature, and may serve as a starting point for the further development of meaningful psychobiological models. First, anxiety disorders are frequently associated with altered autonomic function, although these alterations may vary considerably across nosological categories, and among individuals within a given category. Second, autonomic reactions often mirror the pattern of exaggerated affective/behavioral response, rather than reflecting a primary abnormality in autonomic regulation. Third, enhanced autonomic reactivity is most often apparent in phasic responses to specific stimuli or contexts, rather than in basal measures.

There continue to be reports of enhanced autonomic reactivity to experimental stimuli in patients with anxiety disorders, consistent with the view that anxiety may be associated with exaggerated autonomic reactivity [102]. This is by no means a universal finding, however, as a number of studies have not observed enhanced autonomic responding, or in fact report reduced responses in anxiety disorders [103–105, 214]. In some cases, a reduction in autonomic reactivity may be related to elevated baselines or to autonomic adaptation in chronic anxiety states. Either of these factors could contribute to a reduced magnitude of autonomic response, although exaggerated reactivity may still be reflected in retarded habituation [100, 127, 213].

The available data continue to reveal considerable diversity in the patterns of autonomic control in anxiety disorders. Two general trends have emerged, however, and offer some organization to the literature. First, among the clearest instances of exaggerated autonomic reactivity are in specific phobias, where anxiety is associated with a particular stimulus or context [170]. In contrast, exaggerated reactivity is less apparent in more global anxiety states such as generalized anxiety disorder [102]. Second, behavioral and autonomic responses are often highly concordant in specific phobias, but may be relatively uncorrelated in multi-phobics or more global anxiety states, such as generalized anxiety disorder [170].

Specific phobias (simple phobias) are common disorders, with a lifetime incidence estimated to be greater than 10% [148]. Specific phobias are characterized by an exaggerated fear of a particular stimulus or context. These patients may not show a prevalent alteration in basal autonomic measures [102, 170, 244], nor do they generally show a global increase in either behavioral or autonomic reactivity to experimental stimuli. Rather, enhanced autonomic reactivity is displayed primarily in the presence of the specific feared stimulus or context [46, 102, 155, 170]. McNeil et al. [170] report that specific phobics show normal resting heart rates and typical heart rate responses to non-phobic stimuli, but an exaggerated tachycardia to fear-relevant stimuli. These authors further report a significant correlation between subjective distress and the pattern of exaggerated autonomic response to fear stimuli in "simple" phobias [46, 170]. A further illustration of the potential specificity of phobias comes from the demonstration that phobic subjects show a selective disposition to acquire a conditioned aversive autonomic response to feared, but not to nonfeared objects [186].

Individual differences are apparent within the general category of specific phobias. Rather than a characteristic sympathetic-like tachycardia to the feared stimulus, for example, blood-injury phobics often show a transient tachycardia followed by a profound vagal-like bradycardia and syncope [102, 156]. In addition, although subjective distress and autonomic responses may be closely associated in specific phobias, this relationship may not hold for more general phobic anxiety conditions, such as social phobias or multiple phobias [46, 170].

The literature on posttraumatic stress disorder (PTSD) is somewhat more complex. Based on a review of the existing literature, Hoehn-Saric and McLeod [102] conclude that PTSD patients may not be generally over reactive, but rather show an exaggerated autonomic reactivity to stimuli or contexts reminiscent of precipitating traumatic events. Like many specific phobics, PTSD patients may display a pattern of autonomic response roughly paralleling their pattern of behavioral/affective reactivity. Although these authors note that baseline autonomic measures are sometimes elevated in PTSD, they point out the difficulty of achieving "true" baseline levels as laboratory contexts may themselves be anxiogenic.

The recent literature on PTSD is in general accord with these perspectives. Baseline heart rate and other autonomic measures are not invariably elevated, but exaggerated behavioral and autonomic reactivity to trauma-relevant stimuli are characteristic of this disorder [78, 164, 234, 235]. This enhanced reactivity appears to be somewhat more generalized than for specific phobics, however, and may not be limited exclusively to trauma-relevant stimuli. Subjects with PTSD may show more generalized avoidance or withdrawal tendencies, and have been reported to display exaggerated cardioacceleratory responses to nonsignal auditory stimuli [188, 189, 234], as well as enhanced basal somatic startle and especially fear potentiated startle responses [176, 177, 188].

Panic disorder is characterized by powerful, episodic fear-like reactions, typically associated with exaggerated cardiovascular responses [8, 9]. Panic has been considered to parallel features of fear, including a potent fight/flight action disposition, although panic reactions can be seen in the absence of an explicit cue [9]. Elevated basal autonomic measures such as heart rate are sometimes reported in laboratory studies on panic patients, but ambulatory monitoring studies in natural settings generally have not reported baseline differences in autonomic functions in the absence of anxiety episodes [102]. Although basal differences may exist on indirect measures such as plasma epinephrine [262] and cerebrovascular control [65], the notable autonomic features of panic disorders are associated with phasic reactions. Striking increases in heart rate, disproportionate to associated activity changes, have been reported generally during panic attacks [44, 72, 80, 253]. However, spontaneous panic attacks occurring in the absence of an explicitly evocative context have been reported in some cases to be associated with minimal heart rate changes [154].

Earlier studies suggested that panic disorder patients may evidence larger autonomic responses and/or slower habituation rates to a range of environmental stimuli [102]. Exaggerated cardiovascular responses and delayed habituation of the skin conductance response in panic disorder patients have been reported [106, 213], although these findings are not uniform [214]. Panic disorder patients may be more likely to panic in laboratory testing contexts, but otherwise they may show relatively normal patterns of autonomic reactivity and habituation to labo- ratory stressors [4, 105]. Moreover, patients with panic disorders do not show a generalized in- crease in either the somatic [88] or cardiovascular [215] components of startle. Rather, the primary autonomic characteristic of panic disorder is the exaggerated cardiovascular response associated with precipitated panic attacks.

A final category to be considered is general anxiety disorder (GAD), one of the more com- mon anxiety disorders, characterized by chronic global anxiety [3, 101]. Like panic disorder, GAD does not appear to be associated with general- ized elevations of basal autonomic activity [104, 158, 168]. A decrease in parasympathetic cardiac control, as indexed by respiratory sinus arrhyth- mia, has been reported for GAD patients [254], although this is not a universal finding [135]. Similarly, GAD patients generally have not been reported to display enhanced reactivity to typical laboratory stressors, and may even show smaller responses, although responses may be slower to habituate [101, 104]. This has led to the con- struct of an autonomic restriction or inflexibility in GAD [104, 254]. Exaggerated cardiovascular reactivity, however, has been suggested to char- acterize a subgroup of GAD patients with car- diovascular complaints [105].

3.3 Summary

The literature on autonomic functions in anxi- ety disorders is complex, but altered autonomic measures are frequently reported in this class of disorders. These differences are generally more apparent in reactive responses than in baseline measures, and often entail a pattern of enhanced autonomic response. Although baseline differ- ences in autonomic state have been reported, these findings are difficult to interpret given the inherent stress of laboratory contexts, and the enhanced autonomic reactivity observed in many anxiety disorders. Apparent basal differences may disappear with adaptation, and are often not ob- served during sleep or nonstressful contexts in ambulatory monitoring studies. Second, auto- nomic reactivity may vary between subjects and categories, and is often related to the broader pattern of behavioral and affective reaction. The literature on more global anxiety states, such as generalized anxiety disorder, is more difficult to fit within a general organizing scheme. In fact in some anxiety states, diminished reactivity or reduced autonomic variability may be manifest [103, 105, 254]. While it is apparent that auto- nomic functions may be altered in anxiety states, the relations between anxiety and autonomic functions are not simple. In the next section we consider some perspectives that offer an organiz- ing framework.

4 Emerging Views and Organizing Perspectives

4.1 Autonomic Regulation and Functional Reactions

Behavioral manifestations can vary widely among subcategories of anxiety disorders, and even between subjects within a given category, and there may be multiple central systems and processes that are differentially involved in varied anxiety states. Hence, it may be unreal- istic to expect a uniform pattern of altered auto- nomic function or reactivity in anxiety states. Based on the neuropsychological model of Gray [83], Fowles [71] has suggested that many incon- sistencies in autonomic function associated with anxiety may be due to an infelicitous concep- tualization of autonomic reactivity. Rather than reflecting simple and rigid stimulus-response relationships, autonomic responses may corre- spond more closely to the pattern of functional reaction to a stimulus. Moreover, the reaction to a given aversive stimulus may be dependent on the paradigm or testing context, and may entail either a general pattern of behavioral activation (e.g. escape/avoidance) or behavioral inhibi- tion (e.g. freezing). According to Fowles, a given stimulus or context will yield cardioacceleration to the extent to which it activates the behavioral approach system of Gray (BAS), whereas diminished BAS activity associated with activation of the behavioral inhibition system (BIS) would be expected to result in cardiodeceleration. Consistent with this suggestion, Martin and Fitzgerald [157] report that restrained rats respond to a shock CS with freezing and bradycardia, whereas unrestrained rats display tachycardia. This may reflect fundamental differences in the adaptive response of the organism in distinct contexts. Although bradycardia may be associated with behavioral inhibition, the observed heart rate changes in behavioral paradigms cannot be accounted for on the basis of simple metabolic consequences of the response [69]. The heart rate response to laboratory stressors typically exceeds that associated with metabolic demands [139, 185, 258], and typical conditioned and unconditioned cardiac responses can be seen in curarized animals [60] and paralyzed humans [14] in the absence of somatic activity.

Although further work is necessary to clarify the relations between psychological states and autonomic reactions, it is clear that autonomic responses are often more closely associated with the pattern of functional response than with the specific physical features of the stimulus. A novel stimulus that evokes a typical orienting-like bradycardia in a familiar environment, for example, may trigger no cardiac response in a novel context where other stimuli compete for attention [216]. This differential pattern of response to the identical stimulus indicates that autonomic responses may correspond more closely to the organism's reactions to the stimulus, rather than the physical characteristics of the stimulus, per se. In this regard, specific phobics can show normal basal autonomic states, and typical cardiac responses even to negative or aversive stimuli. In accord with their enhanced psychological reactions, however, exaggerated autonomic responses are displayed to stimuli associated with the specific phobia of the subject [90, 131].

4.2 Level of Processing of Anxiogenic Stimuli

Aversive or anxiogenic stimuli can be processed at multiple levels of the neuraxis, and these multiple processing substrates may have differential links with central autonomic mechanisms. Pain stimuli can trigger sympathetic reflexes even at the level of the isolated spinal cord [220], and decerebrate organisms with only an intact brainstem show characteristic evoked cardiovascular responses to a wide range of sensory stimuli [212, 257]. These findings document inherent links between environmental stimuli and central autonomic mechanisms, organized at the lowest levels of the neuraxis. Higher neural structures, such as the amygdala have been shown to be more important for classically conditioned fear responses, as amygdalar lesions can block the acquisition and expression of conditioned autonomic responses to a fear CS [125, 142, 217]. In fact, a direct pathway from the thalamic auditory relay nucleus (medial geniculate) to the lateral nucleus of the amygdala appears to be sufficient for the development of a conditioned fear response to a simple auditory stimulus, in the absence of higher cortical processing of the auditory signal [142]. Similarly, presentations of photographs of phobic objects followed by a visual masking stimulus can evoke characteristic autonomic reactions in phobic subjects, despite the fact that subjects are unable to describe or identify the phobic stimulus [186]. These findings indicate that anxiogenic stimuli can be evaluated by lower processing substrates, in the absence of cognitive mediation or even awareness.

On the other hand, cortical mechanisms appear to be critical for the processing of more complex stimuli and for contextual fear conditioning [142, 195]. Indeed, cortical/cognitive processing mechanisms appear to be capable of inducing fear and anxiety even in the absence of a relevant environmental fear stimulus. Mental imagery of aversive or anxiogenic contexts induces cortical activation, especially in limbic, paralimbic and associated cortical areas as evidenced by PET studies [136, 205, 206]. Mental imagery can: (a) trigger autonomic responses [232, 273]; (b) potentiate startle responses in a fashion similar to classically conditioned fear CSs [263]; and (c) trigger anxiety symptoms in patients with phobias or PTSD [170, 205, 206]. These findings attest to the potential importance of cognitive variables in anxiety states—variables that are likely mediated by cortical systems.

In the aggregate, these findings document the multiple processing level for anxiogenic stimuli. They further demonstrate that the multiple levels of evaluative processing may function in at least partial independence from other levels. The existence of multiple processing substrates for anxiogenic stimuli introduces considerable complexity for conceptual models of autonomic function in anxiety states, and likely underlies some of the apparent inconsistencies in the literature.

4.3   Complexities of Autonomic Control

An additional contribution to the complexity of the literature on autonomic function in anxiety is the intricacy of central autonomic control. The historical view of the sympathetic branch as a globally organized, undifferentiated system is no longer tenable. Although a somewhat generalized activation of the sympathetic innervations of diverse organs may be apparent under some conditions, it is now clear that organ-specific patterns of activation are also possible [266]. Consequently, measures of sympathetic control of different organ systems may not always be concordant. Laboratory stressors, for example, can selectively increase activity in forelimb muscle sympathetic nerves without altering activity in hindlimb innervations [266]. Indeed, these findings raise serious questions as to the appropriateness of a global construct of autonomic "hyperactivity."

Moreover, the traditional concept of a reciprocal central control of the two autonomic branches has undergone considerable qualification in the light of contemporary findings, and

it is now clear that the two autonomic branches can vary reciprocally, coactively, or independently [17, 18, 21, 134]. Many basic reflexes such as baroreceptor reflexes do exert powerful reciprocal control over the autonomic branches, but descending influences can inhibit or otherwise modulate baroreceptor reflexes [122, 243]. These include peptidergic systems, such as hypothalamic neurons containing corticotropin releasing hormone or vasopressin that can alter the baroreflex set point or otherwise modulate autonomic outflow [53, 93]. In fact, hypothalamic stimulation can evoke all of the basic modes of reciprocal, coactive, or independent changes in the activity of the autonomic branches [130, 133, 197]. Descending influences from rostral neural systems are capable of generating highly flexible patterns of autonomic outflow.

The findings outlined above introduce considerable complexity in the quantification and interpretation of autonomic control. Autonomic control cannot be viewed as lying along a single, reciprocal autonomic continuum extending from sympathetic dominance at one end to parasympathetic dominance at the other. Rather, autonomic control of dually innervated organs is more appropriately represented by a bivariate autonomic plane, consisting of orthogonal sympathetic and parasympathetic axes. This is illustrated by the model of the autonomic plane and the overlying cardiac effector surface in Fig. 29.1, which depicts the chronotropic state of the heart for any given combination of sympathetic and parasympathetic activities.

The relative lengths of the sympathetic and parasympathetic axes are proportional to the overall dynamic ranges of the two autonomic branches, and reflect the considerably greater dynamic range of the parasympathetic division (for development and review of this model see [18] for the human, and [21] for the rat). The shape of the parasympathetic marginal function is based on the almost universal finding that vagal nerve frequency is linearly related to cardiac chronotropic state, when expressed in heart

Cardiac Chronotropic Surface

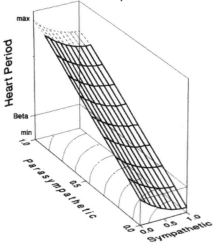

Figure 29.1
Autonomic plane and overlying cardiac effector surface. The effector surface depicts the relative chronotropic state of the heart for all possible combinations of sympathetic and parasympathetic activities. The length of the autonomic axes are proportional to the relative dynamic ranges of the autonomic branches, and beta is the intrinsic heart period level in the absence of autonomic influences. The dashed lines at the highest levels of vagal control represent the ambiguity in the shape of the surface at the highest levels of vagal control. The curved lines on the autonomic plane depict isofunctional contours, along which varied combinations of sympathetic and parasympathetic activities yield comparable heart period levels.

period, as documented by neurophysiological recordings and direct nerve stimulation [20, 21].[3,4] In contrast, the sympathetic function is somewhat less linear, with diminishing effects at higher frequencies [20, 21]. The effector surface of Fig. 29.1 depicts only the simple additive effects of the autonomic branches, although potential interactions may occur between the branches at higher levels of co-activation [145].[5] Because these interactions and the precise quantitative features of the effector surface do not appreciably alter the

implications of the present model, they will not be further considered here (for further discussion see [200]).

An important feature of the bivariate model of autonomic control is the fact that a given chronotropic level can be produced by varied combinations of sympathetic and parasympathetic activities. Hence, the chronotropic state of the heart is ambiguous with regard to its autonomic origins. This is illustrated by the curved lines on the autonomic plane of Fig. 29.1. These lines represent isofunctional contours that depict the multiple combinations of sympathetic and parasympathetic activities that yield equivalent effects on the chronotropic state of the heart. This ambiguity can cloud interpretations of basal chronotropic state and reactive response.

As suggested above, descending influences from rostral systems appear particularly likely to yield nonreciprocal modes of autonomic outflow in behavioral contexts. This is illustrated by a comparison of the autonomic response of human subjects to an orthostatic stress (assumption of an upright posture) compared with their response to typical psychological stressors such as mental arithmetic and a speeded reaction time task [16, 30]. Quantitative estimates of the sympathetic and parasympathetic contributions to cardiac responses were derived from single and dual autonomic blockade studies [16, 19, 30]. At the group level, the orthostatic and psychological stressors yielded an essentially equivalent pattern of heart rate increase, associated with sympathetic activation and parasympathetic withdrawal. For the orthostatic stressor, the cardiac response reflected a relatively tight reciprocal central control of the autonomic branches, as evidenced by the significant negative correlation between the responses of the autonomic branches across subjects ($r = -0.71$). Although the group response to psychological stressors was similar, there were considerable individual differences in the pattern of autonomic response, and there was no significant correlation between responses of the two branches across subjects ($r = 0.09$). Although the

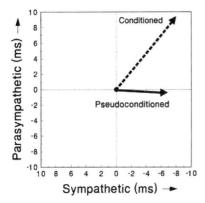

Figure 29.2
Autonomic response vectors to a conditioned stimulus, for conditioned and pseudoconditioned animals. Axes represent a segment of the cardiac effector surface of Figure 29.1, with the basal (prestimulus) position depicted at the 0,0 point on the axes. The arrowheads represent the change in autonomic state at the peak of the response, depicted as milliseconds of heart period change derived from selective pharmacological blockades of the autonomic branches. (Data derived from ref. 116.)

individual modes of response were highly reliable across different psychological stressors, subjects differed considerably in their pattern of response. Some subjects showed primarily sympathetic activation, some reciprocal sympathetic activation and parasympathetic withdrawal, and others, primarily parasympathetic withdrawal.

Importantly, the distinct modes of autonomic control may not be apparent in simple measures of end organ state. Iwata and LeDoux [116], for example, observed equivalent cardioacceleratory responses to a fear CS in both conditioned and pseudoconditioned rats. This might lead to the erroneous conclusion that autonomic cardiac control is not sensitive to the learning history of the subjects. As illustrated in Fig. 29.2, the application of selective pharmacological blockades of the sympathetic and parasympathetic innervations of the heart, however, revealed that the

similar cardioacceleratory responses of the two groups of animals arose from distinct modes of autonomic control. Blockade analyses revealed that the tachycardia of pseudoconditioned animals arose largely from selective sympathetic activation, as it was virtually eliminated by β-adrenergic blockade and unaffected by atropine. In contrast, the cardioacceleratory response of conditioned animals was enhanced by vagal blockade, being significantly larger than that of pseudoconditioned animals under identical blockade conditions. This suggests that, in the unblocked state, vagal responses opposed the larger sympathetic effects on the heart in the conditioned animals. Consistent with this interpretation, β-adrenergic blockade not only eliminated the cardioacceleratory response in this group, but unmasked a sizeable deceleratory response of putative vagal origin. These findings suggest that the sympathetic response of conditioned animals was appreciably larger than that of pseudoconditioned animals, but that the cardiac manifestations were dampened by a coactivation of the parasympathetic branch. Importantly, this differential pattern of autonomic control was not apparent in simple measures of end-organ state.

In the Iwata and LeDoux study, the similar (unblocked) cardiac response in conditioned and pseudoconditioned animals failed to reveal the autonomic differentiation associated with distinct behavioral processes. Measures of the cardiac chronotropic response may similarly fail to reveal lawful psychosomatic relationships. There is now considerable literature suggesting that individual differences in cardiovascular reactivity to laboratory stressors may be associated with differential risk for cardiovascular and other diseases [161, 258]. Cardioacceleratory responses to laboratory stressors, however, can arise from distinct autonomic modes of control, as an increase in heart rate may result from sympathetic activation, parasympathetic withdrawal, or both. This differentiation is important, as endocrinological and immune functions have been shown to be more closely related to the sympathetic component of the cardioacceleratory response than to the overall heart rate reactivity [29]. These findings are in accord with the report that immunologic consequences of acute cognitive stressors may be prevented by sympathetic blockade with β-adrenergic antagonists [13].

In summary, these findings suggest that the mode of autonomic control may be more closely related to behavioral states and processes than are simple measures of end-organ state. It is likely that many of the inconsistencies and ambiguities in the literature on anxiety and cardiovascular regulation may be resolved by closer attention to the underlying patterns of autonomic control. This applies not only to patterns of reactive response of the autonomic branches, but to potential differences in basal autonomic state.

4.4 Overview and Implications

Anxiety disorders are diverse, and vary widely along the dimension of specificity generality, the nature and range of the evocative contexts, and psychological or behavioral manifestations. Hence, it should not be surprising that the literature fails to reveal simple, universal relationships with autonomic function. At the same time, many apparent inconsistencies in the literature likely relate to limitations of conceptual models, rather than the lack of lawful relationships between anxiety states and autonomic control. One possible strategy for disentangling the complex interactions between psychological and physiological processes in anxiety is through the use of pharmacological models.

5 Benzodiazepine Receptor Ligands as Anxiolytics/Anxiogenics

In humans, benzodiazepine receptor (BZR) agonists effectively reduce the symptoms of anxiety. Likewise, in animals, BZR agonists potently attenuate the behavioral manifestations of fear

and anxiety in a variety of paradigms [75, 183, 218]. Despite almost 40 years of clinical use and research on BZR agonists, however, the behavioral/cognitive mechanisms mediating the anxiolytic effects of these compounds have remained unclear. The complexities inherent in attempts to conceptualize anxiety in behavioral or cognitive terms may have contributed to the rather limited research on the mechanisms underlying the attenuation of anxiety by BZR agonists [86, 87].[6] Gray's neuropsychological model of anxiety explains the antianxiety effects of drugs by antagonizing the actions of a "behavioral inhibition system." This system normally responds to signals of punishment, non reward, and novelty by inhibiting ongoing behavior and by increased arousal and attention to anxiety related stimuli [84]. It may be speculated that, conversely, drug-induced anxiogenesis results from an augmentation of the actions of the "behavioral inhibition system" which would be characterized predominantly by hyperarousal and hyperattentional processing of fear and anxiety associated stimuli. As chronic anxiety is associated with an emerging bias toward the selection and processing of fear or threat associated stimuli [11, 159, 169], drug-induced augmentation of that processing may be a primary mechanism mediating drug-induced potentiation of fear and anxiety [184].

Cognitive theories of anxiety have consistently stressed attentional dysfunctions as a major component in the development and persistence of anxiety disorders. Eysenck [64] describes anxious groups as more likely to attend to threat-related stimuli and having more narrowly focused attention. According to this theory of anxiety, antianxiety drugs are hypothesized to produce therapeutic effects largely via their attention-reducing properties [47, 132, 167].

BZR agonists exert their anxiolytic actions by an allosteric interaction with the BZR–GABA receptor complex, and the resulting enhancement of GABAergic transmission. In contrast, BZR inverse agonists and partial inverse agonists attenuate GABAergic transmission, and have effects that are generally opposite those of the BZR agonists. These agents, for example, have been shown to enhance the punishing effects of shock [59], to parallel the behavioral and analgesic effects of inescapable shock [58, 98], to enhance corticosterone levels in a novel environment [193], and to increase fear-like behaviors and central catecholamine responses of monkeys in threat contexts [124]. In accord with the present view, the anxiogenic effects of BZR inverse agonists may derive, at least in part, from their effects on cortical information processing. Specifically, these anxiogenic agents may promote an overprocessing of stimuli and contexts associated with fear and anxiety [107, 229].

Clearly, such a theoretical perspective remains limited and oversimplifies the role of cognitive variables in anxiety and drug-induced alterations of anxiety states. In particular, the long-term and dynamic effects of biased attentional processes for the mnemonic aspects of anxiety rarely have been conceptualized. However, numerous studies [147] demonstrate that subjects suffering from phobia and panic attacks show a recall bias for fear- and anxiety-associated information. Such memorial biases would be expected to further escalate the preoccupation with and processing of fear- and anxiety-related stimuli. The hypothesis that attentional and associated mnemonic biases contribute to the development and persistence of anxiety disorders provides a fruitful basis for experimental approaches to the neural and psychophysiological mechanisms of anxiety.

The available studies on the anxiogenic effects of BZR inverse agonists, and the prototype anxiogenic partial inverse agonist FG 7142, were not designed to determine the specific behavioral or cognitive components of drug-induced anxiety. Consequently, they do not permit a critical evaluation of the hypothesis that drug-induced augmentation of the processing of fear- and anxiety-related information contributes to the emergence of anxiety-like symptoms.

The original report on the anxiogenic effects of FG 7142 in healthy volunteers [57] was based on an open trial. Moreover, as discussed by Thiebot et al. [256], self-reports about severe anxiety may have been biased by uncontrolled experimental variables, as the volunteers were instructed to expect symptoms of anxiety [256] (p. 453). In the study by Dorow et al., FG 7142 produced marked peripheral effects (e.g. increases in blood pressure, pulse rate, and muscular tension) as well as self-reports of anxiety. Nevertheless, the available evidence from human and animal studies collectively supports the hypothesis that FG 7142 and other BZR partial inverse agonists can induce or potentiate anxiety [76, 77, 219, 256].

6 Central Cholinergic Systems: Lessons from FG 7142

As considered above, BZR inverse agonists have been reported to have potent anxiogenic actions. An especially important subclass of these compounds is represented by the BZR partial inverse agonists, which display a differential potency for the multiple actions of the inverse agonists. An example is the β-carboline FG 7142, which has potent proconflict and anxiogenic effects, but minimal convulsive actions when compared with full inverse agonists. Anxiogenic effects of FG are suggested by the fact that it decreases open arm entries in the elevated plus maze [45, 211], enhances measures of anxiety in social interaction tests [12, 67, 207], and mimics the effects of inescapable shock on social processes [238]. Moreover, the physiological state induced by FG 7142 generalizes to novelty and shock conditions in a drug discriminative paradigm [143]. In comparison to other compounds assumed to produce anxiogenic effects (e.g. sodium lactate or yohimbine), the behavioral effects of FG are relatively specific and do not reflect the rather global behavioral consequences of a drug-induced state of "stress." Thiebot et al. [255] report that in an

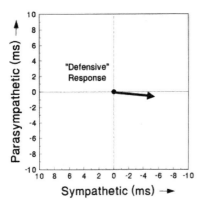

Figure 29.3
Autonomic response vector depicting the defensive-like cardioacceleratory response to a moderate intensity, nonsignal stimulus. Axes represent a segment of the cardiac effector surface of Figure 29.1, with the basal (prestimulus) position depicted at the 0,0 point on the axes. The arrowhead represents the change in autonomic state at the peak of the response, depicted as milliseconds of heart period change derived from selective pharmacological blockades of the autonomic branches.

operant task, relatively small doses of FG enhance the behavioral suppressive effects of withdrawal of a "safety signal" (from shock), but do not affect appetitively-motivated responding during safety periods. Lending further support for FG 7142 as a pharmacological model for anxiety is the fact that the apparent anxiogenic effects of this agent can be blocked by anti-panic drugs such as clonidine, imipramine and adinazolam [68, 123, 193, 194].

More recently, we have found that FG 7142 yields a notable potentiation of the cardioacceleratory response to a moderately intense, nonsignal acoustic stimulus in rats. As illustrated in Fig. 29.3, this cardioacceleratory response is mediated by sympathetic activation, and based on the stimulus characteristics and response features, is consistent with a defensive response [82].

The FG-induced potentiation of this cardioacceleratory response is in general accord with the enhanced cardiovascular reactivity after FG, as reported for humans [57] and monkeys [180]. The exaggerated cardioacceleratory response observed after FG is reminiscent of a defensive response, and is similar to the effects of increasing stimulus intensity or contextual aversive conditioning [199].

Among the more general effects of BZR agonists and inverse agonists is the bidirectional modulation of cortical information processing [225, 229]. BZR agonists inhibit, and inverse agonists enhance, basal forebrain-cortical cholinergic activity [174, 175, 222], and recent findings suggest that the basal forebrain cholinergic system may mediate the FG-induced enhancement of the cardioacceleratory response. This is evidenced by the following: (a) the FG-induced enhancement of the cardioacceleratory responses is paralleled by intracerebroventricular administration of the cholinergic agonist carbachol; (b) the effects of both FG and carbachol were blocked by intracerebroventricular pretreatment with the cholinergic antagonist atropine; and (c) FG no longer potentiated the cardiac response after selective immunotoxic lesions (192 IgG-saporin) of basal forebrain cholinergic neurons [22]. Although basal forebrain cholinergic projections terminate in the amygdala, as well as the cortex, additional considerations implicate the cortical projections in the effects of FG on the cardiovascular defensive response. The neurotoxin 192 IgG-saporin specifically targets the p75 low affinity nerve growth factor receptors that reside on cortically projecting basal forebrain neurons. The subset of cholinergic neurons that project to the amygdala, however, seems not to bear these receptors and hence is largely spared by the immunotoxic lesion [97]. Consequently, the lack of effect of FG on the cardiac defensive response, after the basal forebrain lesions, appears to have resulted from the selective loss cortical cholinergic projections.

The above findings implicate basal forebrain cortical cholinergic projections in the cardiovascular actions of FG 7142, and suggest a hypothesis concerning the behavioral origins of anxiogenic effects of this agent. Because the cortical cholinergic innervation appears to enhance or amplify ongoing cortical processing [172, 223], alterations in cortical acetylcholine might be expected to selectively impact on cognitive processes that are heavily dependent on cortical substrates. In this regard, BZR agonists such as chlordiazepoxide impede cognitive and attentional processing of a broad range of stimuli [167, 229], and their anxiolytic effects may well be due to the reduction in the exaggerated cortical processing of anxiogenic stimuli [64]. In contrast, BZR inverse agonists or partial inverse agonists such as FG 7142, can enhance cognitive and attentional processing [225, 229], and their anxiogenic effects may be attributable in part to an exaggerated processing of fear or anxiety relevant stimuli.

FG, however, may not potentiate all features of anxiety. Although FG consistently enhances the cardiac response to a nonsignal stimulus, it does not increase and may even suppress the somatic and cardiovascular components of the startle response [23, 24]. Similarly, FG does not enhance fear-potentiated startle [95] a commonly reported feature of anxiety states. These findings support the view that anxiogenic stimuli may be processed at multiple levels of neuraxial organization, and suggest a potentially important dimension of differentiation in the neural substrates of anxiety. We hypothesize that the basal forebrain cholinergic projection is primarily involved in aspects of anxiety that arise from or depend on cortical processing of fear and anxiety-associated stimuli and associations.

This hypothesis offers an explanation for the differential effects of FG on startle and defensive responses. The basic startle circuit is largely organized at the level of the brainstem, and is not dependent on cortical or other forebrain systems [51]. Hence, startle responses might not be expected to be potentiated by BZR agents that enhance cortical cholinergic activity. In contrast, defensive-like responses to a novel nonsignal stimulus likely arise from an active cognitive/affective evaluation of the stimulus, that would be expected to be highly dependent on cortical processing substrates. This may be the basis for the selective effect of FG on the defensive response.

Although the basic startle circuit is organized at a brainstem level, the amygdala contributes importantly to conditioned fear and to fear-potentiated startle [34, 50, 52, 125, 142, 159], and this structure also receives cholinergic projections from the basal forebrain. In this regard, FG not only fails to potentiate basal startle responses, but also does not enhance fear-potentiated startle [95]. Again, the primary locus of FG-induced anxiogenesis may be within cortical processing substrates, as the cortical cholinergic projections of the basal forebrain specifically are implicated in the FG-induced potentiation of the cardiovascular defensive response. Although the amygdala may be critically involved in fear-potentiated startle, cortical systems may not be pivotal, at least for fear-potentiated startle based on a simple conditioned fear CS. In keeping with this view, although lesions of the nucleus basalis may impair acquisition of conditioned heart rate responses to an aversive stimulus, perhaps by an attentional mechanism, they do not block the expression of conditioned fear responses [79].

In the aggregate, studies outlined above suggest a special role for basal forebrain cortical cholinergic projections in the anxiogenic effects of the BZR partial inverse agonist FG 7142. These findings raise a potentially important distinction between features of fear and anxiety that derive from cortical processing and those that may be mediated largely by subcortical structures. This differentiation is not likely to be absolute, but is offered as a conceptual heuristic that may serve to organize empirical findings and guide subsequent theoretical developments.

7 Cardiovascular Reactivity and Cortical Acetylcholine: Anatomy and Function

The discussion above provides the basis for the formulation of several hypotheses. (1) Cognitive evaluation of fear- and anxiety-associated stimuli and contexts represent an important component in the emergence of anxiety. (2) There is a relationship between the manifestation of enhanced autonomic, specifically cardiovascular reactivity and the degree to which anxiety-related stimuli or contexts are cognitively evaluated. The intensity of the actual affective state or the amplitude of the behavioral response considered to reflect such a state is less clearly related to autonomic reactivity changes. (3) The cognitive evaluation of anxiety-related stimuli and contexts depends on the integrity of the basal forebrain cholinergic system, and cardiovascular reactivity changes indirectly modulate basal forebrain cholinergic neuronal excitability and thus the processing of fear- and anxiety-associated information.

Cardiovascular–basal forebrain interactions will be conceptualized in terms of the ascending and descending components of these interactions. Specifically, the ascending modulation of basal forebrain cholinergic activity by cardiovascular reactivity changes is hypothesized to enhance the evaluative processing of anxiety-related stimuli and contexts. Conversely, the descending system mediates the expression of anxiety and, in addition, initiates autonomic responses. The traditional neuronal circuits implicated in fear and anxiety, specifically, the amygdala and its descending projections to brainstem nuclei, represent an integral part of the descending limb of this model. Finally, several predictions based on this model will be discussed in terms of available evidence and experimental approaches.

7.1 The Expression of Anxiety and Modulation of Cardiovascular Reactivity by Cortical ACh

The descending branch of the present model system (Fig. 29.4) describes primary components of the network mediating the expression of anxiety, and associated autonomic reactions. These autonomic responses, in turn, may modulate the processing of anxiety- and fear-associated stimuli, via ascending influences discussed below (see Section 7.2). Existing neural models of anxiety represent essential components of this descending system. These traditional models have focused generally on the descending connections of the amygdala and have rarely attempted to integrate the role of cognitive processes in psychological and neuronal theories of anxiety [52, 142]. The available evidence supports the role of telencephalic, including cortical mechanisms in the expression of anxiety and the regulation of cardiovascular reactivity and provides the basis for a detailed description of the functional significance of descending branch of the present model (Fig. 29.4).

Stimulation of the amygdala has been known for over half a century to elicit fear- and anxiety-like states and sympatho-excitatory effects [50, 52, 248]. The attribution of emotional, particularly anxiety- and fear-associated qualities to sensory stimuli has been traditionally assigned to amygdaloid circuits [227, 228]. Furthermore, the sympathetic and behavioral effects of conditioned stimuli for anxiety and fear are blocked by central amygdala lesions, suggesting a crucial role for this component of telencephalic/limbic circuits in the mediation of fear and anxiety [142, 146, 192, 275].

Several models emphasize additional projections of the amygdala to the lateral and paraventricular hypothalamus as well as to the midbrain central gray as critical for the mediation of particular aspects of defensive responses and autonomic regulation [2, 52, 81, 142, 227, 236, 241, 242]. For example, stress-related increases in plasma corticosterone can be blocked by lesions of the stria terminalis which links the amygdala with the paraventricular nucleus of the hypothalamus [50]. Although the exact contribution of direct and indirect amygdalofugal projections in the acquisition and expression of anxiety

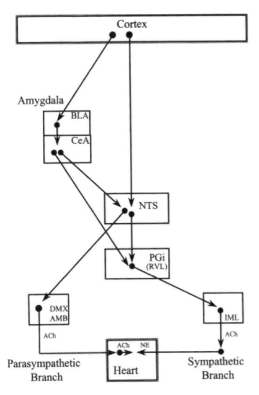

Figure 29.4
Descending branch of the anatomical model of neuronal substrates by which cortical/cognitive processes
may contribute to the development and expression of
anxiety and its autonomic features. The model is not
intended to present an anatomically complete description of relevant circuits and transmitters; rather it is
conceptually driven and focuses on hypotheses derived
in part from experimental evidence (see text and ref.
22). Abbreviations: ACh, acetylcholine; AMB, nucleus
ambiguus; BLA, basolateral amygdala; CeA, central
nucleus of the amygdala; DMX, dorsal motor nucleus
of the vagus; IML, sympathetic preganglionic neurons
of the intermediolateral cell column; NE, norepinephrine; NTS, nucleus tractus solitarius; PGi, nucleus paragigantocellularis; RVL, rostral ventrolateral
medullary "pressor" area [89, 108, 243].

and fear and sympatho-excitation is unclear, the
direct descending projection (Fig. 29.4) of the
central amygdala to the NTS represents a sufficient pathway for the regulation of autonomic
state by telencephalic structures [99, 115, 146,
162, 196, 217, 220, 231, 280]. The NTS also
receives direct input from the medial prefrontal
cortex [260], an area that has been implicated in
anxiety and affective processes [119, 138], as well
as cardiovascular regulation [39, 261]. Stimulation of the medial prefrontal and other cortical
areas potently alters heart rate and blood pressure [39, 91, 92, 187], and lesion studies revealed
the involvement of the medial prefrontal cortex
in the acquisition of autonomic adjustments [74,
179, 198]. Thus, the prefrontal cortex can execute
direct and indirect (via the amygdala) control of
behavior-associated autonomic, particularly cardiovascular reactivity (Fig. 29.4). Other cortical
areas, such as the insular cortex, may also be
involved in anxiety and cardiovascular control
[39, 204, 261]. The role of the septohippocampal
system in anxiety and contextual fear conditioning has been recognized widely, and the hippocampus in turn projects to structures such as the
amygdala, hypothalamus and bed nucleus of the
stria terminalis that can modulate autonomic
functions [38, 53, 85, 152, 169, 195]. The model
presented in Fig. 29.4 is intended to be illustrative rather than exhaustive.

Collectively, a substantial amount of evidence
supports the long-standing hypotheses about the
role of the amygdala in the emotional coloring of
sensory stimuli in general and in the acquisition
and expression of anxiety in particular [1, 227,
228]. Major cortical inputs to the amygdala can
supply the sensory stimuli and associations which
may then gain emotional significance via processing within amygdalo–telencephalic circuits
[34, 40, 153, 227, 228]. The efficiency of processing of such stimuli and associations through
telencephalic/amygdaloid circuits would be expected to depend, in part, on cortical ACh (Fig.
29.5; see also Section 6; for a detailed discussion
of the cognitive functions of cortical ACh, see

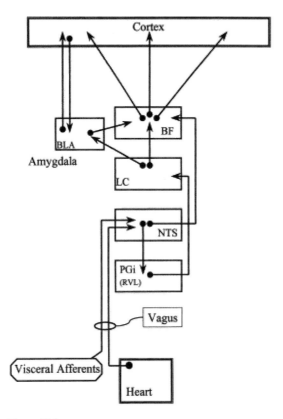

Figure 29.5
Ascending branch of the anatomical model of neuronal substrates by which cortical/cognitive processes may contribute to the development and expression of anxiety and its autonomic features. Ascending pathways illustrate the potential routes by which sympathetic activity and visceral afference may modulate rostral systems. Abbreviations: BF, basal forebrain cortical cholinergic system; BLA, basolateral amygdala; LC, locus coeruleus; NTS, nucleus tractus solitarius; PGi, nucleus paragigantocellularis; RVL, rostral ventrolateral medullary "pressor" area [89, 108, 243].

[223]). In this fashion, basal forebrain cortical-cholinergic activity would modulate the descending circuit (Fig. 29.4) implicated in the acquisition and expression of fear and anxiety. Moreover, this cortical cholinergic activity would contribute directly and indirectly to the regulation of autonomic reactivity via cortical efferents to the amygdala, the NTS, and directly to lower autonomic motor nuclei [25, 26, 39, 109]. It is in this context that we have interpreted the effects of basal forebrain cholinergic lesions on the cardiovascular effects of the anxiogenic FG 7142 [22, 23, 79].

7.2 Modulation of Basal Forebrain Cholinergic Neuronal Excitability by Cardiovascular Responses

Basal forebrain cholinergic neurons that are situated in the substantia innominata and the nucleus basalis Meynert in the basal forebrain innervates all cortical areas and layers, suggesting a uniform modulatory function of acetylcholine on cortical information processing [223]. Several lines of evidence, including in vivo measures of cortical ACh release in task-performing animals [225] and investigations of the cognitive effects of lesions of this system [166], collectively suggested a crucial role of cortical ACh in the detection and selection of relevant stimuli and in the capacity to subject such stimuli to extended processing, i.e. in attentional functions [223].

The cholinergic neurons in the basal forebrain receive several afferent projections which modulate the activity of the cortical cholinergic projection [222]. A major afferent projection to basal forebrain neurons originates in the locus coeruleus and employs noradrenaline as a transmitter [121]. The direct innervation of basal forebrain cholinergic neurons by ascending noradrenergic projections has been extensively described [41, 275–278]. In contrast, functional data on basal forebrain catecholaminergic–cholinergic interactions are rather rare (for indirect evidence see [10, 210, 252]). However, noradrenaline (NA)

depolarizes cholinergic cells in the basal forebrain via α_1 receptors [70] and thus would be expected to increase cortical ACh release. The exact effects of NA at basal forebrain cholinergic neurons may be more complex, however, as they are modulated by other inputs to the basal forebrain cholinergic neurons, particularly the inhibitory GABAergic projection from the nucleus accumbens [222] and the excitatory afferents from several telencephalic areas. In essence, however, increases in activity in the LC ascending NA projection are expected to increase the excitability of cortical cholinergic inputs.

The LC also projects directly to the cortex [191]. The present model, however, centers around our experimental data on the basal forebrain cholinergic system, and hence emphasizes the LC innervation of basal forebrain cholinergic neurons. The regulation of cortical ACh by basal forebrain noradrenergic afferents represents an important route by which ascending noradrenergic projections could mediate potential feedback effects of cardiovascular reactivity in the modulation of cortical processing and ultimately, anxiety.

The electrophysiological experiments of Aston-Jones and co-workers cumulated in the hypothesis that LC ascending projections mediate emotional activation [5]. These and other researchers observed that LC neuronal activity robustly increases in response to the presentation of stress-, fear- and anxiety-inducing stimuli, but also to stimuli that are associated with rewarding events, suggesting that emotionally significant stimuli activate the LC ascending system regardless of the affective valence (see also [203]). Aston-Jones further stressed that the generality of the LC response to all classes of emotional stimuli indicates that the quality of the emotion is not encoded into LC activation. Rather, LC activation represents a state-setting mechanism which facilitates the processing of more specific contexts and stimuli of discrete emotional quality by more rostral structures efferent to the noradrenergic bundle. The basal forebrain cholinergic system represents a major component mediating the processing of such contexts and stimuli, and the amygdala may represent an important switch for determination of the valence of the affective response.

The ability of emotional stimuli to activate the noradrenergic ascending system appears to be a direct function of the state of the sympathetic branch of the autonomic nervous system [208, 239]. For example, sympathetic activation induced by nitroprusside-hypotension was found to be associated with increases in LC firing, and this effect was shown to be mediated via visceral afferents from the cardiac atrial volume receptors [62].

The anatomical basis that allows the LC to monitor sympatho-excitatory events is straightforward. One major afferent connection to the LC originates from the nucleus paragigantocellularis (PGi) in the medulla, and involves several transmitters, including excitatory amino acids, adrenaline and enkephalin [6]. The PGi, in turn, receives information from a variety of sources in the brain stem and spinal cord, including the NTS, which collectively suggests that the PGi projections to the LC transmit information reflecting autonomic activity and visceral afference. The PGi is partially coextensive with the rostral ventrolateral medullary pressor area, a region that directly innervates sympathetic motor neurons of the intermediolateral cell column of the cord [89, 108]. These findings suggest that PGi neurons activate in parallel the LC and sympathetic motor neurons, and thus modulate the autonomic and cognitive (via the LC) aspects of emotional activation [7, 239]. In addition, the medial prefrontal cortex exerts a potent excitatory influence on the LC [120], which could provide for top-down activation of this system. While our model suggests that the autonomic modulation of basal forebrain cholinergic neuronal activity is mediated via the noradrenergic LC projections to the basal forebrain, it should be noted that evidence for a direct innervation of the basal forebrain by adrenergic or noradrener-

gic neurons of the NTS suggests an even more direct influence of autonomic states on cortical information processing [233].

The anatomy-driven model shown in Fig. 29.5 attributes the evaluative processing of anxiety-related stimuli to an ascending system which also serves to integrate the modulatory effects of autonomic state [6, 7]. Several issues require further clarification. An obvious, though frequently neglected, question arises concerning the causal sequence of events in emotional activation. Clearly, ascending modulation of cognitive processing by autonomic reactions requires an initiation (via descending projections) of such reactivity changes (see discussion below and [31]). The reciprocal telencephalic connections of the basolateral amygdala are essential in mediating the classification and processing of stimuli associated with anxiety or fear and are therefore integral parts of both the ascending (anxiety modulating) and descending (anxiety expressing) components of the present model (Figs. 29.4 and 29.5) [226]. In addition, neuronal circuits which include the connections between the amygdala and the hippocampal formation (subiculum; not shown in Fig. 29.5) have been speculated to mediate the evaluation of anxiety contexts and the cognitive biases which characterize pathological states of anxiety [142, 195]. Thus several limbic circuits which are organized in parallel with the ascending network illustrated in Fig. 29.5 are essential for the cognitive processing of anxiety-associated stimuli and associations. Importantly, however, this model hypothesizes that the ascending recruitment of these limbic circuits, primarily via noradrenergic-cholinergic activation, serves to prime these rostral substrates for processing of the cognitive aspects fear and anxiety. Moreover, the model is permissive of a cognitively-driven, top-down activation of the descending arm of this system. The importance of this possibility is that such a top-down activation might be expected to trigger a feedback cascade associated with the ascending component of the system. Indeed, there is an intriguing compatibility of this view with the irrationality of much anxiety-related ideation in anxiety disorders.

Although ascending and descending limbs of our model are separated for conceptual and descriptive clarity, the functional significance of the model lies in the interactions between the ascending and descending branches. The ascending component shown in Fig. 29.5 suggests that alterations in cardiovascular reactivity are able to modulate the efficacy of cortical information processing. As considered above, the available data suggest that LC discharge, and consequent cortical cholinergic activity, may be modulated by the NTS-PGi circuit in accord with visceral afference. Thus, increases in cardiovascular activity may bias cortical cholinergic inputs toward increased reactivity and an enhanced processing of affective stimuli. Functional evidence to directly link cardiovascular reactivity with modulations in cortical stimulus processing, specifically entailing cortical cholinergic afferents, is limited [22, 118, 173]. As discussed above, however, a relatively extensive literature has consistently implicated the locus coeruleus and the ascending noradrenergic system in the development of anxiety. Additional data suggest links between LC activity, anxiety, and BZR systems, as stimulation of the LC results in anxiety-like behaviors in monkeys which can be blocked by anxiolytic BZR agonists [27]. Similarly, stress- and anxiety-induced increases in NA turnover in telencephalic target regions of the LC are blocked by BZR agonists [111]. Moreover, the anxiety-inducing effects of so-called "anxiogenic" agents, such as CRF and yohimbine, are associated with increases in the activity of the ascending noradrenergic system, and FG 7142 also activates ascending noradrenergic systems [28, 42, 110, 251, 270, 274]. In fact, the robust increases in cortical ACh release produced by FG 7142 [175] may be due, at least in part, to noradrenergic driving of basal forebrain cholinergic neurons, coupled with an attenuation of local GABAergic inhibition. These findings suggest a close functional

relationship between central adrenergic activity, BZR/GABAergic mechanisms, basal forebrain cortical cholinergic projections, and anxiety.

7.3 Model-derived Predictions

The present model provides fertile ground for experimental predictions. The descending system has been more extensively studied than has the potential influence of the ascending arm on cortical cognitive processing. Three predictions based on the present model, serve to integrate the potential ascending and descending influences, and illustrate the heuristic potential of the proposed system.

7.3.1 Increases in Cortical ACh Release Augment the Expression of Fear and Anxiety, as well as Associated Autonomic Changes

As discussed above, the anxiogenic drug FG 7142 augments cortical ACh release [175, 222], and enhances the defensive-like cardioacceleratory responses [22, 201]. In this respect, it is intriguing that organophosphate anticholinesterase exposure has been reported to induce anxiety, even at exposure levels that do not yield standard clinical signs of toxicity [144, 171]. The latter is only consistent with the cholinergic model, as it has not been shown that putative anticholinesterase-induced anxiety arises from cortical cholinergic effects. Moreover, the generality of pharmacological models clearly needs to be demonstrated by extensions to more natural behavioral models of anxiety and anxiogenic conditions.

A secondary issue that warrants attention in this context relates to the hypothesis that BZR inverse agonists enhance certain cognitive functions [223–225]. The possibility of drug-induced cognition enhancement, particularly in subjects suffering from the partial loss of cortical cholinergic inputs is conceptually related to the potential of these drugs to augment the processing of anxiety-related information. In fact, it is difficult to conceive of a potential "cognition enhancer" which does not also augment a pathologically pre-biased, anxiety-focused selection of stimuli and contexts for extended evaluation, particularly in intact subjects.

7.3.2 Reduction or Normalization of Increased Cortical Cholinergic Transmission Should Reduce Symptoms of Anxiety and Anxiety-related Cardiovascular Reactions

Our previous studies demonstrated that the enhanced sympathetic reactivity to a defensive stimulus after FG 7142 can be blocked by specific lesions of the basal forebrain-cortical cholinergic projection [22]. The effects of intraventricular infusions of cholinergic agonists and antagonists further supported the critical role of forebrain muscarinic receptors in the effects of FG on the cardioacceleratory response. Moreover, the anxiolytic benzodiazepine receptor agonists potently reduce cortical ACh release [112, 175, 222], raising the possibility that their therapeutic effects are mediated in part via decreases in cortical ACh release. This, of course, does not imply that muscarinic cholinergic receptor blockers should be therapeutically effective in anxiety, as blockade of cholinergic transmission is not equivalent to a normalization of an enhanced level of transmission. Consequently, therapeutic effects of receptor blockers would not be expected necessarily.

Less evidence is available as to the direct role of cortical ACh in the natural expression of fear and anxiety. Some studies, however, do bear on this issue. Stoehr and Wenk [249] demonstrated that lesions of the basal forebrain area attenuate conditioned freezing to an environmental context. This suggests that the integrity of the basal forebrain cholinergic system is important for the expression of context-dependent aversive reactions, which have been suggested to be cortically dependent phenomena [142, 195]. Also consistent with the present model is the finding that patients with Alzheimer's disease, which is associated with degeneration of the basal forebrain cholinergic system, display less severe anxiety symptoms than patients with vascular dementias (matched for education, age, and severity of dementia) [250].

Clearly, a normalization of increased cortical ACh release as a component of anxiolytic mechanisms represents a testable hypothesis. As considered above, however, no such role would be expected in models assessing spontaneous fear- and anxiety-related responses that do not involve cognitive appraisal of stimuli and/or contexts. The degree to which cortical ACh contributes to fear and anxiety is conceptualized as a function of the role of cognitive variables in anxiety. This leads to clear predictions. For example, the potentiation of startle responding by simple conditioned stimuli may not require cortical processing, and hence may not be substantially affected by the basal forebrain cholinergic system. On the other hand, startle potentiation based on negative imagery [263] likely entails cortical processing, and hence would be expected to be highly sensitive to basal forebrain cholinergic activity.

7.3.3 Increases in Autonomic, Particular Cardiovascular Reactivity Increases Cortical ACh Release via Adrenergic Receptor Stimulation in the Basal Forebrain

Direct evidence for this crucial hypothesis is lacking, although some relevant literature on the role of visceral afference in emotion will be considered in the next section. As discussed above, the afferent inputs to the LC, and the effects of stressors on autonomic reactivity and activity in the ascending noradrenergic bundle provide circumstantial evidence in support of this central aspect of the model. However, the assumption that increased autonomic activity invariably translates into activation of cortical cholinergic afferents may be invalid. As emphasized above, the ability of noradrenaline to increase the excitability of basal forebrain cholinergic neurons may depend on interactions with other converging afferents, particularly from the amygdala and the nucleus accumbens to basal forebrain neurons. In functional terms, such interactions may restrict the ascending effects on autonomic reactivity to situations which involve activation of amygdaloid circuits, or more generally, of rostral limbic areas. In other words, autonomic reactivity changes may affect cortical processing predominately in situations characterized by strong emotional-cognitive appraisal processes. To the extent this hypothesis is correct, it would imply that the functional significance of autonomic reactivity differs substantially between control subjects and those with a pathological bias toward fear- and anxiety-related information processing.

8 Anxiety and Autonomic Function: The Role of Visceral Afference

8.1 Historical Background

Scientific interest in the somatovisceral substrates of emotions (e.g. Darwin [49]) was aroused when William James [117] argued that emotional feelings were consequences rather than antecedents of peripheral physiological changes brought about by some external stimulus. Limiting attention to emotions "that have a distinct bodily expression" (p. 189), James [117] maintained that discrete emotional experiences could be identified with unique patterns of peripheral physiological changes, and that the perception of these specific patterns of response constituted the emotional experience. James' theory has stimulated debate and research for more than a century.

In contrast, Walter Cannon [35] argued that peripheral autonomic reactions did not contribute to emotions, based on five facts: (1) separation of the viscera from the central nervous system does not alter emotional behavior; (2) the same visceral changes occur in very different emotional as well as non-emotional states; (3) the viscera are relatively insensitive structures; (4) visceral changes are too slow to be a source of emotional feeling; and (5) artificial induction of the visceral changes typical of strong emotions

does not evoke these emotions. Based on these considerations, Cannon relegated autonomic activity to a rather cursory role in emotions, and this view dominated the literature for more than three decades.

8.2 Contemporary Perspectives and Empirical Data

Research on emotions in patients with high spinal cord transections [43], and on the influence of cognitive appraisals in emotion [240, 259] suggests that afferent information from peripheral autonomic activity is not a necessary condition for emotional experiences. Moreover, despite occasional claims that discrete emotions are associated with distinctive autonomic patterns [61], meta-analyses have not supported the strong version of this hypothesis [32]. These findings do not lend support to James' theory, but they do not rule out a potentially important contribution of visceral afference to affective reactions.

Although there may not be highly unique patterns of autonomic response and visceral afference associated with different emotional states, visceral afferents may play an important role in priming affective responses. Administration of epinephrine, for example, has been reported to potentiate discrete and divergent emotional states, dependent on the cognitive context [209, 230]. Thus, a relatively undifferentiated visceral activity and afference may prime affective reactivity generally, with the specific nature of the response determined by environmental cues. Alternatively, top-down perceptual biases could lead to divergent affective consequences even from a relatively undifferentiated pattern of visceral afference [31]. Such a bias may be operating, for example, when perception of an increase in heart rate triggers a panic attack.

Research in two areas suggests the importance of visceral afference in emotion and cognition, and the significance of interactions between the brain and visceral afference in the response to stress. Systemic administration of the β-blocker propranolol has been shown to selectively impair emotional memories, without a general effect on memory performance [33]. In addition, systemic administration of epinephrine or substance P has been reported to potentiate "emotional" memories in rats, and these effects can be blocked or attenuated by inactivation of the NTS or subdiaphragmatic vagotomy, or by direct infusions of β-blockers into rostral affective substrates such as the amygdala [165, 181, 272]. Further work is clearly needed in this area, but the existing data are in accord with the bidirectional interaction between rostral and caudal central substrates in the control of emotional and autonomic reactivity.

A second literature on brain–immune interactions further supports the potential importance of visceral afference in emotional states and the response to stress. There are common elements to the physiological response to a wide range of stressors. Pathogens, for example, result in pituitary-adrenocortical and sympathetic activation, characteristic of the response to psychological stress, and psychological stressors may trigger features of the "illness" response to pathogens, including anorexia and fever [150, 268, 269]. The cytokine, interleukin-1-β (IL-1) appears to mediate many of the neural, endocrine, immunological, and behavioral consequences of injury and infection [149]. The fever associated with pathogens may be due to central actions of IL-1, as it can be mimicked by ICV infusions of IL-1, and blocked by ICV infusions of IL-1 antagonists [150, 268]. Similarly, IL-1 antagonists block the enhanced fear conditioning and impaired escape learning produced by inescapable shock [149]. These central components of the stress response appear to be dependent on visceral afferent signals, as subdiaphragmatic vagotomy largely blocks the increase in body temperature and pain sensitivity associated with pathogens and with psychological stressors [150, 268, 269].[7]

The precise implications of the latter findings for anxiety are unclear, but these studies serve to illustrate the powerful peripheral/central inter-

actions that are mediated by visceral afference. At the present time, the role of visceral afference in anxiety remains largely speculative, although the model of Fig. 29.5 clearly reveals a basis for such an afferent influence. The role of visceral afference in anxiety and anxiety disorders is an especially important area for future research.

9 Overview

The relations between anxiety and autonomic function are far from simple. To some extent, the complexity in the literature likely derives from the diversity of anxiety disorders, the intricacies of central autonomic control, and the multiple neural systems and processes involved in anxiety states. The proposed model is offered to provide a more comprehensive neurobiological organizing framework, to facilitate the elucidation of the relations between anxiety states, central mechanisms, and autonomic functions. The model is intended to expand and develop, rather than supplant, existing perspectives. Two important features of the present model are the involvement of the basal forebrain cholinergic system in the cognitive aspects of anxiety, and the detailing of ascending routes by which visceral afference may modulate rostral components of the system.

The proposed model, of course, does not provide a complete account of systems and structures involved in anxiety and autonomic control. Indeed, we included only enough detail to illustrate potential bases for the cognitive contributions to anxiety and autonomic control, the relationships with existing neural models, and the possible routes by which visceral afference may modulate activity in these central substrates.

There are several directions that will be important in future development of the model, and further illumination of the relations between behavioral states and autonomic function. First, it will be important to clarify behavioral features and implications of the model. This includes an elucidation of the specific range of psychological/

behavioral processes that are influenced by the basal forebrain cholinergic system, as well as the precise nature of this influence. Similarly, there is a need for refinement in our understanding of behavioral-autonomic relations, and the specific classes, features or dimensions of anxiety states that are associated with patterns of autonomic control. Second, further research is necessary to illuminate the autonomic components of the model. This will require attention to the multiple modes of autonomic control, including the potential origins of these autonomic patterns and their relations to behavioral states and processes. This includes clarification of the role of visceral afference in anxiety and cognition, at both neural and behavioral levels. Finally, it will be important to further specify the multiple neural systems and structures underlying fear and anxiety, and the mechanisms underlying these contributions.

The relations between neural systems, anxiety and autonomic control are intricate indeed, and the literature on autonomic function in anxiety states is at times bewildering. The nature and origin of these relations are of sufficient importance, however, that further research and especially the development of organizing perspectives will be well worthwhile.

Acknowledgements

Preparation of this manuscript was supported in part by a grant from the NHLBI (HL52321) and by a Research Scientist Development Award to M. S. (KO2MH01072).

Notes

1. There have been varied conceptualizations of the relations between fear and anxiety, although fear is often considered a more direct action disposition to explicit proximal stimuli (e.g. those paired with pain), whereas anxiety is characterized by a more generalized reaction to a broader range of contextual stimuli or a more global apprehension [9, 53, 170]. Of additional relevance to the present consideration is the relation between transient, experimentally induced anxiety and chronic anxiety disorders. It would appear that patients with chronic anxiety disorders are characterized by a more potent disposition toward anxiety reactions than subjects merely experiencing transient, situationally induced anxiety [9]. Although there may be distinctions between transient and chronic anxiety states, and between different anxiety disorders, all serious neurobiological models of anxiety recognize some commonality to substrates underlying these disparate manifestations [5, 6, 53, 84, 85, 142]. This is supported by brain imaging studies in anxiety patients that reveal areas of cortical and subcortical activation in structures and systems that have been implicated in laboratory models of transient fear and anxiety [55, 204]. Although a detailed neuropsychological model of the relative contributions of neural systems and functional processes underlying distinct aspects of anxiety disorders will be important ultimately, it is beyond the scope of the present chapter.

2. The concepts of allostatic (allo meaning "other") and allodynamic regulation represent expansions of the homeostatic model, in recognition of the contribution of rostral neural systems in the broader integration and orchestration of behavioral, autonomic and neuroendocrine reactions to adaptive challenge [15, 163, 247]. These reactions may entail direct modulations of central autonomic outflows, alterations of homeostatic setpoints and compensatory adjustments among interacting systems that do not adhere to the simple homeostatic model.

3. Linear functions in biological systems are uncommon. The quantitative biophysical model of Dexter et al. [54], however, suggest that the essential linearity of the vagal effect on heart period is a resultant of two nonlinear processes. The first is a negatively accelerating function relating vagal frequency to the quantity of acetylcholine released at the sinus node, and the second is a positively accelerating function relating the concentration of acetylcholine in the synaptic region to the prolongation of the sinus rhythm.

4. There may be species- and even individual-differences in the maximal effects of vagal activity. Some studies suggest a plateau in vagal effects, whereas others report a relative linearity to the point of cardiac arrest.

5. The chronotropic effects of sympathetic activation have been reported to be enhanced by concurrent vagal activity, a phenomenon termed accentuated antagonism that is assumed to represent an interaction among the autonomic innervations of the sinoatrial node [145]. The magnitude of this interaction, however, may be substantially overestimated by the common use of heart rate rather than heart period in this literature [200]. Considerable species differences have been reported in autonomic interactions, and accentuated antagonism has not yet been documented in human subjects. More recently, neuropeptide Y which is co-localized with norepinephrine in many sympathetic terminals, has been found to be released with high frequency activation and may produce a profound effect of vagal chronotropic control [267]. Consequently, there remains some ambiguity in the precise form of the upper right corner of the effector surface of Fig. 29.1.

6. Behavioral drug effects are often "explained" by their neurochemical effects, e.g. the anxiolytic effects of BZR agonists are "explained" by their allosteric effects on GABAergic transmission. Such an attempt, of course, violates the doctrine that a behavioral effect first requires an explanation and reduction in the behavioral domain. To continue with an example used by Frith [73], the idea that "alien thoughts are caused by inappropriate firing of dopamine neurons" (p. 26) is unlikely to describe a productive isomorphism between the (mal)operations of neuronal circuits and function [221]. Neuropsychopharmacological theories of "anti-anxiety" effects require reductionist explanations in behavioral or cognitive terms which are presumably closer to the entities of information processing by neuronal networks of interest. In this context, it should also be noted that, as neuronal systems process information rather than emotional qualities, it is difficult to see the basis for a productive dissociation between cognition and emotion [190], although LeDoux takes a more practical approach to maintain a dissociation between cognitive and emotional variables [142].

7. The origins of the vagal signals for the common central effects of pathogens and psychological stressors is uncertain, but they may arise from vagal paraganglia, which are small clusters of neural crest-derived cells distributed along the vagus. These paraganglia appear to have chemoreceptor-like functions, have a high concentration of IL-1 receptors, and give rise to and/or synapse on vagal afferent fibers [268].

References

[1] Adolphs R, Tranel D, Damasio H, Damasio AR. Fear and the human amygdala. J Neurosci 1995; 15:5879–91.

[2] Allen GY, Cechetto DF. Functional and anatomical organization of cardiovascular pressor and depressor sites in the lateral hypothalamic area: I. Descending projections. J Comp Neurol 1992; 315:313–32.

[3] American Psychiatric Association. Diagnostic and Statistical Manual of Mental Disorders, 4th ed. Washington: American Psychiatric Association, 1994.

[4] Asmundson GJ, Stein MB. Vagal attenuation in panic disorder: an assessment of parasympathetic nervous system function and subjective reactivity to respiratory manipulations. Psychosom Med 1994; 56:187–93.

[5] Aston-Jones G, Rajkowski J, Kubiak P, Valentino RJ, Shipley MT. Role of the locus coeruleus in emotional activation. Prog Brain Res 1996; 107:379–402.

[6] Aston-Jones G, Shipley MT, Chouvet G, Ennis M, van Bockstaele E, Pieribone V, Shiekhattar R, Akaoka H, Drolet G, Astier B, Charlety P, Valentino RJ, Williams JT. Afferent regulation of locus coeruleus neurons: anatomy, physiology and pharmacology. In: Barnes CD, Pompeiano O, editors. Progress in Brain Research, vol. 88. Amsterdam: Elsevier, 1991:47–75.

[7] Aston-Jones G, Chiang C, Alexinsky T. Discharge of noradrenergic locus coeruleus neurons in behaving rats and monkeys suggests a role in vigilance. In: Barnes CD, Pompeiano O, editors. Progress in Brain Research, vol. 88. Amsterdam: Elsevier, 1991:501–20.

[8] Ballenger JC, editor. Neurobiology of Panic Disorder. New York: Wiley, 1990.

[9] Barlow DH, Chorpita BF, Turnovsky J. Fear, panic, anxiety, and disorders of emotion. Nebraska Symp Motiv 1996; 43:251–328.

[10] Beani L, Tanganelli S, Antonelli T, Bianchi C. Noradrenergic modulation of cortical acetylcholine release is both direct and γ-aminobutyric acid-mediated. J Pharmacol Exp Ther 1986; 236:230–6.

[11] Beck AT, Emery G. Anxiety Disorders and Phobias: A Cognitive Perspective. New York: Basic Books, 1985.

[12] Beck CHM, Cooper SJ. The effect of the β-carboline FG 7142 on the behavior of male rats in a

living cage: An ethological analysis of social and non-social behaviour. Psychopharmacology 1986; 89:203–7.

[13] Benschop RJ, Nieuwenhuis EES, Tromp EAM, Godart GLR, Ballieux RE, van Doornen LPJ. Effects of β-adrenergic blockade on immunologic and cardiovascular changes induced by mental stress. Circulation 1994; 89:762–9.

[14] Berntson GG, Boysen ST. Cardiac indices of cognition in infants, children and chimpanzees. In: Rovee-Collier C, Lipsitt L, editors. Advances in Infancy Research, vol. 6. New York: Ablex, 1990:187–220.

[15] Berntson GG, Cacioppo JT. From homeostasis to allodynamic regulation. In: Cacioppo JT, Tassinary LG, Berntson GG, editors. Handbook of Psychophysiology. Cambridge: Cambridge University Press, 1999: in press.

[16] Berntson GG, Cacioppo JT, Binkley PF, Uchino BN, Quigley KS, Fieldstone A. Autonomic cardiac control: III. Psychological stress and cardiac response in autonomic space as revealed by pharmacological blockades. Psychophysiology 1994; 31:599–608.

[17] Berntson GG, Cacioppo JT, Quigley KS. Autonomic determinism: The modes of autonomic control, the doctrine of autonomic space, and the laws of autonomic constraint. Psychol Rev 1991; 98:459–87.

[18] Berntson GG, Cacioppo JT, Quigley KS. Cardiac psychophysiology and autonomic space in humans: Empirical perspectives and conceptual implications. Psychol Bull 1993; 114:296–322.

[19] Berntson GG, Cacioppo JT, Quigley KS. Autonomic cardiac control. I. Estimation and validation from pharmacological blockades. Psychophysiology 1994; 31:572–85.

[20] Berntson GG, Cacioppo JT, Quigley KS. The metrics of cardiac chronotropism: biometric perspectives. Psychophysiology 1995; 32:162–71.

[21] Berntson GG, Cacioppo JT, Quigley KS, Fabro VJ. Autonomic space and psychophysiological response. Psychophysiology 1994; 31:44–61.

[22] Berntson GG, Hart S, Ruland S, Sarter M. A central cholinergic link in the cardiovascular effects of the benzodiazepine receptor partial inverse agonist FG 7142. Behav Brain Res 1996; 74:91–103.

[23] Berntson GG, Hart S, Sarter M. The cardiovascular startle response: anxiety and the benzodiazepine receptor complex. Psychophysiology 1997; 34:348–57.

[24] Berntson GG, Sarter M, Ruland S, Hart S, Ronis V. Benzodiazepine receptor agonists and inverse agonists yield concordant rather than opposing effects on startle responses. J Psychopharmacol 1996; 10:309–12.

[25] Brezenoff HE, Giuliano R. Cardiovascular control by cholinergic mechanisms in the central nervous system. Ann Rev Pharmacol Toxicol 1982; 22:341–81.

[26] Buchanan SL, Thompson RH, Maxwell BL, Powell DA. Efferent connections of the medial prefrontal cortex in the rabbit. Exp Brain Res 1994; 100:469–83.

[27] Bunney WE Jr., Tallman JF. New biological research relevant to anxiety. Pharmacopsychiatr Neuro-Psychopharmacol 1980; 13:273–6.

[28] Butler PD, Weiss JM, Stout JC, Nemeroff CB. Corticotropin-releasing factor produces fear-enhancing and behavioral activating effects following infusions into the locus coeruleus. J Neurosci 1990; 10:176–83.

[29] Cacioppo JT. Social neuroscience: autonomic, neuroendocrine, and immune responses to stress. Psychophysiology 1994; 31:113–28.

[30] Cacioppo JT, Berntson GG, Binkley PF, Quigley KS, Uchino BN, Fieldstone A. Autonomic cardiac control. II. Basal response, noninvasive indices, and autonomic space as revealed by autonomic blockades. Psychophysiology 1994; 31:586–98.

[31] Cacioppo JT, Berntson GG, Klein DJ. What is an emotion? The role of somatovisceral afference, with specific emphasis on somatovisceral "illusions." Rev Pers Social Psychol 1992; 14:63–98.

[32] Cacioppo JT, Berntson GG, Klein DJ, Poehlmann KM. The psychophysiology of emotion across the lifespan. Ann Rev Gerontol Geriatr 1998; 17:27–74.

[33] Cahill L, Prins B, Weber M, McGaugh JL. β-Adrenergic activation and memory for emotional events. Nature 1994; 371:702–4.

[34] Campeau S, Davis M. Involvement of subcortical and cortical afferents to the lateral nucleus of the amygdala in fear conditioning measured with fear-potentiated startle in rats trained concurrently with auditory and visual conditioned stimuli. J Neurosci 1995; 15:2312–27.

[35] Cannon WB. The James–Lange theory of emotions: a critical examination and an alternative theory. Am J Psychol 1927; 39:106–24.

[36] Cannon WB. The mechanism of emotional disturbance of bodily functions. New Engl J Med 1928; 198:877–84.

[37] Cannon WB. The Wisdom of the Body. New York: Norton, 1932.

[38] Canteras NS, Swanson L. Projections of the ventral subiculum to the amygdala, septum, and hypothalamus: a PHAL anterograde tract-tracing study in the rat. J Comp Neurol 1992; 324:180–94.

[39] Cechetto DF, Saper CB. Role of the cerebral cortex in autonomic function. In: Loewy AD, Spyer KM, editors. Central Regulation of Autonomic Function. New York: Oxford University Press, 1990:208–23.

[40] Chachich M, Penney J, Powell DA. Subicular lesions disrupt but do not abolish classically conditioned bradycardia in rabbits. Behav Neurosci 1996; 110:707–10.

[41] Chang HT. Noradrenergic innervation of the substantia innominata: a light and electron microscopic analysis of dopamine β-hydroxylase immunoreactive elements in the rat. Expl Neurol 1989; 104: 101–12.

[42] Chen MF, Chiu TH, Lee EH. Noradrenergic mediation of the memory-enhancing effect of corticotropin-releasing factor in the locus coeruleus of rats. Psychoneuroendocrinology 1992; 17:113–24.

[43] Chwalisz K, Diener E, Gallagher D. Autonomic arousal feedback and emotional experience: evidence from the spinal cord injured. J Pers Soc Psychol 1988; 54:820–8.

[44] Clark DB, Taylor CB, Hayward C, King R, Margraf J, Ehlers A, Roth WT, Agras WS. Motor activity and tonic heart rate in panic disorder. Psychiatr Res 1990; 32:45–53.

[45] Cole BJ, Hillmann M, Seidelmann D, Klewer M, Jones GH. Effects of the BZR partial inverse agonists in elevated plus maze test of anxiety. Psychopharmacology 1995; 121:118–26.

[46] Cook EW, Melamed BG, Cuthbert BN, McNeil DW, Lang PJ. Emotional imagery and the differential diagnosis of anxiety. J Consult Clin Psychol 1988; 58:734–40.

[47] Curran VH. Benzodiazepines, memory and mood: a review. Psychopharmacology 1991; 105:1–8.

[48] Danielsen EH, Magnuson DJ, Gray TS. The central amygdaloid nucleus innervation of the dorsal vagal complex in rat: a Phaseolus vulgaris leucoagglutinin

lectin anterograde tracing study. Brain Res Bull 1989; 22:705–15.

[49] Darwin C. The Expression of Emotions in Man and Animals. New York: Appelton, 1873. Originally published in 1872.

[50] Davis M. The role of the amygdala in fear and anxiety. Ann Rev Neurosci 1992; 15:353–75.

[51] Davis M, Gendelman DS, Tischler MD, Gendelman PM. A primary acoustic startle circuit: lesion and stimulation studies. J Neurosci 1982; 2:791–805.

[52] Davis M, Rainne D, Cassell M. Neurotransmission in the rat amygdala related to fear and anxiety. Trends Neurosci 1994; 17:208–14.

[53] Davis M, Walker DL, Lee Y. Roles of the amygdala and the bed nucleus of the stria terminalis in fear and anxiety measured with the acoustic startle reflex. Possible relevance to PTSD. Ann NY Acad Sci 1998: in press.

[54] Dexter F, Levy MN, Rudy Y. Mathematical model of the changes in heart rate elicited by vagal stimulation. Circulation Res 1989; 65:1330–9.

[55] Diedrich O, Grodd W, Weiss U, Schneider F, Flor H, Birbaumer N. Amygdala activation in social phobics during Pavlovian conditioning detected by functional MRI. Psychophysiology 1997; 34(Suppl.):30.

[56] Ditto B, France C. Carotid baroreflex sensitivity at rest and during psychological stress in offspring of hypertensives and non-twin sibling pairs. Psychosom Med 1990; 52:610–20.

[57] Dorow R, Horowski R, Paschelke G, Amin M, Braestrup C. Severe anxiety induced by FG 7142, a β-carboline ligand for benzodiazepine receptors. Lancet 1983; 8:98–9.

[58] Drugan RC, Maier SF, Skolnick P, Paul SM, Crawley JN. An anxiogenic benzodiazepine receptor ligand induces learned helplessness. Eur J Pharmacol 1986; 113:453–7.

[59] Duka T, Stevens DN. Potentiation of the propunishment but not the convulsant action of the β-carboline DMCM by naltrexone. Pharmacol Biochem Behav 1986; 25:595–8.

[60] Dworkin BR, Dworkin S. Learning of physiological responses: I. Habituation, sensitization, and classical conditioning. Behav Neurosci 1990; 104:298–319.

[61] Ekman P, Levenson RW, Friesen WV. Autonomic nervous system activity distinguishes among emotions. Science 1983; 221:1208–10.

[62] Elam M, Svensson TH, Thoren P. Differentiated cardiovascular afferent regulation of locus coeruleus neurons and sympathetic nerves. Brain Res 1985; 358: 77–84.

[63] Eysenck HJ. The Biological Basis of Personality. Springfield: Thomas, 1967.

[64] Eysenck MW. Cognitive factors in clinical anxiety: potential relevance to therapy. In: Briley M, File SE, editors. New Concepts in Anxiety. Boca Raton, FL: CRC Press, 1991:418–33.

[65] Faravelli C, Marinoni M, Spiti R, Ginanneschi A, Serena A, Fabbri C, Di Matteo C, Del Mastio M, Inzitari D. Abnormal brain hemodynamic responses during passive orthostatic challenge in panic disorder. Am J Psychiatr 1997; 154:378–83.

[66] Felder RB, Mifflin SW. Baroreceptor and chemoreceptor afferent processing in the solitary tract nucleus. In: Barraco IRA, editor. Nucleus of the Solitary Tract. Boca Raton, FL: CRC Press, 1994:169–85.

[67] File SE, Pellow S. The anxiogenic action of FG 7142 in the social interaction test is reversed by CDP and Ro 15-1788 but not CGS 8216. Arch Int Pharmacodyn 1984; 271:198–205.

[68] File SE, Pellow S. Triazolobenzodiazepines antagonize the effects of anxiogenic drugs mediated at three central nervous system sites. Neurosci Lett 1985; 61:115–9.

[69] Fitzgerald RD, Stainbrook GL, Francisco D. Classically conditioned bradycardia and skeletal-motor activity in restrained rats. Physiol Psychol 1985; 13:211–6.

[70] Fort P, Khateb A, Pegna A, Mühlethaler M, Jones BE. Noradrenergic modulation of cholinergic nucleus basalis neurons demonstrated by an in vitro pharmacological and immunohistochemical evidence in the guinea-pig brain. Eur J Neurosci 1995; 7:1502–11.

[71] Fowles DC. Heart rate as an index of anxiety: failure of a hypothesis. In: Cacioppo JT, Petty RE, editors. Perspectives in cardiovascular psychophysiology. New York: Guilford, 1982:93–127.

[72] Freedman RR, Ianni P, Ettedgui E, Puthezhath N. Ambulatory monitoring of panic disorder. Arch Gen Psychiatr 1985; 42:244–8.

[73] Frith CD. The Cognitive Neuropsychology of Schizophrenia. Hove, UK: Lawrence Erlbaum, 1991.

[74] Frysztak RJ, Neafsey EJ. The effect of medial frontal cortex lesions on cardiovascular conditioned emotional responses in the rat. Brain Res 1994; 643:181–93.

[75] Gardner CR, Tully WR, Gedecock JR. The rapidly expanding range of neuronal benzodiazepine receptor ligands. Prog Neurobiol 1992; 40:1–61.

[76] Gentil V, Gorenstein C, Camargo C, Singer JM. Effects of flunitrazepam on memory and their reversal by two antagonists. J Clin Pharmacol 1989; 9:191–7.

[77] Gentil V, Tavares S, Gorenstein C, Bello C, Mathias L, Gronich G, Singer J. Acute reversal of flunitrazepam effects by Ro15-1788 and Ro15-3505 inverse agonism, tolerance, and rebound. Psychopharmacology 1990; 100:54–9.

[78] Gerardi RJ, Keane TM, Cahoon BJ, Klauminzer GW. An in vivo assessment of physiological arousal in posttraumatic stress disorder. J Abnorm Psychol 1994; 103:825–7.

[79] Ginn SR, Powell DA. Nucleus basalis lesions attenuate acquisition, but not retention, of Pavlovian heart rate conditioning and have no effects on eyeblink conditioning. Exp Brain Res 1992; 89:501–10.

[80] Goetz RR, Klein DF, Gully R, Kahn J, Liebowitz MR, Fryer AJ, Gorman JM. Panic attacks during placebo procedures in the laboratory. Physiology and symptomatology. Arch Gen Psychiatr 1993; 50:280–5.

[81] Graeff F, Silveira MCL, Nogueira RL, Audi EA, Oliveira RMW. Role of the amygdala and periaqueductal gray in anxiety and panic. Behav Brain Res 1993; 58:123–31.

[82] Graham FK. An affair of the heart. In: Coles MGH, Jennings JR, Stern JA, editors. Psychophysiological Perspectives: Festschrift for Beatrice and John Lacey. New York: Van Nostrand Reingold, 1984:171–87.

[83] Gray JA. The neuropsychology of anxiety. Br J Psychol 1978; 69:417–34.

[84] Gray JA. The Psychology of Fear and Stress. Cambridge: Cambridge University Press, 1987.

[85] Gray JA, McNaughton N. The neuropsychology of anxiety: reprise. Nebraska Symp Motiv 1996; 43:61–134.

[86] Gray JA, Whattley SA, Snape M. The neuropsychology of anxiety and tolerance for stress. In: Briley M, File SE, editors. New Concepts in Anxiety. Boca Raton, FL: CRC Press, 1991:13–38.

[87] Green S. Benzodiazepines, putative anxiolytics and animal models of anxiety. Trends Neurosci 1991; 14:101–4.

[88] Grillon C, Ameli R, Goddard A, Woods SW, Davis M. Baseline and fear-potentiated startle in panic disorder patients. Biol Psychiatr 1994; 35:431–9.

[89] Guyenet PG. Role of the ventral medulla oblongata in blood pressure regulation. In: Loewy AD, Spyer KM, editors. Central Regulation of Autonomic Function. New York: Oxford, 1990:145–67.

[90] Hamm AO, Cuthbert BN, Globisch J, Vaitl D. Fear and the startle reflex: blink modulation and autonomic response patterns in animal and mutilation fearful subjects. Psychophysiology 1997; 34:97–107.

[91] Hardy SGP, Holmes DE. Prefrontal stimulus-produced hypotension in rat. Exp Brain Res 1988; 73:249–55.

[92] Hardy SGP, Mack SM. Brainstem mediation of prefrontal stimulus-produced hypotension. Exp Brain Res 1990; 79:393–9.

[93] Harris MC, Loewy AD. Neural regulation of vasopressin-containing hypothalamic neurons and the role of vasopressin in cardiovascular function. In: Loewy AD, Spyer KM, editors. Central Regulation of Autonomic Function. New York: Oxford University Press, 1990:224–46.

[94] Hart JD. Physiological responses of anxious and normal subjects to simple signal and non-signal auditory stimuli. Psychophysiology 1974; 14:443–51.

[95] Hart S, Sarter M, Berntson GG. Cardiovascular and somatic startle and defense: concordant and discordant actions of benzodiazepine receptor agonists and inverse agonists. Behav Brain Res 1998; 90:175–86.

[96] Hayward C. Psychiatric illness and cardiovascular disease risk. Epidemiol Rev 1995; 17:129–38.

[97] Heckers S, Ohtake T, Wiley RG, Lappi DA, Geula C, Mesulam M-M. Complete and selective cholinergic denervation of rat neocortex and hippocampus but not amygdala by an immunotoxin against the p75 receptor. J Neurosci 1994; 14:1271–89.

[98] Helmstetter FJ, Calcagnetti J, Fanselow MS. The β-carboline DMCM produces hypoalgesia after central administration. Psychobiology 1990; 18:293–7.

[99] Hitchcock JM, Sananes CB, Davis M. Sensitization of the startle reflex by footshock: blockade by lesions of the central nucleus of the amygdala or its efferent pathway to the brainstem. Behav Neurosci 1989; 103:509–18.

[100] Hoehn-Saric R, McLeod DR. The peripheral sympathetic nervous system: its role in pathological anxiety. Psychiatr Clin North Am 1988; 11:375–86.

[101] Hoehn-Saric R, McLeod DR. Generalized anxiety disorder in adulthood. In: Hersen M, Last CG, editors. Handbook of Child and Adult Psychopathology. New York: Pergamon, 1990:247–60.

[102] Hoehn-Saric R, McLeod DR. Somatic manifestations of normal and pathological anxiety. In: Hoehn-Saric R, McLeod DR, editors. Biology of Anxiety Disorders. Washington: American Psychiatric Press, 1993.

[103] Hoehn-Saric R, McLeod DR, Hipsley P. Is hyperarousal essential to obsessive-compulsive disorder? Diminished physiologic flexibility, but not hyperarousal, characterizes patients with obsessive-compulsive disorder. Arch Gen Psychiatr 1995; 52:688–93.

[104] Hoehn-Saric R, McLeod DR, Zimmerli WD. Somatic manifestations in women with generalized anxiety disorder: psychophysiological responses to psychological stress. Arch Gen Psychiatr 1989; 46:1113–9.

[105] Hoehn-Saric R, McLeod DR, Zimmerli WD. Symptoms and treatment responses of generalized anxiety disorder patients with high versus low levels of cardiovascular complaints. Am J Psychiatr 1989; 146:854–9.

[106] Hoehn-Saric R, McLeod DR, Zimmerli WD. Psychophysiological response patterns in panic disorder. Acta Psychiatr Scand 1991; 83:4–11.

[107] Holley LA, Turchi J, Apple C, Sarter M. Dissociation between the attentional effects of infusions of a benzodiazepine receptor agonist and an inverse agonist into the basal forebrain. Psychopharmacology 1995; 120:99–108.

[108] Hopkins DA, Ellenberger HH. Cardiorespiratory neurons in the medulla oblongata: input and output relationships. In: Armour JA, Ardell JC, editors. Neurocardiology. New York: Oxford University Press, 1994:277–307.

[109] Hurley KM, Herbert H, Moga MM, Saper CB. Efferent projections of the infralimbic cortex of the rat. J Comp Neurol 1991; 308:249–76.

[110] Ida Y, Elsworth JD, Roth RH. Anxiogenic β-carboline FG 7142 produces activation of nor-

adrenergic neurons in specific brain regions of rats. Pharmacol Biochem Behav 1991; 39:791–3.

[111] Ida Y, Tanaka M, Tsuda A, Tsujimaru S, Nagasaki N. Attenuating effect of diazepam on stress-induced increases in noradrenaline turnover in specific brain regions of rats: antagonism by Ro 15-1788. Life Sci 1985; 37:2491–8.

[112] Impaerato A, Dazzi L, Serra M, Gessa GL, Biggio G. Differential effects of abecarnil on basal release of acetylcholine and dopamine in the rat brain. Eur J Pharmacol 1994; 261:205–8.

[113] Inui K, Murase S, Nosaka S. Facilitation of the arterial baroreflex by the ventrolateral part of the midbrain periaqueductal grey matter in rats. J Physiol 1994; 477:89–101.

[114] Inui K, Nomura J, Murase S, Nosaka S. Facilitation of the arterial baroreflex by the preoptic area in anaesthetized rats. J Physiol 1995; 488:521–31.

[115] Iwata J, Chida K, LeDoux JE. Cardiovascular responses elicited by stimulation of neurons in the central amygdaloid nucleus in awake but not anesthetized rats resemble conditioned emotional responses. Brain Res 1987; 418:183–8.

[116] Iwata J, LeDoux JE. Dissociation of associative and nonassociative concomitants of classical fear conditioning in the freely behaving rat. Behav Neurosci 1988; 102:66–76.

[117] James W. What is an emotion? Mind 1884; 9:188–205.

[118] Jhamandas JH, Renaud LP. Diagonal band neurons may mediate arterial baroreceptor input to hypothalamic vasopressin-secreting neurons. Neurosci Lett 1986; 65:214–8.

[119] Jinks AL, McGregor IS. Modulation of anxiety-related behaviours following lesions of the prelimbic or infralimbic cortex in the rat. Brain Res 1997; 772:181–90.

[120] Jodo E, Chiang C, Aston-Jones G. Potent excitatory influence of prefrontal cortex activity on noradrenergic locus coeruleus neurons. Neuroscience 1998; 83:63–79.

[121] Jones BE, Yang TZ. The efferent projections from the reticular formation and the locus coeruleus studied by anterograde and retrograde axonal transport in the rat. J Comp Neurol 1985; 242:56–92.

[122] Hopkins DA, Ellenberger HH. Cardiorespiratory neurons in the medulla oblongata: input and output relationships. In: Armour JA, Ardell JC, editors. Neurocardiology. New York: Oxford University Press, 1994:277–307.

[123] Kalin NH, Shelton SE, Turner JG. Effects of alprazolam on fear-related behavioral, hormonal, and catecholamine responses in infant rhesus monkeys. Life Sci 1991; 49:2031–44.

[124] Kalin NH, Shelton SE, Turner JG. Effects of β-carboline on fear-related behavioral and neurohormonal responses in infant rhesus monkeys. Biol Psychiatr 1992; 31:1008–19.

[125] Kapp BS, Pascoe JP, Bixler MA. The amygdala: a neuroanatomical systems approach to its contribution to aversive conditioning. In: Squire LR, Butters N, editors. The Neuropsychology of Memory. New York: Guilford, 1984:473–88.

[126] Kawachi I, Colditz GA, Ascherio A, Rimm EB, Giovannucci E, Stampfer MJ, Willett WC. Prospective study of phobic anxiety and risk of coronary heart disease in men. Circulation 1994; 89:1992–7.

[127] Kelly D. Anxiety and emotions: physiological basis and treatment. Springfield: Thomas, 1980.

[128] Kelly D, Brown CC, Shaffer JW. A comparison of physiological measurements on anxious patients and normal controls. Psychophysiology 1970; 6:429–41.

[129] Kessler RC, Sonnega A, Bromet E, Hughes M, Nelson CB. Posttraumatic stress disorder in the national comorbidity survey. Arch Gen Psychiatr 1995; 52:1048–60.

[130] Kimura A, Sato A, Sato Y, Trzebski A. Role of the central and arterial chemoreceptors in the response of gastric tone and motility to hypoxia, hypercapnia and hypocapnia in rats. J Autonom Nerv Syst 1993; 45:77–85.

[131] Klorman R, Weissberg RP, Wiesenfeld AR. Individual differences in fear and autonomic reactions to affective stimulation. Psychophysiology 1977; 14:45–51.

[132] Koelega HS. Benzodiazepines and vigilance performance: a review. Psychopharmacology 1989; 98:145–56.

[133] Koizumi K, Kollai M. Control of reciprocal and non-reciprocal action of vagal and sympathetic efferents: study of centrally induced reactions. J Autonom Nerv Syst 1981; 3:483–501.

[134] Koizumi K, Kollai M. Multiple modes of operation of cardiac autonomic control: development of the

ideas from Cannon and Brooks to the present. J Autonom Nerv Syst 1992; 41:19–30.

[135] Kollai M, Kollai B. Cardiac vagal tone in generalized anxiety disorder. Br J Psychiatr 1992; 161:831–5.

[136] Kosslyn SM, Shin LM, Thompson WL, McNally RJ, Rauch SL, Pitman RK, Albert NM. Neural effects of visualizing and perceiving aversive stimuli: a PET investigation. Neuroreport 1996; 7:1569–76.

[137] Lader MH, Wing I. Physiological Measures, Sedative Drugs, and Morbid Anxiety. Oxford, London: Maudsley Monograph # 14, 1966.

[138] Lane RD, Reiman EM, Bradley MM, Lang PJ, Ahern GL, Davidson RJ, Schwartz GE. Neuroanatomical correlates of pleasant and unpleasant emotion. Neuropsychologia 1997; 35:1437–44.

[139] Langer AW, McCubbin JA, Stoney CM, Hutcheson JS, Charleton JD, Obrist PA. Cardiopulmonary adjustments during exercise and an aversive reaction time task. Effects of β-adrenoreceptor blockade. Psychophysiology 1985; 22:59–68.

[140] Langley JN. The Autonomic Nervous System. Cambridge: Heffler, 1921.

[141] Lawler JE, Sanders BJ, Cox RH, O'Connor EF. Baroreflex function in chronically stressed borderline hypertensive rats. Physiol Behav 1991; 49:539–42.

[142] LeDoux JE. Emotion: clues from the brain. Ann Rev Psychol 1995; 46:209–35.

[143] Leidenheimer NJ, Schechter MD. Discriminative stimulus control by the anxiogenic β-carboline FG 7142: generalization to a physiological stressor. Pharmacol Biochem Behav 1988; 30:351–5.

[144] Levin HS, Rodnitzky RL, Mick DL. Anxiety associated with exposure to organophosphate compounds. Arch Gen Psychiatr 1976; 33:225–8.

[145] Levy MN. Cardiac sympathetic-parasympathetic interactions. Fed Proc 1984; 3:2598–602.

[146] Lewis SJ, Verberne AJM, Robinson TG, Jarrott B, Louis WJ, Beart PM. Excitotoxin-induced lesions of the central but not basolateral nucleus of the amygdala modulate the baroreceptor heart rate reflex in conscious rats. Brain Res 1989; 494:232–40.

[147] Lister RG. Anxiety and cognition. In: Briley M, File SE, editors. New Concepts in Anxiety. Boca Raton, FL: CRC Press, 1991:406–17.

[148] Magee WJ, Eaton WW, Wittchen H-C, McGonagle KA, Kessler RC. Agoraphobia, simple phobia, and social phobia in the national comorbidity survey. Arch Gen Psychiatr 1996; 53:159–68.

[149] Maier SF, Watkins LR. Intracerebroventricular interleukin-1 receptor antagonist blocks the enhancement of fear conditioning and interference with escape produced by inescapable shock. Brain Res 1995; 695:279–82.

[150] Maier SF, Watkins LR, Fleshner M. Psychoneuroimmunology: the interface between behavior, brain, and immunity. Am Psychol 1994; 49:1004–17.

[151] Malmo RB. On Emotions, Needs, and our Archaic Brain. New York: Holt, Rinehart and Winston, 1975.

[152] Maren S, Fanselow MS. Electrolytic lesions of the fimbria/fornix, dorsal hippocampus, or entorhinal cortex produce anterograde deficits in contextual fear conditioning in rats. Neurobiol Learn Mem 1997; 67:142–9.

[153] Maren S, Aharonov G, Fanselow MS. Retrograde abolition of conditional fear after excitotoxic lesions in the basolateral amygdala of rats: absence of a temporal gradient. Behav Neurosci 1996; 110:718–26.

[154] Margraf J, Taylor CB, Ehlers A, Roth WT, Agras WS. Panic attacks in the natural environment. J Nerv Ment Dis 1987; 175:558–65.

[155] Marks IM. Fears, Phobias, and Rituals. New York: Oxford University Press, 1987.

[156] Marks IM. Blood-injury phobia: a review. Am J Psychiatr 1988; 145:1207–13.

[157] Martin GK, Fitzgerald RD. Heart rate and somatomotor activity in rats during signalled escape and yoked classical conditioning. Physiol Behav 1980; 25:519–26.

[158] Mathew RJ, Ho BT, Frances DJ, Taylor DL, Weinman ML. Catecholamines and anxiety. Acta Psychiatr Scand 1982; 65:142–7.

[159] Mathews AM. Anxiety and the processing of threatening information. In: Hamilton V, Bower GH, Frijda NH, editors. Cognitive Perspectives on Emotion and Motivation (Behavioral and Social Sciences), vol. 44. Dordrecht: Kluwer, 1988:265–84.

[160] Mathews AM, Lader MH. An evaluation of forearm blood flow as a psychophysiological measure. Psychophysiology 1971; 8:509–24.

[161] Matthews KA, Woodall KL, Allen MT. Cardiovascular reactivity to stress predicts future blood pressure status. Hypertension 1993; 22:479–85.

[162] McCabe PM, Gentile CG, Markgraph CG, Teich AH, Schneiderman N. Ibotenic acid lesions of the amygdaloid central nucleus but not the lateral subthalamic area prevent the acquisition of differential Pavlovian conditioning of bradycardia in rabbits. Brain Res 1992; 580:155–63.

[163] McEwen BS, Stellar E. Stress and the individual: mechanisms leading to disease. Arch Int Med 1993; 153:2093–101.

[164] McFall ME, Murburg MM, Ko GN. Autonomic responses to stress in Vietnam combat veterans with posttraumatic stress disorder. Biol Psychiatr 1990; 27:1165–75.

[165] McGaugh JL, Cahill L, Roozendaal B. Involvement of the amygdala in memory storage: interaction with other brain systems. Proc Nat Acad Sci 1996; 93:13508–14.

[166] McGaughy J, Kaiser T, Sarter M. Behavioral vigilance following infusions of 192 IgG-saporin into the basal forebrain: selectivity of the behavioral impairment and relation to cortical AChE-positive fiber density. Behav Neurosci 1996; 110:247–65.

[167] McGaughy J, Sarter M. Behavioral vigilance in rats: task validation and effects of age, amphetamine, and benzodiazepine receptor ligands. Psychopharmacology 1995; 117:340–57.

[168] McLeod DR, Hoehn-Saric R, Porges SW, Zimmerli WD. Effects of alprazolam and imipramine on parasympathetic cardiac control in patients with generalized anxiety disorder. Psychopharmacology 1992; 107:535–40.

[169] McNaughton N. Cognitive dysfunction resulting from hippocampal hyperactivity—a possible cause of anxiety disorder? Pharmacol Biochem Behav 1997; 56:603–11.

[170] McNeil DW, Vrana SR, Melamed BG, Cuthbert BN, Lang PJ. Emotional imagery in simple and social phobia: fear versus anxiety. J Abnorm Psychol 1993; 102:212–25.

[171] Mearns J, Dunn J, Lees-Haley PR. Psychological effects of organophosphate pesticides: A review and call for research by psychologists. J Clin Psychol 1994; 50:286–94.

[172] Metherate R, Weinberger NM. Cholinergic modulation of responses to single tones produces tone-specific receptive field alterations in cat auditory cortex. Synapse 1990; 6:133–45.

[173] Middleton HC, Coull JT, Sahakian BJ, Robbins TW. Clonidine-induced changes in the spectral distribution of heart rate variability correlate with performance on a test of sustained attention. J Psychopharmacol 1994; 8:1–7.

[174] Moore H, Sarter M, Bruno JP. Bidirectional modulation of stimulated cortical acetylcholine release by benzodiazepine receptor inverse agonists. Brain Res 1993; 627:267–74.

[175] Moore H, Stuckman S, Sarter M, Bruno JP. Stimulation of cortical acetylcholine efflux by FG 7142 measured with repeated microdialysis sampling. Synapse 1995; 21:324–31.

[176] Morgan CA, Grillon C, Southwick SM, Davis M, Charney DS. Fear-potentiated startle in posttraumatic stress disorder. Biol Psychiatr 1995; 38:378–85.

[177] Morgan CA, Grillon C, Southwick SM, Davis M, Charney DS. Exaggerated acoustic startle reflex in Gulf War veterans with posttraumatic stress disorder. Am J Psychiatr 1996; 153:64–8.

[178] Nakata T, Berard W, Kogosov E, Alexander N. Effects of environmental stress on release of norepinephrine in posterior nucleus of the hypothalamus in awake rats: role of sinoaortic nerves. Life Sci 1991; 48:2021–6.

[179] Neafsey EJ. Prefrontal cortical control of the autonomic nervous system: anatomical and physiological observations. Prog Brain Res 1990; 85:147–66.

[180] Ninan PT, Insel TM, Cohen RM, Cook JM, Skolnick P, Saul SM. Benzodiazepine receptor-mediated experimental "anxiety" in primates. Science 1982; 218:1332–4.

[181] Nogueira PJ, Tomaz C, Williams CL. Contribution of the vagus nerve in mediating the memory-facilitating effects of substance P. Behav Brain Res 1994; 62:165–9.

[182] Nosaka S, Nakase N, Murata K. Somatosensory and hypothalamic inhibitions of baroreflex vagal bradycardia in rats. Pflugers Arch 1989; 413:656–66.

[183] Nutt DJ. Anxiety and its therapy: today and tomorrow. In: Briley M, File SE, editors. New Concepts in Anxiety. Boca Raton, FL: CRC Press, 1991:1–12.

[184] Nutt DJ, Glue P, Lawson C, Wilson S. Flumazenil provocation of panic attacks. Arch Gen Psychiatr 1990; 47:917–25.

[185] Obrist PA. Cardiovascular Psychophysiology: A Perspective. New York: Plenum, 1981.

[186] Öhman A. Preferential preattentive processing of threat in anxiety: preparedness and attentional biases. In: Rapee RM, editor. Current Controversies in the Anxiety Disorders. New York: Guilford, 1996:253–90.

[187] Oppenheimer SM, Cechetto DF. Cardiac chronotropic organization of the rat insular cortex. Brain Res 1990; 533:66–72.

[188] Orr SP, Lasko NB, Shalev AY, Pitman RK. Physiologic responses to loud tones in Israeli patients with posttraumatic stress disorder. J Abnorm Psychol 1995; 104:75–82.

[189] Paige SR, Reid GM, Allen MG, Newton JEO. Psychophysiological correlates of posttraumatic stress disorder in Vietnam veterans. Biol Psychiatr 1990; 27:419–30.

[190] Panksepp J. A proper distinction between affective and cognitive process is essential for neuroscientific progress. In: Ekman P, Davidson RJ, editors. The Nature of Emotion. New York: Oxford University Press, 1994:224–6.

[191] Papadopoulos GC, Parnavelas JG. Monoamine systems in the cerebral cortex: evidence for anatomical specificity. Progr Neurobiol 1991; 36:195–200.

[192] Pascoe JP, Bradley DJ, Spyer KM. Interactive responses to stimulation of the amygdaloid central nucleus and baroreceptor afferent activation in the rabbit. J Autonom Nerv Syst 1989; 26:157–67.

[193] Pellow S, File SE. The effects of putative anxiogenic compounds (FG 7142, CGS 8216 and Ro 15-1788) on the rat corticosterone response. Physiol Behav 1985; 35:587–90.

[194] Pellow S, File SE. Can anti-panic drugs antagonise anxiety produced in the rat by drugs acting at the GABA-benzodiazepine receptor complex? Neuropsychobiology 1987; 17:60–5.

[195] Phillips RG, LeDoux JE. Differential contribution of amygdala and hippocampus to cues and contextual fear conditioning. Behav Neurosci 1992; 106:274–85.

[196] Pickel VM, Van Bockstaele EJ, Chan J, Cestari DM. GABAergic neurons in rat nuclei of solitary tracts receive inhibitory-type synapses from amygdaloid efferents lacking detectable GABA-immunoreactivity. J Neurosci Res 1996; 44:436–58.

[197] Powell DA, Goldberg SR, Dauth GW, Schneiderman E, Schneiderman N. Adrenergic and cholinergic blockade of cardiovascular responses to subcortical electrical stimulation in unanesthetized rabbits. Physiol Behav 1972; 8:927–36.

[198] Powell DA, Watson K, Maxwell B. Involvement of subdivisions of the medial prefrontal cortex in learned cardiac adjustments in rabbits. Behav Neurosci 1994; 108:294–307.

[199] Quigley KS, Berntson GG. Autonomic origins of cardiac responses to nonsignal stimuli in the rat. Behav Neurosci 1990; 104:751–62.

[200] Quigley KS, Berntson GG. Autonomic interactions and chronotropic control of the heart: heart period vs. heart rate. Psychophysiology 1996; 33:605–11.

[201] Quigley KS, Sarter MF, Hart SL, Berntson GG. Cardiovascular effects of the benzodiazepine receptor partial inverse agonist FG 7142 in rats. Behav Brain Res 1994; 62:11–20.

[202] Raskin M. Decreased skin conductance response habituation in chronically anxious patients. Biol Psychol 1975; 2:309–19.

[203] Rasmussen K, Jacobs BL. Single unit activity of locus coeruleus neurons in the freely moving cat: II. Conditioning and pharmacologic studies. Brain Res 1986; 23:335–44.

[204] Rauch SL, Savage CR, Alpert NM, Fischman AJ, Jenike MA. The functional neuroanatomy of anxiety: a study of three disorders using positron emission tomography and symptom provocation. Biol Psychiatr 1997; 42:446–52.

[205] Rauch SL, Savage CR, Alpert NM, Miguel EC, Baer L, Breiter HC, Fischman AJ, Manzo PA, Moretti C, Jenike MA. A positron emission tomographic study of simple phobic symptom provocation. Arch Gen Psychiatr 1995; 52:20–8.

[206] Rauch SL, van der Kolk BA, Fisler RE, Alpert NM, Orr SP, Savage CR, Fischman AJ, Jenike MA, Pitman RK. A symptom provocation study of posttraumatic stress disorder using positron emission tomography and script-driven imagery. Arch Gen Psychiatr 1996; 53:380–7.

[207] Rawleigh JM, Kemble ED. Test specific effects of FG 7142 on isolation-induced aggression in mice. Pharmacol Biochem Behav 1992; 42:317–21.

[208] Reiner PB. Correlational analysis of central noradrenergic neuronal activity and sympathetic tone in behaving cats. Brain Res 1986; 378:86–96.

[209] Reisenzein R. The Schachter theory of emotion: two decades later. Psychol Bull 1983; 94:239–64.

[210] Robinson SE. 6-Hydroxydopamine lesion of the ventral noradrenergic bundle blocks the effect of amphetamine on hippocampal acetylcholine release. Brain Res 1986; 397:181–4.

[211] Rodgers RJ, Cole JC, Aboualfa K, Stephenson LH. Ethopharmacological analysis of the effects of putative "anxiogenic" agents in the mouse elevated plus-maze. Pharmacol Biochem Behav 1995; 52:805–13.

[212] Ronca AE, Berntson GG, Tuber DA. Cardiac orienting and habituation to auditory and vibrotactile stimuli in the infant decerebrate rat. Dev Psychobiol 1986; 18:79–83.

[213] Roth WT, Ehlers A, Taylor CB, Margraf J, Agras WS. Skin conductance habituation in panic disorder patients. Biol Psychiatr 1990; 27:1231–43.

[214] Roth WT, Margraf J, Ehlers A, Taylor CB, Maddock RJ, Davies S, Agras WS. Stress test reactivity in panic disorder. Arch Gen Psychiatr 1992; 49:301–10.

[215] Roth WT, Telch MJ, Taylor CB, Sachitano JA, Gallen CC, Kopell ML, McClenahan KL, Agras WS, Pfefferbaum A. Autonomic characteristics of agoraphobia with panic attacks. Biol Psychiatr 1986; 21:1133–54.

[216] Saiers JA, Richardson R, Campbell BA. Disruption and recovery of the orienting response following shock or context change in preweanling rats. Psychophysiology 1990; 27:45–56.

[217] Sananes CB, Campbell BA. Role of central nucleus of the amygdala in olfactory heart rate conditioning. Behav Neurosci 1989; 103:519–25.

[218] Sanger DJ. Animal models of anxiety and the screening and development of novel antianxiety drugs. In: Boulton A, Baker G, Martin-Iverson M, editors. Animal Models in Psychiatry, vol. II. Clifton, NJ: Human Press, 1991:147–98.

[219] Sanger DJ, Cohen C. Fear and anxiety induced by benzodiazepine receptor inverse agonists. In: Sarter M, Nutt DJ, Lister RG, editors. Benzodiazepine Receptor Inverse Agonists. New York: Wiley-Liss, 1995:185–212.

[220] Santajuliana D, Zukowska-Grojec Z, Osborn JW. Contribution of α- and β-adrenoceptors and neuropeptide-y to autonomic dysreflexia. Clin Autonom Res 1995; 5:91–7.

[221] Sarter M, Berntson GG, Cacioppo JT. Brain imaging and cognitive neuroscience: toward strong inference in attributing function to structure. Am Psychol 1996; 51:13–21.

[222] Sarter M, Bruno JP. Cognitive functions of cortical ACh [acetylcholine]: lessons from studies on the trans-synaptic modulation of activated efflux. Trends Neurosci 1994; 17:217–21.

[223] Sarter M, Bruno JP. Cognitive functions of cortical acetylcholine: toward a unifying hypothesis. Brain Res Rev 1997; 23:28–46.

[224] Sarter M, Bruno JP. Trans-synaptic stimulation of cortical acetylcholine and enhancement of attentional functions: A rational approach for the development of cognition enhancers. Behav Brain Res 1997; 83:7–15.

[225] Sarter M, Bruno JP, Himmelheber AM. Cortical acetylcholine and attention: neuropharmacological and cognitive principles directing treatment strategies for cognitive disorders. In: Brioni JE, Decker MW, editors. Pharmacological Treatment of Alzheimer's Disease: Molecular and Neurobiological Foundations. New York: Wiley-Liss, 1997:105–28.

[226] Sarter M, Markowitsch HJ. Collateral innervation of the medial and lateral prefrontal cortex by amygdaloid, thalamic and brain-stem neurons. J Comp Neurol 1984; 224:445–60.

[227] Sarter M, Markowitsch HJ. Involvement of the amygdala in learning and memory: a critical review with emphasis on anatomical relations. Behav Neurosci 1985; 99:342–80.

[228] Sarter M, Markowitsch HJ. The amygdala's role in human mnemonic processing. Cortex 1985; 21:7–24.

[229] Sarter M, McGaughy J, Holley LA, Dudchenko P. Behavioral facilitation and cognition enhancement. In: Sarter M, Nutt DJ, Lister RG, editors. Benzodiazepine Receptor Inverse Agonists. New York: Wiley-Liss, 1995:213–42.

[230] Schachter S, Singer JE. Cognitive, social, and physiological determinants of emotional state. Psychol Rev 1962; 69:379–99.

[231] Schwaber JS, Kapp BS, Higgins GA, Rapp PR. Amygdaloid and basal forebrain direct connections with the nucleus of the solitary tract and the dorsal motor nucleus. J Neurosci 1982; 10:1424–38.

[232] Schwartz GE, Weinberger DA, Singer JA. Cardiovascular differentiation of happiness, sadness, anger, and fear following imagery and exercise. Psychosom Med 1981; 43:343–64.

[233] Semba K, Reiner PB, McGerr EG, Fibiger HC. Brainstem afferents to the magnocellular basal forebrain studied by axonal transport, immunohistochemistry, and electrophysiology in the rat. J Comp Neurol 1988; 267:433–53.

[234] Shalev AY, Orr SP, Pitman RK. Psychophysiologic response during script-driven imagery as an outcome measure in posttraumatic stress disorder. J Clin Psychiatr 1992; 53:324–6.

[235] Shalev AY, Orr SP, Pitman RK. Psychophysiologic assessment of traumatic imagery in Israeli civilian patients with posttraumatic stress disorder. Am J Psychiatr 1993; 150:620–4.

[236] Shekar A, Sims LS, Bowsher RR. GABA receptors in the region of the dorsomedial hypothalamus of rats regulate anxiety in the elevated plus-maze test. II. Physiological measures. Brain Res 1993; 627:17–24.

[237] Shih CD, Chan SH, Chan JY. Participation of hypothalamic paraventricular nucleus in the locus coeruleus-induced baroreflex suppression in rats. Am J Physiol 1995; 269:H46–52.

[238] Short KR, Maier SF. Stressor controllability, social interaction and benzodiazepine systems. Pharmacol Biochem Behav 1993; 45:827–35.

[239] Singewald N, Zhou GY, Schneider C. Release of excitatory and inhibitory amino acids from the locus coeruleus of conscious rats by cardiovascular stimuli and various forms of acute stress. Brain Res 1995; 704:42–50.

[240] Smith CA, Ellsworth PC. Patterns of appraisal and emotion related to taking an exam. J Pers Soc Psychol 1987; 52:475–88.

[241] Smith OA, Astley CA, Devito JL, Stein JM, Walsh RE. Functional analysis of hypothalamic control of the cardiovascular responses accompanying emotional behavior. Fed Proc 1980; 39:2487–94.

[242] Spyer KM. Neural mechanisms involved in cardiovascular control during affective behavior. Trends Neurosci 1989; 12:506–13.

[243] Spyer KM. The central nervous organization of reflex circulatory control. In: Loewy AD, Spyer KM, editors. Central Regulation of Autonomic Function. New York: Oxford University Press, 1990:1168–88.

[244] Stein MB, Tancer ME, Uhde TW. Heart rate and plasma norepinephrine responsivity to orthostatic challenge in anxiety disorders. Arch Gen Psychiatr 1992; 49:311–7.

[245] Stephensen RB, Smith OA, Scher AM. Baroreflex regulation of heart rate in baboons during different behavioral states. Am J Physiol 1981; 241:277–85.

[246] Steptoe A, Sawada Y. Assessment of baroreceptor reflex function during mental stress and relaxation. Psychophysiology 1989; 26:140–7.

[247] Sterling P, Eyer J. Allostasis: a new paradigm to explain arousal pathology. In: Fisher S, Reason J, editors. Handbook of Life Stress, Cognition and Health. New York: Wiley, 1988:629–49.

[248] Stock G, Schlör Y, Heidt H, Russ J. Psychomotor behavior and cardiovascular patterns during stimulation of the amygdala. Pflügers Arch 1978; 376:177–84.

[249] Stoehr JD, Wenk GL. Effects of age and lesions of the nucleus basalis on contextual fear conditioning. Psychobiology 1995; 23:173–7.

[250] Sultzer DL, Levin HS, Mahler ME, High WM, Cummings JL. A comparison of psychiatric symptoms in vascular dementia and Alzheimer's disease. Am J Psychiatr 1993; 150:1806–12.

[251] Swiergiel AH, Takahashi LK, Rubin WW, Kalin NH. Antagonism of corticotropin-releasing factor receptors in the locus coeruleus attenuates shock-induced freezing in rats. Brain Res 1992; 7:263–8.

[252] Szerb JC. Cortical acetylcholine release and electroencephalographic arousal. J Physiol 1967; 192:329–43.

[253] Taylor CB, Sheikh J, Agras S, Roth WT, Margraf J, Ehlers A, Maddock RJ, Gossard D. Ambulatory heart rate changes in patients with panic attacks. Am J Psychiatr 1986; 143:478–84.

[254] Thayer JF, Friedman BH, Borkovec TD. Autonomic characteristics of generalized anxiety disorder and worry. Biol Psychiatr 1996; 39:255–66.

[255] Thiebot MH, Dangoumau L, Richard G, Puech AJ. Safety signal withdrawal: a behavioral paradigm sensitive to both "anxiolytic" and "anxiogenic" drugs under identical experimental conditions. Psychopharmacology 1991; 103:415–24.

[256] Thiebot MH, Soubrie P, Sanger D. Anxiogenic properties of beta-CCE and FG 7142: a review of promises and pitfalls. Psychopharmacology 1988; 94:452–63.

[257] Tuber DS, Berntson GG, Bachman DS, Allen JN. Associative learning in premature hydranencephalic and normal twins. Science 1980; 210:1035–7.

[258] Turner JR. Cardiovascular Reactivity and Stress: Patterns of Physiological Response. New York: Plenum, 1994.

[259] Valins S. Cognitive effects of false heart-rate feedback. J Pers Soc Psychol 1966; 4:400–8.

[260] Van der Kooy D, Koda LY, McGinty JF, Gerfen CR, Bloom FE. The organization of projections from the cortex, amygdala, and hypothalamus to the nucleus of the solitary tract in rat. J Comp Neurol 1984; 224:1–24.

[261] Verberne AJM, Owens NC. Cortical modulation of the cardiovascular system. Prog Neurobiol 1998; 54:149–68.

[262] Villacres EC, Hollifield M, Katon WJ, Wilkinson CW, Veith RC. Sympathetic nervous system activity in panic disorder. Psychiatr Res 1987; 21:313–21.

[263] Vrana SR. Emotional modulation of skin conductance and eyeblink responses to startle probe. Psychophysiology 1995; 32:351–7.

[264] Wachtel PI. Concepts of broad and narrow attention. Psychol Bull 1967; 68:417–29.

[265] Wallace DM, Magnuson DJ, Gray TS. Organization of amygdaloid projections to brainstem dopaminergic, noradrenergic, and adrenergic cell groups in the rat. Brain Res Bull 1992; 28:447–54.

[266] Wallin BG, Fagius J. Peripheral sympathetic neural activity in conscious humans. Ann Rev Physiol 1988; 50:565–76.

[267] Warner MR, Levy MN. Neuropeptide Y as a putative modulator of the vagal effects on heart rate. Circulation Res 1989; 64:882–9.

[268] Watkins LR, Maier SF, Goehler LE. Immune activation: the role of pro-inflammatory cytokines in inflammation, illness responses and pathological pain states. Pain 1995; 63:289–302.

[269] Watkins LR, Maier SF, Goehler LE. Cytokine-to-brain communication: a review and analysis of alternative mechanisms. Life Sci 1995; 57:1011–26.

[270] Weiss JM, Stout JC, Aaron MF, Quan N, Owens MJ, Butler PD, Nemeroff CB. Depression and anxiety: role of the locus coeruleus and corticotropin-releasing factor. Brain Res Bull 1994; 35:561–72.

[271] Wenger MA. Studies of autonomic balance: a summary. Psychophysiology 1966; 2:173–86.

[272] Williams CL, McGaugh JL. Reversible lesions of the nucleus of the solitary tract attenuate the memory-modulating effects of posttraining epinephrine. Behav Neurosci 1993; 107:955–62.

[273] Witvliet CV, Vrana SR. Psychophysiological responses as indices of affective dimensions. Psychophysiology 1995; 32:436–43.

[274] Yang XM, Luo ZP, Zhou JH. Behavioral evidence for the role of noradrenaline in the putative anxiogenic actions of the inverse benzodiazepine receptor agonist methyl-4-ethyl-6,7-dimethoxy-β-carboline-3-carboxylate. J Pharmacol Exp Ther 1989; 250:358–63.

[275] Young BJ, Leaton RN. Amygdala central nucleus lesions attenuate acoustic startle stimulus-evoked heart rate changes in rats. Behav Neurosci 1996; 110:228–37.

[276] Zaborszky L. Synaptic organization of basal forebrain cholinergic projection neurons. In: Levin ED, Decker MW, Butcher LL, editors. Neurotransmitter Interactions and Cognitive Function. Boston: Birkhäuser, 1992:27–65.

[277] Zaborszky L, Cullinan WE. Direct catecholaminergic-cholinergic interactions in the basal forebrain. I. Dopamine-β-hydroxylase and tyrosine hydroxylase input to cholinergic projection neurons. J Comp Neurol 1996; 374:535–54.

[278] Zaborszky L, Cullinan WE, Luine VN. Catecholaminergic-cholinergic interaction in the basal forebrain. In: Cuello AC, editor. Progress in Brain Research, vol. 98. Amsterdam: Elsevier, 1993:31–49.

[279] Zardetto-Smith AM, Gray TS. Catecholamine and NPY efferents from the ventrolateral medulla to the amygdala in the rat. Brain Res Bull 1995; 38:253–60.

[280] Zhang JX, Harper RM, Ni H. Cryogenic blockade of the central nucleus of the amygdala attenuates aversively conditioned blood pressure and respiratory responses. Brain Res 1986; 386:136–45.

30

A Motivational Analysis of Emotion: Reflex–Cortex Connections

Peter J. Lang, Margaret M. Bradley, and Bruce N. Cuthbert

From the perspective of psychobiology, motivation has traditionally been defined by two basic parameters—behavioral direction and energy (Hebb, 1949). In his classic theory of learning, Hull (1943) postulated a single energy dimension of drive, having a multiplicative effect on all behaviors. More physiologically oriented thinkers (Duffy, 1957) similarly embraced the concept of general activation, linking the energetics of behavior to the brain stem reticular formation. Behavioral direction was determined by separate incentive systems, accommodating the many survival needs of fight-flight, hunger, and sex, or even a broader list including exploration and nurturance.

Pondering these same issues, Konorski (1948, 1967) proposed a theoretical reduction that integrated direction and drive, based on a classification of mammalian exteroceptive reflexes. In his view, all reinforcers were presumed to have both motivational and sensory-behavioral attributes. The latter attributes were many and unique to each reflex (e.g., modality of the evoking stimulus, specific efferent pattern), but the motivational attributes (responsible for reinforcement) were of only two types—either appetitive or aversive. Konorski went on to postulate two general motivational systems for all behavior: The aversive system served all protective and defensive functions; the appetitive system collectively embodied alimentary, nurturant, and procreative needs. Both were considered to be arousal systems, but their actions were reciprocal: Aversive activity decreased appetitive responses, and vice versa.

As with reflexes, emotional states and affect-evoking stimuli naturally fall into one of two classes—pleasant or unpleasant. It is suggested that pleasant states are driven by the appetitive system and unpleasant states by the aversive motivation system; energy may be mobilized equally by either system. Thus, an abstract motivational space can be defined by the orthogonal parameters of valence (pleasant/appetitive vs. unpleasant/defensive) and arousal (calm vs. excitatory), as shown in Figure 30.1 (see also Lang, Bradley, & Cuthbert, 1990). This organization parallels multivariate studies of affective language (Russell & Mehrabian, 1977). Specific emotion states (fear, anger, joy, sadness, etc.) are located in this space according to the directional properties of the implied affective action (appetitive approach vs. defensive withdrawal) and its predominantly ergotropic or trophotropic character.

This analysis is not meant to imply that emotional states differ only in their motivational characteristics. Paralleling the two attributes of reflexes, a distinction can be made between an affect's strategic motivational properties (appetitive or aversive valence and activation strength) and the tactical response patterns to a specific cue or context. These latter behaviors are highly varied and sometimes paradoxical. Thus, for example, while withdrawal is the primitive behavioral characteristic of aversive states, the tactical response to a stressor in evolved mammals can be attack (i.e., physical approach), immobility, or a displacement activity, as well as flight; however, in all cases, the aversive-defense system is presumed to be dominant. This analysis also implies that outwardly similar behaviors (e.g., predator aggression and defensive attack) can be driven by different motivational strategies.

The focus here is on the strategic motivational

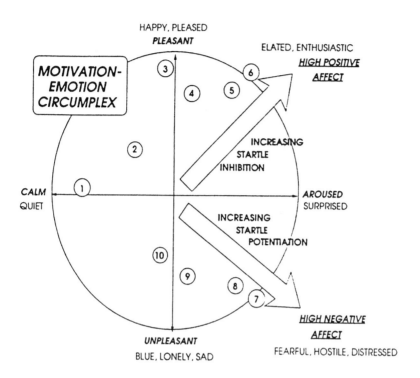

HAPPY, PLEASED
PLEASANT

ELATED, ENTHUSIASTIC
HIGH POSITIVE AFFECT

MOTIVATION-EMOTION CIRCUMPLEX

INCREASING STARTLE INHIBITION

CALM
QUIET

AROUSED
SURPRISED

INCREASING STARTLE POTENTIATION

HIGH NEGATIVE AFFECT

FEARFUL, HOSTILE, DISTRESSED

UNPLEASANT
BLUE, LONELY, SAD

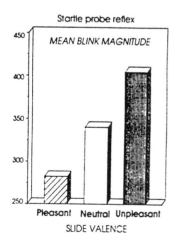

Startle probe reflex

MEAN BLINK MAGNITUDE

450

400

350

300

250

Pleasant   Neutral   Unpleasant
SLIDE VALENCE

variables that link together and organize the varying expressions of emotion, rather than on tactical affective diversity. A basic principle of this analysis is that responses activated by the same motivational system (appetitive or aversive) are synergistically augmenting, and that responses activated by different systems are mutually inhibiting. If we assume this is a general property of organisms (reliable at all levels of behavioral complexity), a simple unconditioned stimulus can become a tool for probing the underlying motivational status of emotional expression.

The reflex probe employed in our research is a startle-inducing stimulus, which prompts a protective-defensive reflex and, in theory, activates the aversive motivational system. Consistent with the above considerations, it is hypothesized that startle reflexes evoked during an ongoing appetitive emotional state (a reflex–affect mismatch) will be inhibited; startle reflexes evoked during an aversive state (a reflex–affect match) will be markedly augmented. Thus, presentation of a brief startle stimulus during a foreground task permits an affective-motivational analysis of the task's effect on the organism, and one that is not confounded by tactical differences in behavior or peripheral physiology. The procedure is straightforward, and can be accomplished in the blink of an eye.

The Probe Startle Reflex

Abruptness is the key to startle elicitation: Ideally, the risetime of the startle stimulus should be instantaneous. Although strong stimuli generate larger and more reliable reflexes than weak stimuli, high stimulus intensity is not necessary to evoke a reaction. The startle response is a progressive flexor movement, involving the entire body, and is grossly similar across mammalian species. In research with rats, the whole-body startle response is recorded as the displacement of a stabilimeter cage floor. Sudden closure of the eyelids is one of the first, fastest (occurring within 30 to 50 ms after startle stimulus onset), and most stable elements in the reflex sequence, and in recent studies of human beings, only this blink component is typically monitored. Electromyograph electrodes placed just beneath the eye (see Anthony, 1985; Lang et al., 1990) sense the bioelectric potentials produced by *orbicularis oculi* contraction, and the onset latency and magnitude of this muscle activity are recorded.

Startle Potentiation

Reflexes are, by definition, obligatory events, but it has long been known that reflex strength varies with psychological factors. Brown, Kalish, and

Figure 30.1
An emotion circumplex, defined by the dimensions of arousal and affective valence, is presented in the left panel. The open arrows show the direction of Tellegen's Positive and Negative Affect dimensions (Watson & Tellegen, 1985), which data suggest may be the paths of increasing startle inhibition and potentiation, respectively (Lang, Bradley, Cuthbert, & Patrick, in press). The numbered circles represent the approximate rated locations of photographic slides from the International Affective Picture System: 1, wicker basket; 2, nature scene; 3, happy baby; 4, chocolate sundae; 5, water skier; 6, erotic couple; 7, violent death; 8, aimed gun; 9, AIDS patient; 10, cemetery. Differences in mean startle probe magnitudes (in analog-to-digital units) for pleasant, low-arousal neutral, and unpleasant slides are presented in the right panel of the figure (from Bradley, Cuthbert, & Lang, 1990).

Farber (1951), noting that anxiety patients often show exaggerated startle responses, hypothesized that a high drive state may lead to increases in startle magnitude (Hull, 1943). Thus, animals conditioned to be fearful should show enhanced reflexes when startle probes are presented in the context of a stimulus earlier paired with electric shock. The results Brown et al. obtained conformed to expectation: Larger reflexes were evoked for probes presented in the context of conditioned stimuli, relative to control stimuli. These general findings were subsequently replicated in animals and, using the blink reflex, in human subjects (Ross, 1961).

In recent years, Davis and his associates (see Davis, 1989a, for an excellent review) have explored the neural mechanisms of this fear-potentiated startle effect in rats. Acoustic startle probes initially activate the cochlear nucleus of the brain, relaying impulses to the lateral lemniscus, and then on to the reticular formation; the output path proceeds from the reticularis pontis caudalis through spinal neurons to the reflex effectors. This is the basic obligatory circuit, directly driven by the parameters of the input stimulus (e.g., stimulus intensity, frequency, risetime). Startle potentiation by conditioned fear implies, however, a secondary circuit that connects with, and modulates, the primary pathway. Berg and Davis (1985) searched for this site by intervening directly in the neural path of the primary circuit, applying an electrical stimulus with a micro-electrode to evoke the startle response. Obligatory reflexes were obtained along the entire pathway. However, augmentation of the response due to fear conditioning was observed only when the point of electrical stimulation was earlier in the circuit than the nucleus reticularis pontis caudalis, suggesting that the modulatory and obligatory circuits intersect at this site.

Various lines of evidence indicate that, the nuclei of the amygdala may figure significantly in the second, modulatory circuit producing fear-potentiated startle. First, there are direct, monosynaptic projections from the amygdala nuclei to the reticular site; second, electrical stimulation of the amygdala (below the level for kindling) directly enhances startle reflex amplitude; finally, lesions abolish conditioned startle enhancement (see Davis, 1989a).

The amygdala receives projections from both sensory and cortical association areas, and its stimulation in humans prompts reports of tension-laden images (Halgren, 1981). In amygdala-lesioned animals trained using appetitive (sucrose) or aversive (shock) unconditioned stimuli, Cahill and McGaugh (1990) found a performance deficit only for the aversive learning task. These authors stressed that the amygdala specifically relays effects of arousal and "the release of stress-related hormones" (p. 541), and is thus part of a motivational circuit—rather than a site specific to associative linkage, as some have maintained. Attribution of motivational significance to the amygdala accords with fear sensitization studies, in which startle reflexes are potentiated without conditioning by simply administering foot shocks, prompting a general aversive state (Davis, 1989b).

Ablation and stimulation of the amygdala appear to inhibit and activate a variety of emotional states (in addition to fear) in animals, primarily those of a nocent or defensive character (Halgren, 1981). Furthermore, the amygdala projects to most visceral and somatic effector systems (e.g., respiratory, cardiovascular, facial) generally associated with emotional arousal. Thus, the amygdala-startle circuit may be the pathway of a broader aversive motivational system. At this time, however, there is essentially no animal literature on the neurophysiology of the startle phenomenon in which aversive reinforcers other than shock are employed (e.g., frustration, conflict, toxins), or in which startle probes were administered during emotional states that could not be defined as primarily fearful.

Startle Inhibition

Reward and Drive

The hypothesis that startle reflex potentiation indexes Hull's (1943) generalized Drive (D) factor prompted investigators to examine appetitive, as well as aversive, motivational states. Merryman (1952, described in Brown, 1961) recorded startle responses in fear-conditioned rats (using shock), following food deprivation. Rats who were both fearful and hungry reacted more strongly than fear-only or hungry-only animals. Brown interpreted these results as supporting the concept of generalized activation—assuming aversive and appetitive drive strengths were additive. However, subsequent studies of the startle response during food or water deprivation—which did not include fear conditioning—failed to find the expected reflex increases (Trapold, 1962), failed to replicate initial potentiation results, or, more often, found significant startle attenuation (Ison & Krauter, 1975).

Contrary to the expectations of drive theorists, startle reflexes are not typically augmented when presented in the context of conditioned positive incentives. Rather, several studies have found significantly smaller responses during presentation of cues that signaled food or water (Armus, Carlson, Guinan, & Crowell, 1964). In effect, pairing a conditioned stimulus (CS) with an appetitive unconditioned stimulus (UCS) modulates startle in a way opposite to that of pairing it with an aversive, shock UCS: In the appetitive case, probe responses tend to be inhibited during posttraining CS presentations. Furthermore, when the appetitive context is then rendered aversive, by presenting cues that are associated with the withholding of rewards and frustration (Wagner, 1963), startle amplitude is augmented, as with a punitive shock. While the findings are complex, the animal research supports the general view that startle is modulated by positive, as well as aversive, motivational systems. Unfortunately, unlike aversive startle potentiation, the neural circuitry underlying appetitive system inhibition has yet to be explored.

Attention and Emotion

In recent experiments with human subjects that demonstrate startle inhibition, the focus of investigation has been on attention rather than motivation (Anthony & Graham, 1985). Simons and Zelson (1985) obtained smaller blink reflexes to an acoustic startle probe presented while the subject viewed interesting slides (i.e., attractive nude men and women), relative to reflexes elicited during presentation of a dull slide (i.e., a basket). Whereas their explanatory hypothesis was sensory (i.e., in terms of the amount of visually directed attentional resources), it is clear that these interesting stimuli are not motivationally neutral. Pictures of attractive nudes are reliably classified as both highly pleasant and arousing (Greenwald, Cook, & Lang, 1989). As the animal research suggests, cues associated with positive incentives often prompt inhibition of probe startle responses. Thus, these effects are potentially accounted for by the mismatch between motivational systems activated by a pleasant foreground and an aversive startle probe.

Probing Human Emotion

Looking at Pictures

A study (Vrana, Spence, & Lang, 1988) exploring the general hypothesis that startle responses are inhibited for pleasant affects, and that aversive affects augment the same startle reflex, used an adaptation of Simons and Zelson's (1985) paradigm. The subject viewed a series of photographic slides while acoustic startle probes were randomly presented. The slide stimuli were selected from the International Affective Picture System (IAPS; see Lang, Öhman, & Vaitl, 1988) on the basis of normative affective ratings (see Fig. 30.1) and organized into three affective classes: unpleasant (e.g, poisonous snakes, aimed guns, pictures of violent death), pleasant (e.g., happy babies, appetizing food, attractive nudes), and neutral (e.g., umbrellas, hair dryer, other common household objects). As shown in the Figure 30.1 inset, a significant linear trend was observed over slide valence categories, with the largest startle blink responses occurring during unpleasant content and the smallest during pleasant content.

Subsequent replication in several independent experiments has confirmed that the phenomenon involves both a significant potentiation of responding during unpleasant slides and a significant inhibition during pleasant pictures relative to neutral content (see Lang et al., 1990; Lang, Bradley, Cuthbert, & Patrick, in press). The phenomenon was replicated using monaural, rather than binaural, acoustic probes, and this study obtained evidence that the affect-startle effect may be lateralized (i.e., left-ear probes, presumably conferring an advantage in right-brain processing, showed the strongest relationship with affective valence) (Bradley, Cuthbert, & Lang, 1991). Jansen and Frijda (1991), using evocative video film clips, and Hamm, Stark, and Vaitl (1990), using the IAPS slides, obtained the affect-startle effect in European subjects. Finally, we (Bradley, Cuthbert, & Lang, 1990) found the same pattern of affective modulation using visual rather than acoustic startle probes, disconfirming an alternative hypothesis that affective differences were secondary to differences in modality-directed attention (Anthony & Graham, 1985).

Other data from the above research (Bradley et al., 1990, 1991) further support the view that the affect-startle effect is specific to emotional valence. Thus, both pleasant and unpleasant slides elicited similar large skin conductance responses, and reports of greater arousal and interest value, than did neutral slides. Furthermore, subjects spent more time looking at both types of affective slides than neutral pictures when allowed to control viewing time. Only the startle blink varied linearly over slide valence categories, increasing monotonically in magnitude from pleasant, to neutral, to unpleasant contents, supporting the hypothesis that the startle reflex is potentiated or inhibited, depending specifically on whether it matches the valence of ongoing emotional perception.

Mood and Emotional Imagery

If startle modulation is determined by motivational state, rather than by sensory factors, foreground stimulation should not be necessary to show the effect. In a recent experiment (Lang et al., in press), we used a blocked stream of pleasant or unpleasant slides to establish a persisting positive or negative mood state. Probe startle responses confirmed the effectiveness of the mood induction method: Reflexes were smallest during pleasant states and largest during unpleasant states, even though probes were presented only during interstimulus intervals and not during actual slide exposure.

In a study of probe responses during emotional memories (i.e., with no proximal affective stimulus) (Vrana & Lang, 1990), reflex responses were larger when subjects remembered sentences with fearful, unpleasant content than when neutral sentences were recalled. Furthermore, this effect was enhanced in subjects instructed to vividly imagine the sentence content. Cook, Hawk, Davis, and Stevenson (1991) have replicated this affect-startle effect during emotional imagery.

Clinical Theory and Applications

Emotion and Psychopathology

Fear and anticipatory anxiety reliably potentiate the startle response. To the extent that these affects define phobic disorders, the phenomenon might be accentuated in the phobic population. Consistent with this view, Cook et al. (1991), studying imagery, observed a significantly stronger affect-startle effect for subjects reporting more frequent and intense fears. Preliminary evidence suggests that larger startle reflexes are obtained for panic patients, relative to other anxious patients (Lang et al., in press). Finally, Vrana and Constantine (1990) found a systematic reduction in potentiated blink reflexes during phobia-related imagery after desensitization therapy. These preliminary results encourage the view that startle probe analyses may be useful in assessing fear change and in discriminating among anxiety pathologies.[1]

Startle probe analysis can also be used to explore clinically significant affective deficits. Psychopaths have been described as deficient in affective response, particularly in the context of aversion and punishment (Hare, 1978). A recent study of a prison population explored the hypothesis that psychopaths should show a reduced potentiated startle to unpleasant stimuli (Patrick, Bradley, & Lang, 1991). Nonpsychopathic prisoners, like college students, showed a monotonic increase in startle magnitude from pleasant to unpleasant photographic slides. In contrast, psychopaths did not show potentiation to aversive materials—although they showed the same startle inhibition during pleasant slides as the other subjects. Differences in these startle patterns occurred despite the fact that both psychopaths and nonpsychopaths reported the unpleasant slides to be highly aversive and arousing.

Neurological Disorder

The startle probe methodology suggests at least two lines of investigation pertinent to the study of the damaged brain. First, the animal data clearly show the significance of the amygdala in the neural circuit modulating the startle response. Nearly all the basic behavioral phenomena observed in the animal research that support this analysis have been replicated in human subjects. Thus, several studies demonstrate significant startle potentiation following aversive conditioning using shock (see the discussion in Lang et al., in press), while Hamm et al. (1990), using a nonaversive UCS, found no potentiated startle effects, although skin conductance conditioning was demonstrated. Subsequent studies have shown that brief shock exposure or instructions that shock will be administered (Grillon, Ameli, Woods, Merikangas, & Davis, in press) produce the same sensitization and potentiated startle effects found in studies using rats. Use of these probe paradigms with human subjects who have suffered damage to the amygdala and associated structures will be important in determining commonalities in pathways and functions between species.

Second, the demonstration that the affect-startle effect may be stronger for left-ear than right-ear probes (Bradley et al., 1991) has significant implications for studies of brain lateralization in emotion. Two hypotheses encompass current theorizing: One holds that the right brain is dominant in processing all affects (Heilman & Bowers, 1990), whereas the other suggests that the anterior right brain is specialized in the production of aversive affects, while the left brain is specialized for positive affect (Davidson, 1984, this issue). The left-monaural startle data to date show a linear valence–reflex relationship, but are insufficient to determine whether the effect is both inhibitory and facilitatory—or stronger for either pleasant or unpleasant stimuli. If the superiority of left-ear probes is shown to pertain only to enhanced potentiation during aversive stimulation (and not appetitive inhibition), the data would encourage the second, lateralized affect-production hypothesis. Balanced modulation, however, would be consistent with the theory relating affective perception in general to right-brain processing.[2]

Conclusions: Theoretical Issues

Of immediate importance are the related problems of clarifying the role of emotional intensity in modulating probe reflex responses and of determining if startle modulation occurs generally for all positive and aversive emotions. The first issue was recently addressed by covarying valence and arousal: Probe responses were examined for equivalently pleasant slides that were high and low in arousal; a similar comparison was made for unpleasant slides (see Lang et al., in press). Skin conductance, a useful measure of sympathetic activation, increased monotonically with reported arousal, irrespective of valence. Startle modulation also increased with arousal, but the direction of effect was again specific to emotional valence. Thus, greater reflex inhibition was found for the most arousing pleasant stimuli; for unpleasant stimuli, reflex potentiation increased with arousal.

These data are consonant with Konorski's (1948) conception of opponent aversive and appetitive arousal systems, in that the different reflex modulation patterns are enhanced by increases in excitation of either affective type. The data also follow Watson and Tellegen's (1985) positive and negative affect dimensions, defined by a 45° rotation of the valence-arousal circumplex (see Fig. 30.1). This model suggests that magnitude might increase for action affects such as fear and anger, but

would be less influenced by sadness, helplessness, or depression, which are equally unpleasant, but may involve low activation. Similarly, little reflex inhibition would be found in contented relaxation, whereas sexual pleasure, elation, or enthusiasm should produce clear reflex attenuation.[3]

Regardless of the ultimate resolution of these issues, the startle probe has already demonstrated its value in exploring the organization of emotion. Preliminary success in differentiating clinical groups suggests, furthermore, that it may prove useful in examining individual differences in temperament. Startle probes have been employed with infants in research on attention (Anthony & Graham, 1985). We do not yet know, however, the developmental course of the affect-startle effect, or whether early response patterns might be different, for example, in shy, fearful children than in children who are more action oriented and socially outgoing (Kagan, Reznick, & Snidman, 1989). Indeed, an important virtue of the startle probe methodology is its suitability for a broad variety of populations—with or without language skills, and including the functionally disordered and neurologically impaired. This same paradigmatic generality links human research to animal models, confirming the evolutionary continuity of basic motivational variables, connecting complex human affects to basic reflexes, and guiding investigation of the relevant emotion structures and circuits in the brain.

Acknowledgments

Preparation of this article and much of the research described were supported in part by National Institute of Mental Health Grants MH37757, MH41950, and MH43975 and Grant AG09779 from the National Institute of Aging to Peter J. Lang.

Notes

1. Posttraumatic stress disorder is of particular interest as the clinical diagnosis is determined in part by the clinical judgment that exaggerated startle reactions are present.

2. A recent neurological case study (Morris, Bradley, Bowers, Lang, & Heilman, 1991) is interesting in this respect. The patient in question underwent a right anterior temporal lobectomy (including the amygdala) for removal of an arteriovenous malformation. His skin conductance responses to pleasant, arousing slides were larger than to neutral content, as for normal subjects; however, the parallel, normal enhanced response to arousing pictures that were aversive was not observed. These data suggest lateralized deficits specific to affective valence, and encourage efforts at replication and extension with a larger sample of patients.

3. The startle probe is only one tool for exploring a biphasic model of emotion. For example, a complementary *appetitive* probe (e.g., an olfactory stimulus that prompts salivation), used in conjunction with the same emotional perception and memory imagery paradigms already studied, would be a valuable addition. Furthermore, with respect again to the startle reflex, the neural circuit underlying modulation by the appetitive system has yet to be defined, and could be quite different from that found for aversive states—perhaps involving the attentive and preattentive mechanisms considered in studies of attention allocation. Finally, while we have speculated about activation and startle modulation, and the apparent stability of the affect-startle effect with variation in tactical affective physiologies (e.g., see Vrana & Lang, 1990, p. 195), there are as yet few data on the effects of specific behavioral dispositions and probe response, for example, during overt approach or withdrawal, in states of inhibition or restraint, with active or passive coping—all of which have interesting theoretical implications.

References

Anthony, B. J. (1985). In the blink of an eye: Implications of reflex modification for information processing. In P. K. Ackles, J. R. Jennings, & M. G. H. Coles (Eds.), *Advances in psychophysiology* (Vol. 1, pp. 167–218). Greenwich, CT: JAI Press.

Anthony, B. J., & Graham, F. (1985). Blink reflex modification by selective attention: Evidence for the modulation of "automatic" processing. *Biological Psychology,* 21, 43–59.

Armus, H. L., Carlson, K. R., Guinan, J. F., & Crowell, R. A. (1964). Effect of a secondary reinforcement stimulus on the auditory startle response. *Psychological Reports,* 14, 535–540.

Berg, W. K., & Davis, M. (1985). Associative learning modifies startle reflexes at the lateral lemniscus. *Behavioral Neuroscience,* 99, 191–199.

Bradley, M. M., Cuthbert, B. N., & Lang, P. J. (1990). Startle reflex modification: Attention or emotion? *Psychophysiology,* 27, 513–523.

Bradley, M. M., Cuthbert, B. N., & Lang, P. J. (1991). Startle and emotion: Lateral acoustic stimuli and the bilateral blink. *Psychophysiology,* 28, 285–296.

Brown, J. S. (1961). *The motivation of behavior.* New York: McGraw-Hill.

Brown, J. S., Kalish, H. I., & Farber, I. E. (1951). Conditioned fear as revealed by magnitude of startle response to an auditory stimulus. *Journal of Experimental Psychology,* 32, 317–328.

Cahill, L., & McGaugh, J. L. (1990). Amygdaloid complex lesions differentially affect retention of tasks using appetitive and aversive reinforcement. *Behavioral Neuroscience,* 104, 532–543.

Cook, E. W., III, Hawk, L. W., Jr., Davis, T. L., & Stevenson, V. E. (1991). Affective individual differences and startle reflex modulation. *Journal of Abnormal Psychology,* 100, 5–13.

Davidson, R. J. (1984). Affect, cognition, and hemispheric specialization. In C. E. Izard, J. Kagan, & R. Zajonc (Eds.), *Emotion, cognition, and behavior* (pp. 320–365). New York: Cambridge University Press.

Davis, M. (1989a). Neural systems involved in fear-potentiated startle. *Annals of the New York Academy of Sciences,* 563, 165–183.

Davis, M. (1989b). Sensitization of the acoustic startle reflex by footshock. *Behavioral Neuroscience,* 103, 495–503.

Duffy, E. (1957). The psychological significance of the concept of "arousal" and "activation." *Psychological Review*, 64, 265–275.

Greenwald, M. K., Cook, E. W., & Lang, P. J. (1989). Affective judgment and psychophysiological response: Dimensional covariation in the evaluation of pictorial stimuli. *Journal of Psychophysiology*, 3, 51–64.

Grillon, C., Ameli, R., Woods, S. W., Merikangas, K., & Davis, M. (in press). Fear-potentiated startle in humans: Effects of anticipatory anxiety on the acoustic blink reflex. *Psychophysiology*.

Halgren, E. (1981). The amygdala contribution to emotion and memory: Current studies in humans. In Y. Ben-Ari (Ed.), *The amygdaloid complex* (pp. 395–408). Amsterdam: North-Holland Elsevier.

Hamm, A., Stark, R., & Vaitl, D. (1990). Startle reflex potentiation and electrodermal response differentiation: Two indicators of two different processes in Pavlovian conditioning [Abstract]. *Psychophysiology*, 27, S37.

Hare, R. D. (1978). Electrodermal and cardiovascular correlates of psychopathy. In R. D. Hare & D. Schalling (Eds.), *Psychopathic behavior: Approaches to research* (pp. 107–143). Chichester, England: Wiley.

Hebb, D. O. (1949). *The organization of behavior: A neuropsychological theory*. New York: Wiley.

Heilman, K., & Bowers, D. (1990). Neuropsychological studies of emotional changes induced by right and left hemisphere lesions. In N. Stein, B. Leventhal, & T. Trabasso (Eds.), *Psychological and biological approaches to emotion* (pp. 97–114). Hillsdale, NJ: Erlbaum.

Hull, C. L. (1943). *Principles of behavior*. New York: Appleton-Century.

Ison, J. R., & Krauter, E. E. (1975). Acoustic startle reflexes in the rat during consummatory behavior. *Journal of Comparative and Physiological Psychology*, 89, 39–49.

Jansen, D. M., & Frijda, N. (1991). *Modulation of acoustic startle response by film-induced fear and sexual arousal*. Manuscript submitted for publication.

Kagan, J., Reznick, J. S., & Snidman, N. (1989). Issues in the study of temperament. In G. A. Kohnstamm, J. E. Bates, & M. K. Rothbart (Eds.), *Temperament in childhood* (pp. 133–144). Chichester, England: Wiley.

Konorski, J. (1948). *Conditioned reflexes and neuron organization*. Cambridge, England: Cambridge University Press.

Konorski, J. (1967). *Integrative activity of the brain: An interdisciplinary approach*. Chicago: University of Chicago Press.

Lang, P. J., Bradley, M. M., & Cuthbert, B. N. (1990). Emotion, attention, and the startle reflex. *Psychological Review*, 97, 377–398.

Lang, P. J., Bradley, M. M., Cuthbert, B. N., & Patrick, C. J. (in press). Emotion and psychopathology: A startle probe analysis. In L. Chapman & D. Fowles (Eds.), *Progress in experimental personality and psychopathology research: Models and methods of psychopathology*. New York: Springer.

Lang, P. J., Öhman, A., & Vaitl, D. (1988). *The International Affective Picture System* [Photographic slides]. Gainesville, FL: University of Florida, Center for Research in Psychophysiology.

Morris, M., Bradley, M., Bowers, D., Lang, P., & Heilman, K. (1991). Valence-specific hypoarousal following right temporal lobectomy [Abstract]. *Journal of Clinical and Experimental Neuropsychology*, 13, 42.

Patrick, C. J., Bradley, M. M., & Lang, P. J. (1991). *Emotion in the criminal psychopath: Startle reflex modification*. Manuscript submitted for publication.

Ross, L. E. (1961). Conditioned fear as a function of CS-UCS and probe stimulus intervals. *Journal of Experimental Psychology*, 61, 265–273.

Russell, J. A., & Mehrabian, A. (1977). Evidence for a three-factor theory of emotions. *Journal of Research in Personality*, 11, 273–294.

Simons, R. F., & Zelson, M. F. (1985). Engaging visual stimuli and reflex blink modification. *Psychophysiology*, 22, 44–49.

Trapold, M. A. (1962). The effect of incentive motivation on an unrelated reflex response. *Journal of Comparative Physiological Psychology*, 55, 1034–1039.

Vrana, S. R., & Constantine, J. A. (1990). The startle reflex as an outcome measure in the treatment of simple phobia [Abstract]. *Psychophysiology*, 27, S74.

Vrana, S. R., & Lang, P. J. (1990). Fear imagery and the startle probe reflex. *Journal of Abnormal Psychology*, 99, 189–197.

Vrana, S. R., Spence, E. L., & Lang, P. J. (1988). The startle probe response: A new measure of emotion? *Journal of Abnormal Psychology, 97,* 487–491.

Wagner, A. R. (1963). Conditioned frustration as a learned driver. *Journal of Experimental Psychology, 66,* 142–148.

Watson, D., & Tellegen, A. (1985). Toward a consensual structure of mood. *Psychological Bulletin, 98,* 219–235.

31   The Functional Neuroanatomy of Emotion and Affective Style

Richard J. Davidson and William Irwin

This chapter presents an overview of recent research on the functional neuroanatomy of human affective processes, focusing on studies using positron emission tomography (PET) or functional magnetic resonance imaging (fMRI). Where relevant, some studies on patients with discrete lesions are also included, as well as animal studies that provide much of the foundation for the modern human work. Research on patients with mood and anxiety disorders is, for the most part, not included as such studies have been extensively reviewed in a number of recent publications.[1–6] Over the past 10 years, there has been an enormous increase in animal research that has provided a detailed foundation for understanding the neural circuitry of several basic emotional processes.[7] This corpus of literature has helped to make emotion a tractable problem in the neurosciences and has led to the development of affective neuroscience.[8] With recent advances in functional brain imaging, the circuitry underlying emotion in the human brain can now be studied with unprecedented precision (see Box 31.1).

The Functional Neuroanatomy of Approach and Withdrawal-related Emotion

Two basic systems mediating different forms of motivation and emotion have been proposed.[9–12] Although the descriptors chosen by different investigators varies and the specifics of the proposed anatomical circuitry is presented in varying levels of detail, the essential characteristics of each system are similar across conceptualizations. The *approach* system facilitates appetitive behavior and generates certain types of positive affect that are approach-related, for example, enthusiasm, pride, etc.[13] This form of positive affect is usually generated in the context of moving toward a desired goal (see Refs. 14, 15 for

theoretical accounts of emotion that place a premium on goal states). There appears to be a second system concerned with the neural implementation of *withdrawal*. This system facilitates the withdrawal of an individual from sources of aversive stimulation and generates certain forms of negative affect that are withdrawal-related. For example, both fear and disgust are associated with increasing the distance between the organism and a source of aversive stimulation. A variety of evidence drawn from multiple sources suggests the view that the systems that support these forms of positive and negative affect are implemented in partially separable neural circuits. The key elements of the circuitry are reviewed below.

Prefrontal Cortex

A large body of lesion, neuroimaging and electrophysiological data supports the view that the prefrontal cortex (PFC) is an important part of the circuitry that implements both positive and negative affect. There are several important subdivisions of the PFC that are critical to note with respect to affective processing. First are the distinctions among the dorsolateral, ventromedial and orbitofrontal sectors and the second is the distinction between left and right sectors within each of these regions of PFC (see Fig. 31.1).

A number of early studies that evaluated mood subsequent to brain damage suggested that patients with damage to the left hemisphere, particularly in PFC, were more likely to develop depressive symptoms compared with patients having lesions in homologous regions of the right hemisphere.[16–18] Most of the lesions in these studies are large and include more than one sector of PFC. However, dorsolateral PFC is affected in the majority of patients represented in these studies. The general finding of left dorso-

Box 31.1
Conceptual and methodological complexities in neuroimaging studies of human emotion

PET and fMRI provide powerful and complementary information that has not been possible to acquire with other methods. These techniques enable scientists to examine regional patterns of activation in normal intact humans with considerable spatial precision and, in the case of fMRI, with temporal resolution on the order of seconds. With PET, in addition to its use as a measure of hemodynamic or metabolic activity, it can also be used to probe components of neurotransmission *in vivo* in relation to behavioral performance (Ref. a). The application of these methods to the study of emotion has burgeoned over the past several years and has generated a new body of literature on the circuitry associated with selective features of emotional responding and affective traits. There are a number of critical conceptual and methodological issues that are fundamental to neuroimaging studies of emotion:

(1) The perception of emotional information must be carefully distinguished from the production of emotion. There are many studies that present as stimuli to subjects, facial expressions of emotion. The presentation of facial expressions of emotion does not necessarily (nor even likely) elicit any emotion. Thus, when investigators use this procedure it is important that it is described as a study of the perception of emotional faces and not a study about emotion *per se* (Refs b,c).

(2) The control conditions against which emotion activation is compared crucially influences the nature of the data obtained. When using subtractive methodology, it is helpful to control for as much of the stimulus content as possible to isolate the effects of emotion itself. For example, the comparison of a condition during which subjects were self-generating emotional imagery to a resting baseline would be problematic (Ref. d) because any effects observed might not be a function of the particular emotion that was aroused, but rather the cognitive processes involved in retrieving information from memory and voluntarily generating visual imagery. It is good practice to include more than one emotion condition (e.g. both positive

and negative), as any effect produced as a consequence of simply generating emotion *per se* should be common to the two emotions, while differences between conditions can be attributed to the specific nature of the emotional process elicited.

(3) Stimuli designed to elicit different emotions must be matched on arousal and on physical characteristics. Arousal can be inferred in several different ways including self-report and skin conductance measures (Ref. e). Differences in patterns of activation observed between two emotion conditions that are not matched on intensity or arousal can obviously result from a failure to match appropriately and might be more a function of the arousal differences rather than the emotion differences between conditions (see Ref. f for more extended discussion). A related issue is the need to match stimuli across emotion and control conditions on physical properties, such as color, the presence of faces, spatial frequency, etc. Some differences found between emotion conditions might conceivably be a function of physical differences between the stimuli that have nothing directly to do with emotion. For example, in our fMRI studies of emotion induced with pictures, we have found (Ref. g) that activation of secondary visual cortex by negative pictures compared with neutral pictures may in part be a function of the color differences between these classes of stimuli.

(4) Putatively asymmetric effects must be rigorously statistically interrogated. Many investigators using both PET and fMRI have reported asymmetric changes associated with emotion (Ref. h). In most cases, claims about an activation being asymmetric were made on the basis of voxels in one hemisphere that exceeded statistical threshold while homologous voxels in the opposite hemisphere did not. However, such an analytic strategy, while typical, tests only for the main effects of the condition. To demonstrate an actual difference between the two hemispheres, it is necessary to test the Condition X Hemisphere or Group X Hemisphere interaction. The fact that such tests are rarely performed is largely a function of the fact that software is not

Box 31.1
(continued)

commercially available to perform such analyses for the entire brain volume. If this interaction was not significant, it is not legitimate to claim that an asymmetric finding was observed since the lack of a significant interaction means that the changes found in one hemisphere were not significantly different from those observed in the other, even if the effects were independently significant in one hemisphere but not in the other. Moreover, it is possible for significant interactions to arise in the absence of any significant main effects. As discussed in the main text, very few investigators who have reported asymmetric effects have properly tested for the Condition X Hemisphere interaction.

References

a. Koepp, M. J. et al. (1998) Evidence for striatal dopamine release during a video game *Nature* 393, 266–268.

b. Davidson, R. J. (1993) Cerebral asymmetry and emotion: conceptual and methodological conundrums *Cognition Emotion* 7, 115–138.

c. Davidson, R. J. and Irwin, W. Functional MRI in the Study of Emotion, in *Medical Radiology—Diagnostic Imaging and Radiation Oncology: Functional MRI* (Moonen, C. and Bandettini, P. A., eds), Springer-Verlag (in press).

d. Pardo, J. V., Pardo, P. J. and Raichle, M. E. (1993) Neural correlates of self-induced dysphoria *Am. J. Psychiatry* 150, 713–719.

e. Lang, P. J., Bradley, M. M. and Cuthbert, B. N. (1990) Emotion, attention and the startle reflex *Psychol. Rev.* 97, 377–398.

f. Davidson, R. J. et al. (1990) Approach–withdrawal and cerebral asymmetry: emotional expression and brain physiology: I *J. Pers. Social Psychol.* 58, 330–341.

g. Irwin, W. et al. (1997) Positive and negative affective responses: neural circuitry revealed using functional magnetic resonance imaging *Soc. Neurosci. Abstr.* 23, 1318.

h. Morris, J. S., Ohman, A. and Dolan, R. J. (1998) Conscious and unconscious emotional learning in the human amygdala *Nature* 393, 467–470.

lateral PFC damage increasing the likelihood of depressive symptoms has been interpreted to reflect the contribution of this cortical territory to certain features of positive affect, which, when disrupted, increases the probability of depressive symptomatology. This line of reasoning is consistent with the idea that depression is associated with deficits in positive affect.[19] Recent reviews of the modern literature on this topic[20] have largely supported these earlier studies, though some inconsistencies have been reported[21,22] (see Ref. 23 for discussion of conceptual issues in this literature). Morris et al.,[24] in a study with the largest sample size yet for research of this kind (N = 193) and with patients who were in the acute stage of stroke (all patients were tested between 7 and 10 days post-stroke), found that it

was only among patients with small-sized lesions that the relation between left PFC damage and depressed mood was found. Larger lesions probably intrude on other cortical sectors and may obscure the relationship between left PFC damage and depression.

Bechara and colleagues have amassed considerable evidence over the past several years that patients with bilateral lesions of the ventromedial PFC cannot anticipate future positive or negative consequences of their actions, although immediately available rewards and punishments do influence their behavior.[25] Such patients also fail to show anticipatory electrodermal responses when confronted by a risky choice whereas normal controls generate such anticipatory autonomic responses even before they explicitly knew

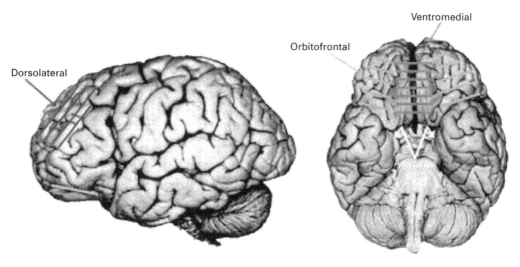

Figure 31.1
Sectors of human prefrontal cortex. (Left) Lateral view indicating dorsolateral (blue), ventromedial (red) and orbitofrontal (green) cortical territories. (Right) ventral view indicating ventromedial (red) and orbitofrontal (green) cortical territories. Also indicated are the amygdalae located on the medial margin of the temporal lobes, just dorsal to the unci which are identified by the tips of the arrowhead (yellow; see Fig. 31.2). (Adapted from Ref. 93.)

it was a risky choice.[26,27] Recently, this group[28] demonstrated a double dissociation whereby patients with anterior ventromedial PFC damage were impaired on a gambling task that assesses anticipation of future positive and negative consequences while performing normally on a working memory task (delayed non-matching to sample). Patients with right dorsolateral PFC damage were impaired on the working memory task while performing normally on the gambling task. Whether separable influences on the anticipation of positive or negative consequences would result from unilateral left- versus right-sided ventromedial damage respectively, has never been studied.

The differential involvement of the left and right PFC in certain forms of positive and negative emotion is supported by electrophysiological measures of regional activation in normal subjects exposed to stimuli that elicit emotion.[12,29–31] These studies find increased left anterior activation during positive affect and increased right-sided anterior activation during negative affect. A major limitation of these studies is the lack of spatial resolution afforded by the electrophysiological measures.

Using an extended-picture-presentation paradigm to induce consistent changes in positive or negative mood,[32] we measured regional glucose metabolism using PET while we independently and objectively verified the presence of the intended emotional states using emotion-modulated startle and facial electromyography.[33] During the production of negative affect, we found right-sided increases in metabolic rate in both inferior and superior regions of the PFC including the anterior orbital, inferior frontal, middle frontal and superior frontal gyri. During the production of positive affect, a pattern of predominantly left-sided activation was observed with a somewhat more posterior distribution compared with negative affect. During positive affect, left-sided metabolic increases were observed in the region of the pre- and post-central gyri. In addition, increases were observed in the region of the left nucleus accumbens (discussed below).

Relatively few other neuroimaging studies have compared objectively verified positive and negative affect in the same subjects. Some studies have examined patterns of activation that were common across emotions in comparison with a neutral baseline condition.[34] In this latter study, Lane et al. reported that the emotion conditions produced significantly greater activation in the medial PFC compared with the neutral control condition. A very similar finding was obtained in an independent sample of subjects exposed to pleasant, unpleasant and neutral pictures, with the emotional pictures producing increased activation in medial PFC compared with the neutral pictures.[35]

Many other studies that have used PET to measure regional cerebral blood flow or metabolism have observed emotion-related alterations in PFC activation. A common method for the experimental production of aversive emotion has been to use anxiety-disordered patients exposed to stimuli that provoke anxiety (e.g. pictures of spiders for spider phobics). Pooling across data from three different anxiety disordered groups (obsessive–compulsive disorder, simple phobia, and post-traumatic stress disorder) Rauch and colleagues[36] found a group of structures commonly activated across these disorders during the experimental provocation of anxiety. Two regions within the PFC were strongly activated across groups: right inferior PFC and right medial orbital PFC. In an fMRI study of symptom provocation among patients with obsessive–compulsive disorder, Breiter and colleagues[37] observed bilateral activation of anterior and posterior orbitofrontal cortex.

Several investigators have used classical aversive conditioning to study the neural substrates of the acquisition and extinction of emotional learning. Most studies have focused on the amyg-dala and they will be reviewed below. However, in the present context, we note that Hugdahl et al.[38,39] reported a significant increase in widespread zones of the right PFC including the orbitofrontal and dorsolateral cortices and inferior and superior frontal cortices during extinction compared to habituation.

Various studies have reported significant decreases in PFC blood flow associated with the activation of particular emotional states, with induced happiness resulting in a reduction in activation in the right superior PFC and visually induced recall of an aversive emotional episode being associated with a significant reduction in left-sided PFC activation in the region of Broca's area and the operculum.[40,41]

In summary, there is growing consistency between the lesion data on the mood consequences of small unilateral lesions and the findings from neuroimaging studies in supporting the view of right-sided activation in several regions within PFC during the experimental arousal of negative emotion. Less evidence is available on the prefrontal changes associated with positive affect, in part because much of the literature on negative affect is derived from the study of patients with anxiety and mood disorders. Systematic study of comparable subjects who are predisposed to positive affect has never been undertaken though certainly could be based upon available evidence.[31,42] It must be noted that some of the neuroimaging evidence for lateralized changes in PFC activation during emotion is derived from studies that have not rigorously tested the interaction of condition with hemisphere and thus, must be regarded with some caution until additional studies using more appropriate analytic procedures have been performed.

Bechara and colleagues' studies on the ventromedial PFC strongly suggest that this neural sector is involved in the anticipation of future affective consequences because patients with damage to this region fail to generate the normal anticipatory electrodermal responses to affectively salient cues. It will be of great interest in the future to carefully examine whether asymmetries in the representation of valence are present in this region. The evidence to date is derived from patients with bilateral lesions.

Many theoretical accounts of emotion assign it an important role in guiding action and organizing behavior in a motivationally consistent manner.[43] To accomplish this, it is essential that the organism have some means of representing affect in the absence of immediate elicitors—an affective working memory. It is likely that the PFC plays a crucial role in this process. Damage to specific sectors of the PFC appears to impair a person's ability to sustain emotion and to use it to guide behavior in an adaptive fashion. Note that such damage would not impair immediate reactivity to incentives, but only the capacity to sustain and anticipate such reactions when the immediate elicitors are not present. The ventromedial sector of the PFC is probably most directly involved in the representation of elementary positive and negative states in the absence of immediately present incentives, while the dorsolateral PFC is probably most directly involved in the representation of the goal states toward which these more elementary positive and negative states are directed. This formulation must be tested explicitly in future research.

Amygdala

A growing body of data from a small group of human patients with discrete lesions in the amygdala highlight the importance of this region for both the perception and production of negative affect and associative aversive learning (see Ref. 7 for general review and Ref. 44 for review of animal studies on the amygdala and emotional memory) (see Fig. 31.2). Adolphs and his colleagues[45,46] have demonstrated that the recognition of facial signs of fear was impaired in patients with bilateral amygdala damage while recognition of other facial expressions was intact. A specific deficit in the recognition of facial

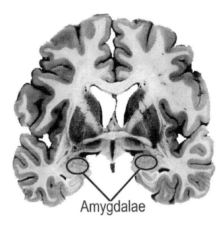

Figure 31.2
Human amygdalae. Coronal section of the human brain indicating the location of the amygdalae (yellow) deep within the temporal lobes. (Adapted from ref. 93.)

expressions of fear in patients with amygdala damage has been demonstrated in two additional studies using a different methodology for the assessment of facial expression recognition.[47,48] It is likely that the deficit in the perception of expressive signs of fear in patients with amygdala damage is not specific to facial expressions since Scott et al.[49] demonstrated a deficit in the recognition of vocalic expressions of fear and anger in a patient with bilateral amygdala damage.

Bechara and colleagues[50] have demonstrated a crucial double dissociation by comparing a patient with selective bilateral amygdala damage to one with selective bilateral hippocampal damage on a conditioning task during which electrodermal measures of affective aversive association were obtained, along with measures of declarative knowledge of the conditioning contingencies. It was found that the patient with amygdala damage was impaired in electrodermal conditioning but showed intact declarative knowledge of the task contingencies while the patient with hippocampal damage and an intact amygdala demonstrated reliable electrodermal conditioning but showed no declarative knowledge of the conditioning contingencies. A patient with bilateral damage to both structures was impaired on both sets of measures. Other evidence suggests that declarative memory for complex emotional material is selectively disrupted in patients with bilateral amygdala damage.[51]

Angrilli and colleagues[52] studied the startle responses of a patient with a benign tumor of the right amygdala in comparison with a group of controls. Among control subjects, they replicated the well-known effect of aversive stimuli potentiating startle magnitude. However, in the patient with the right amygdala lesion, no startle potentiation was observed in response to aversive versus neutral stimuli. These data are consistent with the view that the amygdala is crucial for normal negative-affect potentiated startle in humans. In a very recent study that required subjects to make judgements of the trustworthiness and approachability of unfamiliar individuals from facial photographs, patients with bilateral damage to the amygdala judged the unfamiliar individuals to be more approachable and more trustworthy than did control subjects.[53] Collectively, the studies of patients with damage to the amygdala suggest that this structure plays an important role in both the perception and production of certain forms of negative emotion. The extent to which the human amygdala also plays a role in positive affect is unanswered by extant lesion studies. Moreover, the lesion studies need to be complemented by neuroimaging studies that examine activation in the amygdala in intact subjects in response to affective challenges since damage to the amygdala can have functional consequences in territories far removed from the site of the actual lesion.

A growing body of neuroimaging literature using both PET and fMRI have reported on changes in the human amygdala in response to emotional stimuli. These studies are helping to clarify the functional role of the amygdala in various components of emotional processing. However, it is necessary to underline the func-

tional heterogeneity of the amygdala. So significant is this heterogeneity that some anatomists have been led to question whether the amygdala should properly be regarded as a discrete, unitary structure (see Ref. 54 for a compelling statement of this position). Unfortunately, because of its relatively coarse spatial resolution, it is not likely that PET will enable investigators to differentiate among different subnuclei of the amygdala. It is more likely that fMRI will have sufficient spatial resolution, particularly at higher field strengths, to resolve different regions within the amygdala, although there have not yet been attempts to manipulate task variables systematically in order to determine whether differential activation of regions of the amygdala can be detected.

A number of PET and fMRI studies have been performed with patients having one of several different anxiety disorders and examining cerebral blood flow in the amygdala and other brain regions in response to the experimental provocation of anxiety. For example, using PET measures of blood flow, Rauch[55] exposed patients with post traumatic stress disorder to imagery scripts that were designed to activate traumatic memories. These were compared to neutral imagery scripts. Activation of the right amygdala was found in this study and remained equally significant when compared to a teeth clenching control condition.[56] Breiter et al.[37] used fMRI to examine regional patterns of activation in patients with obsessive–compulsive disorder exposed to idiographically tailored stimuli designed to provoke the patient's symptoms. In response to such stimuli compared with control stimuli, significant bilateral activation of the amygdala was detected. Birbaumer and colleagues[57] reported bilateral amygdala activation in response to neutral facial expressions (compared with a resting baseline condition) in a group of male social phobics. The amygdalar activation in this group was comparable in magnitude to that elicited by an aversive odor. In a group of controls, they observed amygdalar activation to the aversive odor but not to the neutral faces.

Consistent with the lesion data are studies that find specific activation of the amygdala in response to faces depicting expressions of fear. Using PET, Morris et al.[58] demonstrated that fear faces elicit significantly greater blood flow in the amygdala compared with happy faces. Moreover, the intensity of fear displayed in faces was systematically related to increases in blood flow in the left amygdala. In a subsequent reanalysis of these data, Morris and colleagues[59] found that increased blood flow in the amygdala predicted increased blood flow in extrastriate visual cortex during fear but not during happy presentations. These findings indicate that the pattern of functional connectivity between these regions is altered as a function of emotional expression condition.

Activation of the amygdala in response to fear faces has also been found with fMRI. Because of the better time resolution of fMRI, Breiter et al.[60] were able to examine the temporal changes in amygdalar activation and found that the response to fear faces showed rapid habituation. Phillips et al.[61] replicated this finding and further demonstrated that disgust faces failed to activate the amygdala. Rather, in response to disgust faces, subjects showed activation in a region implicated in processing gustatory stimuli— the anterior insula. Recently, Whalen and colleagues[62] demonstrated activation of the amygdala in response to fear faces that were not consciously perceived. They achieved this by masking the fear faces with neutral faces that were presented contiguously with the offset of the fear faces. Happy faces masked in this way showed significantly less amygdala activation compared with masked fear faces.

Using either pleasant and unpleasant pictures or happy and sad faces accompanied by instructions to generate the emotion depicted on faces, while measuring regional blood flow with PET, investigators have found activation in the left amygdala during unpleasant compared to neutral pictures[63] and during sad compared with happy mood generation.[64] In a conceptual rep-lication of this latter study, the same group used fMRI to detect regional brain activation and again found activation of the left amygdala but this time to both sad and happy conditions compared to the neutral condition.[65] Using fMRI, we presented pleasant and unpleasant pictures and compared them to neutral pictures and found that only unpleasant pictures activated the amygdala.[66,67] LaBar et al.[68] found bilateral activation in the amygdala in response to both unpleasant and pleasant stimuli compared to neutral stimuli. Importantly, the LaBar et al. study included erotic nudes in their positive picture set while our studies did not. It may well be that the inclusion of these stimuli made a crucial difference in the activation of the amygdala during the positive condition. We will return to this issue at the end of this section.

Two recent fMRI studies of classical aversive conditioning[69,70] have reported bilateral amygdala activation during the early phases of acquisition which then habituates rapidly. In a recent PET study of conscious and unconscious conditioning, Morris and colleagues[71] compared the responses to backwardly masked angry faces that had been paired with noise to consciously perceived angry faces paired with noise. Masked presentations of the conditioned angry face elicited activation in the right amygdala while unmasked presentations of the same face elicited activation in the left amygdala.

Several others types of manipulations have been found to enhance neural activity in the amygdala. Exposing normal individuals to an unsolvable anagram task of the sort used to induce learned helplessness produced increased blood flow in the amygdala.[72] Aversive olfactory stimuli were found to produce strong activation in the left amygdala[73] compared to a no odorant control condition, while aversive gustatory stimuli produced activation in the right amygdala.[74]

Individual differences in amygdala activation have been related to various measures of affective style (see Box 31.2).

Box 31.2
The amygdala and affective style

A number of recent studies have examined individual differences in amygdala activation in relation to various features of emotional reactivity and affective style. One of the most striking features of emotion is the profound variability among individuals in the quality and intensity of response to the identical stimulus. Davidson (Ref. a) has outlined a program of future research on affective style that seeks to parse the domain into specific sub-components, with an emphasis on the temporal dynamics of responding. For example, in this scheme, the time required to recover (i.e. return back to baseline) from a negative provocation is an important mechanism governing individual differences in negative affect.

Studies that examine individual differences in amygdala activation and affective style fall into two broad categories. First are studies that examine the correlates of individual differences in baseline blood flow or glucose metabolism in the amygdala. One of the first to perform such an analysis was Drevets and his colleagues (Ref. b) who examined relation between PET measures of resting blood flow and depression severity in a small group of depressed patients. These investigators reported that depressed patients with increased baseline blood flow in the amygdala had higher depression severity ratings. This analysis was based upon a region-of-interest (ROI) created by growing a sphere around a Talairach coordinate for the left amygdala. This approach is likely to include activity from a much larger region than just the amygdala, particularly since the PET data were smoothed to minimize contributions of anatomical variability across subjects in the group analysis. Using MRI coregistration with ROIs drawn on each subject's MRI scan around the amygdala and unsmoothed PET data, we (Ref. c) largely replicated the Drevets et al. (Ref. b) finding in a larger sample of depressed patients using baseline PET measures of regional glucose metabolism (see Figs 31.3 and 31.4A,B) and a psychometrically well-validated measure of dispositional negative affect. Individuals who exhibited elevated levels of glucose metabolism at

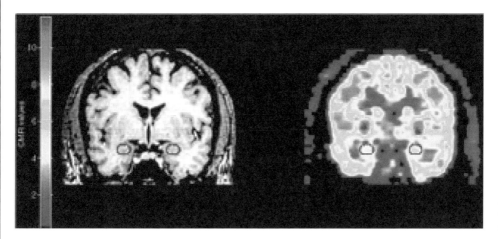

Figure 31.3
Illustration of PET-MRI coregistration and amygdalar RO1 delineation. Representative image planes in coronal section are shown for one participant. The PET image plane is presented besides its corresponding coregistered MRI plane. Units of the PET color scale are in mg/100g/min. (Adapted from Ref. 94.)

Box 31.2
(continued)

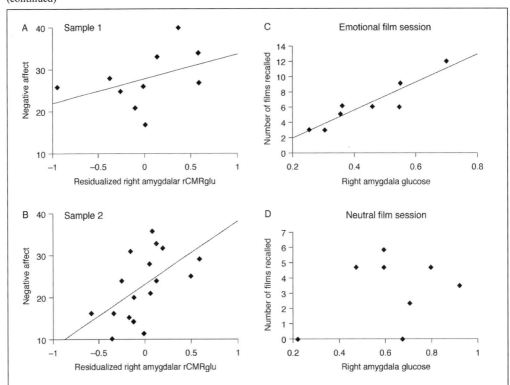

Figure 31.4
Metabolic activity in the right amygdala and individual differences in negative affect. Scatter plots of correlations in depressed groups between dispositional negative affect (assessed with the PANAS Negative Affect
Scale—Trait Version (Ref. i) and glucose metabolism in the right amygdala (rCMRglu = regional cerebral
metabolic rate for glucose, residualized for global metabolic rate) for two samples (**A, B**) of depressed
patients (N = 10 and 17 respectively, tested on different PET scanners). Sample 1, r(8) = 0.41, p = 0.24;
Sample 2, r(15) = 0.56, p = 0.02. (Adapted from Ref. 94.) (**C, D**) Scatter plots of correlations in normal
subjects between the number of negative emotional films recalled (**C**; r = 0.93, p > 0.01) and the number of
neutral films recalled (**D**; r = 0.33, not significant) and metabolic rate in the right amygdala derived from
PET during the respective film clips. (Adapted from Ref. 95.)

Box 31.2
(continued)

baseline reported significantly higher levels of dispositional negative affect.

The second type of study examines the relation between individual differences in reactivity of amygdala blood flow or metabolism to an emotional challenge and other behavioral or self-report indices of emotional reactivity. Cahill and colleagues (Ref. d) reported that subjects with higher levels of amygdala metabolic rate in response to negative emotional films showed better free recall of these films three weeks following their presentation. Glucose metabolism in the amygdala showed no relation to recall of neutral film clips (see Fig. 31.4C,D). We recently found that subjects showing greater MR signal change in the amygdala in response to negative compared with neutral pictures reported significantly higher levels of dispositional negative affect on a self-report measure (Ref. e). Fredrikson and his colleagues reported that those subjects showing greater increases in amygdala blood flow (particularly on the right side) detected with PET during extinction compared with habituation in a classical conditioning paradigm also showed greater evidence of electrodermal conditioning (Ref. f). LaBar et al. conceptually replicated this finding using fMRI (Ref. g), though in this study, electrodermal measures were obtained during a separate session 1–3 months following the fMRI data collection. Despite the time interval between sessions, a significant positive correlation was obtained between MR signal change in the amygdala during conditioning and magnitude of skin conductance responses obtained 1–3 months later.

Using a pharmacological challenge procedure with the anesthetic procaine, Ketter and colleagues compared those individuals who reported euphoric versus dysphoric responses to the challenge (Ref. h). Subjects with the negative affective response to the procaine had significantly greater activation of the amygdala as detected by PET. Moreover,

amygdala blood flow correlated positively with fear and negatively with euphoria on self-report measures of emotional intensity.

References

a. Davidson, R. J. (1998) Affective style and affective disorders: perspectives from affective neuroscience *Cognition Emotion* 12, 307–320.

b. Drevets, W. C. et al. (1992) A functional-anatomical study of unipolar depression *J. Neurosci.* 12, 3628–3641.

c. Abercrombie, H. C. et al. (1998) Metabolic rate in the right amygdala predicts negative affect in depressed patients *NeuroReport* 9, 3301–3307.

d. Cahill, L. et al. (1996) Amygdala activity at encoding correlated with long-term, free recall of emotional information *Proc. Natl. Acad. Sci. U.S.A.* 93, 8016–8021.

e. Irwin, W. et al. (1997) Relations between human amygdalar activation and self-reported dispositional affect *J. Cogn. Neurosci.* (Suppl. S), 109.

f. Furmark, T. et al. (1997) The amygdala and individual differences in fear conditioning *NeuroReport* 8, 3957–3960.

g. LaBar, K. S. et al. (1998) Human amygdala activation during conditioned fear acquisition and extinction: a mixed-trial fMRI study *Neuron* 20, 937–945.

h. Ketter, T. A. et al. (1996) Anterior paralimbic mediation of procaine-induced emotional and psychosensory experiences *Arch. Gen. Psychiatry* 53, 59–69.

i. Watson, D., Clark, L. A. and Tellegan, A. (1988) Development and validation of brief measures of positive and negative affect: the PANAS Scales *J. Pers. Social Psychol.* 54, 1063–1070.

Issues Raised by the Amygdala Findings

The data reviewed above clearly implicate the amygdala as an important site for the control of emotion in the human brain. However, the results also raise many questions about the precise nature of the role this region plays in emotion. Here we wish to highlight three major issues.

(1) *Affect in general, negative affect in particular, or fear most specifically?* The existing data are equivocal on this issue. Many studies find greater amygdala activation in response to negative elicitors compared with positive elicitors. Some studies find that the greater the reported or autonomically displayed negative affect, the greater the activation in the amygdala. Other studies have found amygdala activation in response to both negative and positive emotional challenges. For example, LaBar et al.[68] observed bilateral MR signal increases in the amygdala in response to both negative and positive pictures compared with neutral pictures. As we noted above, this latter study included erotic nudes among the positive picture set while our study,[67] which revealed amygdala activation only in response to negative versus neutral pictures, did not. It is noteworthy that the Breiter et al. fMRI study of the effects of cocaine in cocaine addicts (Ref. 75, discussed in more detail below) found significant deactivation of the amygdala during cocaine-induced "highs."

The studies that have compared activation of the amygdala in response to facial expressions depicting different emotions have consistently found the greatest activation of the amygdala in response to fear faces. It is conceivable that these data could be subsumed under a model of amygdala function that assigned a premium role to the detection of ambiguity (see Ref. 76 for a discussion of this theory). On this view, the preferential activation of the amygdala in response to fear compared with angry faces, for example, is explained by the fact that angry faces provide information about the presence of threat as well as

the source of threat while fear faces provide information about the former but not the latter. Erotic stimuli may be interpreted as ambiguous for many different reasons (e.g. they might automatically elicit approach, but also could activate avoidance responses because of moral considerations etc.). Inconsistent with this view, however, are the data on the recognition of vocal affect in a patient with bilateral amygdala damage which indicated impaired recognition of both fear and anger.[49] What is required is to manipulate the valence of emotion while carefully matching conditions on variables that might be associated with ambiguity. Alternatively, ambiguity can be parametrically varied (e.g. by altering the probability of a shock appearing during the presence of a particular CS) to determine if amygdala activation tracked variations in manipulated ambiguity.

(2) *Left, right or both?* During the experimental arousal of negative affect, some studies report changes in left amygdala activation,[65] others report changes in right amygdala activation,[55] while still others report bilateral changes.[66] Adding to this complexity is the recent report by Morris et al.[71] who observed right amygdala activation to unconsciously presented aversively conditioned angry faces and left amygdala activation to conscious presentations of the same face. It is essential to stress the importance of proper statistical analysis of laterality effects in neuroimaging studies (see Box 31.1 and Ref. 77 for a more in depth discussion). Until these procedures are followed more rigorously, it will not be possible to sort out whether asymmetric activation in the amygdala is associated with different patterns of affective response.

(3) *Can the amygdala be treated as a homogeneous structure?* Of course, the obvious answer to this question is a resounding no, yet most investigators continue to treat this region as if it were a unitary structure. Unfortunately, this state of affairs is not likely to change until studies are

completed on MRI scanners with field strengths higher than conventional scanners (i.e. more than 2T). When such studies are performed, it is likely that the region of the amygdala that is activated in response to faces will differ from the region activated during the expression of a negative emotional response. Uneven sampling of the amygdala and partial volume effects with other adjacent structures due to the relatively coarse resolution of most fMRI and all PET studies probably accounts for some of the variability among studies. Future fMRI studies at higher field strength hold great promise in elucidating the functional specialization of different amygdaloid regions.

Other Brain Regions

While most of the extant literature has focused on PFC and amygdala as two critical components of a circuit involved in human emotion processing, many studies have offered evidence of other brain regions participating in affective responding. One key region that has emerged mostly from behavioral, lesion and electrophysiological data is posterior right hemisphere involvement in both the perception of emotional information as well as in the arousal component of emotion. This literature is not reviewed here because it has been recently reviewed elsewhere.[78–80] In addition, precise anatomical specification of the locus of these effects is not available because the methods that have been used for their study provide only course localizing information. Here we briefly review data on three other regions that have been most consistently implicated in emotional processing in recent neuroimaging studies.

Ventral Striatum

Breiter et al.[75] examined the effects of cocaine infusion in cocaine addicts on MR signal change in comparison to saline infusion. They found activation in a distributed circuit that included cortical and subcortical regions. Of note is the strong activation observed in regions of the ventral striatum which includes the caudate, putamen and the nucleus accumbens. Activation in this latter region is consistent with a large corpus of non-human data demonstrating the critical role played by the mesolimbic dopaminergic pathway in positive affect and addictive behaviors.[81,82] Stein et al.[83] in the first fMRI study of the effects of nicotine on regional brain activation in cigarette smokers also found activation of the nucleus accumbens during infusion of nicotine compared with saline. In our PET study described above that used pleasant and unpleasant pictures in an extended picture paradigm,[33] we observed activation in a region including the nucleus accumbens during the picture-induced positive affect.

Anterior Cingulate

Many neuroimaging studies that have compared an emotional to a neutral condition have reported activation in the anterior cingulate cortex (ACC). Theoretical and empirical analyses suggest that the ACC plays an important role in aspects of attentional processing.[84] In a recent study that was designed to better understand the role of the ACC in emotion, Lane et al.[63] exposed subjects to emotional pictures under two conditions: during one condition subjects were asked to attend to their subjective emotional responses and indicate whether the picture evoked a pleasant, unpleasant or neutral feeling, while in a second condition (during exposure to similar pictures), they were asked to indicate whether the picture depicted a scene that was indoors, outdoors or either. They observed a significant focus of activation in the ACC during the condition requiring attention to subjective emotional responses compared with the condition requiring attention to the context of the stimulus (see also Ref. 85).

Insular Cortex

Activation of the insular cortex has also been reported in many neuroimaging studies that have manipulated emotion, ranging from studies of symptom provocation in anxiety-disordered patients[86] to studies of emotion activation in normal individuals[34] and to pharmacologically manipulated emotion.[75] The fact that a very diverse range of manipulations produce activation in the insular cortex is consistent with the idea that this cortical territory plays a critical role in visceral representation.[87] The insular cortex receives afferents from several major autonomic regions and sends efferents to a number of brain regions that play a critical role in regulating autonomic responses that accompany emotion including the central nucleus of the amygdala and the lateral hypothalamus. The insular cortex is topographically organized and includes a major zone dedicated to gustatory processing. This latter fact is probably responsible for the significant insular activation detected with fMRI in response to disgust faces,[61] which can be understood as signifying distasteful stimuli (see recent discussions by Rozin and Young et al.[88,89]).

To summarize the findings from these other brain regions, activation of ventral striatum has most consistently appeared in studies that manipulated positive affect. This region is richly innervated by dopaminergic neurons and a recent human PET study has found increases in dopamine turnover in this general region during the playing of an enjoyable video game.[90] The mesolimbic dopamine system has been implicated in incentive reward motivation[13] and it is likely that this system plays an important role in what Davidson[91] has previously described as "pre-goal attainment positive affect," that form of positive affect that arises as one moves progressively closer toward a desired goal.

The anterior cingulate region has been reported to be activated in most neuroimaging studies of emotion when an emotion condition is compared with a neutral control condition. This region might play an important role in mediating the attentional effects of affective arousal. When emotion is evoked it is usually attentionally salient. It would be informative in future research to compare emotion evoked non-consciously versus consciously[71] and determine if activation of the ACC occurs during the latter but not the former.

Based upon its known inputs and outputs, activation of the insular cortex during emotion is probably associated with the autonomic changes that typically occur when emotion is evoked. However, from the extant evidence, we do not know if the insular activation is primarily a function of visceral afferent feedback or rather is produced by the insular cortex issuing efferent commands for autonomic change. The use of peripheral beta blockers to attenuate peripheral autonomic activity during emotional arousal[92] in conjunction with neuroimaging would permit the determination of whether insular activation was primarily driven by visceral feedback to the insular or rather insular participation in the efferent control of autonomic function.

Conclusions

Just as cognitive neuroscience has taught us the importance of decomposing global cognitive constructs into more elementary constituents whose neural substrates could be identified, so too modern research in affective neuroscience underlines the importance of identifying specific subcomponents of emotion whose anatomical bases may be examined. In this article we have relied on three primary sources of data to make inferences about the circuitry underlying positive and negative emotion in the human brain: lesion, PET and fMRI studies. This corpus of work underlines the importance of several interconnected regions comprising a circuit for human affective responding: the ventromedial and dorsolateral PFC, amygdala, ventral striatum, anterior cingulate and insular cortex. Each of these regions appears to play a separate function in emotion although very few studies have been designed to manipulate these emotion subcomponents specifically in order to demonstrate rigorously such specificity. Evidence for the lateralization for emotional valence was also summarized, which supports the view of regions of the right PFC specifically implementing components of aversive emotional responding. As we develop more reliable methods to investigate emotion in the laboratory and to study its interaction with various cognitive processes, these procedures, combined with neuroimaging technologies, will allow us to address questions about brain mechanisms in ways that were previously approachable only through research on non-human species. This new information will provide a compelling foundation for theoretical advances in the basic understanding of the constituents of emotion and for practical advances in the treatment of affective dysfunction.

Acknowledgements

Supported by NIMH grants MH43454, MH40747, Research Scientist Award K05-MH00875, and P50-MH52354 to the Wisconsin Center for Affective Science (R. J. Davidson, Director), by a NARSAD Established Investigator Award, and by a grant from the John D. and Catherine T. MacArthur Foundation. We thank the many individuals in our laboratory who have contributed importantly to this research over the years, including Andy Tomarken, Steve Sutton, Daren Jackson, Heather Abercrombie, Jeff Henriques, Chris Larson, Stacey Schaefer, Terry Ward, Terry Oakes, Isa Dolski, Alex Shackman, Jack Nitschke, John Koger, Adrian Pederson as well as the many collaborators outside the lab too numerous to name.

References

1. Drevets, W. C. and Raichle, M. E. (1995) PET imaging studies of human emotional disorders, in *The Cognitive Neurosciences* (Gazzaniga, M. S., ed.), MIT Press.

2. Frith, C. and Dolan, R. J. (1998) Images of psychopathology *Curr. Opin. Neurobiol.* 8, 259–262.

3. Rauch, S. L. and Renshaw, P. F. (1995) Clinical neuroimaging in psychiatry *Harvard Rev. Psychiatry* 2, 297–312.

4. Reiman, E. M. (1997) The application of positron emission tomography to the study of normal and pathologic emotions *J. Clin. Psychiatry* 58, 4–12.

5. Dolan, R. J. (1997) Mood disorders and abnormal cingulate cortex *Trends Cognit. Sci.* 8, 283–284.

6. Drevets, W. C. (1997) Mood disorders and abnormal cingulate cortex. Response from Drevets *Trends Cognit. Sci.* 8, 284–286.

7. LeDoux, J. E. (1996) *The Emotional Brain,* Simon and Schuster.

8. Davidson, R. J. and Sutton, S. K. (1995) Affective neuroscience: the emergence of a discipline *Curr. Opin. Neurobiol.* 5, 217–224.

9. Cacioppo, J. T. and Gardner, W. L. Emotion *Annu. Rev. Psychol.* 50 (in press).

10. Gray, J. A. (1994) Three fundamental emotion systems, in *The Nature of Emotion: Fundamental Questions* (Ekman, P. and Davidson, R. J., eds), pp. 243–247, Oxford University Press.

11. Lang, P. J., Bradley, M. M. and Cuthbert, B. N. (1990) Emotion, attention and the startle reflex *Psychol. Rev.* 97, 377–398.

12. Davidson, R. J. (1995) Cerebral asymmetry, emotion and affective style, in *Brain Asymmetry* (Davidson, R. J. and Hugdahl, K., eds), pp. 361–387, MIT Press.

13. Depue, R. A. and Collins, P. F. Neurobiology of the structure of personality: dopamine, incentive motivation and extroversion *Behav. Brain Sci.* (in press).

14. Lazarus, R. S. (1991) *Emotion and Adaptation,* Oxford University Press.

15. Stein, N. L. and Trabasso, T. (1992) The organization of emotional experience: creating links among emotion, thinking, language and intentional action *Cognition Emotion* 6, 225–244.

16. Gainotti, G. (1972) Emotional behavior and hemispheric side of lesion *Cortex* 8, 41–55.

17. Sackeim, H. A. et al. (1982) Pathological laughter and crying: functional brain asymmetry in the expres-

sion of positive and negative emotions *Arch. Neurol.* 39, 210–218.

18. Robinson, R. G. et al. (1984) Mood disorders in stroke patients: importance of location of lesion *Brain* 107, 81–93.

19. Mineka, S., Watson, D. and Clark, L. A. (1998) Comorbidity of anxiety and unipolar mood disorders *Annu. Rev. Psychol.* 49, 377–412.

20. Robinson, R. G. and Downhill, J. E. (1995) Lateralization of psychopathology in response to focal brain injury, in *Brain Asymmetry* (Davidson, R. J. and Hugdahl K., eds), pp. 693–711, MIT Press.

21. House, A. et al. (1990) Mood disorders after stroke and their relation to lesion location: a CT scan study *Brain* 113, 1113–1129.

22. Gainotti, G. et al. (1997) Relation of lesion location to verbal and nonverbal mood measures in stroke patients *Stroke* 28, 2145–2149.

23. Davidson, R. J. (1993) Cerebral asymmetry and emotion: conceptual and methodological conundrums *Cognition Emotion* 7, 115–138.

24. Morris, P. L. P. et al. (1996) Lesion characteristics and depressed mood in the stroke data bank study *J. Neuropsychiatry Clin. Neurosci.* 8, 153–159.

25. Bechara, A. et al. (1994) Insensitivity to future consequences following damage to human prefrontal cortex *Cognition* 50, 7–15.

26. Bechara, A. et al. (1997) Deciding advantageously before knowing the advantageous strategy *Science* 275, 1293–1295.

27. Bechara, A. et al. (1996) Failure to respond autonomically to anticipated future outcomes following damage to prefrontal cortex *Cereb. Cortex* 6, 215–225.

28. Bechara, A. et al. (1998) Dissociation of working memory from decision making within the human prefrontal cortex *J. Neurosci.* 18, 428–437.

29. Davidson, R. J. et al. (1990) Approach–withdrawal and cerebral asymmetry: emotional expression and brain physiology: I *J. Pers. Social Psychol.* 58, 330–341.

30. Davidson, R. J. (1992) Emotion and affective style: hemispheric substrates *Psychol. Sci.* 3, 39–43.

31. Davidson, R. J. (1998) Affective style and affective disorders: perspectives from affective neuroscience *Cognition Emotion* 12, 307–320.

32. Sutton, S. K. et al. (1997) Manipulating affective state using extended picture presentation *Psychophysiology* 34, 217–226.

33. Sutton, S. K. et al. (1997) Asymmetry in prefrontal glucose metabolism during appetitive and aversive emotional states: an FDG–PET study *Psychophysiology* 34, S89.

34. Lane, R. D. et al. (1997) Neuroanatomical correlates of happiness, sadness and disgust *Am. J. Psychiatry* 154, 926–933.

35. Lane, R. D. et al. (1997) Neuroanatomical correlates of pleasant and unpleasant emotion *Neuropsychologia* 35, 1437–1444.

36. Rauch, S. L. et al. (1997) The functional neuroanatomy of anxiety: a study of three disorders using positron emission tomography and symptom provocation *Biol. Psychiatry* 42, 446–452.

37. Breiter, H. C. et al. (1996) Functional magnetic resonance imaging of symptom provocation in obsessive–compulsive disorder *Arch. Gen. Psychiatry* 53, 595–606.

38. Hugdahl, K. et al. (1995) Brain mechanisms in human classical conditioning: a PET blood flow study *NeuroReport* 6, 1723–1728.

39. Hugdahl, K. (1998) Cortical control of human classical conditioning: autonomic and positron emission tomography data *Psychophysiology* 35, 170–178.

40. George, M. S. et al. (1995) Brain activity during transient sadness and happiness in healthy women *Am. J. Psychiatry* 152, 341–351.

41. Fischer, H., Wik, G. and Fredrikson, M. (1996) Functional neuroanatomy of robbery re-experience: affective memories studied with PET *NeuroReport* 7, 2081–2086.

42. Sutton, S. K. and Davidson, R. J. (1997) Prefrontal brain asymmetry: a biological substrate of the behavioral approach and inhibition systems *Psychol. Sci.* 8, 204–210.

43. Frijda, N. H. (1988) The laws of emotion *Am. Psychol.* 43, 349–358.

44. Cahill, L. and McGaugh, J. L. (1998) Mechanisms of emotional arousal and lasting declarative memory *Trends Neurosci.* 21, 273–313.

45. Adolphs, R. et al. (1995) Fear and the human amygdala *J. Neurosci.* 15, 5879–5892.

46. Adolphs, R. et al. (1996) Cortical systems for the recognition of emotion in facial expressions *J. Neurosci.* 16, 7678–7687.

47. Calder, A. J. et al. (1996) Facial emotion recognition after bilateral amygdala damage: differentially severe impairment of fear *Cognit. Neuropsychol.* 13, 699–745.

48. Broks, P. et al. (1998) Face processing impairments after encephalitis: amygdala damage and recognition of fear *Neuropsychologia* 36, 59–70.

49. Scott, S. K. et al. (1997) Impaired auditory recognition of fear and anger following bilateral amygdala lesions *Nature* 385, 254–257.

50. Bechara, A. et al. (1995) Double dissociation of conditioning and declarative knowledge relative to the amygdala and hippocampus in humans *Science* 269, 1115–1118.

51. Adolphs, R. et al. (1997) Impaired declarative memory for emotional material bilateral amygdala damage in humans *Learn. Mem.* 4, 291–300.

52. Angrilli, A. et al. (1996) Startle reflex and emotion modulation impairment after a right amygdala lesion *Brain* 119, 1991–2000.

53. Adolphs, R., Tranel, D. and Damasio, A. R. (1998) The human amygdala in social judgment *Nature* 393, 470–474.

54. Swanson, L. W. and Petrovich, G. D. (1998) What is the amygdala? *Trends Neurosci.* 21, 323–331.

55. Rauch, S. L. et al. (1996) A symptom provocation study of post-traumatic stress disorder using positron emission tomography and script-driven imagery *Arch. Gen. Psychiatry* 53, 380–387.

56. Drevets, W. C. et al. (1992) PET images of blood changes during anxiety: correction *Science* 256, 1696.

57. Birmbaumer, N. et al. (1998) fMRI reveals amygdala activation to human faces in social phobics *NeuroReport* 9, 1223–1226.

58. Morris, J. S. et al. (1996) A differential neural response in the human amygdala to fearful and happy facial expressions *Nature* 383, 812–815.

59. Morris, J. S. et al. (1998) A neuromodulatory role for the human amygdala in processing emotional facial expressions *Brain* 121, 42–57.

60. Breiter, H. C. et al. (1996) Response and habituation of the human amygdala during visual processing of facial expression *Neuron* 17, 875–887.

61. Phillips, M. L. et al. (1997) A specific neural substrate for perceiving facial expressions of disgust *Nature* 389, 495–498.

62. Whalen, P. J. et al. (1998) Masked presentations of emotional facial expressions modulate amygdala activity without explicit knowledge *J. Neurosci.* 18, 411–418.

63. Lane, R. D. et al. (1997) Neural activation during selective attention to subjective emotional responses *NeuroReport* 8, 3969–3972.

64. Schneider, F. et al. (1995) Mood effects on limbic blood flow correlate with emotional self-ratings: a PET study with oxygen-15 labeled water *Psychiatry Res. (Neuroimaging)* 61, 265–283.

65. Schneider, F. et al. (1997) Functional MRI reveals left amygdala activation during emotion *Psychiatry Res. (Neuroimaging)* 76, 75–82.

66. Irwin, W. et al. (1996) Human amygdala activation detected with echo-planar functional magnetic resonance imaging *NeuroReport* 7, 1765–1769.

67. Irwin, W. et al. (1997) Positive and negative affective responses: neural ciruitry revealed using frontal magnetic resonance imaging *Soc. Neurosci. Abstr.* 23, 1318.

68. LaBar, K. S. et al. (1998) Role of the amygdala in emotional picture evaluation as revealed by fMRI *J. Cogn. Neurosci.* (Suppl. S), 108.

69. Buchel, C. et al. (1998) Brain systems mediating aversive conditioning: an event-related fMRI study *Neuron* 20, 947–957.

70. LaBar, K. S. et al. (1998) Human amygdala activation during conditioned fear acquisition and extinction: a mixed-trial fMRI study *Neuron* 20, 937–945.

71. Morris, J. S., Ohman, A. and Dolan, R. J. (1998) Conscious and unconscious emotional learning in the human amygdala *Nature* 393, 467–470.

72. Schneider, F. et al. (1996) Cerebral blood flow changes in limbic regions induced by unsolvable anagram tasks *Am. J. Psychiatry* 153, 206–212.

73. Zald, D. H. and Pardo, J. V. (1997) Emotion, olfaction and the human amygdala: amygdala activation during aversive olfactory stimulation *Proc. Natl. Acad. Sci. U. S. A.* 94, 4119–4124.

74. Zald, D. H. et al. (1998) Aversive gustatory stimulation activates limbic circuits humans *Brain* 121, 1143–1154.

75. Breiter, H. C. et al. (1997) Acute effects of cocaine on human brain activity and emotion *Neuron* 19, 591–611.

76. Whalen, P. Fear, vigilance and ambiguity: initial neuroimaging studies of the human amygdala *Curr. Dir. Psychol. Sci.* (in press).

77. Davidson, R. J. and Irwin, W. Functional MRI in the study of emotion, in *Medical Radiology—Diagnostic Imaging and Radiation Oncology: Functional MRI* (Moonen, C. and Bandettini, P. A., eds), Springer (in press).

78. Borod, J. (1993) Cerebral mechanisms underlying facial, prosodic and lexical emotional expression: a review of neuropsychological studies and methodological issues *Neuropsychology* 7, 445–463.

79. Heller, W. and Nitschke, J. B. (1997) Regional brain activity in emotion: a framework for understanding cognition in depression *Cognition Emotion* 11, 637–661.

80. Heller, W. and Nitschke, J. B. (1998) The puzzle of regional brain activity in depression and anxiety: the importance of subtypes and co-morbidity *Cognition Emotion* 12, 421–447.

81. Koob, G. F. (1992) Neurobiological mechanisms of cocaine and opiate dependence, in *Addictive States* (O'Brien, C. P. and Faffe, J. H., eds), pp. 171–191, Raven Press.

82. Koch, M., Schmid, A. and Schnitzler, H-U. (1996) Pleasure-attentuation of startle is disrupted by lesions of the nucleus accumbens *NeuroReport* 7, 1442–1446.

83. Stein, E. A. et al. (1998) Nicotine-induced limbic cortical activation in the human brain: a functional MRI study *Am. J. Psychiatry* 155, 1009–1015.

84. Posner, M. (1995) Neuropsychology: modulation by instruction *Nature* 373, 198–199.

85. Davis, K. D. et al. (1997) Functional MRI of pain- and attention-related activations in the human cingulate cortex *J. Neurophysiol.* 77, 3370–3380.

86. Rauch, S. L. et al. (1995) A positron emission tomographic study of simple phobic symptom provocation *Arch. Gen. Psychiatry* 52, 20–28.

87. Cechetto, D. F. and Saper, C. B. (1990) Role of the cerebral cortex in autonomic function, in *Central Regulation of Autonomic Functions* (Loewy, A. D. and Spyer, K. M., eds), pp. 208–223, Oxford University Press.

88. Rozin, P. (1997) Disgust faces, basal ganglia and obsessive–compulsive disorder: some strange brainfellows *Trends Cognit. Sci.* 1, 321–322.

89. Young, A. W. et al. (1997) Disgust faces, basal ganglia and obsessive–compulsive disorder: some strange brainfellows. Response from Young, Sprengelmeyer, Phillips and Calder *Trends Cognit. Sci.* 1, 322–325.

90. Koepp, M. J. et al. (1998) Evidence for striatal dopamine release during a video game *Nature* 393, 266–268.

91. Davidson, R. J. (1994) Asymmetric brain function, affective style and psychopathology: the role of early experience and plasticity *Dev. Psychopathol.* 6, 741–758.

92. Cahill, L. et al. (1994) β-Adrenergic activation and memory for emotional events *Nature* 371, 702–704.

93. DeArmond, S. J., Fusco, J. F. and Dewy, M. M. (1989) *Structure of the Human Brain: a Photographic Atlas* (3rd edn), Oxford University Press.

94. Abercrombie, H. C. et al. (1998) Metabolic rate in the right amygdala predicts negative affect in depressed patients *NeuroReport* 9, 3301–3307.

95. Cahill, L. et al. (1996) Amygdala activity at encoding correlated with long-term, free recall of emotional information *Proc. Natl. Acad. Sci. U. S. A.* 93, 8016–8021.

IV SOCIAL NEUROSCIENCE OF MOTIVATION, EMOTION, AND ATTITUDES

B. Social Applications

i. Motivation and Emotion

32 The Affect System Has Parallel and Integrative Processing Components: Form Follows Function

John T. Cacioppo, Wendi L. Gardner, and Gary G. Berntson

Affect in personality and social psychology has traditionally been treated as the conscious subjective aspect of an emotion considered apart from bodily changes (e.g., Osgood, Suci, & Tannenbaum, 1957; Thurstone, 1931). Like the organization and processes underlying the undeniable percept that the sun circles the earth, however, the organization and processes underlying affective experiences may be far subtler than their apparent manifestations might lead one to suspect. Although rich in emotional terms (Clore, Ortony, & Foss, 1987; Frijda, Markam, Sato, & Wiers, 1995; Ortony, Clore, & Foss, 1987; Russell, 1978), language sometimes fails to capture affective experiences—especially intense affective experiences—so metaphors become more likely vehicles for rendering these conscious states of mind (Fainsilber & Ortony, 1987; Hoffman, Waggoner, & Palermo, 1991; Ortony & Fainsilber, 1989).

Affective reports have also long been recognized as subject to a host of motivational influences (e.g., Abelson et al., 1968; Brehm, 1956) and contextual distortions (e.g., Fabrigar, Visser, & Browne, 1997; Irvine, 1995; Ostrom & Upshaw, 1968; Schwarz & Strack, in press) as well as being only modestly related to other aspects of affective reactions, such as physiology and behavior (e.g., Cook & Selltiz, 1964; Lang, 1971; Nisbett & Wilson, 1977). Furthermore, recent investigations in personality and social psychology have characterized affect as capable of being elicited quickly, effortlessly, automatically, or even unconsciously, on exposure to the stimulus (e.g., Bargh, Chaiken, Govender, & Pratto, 1992; Pratto & John, 1991; see Tesser & Martin, 1996). Investigations of the structure of affective words and of self-reports of affect are, therefore, important but may be incomplete. Our goal here is to review selective evidence ranging from neural mechanisms to political behavior to explore some of the properties and features of the system

underlying affective appraisals, experiences, and actions.[1] As we will see, the structure of the affect system depends on function, which varies across the level of the nervous system (neuraxis).

The Affect System

The affect system has been sculpted by the hammer and chisel of adaptation and natural selection to differentiate hostile from hospitable stimuli and to respond accordingly. Although specific behaviors may differ depending on the stimulus and context, there is an underlying commonality to these behaviors. Affective categorizations and responses are so critical that all enduring species have rudimentary reflexes for categorizing and approaching or withdrawing from certain classes of stimuli and for providing metabolic support for these actions (e.g., Berntson, Boysen, & Cacioppo, 1993; Davis, 1997; LeDoux, 1995). These rudimentary processes are evident in humans as well, but a remarkable feature of humans is the extent to which the affective categorizations are shaped by learning and cognition (Berntson et al., 1993; Kahneman, Diener, & Schwarz, in press). As various authors have noted, an additional adaptive advantage is conferred on species whose individual members have the capacity to learn on the basis of the unique environmental contingencies to which they are exposed, to represent and predict events in their environment, to manipulate and plan on the basis of representations, and to exert some control over their attentional and cognitive resources.

Zajonc's (1980) influential article, "Preferences Need No Inferences," underscored the utility of the affect system as an object of study in its own right. Such a focus is not to deny the inextricable links between affect and cognition. Affect directs attention, guides decision making, stimulates learning, and triggers behavior (e.g., Damasio,

1994). Evolutionary forces, however, do not value knowledge or truth per se but rather species survival. Evidence that the neural circuitry involved in computing the affective significance of a stimulus (i.e., evaluative processing) diverges at least in part from the circuitry involved in identification and discrimination (i.e., nonevaluative processing) was provided by Shizgal (in press) in a series of studies involving brain stimulation in rats and by Cacioppo, Crites, and Gardner (1996; Crites & Cacioppo, 1996; Gardner & Cacioppo, in press) in a series of studies of event-related brain potential (ERP) topographies in humans. For instance, investigations of the spatial distribution of late positive potentials (LPP) across the scalp have revealed a right lateralization of affective categorizations, whereas the spatial distribution of the LPP associated with nonaffective categorizations is more symmetrical (Cacioppo et al., 1996). Whether individuals performed affective or nonaffective categorizations of stimuli was manipulated by Crites and Cacioppo (1996), who similarly obtained a symmetrical topography of LPPs when a nonaffective categorization is performed (e.g., deciding whether a food item is a vegetable) but a right lateralized topography of LPPs with an affective categorization (e.g., deciding whether a food item is positive). This asymmetrical activation is consistent with the importance of the right hemisphere in emotion (see Tucker, 1981; Tucker & Frederick, 1989). However, considerable similarities in the ERPs were observed as well, consistent with the notion that affective and nonaffective appraisals rely on a number of common information-processing operations. In the next section we examine the form of the activation functions that characterize the operation of the affect system.

Activation (Currency) Functions

Stimuli and events in the world are diverse, complex, and multidimensional—in short, seemingly incomparable. Yet each perceptual system has

evolved to be tuned to specific features, resulting in the expression of these stimuli on a common metric (Tooby & Cosmides, 1990; see also Ohman, Hamm, & Hugdahl, in press). People have little difficulty doing cross-modal matching, in which they express variations in the intensity of a visual stimulus in terms of sound or touch. Seemingly incomparable stimuli and events are also expressed on common valuation metrics or "currency functions" (Shizgal, in press). The perceptual systems are important not for the description they give of the environment but for the adaptive implications of the stimuli that pass through their bandwidths. As Ohman et al. (in press) noted,

Evolution has primed organisms to be responsive to stimuli that more or less directly are related to the overall task of promoting one's genes to prosper in subsequent generations. Such stimuli include those related to the survival tasks ... stimuli of these types are embedded within emotional systems that help regulate behavior within critical functional domains.

An *activation function* refers to the mathematical relationship between the full range of inputs to a system and the outputs obtained from that system. The activation functions for hedonic inputs can be thought of as currency functions. Information is lost in the translation of a multidimensional representation of a stimulus onto a currency function. As Shizgal (in press) noted,

One cannot recover the temperature, sweetness, or texture of a gustatory stimulus from a currency value representing its instantaneous utility. However, the information lost due to the collapsing of multiple dimensions is essential for identifying the stimulus and distinguishing it from others. Thus, the circuitry that computes instantaneous utility must diverge from the perceptual circuitry subserving identification and discrimination.

Indeed, it is features such as these that make it useful to think of the affect system as an entity intimately related to yet distinguishable from the cognitive system.

Perceptual activation functions tend to be negatively accelerating, and currency functions appear to be negatively accelerating as well (Boysen, Berntson, Hannan, & Cacioppo, 1996; Kemp, Lea, & Fussell, 1995). Boysen et al. (1996), for instance, tested chimpanzees (*Pan troglodytes*) with training in counting and numerical skills. The chimps performed a reverse contingency task in which they selected between two appetitive stimuli, represented either as arrays of different amounts of candies or, more symbolically, by two Arabic numerals. Performance on the task was highly sensitive not to the objective value (e.g., number of candies) of the array stimuli but to the numerical disparity between the arrays. However, the chimps did not appear to be making absolute disparity judgments. Instead, the effects of disparity were qualified by the overall size of the stimulus arrays, with a given disparity yielding smaller effects with larger overall array sizes. That is, the chimpanzees' judgments of the differential incentive values of the stimuli were reminiscent of microeconomic marginal utility functions in which the relative effectiveness of a given increment in payoff diminishes as the base size of the payoff increases. This suggests that the currency functions for the affect system may best be depicted as negatively accelerating when characterizing their full range of activation. Linear functions are reasonable approximations when dealing with more restricted ranges of activation, such as that observed in psychological laboratories in response to pictures (Ito, Cacioppo, & Lang, 1998).

Stages of Evaluative Processing

One distinction between the evaluative channels of the affect system and the perceptual channels of the perceptual system is that the former is constructed not to return objective properties of the stimulus but to provide a subjective estimate of the current significance of these properties (Cacioppo & Gardner, 1999; Shizgal, in press;

Zajonc, 1980).[2] How many evaluative channels are there in the affect system? Most researchers have posited one in which subjective, valent information is derived from the flow of sensation (e.g., D. P. Green, Salovey, & Truax, 1999; Russell & Carroll, 1999; Russell & Feldman Barrett, 1999). Research on the conceptual organization of emotion is consistent with the notion that people's knowledge about emotions is hierarchically organized and that a superordinate division is between positivity and negativity (e.g., Russell, 1983; Russell & Mehrabian, 1977; see Tesser & Martin, 1996; Watson & Tellegen, 1985).

Physical constraints generally restrict behavioral manifestations to bivalent actions (approach–withdrawal). It is true that one can stay motionless or circle a stimulus at a constant distance. Evolution, however, favors the organism that can learn, represent, and access rapidly whether approach or withdrawal is adaptive when confronted by a stimulus. There is also a behavioral efficiency, a conservation of limited cognitive resources, and a reduction in physiological stress that is served by mental representations of general and enduring net action predispositions toward classes of stimuli (Blascovich et al., 1993; Fazio, Blascovich, & Driscoll, 1992; Lingle & Ostrom, 1981). Accordingly, mental guides for one's actions in future encounters with the target stimuli, such as attitudes (e.g., Cacioppo & Berntson, 1994; Fishbein & Ajzen, 1975) and preferences (e.g., Kahneman, in press), may tend to be more expected and stable when organized in terms of a bipolar evaluative dimension. Indeed, Brehm (1956) found individuals to amplify the positive features and diminish the negative features of a chosen alternative and to magnify the negative features and minimize the positive features of an unchosen alternative. This motivational push toward affective bipolarity was especially compelling when individuals initially regarded the alternatives to be similarly appealing. The bipolar (positive-negative) structure that comes from the spreading of alternatives represents a stable endpoint, however, not the states or processes that preceded this endpoint.

The fact that approach and withdrawal are reciprocally activated behavioral manifestations does not mean that they were derived from a single bipolar evaluative channel. Nor does the fact that positive and negative affect have antagonistic effects on approach or withdrawal behavior mean that the affective inputs are invariably reciprocally activated (e.g., see Edwards & Ostrom, 1971). They mean only that the outputs of the evaluative processors composing the affect system are combined in order to compute bivalent action tendencies and actions (Cacioppo & Berntson, 1994). Such an organization fosters function: free and swift approach to appetitive stimuli and rapid and unfettered withdrawal from aversive stimuli. This organization is patent in the neural architecture of spinal cord reflexes—the so-called final common pathway for behavior—where activation of flexor reflexes reciprocally inhibits extensor antagonists and vice versa (Sherrington, 1906). This introduces a reciprocal bias in motor outputs, but this peripheral organization does not preclude the activation of both flexors and extensors (e.g., isometric contractions) via input from rostral brain areas (e.g., through voluntary efforts). The affect system may be organized similarly, perhaps not by accident, because the affect system—constituted largely of reflexes and fixed action patterns in simple organisms—evolved to direct behavior in a way that fosters species survival.

Various theorists have posited that the theoretical module in the affect system that computes attitudes, preferences, and actions derives input from at least two specialized evaluative channels that process information in parallel: one in which threat-related (i.e., negative) information is derived from the flow of sensory inputs and its associations and a second in which safety and appetitive (i.e., positive) information is derived (e.g., Cacioppo & Berntson, 1994; Cacioppo, Gardner, & Berntson, 1997; Gilbert, 1993; Gray,

1994; Lang, Bradley, & Cuthbert, 1990; Marcus & Mackuen, 1993; Marcus, Sullivan, Theiss-Morse, & Wood, 1995; Watson, Wiese, Vaidya, & Tellegen, 1999; Zautra, Potter, & Reich, 1997). In an important and integrative article, Lang et al. (1990) summarized the behavioral evidence for distinguishing between approach and withdrawal reflexes or behaviors, with negatively valent behaviors organized in terms of an "aversive" or "defensive motivational system" and positively valent behaviors organized in terms of an "appetitive motivational system" (Konorski, 1967; Masterson & Crawford, 1982; Miller, 1961; Schneirla, 1959). Lang and colleagues (e.g., Lang et al., 1990; Lang, Bradley, & Cuthbert, 1992) have incorporated appetitive and aversive motivational systems into a theory of emotion:

It is proposed that two motive systems exist in the brain—appetitive and aversive—accounting for the primacy of the valence dimension. Arousal is not viewed as having a separate substrate, but rather, as reflecting variations in the activation (metabolic and neural) of either or both systems. (Lang, 1995, p. 374)

Individuals approach, acquire, or ingest certain classes of stimuli and withdraw from, avoid, or reject others. Many behaviors that do not fall at these extremes can nevertheless be placed along an approach–withdrawal continuum. Because behavior is often constrained by the mutual exclusivity of the various options, Lang and colleagues posited that appetitive and aversive motivational systems were uniformly reciprocally activated. That is, emotions are viewed by Lang et al. (1990, 1992) as evolving from simple action tendencies that directly reflect activation of aversive or appetitive systems.[3] The appetitive and aversive motivational systems are reducible to a single valence (good–bad) dimension in Lang's theory because these motivational systems were assumed explicitly to be reciprocally activated. Given that Lang et al. (1990, 1992) were focused on defensive reflexes, where reciprocal activation is the rule, Lang's formulation serves as a principal example of form following function. Startle reflex modulation does indeed seem to be organized in a bipolar structure, reflecting the net reciprocal activation at this level of the aversive and appetitive motivational systems (Lang, 1995).

When thinking about the human affect system as a whole, no single structure appears to apply; rather, the shape of the affective system appears to reflect the goal of the affective processing at any given level. According to our model of evaluative space (Cacioppo & Berntson, 1994; Cacioppo et al., 1997), when the appetitive and aversive features of stimuli are being determined, these rapid, critical evaluations can occur at least in part in parallel, and the potential affective space can be depicted as being at least bivariate. The form of these early stages of information processing, which involves subcortical and cortical circuits (see *Neural Substrates,* below), is functionally adaptive in that it fosters the extraction and evaluation of hedonic inputs. The greater the appetitive inputs the greater the activation of positivity (appetitive motivational force), whereas the greater the aversive inputs the greater the activation of negativity (aversive motivational force).[4] The world and life experiences are complex, so a given stimulus can have very different effects on different individuals (or the same individual in different circumstances), and a given stimulus can have similar or different effects on the activation of positivity and the activation of negativity. Stimuli that activate neither positivity nor negativity elicit indifference, whereas stimuli that strongly activate both positivity and negativity elicit intense ambivalence. A two-dimensional representation of the activation of positivity and negativity, therefore, may provide a more comprehensive formulation for depicting these operations. This two-dimensional space, which is depicted as the bottom plane in Figure 32.1, is termed the *evaluative plane or space.*

Given that the affect system evolved to guide behavior, information processed by the affect system does not stop with its registration on the evaluative space. Instead, the antagonistic effects of the activation of positivity and negativity are integrated into a net affective predisposition or action, which can be represented as an overlying bipolar response surface (see Figure 32.1).[5]

Modes of Evaluative Activation

Our questioning of the assumption that the motivational systems (i.e., evaluative channels) are invariably reciprocally activated derives from the notion of evolutionary economy. Two evaluative channels (i.e., positivity and negativity, relating to the appetitive and aversive motivational systems, respectively) can be construed as having three activational states each: decreasing activation, no change in activation, and increasing activation. If the positive and negative evaluative channels are orchestrated such that they are always reciprocally activated, the dynamic range of the affect system as a whole is enhanced, but the two evaluative channels still have only three activational states: increased positivity–decreased negativity, no change, and decreased positivity–increased negativity. Separable evaluative channels would not need to have evolved if their actions were always reciprocally organized, because a single evaluative channel ranging from positivity to negativity would have sufficed. Why, then, might appetitive and aversive motivational systems have evolved as orchestrated but distinguishable assemblages? If the mode of activation of these two evaluative channels varies, the combinations of evaluative input from these two channels expands from three to nine, with a consequent expansion of response properties (e.g., directional stability, dynamic range, and response lability; see Cacioppo & Berntson, 1994, Table 1). This leads to the concept of multiple *modes of evaluative activation* underlying behavioral predispositions and actions: (a) reciprocal activation occurs when a stimulus has opposing effects on the activation of positivity and negativity, (b) uncoupled activation occurs when a stimulus affects only positive or only

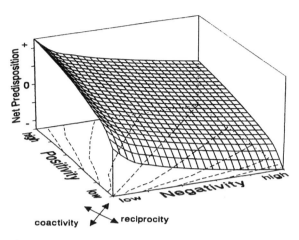

Figure 32.1

Illustrative bivariate evaluative space and its associated affective response surface. This surface represents the net predisposition of an individual toward (+) or away (−) from the target stimulus. This net predisposition is expressed in relative units, and the axis dimensions are in relative units of activation. The point on the surface overlying the left axis intersection represents a maximally positive predisposition, and the point on the surface overlying the right axis intersections represents a maximally negative predisposition. Each of the points overlying the dashed diagonal extending from the back to the front axis intersections represent the same middling predisposition. Thus, the non-reciprocal diagonal on the evaluative plane—which represents different evaluative processes (e.g., neutrality to ambivalence)—yields the same middling expression on the affective response surface. Dashed lines (including the coactivity diagonal) represent isocontours on the evaluative plane, which depict many-to-one mappings between the affective response surface and the underlying evaluative space. These isocontours are illustrative rather than exhaustive. (From "Relationship Between Attitudes and Evaluative Space: A Critical Review, With Emphasis On the Separability of Positive and Negative Substrates," by J. T. Cacioppo and G. G. Berntson, 1994, *Psychological Bulletin, 115*, p. 412. Copyright 1994 by the American Psychological Association.)

negative evaluative activation, and (c) non-reciprocal activation occurs when a stimulus increases (or decreases) the activation of both positivity and negativity.[6]

The bivariate evaluative space presented in Figure 32.1 accommodates all possible combinations of positive and negative affective activation: The reciprocal mode of evaluative activation is represented as one diagonal vector that ranges from maximal positivity–minimal negativity to maximal negativity–minimal positivity, the non-reciprocal mode of evaluative activation is represented as the alternate diagonal that ranges from minimal positivity and negativity to maxi-

mal positivity and negativity, and the uncoupled modes of evaluative activation are represented as vectors lying along the axes. The family of vectors parallel to those above represents the general categories, or modes, of evaluative activation expressed from varying starting points within the two-dimensional plane depicted in evaluative space. As noted above, low activation of both positivity and negativity by a stimulus reflects neutrality or indifference, whereas high activation of positivity and negativity reflects ambivalence. Note that although indifference and ambivalence represent two very different affective substrates, their mapping onto the overlying surface yields similarly middling (e.g., neither approach nor avoidance) responses. Thus, knowledge of the position of a response on the overlying bipolar affective surface does not provide definitive information about underlying processes or mechanisms. This is one of the reasons that knowledge of an individual's net affective predisposition is not sufficient to understand fully the state of the affect system.

In reciprocal evaluative activation, changes in behavioral predispositions and behavior are fueled consistently by the changes in the positive and negative evaluative processes underlying these endpoints. For instance, an individual's preference for or behavior toward a stimulus would become more positive if the stimulus evokes positive evaluative processes and diminishes negative evaluative processes. Variations in the magnitude of their reciprocal activation, although affecting the magnitude of the change in preference, would not be expected to alter the basic direction of the change. Of course, positive and negative evaluative processes could be reciprocally activated with the negativity evoked by a stimulus increasing and the positivity evoked by the stimulus decreasing rather than vice versa. In contrast, nonreciprocal modes (coactivation or coinhibition) have an inherently variable or unstable effect on the *direction* of behavioral predispositions or behavior while the range of response is constrained. In coactivation, for instance, both positive and negative evaluative processing are increasing; however, changes in the activation of positivity and negativity have functionally opposite effects on the consequent predisposition or approach–withdrawal behavior. Minor variations in the magnitude of the relative activation of positivity or negativity, therefore, can lead to a more positive predisposition, a more negative predisposition, or no manifest change in predisposition toward the stimulus, depending on which evaluative substrate dominates. The directional instability of ambivalent attitudes, for instance, has been noted (e.g., Katz, Wackenhut, & Hass, 1986) and is explicable as a for-

mal property of the coactivation of opposing evaluative activation functions.

Note, too, that this conceptualization of the affect system does not reject the bipolar conceptualization but rather subsumes it in two ways: (a) as the reciprocal diagonal and the family of vectors parallel to this diagonal within the evaluative space and (b) as the net response predisposition represented by the overlying surface (see Figure 32.1). One of the unique implications of this framework is that the question should be not whether positive and negative affective processes are reciprocally activated but rather under what conditions are they reciprocally, nonreciprocally, or independently activated.

Evidence for the existence of multiple modes of evaluative activation has been observed across all levels of analysis (cf. Cacioppo & Berntson, 1994). For instance, Hoebel (in press) reviewed evidence that food restriction alters neurochemical effects underlying approach behavior in an uncoupled fashion, whereas morphine has reciprocal effects on neurochemical processes underlying approach and withdrawal behavior. The separable activation of positivity and negativity at the verbal level is evident in a study by Goldstein and Strube (1994) in which self-reported positive and negative affect were collected from students at the beginning and end of three consecutive class periods. Although a bipolar model would predict reciprocal activation of positive and negative affect, as evidenced by negative within-subject correlations between the intensity of positive and negative reactions on a particular day, the reactions were in fact uncorrelated. Moreover, exam feedback activated positivity and negativity differently. Students who scored above the mean on the exam showed an increase in positive affect relative to their beginning-of-class level, whereas their level of negative affect remained unchanged within the class period. Similarly, students who scored below the mean on the exam showed an increase in negative affect but no change in positive affect within the class period. Distinctions between positive and negative affective processes have also been observed in uplifts and hassles (Gannon, Vaux, Rhodes, & Luchetta, 1992; Zautra, Reich, & Gaurnaccia, 1990), mood states (Lawton, Kleban, Dean, Rajagopal, & Parmelee, 1992; Watson & Tellegen, 1985; Zautra, Potter, & Reich, 1997), organization of self-knowledge (e.g., Showers, 1995; Showers & Kling, 1996), self-regulatory focus (e.g., Higgins, 1997), self-efficacy (Zautra, Hoffman, & Reich, 1997), personality processes (Depue, 1996; Diener & Lucas, in press; Robinson-Whelen, Kim, MacCallum, & Kiecolt-Glaser, 1997; Rusting & Larsen, 1998; Watson, Clark, McIntyre, & Hamaker, 1992), achievement motivations (Elliot & Church, 1997; Elliot & Harackiewicz, 1996), organ donations (Cacioppo & Gardner, 1993), emotional expressivity (Gross & John, 1997), interpersonal relationships (Berry & Hansen, 1996; Cacioppo et al., 1997), affect toward political leaders (Marcus & Mackuen, 1993), and inter-group discrimination (Blanz, Mummendey, & Otten, 1997; Brewer, 1996; Mummendey, 1994).

Watson and Clark (1991, 1992; Watson & Tellegen, 1985) proposed that positive and negative affect were separate dimensions and that negative affect can be represented at two distinct structural levels.[7] At the higher level of abstraction, a general negative factor accounts for shared variance across the negative affects, whereas at the lower level of abstraction the negative affects (e.g., fear, hostility, sadness, and guilt) are distinct and exhibit unique variance. Much of the research on Watson and Clark's proposed two-factor structure of affective space has centered on methodological or statistical issues. D. P. Green, Goldman, and Salovey (1993; D. P. Green & Citrin, 1994), for instance, questioned the notion that positive and negative affect were separable on methodological grounds (see also Bagozzi, 1993; Marsh, 1996; Suh, Diener, & Fujita, 1996; Watson & Clark, 1997). Specifically, they argued that measures of affect typically rely on similarly worded scales with identical endpoints. This fea-

ture, they argued, leads to a similarity in responses to the positive and negative scale items (i.e., positively correlated measurement error), which would suppress the magnitude of the true negative correlation between positive and negative affective states. In an interesting analysis of data on the public perceptions of Hispanics, D. P. Green and Citrin (1994) demonstrated that nonrandom measurement error in survey questions (e.g., error attributable to the common format and response options) can diminish the correlation between positively and negatively valenced statements.[8]

A recent investigation by Nelson (in press) addressed the methodological concerns of D. P. Green and colleagues and found evidence for the operation of multiple modes of evaluative activation. Nelson used a structural modeling approach to examine the structure of affect toward two different social categories—African Americans and the poor—while accounting for correlated measurement error among the observed variables. Nelson's analyses of the structure of the non-poor students' emotional responses toward the poor revealed substantial independence between positive and negative factors. This two-factor model was significantly better than the bipolar model, even when the effects of correlated measurement error were extracted. This result is precisely what one would expect if positive and negative affect were separate dimensions at the most abstract level, as posited by Watson and Clark (1991, 1992). Nelson's analyses of the structure of the students' emotional responses toward African Americans, however, revealed a bipolar model to be sufficient when the effects of correlated measurement error were considered. This latter result illustrates that affect as a subjective state or response disposition does not invariably manifest in a bipolar or a bivariate structure but rather its manifest structure is influenced by the mode of evaluative activation elicited by the stimulus (Cacioppo & Berntson, 1994). That is, conceptualizations of positivity and negativity as the opposite endpoints of a single bipolar evaluative channel do not provide a comprehensive account.

Although Nelson's (in press) demonstration is notable for its theoretical import, we are not suggesting that the nonreciprocal modes of evaluative activation are common. To the contrary, the clearest guides to behavior are provided when a stimulus elicits reciprocal activation (Cacioppo et al., 1997). The most salient structural feature of predispositions to respond that are stored in memory—for instance, for simple and familiar stimuli toward which one has acted previously (e.g., Brehm, 1956)—is therefore likely to be bipolarity. Consider the International Affective Picture System (IAPS; Lang, Bradley, & Cuthbert, 1995), a set of several hundred photographs that have been scaled in terms of their valence, arousal, and dominance. Included among these pictures are items people are likely to encounter in everyday life, such as cute dogs, delectable foods, dirty dishes, and scenes with trash. We recently scaled these pictures using unipolar positivity, negativity, and ambivalence ratings and bipolar valence, dominance, and arousal ratings (Ito, Cacioppo, & Lang, 1998). The vast majority of these pictures were characterized by reciprocal activation, and the set as a whole elicited reciprocal activation. Moreover, when participant rather than picture was used as the unit of analysis, individuals generally showed reciprocal activation.[9] This is to be expected (Cacioppo et al., 1997; see also D. P. Green et al., 1999; Russell & Carroll, 1999). The best tests of theories are crucial tests, however. If reciprocal activation were the only mode of evaluative activation, then one should never find evidence of nonreciprocal or uncoupled activation. This is why studies ranging from Brehm (1956) to Nelson (in press), why the emergence of any stimulus in the IAPS that appeared to elicit nonreciprocal activation (Ito, Cacioppo, & Lang, 1998), and why affective states such as bittersweetness and ambivalence, are so informative.

In sum, if the activation of positive and negative evaluative processes were inevitably reciprocally coupled, then detailing separable positive and negative evaluative channels would not enhance prediction of the resulting affective responses. However, theory and research from areas ranging from the conceptual organization of emotion through sociopolitical issues to unconditioned responses indicate that positive and negative evaluative processes have some nonoverlapping operating components (e.g., functional independence), are opposing in their effects on attitudes or behavior, and are capable of being differentially activated. There is evidence that reciprocal modes of evaluative activation are more likely to manifest postdecisionally (see Cacioppo et al., 1997), at high levels of emotional (particularly negative) intensity (Zautra, Potter, & Reich, 1997), and as one moves down the level of the neuraxis (Berntson et al., 1993; Ito & Cacioppo, in press), but additional research is needed on the factors governing the mode of evaluative activation. Even though these questions remain, the concept of modes of evaluative activation appears to be useful in thinking about the operation and structure of the affect system.

Neural Substrates

The extant neurophysiological data cannot resolve the nature and structure of the affect system. Research on the neural substrates of emotion, however, can contribute to social psychological theory and research by inspiring new concepts and relationships, providing supportive or nonsupportive evidence on predicted structural relations, and adding realistic constraints to theoretical conjectures (Cacioppo & Berntson, 1992). All thoughts, motives, affects, and actions are organized and orchestrated by the central nervous system (CNS). Although the complexity of the CNS may at times seem bewildering, central neural substrates evidence general principles of organization that are common features across distinct systems and mechanisms. These principles offer a framework for understanding not only spinal reflexes and somatic motor actions but also psychological and behavioral processes. As mentioned above, one general principle of neural organization is the reciprocal innervation of opponent effector systems (Sherrington, 1906). This is based on the spinal organization of reflex controls of antagonistic flexor and extensor muscles, by which activation of one effector system was accompanied by inhibition of the other, opposing system. The neural circuitry underlying spinal somatomotor control now is fairly well clarified, including the specific motoneuron pools and the interneuronal pathways underlying the reciprocal innervation. Although derived from the study of spinal reflexes, the principle of reciprocal innervation is recognized to be a far more pervasive feature of central neural systems (Sherrington, 1906; for a synopsis, see Berntson et al., 1993).

The functional organization of the somatomotor system may be instructive in considering the central substrates of affective systems and approach–avoidance reactions in general. Flexors (e.g., biceps) and extensors (e.g., triceps) have directly opposing actions, and the joint outcome of these actions can yield varying degrees of either flexion or extension of the forearm, but not both. That is, the output of this opponent system is bipolar, varying along a continuum from extreme flexion to extreme extension, as constrained by the musculoskeletal structure of the arm. In the organization of simple reflexes, such as the flexor (pain) withdrawal reflex, reciprocal innervation of the flexor and extensor motoneurons can be highly adaptive. The pain stimulus that triggers flexor contraction synergistically inhibits extensor activity and promotes flexor withdrawal.

Despite the pattern of reciprocal innervation of antagonistic motor neuron pools at the reflex level, the neural organization of flexor–extensor control cannot be viewed along a simple bipolar continuum. Rostral motor systems exert potent descending control not only over reciprocally organized spinal reflex circuits but also directly on lower motor neurons. Moreover, rostral motor systems controlling extensors and flexors have separate cortical representations (see classic work by Asanuma, 1975). Rostral systems are able to inhibit or override reciprocal spinal organizations and can coactivate both extensor and flexor lower motoneuron pools. This is important in postural support reactions, balance, and dynamic motor adjustments. It also provides the neurological substrate for volitional increases in tension in both biceps and triceps muscles (e.g., in stiffening the arm) and for the ability to inhibit basic flexor withdrawal reflexes (e.g., in suppression of pain withdrawal in the cold pressor test). These phenomena document central bivariate control of flexors and extensors despite the fact that this bivariate central control is physically constrained into bipolar manifestations.

Although the pattern of reciprocal inhibition does tend to promote a bipolar output, the fundamental bipolar nature of forearm flexion and extension arises from the physical constraints of the musculoskeletal system, not from central motor substrates. This poses an important caveat for conceptualizations of central affective networks. Although there may be interactions among positive and negative affective systems, the fact that conceptual organizations of emotion and behavioral outputs tend toward a bipolar structure does not imply that central mechanisms adhere to the same structure. Indeed, emerging data on central substrates for positive and negative affect suggest the existence of at least partially distinct neural mechanisms.

Early work on the neural systems mediating reward and aversion revealed that reinforcing and punishing effects could be induced by stimulation of differentiated brain areas (Delgado, Roberts, & Miller, 1958; Olds & Milner, 1954). This work spearheaded efforts to elucidate the neural and neurochemical substrates of hedonic processes. Recent studies have focused on the role of the mesolimbic dopamine pathway in reward (Wise, 1996) and on the amygdala as a substrate for aversion (Davis, 1992b; LeDoux, 1992).

The mesolimbic dopamine pathway originates in the ventral tegmental area of the midbrain and projects to the nucleus accumbens. Activation of this system has been shown to function as a reward, and animals will perform an arbitrary operant in order to self-administer stimulation of this pathway (Wise, 1996). Like natural rewards, this stimulation triggers release of dopamine in the nucleus accumbens, which appears to contribute importantly to reward (Hoebel, Hernandex, Mark, & Pothos, 1992). Similarly, administration of addictive drugs, such as cocaine, induces dopamine release in the nucleus accumbens, and blockade of dopamine receptors in this area has been reported to attenuate the rewarding effects of addictive drugs as well as natural rewards (Hoebel et al., 1991; Wise, 1996). Moreover, animals will self-administer dopamine receptor agonists into the nucleus accumbens, as well as drugs that release endogenous dopamine. These and other findings have led to the view that the mesolimbic dopamine pathway is a crucial central substrate for reward. Although invasive studies are obviously precluded in humans, indirect findings are in accord with this view. Drugs that potentiate dopamine activity, such as amphetamine and cocaine, can be highly euphoric and can enhance natural rewards, whereas agents that block dopamine action have been reported to attenuate reward (Wise, 1996).

In contrast, the amygdala has been implicated in negative affect (Adolphs, Tranel, Damasio, & Damasio, 1995; Davis, 1992a, 1992b; LeDoux, 1992). Aversive reactions and punishment effects can be evoked by stimulation of the amygdala (Halgren, 1982). Although somewhat similar results can be obtained by stimulation of central pain transmission pathways, the effects of amygdalar stimulation do not appear to reflect pain per se. The amygdala is not part of the primary pain projection system, and lesions of this structure do not eliminate simple unconditioned responses to pain stimuli (LeDoux, 1992). Rather, lesions appear to selectively attenuate affective reactions to aversive stimuli, particularly responses to conditioned aversive stimuli (Davis, 1992a; Killcross, Robbins, & Everitt, 1997; LeDoux, 1992). Consistent with inferences derived from animal research, brain imaging studies in humans have revealed activation of the amygdala in response to negative affective stimuli (Irwin et al., 1996) and during aversive conditioning (Diedrich et al., 1997). Moreover, fear and other negative emotions in humans have been reported frequently with amygdaloid stimulation or abnormal epileptic activity (Cendes et al., 1994; Halgren, 1982). The difference is not absolute, however, as specific amygdalar circuits may also play some role in positive affect.

The focus on the amygdala and nucleus accumbens does not adequately reflect the complexity and multiplicity of central evaluative substrates.[10] The nucleus accumbens and the amygdala represent critical nodal points in affective mechanisms, but reward and aversion can be evoked by stimulation of widely distributed, but differentiated, central systems. These systems defined by stimulation and lesion methods closely correspond to relevant substrates identified during naturally induced affective states by metabolic or gene markers that reflect neural activation (Gomita, Moriyama, Ichimaru, & Araki, 1988; Sandner et al., 1993; Yeomans, 1990). Despite partial overlap and interaction among these systems, positive and negative affective reactions appear to be associated with separable neural circuits. Even in overlapping areas that can yield both self-stimulation and escape behavior, the rewarding and aversive consequences of stimulation appear to be mediated by distinct neural populations (Anderson, Diotte, & Miliaressis, 1995; Bielajew & Shizgal, 1980), indicating a simple algebraic summation of independent contributions (Anderson et al., 1995).

Dissociation between stimulation-induced approach and escape reactions have also been reported with drug administration. Morphine, for example, has been shown to elevate stimulation thresholds for escape behavior without altering self-stimulation (Carr, Bonnet, & Simon, 1982; Ichitani & Iwasaki, 1986). Similarly, the benzodiazepine receptor agonist diazepam was found to reduce the punishing effects of foot shock on operant performance, again without altering self-stimulation (Gomita & Ueki, 1981). Moreover, the rewarding effects of opiates are disrupted by lesions of the nucleus accumbens, whereas the aversive effects of cocaine withdrawal are unaltered; in contrast, lesions of the amygdala attenuate the aversive effects of withdrawal without attenuating the rewarding effects of opiate administration (Kelsey & Arnold, 1994). These findings reveal that central mechanisms for reward and aversion can be independently manipulated, again indicating a fundamental dissociability of brain systems subserving positive and negative affect.

Although we have considered some findings on the amygdala and nucleus accumbens, this discussion is not about particular brain structures but about the fundamental separability of positive and negative substrates. Central systems for positive and negative affect are vast and complex (Berridge, 1996). Studies on both decerebrate humans and animals reveal basic, stereotyped orofacial intake-rejection reflexes to positive and aversive tastes (for a review see Berridge, 1996; Berridge & Pecina, 1995). Higher systems, such as the amygdala and nucleus accumbens, appear to play a more important role in appetitive aspects of food intake and in acquired taste aversions (Berridge, 1996; Roldan & Bures, 1994; Schafe & Bernstein, 1996). Even at the most basic level of organization, however, intake-rejection reflexes are not organized reciprocally. Experimental manipulations at the level of the brain stem can selectively potentiate intake responses without altering aversive-rejection responses (Berridge & Pecina, 1995). Moreover, these basic reflexes are sensitive to distinct taste qualities. Intake responses are selectively poten-

tiated with sucrose, whereas rejection responses are preferentially enhanced with quinine. When a combined solution of sucrose and quinine is presented, one does not see an attenuation of both intake and rejection in rats. Quite the contrary: Both reflexes are potentiated, and one sees an alternation of vigorous, opposing orofacial patterns (Berridge & Grill, 1984). Rostral neural systems likely add considerable flexibility in food intake patterns, and multiple substrates may be involved in distinct aspects of food intake. Despite the fact that differential patterns of neural activity may underlie different aspects of food intake—or different affective states, for that matter—there remains a basic commonality in the approach–avoidance systems. A neutral stimulus (conditioned stimulus [CS], e.g., Pavlov's bell) paired with an unconditioned stimulus (US, e.g., food powder) can yield a new association such that the CS comes to evoke conditioned responses (CRs) such as approach, salivation, and so on, similar to those of the US (i.e., unconditioned responses [URs]). In this case of food, the basic US–UR relation appears to be intrinsically organized at brain stem levels, whereas the CS–CR link requires higher neural mechanisms. Nevertheless, they operate on a common appetitive substrate, as evidenced by the fact that degrading the US–UR relation (e.g., by adding a foul taste to the food) results in an associated degradation of a previously established CS–CR link (see MacIntosh, 1983).

Although they are separable, central systems for positive and negative affect do appear to interact naturally, in accord with the principle of reciprocal innervation. Noncontingent stimulation of "reward" sites in the hypothalamus, for example, appears to generally facilitate approach behaviors while suppressing escape or withdrawal responses. Conversely, stimulation of "aversive" systems is associated with an enhancement of escape reactions generally and inhibition of approach responses (Stellar, Brooks, & Mills, 1979). Moreover, as is the case for extensor and flexor activity, behavioral constraints may further bias toward bipolar manifestations of affective processes. By the use of experimental paradigms that permit concurrent expression of positive and negative affective processes, the studies outlined above reveal that central affective systems can be independently manipulated. Although overt affective expression may tend toward bipolarity, a bivariate model of central affective processes is necessary to accommodate these results.

Distinctions Between the Currency Functions for Positivity and Negativity

The effects of the activation of positivity and negativity are not mirror opposites. Active forms of coping, such as problem solving, influence positive affective states more than negative affective states in chronic pain patients (Zautra, Burleson, et al., 1995; Zautra, Reich, & Newsom, 1995). Classroom performance motivated by the desire for mastery or for social approval (approach motivations), in contrast to a fear of failure (avoidance motivation), is associated with better grades and more durable intrinsic motivation (Elliot & Church, 1997). In research on social interactions, positive and negative affectivity have each been related to the number of social interactions in which individuals engage and the amount of time spent engaged in social contact, but positive (and not negative) affectivity has predicted the pleasantness of the social interactions, whereas negative affectivity has predicted the frequency of relatively superficial dyadic same-sex interactions (Berry & Hansen, 1996). On the basis of research suggesting that positive and negative interracial attitudes and behaviors were related to different factors, Schofield (1991) reasoned that practices designed to increase positive interaction among Black and White students may not substantially decrease negative interaction. Schofield's hypothesis is provocative because it suggests that theory and research on promoting positive interracial affect and behaviors may not have the intended reciprocal effect on negative interracial affect and behaviors. Similarly, investigators have been perplexed by why so few people who feel positively about donor behaviors are themselves donors (Sarason, Sarason, Pierce, Shearin, & Sayers, 1991; Sarason et al., 1993). Part of the answer may lie in the findings that the positive and negative evaluative processes underlying donor attitudes and behaviors are separable and that the negative substrate represents a powerful impediment (Parisi & Katz, 1986; see Cacioppo & Gardner, 1993; Gardner & Cacioppo, 1995).

Evolution can genetically endow only limited fixed adaptive responses relative to the potential range of circumstances an organism could encounter. Therefore, there is an evolutionary pressure to maximize flexibility. The partial segregation of the positive and negative evaluative channels in the affect system confers the additional flexibility of orchestrating appetitive and aversive motivational forces via modes of evaluative activation, which in turn affords greater flexibility for learned dispositions. It also affords evolution the opportunity to sculpt distinctive activation (i.e., currency) functions for positivity and negativity. Interest in differences in the impact of positive versus negative information has grown substantially in recent years. Numerous articles and several major reviews on the topic have appeared (e.g., Cacioppo & Berntson, 1994; Levy, 1992; Peeters & Czapinski, 1990; Skowronski & Carlston, 1989; Taylor, 1991), and the two final issues of the *European Journal of Social Psychology* in 1990 were devoted to the topic. Of particular interest here is the research on affective asymmetries (e.g., appetitive vs. aversive stimuli) rather than cognitive asymmetries (e.g., presence vs. absence of a feature) in positive and negative information processing (McGuire & McGuire, 1996). The extant data suggest at least two differences in these currency functions: (a) a positivity offset—the output of positivity is higher than the output of negativity at very low levels of affective input and (b) a negativity bias—the increase in output per quantum of input is greater for negativity than for positivity.

Positivity Offset

The *positivity offset* is the tendency for there to be a weak positive (approach) motivational output at zero input. In other words, the level of positive output is higher at the intercept than is the level of negative output. As a consequence of the positivity offset, the motivation to approach is stronger than the motivation to avoid at very low levels of evaluative activation. What might be the possible evolutionary significance of the positivity offset? Without a positivity offset, an organism in a neutral environment may be unmotivated to approach novel objects, stimuli, or contexts. The neophobic response to foreign stimuli that characterizes most species permits an initial period of observation. With no negative outcomes, this exposure allows the initial neophobic response to habituate, thereby allowing exploratory behavior to manifest. In the absence of such a motivation to explore, organisms would learn little about novel or neutral-appearing environments and their potential reward value. With a positivity offset, however, an organism facing neutral or unfamiliar stimuli would be weakly motivated to approach and, with the quick habituation of the initial fear response, to engage in exploratory behavior. Such a pairing of initial neophobic and subsequent exploratory tendencies may have important survival value, at least at the level of a species. A positivity offset also fosters social cohesion even in the absence of other information about conspecifics.

If this reasoning is correct, one might expect such a tendency to manifest itself in the human cognitive system in several ways. First, individuals may exhibit relatively positive rather than neutral expectations for unknown future events. Several recent studies have found this to be the case. Pulford and Colman (1996) found that people overestimated the likelihood that they would experience positive and negative outcomes in the coming week, with this overestimation being greater for positive than for negative outcomes. Hoorens and Buunk (1993) found that people attributed lower health risks to them-

selves than to others. Brinthaupt, Moreland, and Levine (1991) found that students interested in joining campus groups expected membership to lead to more rewards and fewer costs for them than others (for whom expected rewards and costs were more equally distributed). Diener and colleagues have reported extensive evidence demonstrating that the normative human experience seems to involve a state of mildly positive affect (e.g., Diener & Diener, 1996). Finally, Regan, Snyder, and Kassin (1995) reported two experiments in which individuals held more positive expectations about their own futures than those of an aggregate of same-sex peers or other individual social objects. As Regan et al. noted: "Indeed, most of us remain firmly encased in the solipsistic belief that negative life events or outcomes are less likely to happen to us than to others and that positive events are more likely to happen to us than to others" (p. 1073).

In addition to imparting an optimistic glow to future expectations, the positivity offset should also sway attitude and impression *formation*. Indeed, a robust "positivity bias" in impression formation is evident in the literature (Adams-Weber, 1979; Benjafield, 1985; Kaplan, 1973; Klar & Giladi, 1997; Sears, 1983). Boucher and Osgood (1969) first documented the tendency to form positive impressions of unknown others, christening it the *Pollyanna bias;* they asserted that this bias reflected unrealistically optimistic assumptions about human nature. This tendency toward generosity in our evaluations of others has been attributed variously to impression management on the part of the research participant (Bruner & Tagiuri, 1954), the manifestation of the "golden section" ratio in the use of positive versus negative descriptors (Benjafield, 1985), the attributional implications of the behaviors used (e.g., neutral descriptors implying a lack of negative features; Jones & Davis, 1965), and the "bonus" attraction that results from an individual's fundamental similarity with any conspecific (Byrne, 1971; Sears, 1983). Although all of these processes have been shown to affect the magnitude of the positivity bias, none of them has been shown to erase it completely. Gardner (1996) hypothesized that the robust "positivity bias" in impression formation reflected the more general positivity offset in the evaluative system. In four studies, Gardner found evidence of a positivity offset in impression formation that was not limited by the social desirability concerns of the participants, by the type of neutral behaviors used, or by the similarity between target and participant. Indeed, the positivity offset was observed not only in impressions of human targets but also with impressions of novel fish and insects. The positivity offset demonstrated in this work, then, could not have been a result of the neutral behaviors implying the absence of negative attributes. Neither could it have merely reflected the process of similarity leading to attraction, as Sears's (1983) "person positivity bonus" would have predicted. Instead, the positivity offset appeared to be a more general operating characteristic of the affect system. We turn next to what we believe to be another general operating characteristic of the affect system: the negativity bias.

Negativity Bias

Human taste buds respond to sweet, salty, sour, and bitter stimuli. Most can detect sweetness in approximately 1 part in 200, saltiness in 1 part in 400, sourness in 1 in 130,000, and bitterness in 1 in 2,000,000. From the perspective of the affect system, a given amount of a negative or threat-related gustatory stimulus (e.g., most poisons taste bitter) activates a stronger affective response than the same amount of a positive (e.g., sweet) gustatory stimulus. This may be more than an epicurean curiosity; it may represent differences in the currency functions for positive and negative affects that is so pervasive it has been termed the *negativity bias* (see reviews by Cacioppo & Berntson, 1994; Cacioppo et al., 1997; Peeters & Czapinski, 1990; Skowronski & Carlston, 1989; Taylor, 1991). Among the earliest evidence for a negativity bias is Miller's (1959) study, in

which he determined that the slope for the avoidance gradient in his rodent research on conflict behavior was steeper than the slope for the approach gradient. Skowronski and Carlston (1989) reviewed research on impression formation and found support for a negativity bias in impression formation, and Cacioppo and Gardner (1993) found evidence for the negativity bias in their review of research on attitudes toward blood and organ donations. Recent work has also found evidence of a negativity bias in individuals of various ages and in nonlaboratory settings (e.g., Aloise, 1993; Robinson-Whelen et al., 1997). Aloise (1993), for instance, asked children in grades 3–5 and college students how many behaviors they require before attributing positive or negative traits to other people. Regardless of age, individuals tended to require fewer behaviors to infer negative than positive traits. Walden (1993) examined reactions of children (ages 27–95 months) to an ambiguous stimulus that had not been described or had been described as fearful, neutral, or positive. Negative expectations had a stronger impact on the children's behavior than positive expectations, and this effect was magnified in younger children. The negativity bias can also be seen in the assessments of utility by accounting for what has been called *loss aversion* (Kahneman & Tversky, 1984). Observing that losses loom larger than gains, Kahneman and Tversky (1984) argued that the value function relating negative events to subjective value has a steeper slope than the one relating positive events to subjective value.

Klein (1991) observed a negativity bias in the political domain as well. More than 3,000 respondents rated presidential candidates on several personality traits in national election surveys from 1984 to 1988. Results revealed that negative personality characteristics were more predictive of overall evaluations and voting behavior than were positive traits. These results were replicated by Klein (1996) in a study of the voters' impressions of Bill Clinton and George Bush in the 1992 presidential election. Taylor (1991) summarized a wide range of evidence showing that negative events in a context evoke stronger and more rapid physiological, cognitive, emotional, and social responses than neutral or positive events (see also Cacioppo, Berntson, Larsen, & Poehlmann, in press; Westermann, Spies, Stahl, & Hesse, 1996).

Several factors have been identified as accounting for the fact that negative information receives more weight than positive information does. A dominant explanation in the impression formation literature rests on the differential diagnosticity of negative versus positive behaviors (Reeder & Brewer, 1979; Skowronski & Carlston, 1989). In short, this theory argues that impressions depend on the diagnosticity of a given behavior in exemplifying a trait category (e.g., honest, athletic). The diagnosticity of a behavior is determined by both the valence of the behavior and the applicability of the behavior to either a morality or an ability domain. In morality-relevant domains, when people are judging others for their honesty or kindness, negative behaviors provide a higher level of diagnosticity, because moral individuals are necessarily constrained from exhibiting immoral acts (e.g., an honest person never cheats), but immoral individuals are free to display either moral or immoral behavior. Ability-relevant domains, in which judgments concern athleticism or intelligence, are restricted in the reverse fashion. Individuals high in ability can exhibit behavior either high or low in ability (e.g., even Tiger Woods may have a bad game now and then), but low-ability individuals cannot exhibit high-ability behaviors; positive behaviors should thus be weighted more heavily in ability-relevant impressions.

To the extent that much of the impression literature has investigated morality-relevant domains, it is difficult to unravel whether evidence of a negativity bias results from an operating feature of the affective system or reflects attributional analyses of behavioral diagnosticity. However, Gardner (1996) found evidence of a negativity bias even when only ability-relevant

behaviors were presented in an impression task. Furthermore, Ganzach (1995) found that greater weight was given to negative attributes than to positive attributes in an analysis of three real-world data sets of performance evaluation, and Rowe (1989) observed conceptually similar results in employment decisions. Given that performance and employment decisions represent judgments of ability, it appears that explanations of the negativity bias that rest on diagnosticity calculations alone cannot fully account for the empirical evidence.

Furthermore, evidence for the negativity bias (as well as for the positivity offset) has been found in paradigms in which diagnosticity and morality–competence are irrelevant. Miller's (1959) studies of learning in rats is a case in point. In humans, Ito, Cacioppo, and Lang (1998) measured the positive and negative feelings evoked by 472 slides selected to represent the full affective space captured by the IAPS (Lang et al., 1995). Arousal ratings were used to index the intensity of the affective stimulus (they were plotted on the abscissa), and the unipolar positivity and unipolar negativity ratings were used to index the magnitude of the affective response (they were plotted on the ordinate). Analyses revealed that the intercept was significantly higher for ratings of positive than for negative stimuli (i.e., a positivity offset). Results also revealed that the slope of the regression line for the ratings of the negative stimuli was significantly steeper than that of the regression line for the ratings of the positive stimuli (i.e., the negativity bias). That is, positive stimuli have a greater effect on affect than negative stimuli do at comparably low levels of activation, but the opposite is the case at comparably high levels of activation. A conceptually similar pattern of results was reported by Wojciszke, Brycz, and Borkenau (1993), who investigated reactions to moderately or extremely positive and negative behaviors of fictitious targets.

Evidence for the negativity bias has also been found in studies of electrocortical potentials, as well. We have developed a paradigm using ERPs to investigate evaluative processes independent of behavioral responses (Cacioppo et al., 1996; Crites & Cacioppo, 1996). In an illustrative study, Cacioppo et al. (1996) recorded ERPs as participants were exposed to a series of positive, neutral, and negative stimuli (e.g., trait words). To maximize the likelihood that participants were categorizing the stimuli along evaluative dimensions, the stimuli were presented within sequences of six, and participants were asked to count silently the number of positive (or negative, counterbalanced) stimuli that appeared in each sequence. The majority of the stimuli within each sequence were drawn from a single evaluative category (e.g., all positive or all negative). In some sequences, for instance, all six stimuli were drawn from this same evaluative category, but in others one of the six stimuli was drawn from the other evaluative category (e.g., a positive food embedded within a sequence of negative foods). This made it possible to record the ERPs associated with the appraisal of evaluatively consistent and evaluatively inconsistent target stimuli. Cacioppo et al. found a larger amplitude LPP (a P300-like component) with a mean latency of approximately 650 ms to evaluatively inconsistent stimuli (e.g., a negative stimulus embedded in a sequence of positive stimuli) than to evaluatively consistent stimuli (e.g., a positive stimulus embedded in a sequence of positive stimuli). This LPP enhancement was found regardless of whether the evaluatively inconsistent stimulus was positive or negative. Subsequent studies demonstrated that the LPP amplitudes associated with evaluative processes are maximal over central–parietal regions, vary as a function of the degree of evaluative inconsistency (e.g., LPP amplitudes are larger to extremely negative stimuli than to moderately negative stimuli embedded in a sequence of positive stimuli), and vary more as a function of evaluative categorizations than response selection or execution (Cacioppo, Crites, Gardner, & Berntson, 1994; Crites, Cacioppo, Gardner, & Berntson, 1995).

In Study 1, Crites et al. (1995) presented positive, neutral, and negative stimuli in series of predominantly positive stimuli, whereas in Study 2 they presented positive, neutral, and negative stimuli in series of predominantly negative stimuli. A reexamination of data from Crites et al. revealed larger LPP amplitudes to negative stimuli embedded in a series of positive stimuli ($M = 8.93$ μV) as compared to positive stimuli embedded in a series of negative stimuli ($M = 6.70$ μV). Ito, Larsen, Smith, and Cacioppo (1998) explicitly tested whether the negativity bias operates at the evaluative categorization stage in two experiments using ERPs. The LPP, which is differentially sensitive to the evaluative categorization but not the response output stage (Cacioppo et al., 1994; Crites et al., 1995; Gardner & Cacioppo, in press), was recorded to positive, negative, and neutral pictures embedded within sequences of other neutral pictures. Results confirmed that (a) the evaluative categorization of positive or negative stimuli in sequences of neutral stimuli was associated with larger amplitude late positive brain potentials over central–parietal regions and (b) the evaluative categorization of negative stimuli was associated with a larger amplitude LPP than was the evaluative categorization of equally probable, equally evaluatively extreme, and equally arousing positive stimuli. Because the degree of evaluative consistency and inconsistency was equivalent for positive and negative targets in these studies, the larger LPPs evoked by negative than positive stimuli is consistent with the notion that the currency function for negativity is steeper than the currency function for positivity.

In sum, exploratory behavior can provide useful information about an organism's environment, and the positivity offset fosters such behavior. But exploration can also place an organism in proximity to hostile stimuli. Because it is more difficult to reverse the consequences of an injurious or fatal assault than those of an opportunity not pursued, the process of natural selection may have resulted in distinguishable motivational organizations for positivity and negativity with the propensity to react more strongly to proximate negative events than to positive or neutral events. Species with a positivity offset and a negativity bias enjoy the benefits of exploratory behavior and the self-preservative benefits of a predisposition to avoid or withdraw from threatening events. Negative emotion has been depicted previously as playing a fundamental role in calibrating psychological systems; it serves as a call for mental or behavioral adjustment, whereas positive emotion serves as a cue to stay the course. These characterizations may also help account for evolutionary forces sculpting separable substrates and distinctive currency functions for positive and negative affect.

The focus of our model is more on the architecture and operating characteristics of the affect system than on the antecedent conditions for arousing positive or negative affect. Like the phenomenon of color perception, however, affect is not an invariant property of the stimulus but a product of neural transformations of the stimulus input within an array of contextual information. Work on the relativity of emotion, for instance, has demonstrated that cognitive factors and physiological states can influence the extent to which appetitive or defensive motivations are aroused (see Cacioppo & Gardner, 1999). Brendl and Higgins (1995), for example, provided evidence that an incentive is greater when it is compatible with a person's self-regulatory focus and goal (see also Shah, Higgins, & Friedman, 1998). These models complement the present by identifying factors that influence the degree to which appetitive or defensive motivations are aroused.

Conclusion

When asked to define poetry, A. E. Houseman said "I could no more define poetry than a terrier can a rat, but I thought we both recognized the object by the symptoms which it provokes in us"

(Ackerman, 1990, p. 295). The same might be said about affect. It is understandable, therefore, why the structure of affect has tended to be defined in terms of the symptoms it provokes (i.e., the words used to describe these feelings; D. P. Green et al., 1999; Russell & Feldman Barrett, 1999; Watson et al., 1999). We have also suggested that this approach, although important, may paint an incomplete picture of the affect system. As research on automatic emotional processing has so nicely shown, it is important to go beyond the traditional boundaries of conscious mental states in theories of the affect system.

The prior literature on the structure of affect and moods has tended both to focus on people's verbal reports of feeling states and to cast the question as whether positive and negative feelings are organized in a bipolar or bivariate structure (e.g., Russell & Carroll, 1999). We do not believe this approach to be productive any longer, and we have suggested several revisions.

First, we have suggested that the structure of verbally expressed moods and feelings is important to understand as a psychological phenomenon but that we should not confuse this with the task of understanding the form and function of the underlying affect system. What are needed are psychological models of the affect system that do not merely speculate about mediating psychological processes but that instead specify them in detailed, empirically meaningful ways. Additionally, these models and specifications would not rely solely on self-report evidence of psychological processes but would be based also on more rigorous experimental techniques—including approaches from the cognitive sciences and the neurosciences—for uncovering mediating mechanisms.

Second, and relatedly, the stimuli and scales that are used in studies can bias the results that are obtained. R. F. Green and Goldfried (1965) long ago noted that when affect is defined as consciously accessible elemental feelings of pleasure and activation, and the experimental stimuli and scales are selected to differ in terms of valence and arousal, it is not surprising to find evidence that affect is organized in terms of valence and arousal. Watson et al. (1999) noted that high negative affectivity is marked by more terms (*distressed, fearful, hostile, jittery, nervous,* and *scornful*) than low negative affect (*calm, at rest, placid,* and *relaxed*). Terms such as *quiet, hushed, reposed, peaceful, tranquil, undisturbed,* and *serene* appear not to have been among the experimental stimuli, however. It is unclear whether the relative dearth of linguistic markers at the lower end of the continua is a function of the stimulus set(s) used in these studies or a reflection of the structure of affective experience.

Third, the issue may be not either–or but under what conditions and at what stage of affective processing are positivity and negativity organized in a bipolar versus bivariate (or even more complex) fashion. Physical limitations constrain behavioral expressions and incline behavioral guides toward bipolar (good–bad; approach–withdraw) dispositions while cognitive economies incline conceptual organizations toward a similar structure. These endpoints do not imply that the form of the underlying processes is similarly structured, however. We have suggested that the common metric governing approach–withdrawal is generally bipolar at response stages but that this response organization is the consequence of two intervening metrics: the activation function for positivity (appetition) and the activation function for negativity (aversion), at an earlier stage of affective processing. A two-dimensional representation of the activation of positivity and negativity may therefore provide a more comprehensive formulation for depicting the affective processes that predispose and culminate in an affective (e.g., approach–withdrawal) predisposition or response. This net action tendency can then be represented as an overlying bipolar response surface (see Figure 32.1). Inherent in this framework is the concept of modes of evaluative activation, which accommodates all possible combinations of positive and negative evaluative

activation. Thus, in this conceptualization of the affect system the bipolar conceptualization is subsumed in two ways: (a) as the reciprocal diagonal and the family of vectors parallel to this diagonal in evaluative space and (b) as the overlying surface representing the net predisposition to respond.

D. P. Green et al. (1999) noted that biases that are due to random and nonrandom measurement error can mask bipolar structure in mood ratings. This is an important point for investigators to recognize in studies of affective ratings. There are other rating biases that also should be considered, of course. Thompson, Zanna, and Griffin (1995), for instance, highlighted biases that can make affective ratings appear more rather than less bipolar than they actually are. It is important, though, that demonstrations that bipolarity in affective ratings can be masked by methodological biases do not logically imply that affective processes or experiences are necessarily organized in a bipolar fashion. D. P. Green et al. acknowledged this point but appear to argue that pleasant and unpleasant states are best understood using a bipolar framework, because in most circumstances these feelings are experienced inversely. What is true in most circumstances is not necessarily the most important or relevant data from a theoretical perspective. Experimental social psychologists have long recognized the importance of artificial environments to obtain theoretical insights. Most of the data to date, for instance, still favor the view that self-perception and cognitive dissonance theories can account for changes that follow attitude-discrepant behaviors. But this theoretical question was essentially resolved in a single study by Fazio, Zanna, and Cooper (1977), who showed that neither theory could account entirely for their results but instead that each theory had a unique domain of application. Physicists, too, have long recognized the need to create quite artificial circumstances—events that are so infrequent as to not be observable in the normal course of daily events—to test theories about the structure (nature, elements) and forces underlying physical phenomena. One therefore does not need the majority of studies to yield results inconsistent with bipolarity to question the adequacy of a bipolar model of affect. Even were deviations from bipolarity to be fleeting (but see lingering states of ambivalence), it would not mean they were unimportant. Cognitive dissonance, for instance, is typically a rather fleeting state, but its short- and long-term consequences can be rather dramatic. Thus, we agree that bipolarity may frequently describe people's affective ratings, but we disagree that this means that the structure of the affect system can be captured comprehensively or parsimoniously by bipolarity.

One might question the utility of placing all "pleasant" goal states into one positive category and all "unpleasant" goal states into one negative category. We would agree that there is substantial value in retaining categorical conceptualizations of emotion (e.g., happy, sad, fear, anger, disgust). We would further contend, however, that there is substantial and unique insight to be gained by the present framework. As Marr (1982) noted, different data representations render certain mental operations simple and others complex. The literature on emotion is replete with examples of the utility of both categorical (i.e., discrete) and dimensional perspectives, and there is precedence for such an approach in other sciences (e.g., particle vs. wave theories of light). The issue, therefore, may be not whether all pleasant states should be placed into one positive category and all unpleasant states into a negative category but what new or unique insights, understandings, and testable hypotheses are obtained by such a conceptualization.

Indeed, the value of considering the additional complexities introduced by multiple evaluative channels and modes of evaluative activation derives in large part from the data it explains, the questions it generates, and the bridges it builds across empirical literatures previously thought to be separate. Data from the neurosciences to the

social sciences suggest the separability of positive and negative affective processes. Self-report and ERP data suggest distinctive currency functions for positivity and negativity. These currency functions represent multifarious appetitive and aversive inputs, respectively, along common metrics. Research using multiple operationalizations suggests a positivity offset and a negativity bias in these currency functions. There is also evidence that reciprocal modes of evaluative activation are more likely to manifest postdecisionally (see Cacioppo et al., 1997), at high levels of emotional (particularly negative) intensity (Zautra, Potter, & Reich, 1997), and as one moves down the level of the neuraxis (Berntson et al., 1993), but additional research is needed on the factors governing the modes of evaluative activation. The greater likelihood of reciprocal relations between positivity and negativity as one moves from the determination of the appetitive and aversive qualities of a stimulus to action in response to the stimulus is consistent with the physical constraints that generally restrict behavioral manifestations to bivalent actions and the role of the somatic and autonomic nervous system in carrying out the results of appraisals to achieve these actions. This formulation may also provide a useful heuristic for investigating individual differences in motivational orientation. For instance, the magnitude of the positivity offset and negativity bias may be expected to differ across individuals. Research to explore the stability and predictive utility of these parameters, as well as their relation to affective disorders, may therefore be worthwhile.

We previously used temperature (hot and cold) to illustrate the activation functions that would be expected from entities at the opposite ends of a whole bipolar dimension (Cacioppo et al., 1997). Note that we were not speaking of people's perceptions of temperature but rather the physics of temperature. Cold is the absence of heat. The structure of people's perceptions of temperature are considerably more complicated, as is apparent when one feels both feverish and chilly. Thus, studies of people's perceptions of temperature (e.g., see Russell & Carroll, 1999) may tell us more about the nonbipolarity of people's perceptions of temperature than of how complex data from a bipolar dimension may look.

Finally, and perhaps most important, most of the research on the structure of affect has relied on correlational procedures. Theory and research on the structure of affect could benefit considerably from a greater reliance on experimental methods. For example, we have manipulated the extent of positive and negative information about an object as one means of determining the activation functions for positivity and for negativity (Gardner, 1996). Similarly, Edwards and Ostrom (1971) used an experimental approach in their study of the limitations of bipolarity. To the extent that bipolar, circumplex, and evaluative space conceptualizations make the same predictions, distinguishing between them is moot. To the extent that they make different predictions, a focused experimental test of these predictions is best. For instance, the model of evaluative space offered the novel prediction that ambivalence is asymmetrical in that not only is ambivalence perceived to be more negative than positive but also that negative components are weighted more heavily than positive components. Experimental tests supported this hypothesis (Cacioppo et al., 1997). It is important that experimental methods do not bias the answer about the structure of affect one way or another; they simply eliminate some of the biases (e.g., subject-selection artifacts) that can be introduced when relying on correlational methods, and they allow more sharply focused empirical tests among theories.

Notes

1. Discussion of the factors that lead to more or less activation of the affect system is beyond the scope of this article (but see Brendl & Higgins, 1995, or Cacioppo & Gardner, 1999, for a review).

2. This distinction has long been recognized in social psychology and has served, for instance, as a rationale for social comparison processes (Festinger, 1954).

3. Lang et al. (1990, 1992) acknowledged that there are many emotions but posited that these discrete emotions are organized by their motivational determinants and can be construed as ordered along strategic dimensions of valence and arousal.

4. The term *positivity* is used here to refer to an abstract entity that includes appetitive motivational substrates, processes, and outputs, whereas the term *negativity* is used to refer to the abstract entity including aversive motivational substrates, processes, and outputs. In our formulation, positivity (and negativity) can range from inactive to fully activated (cf. Konorski, 1967; Lang et al., 1990; Masterson & Crawford, 1982; Miller, 1961; Schneirla, 1959). Thus, our use of these terms differs from that of Watson and colleagues. For instance, high levels of positivity and negativity yield ambivalence in our formulation, whereas high positive affectivity and negative affectivity in Watson and Tellegen's (1985) formulation are characterized by arousal, astonishment, and surprise. This is due to differences in the conceptualizations of positivity and negativity.

5. The positivity × negativity plane depicted in Figure 32.1 represents the status in what we have termed *evaluative space* because it describes the level of activation of the underlying positive and negative inputs to a bivalent affective response. The resulting behavioral predisposition to approach or withdraw can be represented in terms of an overlying surface. It is possible to derive this overlying surface for all combinations of positivity and negativity. The exact shape of the attitudinal surface is dependent on the form of the activation functions, the relative value of the weighting coefficients, and the scaling of the axes (see Cacioppo & Berntson, 1994). For purposes of approximation, the currency functions for positivity and negativity were designated as negatively accelerating, with the exponent for negativity being larger than the exponent for positivity and the intercept being larger for positivity than for negativity (Cacioppo & Berntson, 1994; Cacioppo et al., 1997).

6. It is important to note that the activation of positivity and negativity is assumed generally to have antagonistic effects on behavior regardless of mode. *Modes of evaluative activation* refer not to whether positivity, for instance, fosters approach and negativity

fosters withdrawal but to the level (e.g., increase, no change, decrease) of positivity and negativity elicited by an event or stimulus. Note, too, that the model does not specify why positivity or negativity is activated but rather it specifies the form of their activation, the modes and effects of their activation, and so forth (see Cacioppo et al., 1997).

7. Watson and colleagues (e.g., Watson & Clark, 1991) conceptualized these two dimensions as bipolar rather than as unipolar (cf. Cacioppo & Berntson, 1994). Watson et al. (1999) recently revised their formulation such that there is now agreement between their model and ours on this feature.

8. In a related program of research, Thompson et al. (1995) suggested that methodological artifacts (e.g., carryover between unipolar positive and negative rating scales) could inflate the negative correlation between positive and negative rating scales. They recommended segregating self-report measures of positive and negative affect to avoid self-presentational biases.

9. These results were generally replicated when using a structural modeling approach to analyze these data (P. Salovey, personal communication, October 23, 1998).

10. The precise role of these structures in reward processes has yet to be fully explicated. Stressors, for example, have also been found to trigger dopamine (DA) release from the nucleus accumbens (Salamone, Cousins, & Snyder, 1997). This may be consistent with the role of DA in reward, as aversive contexts motivate behavior and set the stage for reinforcement of responses that lead to escape or otherwise reduce the aversive context. Current models emphasize the role of the mesolimbic DA system in incentive motivation and the link to behavioral action (Salamone et al., 1997; Wickelgren, 1997). This view is also consistent with recent data on drug addiction. Many drugs of abuse, such as cocaine, amphetamine, and morphine, are potent releasers of DA in the nucleus accumbens and can be highly euphoric. Drug consequences such as euphoria, however, may be of secondary importance in addiction. Drug addicts are often driven more by the desire for a drug, even though they report minimal pleasure on drug delivery (Berridge & Robinson, 1995; Wickelgren, 1997). These latter phenomena are in keeping with the potential role of the nucleus accumbens in incentive dispositions and associated attentional and cognitive biases toward drug-related stimuli and actions.

References

Abelson, R. P., Aronson, E., McGuire, W. J., Newcomb, T. M., Rosenberg, M. J., & Tannenbaum, P. H. (1968). *Theories of cognitive consistency: A sourcebook.* Skokie, IL: Rand-McNally.

Ackerman, D. (1990). *A natural history of the senses.* New York: Vintage Books.

Adams-Weber, J. R. (1979). *Personal construct theory: Concepts and applications.* Chichester, England: Wiley.

Adolphs, R., Tranel, D., Damasio, H., & Damasio, A. R. (1995). Fear and the human amygdala. *Journal of Neuroscience,* 15, 5879–5891.

Aloise, P. A. (1993). Trait confirmation and disconfirmation: The development of attribution biases. *Journal of Experimental Child Psychology,* 55, 177–193.

Anderson, R., Diotte, M., & Miliaressis, E. (1995). The bidirectional interaction between entral tegmental rewarding and hindbrain aversive stimulation effects in the rat. *Brain Research,* 688, 15–20.

Asanuma, H. (1975). Recent developments in the study of the columnar arrangement of neurons within the motor cortex. *Physiological Reviews,* 55, 143–156.

Bagozzi, R. P. (1993). An examination of the psychometric properties of measures of negative affect in the PANAS-X scales. *Journal of Personality and Social Psychology,* 65, 836–851.

Bargh, J. A., Chaiken, S., Govender, R., & Pratto, F. (1992). The generality of the automatic attitude activation effect. *Journal of Personality and Social Psychology,* 62, 893–912.

Benjafield, J. (1985). Review of recent research on the golden section. *Empirical Studies of the Arts,* 3, 117–134.

Berntson, G. G., Boysen, S. T., & Cacioppo, J. T. (1993). Neurobehavioral organization and the cardinal principle of evaluative bivalence. *Annals of the New York Academy of Sciences,* 702, 75–102.

Berridge, K. C. (1996). Food reward: Brain substrates of wanting and liking. *Neuroscience Biobehavioral Review,* 20, 1–25.

Berridge, K. C., & Grill, H. J. (1984). Isohedonic tastes support a two-dimensional hypothesis of palatability. *Appetite,* 5, 221–231.

Berridge, K. C., & Pecina, S. (1995). Benzodiazepines, appetite, and taste palatability. *Neuroscience Biobehavioral Review,* 19, 121–131.

Berridge, K. C., & Robinson, T. E. (1995). The mind of an addicted brain: Neural sensitization of wanting versus liking. *Current Directions in Psychological Science,* 4, 71–76.

Berry, D. S., & Hansen, J. S. (1996). Positive affect, negative affect, and social interaction. *Journal of Personality and Social Psychology,* 71, 796–809.

Bielajew, C., & Shizgal, P. (1980). Dissociation of the substrates for medial forebrain bundle self-stimulation and stimulation-escape using a two-electrode stimulation technique. *Physiology and Behavior,* 25, 707–711.

Blanz, M., Mummendey, A., & Otten, S. (1997). Normative evaluations and frequency expectations regarding positive versus negative outcome allocations between groups. *European Journal of Social Psychology,* 27, 165–176.

Blascovich, J., Ernst, J. M., Tomaka, J., Kelsey, R. M., Salomon, K. L., & Fazio, R. H. (1993). Attitude accessibility as a moderator of autonomic reactivity during decision making. *Journal of Personality and Social Psychology,* 64, 165–176.

Boucher, J., & Osgood, C. E. (1969). The Pollyanna hypothesis. *Journal of Verbal Learning and Verbal Behavior,* 8, 1–8.

Boysen, S. T., Berntson, G. G., Hannan, M. B., & Cacioppo, J. T. (1996). Quantity-based choices: Interference and symbolic representations in chimpanzees (*Pan troglodytes*). *Journal of Experimental Psychology: Animal Behavior Processes,* 22, 76–86.

Brehm, J. W. (1956). Post-decision changes in desirability of alternatives. *Journal of Abnormal and Social Psychology,* 52, 384–389.

Brendl, C. M., & Higgins, E. T. (1995). Principles of judging valence: What makes events positive or negative? *Advances in Experimental Social Psychology,* 28, 95–160.

Brewer, M. B. (1996). In-group favoritism: The subtle side of intergroup discrimination. In D. M. Messick & A. E. Tenbrunsel (Eds.), *Codes of conduct: Behavioral research into business ethics* (pp. 160–170). New York: Russell Sage Foundation.

Brinthaupt, L. J., Moreland, R. L., & Levine, J. M. (1991). Sources of optimism among prospective group members. *Personality and Social Psychology Bulletin,* 17, 36–43.

Bruner, J. S., & Tagiuri, R. (1954). The perception of people. In G. Lindzey (Ed.), *Handbook of social psychology* (pp. 634–654). Reading, MA: Addison-Wesley.

Byrne, D. (1971). *The attraction paradigm.* New York: Academic Press.

Cacioppo, J. T., & Berntson, G. G. (1992). Social psychological contributions to the decade of the brain: The doctrine of multilevel analysis. *American Psychologist,* 47, 1019–1028.

Cacioppo, J. T., & Berntson, G. G. (1994). Relationship between attitudes and evaluative space: A critical review, with emphasis on the separability of positive and negative substrates. *Psychological Bulletin,* 115, 401–423.

Cacioppo, J. T., Berntson, G. G., Larsen, J. T., & Poehlmann, K. M. (in press). The psychophysiology of emotion. In R. Lewis & J. M. Haviland (Eds.), *Handbook of emotion* (2nd ed.). New York: Guilford Press.

Cacioppo, J. T., Crites, S. L., Jr., & Gardner, W. L. (1996). Attitudes to the right: Evaluative processing is associated with lateralized late positive event-related brain potentials. *Personality and Social Psychology Bulletin,* 22, 1205–1219.

Cacioppo, J. T., Crites, S. L., Jr., Gardner, W. L., & Berntson, G. G. (1994). Bioelectrical echoes from evaluative categorizations: I. A late positive brain potential that varies as a function of trait negativity and extremity. *Journal of Personality and Social Psychology,* 67, 115–125.

Cacioppo, J. T., & Gardner, W. L. (1993). What underlies medical donor attitudes and behavior? *Health Psychology,* 12, 269–271.

Cacioppo, J. T., & Gardner, W. L. (1999). Emotion. *Annual Review of Psychology,* 50, 191–214.

Cacioppo, J. T., Gardner, W. L., & Berntson, G. G. (1997). Beyond bipolar conceptualizations and measures: The case of attitudes and evaluative space. *Personality and Social Psychology Review,* 1, 3–25.

Carr, K. D., Bonnet, K. A., & Simon, E. J. (1982). Mu and kappa opioid agonists elevate brain stimulation threshold for escape by inhibiting aversion. *Brain Research,* 245, 389–393.

Cendes, F., Andermann, F., Gloor, P., Gambardella, A., Lopes-Cendes, I., Watson, C., Evans, A., Carpenter, S., & Olivier, A. (1994). Relationship between atrophy of the amygdala and ictal fear in temporal lobe epilepsy. *Brain*, 117, 739–746.

Clore, G. L., Ortony, A., & Foss, M. A. (1987). The psychological foundations of the affective lexicon. *Journal of Personality and Social Psychology*, 53, 751–766.

Cook, S. W., & Selltiz, C. A. (1964). A multiple-indicator approach to attitude measurement. *Psychological Bulletin*, 62, 36–55.

Crites, S. L., Jr., & Cacioppo, J. T. (1996). Electrocortical differentiation of evaluative and nonevaluative categorizations. *Psychological Science*, 7, 318–321.

Crites, S. L., Jr., Cacioppo, J. T., Gardner, W. L., & Berntson, G. G. (1995). Bioelectrical echoes from evaluative categorizations: II. A late positive brain potential that varies as a function of attitude registration rather than attitude report. *Journal of Personality and Social Psychology*, 68, 997–1013.

Damasio, A. R. (1994). *Descartes' error: Emotion, reason, and the human brain*. New York: Grossett/Putnam.

Davis, M. (1992a). The role of the amygdala in conditioned fear. In J. P. Aggleton (Ed.), *The amygdala: Neurobiological aspects of emotion, memory and mental dysfunction* (pp. 255–306). New York: Wiley Liss.

Davis, M. (1992b). The role of the amygdala in fear and anxiety. *Annual Review of Neuroscience*, 15, 353–375.

Davis, M. (1997). The neurophysiological basis of acoustic startle modulation: Research on fear motivation and sensory gating. In P. J. Lang, R. F. Simons, & M. Balaban (Eds.), *Attention and orienting* (pp. 69–96). Mahwah, NJ: Erlbaum.

Delgado, J. M. R., Roberts, W. W., & Miller, N. E. (1954). Learning motivated by electrical stimulation of the brain. *American Journal of Physiology*, 179, 587–593.

Depue, R. A. (1996). A neurobiological framework for the structure of personality and emotion: Implications for personality disorders. In J. F. Clarkin & M. F. Lenzenweger (Eds.), *Major theories of personality disorder* (pp. 347–390). New York: Guilford Press.

Diedrich, O., Grodd, W., Weiss, U., Schneider, F., Flor, H., & Birbaumer, N. (1997). Amygdala activation in social phobics during Pavlovian conditioning detected by functional MRI. *Psychophysiology*, 34, S30.

Diener, E., & Diener, C. (1996). Most people are happy. *Psychological Science*, 7, 181–185.

Diener, E., & Lucas, R. E. (in press). Personality and subjective well-being. In D. Kahneman, E. Diener, & N. Schwarz (Eds.), *Well-being: The foundations of hedonic psychology*. New York: Cambridge University Press.

Edwards, J. D., & Ostrom, T. M. (1971). Cognitive structure and neutral attitudes. *Journal of Experimental Social Psychology*, 7, 36–47.

Elliot, A. J., & Church, M. A. (1997). A hierarchical model of approach and avoidance achievement motivation. *Journal of Personality and Social Psychology*, 72, 218–232.

Elliot, A. J., & Harackiewicz, J. M. (1996). Approach and avoidance achievement goals and intrinsic motivation: A mediational analysis. *Journal of Personality and Social Psychology*, 70, 461–475.

Fabrigar, L. R., Visser, P. S., & Browne, M. W. (1997). Conceptual and methodological issues in testing the circumplex structure of data in personality and social psychology. *Personality and Social Psychology Review*, 1, 184–203.

Fainsilber, L., & Ortony, A. (1987). Metaphorical uses of language in the expression of emotions. *Metaphor and Symbolic Activity*, 2, 239–250.

Fazio, R. H., Blascovich, J., & Driscoll, D. M. (1992). On the functional value of attitudes: The influence of accessible attitudes on the ease and quality of decision making. *Personality and Social Psychology Bulletin*, 18, 388–401.

Fazio, R. H., Zanna, M. P., & Cooper, J. (1977). Dissonance versus self-perception: An integrative view of each theory's proper domain of application. *Journal of Experimental Social Psychology*, 13, 464–479.

Festinger, L. A. (1954). A theory of social comparison processes. *Human Relations*, 7, 117–140.

Fishbein, M., & Ajzen, I. (1975). *Belief, attitude, intention, and behavior: An introduction to theory and research*. Reading, MA: Addison-Wesley.

Frijda, N. H., Markam, S., Sato, K., & Wiers, R. (1995). Emotions and emotion words. In J. A. Russell, J. Fernandez-Dols, A. S. R. Manstead, & J. C. Wellenkamp (Eds.), *Everyday conceptions of emotion: An introduction to the psychology, anthropology and linguistics of emotion* (NATA ASI Series D: Behavioural and social sciences, Vol. 81, pp. 121–143). Dordrecht, The Netherlands: Kluwer Academic.

Gannon, L., Vaux, A., Rhodes, K., & Luchetta, T. (1992). A two-domain model of well-being: Everyday events, social support, and gender-related personality factors. *Journal of Research in Personality, 26*, 288–301.

Ganzach, Y. (1995). Negativity (and positivity) in performance evaluation: Three field studies. *Journal of Applied Psychology, 80*, 491–499.

Gardner, W. L. (1996). *Biases in impression formation: A demonstration of a bivariate model of evaluation.* Unpublished doctoral dissertation, Ohio State University.

Gardner, W. L., & Cacioppo, J. T. (1995). Multigallon blood donors: Why do they give? *Transfusion, 35*, 795–798.

Gardner, W. L., & Cacioppo, J. T. (in press). A brain based index of evaluative processing: A late positive brain potential reflects individual differences in the extremity of a negative evaluation. *Social Cognition.*

Gilbert, P. (1993). Defence and safety: Their function in social behaviour and psychopathology. *British Journal of Clinical Psychology, 32*, 131–153.

Goldstein, M. D., & Strube, M. J. (1994). Independence revisited: The relation between positive and negative affect in a naturalistic setting. *Personality and Social Psychology Bulletin, 20*, 57–64.

Gomita, Y., Moriyama, M., Ichimaru, Y., & Araki, Y. (1988). Neural systems activated by the aversive stimulation of dorsal central gray. *Japanese Journal of Pharmacology, 48*, 137–141.

Gomita, Y., & Ueki, S. (1981). "Conflict" situation based on intracranial self-stimulation behavior and the effect of benzodiazepines. *Pharmacology, Biochemistry and Behavior, 14*, 219–222.

Gray, J. A. (1994). Personality dimensions and emotion systems. In P. Ekman & R. J. Davidson (Eds.), *The nature of emotion: Fundamental questions* (pp. 329–331). New York: Oxford University Press.

Green, D. P., & Citrin, J. (1994). Measurement error and the structure of attitudes: Are positive and negative judgments opposites? *American Journal of Political Science, 38*, 256–281.

Green, D. P., Goldman, S. L., & Salovey, P. (1993). Measurement error masks bipolarity in affect ratings. *Journal of Personality and Social Psychology, 64*, 1029–1041.

Green, D. P., Salovey, P., & Truax, K. M. (1999). Static, dynamic, and causative bipolarity of affect.

Journal of Personality and Social Psychology, 76, 856–867.

Green, R. F., & Goldfried, M. R. (1965). On the bipolarity of semantic space. *Psychological Monographs, 79* (6, Whole No. 599).

Gross, J. J., & John, O. P. (1997). Revealing feelings: Facets of emotional expressivity in self-reports, peer ratings, and behavior. *Journal of Personality and Social Psychology, 72*, 435–448.

Halgren, E. (1982). Mental phenomena induced by stimulation in the limbic system. *Human Neurobiology, 1*, 251–260.

Higgins, E. T. (1997). Beyond pleasure and pain. *American Psychologist, 52*, 1280–1300.

Hoebel, B. G. (in press). Neural systems for reinforcement and inhibition of behavior: Relevance to eating, addiction and depression. In D. Kahneman, E. Diener, & N. Schwarz (Eds.), *Well-being: The foundations of hedonic psychology.* New York: Cambridge University Press.

Hoebel, B. G., Herndandez, L., Mark, G. P., & Pothos, E. (1992). Microdialysis in the study of psychostimulants and the neural substrate for reinforcement: Focus on dopamine and serotonin. *NIDA Research Monograph, 124*, 1–34.

Hoffman, R. R., Waggoner, J. E., & Palermo, D. S. (1991). Metaphor and context in the language of emotion. In R. R. Hoffman & D. S. Palermo (Eds.), *Cognition and the symbolic processes: Applied and ecological perspectives* (pp. 163–185). Hillsdale, NJ: Erlbaum.

Hoorens, V., & Buunk, B. P. (1993). Social comparison of health risks: Locus of control, the person-positivity bias, and unrealistic optimism. *Journal of Applied Social Psychology, 23*, 291–302.

Ichitani, Y., & Iwasaki, T. (1986). Approach and escape responses to mesencephalic central gray stimulation in rats: Effects of morphine and naloxone. *Behavioural Brain Research, 22*, 63–73.

Irvine, J. T. (1995). A sociolinguistic approach to emotion concepts in a Senegalese community. In J. A. Russell, J. Fernandez-Dols, A. S. R. Manstead, & J. C. Wellenkamp (Eds.), *Everyday conceptions of emotion: An introduction to the psychology, anthropology and linguistics of emotion* (NATA ASI Series D: Dehavioural and social sciences, Vol. 81, pp. 251–265). Dordrecht, The Netherlands: Kluwer Academic.

Irwin, W., Davidson, R. J., Lowe, M. J., Mock, B. J., Sorenson, J. A., & Turski, P. A. (1996). Human amygdala activation detected with echo-planar functional magnetic resonance imaging. *Neuroreport,* 7, 1765–1769.

Ito, T. A., & Cacioppo, J. T. (in press). The psychophysiology of utility appraisals. In D. Kaheman, E. Diener, & N. Schwarz (Eds.), *Well-being: The foundations of hedonic psychology.* New York: Cambridge University Press.

Ito, T. A., Cacioppo, J. T., & Lang, P. J. (1998). Eliciting affect using the International Affective Picture System: Trajectories through evaluative space. *Personality and Social Psychology Bulletin,* 24, 855–879.

Ito, T. A., Larsen, J. T., Smith, N. K., & Cacioppo, J. T. (1998). Negative information weighs more heavily on the brain: The negativity bias in evaluative categorizations. *Journal of Personality and Social Psychology,* 75, 887–900.

Jones, E. E., & Davis, K. E. (1965). From acts to dispositions: The attribution process in person perception. In L. Berkowitz (Ed.), *Advances in experimental social psychology* (Vol. 2, pp. 220–266). New York: Academic Press.

Kahneman, D. (in press). Objective happiness. In D. Kahneman, E. Diener, & N. Schwarz (Eds.), *Well-being: The foundations of hedonic psychology.* New York: Cambridge University Press.

Kahneman, D., Diener, E., & Schwarz, N. (in press). *Well-being: the foundation of hedonic psychology.* New York: Cambridge University Press.

Kahneman, D., & Tversky, A. (1984). Choices, values, and frames. *American Psychologist,* 39, 341–350.

Kaplan, K. J. (1973). On the ambivalence–indifference problem in attitude theory and measurement: A suggested modification of the semantic differential technique. *Psychological Bulletin,* 77, 361–372.

Katz, I., Wackenhut, J., & Hass, R. G. (1986). Racial ambivalence, value duality and behavior. In J. F. Dovidio & S. L. Gaetner (Eds.), *Prejudice, discrimination, and racism* (pp. 35–59). New York: Academic Press.

Kelsey, J. E., & Arnold, S. R. (1994). Lesions of the dorsomedial amygdala, but not the nucleus accumbens, reduce the aversiveness of morphine withdrawal in rats. *Behavioral Neurosciences,* 108, 1119–1127.

Kemp, S., Lea, S. E. G., & Fussell, S. (1995). Experiments on rating the utility of consumer goods: Evidence supporting microeconomic theory. *Journal of Economic Psychology,* 16, 543–561.

Killcross, S., Robbins, T. W., & Everitt, B. J. (1997). Different types of fear-conditioned behaviour mediated by separate nuclei within amygdala. *Nature,* 388, 377–380.

Klar, Y., & Giladi, E. E. (1997). No one in my group can be below the group's average: A robust positivity bias in favor of anonymous peers. *Journal of Personality and Social Psychology,* 73, 885–901.

Klein, J. G. (1991). Negativity effects in impression formation: A test in the political arena. *Personality and Social Psychology Bulletin,* 17, 412–418.

Klein, J. G. (1996). Negativity in impressions of presidential candidates revisited: The 1992 election. *Personality and Social Psychology Bulletin,* 22, 288–295.

Konorski, J. (1967). *Integrative activity of the brain.* Chicago: University of Chicago Press.

Lang, P. J. (1971). The application of psychophysiological methods to the study of psychotherapy and behavior change. In A. E. Bergin & S. L. Garfield (Eds.), *Handbook of psychotherapy and behavior change: An empirical analysis* (pp. 75–125). New York: Wiley.

Lang, P. J. (1995). The emotion probe: Studies of motivation and attention. *American Psychologist,* 50, 372–385.

Lang, P. J., Bradley, M. M., & Cuthbert, B. N. (1990). Emotion, attention, and the startle reflex. *Psychological Review,* 97, 377–395.

Lang, P. J., Bradley, M. M., & Cuthbert, B. N. (1992). A motivational analysis of emotion: Reflec–cortical connections. *Psychological Science,* 3, 44–49.

Lang, P. J., Bradley, M. M., & Cuthbert, B. N. (1995). *International affective picture system (IAPS): Technical menual and affective ratings.* Gainesville: NIMH Center for the Study of Emotion and Attention, University of Florida.

Lawton, M. P., Kleban, M. H., Dean, J., Rajagopal, D., & Parmelee, P. A. (1992). The factorial generality of brief positive and negative affect measures. *Journal of Gerontology: Psychological Sciences,* 47, 228–237.

LeDoux, J. E. (1992). Emotion in the amygdala. In J. P. Aggelton (Ed.), *The amygdala: Neurobiological aspects of emotion, memory and mental dysfunction* (pp. 339–351). New York: Wiley Liss.

LeDoux, J. E. (1995). Emotion: Clues from the brain. *Annual Review of Psychology,* 46, 209–235.

Levy, J. S. (1992). An introduction to prospect theory. *Political Psychology,* 13, 171–186.

Lingle, J. H., & Ostrom, T. M. (1981). Principles of memory and cognition in attitude formation. In R. E. Petty, T. M. Ostrom, & T. C. Brock (Eds.), *Cognitive responses in persuasion* (pp. 399–420). Hillsdale, NJ: Erlbaum.

MacIntosh, N. J. (1983). *Conditioning and associative learning.* New York: Oxford University Press.

Marcus, G. E., & Mackuen, M. B. (1993). Anxiety, enthusiasm, and the vote: The emotional underpinnings of learning and involvement during presidential campaigns. *American Political Science Review,* 87, 672–685.

Marcus, G. E., Sullivan, J. L., Theiss-Morse, E., & Wood, S. L. (1995). *With malice toward some.* New York: Cambridge University Press.

Marr, D. (1982). *Vision: A computational investigation into the human representation and processing of visual information.* New York: Freeman.

Marsh, H. W. (1996). Positive and negative global self-esteem: A substantively meaningful distinction of artifactors? *Journal of Personality and Social Psychology,* 70, 810–819.

Masterson, F. A., & Crawford, M. (1982). The defense motivation system: A theory of avoidance behavior. *Behavioral and Brain Sciences,* 5, 661–696.

McGuire, W. J., & McGuire, C. V. (1996). Enhancing self-esteem by directed-thinking tasks: Cognitive and affective positivity asymmetries. *Journal of Personality and Social Psychology,* 70, 1117–1125.

Miller, N. E. (1959). Liberalization of basic S–R concepts: Extensions to conflict behavior, motivation and social learning. In S. Koch (Ed.), *Psychology: A study of a science, Study 1* (pp. 198–292). New York: McGraw-Hill.

Miller, N. E. (1961). Some recent studies on conflict behavior and drugs. *American Psychologist,* 16, 12–24.

Mummendey, A. (1994). Positive distinctiveness and social discrimination: An old couple living in divorce. *European Journal of Social Psychology,* 25, 657–670.

Nelson, T. E. (in press). Group affect and attribution in social policy opinion. *Journal of Politics.*

Nisbett, R. E., & Wilson, T. D. (1977). Telling more than we can know: Verbal reports on mental processes. *Psychological Review,* 84, 231–259.

Ohman, A., Hamm, A., & Hugdahl, K. (in press). Cognition and the autonomic nervous system: Orienting, anticipation, and conditioning. In J. T. Cacioppo, L. G. Tassinary, & G. G. Berntson (Eds.), *Handbook of psychophysiology.* New York: Cambridge University Press.

Olds, J., & Milner, P. (1954). Positive reinforcement produced by electrical stimulation of septal area and other regions. *Journal of Comparative and Physiological Psychology,* 47, 419–427.

Ortony, A., Clore, G. L., & Foss, M. A. (1987). The referential structure of the affective lexicon. *Cognitive Science,* 11, 341–364.

Ortony, A., & Fainsilber, L. (1989). The role of metaphors in descriptions of emotions. In Y. Wilks (Ed.), *Theoretical issues in natural language processing* (pp. 178–182). Hillsdale, NJ: Erlbaum.

Osgood, C. E., Suci, G. J., & Tannenbaum, P. H. (1957). *The measurement of meaning.* Urbana: University of Illinois Press.

Ostrom, T. M., & Upshaw, H. S. (1968). Psychological perspective and attitude change. In A. G. Greenwald, T. C. Brock, & T. M. Ostrom (Eds.), *Psychological foundations of attitudes* (pp. 217–242). New York: Academic Press.

Parisi, N., & Katz, I. (1986). Attitudes toward posthumous organ donation and commitment to donate. *Health Psychology,* 5, 565–580.

Peeters, G., & Czapinski, J. (1990). Positive–negative asymmetry in evaluations: The distinction between affective and informational negativity effects. In W. Stroebe & M. Hewstone (Eds.), *European review of social psychology* (Vol. 1, pp. 33–60). New York: Wiley.

Pratto, F., & John, E. (1991). Automatic vigilance: The attention-grabbing power of negative social information. *Journal of Personality and Social Psychology,* 61, 380–391.

Pulford, B. D., & Colman, A. M. (1996). Overconfidence, base rates and outcome positivity/negativity of predicted events. *British Journal of Psychology,* 87, 431–445.

Reeder, G. D., & Brewer, M. B. (1979). A schematic model of dispositional attribution in interpersonal perception. *Psychological Review,* 86, 61–79.

Regan, P. C., Snyder, M., & Kassin, S. M. (1995). Unrealistic optimism: Self-enhancement or person positivity? *Personality and Social Psychology Bulletin,* 21, 1073–1082.

Robinson-Whelen, S., Kim, C., MacCallum, R. C., & Kiecolt-Glaser, J. K. (1997). Distinguishing optimism from pessimism in older adults: Is it more important to be optimistic or not to be pessimistic? *Journal of Personality and Social Psychology,* 73, 1345–1353.

Roldan, G., & Bures, J. (1994). Tetrodotoxin blockade of amygdala overlapping with poisoning impairs acquisition of conditioned taste aversion in rats. *Behavioural Brain Research,* 65, 1345–1353.

Rowe, P. M. (1989). Unfavorable information and interview decisions. In R. W. Eder & G. R. Ferris (Eds.), *The employment interview: Theory, research, and practice* (pp. 77–89). Newbury Park, CA: Sage.

Russell, J. A. (1978). Evidence of convergent validity on the dimensions of affect. *Journal of Personality and Social Psychology,* 36, 1152–1168.

Russell, J. A. (1983). Pancultural aspects of the human conceptual organization of emotions. *Journal of Personality and Social Psychology,* 45, 1281–1288.

Russell, J. A., & Carroll, J. M. (1999). On the bipolarity of positive and negative affect. *Psychological Bulletin,* 125, 3–30.

Russell, J. A., & Feldman Barrett, L. (in press). Core affect, prototypical emotional episodes, and other things called *emotion:* Dissecting the elephant. *Journal of Personality and Social Psychology,* 76, 805–819.

Russell, J. A., & Mehrabian, A. (1977). Evidence for a three-factor theory of emotions. *Journal of Research in Personality,* 11, 273–294.

Rusting, C. L., & Larsen, R. J. (1998). Personality and cognitive processing of affective information. *Personality and Social Psychology Bulletin,* 24, 200–213.

Salamone, J. D., Cousins, M. S., & Snyder, B. J. (1997). Behavioral functions of nucleus accumbens dopamine: Empirical and conceptual problems with the anhedonia hypothesis. *Neuroscience and Biobehavioral Reviews,* 21, 341–359.

Sandner, G., Oberling, P., Silveira, M. C., Di Scala, G., Rocha, B., Bagri, A., & Depoortere, R. (1993). What brain structures are active during emotions? Effects of brain stimulation elicited aversion on c-fos immunoreactivity and behavior. *Behavioural Brain Research,* 58, 9–18.

Sarason, I. G., Sarason, B. R., Pierce, G. R., Shearin, E. N., & Sayers, M. H. (1991). A social learning approach to increasing blood donations. *Journal of Applied Social Psychology,* 21, 896–918.

Sarason, I. G., Sarason, B. R., Slichter, S. J., Beatty, P. G., Meyer, D. M., & Bolgiano, D. C. (1993). Increasing participation of blood donors in a bone-marrow registry. *Health Psychology,* 12, 272–276.

Schafe, G. E., & Bernstein, I, LL. (1996). Forebrain contribution to the induction of a brainstem correlate of conditioned taste aversion: I. The amygdala. *Brain Research,* 741, 109–116.

Schneirla, T. C. (1959). An evolutionary and developmental theory of biphasic processes underlying approach and withdrawal. In M. Jones (Ed.), *Nebraska Symposium on Motivation: 1959* (pp. 1–42). Lincoln: University of Nebraska Press.

Schofield, J. W. (1991). School desegregation and intergroup relations. In G. Grant (Ed.), *Review of research in education* (Vol. 17, pp. 335–409). Washington, DC: American Educational Research Association.

Schwarz, N., & Strack, F. (in press). Reports of subjective well-being: Judgmental processes and their methodological implications. In D. Kahneman, E. Diener, & N. Schwarz (Eds.), *Well-being: The foundations of hedonic psychology.* New York: Cambridge University Press.

Sears, D. O. (1983). The person positivity bias. *Journal of Personality and Social Psychology,* 44, 233–249.

Shah, J., Higgins, E. T., & Friedman, R. S. (1998). Performance incentives and means: How regulatory focus influences goal attainment. *Journal of Personality and Social Psychology,* 74, 285–293.

Sherrington, C. A. (1906). *The integrative actions of the nervous system.* New York: Scribner's.

Shizgal, P. (in press). On the neural computation of utility: Implications from studies of brain stimulation reward. In D. Kahneman, E. Diener, & N. Schwarz (Eds.), *Well-being: The foundations of hedonic psychology.* New York: Cambridge University Press.

Showers, C. J. (1995). The evaluative organization of self-knowledge: Origins, processes, and implications for self-esteem. In M. Kernis (Ed.), *Efficacy, agency, and self-esteem* (pp. 101–120). New York: Plenum.

Showers, C. J., & Kling, K. C. (1996). Organization of self-knowledge: Implications for recovery from sad mood. *Journal of Personality and Social Psychology,* 70, 578–590.

Skowronski, J. J., & Carlston, D. E. (1989). Negativity and extremity biases in impression formation: A review of explanations. *Psychological Bulletin,* 105, 131–142.

Stellar, J. R., Brooks, F. H., & Mills, L. E. (1979). Approach and withdrawal analysis of the effects of hypothalamic stimulation and lesions in rats. *Journal of Comparative and Physiological Psychology,* 93, 446–466.

Suh, E., Diener, E., & Fujita, F. (1996). Events and subjective well-being: Only recent events matter. *Journal of Personality and Social Psychology,* 70, 1091–1102.

Taylor, S. E. (1991). Asymmetrical effects of positive and negative events: The mobilization–minimization hypothesis. *Psychological Bulletin,* 110, 67–85.

Tesser, A., & Martin, L. (1996). The psychology of evaluation. In E. T. Higgins & A. W. Kruglanski (Eds.), *Social psychology: Handbook of basic principles* (pp. 400–432). New York: Guilford Press.

Thompson, M. M., Zanna, M. P., & Griffin, D. W. (1995). Let's not be indifferent about (attitudinal) ambivalence. In R. E. Petty & J. A. Krosnick (Eds.), *Attitude strength: Antecedents and consequences* (pp. 361–386). Hillsdale, NJ: Erlbaum.

Thurstone, L. L. (1931). The measurement of attitudes. *Journal of Abnormal Psychology,* 26, 249–269.

Tooby, J., & Cosmides, L. (1990). On the universality of human nature and the uniqueness of the individual: The role of genetics and adaptation. *Journal of Personality,* 58, 17–67.

Tucker, D. M. (1981). Lateral brain function, emotion, and conceptualization. *Psychological Bulletin,* 89, 19–46.

Tucker, D. M., & Frederick, S. L. (1989). Emotion and brain lateralization. In H. Wagner & A. Manstead (Eds.), *Handbook of social psychophysiology* (pp. 27–70). Chichester, England: Wiley.

Walden, T. (1993). Preschool children's responses to affective information about anticipated events. *Journal of Experimental Child Psychology,* 55, 243–257.

Watson, D., & Clark, L. A. (1991). Self- versus peer ratings of specific emotional traits: Evidence of convergent and discriminant validity. *Journal of Personality and Social Psychology,* 60, 927–940.

Watson, D., & Clark, L. A. (1992). Affects separable and inseparable: On the hierarchical arrangement of the negative affects. *Journal of Personality and Social Psychology,* 62, 489–505.

Watson, D., & Clark, L. A. (1997). Measurement and mismeasurement of mood: Recurrent and emergent issues. *Journal of Personality Assessment,* 68, 267–296.

Watson, D., Clark, L. A., McIntyre, C. W., & Hamaker, S. (1992). Affect, personality and social activity. *Journal of Personality and Social Psychology,* 63, 1011–1025.

Watson, D., & Tellegen, A. (1985). Toward a consensual structure of mood. *Psychological Bulletin,* 98, 219–235.

Watson, D., Wiese, D., Vaidya, J., & Tellegen, A. (1999). The two general activation sysems of affect: Structural findings, evolutionary considerations, and psychobiological evidence. *Journal of Personality and Social Psychology,* 76, 820–838.

Westermann, R., Spies, K., Stahl, G., & Hesse, F. W. (1996). Relative effectiveness and validity of mood induction procedures: A meta-analysis. *European Journal of Social Psychology,* 26, 557–580.

Wickelgren, I. (1997, October 3). Getting the brain's attention. *Science,* 278, 35–38.

Wise, R. A. (1996). Addictive drugs and brain stimulation reward. *Annual Review of Neuroscience,* 19, 319–340.

Wojciszke, B., Brycz, H., & Borkenau, P. (1993). Effects of information content and evaluative extremity on positivity and negativity biases. *Journal of Personality and Social Psychology,* 64, 327–335.

Yeomans, J. S. (1990). *Principles of brain stimulation.* New York: Oxford University Press.

Zajonc, R. B. (1980). Feeling and thinking: Preferences need no inferences. *American Psychologist,* 35, 157–193.

Zautra, A. J., Burleson, M. H., Smith, C. A., Blalock, S. J., Wallston, K. F., DeVellis, R. F., DeVellis, B. M., & Smith, T. W. (1995). Arthritis and perceptions of quality of life: An examination of positive and negative affect in rheumatoid arthritis patients. *Health Psychology,* 14, 399–408.

Zautra, A. J., Hoffman, J., & Reich, J. W. (1997). The role of two kinds of efficacy beliefs in maintaining the well-being of chronically stressed older adults. In B.

Gottlieb (Ed.), *Coping with chronic illness* (pp. 245–290). New York: Plenum.

Zautra, A. J., Potter, P. T., & Reich, J. W. (1997). The independence of affects is context-dependent: An integrative model of the relationship between positive and negative affect. *Annual Review of Gerontology and Geriatrics,* 17, 75–103.

Zautra, A. J., Reich, J. W., & Gaurnaccia, C. A. (1990). The everyday consequences of disability and bereavement for older adults. *Journal of Personality and Social Psychology,* 59, 550–561.

Zautra, A. J., Reich, J. W., & Newsom, J. T. (1995). Autonomy and sense of control among older adults: An examination of their effects on mental health. In L. A. Bond, S. J. Cutler, & A. Grams (Eds.), *Promoting successful and productive aging* (pp. 153–168). Thousand Oaks, CA: Sage.

33 Choosing between Small, Likely Rewards and Large, Unlikely Rewards Activates Inferior and Orbital Prefrontal Cortex

Robert D. Rogers, Adrian M. Owen, Hugh C. Middleton, Emma J. Williams, John D. Pickard, Barbara J. Sahakian, and Trevor W. Robbins

Human patients with damage to orbital regions of prefrontal cortex (PFC) are more likely to exhibit personality change and difficulties with social interactions than patients with damage to more dorsal regions of PFC (Stuss and Benson, 1986; Damasio, 1994; Rolls et al., 1994). However, understanding these behavioral changes in terms of compromised cognitive functions supported by orbital PFC has been complicated by clinical evidence that such difficulties in social cognition and real-life decision making are frequently not accompanied by marked changes in many important forms of cognitive function (Eslinger and Damasio, 1985; Saver and Damasio, 1991). Indeed, several of these other cognitive functions, different types of working memory (Goldman-Rakic, 1987, 1994, 1996; Petrides, 1994, 1995), the control of attention (Dias et al., 1996), and behavioral flexibility (Milner, 1964; Berman et al., 1995), have each been proposed to involve dorsolateral regions of PFC, highlighting the possibility that orbital sectors mediate distinctive mechanisms of particular importance to social cognition (Damasio et al., 1990).

Research into these issues has been advanced significantly by the demonstration that patients exhibiting such "acquired sociopathy" after orbital PFC damage also show consistent deficits on a gambling task involving choices between actions that differ in terms of the size and probabilities of their associated punishments and rewards (for review, see Bechara et al., 1994, 1996; Damasio, 1996a). Furthermore, work published recently in this journal (Bechara et al., 1998) found that orbital PFC patients exhibited difficulties with such decision making in the absence of consistent deficits on a modified delayed response task. Because dorsolateral PFC patients showed the opposite pattern of impairment, i.e., deficient delayed response performance but normal decision making, these data appear to confirm the relatively independent contributions made by the orbital and dorsolateral PFC to decision-making and working memory cognition, respectively. Overall, the trend of the clinical and experimental evidence suggests that the orbital PFC, presumably through its rich interconnections with limbic cortices and other neural stations deeply implicated in processes of incentive motivation and reinforcement (Damasio, 1994), represents an important site of contact between emotional or affective information and mechanisms of action selection (for review, see Rolls, 1996).

Although studies with neurological patients have highlighted the role of orbital PFC in decision-making cognition, functional imaging techniques offer the opportunity for specifying more closely which areas of the orbital PFC are particularly involved. The orbital cortex is relatively differentiated in terms of its cytoarchitecture and patterns of interconnectivity (Carmichael et al., 1994, 1995a,b). Moreover, it is likely to be functionally heterogeneous (Rolls, 1996). To address these issues, we used the slow bolus infusion method of water activation ($H_2^{15}O$) to study a novel decision-making task in which subjects were asked to gamble accumulated reward on predictions about which of two mutually exclusive outcomes would occur. Critically, the largest reward was always associated with the least likely of the two outcomes, ensuring that the element of conflict inherent in risk taking was preserved.

Materials and Methods

Subjects

Eight right-handed volunteers, all males, participated. None had a history of psychiatric or

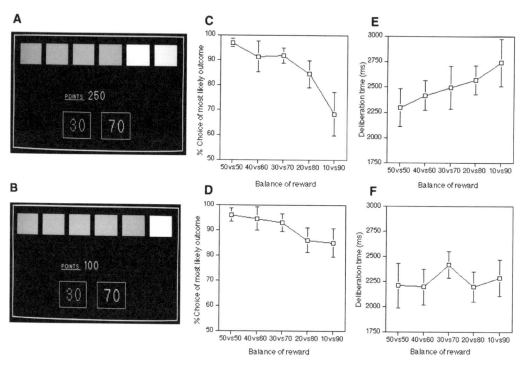

Figure 33.1
Typical displays from the decision-making task, and associated behavioral data across the present study. (A, C, E) Example decision from the 4:2 condition, percentage of choice of the most likely outcome and mean deliberation times as a function of the balance of reward associated with the two outcomes. (B, D, F) Example decision from the 5:1 condition, percentage of choice of the most likely outcome and mean deliberation times as a function of the balance of reward associated with the two outcomes.

neurological illness. Their mean age was 31.9 ± 2.0 (SE) years, whereas their mean verbal IQ, estimated with the National Adult Reading Test (Nelson, 1982), was in the above average range at 120.9 ± 1. Each subject underwent 12 positron emission tomography (PET) scans and one magnetic resonance imaging (MRI) scan within a single session. All subjects gave informed, written consent for participation in the study after its nature and possible consequences had been explained to them. The study was approved by the Local Research and Ethics Committee.

Task Design

Two typical displays from the decision-making task are shown in Figure 33.1, A and B. The subject was told that the computer had hidden a yellow token inside one of the red or blue boxes arrayed at the top of the screen and that he had to decide whether this token was hidden inside a red box or a blue box. However, this decision involved gambling a certain number of points associated with each choice. In these examples, if the subject chose red, then he gained 30 points if the yellow token was indeed hidden inside a red box, but lost 30 points if the token was hidden inside a blue box. On the other hand, if the subject chose blue, then he gained 70 points if the token was hidden inside a blue box, but lost 70 points if it was hidden inside a red box. The subject was told that there was an equal probability that the token would be hidden inside any of the six boxes. The subject indicated his decision by touching one of the two square response panels, located at the bottom of the display, containing the associated "stake" written in either red or blue ink. Immediately after a selection, one of the boxes opened to reveal the location of the token, accompanied by either a "You win!" or a "You lose!" message (written in large yellow Helvetica font). If the subject chose the correct color, the stake associated with that color was added to the total points score; if the subject chose the wrong color, the same stake was subtracted. No monetary significance was attached to the points accumulated by the end of the task.

At the start of each sequence, the subject was given 100 points and instructed to make whatever choices thought necessary to increase this score by as much as possible. It was emphasized that these choices might involve either conservative or risk-taking behavior. The ratio of colored boxes (5:1, 4:2, and 3:3) and the balance between the associated rewards (10 vs 90, 20 vs 80, 30 vs 70, 40 vs 60, and 50 vs 50) varied independently from trial to trial according to a fixed pseudorandom sequence. This sequence ensured that each balance of reward and each ratio of colored boxes co-occurred an equal number of times, with the restriction that on all trials with an unequal ratio of red and blue boxes (i.e., 5:1 or 4:2), the larger reward was always associated with the least likely outcome (i.e., the color with the fewest number of boxes; see Fig. 33.1A,B), thus capturing the conflict inherent in risk-taking situations.

The data analyses centered around two main measures: (1) speed of decision making, i.e., how long it took the subject to decide which color of box was hiding the yellow token as measured by the mean deliberation time (measured in milli-

seconds), and (2) choice of the most likely outcome (associated with the smaller reward).

Design

For 8 of the 12 scans, the subject began working through sequences of decisions 1 min before the scan commenced. However, at the start of the scan window, i.e., when the "head count" began to rise, the experimenter advanced the subject to one of two conditions involving concealed runs of particular ratios of red and blue boxes (see below). After completing this concealed run, the subject was returned to his or her original place in the entire sequence that was then completed. Preliminary pilot tests had shown that each of these hidden runs occupied the typical subject for ~1 min. Because most of the regional cerebral blood flow (rCBF) arising from the cognitive activity associated with any scan window coincides with the steepest increase in head counts (≈ 30 sec; Silbersweig et al., 1993), hidden runs of 1 min were sufficient to ensure that the rCBF data reflected the mental activity associated with the different conditions. On the remaining four scans, the subjects performed a purpose-designed visuomotor control task (see below).

Earlier work had shown that subjects appear to be more sensitive to the balance of reward associated with the two outcomes when the ratio of the colored boxes was 4:2 compared to when it was 5:1. For this reason, our design involved two conditions that allowed us to assess decision making with these different ratios. Thus, in the 4:2 choice conditions, the subject was scanned while making decisions that involved ratios of either 4 red:2 blue or 2 red:4 blue (e.g., Fig. 33.1A), and in which the reward associated with the two outcomes was always one of 30 vs 70, 20 vs 80, and 10 vs 90. As noted above, these choices tend to be particularly associated with reduced choice of the most likely outcome, as well as increased deliberation times, as a function of the balance of reward associated with the two possible outcomes.

In the 5:1 choice conditions, the subject was scanned while making decisions involving ratios of only 5 red:1 blue or 1 red:5 blue (e.g., Fig. 33.1*B*). Although the rewards associated with the two outcomes were the same as in the 4:2 choice conditions, i.e., 30 vs 70, 20 vs 80, and 10 vs 90, these decisions tend to be associated with more consistent choice of the most likely outcome, as well as relatively constant deliberation times. To control for possible differences in the amount of visual and motor processing associated with the 4:2 and 5:1 choice conditions, the presentation rate of trials in each of the 5:1 choice conditions was "yoked" to the latencies of choices in an earlier 4:2 condition. Additionally, because recent evidence has suggested that rCBF changes within orbital PFC and associated limbic circuitry can be seen with changes in reinforcement rate (Elliott et al., 1999), the frequency of reward within the scan windows of the 5:1 choice conditions was also yoked to earlier 4:2 choice conditions. This was achieved by having the computer select the location of the yellow token after the subject had made a response in the 5:1 conditions and thereby permitting the number of wins and losses to be balanced with the 4:2 conditions. In this way, differences in the rCBF in the 4:2 and 5:1 conditions cannot be attributed to gross differences in motor activity or rate of positive or negative feedback across conditions. The subject was not informed about this feature of the study design.

In the control condition, alternative displays showed only all red or all blue boxes with the yellow token already revealed at onset, thus ensuring that subjects were not able to covertly predict which color of box was hiding the yellow token. Moreover, all features of the displays that had previously indicated reward-based information, i.e., the total points score and the size of the rewards associated with two outcomes, were now marked with Xs. The subject was required to monitor the displays until one of the response panels brightened with a white border before touching that panel, the precise delay corre-

sponding to the time required to make earlier decisions in a yoked 4:2 choice condition.

The twelve scans were divided into four runs of three scans each. The first scan in each run was always a 4:2 choice condition, whereas the second and third scans were always either a 5:1 choice condition or a control condition; the order of these two conditions was counterbalanced across scans within and between subjects. To remove linear time effects associated with earlier versus later scans, scan order was entered as a covariate (of no interest) in all analyses of the rCBF data. Before the first scan, but after the subject had been positioned in the scanner, the nature of the task and the task displays were explained to the subject, who was allowed to complete just one sample decision as training.

Scanning Procedure and Statistical Analysis

Each subject was scanned in the presence of low background noise and dimmed ambient lighting. The task displays were presented on a Micro-Touch 20C touch-sensitive screen controlled by a Pentium microcomputer. The screen was mounted at a viewing distance of ∼50 cm so that the subject could touch all areas of the screen with the index finger of the dominant hand, which was rested on the chest between responses.

PET scans were obtained with the General Electrics Advance system, which produces 35 image slices at an intrinsic resolution of ∼5.0 × 5.0 × 5.0 mm. Using the bolus $H_2^{15}O$ methodology, rCBF was measured during four separate scans for each of the three experimental and control conditions (total = 12 scans). For each scan, subjects received a 20 sec intravenous bolus of $H_2^{15}O$ through a forearm cannula at a concentration of 300 MBq/ml^{-1} and a flow rate of 10 ml/min^{-1}. With this method, each scan provided an image of rCBF integrated over a period of 90 sec from when the tracer first entered the cerebral circulation. The twelve PET scans were initially realigned using the first scan as a reference and then again using the mean of the scans as a reference, normalized to a standard brain template that forms part of the Statistical Parametric Mapping 98 (SPM98) software, corrected for global CBF value, and averaged across the eight subjects for each activation state. Then the images were smoothed using an isotropic Gaussian kernel at 16 mm full-width half-maximum (FWHM). Finally, blood flow changes between conditions were estimated for each voxel according to the general linear model, as implemented by Statistical Parametric Mapping (SPM 96; provided by the Wellcome Department of Cognitive Neurology, London, UK).

For each subject, a three-dimensional MRI volume ($1.5 \times 1.5 \times 3.0$ mm) was acquired using a 0.5 T system and Bruker console and resliced to be coregistered with the PET data. Composite stereotaxic MRI and PET volumes were merged to allow direct anatomical localization of regions with statistically significant rCBF change between conditions. Effects at each and every voxel were estimated according to the general linear model (Friston et al., 1995). Condition effects at each voxel were compared using linear contrasts. The resulting set of voxel t statistics constitute a statistical parametric map (SPM {t}). SPM {t} maps were transformed to the unit normal distribution SPM {Z} for display and thresholded at 3.09. The resulting foci were characterized in terms of spatial extent (k) and peak height (u). The significance of each region was estimated using distributional approximations from the theory of Gaussian fields. This characterization is in terms of the probability that the peak height observed (or higher) could occur by chance [$PZ_{max} > u$] over the entire volume analyzed (i.e., a corrected p value).

In the case of comparisons between the decision-making and control scans, all predicted increases in rCBF were tested against a threshold of $p < 0.05$ corrected for multiple comparisons within a volume approximating the size of the orbital PFC. The technique for calculating such a threshold has been described elsewhere

(Worsley et al., 1996). Predicted peaks were confined to orbital PFC in view of the considerable neuropsychological evidence that altered decision making is associated specifically with lesions in these cortical fields (Bechara et al., 1994, 1998; Rogers et al., 1999). To anticipate the results, decision making was exclusively associated with highly significant activations in the orbital PFC, with no evidence of increased activity in other parts of the PFC at either corrected or indeed uncorrected thresholds. Activations (and relative deactivations) beyond the frontal cortex (none of which were predicted a priori) are detailed in the tables and reported only briefly in the text if they survived the additional threshold of $p < 0.05$ corrected for multiple comparisons across the whole brain. As noted above, task-unrelated changes in rCBF associated with linear time effects associated with earlier versus later scans were removed by entering scan position as a covariate (of no interest) in all analyses.

Results

Task Performance

The behavioral data associated with each sequence of decisions (i.e., percentage of choice of the most likely outcome and mean deliberation times) were subject to multifactorial, repeated-measures ANOVA with the following within-subject factors: run (first, second, third, or fourth); ratio (4:2 or 5:1), and balance of reward (50 vs 50, 40 vs 60, 30 vs 70, 20 vs 80, or 10 vs 90). The proportions of trials on which subjects chose the most likely outcome were arcsine-transformed as is appropriate whenever variance is proportional to the mean (Howell, 1987). However, the data shown in the tables and figures represent untransformed values. In those instances in which the additional assumption of homogeneity of covariance in repeated-measures ANOVA was violated, as assessed using the Mauchly sphericity test, the degrees of freedom

Table 33.1
Decision-making performance (i.e., percentage of choice of the most likely outcome and mean deliberation times, plus SEs) as a function of the balance of rewards

	50 vs 50	40 vs 60	30 vs 70	20 vs 80	10 vs 90
Percentage of choice of most likely outcome	96.5 ± 2.1	93.0 ± 5.3	92.4 ± 3.0	85.2 ± 4.3	76.7 ± 7.0
Scanned decisions	—	—	91.6 ± 3.6	84.2 ± 5.2	73.5 ± 7.8
Mean deliberation time (msec)	2254 ± 198	2308 ± 160	2458 ± 162	2385 ± 141	2514 ± 202
Scanned decisions	—	—	2363 ± 199	2335 ± 105	2469 ± 171

Scanned decisions refer to those made during the scan windows of the 4:2 and 5:1 choice conditions.

against which the F term was tested were reduced by the value of the Greenhouse-Geisser epsilon (Howell, 1987). Additional analyses were performed on the mean deliberation times and percentage of choice of the most likely outcome specifically associated with the concealed runs of decisions manipulated in the 4:2 and 5:1 conditions, to check that subjects' behavior during the scan windows was similar to that seen over the entire set of decision-making sequences.

In general, subjects' decision making was markedly influenced by the balance of rewards associated with the most and the least likely outcomes. Specifically, subjects' choice of the most likely outcome was significantly reduced as the size of its reward was diminished in comparison with that of the least likely outcome (Table 33.1; $F_{(4,28)} = 6.97$; $p = 0.001$), whereas the time required to make these choices was significantly increased ($F_{(4,28)} = 3.05$; $p < 0.05$). Moreover, as predicted, the extent to which the balance of rewards influenced subjects' decisions tended to be greater when the ratio of red and blue boxes was 4:2 compared to when it was 5:1, both in terms of choice of the most likely outcome ($F_{(4,28)} = 3.43$; $p < 0.05$) and time required to make decisions ($F_{(4,28)} = 2.89$; $p < 0.05$). Further analysis of simple effects demonstrated that deliberation times were significantly influenced by the balance of rewards with ratios of 4:2 (Fig. 33.1E; $F_{(4,28)} = 3.73$; $p < 0.05$) but not with ratios of 5:1 (Fig. 33.1F; $F_{(4,28)} = 1.85$). Choice

of the most likely outcome was reduced by the changing balance of rewards with both ratios (Fig. 33.1C,D; $F_{(4,28)} = 7.96$; $p < 0.001$; $F_{(4,28)} = 3.58$; $p < 0.05$). Finally, subjects took significantly longer to make their choices with ratios of 4:2 compared to 5:1 (2505 ± 170 msec vs 2263 ± 164 msec; $F_{(1,7)} = 29.30$; $p = 0.001$), especially in the earlier compared to later runs ($F_{(3,21)} = 3.99$; $p < 0.05$). In general, deliberation times were increased in the earlier runs ($F_{(3,21)} = 30.81$; $p < 0.0001$).

Additional analyses were performed on the decisions of the concealed runs constituting the 4:2 and 5:1 conditions (see above). These data were collected during a period beginning at the start of the scan windows and ending 60 sec later. The within-subject factors were unchanged except that the balance of rewards had only three levels instead of five (i.e., 30 vs 70, 20 vs 80, or 10 vs 90). Despite the reduced power available with this much restricted data set, decision-making performance within the scan windows of the 4:2 and 5:1 conditions was typical of the complete sequences. Thus, choice of the most likely outcome was significantly reduced as the size of its associated reward was diminished relative to that associated with the least likely outcome (Table 33.1; $F_{(1,19,14)} = 9.47$; $p < 0.01$). The time required to make decisions also increased, although not significantly ($F_{(2,14)} = 1.3$). Additionally, the balance of rewards influenced subjects' choices more in the 4:2 condition than

Table 33.2
Comparison of the combined rCBF from the 4:2 and 5:1 conditions with the rCBF associated with performance of the visuomotor control task

	BA	L/R	z score	x	y	z
(4:2 + 5:1)—control						
Middle frontal gyrus	10/11	R	4.51	40	54	−8
Inferior frontal gyrus	47	R	4.48	34	20	−4
Orbital frontal gyrus	11	R	4.14	20	42	−28
Fusiform gyrus	18	R	5.21	32	−86	−12
Superior parietal lobule	7	L	5.48	−32	−54	52
Superior parietal lobule	7/40	R	5.78	30	−66	40
Superior parietal lobule	7/40	R	5.41	46	−52	52
Cerebellum	Lateral	L	4.66	−42	−68	−20
Cerebellum	Medial	R	5.23	4	−80	−32
Control—(4:2 + 5:1)						
Medial frontal gyrus	10	L	4.71	−6	54	−16
Medial frontal gyrus	10	M	4.12	0	60	0
Precentral gyrus	4	L	4.37	−12	−20	68
Middle temporal gyrus	39	L	5.22	−46	−72	24
Uncus	28/36	L	4.69	−26	4	−28
Middle temporal gyrus	21	R	4.70	60	−48	8
Superior temporal gyrus	22	R	4.84	64	−44	16
Cerebellum	Lateral	R	4.87	44	−12	−40

A threshold was set at $p < 0.05$ (z score $= 3.83$) corrected for multiple comparisons within the orbital PFC (Worsley et al., 1996); all other reported peaks were significant at $p < 0.05$ corrected across the whole brain.

in the 5:1 condition ($F_{(2, 14)} = 4.46$; $p < 0.05$). Finally, as with the complete sequences, subjects took significantly longer to make their choices in the 4:2 compared to the 5:1 condition (2662 ± 200 msec vs 2373 ± 208 msec; $F_{(1, 7)} = 20.53$; $p < 0.005$), especially within the earlier runs of the study ($F_{(3, 20)} = 4.94$; $p = 0.01$). Deliberation times were significantly increased in the earlier compared to the later runs ($F_{(3, 21)} = 18.25$; $p < 0.0001$).

Regional Cerebral Blood Flow Changes

Decision-making versus Control Conditions
Subtraction of the rCBF associated with the visuomotor control conditions from that asso-

ciated with the 4:2 and 5:1 conditions combined isolated significant and distinct activations in ventral, but not dorsolateral, sectors of the right PFC (Table 33.2). Specifically, there was a highly significant peak positioned along the orbital frontal gyrus [Brodmann area 11 (BA 11); z score $= 4.14$; Fig. 33.2*A*], another positioned more laterally along the most anterior and ventral portion of the middle frontal gyrus (BA 10/11; z score $= 4.51$; Fig. 33.2*B*), and a third significant peak positioned just anterior to the insular cortex, along the ventral part of the inferior frontal gyrus (BA 47; z score $= 4.48$; Fig. 33.2*C*). There were no rCBF increases associated with decision making in other PFC areas.

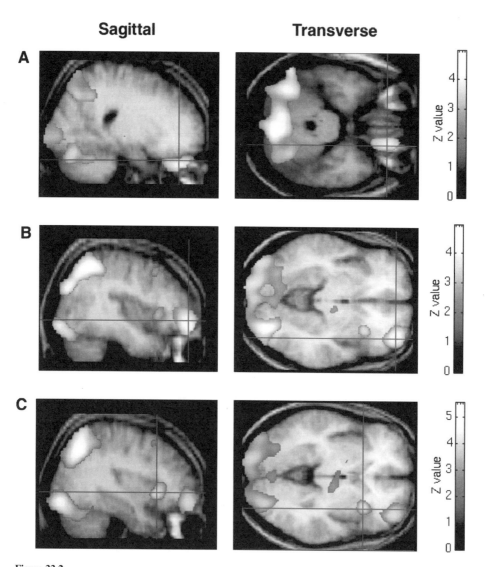

Figure 33.2
Peaks of activity-associated performance of the decision-making task compared to the visuomotor control task rendered onto the averaged MRI scans of the eight volunteer subjects used in the current study (threshold, $p < 0.01$). (A) Peak of activation in orbitomedial PFC (BA 11); (B) peak of activity within orbitolateral PFC (BA 10); (C) activation within the inferior convexity (BA 47).

Table 33.3
Comparison of the rCBF associated with the 4:2 conditions only with the rCBF associated with performance of the visuomotor control task

	BA	L/R	z score	x	y	z
4:2—control						
Middle frontal gyrus	10	R	4.24	42	50	−8
Inferior frontal gyrus	47	R	4.07	34	20	0
Orbital frontal gyrus	11	R	4.42	22	40	−32
Fusiform gyrus	18	R	4.06	30	−84	−12
Superior parietal lobule	7	L	4.70	−28	−58	48
Superior parietal lobule	7	R	5.25	30	−68	40
Cerebellum	Lateral	L	4.50	−42	−68	−20
Cerebellum	Medial	R	4.70	4	−78	−32
Control—4:2						
Orbital frontal gyrus	10	L	4.54	−4	54	−20
Precentral gyrus	4/6	L	5.01	−14	−18	68
Inferior temporal gyrus	21	R	4.32	62	−48	4
Middle temporal gyrus	20	R	4.35	46	−10	−36

A threshold was set at $p < 0.05$ (z score $= 3.83$) corrected for multiple comparisons within the orbital PFC (Worsley et al., 1996); all other reported peaks were significant at $p < 0.05$ corrected across the whole brain.

Additional activations not predicted a priori included a significant rCBF increase along the right fusiform gyrus (Table 33.2; BA 18; z score $= 5.21$). There was also a marked activation within the superior parietal lobule on the left (BA 7; z score $= 5.48$), as well two distinct activations in the same area on the right (BA 7/40; z scores $= 5.78$ and 5.41). Finally, there were significant peaks within the lateral cerebellum on the left (z score $= 4.66$) and the medial cerebellum on the right (z score $= 5.23$).

Subtraction of the combined rCBF of the 4:2 and 5:1 conditions from that of the control conditions also revealed evidence of relatively reduced activation associated with decision making within left anterior PFC; specifically, along the left medial frontal gyrus (Table 33.2; BA 10; z scores $= 4.71$ and 4.12). Additional unpredicted areas of reduced rCBF in the decision-making compared to control conditions were concen-

trated within predominantly temporal lobe areas (Table 33.2) and included the left middle temporal gyrus (BA 39; z score $= 5.22$) and left uncus (BA 28/36; z score $= 4.69$), the right middle and superior temporal gyri (BA 21, z score $= 4.70$; BA 22, z score $= 4.84$), as well as the left precentral gyrus (BA 4; z score $= 4.37$) and lateral cerebellum on the right (z score $= 4.87$).

In general, separate comparisons involving each of the decision-making conditions with the control condition reflected similar patterns of activation in the inferior and orbital PFC, as well as posterior temporal and parietal areas (Tables 33.3, 33.4). In particular, decision making in the 4:2 condition (Fig. 33.3*A*) and the 5:1 condition (Fig. 33.3*B*) activated roughly the same three sites in right orbital PFC: laterally, along the anterior part of the middle frontal gyrus (BA 10/ 11; z scores $= 4.24$ in the 4:2 condition, 3.92 in the 5:1 condition); posteriorly, along the inferior

Table 33.4
Comparison of the rCBF associated with the 5:1 conditions only with the rCBF associated with performance of the visuomotor control task

	BA	L/R	z score	x	y	z
5:1—control						
Middle frontal gyrus	10/11	R	3.92	36	56	−12
Inferior frontal gyrus	47	R	3.89	32	20	−4
Orbital frontal gyrus	11	R	3.81	18	48	−28
Fusiform gyrus	18	R	5.04	32	−86	−12
Superior parietal lobule	7	L	5.14	−32	−54	52
Superior parietal lobule	40	R	5.04	32	−66	44
Inferior parietal lobule	40	R	5.56	48	−54	52
Inferior parietal lobule	40	R	5.00	50	−42	48
Cerebellum	Medial	R	4.70	4	−82	−32
Control—5:1						
Middle temporal gyrus	39	L	4.45	−46	−72	24
Inferior temporal gyrus	20	L	4.44	−46	−16	−28
Uncus	28	L	4.65	−26	4	−28
Superior temporal gyrus	22	R	4.35	64	−44	16

A threshold was set at $p < 0.05$ (z score $= 3.83$) corrected for multiple comparisons within the orbital PFC (Worsley et al., 1996); all other reported peaks were significant at $p < 0.05$ corrected across the whole brain.

frontal gyrus (BA 47; z scores $= 4.07$ in the 4:2 condition, 3.89 in the 5:1 condition); and, medially, in the region of the orbital frontal gyrus (BA 11; z score $= 4.42$ in the 4:2 condition; z score $= 3.81$ in the 5:1 condition).

The two decision-making conditions showed more limited distributions of reduced rCBF in comparison with the control conditions (Tables 33.3, 33.4). Specifically, in orbital PFC areas, only the 4:2 condition showed significantly reduced activity within the left orbital gyrus (BA 11; z score $= 4.54$). However, both conditions were associated with marked deactivations in temporal areas: along the right inferior and middle temporal gyri in the 4:2 conditions (BA 21, z score $= 4.32$; BA 20, z score $= 4.35$), and along the left middle temporal gyrus (BA 39; z score $= 4.45$), left inferior temporal gyrus (BA 20; z score $= 4.44$) and left uncus (BA 28; z score $= 4.65$) in the 5:1 conditions. Additional

rCBF deactivations were evident along the precentral gyrus on the left in the 4:2 condition (BA 4/6; z score $= 5.01$) and along the superior temporal gyrus on the right in the 5:1 condition (BA 22; z score $= 4.35$).

4:2 Condition Minus 5:1 Condition
Direct subtraction of the rCBF associated with the 5:1 conditions from that associated with the 4:2 conditions isolated only modest changes in regional neural activity. Specifically, there was only a limited activation along the orbital frontal gyrus on the left (BA 11; z score $= 3.28$; Table 33.5), as well as a more extensive peak positioned along the anterior cingulate gyrus (BA 24; z score $= 3.62$). There was also some evidence of relatively increased rCBF in the area of the ventral striatum, just adjacent to the nucleus accumbens and putamen (z score $= 3.92$). However, none of these predicted or unpredicted

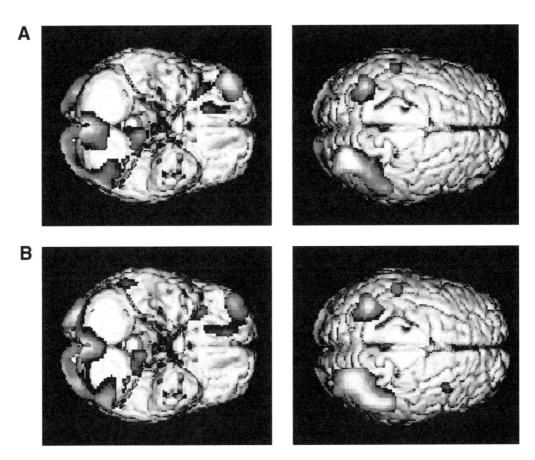

Figure 33.3
Increased rCBF from the two decision-making conditions compared with the visuomotor control task rendered onto
a representative brain (threshold, $p < 0.01$). (A) 4:2 condition—control task; (B) 5:1 condition—control task. Note
the lack of activity within dorsolateral areas of the PFC.

Table 33.5
Direct comparison of the rCBF associated with the 4:2 conditions with the rCBF associated with the 5:1 conditions

	BA	L/R	z score	x	y	z
4:2—5:1						
Orbital frontal gyrus	11	L	3.28	−14	34	−32
Anterior cingulate gyrus	24	L	3.62	−2	28	20
Ventral putamen region		R	3.92	28	−8	−8
5:1—4:2 conditions						
Middle frontal gyrus	6	L	4.26	−34	4	52

A threshold was set at $p < 0.05$ (z score $= 3.88$) corrected for multiple comparisons within the orbital PFC (Worsley et al., 1996); all other reported peaks were significant at $p < 0.05$ corrected across the whole brain.

rCBF changes survived correction for multiple comparisons. Subtraction of the rCBF in the 4:2 conditions from the rCBF in the 5:1 conditions revealed only a single area of changed rCBF along the left middle frontal gyrus (BA 6; z score $= 4.26$).

Covariates of Interest
Further analyses, collapsed across the 4:2 and 5:1 conditions, failed to find any significant association between rCBF in any cortical area and the principal performance measures associated with the scanned sequences: percentage of choice of the most likely outcome, mean deliberation time, mean number of points earned during the scans, and total reward at the end of the scans. Activity within the anterior portion of the right orbital gyrus (BA 11; $x = 14$; $y = 56$; $z = -20$; z score $= 3.66$) did show a positive relationship with the total change in points, i.e., summed losses or wins, from the start of the scan windows through to their completion. However, this increase did not survive correction the threshold set for multiple comparisons within the orbital PFC using the Worsley formula (see above).

Discussion

The behavior of our subjects, across both the entire set of decision-making sequences com-

pleted during the study and the restricted sequences completed within the scan windows of the 5:1 and 4:2 conditions, indicated that the choice of the most likely outcome was significantly reduced when its associated reward was decreased in comparison with that associated with the least likely outcome. Deliberation times associated with these choices were also significantly increased. Thus, these behavioral data (Fig. 33.1C–F) reflect the conflict inherent in "risky choices" in which the probability of relevant outcomes is pitted against the balance of their associated reinforcers. We have shown that, in a sample of healthy young adult males of relatively high intelligence, resolving this conflict in favor of one choice over another is associated with at least three distinct foci of rCBF increase within the inferior and orbital PFC: laterally, in the anterior part of the middle frontal gyrus (BA 10), medially, in the orbital gyrus (BA 11), and posteriorly, in the anterior portion of the inferior frontal gyrus (BA 47).

The multiple activations associated here with choices differing in the likelihood and size of their rewards help to explain the apparently greater incidence of deficient decision making in neurological patients sustaining damage to the orbital PFC compared to those sustaining damage in more dorsolateral and dorsomedial areas (Bechara et al., 1996, 1998, 1999; Rogers et al.,

1999). In view of the current results, it seems that focal lesions of the orbital cortex, as the result of surgery or stroke (Damasio et al., 1996b), are likely to affect cortical areas encompassing the rCBF changes seen here, increasing the probability of deficits in resolving between competing actions on the basis of ambiguous or conflicting information (Bechara et al., 1994, 1996, 1998, 1999; Eslinger and Damasio, 1985).

Choices in this study were not associated with any significant changes in neural activity within those dorsolateral prefrontal areas that have repeatedly been shown to mediate important aspects of the executive control of behavior such as working memory, planning, and attention (Goldman-Rakic, 1987, 1996; Petrides, 1994, 1995; Dias et al., 1996; Roberts et al., 1996). Thus, these results complement both experimental data indicating that impairments in decision making are dissociable from impairments in spatial memory (Bechara et al., 1998) and clinical assessments that ineffective decision making in real-life contexts can be accompanied by relatively normal performance on standard tests of frontal lobe function and measures of visuospatial performance, language, and memory (Eslinger and Damasio, 1985; Saver and Damasio, 1991; Rahman et al., 1999).

Given the intrinsic connectivity within orbital PFC (Barbas and Pandya, 1989; Carmichael and Price, 1995b), the activations of the present study are not likely to be functionally independent. Nevertheless, their distribution within the inferior and orbital cortex reflects the diversity of cell types and connectivity extrinsic to the PFC. Thus, the strong activations around the orbital frontal gyrus fell within an area that, in the primate brain, has a distinctive granular cytoarchitecture (Carmichael and Price, 1994) and receives rich innervation from all major stations of limbic–hippocampal circuitry (Morecroft et al., 1992; Carmichael and Price, 1995a). By contrast, the peaks around the inferior frontal and middle frontal gyri (BA 47 and 10/11) were located in areas that have a relatively agranular composi-

tion (Carmichael and Price, 1994) and receive more pronounced input from distinct sensory association cortices (Jones and Powell, 1970; Barbas, 1988; Morecroft et al., 1992; Carmichael and Price, 1995b). Thus, decision making in this study activated distinct areas of inferior and orbital PFC that have access to heteromodal sources of information and are ideally positioned to integrate sensory and object-based processing of exteroceptive stimuli with processing of their associated reward–punishment valence. Moreover, in addition to its reciprocal connections with medial temporal systems (Jones and Powell, 1970), the orbitomedial and orbitolateral PFC provide important output pathways into the ventral striatum (Haber et al., 1995) and are able to interface such "affective" information with mechanisms of action selection routed through corticostriatal loops (Rolls, 1996).

The orbital PFC is also a prominent target of the monoamine neuromodulatory projections (Thierry et al., 1973). Indeed, the orbital PFC is just one station in an extensive circuitry, incorporating the ventral striatum and amygdala, implicated in processes of reinforcement and incentive motivation and under strong influence from mesocorticolimbic dopamine input (DiChiara and Imperato, 1988; Koob and Bloom, 1988; Wise and Rompré, 1989). Consequently, recent findings that subjects with a history of chronic amphetamine abuse show a pattern of decision-making deficits that closely resembles that shown selectively by patients sustaining damage to orbital PFC suggests that decision-making cognition may be susceptible to altered neuromodulation, perhaps affecting orbital PFC function (Rogers et al., 1999). Converging evidence that this is the case can be seen in the demonstration of marked impairments in the decision making of normal volunteers after acute plasma tryptophan depletion (Rogers et al., 1999), raising the further possibility that reduction in central 5-hydroxytryptamine, itself strongly associated with disorganized, impulsive, and aggressive behavior (Linnoila et al., 1983), is associated with altered decision making in laboratory settings.

The contributions of the orbital PFC to decision making are poorly understood; resolving choices between small, likely rewards and larger, unlikely rewards must recruit several, as yet unspecified, cognitive operations (Bechara et al., 1997; Rogers et al., 1999). However, the proposal that the orbital PFC is involved in the representation of stimulus–reward relationships (for review, see Iversen and Mishkin, 1970; Jones and Mishkin, 1972; Dias et al., 1996; Rolls, 1996) seems especially pertinent because effective real-life decision making must require accurate information about the current reward valence of relevant exteroceptive stimuli. However, the nature of this information remains controversial. On the one hand, the orbital PFC may help to mediate decision making by providing action selection mechanisms with direct information about the reinforcing properties of all types of unconditioned and conditioned stimuli (Rolls, 1996); on the other hand, the orbital PFC may reactivate somatic states previously conditioned to salient features of the choice confronting the subject (Damasio, 1994).

In this context, it is notable that although the reward offered to our subjects, experimenter-defined "points" having no monetary significance, was rather abstract and arbitrary in character, it is clear that the decision making of our subjects was sensitive to the combination of size and probability of rewards associated with the two response options (Fig. 33.1C–F). Moreover, decision making per se over this kind of reward, although effective in activating extensive parts of orbital PFC, did not activate other stations in the circuitry associated with processes of reinforcement such as the ventral striatum and amygdala. Although the detection of rCBF changes in these smaller structures may have been hampered by the width of smoothing filter applied to our data (FWHM = 16 mm), the present results suggest that the orbital PFC is particularly implicated in mediating decision making

over "secondary" reinforcement (i.e., reinforcement conditioned to stimuli associated with "primary" reward; see also Bechara et al., 1999). Exploring whether the orbital PFC participates in a wider network mediating primary reinforcement requires manipulating the type of reinforcement available to subjects in similar tasks.

The strong activations seen in the orbital PFC during the decision-making conditions compared to the control conditions contrasts with the more restricted activity apparent in the direct comparisons between the 4:2 and 5:1 conditions. In general, the decision of the 4:2 conditions were more affected by the balance of reinforcers than those of the 5:1 conditions and were associated with marked increases in deliberation times (Fig. 33.1). Although the limited increase in rCBF seen within the anterior cingulate gyrus is entirely consistent with its proposed role in response selection mechanisms in coordination with interconnected limbic circuitry and orbital PFC (Vogt et al., 1992), the absence of large activations in the orbital PFC itself suggests that this area makes a necessary contribution to decision making that does not depend to any great extent on the degree of conflict inherent in the choice. However, our design deliberately matched reinforcement density across the 4:2 and 5:1 conditions. Recent studies suggest that the activity of the orbital PFC is sensitive to changes in acquired reward (Elliott et al., 1999) and violations of expectations (Nobre et al., 1999). Thus, research into the relationship between decision making, orbital PFC activity, and magnitude of reward also seems warranted.

Finally, appropriate deliberation about the available options in our decision-making task may also have required the temporary suppression of activated or primed responses, for example, those directed toward actions associated with larger but less probable rewards, and this suppression may have been reflected in the activations seen in the inferior convexity during the 4:2 and 5:1 conditions (Kawashima et al., 1996; Konishi et al., 1998; Krams et al., 1998). However, our peaks within the inferior convexity are somewhat ventral to those most recently associated with this inhibitory function (cf. Konishi et al., 1998) and are closer to activations previously seen in working memory studies (Owen et al., 1996; Smith et al., 1996; Courtney et al., 1998). Because it has been proposed that the inferior convexity is involved in the retrieval of information from posterior cortical areas (Petrides, 1994, 1995, 1996; Owen et al., 1996), it is possible that this area contributes to decision making, not by mediating some generic inhibitory function, but by mediating retrieval and/or comparator operations, e.g., over recent reinforcing events, needed for effective choices. Converging evidence that this is the case can be seen in a significant association ($n = 84$; $r = -0.39$; $p < 0.001$) between deliberation times in a decision-making task similar to the one used here and performance on a spatial span task (E. Bazanis, R. D. Rogers, J. H. Dowson, T. W. Robbins, and B. J. Sahakian, unpublished observations) that has previously been shown to activate the same area of ventrolateral PFC as activated in the current study (Owen et al., 1996). Finally, the decision-making deficits of orbital PFC patients do not take the form of impulsive or disinhibited responding (Bechara et al., 1996), but rather slow and ineffective deliberation about the conflicting options for action (Rogers et al., 1999), again suggesting that the contribution of the orbital PFC to decision-making cognition is not the provision of a simple inhibitory mechanism.

Acknowledgments

This work was supported by a Programme Grant from the Wellcome Trust to T.W.R., B.J.E., A.C.R., and B.J.S., and by Technology Foresight (J.D.P.). This is a publication of the Medical Research Council Cooperative on Brain, Behavior, and Neuropsychiatry. We thank Matthew Brett for his advice and help with data analysis.

References

Barbas H (1988) Anatomic organization of basoventral and mediodorsal visual recipient prefrontal regions in the rhesus monkey. J Comp Neurol 276:313–342.

Barbas H, Pandya DN (1989) Architecture and intrinsic connections of the prefrontal cortex in the rhesus monkey. J Comp Neurol 286:353–375.

Bechara A, Damasio AR, Damasio H, Anderson SW (1994) Insensitivity to future consequences following damage to human prefrontal cortex. Cognition 50:7–15.

Bechara A, Tranel D, Damasio H, Damasio AR (1996) Failure to respond autonomically to anticipated future outcomes following damage to prefrontal cortex. Cereb Cortex 6:215–225.

Bechara A, Damasio H, Tranel D, Damasio AR (1997) Deciding advantageously before knowing the advantageous strategy. Science 275:1293–1295.

Bechara A, Damasio H, Tranel D, Anderson SW (1998) Dissociation of working memory from decision-making within human prefrontal cortex. J Neurosci 18:428–437.

Bechara A, Damasio H, Damasio AR, Lee GP (1999) Different contributions of the human amygdala and ventromedial prefrontal cortex to decision-making. J Neurosci 19:5473–5481.

Berman KF, Randolph C, Gold J, Goldberg TE, Coppola R, Ostrem JL, Carson RE, Herscovitch P, Weinberger DR (1995) Physiological activation of a cortical network of the Wisconsin Card Sorting Test: a positron emission tomography study. Neuropsychologia 33:1027–1046.

Carmichael ST, Price JL (1994) Architectonic subdivision of the orbital and medial prefrontal cortex in the macaque monkey. J Comp Neurol 346:366–402.

Carmichael ST, Price JL (1995a) Limbic connections of the orbital cortex and medial prefrontal cortex in macaque monkeys. J Comp Neurol 363:615–641.

Carmichael ST, Price JL (1995b) Sensory and premotor connections of the orbital and medial prefrontal cortex of macaque monkeys. J Comp Neurol 363:642–664.

Courtney SM, Ungerleider LG, Keil K, Haxby JV (1997) Transient and sustained activity in a distributed neural system for human working memory. Nature 386:608–611.

Damasio AR (1994) Descartes' error. New York: Grosset/Putnam.

Damasio AR (1996a) The somatic marker hypothesis and the possible functions of the prefrontal cortex. Philos Trans R Soc Lond B Biol Sci 351:1413–1420.

Damasio H (1996b) Human neuroanatomy relevant to decision-making. In: Neurobiology of decision-making (Damasio AR, ed), pp 1–12. Berlin: Springer.

Damasio AR, Tranel D, Damasio H (1990) Individuals with sociopathic behavior caused by frontal damage fail to respond autonomically to social stimuli. Behav Brain Res 4:81–94.

Dias R, Robbins TW, Roberts AC (1996) Dissociation in prefrontal cortex of affective and attentional shifts. Nature 380:69–72.

DiChiara G, Imperato A (1988) Drugs abused by humans preferentially increase synaptic dopamine concentrations in the mesolimbic system of freely moving rats. Proc Natl Acad Sci USA 85:5274–5278.

Elliott R, Friston KJ, Dolan RJ (1999) Dissociable neural response associated with reward, punishment and risk-taking. NeuroReport 9:S355.

Eslinger PJ, Damasio AR (1985) Severe disturbance of higher cognition after bilateral frontal lobe ablation: patient EVR. Neurology 35:1731–1741.

Friston KJ, Holmes AP, Worsley KJ, Poline J-B, Frith CD, Frackowiak RSJ (1995) Statistical parametric maps in functional imaging: a general approach. Hum Brain Mapp 2:189–210.

Goldman-Rakic PS (1987) Circuitry of primate prefrontal cortex and regulation of behaviour by representational knowledge. In: Handbook of physiology, Vol 5 (Plum F, Mountcastle VB, eds), pp 373–417. Bethesda, MD: American Physiological Society.

Goldman-Rakic PS (1994) The issue of memory in the study of prefrontal functions. In: Motor and cognitive functions of the prefrontal cortex (Thierry AM, Glowinski J, Goldman-Rakic PS, Christen Y, eds), pp 112–122. Berlin: Springer.

Goldman-Rakic PS (1996) The prefrontal landscape: implications of functional architecture for understanding human mentation and the central executive. Philos Trans R Soc Lond B Biol Sci 351:1445–1453.

Haber SN, Kunisho K, Mizobuchi M, Lynd-Balta E (1995) The orbital and medial prefrontal circuit through the primate basal ganglia. J Neurosci 15:4851–4867.

Howell DC (1987) Statistical methods for psychology, Ed 2. Boston: Duxbury.

Iversen SD, Mishkin M (1970) Perseverative interference in monkeys following selective lesions of the inferior prefrontal convexity. Exp Brain Res 11:376–386.

Jones B, Mishkin M (1972) Limbic lesions and the problem of stimulus-reinforcement associations. Exp Neurology 36:362–377.

Jones EG, Powell TPS (1970) An anatomical study of converging sensory pathways within the cerebral cortex of the monkey. Brain 93:793–820.

Kawashima R, Satoh K, Itoh H, Ono S, Furumoto S, Gotoh R, Koyama M, Yoshioka S, Takahashi T, Takahashi K, Yanagisawa T, Fukuda H (1996) Functional anatomy of GO/NO-GO discrimination and response selection—a PET study in man. Brain Res 728:79–89.

Konishi S, Nakajima K, Uchida I, Sekihara K, Miyashita Y (1998) No-go dominant brain activity in human inferior prefrontal cortex revealed by functional magnetic resonance imaging. Eur J Neurosci 10:1209–1213.

Koob GF, Bloom FE (1988) Cellular and molecular mechanisms of drug dependence. Science 242:715–723.

Krams M, Rushworth MFS, Deiber MP, Frackowiak RSJ, Passingham RE (1998) The preparation, execution and suppression of copied movements in the human brain. Exp Brain Res 120:386–398.

Linnoila M, Virkkunen M, Stein M, Nuptial A, Ripon R, Goodwill FK (1983) Low cerebrospinal fluid 5-hydroxyindoleacetic acid differentiates impulsive from nonimpulsive violent behavior. Life Sci 33:2609–2614.

Milner B (1964) Some effects of frontal lobectomy in man. In: The frontal granular cortex and behavior (Warren JM, Akert K, eds). New York: McGraw-Hill.

Morecroft RJ, Geula C, Mesulam M-M (1992) Cytoarchitecture and neural afferents of orbitofrontal cortex in the brain of the monkey. J Comp Neurol 323:341–358.

Nelson HE (1982) National adult reading test (NART) test manual. Windsor: NFER-Nelson.

Nobre AC, Coull JT, Frith CD (1999) Orbitofrontal cortex is activated during breaches of expectation in tasks of visual attention. Nat Neurosci 2:11–12.

Owen AM, Evans AC, Petrides M (1996) Evidence for a two-stage model of spatial working memory within the lateral frontal cortex: a positron emission tomography study. Cereb Cortex 6:31–38.

Petrides M (1994) Frontal lobes and working memory: evidence from investigations of the effects of cortical excision in human primates. In: Handbook of neuropsychology, Vol 9 (Boller F, Grafman J, eds), pp 59–82. Elsevier: Amsterdam.

Petrides M (1995) Functional organisation of the human frontal cortex for mnemonic processing. Ann NY Acad Sci 76:85–96.

Petrides M (1996) Specialized systems for the processing of mnemonic information within the primate frontal cortex. Philos Trans R Soc B Biol Sci 351:1455–1461.

Rahman S, Sahakian BJ, Hodges JR, Rogers RD, Robbins TW (1999) Specific cognitive deficits in mild frontal variant frontotemporal dementia. Brain 122: 1469–1493.

Roberts AC, Robbins TW, Weiskrantz L (1996) Executive and cognitive functions of the prefrontal cortex. Philos Trans R Soc Lond B Biol Sci 351:1387–1527.

Rogers RD, Everitt BJ, Baldacchino A, Blackmore AJ, Swainson R, London M, Deakin JWF, Sahakian BJ, Robbins TW (1999) Dissociating deficits in the decision-making cognition of chronic amphetamine abusers, opiate abusers, patients with focal damage to prefrontal cortex, and tryptophan-depleted normal volunteers: evidence for monoaminergic mechanisms. Neuropsychopharmacology 20:322–329.

Rolls ET, Hornak J, Wade D, McGrath J (1994) Emotion-related learning in patients with social and emotional changes associated with frontal lobe damage. J Neurol Neurosurg Psychiatry 57:1518–1524.

Rolls ET (1996) The orbitofrontal cortex. Philos Trans R Soc Lond B Biol Sci 351:1433–1444.

Saver JL, Damasio AR (1991) Preserved access and processing of social knowledge in a patient with acquired sociopathy due to ventromedial frontal damage. Neuropsychologia 29:1241–1249.

Silbersweig DA, Stern E, Frith CD, Cahill C, Schnorr L, Grootonk S, Spinks T, Clark J, Frackowiak R, Jones T (1993) Detection of thirty-second cognitive activations in single subjects with positron emission tomography: a new low-dose $H_2{}^{15}O$ regional cerebral blood flow three-dimensional imaging technique. J Cereb Blood Flow Metab 13:617–629.

Smith EE, Jonides J, Koeppe RA (1996) Dissociating verbal and spatial and working memory using PET. Cereb Cortex 6:11–20.

Stuss DT, Benson DF (1986) The frontal lobes. New York: Raven.

Thierry AM, Blanc G, Sobel A, Stinus L, Glowinski J (1973) Dopamine terminals in the rat cortex. Science 182:499–501.

Vogt BA, Finch DM, Olson CR (1992) Functional heterogeneity in cingulate cortex: the anterior executive and posterior evaluative regions. Cereb Cortex 2:435–443.

Wise RA, Rompré PP (1989) Brain dopamine and reward. Annu Rev Psychol 40:191–225.

Worsley KJ, Marrett S, Neelin P, Vandal AC, Friston KJ, Evans AC (1996) A unified statistical approach for determining significant signals in images of cerebral activation. Hum Brain Mapp 4:58–73.

34 A Neural Substrate of Prediction and Reward

Wolfram Schultz, Peter Dayan, and P. Read Montague

An adaptive organism must be able to predict future events such as the presence of mates, food, and danger. For any creature, the features of its niche strongly constrain the time scales for prediction that are likely to be useful for its survival. Predictions give an animal time to prepare behavioral reactions and can be used to improve the choices an animal makes in the future. This anticipatory capacity is crucial for deciding between alternative courses of action because some choices may lead to food whereas others may result in injury or loss of resources.

Experiments show that animals can predict many different aspects of their environments, including complex properties such as the spatial locations and physical characteristics of stimuli (1). One simple, yet useful prediction that animals make is the probable time and magnitude of future rewarding events. "Reward" is an operational concept for describing the positive value that a creature ascribes to an object, a behavioral act, or an internal physical state. The function of reward can be described according to the behavior elicited (2). For example, appetitive or rewarding stimuli induce approach behavior that permits an animal to consume. Rewards may also play the role of positive reinforcers where they increase the frequency of behavioral reactions during learning and maintain well-established appetitive behaviors after learning. The reward value associated with a stimulus is not a static, intrinsic property of the stimulus. Animals can assign different appetitive values to a stimulus as a function of their internal states at the time the stimulus is encountered and as a function of their experience with the stimulus.

One clear connection between reward and prediction derives from a wide variety of conditioning experiments (1). In these experiments, arbitrary stimuli with no intrinsic reward value will function as rewarding stimuli after being repeatedly associated in time with rewarding objects—these objects are one form of unconditioned stimulus (US). After such associations develop, the neutral stimuli are called conditioned stimuli (CS). In the descriptions that follow, we call the appetitive CS the sensory cue and the US the reward. It should be kept in mind, however, that learning that depends on CS-US pairing takes many different forms and is not always dependent on reward (for example, learning associated with aversive stimuli). In standard conditioning paradigms, the sensory cue must consistently precede the reward in order for an association to develop. After conditioning, the animal's behavior indicates that the sensory cue induces a prediction about the likely time and magnitude of the reward and tends to elicit approach behavior. It appears that this form of learning is associated with a transfer of an appetitive or approach-eliciting component of the reward back to the sensory cue.

Some theories of reward-dependent learning suggest that learning is driven by the unpredictability of the reward by the sensory cue (3, 4). One of the main ideas is that no further learning takes place when the reward is entirely predicted by a sensory cue (or cues). For example, if presentation of a light is consistently followed by food, a rat will learn that the light predicts the future arrival of food. If, after such training, the light is paired with a sound and this pair is consistently followed by food, then something unusual happens—the rat's behavior indicates that the light continues to predict food, but the sound predicts nothing. This phenomenon is called "blocking." The prediction-based explanation is that the light fully predicts the food that arrives and the presence of the sound adds no new predictive (useful) information; therefore, no association developed to the sound (5). It appears therefore that learning is driven by deviations or "errors" between the predicted time and amount of rewards and their actual experienced times and magnitudes [but see (4)].

Engineered systems that are designed to optimize their actions in complex environments face the same challenges as animals, except that the equivalent of rewards and punishments are determined by design goals. One established method by which artificial systems can learn to predict is called the temporal difference (TD) algorithm (6). This algorithm was originally inspired by behavioral data on how animals actually learn predictions (7). Real-world applications of TD models abound. The predictions learned by TD methods can also be used to implement a technique called dynamic programming, which specifies how a system can come to choose appropriate actions. In this article, we review how these computational methods provide an interpretation of the activity of dopamine neurons thought to mediate reward-processing and reward-dependent learning. The connection between the computational theory and the experimental results is striking and provides a quantitative framework for future experiments and theories on the computational roles of ascending monoaminergic systems (8–13).

Information Encoded in Dopaminergic Activity

Dopamine neurons of the ventral tegmental area (VTA) and substantia nigra have long been identified with the processing of rewarding stimuli. These neurons send their axons to brain structures involved in motivation and goal-directed behavior, for example, the striatum, nucleus accumbens, and frontal cortex. Multiple lines of evidence support the idea that these neurons construct and distribute information about rewarding events.

First, drugs like amphetamine and cocaine exert their addictive actions in part by prolonging the influence of dopamine on target neurons (14). Second, neural pathways associated with dopamine neurons are among the best targets for electrical self-stimulation. In these experiments, rats press bars to excite neurons at the site of an implanted electrode (15). The rats often choose these apparently rewarding stimuli over food and sex. Third, animals treated with dopamine receptor blockers learn less rapidly to press a bar for a reward pellet (16). All the above results generally implicate midbrain dopaminergic activity in reward-dependent learning. More precise information about the role played by midbrain dopaminergic activity derives from experiments in which activity of single dopamine neurons is recorded in alert monkeys while they perform behavioral acts and receive rewards.

In these latter experiments (17), dopamine neurons respond with short, phasic activations when monkeys are presented with various appetitive stimuli. For example, dopamine neurons are activated when animals touch a small morsel of apple or receive a small quantity of fruit juice to the mouth as liquid reward (Fig. 34.1). These phasic activations do not, however, discriminate between these different types of rewarding stimuli. Aversive stimuli like air puffs to the hand or drops of saline to the mouth do not cause these same transient activations. Dopamine neurons are also activated by novel stimuli that elicit orienting reactions; however, for most stimuli, this activation lasts for only a few presentations. The responses of these neurons are relatively homogeneous—different neurons respond in the same manner and different appetitive stimuli elicit similar neuronal responses. All responses occur in the majority of dopamine neurons (55 to 80%).

Surprisingly, after repeated pairings of visual and auditory cues followed by reward, dopamine neurons change the time of their phasic activation from just after the time of reward delivery to the time of cue onset. In one task, a naïve monkey is required to touch a lever after the appearance of a small light. Before training and in the initial phases of training, most dopamine neurons show a short burst of impulses after reward delivery (Fig. 34.1, top). After several days of

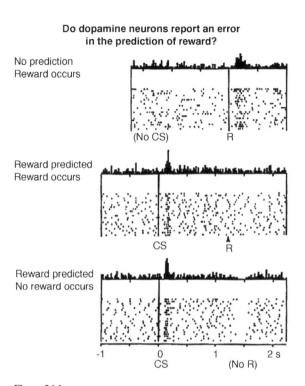

**Do dopamine neurons report an error
in the prediction of reward?**

No prediction
Reward occurs

(No CS)   R

Reward predicted
Reward occurs

CS   R

Reward predicted
No reward occurs

-1   0   1   2 s
CS   (No R)

Figure 34.1
Changes in dopamine neurons' output code for an error in the prediction of appetitive events. (Top) Before learning, a drop of appetitive fruit juice occurs in the absence of prediction—hence a positive error in the prediction of reward. The dopamine neuron is activated by the unpredicted occurrence of juice. (Middle) After learning, the conditioned stimulus predicts reward, and the reward occurs according to the prediction—hence no error in the prediction of reward. The dopamine neuron is activated by the reward-predicting stimulus but fails to be activated by the predicted reward (right). (Bottom) After learning, the conditioned stimulus predicts a reward, but the reward fails to occur because of a mistake in the behavioral response of the monkey. The activity of the dopamine neuron is depressed exactly at the time when the reward would have occurred. The depression occurs more than 1 s after the conditioned stimulus without any intervening stimuli, revealing an internal representation of the time of the predicted reward. Neuronal activity is aligned on the electronic pulse that drives the solenoid valve delivering the reward liquid (top) or the onset of the conditioned visual stimulus (middle and bottom). Each panel shows the perievent time histogram and raster of impulses from the same neuron. Horizontal distances of dots correspond to real-time intervals. Each line of dots shows one trial. Original sequence of trials is plotted from top to bottom. CS, conditioned, reward-predicting stimulus; R, primary reward.

training, the animal learns to reach for the lever as soon as the light is illuminated, and this behavioral change correlates with two remarkable changes in the dopamine neuron output: (i) the primary reward no longer elicits a phasic response; and (ii) the onset of the (predictive) light now causes a phasic activation in dopamine cell output (Fig. 34.1, middle). The changes in dopaminergic activity strongly resemble the transfer of an animal's appetitive behavioral reaction from the US to the CS.

In trials where the reward is not delivered at the appropriate time after the onset of the light, dopamine neurons are depressed markedly below their basal firing rate exactly at the time that the reward should have occurred (Fig. 34.1, bottom). This well-timed decrease in spike output shows that the expected time of reward delivery based on the occurrence of the light is also encoded in the fluctuations in dopaminergic activity (18). In contrast, very few dopamine neurons respond to stimuli that predict aversive outcomes.

The language used in the foregoing description already incorporates the idea that dopaminergic activity encodes expectations about external stimuli or reward. This interpretation of these data provides a link to an established body of computational theory (6, 7). From this perspective, one sees that dopamine neurons do not simply report the occurrence of appetitive events. Rather, their outputs appear to code for a deviation or error between the actual reward received and predictions of the time and magnitude of reward. These neurons are activated only if the time of the reward is uncertain, that is, unpredicted by any preceding cues. Dopamine neurons are therefore excellent feature detectors of the "goodness" of environmental events relative to learned predictions about those events. They emit a positive signal (increased spike production) if an appetitive event is better than predicted, no signal (no change in spike production) if an appetitive event occurs as predicted, and a negative signal (decreased spike production) if an appetitive event is worse than predicted (Fig. 34.1).

Computational Theory and Model

The TD algorithm (6, 7) is particularly well suited to understanding the functional role played by the dopamine signal in terms of the information it constructs and broadcasts (8, 10, 12). This work has used fluctuations in dopamine activity in dual roles: (i) as a supervisory signal for synaptic weight changes (8, 10, 12) and (ii) as a signal to influence directly and indirectly the choice of behavioral actions in humans and bees (9–11). Temporal difference methods have been used in a wide spectrum of engineering applications that seek to solve prediction problems analogous to those faced by living creatures (19). Temporal difference methods were introduced into the psychological and biological literature by Richard Sutton and Andrew Barto in the early 1980s (6, 7). It is therefore interesting that this method yields some insight into the output of dopamine neurons in primates.

There are two main assumptions in TD. First, the computational goal of learning is to use the sensory cues to predict a discounted sum of all future rewards $V(t)$ within a learning trial:

$$V(t) = E[\gamma^0 r(t) + \gamma^1 r(t+1) + \gamma^2 r(t+2) + \cdots]$$
(1)

where $r(t)$ is the reward at time t and $E[\cdot]$ denotes the expected value of the sum of future rewards up to the end of the trial. $0 \leq \gamma \leq 1$ is a discount factor that makes rewards that arrive sooner more important than rewards that arrive later. Predicting the sum of future rewards is an important generalization over static conditioning models like the Rescorla-Wagner rule for classical conditioning (1–4). The second main assumption is the Markovian one, that is, the presentation of future sensory cues and rewards depends only on the immediate (current) sensory cues and not the past sensory cues.

As explained below, the strategy is to use a vector describing the presence of sensory cues $\mathbf{x}(t)$ in the trial along with a vector of adaptable weights $\mathbf{w}$ to make an estimate $\hat{V}(t)$ of the true $V(t)$. The reason that the sensory cue is written as a vector is explained below. The difficulty in adjusting weights $\mathbf{w}$ to estimate $V(t)$ is that the system (that is, the animal) would have to wait to receive all its future rewards in a trial $r(t+1), r(t+2), \ldots$ to assess its predictions. This latter constraint would require the animal to remember over time which weights need changing and which weights do not.

Fortunately, there is information available at each instant in time that can act as a surrogate prediction error. This possibility is implicit in the definition of $V(t)$ because it satisfies a condition of consistency through time:

$$V(t) = E[r(t) + \gamma V(t+1)] \qquad (2)$$

An error in the estimated predictions can now be defined with information available at successive time steps:

$$\delta(t) = r(t) + \gamma \hat{V}(t+1) - \hat{V}(t) \qquad (3)$$

This $\delta(t)$ is called the TD error and acts as a surrogate prediction error signal that is instantly available at time $t+1$. As described below, $\delta(t)$ is used to improve the estimates of $V(t)$ and also to choose appropriate actions.

Representing a Stimulus through Time

We suggested above that a set of sensory cues along with an associated set of adaptable weights would suffice to estimate $V(t)$ (the discounted sum of future rewards). It is, however, not sufficient for the representation of each sensory cue (for example, a light) to have only one associated adaptable weight because such a model would not account for the data shown above—it would not be able to represent both the time of the cue and the time of reward delivery. These experimental data show that a sensory cue can predict

reward delivery at arbitrary times into the near future. This conclusion holds for both the monkeys' behavior and the output of the dopamine neurons. If the time of reward delivery is changed relative to the time of cue onset, then the same cue will come to predict the new time of reward delivery. The way in which such temporal labels are constructed in neural tissue is not known, but it is clear that they exist (20).

Given these facts, we assume that each sensory cue consists of a vector of signals $\mathbf{x}(t) = \{x_1(t), x_2(t), \ldots\}$ that represent the light for variable lengths of time into the future, that is, $x_i(t)$ is 1 exactly i time steps after the presentation of the light in the trial and 0 otherwise (Fig. 34.2B). Each component of $\mathbf{x}(t), x_i(t)$, has its own prediction weight w_i (Fig. 34.2B). This representation means that if the light comes on at time s, $x_1(s+1) = 1, x_2(s+2) = 1, \ldots$ represent the light at $1, 2, \ldots$ time steps into the future and w_1, $w_2, \ldots$ are the respective weights. The net prediction for cue $\mathbf{x}(t)$ at time t takes the simple linear form

$$\hat{V}(t) \equiv \hat{V}(\mathbf{x}(t)) = \Sigma_i w_i x_i(t) \qquad (4)$$

This form of temporal representation is what Sutton and Barto (7) call a complete serial-compound stimulus and is related to Grossberg's spectral timing model (21). Unfortunately, virtually nothing is known about how the brain represents a stimulus for substantial periods of time into the future; therefore, all temporal representations are underconstrained from a biological perspective.

As in trial-based models like the Rescorla-Wagner rule, the adaptable weights $\mathbf{w}$ are improved according to the correlation between the stimulus representations and the prediction error. The change in weights from one trial to the next is

$$\Delta w_i = \alpha_x \Sigma_t x_i(t) \delta(t) \qquad (5)$$

where α_x is the learning rate for cue $\mathbf{x}(t)$ and the sum over t is taken over the course of a trial.

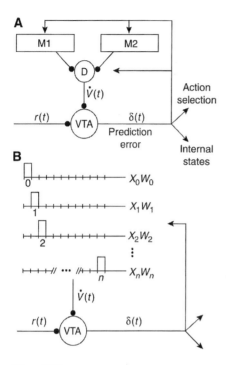

Figure 34.2
Constructing and using a prediction error. (A) Interpretation of the anatomical arrangement of inputs and outputs of the ventral tegmental area (VTA). M1 and M2 represent two different cortical modalities whose output is assumed to arrive at the VTA in the form of a temporal derivative (surprise signal) $V(t)$, which reflects the degree to which the current sensory state differs from the previous sensory state. The high degree of convergence forces $V(t)$ to arrive at the VTA as a scalar signal. Information about reward $r(t)$ also converges on the VTA. The VTA output is taken as a simple linear sum $\delta(t) = r(t) + V(t)$. The widespread output connections of the VTA make the prediction error $\delta(t)$ simultaneously available to structures constructing the predictions. (B) Temporal representation of a sensory cue. A cue like a light is represented at multiple delays $\mathbf{x}_n$ from its initial time of onset, and each delay is associated with a separate adjustable weight $\mathbf{w}_n$. These parameters $\mathbf{w}_n$ are adjusted according to the correlation of activity $\mathbf{x}_n$ and δ and through training come to act as predictions. This simple system stores predictions rather than correlations.

It has been shown that under certain conditions this update rule (Eq. 5) will cause $\hat{V}(t)$ to converge to the true $V(t)$ (22). If there were many different sensory cues, each would have its own vector representation and its own vector of weights, and Eq. 4 would be summed over all the cues.

Comparing Model and Data

We now turn this apparatus toward the neural and behavioral data described above. To construct and use an error signal similar to the TD error above, a neural system would need to possess four basic features: (i) access to a measure of reward value $r(t)$; (ii) a signal measuring the temporal derivative of the ongoing prediction of reward $\gamma\hat{V}(t+1) - \hat{V}(t)$; (iii) a site where these signals could be summed; and (iv) delivery of the error signal to areas constructing the prediction in such a way that it can control plasticity.

It has been previously proposed that midbrain dopamine neurons satisfy features (i), (ii), and (iii) listed above (Fig. 34.2A) (8, 10, 12). As indicated in Fig. 34.2, the dopamine neurons receive highly convergent input from many brain regions. The model represents the hypothesis that this input arrives in the form of a surprise signal that measures the degree to which the current sensory state differs from the last sensory state. We assume that the dopamine neurons' output actually reflects $\delta(t) + b(t)$, where $b(t)$ is a basal firing rate (12). Figure 34.3 shows the training of the model on a task where a single sensory cue predicted the future delivery of a fixed amount of reward 20 time steps into the future. The prediction error signal (top) matches the activity of the real dopamine neurons over the course of learning. The pattern of weights that develops (bottom) provide the model's explanations for two well-described behavioral effects—blocking and secondary conditioning (1). The model accounts for the behavior of the dopamine neurons in a variety of other experiments in monkeys (12). The model also accounts

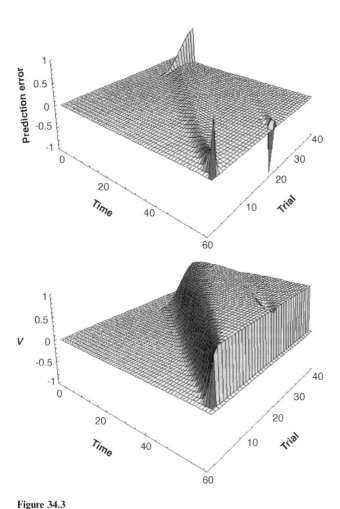

Figure 34.3
Development of prediction error signal through training. (Top) Prediction error (changes in dopamine neuron output) as a function of time and trial. On each trial, a sensory cue is presented at time step 10 and time step 20 followed by reward delivery $[r(t) = 1]$ at time step 60. On trial 0, the presentation of the two cues causes no change because the associated weights are initially set to 0. There is, however, a strong positive response (increased firing rate) at the delivery of reward at time step 60. By repeating the pairing of sensory cues followed in time by reward, the transient response of the model shifts to the time of the earliest sensory cue (time step 10). Failure to deliver the reward during an intermediate trial causes a large negative fluctuation in the model's output. This would be seen in an experiment as a marked decrease in spike output at the time that reward should have been delivered. In this example, the timing of reward delivery is learned well before any response transfers to the earliest sensory cue. (Bottom) The value function $V(t)$. The weights are all initially set to 0 (trial 0). After the large prediction error occurs on trial 0, the weights begin to grow. Eventually they all saturate to 1 so that the only transient is the unpredicted onset of the first sensory cue. The depression in the surface results from the error trial where the reward was not delivered at the expected time.

for changes in dopaminergic activity if the time of the reward is changed (18).

The model makes two other testable predictions: (i) in the presence of multiple sensory cues that predict reward, the phasic activation of the neurons will transfer to the earliest consistent cue. (ii) After training on multiple sensory cues, omission of an intermediate cue will be accompanied by a phasic decrease in dopaminergic activity at the time that the cue formerly occurred. For example, after training a monkey on the temporal sequence light 1 → light 2 → reward, the dopamine neurons should respond phasically only to the onset of light 1. At this point, if light 2 is omitted on a trial, the activity in the neurons will depress at the time that light 2 would have occurred.

Choosing and Criticizing Actions

We showed above how the dopamine signal can be used to learn and store predictions; however, these same responses could also be used to influence the choice of appropriate actions through a connection with a technique called dynamic programming (23). We discuss below the connection to dynamic programming.

We introduce this use with a simple example. Suppose a rat must move through a maze to gain food. In the hallways of the maze, the rat has two options available to it: go forward a step or go backward a step. At junctions, the rat has three or four directions from which to choose. At each position, the rat has various actions available to it, and the action chosen will affect its future prospects for finding its way to food. A wrong turn at one point may not be felt as a mistake until many steps later when the rat runs into a dead end. How is the rat to know which action was crucial in leading it to the dead end? This is called the temporal credit assignment problem: Actions at one point in time can affect the acquisition of rewards in the future in complicated ways.

One solution to temporal credit assignment is to describe the animal as adopting and improving a "policy" that specifies how its actions are assigned to its states. Its state is the collection of sensory cues associated with each maze position. To improve a policy, the animal requires a means to evaluate the value of each maze position. The evaluation used in dynamic programming is the amount of summed future reward expected from each maze position provided that the animal follows its policy. The summed future rewards expected from some state [that is, $V(t)$] is exactly what the TD method learns, suggesting a connection with the dopamine signal.

As the rat above explores the maze, its predictions become more accurate. The predictions are considered "correct" once the average prediction error $\underline{\delta}(t)$ is 0. At this point, fluctuations in dopaminergic activity represent an important "economic evaluation" that is broadcast to target structures: Greater than baseline dopamine activity means the action performed is "better than expected" and less than baseline means "worse than expected." Hence, dopamine responses provide the information to implement a simple behavioral strategy—take [or learn to take (24)] actions correlated with increased dopamine activity and avoid actions correlated with decreases in dopamine activity.

A very simple such use of $\delta(t)$ as an evaluation signal for action choice is a form of learned klinokinesis (25), choosing one action while $\delta(t) > 0$, and choosing a new random action if $\delta(t) \leq 0$. This use of $\delta(t)$ has been shown to account for bee foraging behavior on flowers that yield variable returns (9, 11). Figure 34.4 shows the way in which TD methods can construct for a mobile "creature" a useful map of the value of certain actions.

A TD model was equipped with a simple visual system (two, 200 by 200 pixel retinae) and trained on three different sensory cues (colored blocks) that differed in the amount of reward each contained (blue > green > red). The model

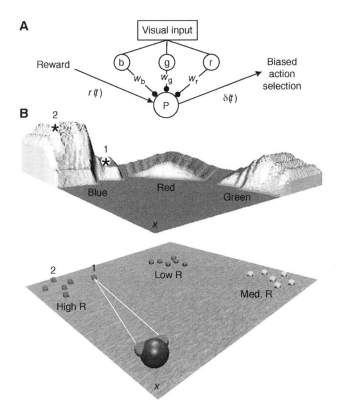

Figure 34.4
Simple cognitive maps can be easily built and used. (A) Architecture of the TD model. Three color-sensitivity units (b, g, r) report, respectively, the percentage of blue, green, and red in the visual field. Each unit influences neuron P (VTA analog) through a single weight. The colored blocks contain varying amounts of reward with blue > green > red. After training, the weights (w_b, w_g, w_r), reflect this difference in reward content. Using only a single weight for each sensory cue, the model can make only one-time step predictions; however, combined with its capacity to move its head or walk about the arena, a crude "value-map" is available in the output $\delta(t)$ of neuron P. (B) Value surface for the arena when the creature is positioned in the corner as indicated. The height of the surface codes for the value $V(x, y)$ of each location when viewed from the corner where the "creature" is positioned. All the creature needs to do is look from one location to another (or move from one position to another), and the differences in value $V(t + 1) - V(t)$ are coded in the changes in the firing rate of P (see text).

had three neurons, each sensitive only to the percentage of one color in the visual field. Each color-sensitive neuron provides input to the prediction unit P (analog of VTA unit in Fig. 34.2) through a single weight. Dedicating only a single weight to each cue limits this "creature" to a one time step prediction on the basis of its current state. After experiencing each type of object multiple times, the weights reflect the relative amounts [of reward in each object, that is, $w_b > w_g > w_r$.] These three weights equip the creature with a kind of cognitive map or "value surface" with which to assay its possible actions (Fig. 34.4B).

The value surface above the arena is a plot of the value function $V(x, y)$ (height) when the creature is placed in the indicated corner and looks at every position (x, y) in the arena. The value $V(x, y)$ of looking at each position (x, y) is computed as a linear function of the weights $[(w_b, w_g, w_r)]$ associated with activity induced in the color-sensitive units. As this "creature" changes its direction of gaze from one position (x_0, y_0) at time t to another position (x_1, y_1) at time $t + 1$, the difference in the values of these two positions $V(t + 1) - V(t)$ is available as the output $\delta(t)$ of the prediction neuron P. In this example, when the creature looks from point 1 to point 2, the percentage of blue in its visual field increases. This increase is available as a positive fluctuation ("things are better than expected") in the output $\delta(t)$ of neuron P. Similarly, looking from point 2 to point 1 causes a large negative fluctuation in $\delta(t)$ ("things are worse than expected"). As discussed above, these fluctuations could be used by some target structure to decide whether to move in the direction of sight. Directions associated with a positive prediction error are likely to yield increased future returns.

This example illustrates how only three stored quantities (weights associated with each color) and the capacity to look at different locations endow this simple "creature" with a useful map of the quality of different directions in the arena. This same model has been given simple card-

choice tasks analogous to those given to humans (26), and the model matches well the human behavior. It is also interesting that humans develop a predictive galvanic skin response that predicts appropriately which card decks are good and which are bad (26).

Summary and Future Questions

We have reviewed evidence that supports the proposal that dopamine neurons in the VTA and the substantia nigra report ongoing prediction errors for reward. The output of these neurons is consistent with a scalar prediction error signal; therefore, the delivery of this signal to target structures may influence the processing of predictions and the choice of reward-maximizing actions. These conclusions are supported by data on the activity changes of these neurons during the acquisition and expression of a range of simple conditioning tasks. This representation of the experimental data raises a number of important issues for future work.

The first issue concerns temporal representations, that is, how is any stimulus represented through time? A large body of behavioral data show that animals can keep track of the time elapsed from the presentation of a CS and make precise predictions accordingly. We adopted a very simple model of this capacity, but experiments have yet to suggest where or how the temporal information is constructed and used by the brain. It is not yet clear how far into the future such predictions can be made; however, one suspects that they will be longer than the predictions made by structures that mediate cerebellar eyeblink conditioning and motor learning displayed by the vestibulo-ocular reflex (27). The time scales that are ethologically important to a particular creature should provide good constraints when searching for mechanisms that might construct and distribute temporal labels in the cerebral cortex.

A second issue is information about aversive events. The experimental data suggest that the dopamine system provides information about appetitive stimuli, not aversive stimuli. It is possible however that the absence of an expected reward is interpreted as a kind of "punishment" to some other system to which the dopamine neurons send their output. It would then be the responsibility of these targets to pass out information about the degree to which the nondelivery of reward was "punishing." It was long ago proposed that rewards and punishments represent opponent processes and that the dynamics of opponency might be responsible for many puzzling effects in conditioning (28).

A third issue raised by the model is the relation between scalar signals of appetitive values and vector signals with many components, including those that represent primary rewards and predictive stimuli. Simple models like the one presented above may be able to learn with a scalar signal only if the scope of choices is limited. Behavior in more realistic environmental situations requires vector signaling of the type of rewards and of the various physical components of the predictive stimuli. Without the capacity to discriminate which stimuli are responsible for fluctuations in a broadcast scalar error signal, an agent may learn inappropriately; for example, it may learn to approach food when it is actually thirsty.

Dopamine neurons emit an excellent appetitive error (teaching) signal without indicating further details about the appetitive event. It is therefore likely that other reward-processing structures subserve the analysis and discrimination of appetitive events without constituting particularly efficient teaching signals. This putative division of labor between the analysis of physical and functional attributes and scalar evaluation signals raises a fourth issue—attention.

The model does not address the attentional functions of some of the innervated structures, such as the nucleus accumbens and the frontal cortex. Evidence suggests that these structures are important for cases in which different amounts of attention are paid to different stimuli. There is, however, evidence to suggest that the required attentional mechanisms might also operate at the level of the dopamine neurons. Their responses to novel stimuli will decrement with repeated presentation and they will generalize their responses to nonappetitive stimuli that are physically similar to appetitive stimuli (29). In general, questions about attentional effects in dopaminergic systems are ripe for future work.

The suggestions that a scalar prediction-error signal influences behavioral choices receives support from the preliminary work on human decision-making and from the fact that changes in dopamine activity fluctuations parallel changes in the behavioral performance of the monkeys (30). In the mammalian brain, the striatum is one site where this kind of scalar evaluation could have a direct effect on action choice, and activity relating to conditioned stimuli is seen in the striatum (31). The widespread projection of dopamine axons to striatal neurons gives rise to synapses at dendritic spines that are also contacted by excitatory inputs from cortex (32). This may be a site where the dopamine signal influences behavioral choices by modulating the level of competition in the dorsal striatum. Phasic dopamine signals may lead to an augmentation of excitatory influences in the striatum (33), and there is evidence for striatal plasticity after pulsatile application of dopamine (34). Plasticity could mediate the learning of appropriate policies (24).

The possibilities in the striatum for using a scalar evaluation signal carried by changes in dopamine delivery are complemented by interesting possibilities in the cerebral cortex. In prefrontal cortex, dopamine delivery has a dramatic influence on working memory (35). Dopamine also modulates cognitive activation of anterior cingulate cortex in schizophrenic patients (36). Clearly, dopamine delivery has important cognitive consequences at the level of the cerebral cortex. Under the model presented here, changes in dopaminergic activity distribute prediction errors to widespread target structures. It seems reasonable to require that the prediction errors be delivered primarily to those regions most responsible for making the predictions; otherwise, one cortical region would have to deal with prediction errors engendered by the bad guesses of another region. From this point of view, one could expect there to be a mechanism that coupled local activity in the cortex to an enhanced sensitivity of nearby dopamine terminals to differences from baseline in spike production along their parent axon. There is experimental evidence that supports this possibility (37).

Neuromodulatory systems like dopamine systems are so named because they were thought to modulate global states of the brain at time scales and temporal resolutions much poorer than other systems like fast glutamatergic connections. Although this global modulation function may be accurate, the work discussed here shows that neuromodulatory systems may also deliver precisely timed information to specific target structures to influence a number of important cognitive functions.

References and Notes

1. A. Dickinson, *Contemporary Animal Learning Theory* (Cambridge Univ. Press, Cambridge, 1980); N. J. Mackintosh, *Conditioning and Associative Learning* (Oxford Univ. Press, Oxford, 1983); C. R. Gallistel, *The Organization of Learning* (MIT Press, Cambridge, MA, 1990); L. A. Real, *Science* 253, 980 (1991).

2. I. P. Pavlov, *Conditioned Reflexes* (Oxford Univ. Press, Oxford, 1927); B. F. Skinner, *The Behavior of Organisms* (Appleton-Century-Crofts, New York, 1938); J. Olds, *Drives and Reinforcement* (Raven, New York 1977); R. A. Wise, in *The Neuropharmacological Basis of Reward*, J. M. Liebeman and S. J. Cooper, Eds. (Clarendon Press, New York, 1989); N. W. White and P. M. Milner, *Annu. Rev. Psychol.* 43, 443 (1992); T. W. Robbins and B. J. Everitt, *Curr. Opin. Neurobiol.* 6, 228 (1996).

3. R. A. Rescorla and A. R. Wagner, in *Classical Conditioning II: Current Research and Theory*, A. H. Black and W. F. Prokasy, Eds. (Appleton-Century-Crofts, New York, 1972), pp. 64–69.

4. N. J. Mackintosh, *Psychol. Rev.* 82, 276 (1975); J. M. Pearce and G. Hall, *ibid.* 87, 532 (1980).

5. L. J. Kamin, in *Punishment and Aversive Behavior*, B. A. Campbell and R. M. Church, Eds. (Appleton-Century-Crofts, New York (1969), pp. 279–296.

6. R. S. Sutton and A. G. Barto, *Psychol. Rev.* 88 (no. 2), 135 (1981); R. S. Sutton, *Mach. Learn.* 3, 9 (1988).

7. R. S. Sutton and A. G. Barto, *Proceedings of the Ninth Annual Conference of the Cognitive Science Society* (Seattle, WA, 1987); in *Learning and Computational Neuroscience*, M. Gabriel and J. Moore, Eds. (MIT Press, Cambridge, MA, 1989). For specific application to eyeblink conditioning, see J. W. Moore et al., *Behav. Brain Res.* 12, 143 (1986).

8. S. R. Quartz, P. Dayan, P. R. Montague, T. J. Sejnowski, *Soc. Neurosci. Abstr.* 18, 1210 (1992); P. R. Montague, P. Dayan, S. J. Nowlan, A. Pouget, T. J. Sejnowski, in *Advances in Neural Information Processing Systems 5*, S. J. Hanson, J. D. Cowan, C. L. Giles, Eds. (Morgan Kaufmann, San Mateo, CA, 1993), pp. 969–976.

9. P. R. Montague, P. Dayan, T. J. Sejnowski, in *Advances in Neural Information Processing Systems 6*, G. Tesauro, J. D. Cowan, J. Alspector, Eds. (Morgan Kaufmann, San Mateo, CA, 1994), pp. 598–605.

10. P. R. Montague and T. J. Sejnowski, *Learn. Mem.* 1, 1 (1994); P. R. Montague, *Neural-Network Approaches to Cognition—Biobehavioral Foundations*, J. Donahoe, Ed. (Elsevier, Amsterdam, in press); P. R. Montague and P. Dayan, *A Companion to Cognitive Science*, W. Bechtel and G. Graham, Eds. (Blackwell, Oxford, in press).

11. P. R. Montague, P. Dayan, C. Person, T. J. Sejnowski, *Nature* 377, 725 (1995).

12. P. R. Montague, P. Dayan, T. J. Sejnowski, *J. Neurosci.* 16, 1936 (1996).

13. Other work has suggested an interpretation of monoaminergic influences similar to that taken above (8–12) [K. J. Friston, G. Tononi, G. N. Reeke, O. Sporns, G. M. Edelman, *Neuroscience* 59, 229 (1994); J. C. Houk, J. L. Adams, A. G. Barto, in *Models of Information Processing in the Basal Ganglia*, J. C. Houk, J. L. Davis, D. G. Beiser, Eds. (MIT Press, Cambridge, MA, 1995)], pp. 249–270. Other models of monoaminergic influences have considered what could

be called attention-based accounts (4) rather than prediction error–based explanations [D. Servan-Schreiber, H. Printz, J. D. Cohen, *Science* 249, 892 (1990)].

14. G. F. Koob, *Semin. Neurosci.* 4, 139 (1992); R. A. Wise and D. C. Hoffman, *Synapse* 10, 247 (1992); G. DiChiara, *Drug Alcohol Depend.* 38, 95 (1995).

15. A. G. Phillips, S. M. Brooke, H. C. Fibiger, *Brain Res.* 85, 13 (1975); A. G. Phillips, D. A. Carter, H. C. Fibiger, *ibid.* 104, 221 (1976); F. Mora and R. D. Myers, *Science* 197, 1387 (1977); A. G. Phillips, F. Mora, E. T. Rolls, *Psychopharmacology* 62, 79 (1979); D. Corbett and R. A. Wise, *Brain Res.* 185, 1 (1980); R. A. Wise and P.-P. Rompré, *Annu. Rev. Psychol.* 40, 191 (1989).

16. R. A. Wise, *Behav. Brain Sci.* 5, 39 (1982); R. J. Beninger, *Brain Res. Rev.* 6, 173 (1983); —— and B. L. Hahn, *Science* 220, 1304 (1983); R. J. Beninger, *Brain Res. Bull.* 23, 365 (1989); M. LeMoal and H. Simon, *Physiol. Rev.* 71, 155 (1991); T. W. Robbins and B. J. Everitt, *Semin. Neurosci.* 4, 119 (1992).

17. W. Schultz, *J. Neurophysiol.* 56, 1439 (1986); R. Romo and W. Schultz, *ibid.* 63, 592 (1990); W. Schultz and R. Romo, *ibid.* p. 607; T. Ljungberg, P. Apicella, W. Schultz, *ibid.* 67, 145 (1992); W. Schultz, P. Apicella, T. Ljungberg, *J. Neurosci.* 13, 900 (1993); J. Mirenowicz and W. Schultz, *J. Neurophysiol.* 72, 1024 (1994); W. Schultz et al., in *Models of Information Processing in the Basal Ganglia,* J. C. Houk, J. L. Davis, D. G. Beiser, Eds. (MIT Press, Cambridge, MA, 1995), pp. 233–248; J. Mirenowicz and W. Schultz, *Nature* 379, 449 (1996).

18. Recent experiments showed that the simple displacement of the time of reward delivery resulted in dopamine responses. In a situation in which neurons were not driven by a fully predicted drop of juice, activations reappeared when the juice reward occurred 0.5 s earlier or later than predicted. Depressions were observed at the normal time of juice reward only if reward delivery was late [J. R. Hollerman and W. Schultz, *Soc. Neurosci. Abstr.* 22, 1388 (1996)].

19. G. Tesauro, *Commun. ACM* 38, 58 (1995); D. P. Bertsekas and J. N. Tsitsiklis, *Neurodynamic Programming* (Athena Scientific, Belmont, NJ, 1996).

20. R. M. Church, in *Contemporary Learning Theories: Instrumental Conditioning Theory and the Impact of Biological Constraints on Learning,* S. B. Klein and R. R. Mowrer, Eds. (Erlbaum, Hillsdale, NJ, 1989), p. 41; J. Gibbon, *Learn. Motiv.* 22, 3 (1991).

21. S. Grossberg and N. A. Schmajuk, *Neural Networks* 2, 79 (1989); S. Grossberg and J. W. L. Merrill, *Cognit. Brain Res.* 1, 3 (1992).

22. P. Dayan, *Mach. Learn.* 8, 341 (1992); P. Dayan and T. J. Sejnowski, *ibid.* 14, 295 (1994); T. Jaakkola, M. I. Jordan, S. P. Singh, *Neural Computation* 6, 1185 (1994).

23. R. E. Bellman, *Dynamic Programming* (Princeton Univ. Press, Princeton, NJ, 1957); R. A. Howard, *Dynamic Programming and Markov Processes* (MIT Press, Cambridge, MA, 1960).

24. A. G. Barto, R. S. Sutton, C. W. Anderson, *IEEE Trans. Syst. Man Cybernetics* 13, 834 (1983).

25. Bacterial klinokinesis has been described in great detail. Early work emphasized the mechanisms required for bacteria to climb gradients of nutrients. See R. M. Macnab and D. E. Koshland, *Proc. Natl. Acad. Sci. U.S.A.* 69, 2509 (1972); N. Tsang, R. Macnab, D. E. Koshland Jr., *Science* 181, 60 (1973); H. C. Berg and R. A. Anderson, *Nature* 245, 380 (1973); H. C. Berg, *ibid.* 254, 389 (1975); J. L. Spudich and D. E. Koshland, *Proc. Natl. Acad. Sci. U.S.A.* 72, 710 (1975). The klinokinetic action-selection mechanism causes a TD model to climb hills defined by the sensory weights, that is, the model will climb the surface defined by the value function V.

26. A. R. Damasio, *Descartes' Error* (Putnam, New York, 1994); A. Bechara, A. R. Damasio, H. Damasio, S. Anderson, *Cognition* 50, 7 (1994).

27. S. P. Perrett, B. P. Ruiz, M. D. Mauk, *J. Neurosci.* 13, 1708 (1993); J. L. Raymond, S. G. Lisberger, M. D. Mauk, *Science* 272, 1126 (1996).

28. S. Grossberg, *Math. Biosci.* 15, 253 (1972); R. L. Solomon and J. D. Corbit, *Psychol. Rev.* 81, 119 (1974); S. Grossberg, *ibid.* 89, 529 (1982).

29. W. Schultz and R. Romo, *J. Neurophysiol.* 63, 607 (1990); T. Ljungberg, P. Apicella, W. Schultz, *ibid.* 67, 145 (1992); J. Mirenowicz and W. Schultz, *Nature* 379, 449 (1996).

30. W. Schultz, P. Apicella, T. Ljungberg, *J. Neurosci.* 13, 900 (1993).

31. T. Aosaki et al., *ibid.* 14, 3969 (1994); A. M. Graybiel, *Curr. Opin. Neurobiol.* 5, 733 (1995); *Trends Neurosci.* 18, 60 (1995). Recent models of sequence generation in the striatum use fluctuating dopamine input as a scalar error signal [G. S. Berns and T. J. Sejnowski, in *Neurobiology of Decision Making,*

A. Damasio, Ed. (Springer-Verlag, Berlin, 1996), pp. 101–113.

32. T. F. Freund, J. F. Powell, A. D. Smith, *Neuroscience* 13, 1189 (1984); Y. Smith, B. D. Bennett, J. P. Bolam, A. Parent, A. F. Sadikot, *J. Comp. Neurol.* 344, 1 (1994).

33. C. Cepeda, N. A. Buchwald, M. S. Levine, *Proc. Natl. Acad. Sci. U.S.A.* 90, 9576 (1993).

34. J. R. Wickens, A. J. Begg, G. W. Arbuthnott, *Neuroscience* 70, 1 (1996).

35. P. S. Goldman-Rakic, C. Leranth, M. S. Williams, N. Mons, M. Geffard, *Proc. Natl. Acad. Sci. U.S.A.* 86, 9015 (1989); T. Sawaguchi and P. S. Goldman-Rakic, *Science* 251, 947 (1991); G. V. Williams and P. S. Goldman-Rakic, *Nature* 376, 572 (1995).

36. R. J. Dolan et al., *Nature,* 378, 180 (1995).

37. P. R. Montague, C. D. Gancayco, M. J. Winn, R. B. Marchase, M. J. Friedlander, *Science* 263, 973 (1994). The mechanistic suggestion requires that local cortical activity (presumably glutamatergic) increases the sensitivity of nearby dopamine terminals to differences from baseline in spike production along their parent axon. This may result from local increases in nitric oxide production. In this manner, baseline dopamine release remains constant in inactive cortical areas while active cortical areas feel strongly the effect of increases and decreases in dopamine delivery due to increases and decreases in spike production along the parent dopamine axon.

We thank A. Damasio and T. Sejnowski for comments and criticisms, and C. Person for help in generating figures. The theoretical work received continuing support from the Center for Theoretical Neuroscience at Baylor College of Medicine and the National Institutes of Mental Health (NIMH) (P.R.M.). P.D. was supported by Massachusetts Institute of Technology and the NIH. The primate studies were supported by the Swiss National Science Foundation, the McDonnell-Pew Foundation (Princeton), the Fyssen Foundation (Paris), the Fondation pour la Recherche Midicale (Paris), the United Parkinson Foundation (Chicago), the Roche Research Foundation (Basel), the NIMH (Bethesda), and the British Council.

35 Selective Enhancement of Emotional, but Not Motor, Learning in Monoamine Oxidase A–Deficient Mice

Jeansok J. Kim, Jean C. Shih, Kevin Chen, Lu Chen, Shaowen Bao, Stephen Maren, Stephan G. Anagnostaras, Michael S. Fanselow, Edward De Maeyer, Isabelle Seif, and Richard F. Thompson

Monoamines, which include catecholamines such as dopamine, norepinephrine (NE), and epinephrine, and indolamines such as serotonin (5-HT), are critically involved in behaviors ranging from sleep to ingestion (1), and aberrant levels of monoamines are correlated with mental dysfunctions (e.g., schizophrenia and depression) and neurological disorders (e.g., Alzheimer and Parkinson diseases) (2–5). The major monoaminergic systems emanate from several brainstem nuclei (e.g., NE in the locus coeruleus, dopamine in the substantia nigra, and 5-HT in the raphe nucleus) and they exert their influences by sending both ascending and descending projections to various regions of the brain and the spinal cord (6).

Recently, mutant mice lacking monoamine oxidase A (MAOA), one of two mitochondrial membrane-bound MAO isoenzymes (the other being MAOB) which degrades monoamines to inert metabolites (7), have been shown to exhibit enhanced aggression (e.g., in the resident-intruder test) and cytoarchitectural changes in their somatosensory cortex (specifically the absence of barrelfield) (8, 9). Similarly to what is observed in normal mice using drugs that block MAOA (10), in MAOA-deficient brains, NE and 5-HT levels were significantly elevated (8). The enhanced aggressive behavior exhibited by the MAOA mutant mice is consistent with the impulsive aggression reported in men from a Dutch family with a complete MAOA deficiency, due to a point mutation in the gene encoding MAOA (11). In addition to abnormal aggressive behavior, these men are also afflicted with borderline mental retardation.

To test whether MAOA-deficient mice also manifest cognitive deficits, we examined learning and memory performance in these animals by using both emotional (classical fear conditioning and step-down inhibitory avoidance) and motor (classical eyeblink conditioning) tasks. Fear conditioning occurs when arbitrary stimuli such as tones, lights, or distinctive environments are paired with aversive unconditioned stimuli (US) such as footshock. Through association formation, arbitrary stimuli become conditioned stimuli (CS) that are capable of eliciting fear responses. In the step-down inhibitory avoidance, the animal must remember that stepping off a safe platform resulted in a footshock. Eyeblink conditioning takes place when a discrete CS (usually tone or light) is paired with a discrete US (usually airpuff or periorbital shock) directed at the eye. The animal initially blinks only to the US; this reflexive eyeblink to the US is known as the unconditioned response. Over the course of training, the animal gradually blinks to the CS; this learned eyeblink to the CS is known as the conditioned response. In addition to learning tasks, species-typical maternal behaviors such as nesting, nursing, and pup retrieval were examined in postparturient MAOA-deficient mice. Finally, monoamine levels were determined in the hippocampus, the frontal cortex, and the cerebellum, structures implicated in some forms of learning and memory (12–14).

Materials and Methods

Subjects

Thirteen MAOA-deficient (4 males and 9 females) and nine wild-type control (5 males and 4 females) mice of C3H/HeJ genetic background (≈ 4 months old) underwent two different types of emotional learning tasks (fear conditioning and step-down avoidance) followed by eyeblink (motor) conditioning. The animals had free access to food and water and all behavioral tests were carried out during the light phase of the light/dark cycle. At the end of the experiment, the genotypes of the mice were reconfirmed by PCR analysis of DNA prepared from tails (8).

Fear Conditioning

For fear conditioning, animals were housed (groups of 1–3 per cage) in the University of California, Los Angeles, Psychology Department vivarium for 2 weeks of adaptation (a 14-hr light/10-hr dark cycle, lights on at 7 A.M.) prior to the start of training. On day 1 of fear conditioning, each mouse was placed in one of four identical experimental chambers (28 × 21 × 22 cm; Lafayette Instruments, North Lafayette, IN) with the floor consisting of 24 stainless steel rods (1-mm diameter) spaced 0.5 cm apart (center-to-center). After 3 min in the chamber, the mice received three tone-footshock pairings (tone: 10 sec, 85 dB, 2 kHz; footshock: 1 sec, 0.5 mA; intertrial interval 1 min apart). One minute after the final footshock, the mice were returned to their home cages. Each chamber was wiped with 5% ammonium hydroxide solution before training. On day 2, fear conditioning to the context was assessed by placing the mice back in the conditioning chamber for an 8-min test, in the absence of any tone and footshock. On day 3, fear conditioning to the tone was measured in observation chambers that were different from those used during conditioning (15). After 2 min in the new chamber, the conditioned tone was presented for a 6-min test. Fear conditioning was assessed during training (day 1), context test (day 2), and tone test (day 3) by measuring the freezing response. Freezing is defined as the absence of all visible movements of the body and vibrissae aside from movement necessitated by respiration. An observer who was blind to the experimental conditions scored each mouse for freezing every 8 sec. The freezing data were transformed to a percentage of total observations, a probability estimate that is amenable to analysis of variance.

Step-Down Avoidance

Promptly following fear conditioning, the animals were transported and individually housed in the University of Southern California, HEDCO Neuroscience Building vivarium (a 12-hr light/12-hr dark cycle, lights on at 7 A.M.). After 2 weeks of adaptation, the mice underwent step-down avoidance training. In this task, each mouse was placed on a 9-cm diameter platform that was elevated 1.5 cm from the grid floor of the experimental chamber (21 × 23 × 26 cm; Ralph Gerbrands, Arlington, MA). Immediately upon stepping down (all four paws on the grid floor), the animals received a single footshock (1 sec, 0.5 mA). After the foot-shock, the animals were returned to their home cage. The mice were placed back on the platform 1, 2, and 7 days following the footshock and step-down latencies were measured; the maximum time allowed on the platform was 3 min.

Eyeblink Conditioning

One week after step-down avoidance testing, animals underwent eyeblink conditioning using a previously described method in mice (16). In brief, under ketamine (80 mg/kg, i.p.) and xylazine (20 mg/kg, i.p.) anesthesia, mice were implanted subcutaneously with four Teflon-coated stainless steel wires (0.003-inch bare, 0.0045-inch coated; A-M Systems, Everett, WA) to the left upper eyelid. The tips of the wires were exposed, and two of the wires were used to record differential electromyograph (EMG) from obicularis oculi, and the remaining two wires were used to deliver periorbital shock. A four-pin strip connector to which the wires were soldered was cemented to the skull of the animal with dental acrylic. Two to 3 days after the surgery, each mouse was placed in one of four identical cylindrical Plexiglas containers (3.75-inch diameter), which was placed inside a sound- and light-attenuating chamber. The strip connector was attached to the mating plug of a commutator with channels to relay EMG signals and to deliver the shock. The daily training consisted of 100 trials grouped in 10 blocks. Each block included one CS alone, one US alone, and eight CS–US paired trials. The CS and US were a 352-msec tone (1000 Hz, 80 dB) and a coterminating 100-msec shock (100-Hz biphasic square pulses), respectively, with a randomized intertrial interval between 20 and 40 sec (mean = 30 sec). The US intensity used was the minimal voltage required to elicit an eyeblink/head turn response (unconditioned response), and the US intensity was adjusted daily for each animal (ranging from 3 to 60 V). After 7 days of paired training, all animals received 4 days of CS-alone extinction trials. The EMG signal was amplified in the band of 300–5,000 Hz and sent to a window discriminator where the number of pulses above the noise envelop was sampled and stored by a computer. The discriminated EMG activity was then analyzed trial by trial using an EMG unit analysis program that made statistical comparisons between pre-CS EMG activity and CS EMG activity (16).

Maternal Behavior

Experimentally naive, postparturient (first litter) MAOA ($n = 4$) and wild-type mice ($n = 4$) (between 3 and 4 months old) were examined for nesting, nursing, and pup retrieval behaviors. The nesting behavior was scored as 0 for no nesting, 1 for incomplete nesting (no enclosing walls), and 2 for complete nesting (enclosing walls). The nursing behavior, defined as crouching and providing milk to the pups, was assigned 0 for the absence and 1 for the presence of the behavior. The pup retrieval behavior was assessed by the average time it took the mother to retrieve displaced pups (the total time required to retrieve all pups/number of pups); the pups were placed on the opposite end of the cage from the nesting area. These maternal behaviors were observed once a day for 5 consecutive days after the pups were born.

Determination of Dopamine, NE, and 5-HT Levels in the Brain Tissue

The frontal cortex, the hippocampus, and the cerebellum were rapidly dissected from the brains of experimentally naive normal and mutant mice and frozen in liquid nitrogen until prepared for HPLC analysis (as described in ref. 17). Each brain region was homogenized in a solution containing 0.1 M trichloroacetic acid, 10 mM sodium acetate, and 0.1 mM EDTA (pH 3.75); 1 μM isoproterenol was used as an internal standard. The homogenates were sonicated for 5 sec (Fisher Sonic Dismembrator, model 300; probe sonicator at setting 60), centrifuged, and the supernatants were divided into aliquots for HPLC analysis. The protein concentrations were determined using the pellet with the method of Lowry (18) with bovine serum albumin as standard.

HPLC analysis was performed using 5-HT and NE (Sigma) as standards. The mobile phase was the same as the homogenization buffer (excluding the isoproterenol) with 15% methanol for detection of 5-HT. NE was quantified separately using 5% methanol in the trichloroacetic acid mobile phase solution. The mobil phases were filtered and deaerated and the pump speed (Shimadzu LC-6A liquid chromatograph) was 1.5 ml per minute. The reverse-phase column used was a Rexchrom S50100-ODS C_{18} column with a length of 25 cm and an internal diameter of 4.6 mm (Regis, Morton Grove, IL). The compounds were measured at +0.7 V using a Shimadzu L-ECD-6A electrochemical detector. Standard curves were determined for 5-HT and NE and the amount of the different compounds in each sample was determined by comparison with the standard curve taking into account a correction factor based upon the amount of the internal standard isoproterenol in the sample.

Kim et al.

Kim et al.

Kim et al.

558

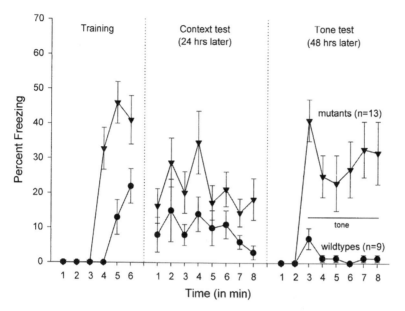

Figure 35.1

Mean ($\pm$ SEM) freezing level during training, context test, and tone test. In the training, 1, 2, and 3 denote 3 min of baseline (pretone footshock) and 4, 5, and 6 represent three posttone footshock intervals. The context test was for 8 min. In the tone test, 1 and 2 signify 2 min of baseline (in a new context) prior to 6 min of tone onset. Freezing scores are expressed as the percentage of total observation.

Results

The freezing, step-down avoidance latency, and eyeblink-conditioned response data were pooled across sex, since there were no differences between males and females, in both MAOA mutant and wild-type mice.

As shown in Fig. 35.1, fear conditioning (percent freezing) was significantly elevated in the MAOA-deficient mice, in comparison to the wild-type mice, during training [immediate postshock freezing during minutes 4, 5, and 6; $F(1,21) = 19.97$; $P < 0.01$], context test [$F(1,21) = 5.86$; $P < 0.05$], and tone test [$F(1,21) = 17.32$; $P < 0.01$]. Prior to the footshock (minutes 1, 2, and 3), neither the MAOA or wild-type mice displayed any freezing behavior.

The MAOA-deficient mice also demonstrated significantly enhanced step-down avoidance latencies on day 1 [$F(1,21) = 7.37$; $P < 0.05$], day 2 [$F(1,21) = 27.63$; $P < 0.01$], and day 7 [$F(1,21) = 24.26$; $P < 0.01$] of training-test intervals when compared with the wild types (Fig. 35.2). Although there was a trend of MAOA-deficient mice having a longer latency than the wild types to step-down from the platform prior to the shock (baseline), this difference was not statistically significant [$F(1,21) = 3.82$; $P > 0.05$]. However, there was no reliable group x training-test interval interaction with the baseline [$F(3,66) = 1.52$; $P > 0.05$].

In contrast to fear conditioning and step-down inhibitory avoidance, there was no statistically reliable difference between the MAOA mutant and the wild-type mice in eyeblink condition-

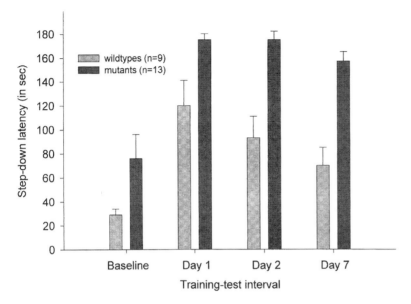

Figure 35.2
Mean ($\pm$ SEM) latency to step down from the platform prior to the footshock (baseline), 1 day after training (day 1), 2 days after training (day 2), and 7 days after training (day 7).

ing ($P > 0.05$) (Fig. 35.3*A*). Both groups showed gradual acquisition of eyeblink conditioned responses over 7 days of CS–US paired training, and demonstrated extinction during the 4 days of CS-alone trials. However, the MAOA mutants appear to be less sensitive to the periorbital shock US since the minimal US intensity (voltage) required to elicit an eyeblink/head turn response was significantly higher in the MAOA-deficient mice than in normal mice across the 7 days of training [group $\times$ day interaction; $F(6, 132) = 4.72$; $P < 0.01$] (Fig. 35.3*B*).

There were no noticeable differences in the species-typical maternal behavior exhibited by postparturient MAOA-deficient and wild-type mice (Table 35.1). Both groups demonstrated comparable nesting, nursing, and pup-retrieval behaviors to their first litter.

When compared with the wild types, the MAOA mutants showed significantly elevated

levels of NE and 5-HT in the hippocampus, the frontal cortex, and the cerebellum (Table 35.2).

Discussion

We found that mice deficient in MAOA enzymatic activity have elevated levels of monoamines (specifically NE and 5-HT) in the brain and display an enhancement in emotional (fear) learning. In the fear conditioning task, neither the MAOA mutants nor the wild types exhibited any freezing behavior prior to the first footshock. However, the MAOA-deficient mice exhibited heightened freezing responses during training (immediate postshock periods), context test (24 hr later), and tone test (48 hr later) in comparison to normal mice. Similarly, the MAOA-deficient mice manifested longer latencies to step down from a safe platform than the normal mice

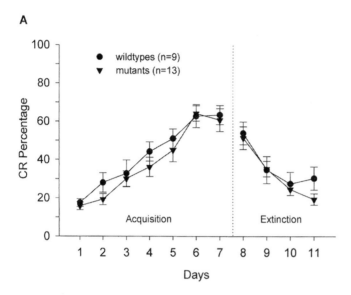

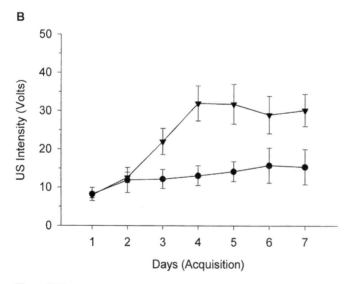

Figure 35.3
(A) Mean (± SEM) percentage of conditioned responses exhibited by MAOA-deficient and wild-type mice during 7 days of acquisition and 4 days of extinction. (B) Mean (± SEM) periorbital shock (US) intensity used for eyeblink conditioning in MAOA and wild-type mice during 7 days of acquisition. The US intensity, the minimal voltage required to elicit an eyeblink/head turn response, was adjusted daily for each animal.

Table 35.1
Maternal behaviors of wild-type and MAOA mutant mice

Genotype	Nesting	Nursing	Pup retrieval
Wild type	1.35 ± 0.19	0.8 ± 0.08	12.7 ± 2.69
MAOA	1.50 ± 0.19	0.19 ± 0.10	14.4 ± 2.94

Values are shown by mean $\pm$ SEM. Nesting: 0, no nesting; 1, incomplete nesting; and 2, complete nesting. Nursing: 0, no nursing; 1, nursing. Pup retrieval, the average time (seconds) it took the mother to retrieve displaced pups. Wild-type mice ($n = 4$); MAOA mice ($n = 4$).

in the inhibitory avoidance learning. Thus, it appears that fear learning is generally enhanced in these mutants.

The enhancement of fear learning observed in MAOA-deficient mice may be due to elevated catecholamine levels, because injections of catecholamines into the brains of mice enhances fear memory formation (19), whereas drugs that lower the levels of catecholamines impair it (20). Since the amygdala is critically involved in both fear conditioning and inhibitory avoidance learning (e.g., refs. 21–24), it is possible that the alteration of catecholamine levels in the amygdala is responsible for the enhancement of fear learning observed in the MAOA mutant mice. Other pharmacological studies indicate that treatments that increase the noradrenergic transmission in the amygdala (e.g., infusions of NE into the amygdala) enhance fear learning, whereas treatments that decrease noradrenergic transmission impair fear learning (e.g., infusions of noradrenergic antagonists) (25, 26). It is conceivable then that the enhancement of emotional learning exhibited by the MAOA-deficient mice is due to the elevation of NE in the amygdala. Although the NE level was not examined specifically in the amygdala, since the locus coeruleus is known to innervate the amygdala (1), the absence of MAOA activity would most likely result in the elevation of NE level in the amygdala. Consis-

tent with this view, the NE level was elevated in other brain structures innervated by the locus coeruleus, such as the frontal cortex, the hippocampus, and the cerebellum.

The effect on emotional learning appears to be reasonably selective, since maternal behavior and eyeblink conditioning were not affected. For instance, there were no observable differences in the species-typical maternal behavior displayed by postparturient MAOA-deficient and wild-type mice. Both groups exhibited comparable nesting, nursing, and pup-retrieval behaviors to their first litter. The lack of effect on eyeblink conditioning was surprising given that monoaminergic afferents constitute one of the three major afferent systems in the cerebellum (the others are the mossy fiber and climbing fiber afferents) (27). The monoaminergic inputs include well-defined noradrenergic and serotonergic afferents from the locus coeruleus and raphe nucleus, respectively. The functional roles of these monoaminergic afferents are not clear, but there is evidence that they modulate synaptic transmission in Purkinje cells and other cerebellar cortical neurons. For instance, iontophoretic application of NE to Purkinje cells results in an enhancement of both excitatory and inhibitory responses of Purkinje cells, both to mossy fiber and climbing fiber inputs (28). In eyeblink conditioning, there is evidence indicating that the mossy fibers and the climbing fibers relay information about the CS and the US, respectively (14). Because MAOA-deficient mice showed a normal rate of acquisition of eyeblink conditioning, either monoaminergic systems are not involved in eyeblink conditioning, the monoamine levels were not sufficiently elevated to influence eyeblink conditioning, or the elevated monoamine levels resulted in some form of developmental compensation. Thus, the lack of an eyeblink conditioning effect in MAOA-deficient mice cannot rule out the involvement of monoamine systems in the normal eyeblink conditioning situation.

Interestingly, there was a significant difference in the minimal periorbital shock US intensity

Kim et al. 562

Table 35.2
Concentrations of neurotransmitters in various brain regions of the wild-type and MAOA mutant mice

Brain region	Neurotransmitters	Wild types	MAOA mutants
Cerebellum	5-HT	17.12 ± 3.06	45.39 ± 3.33**
	NE	10.29 ± 2.08	16.88 ± 4.53*
Frontal cortex	5-HT	17.73 ± 3.10	38.24 ± 6.81*
	NE	8.22 ± 0.97	16.62 ± 2.06**
Hippocampus	5-HT	25.02 ± 13.28	70.43 ± 8.27**
	NE	12.08 ± 3.47	19.42 ± 4.01*

Concentrations are in pmol/mg protein. Values are shown by mean ± SD. For 5-HT, $n = 4$ in wild-type and $n = 4$ in MAOA mutant mice. For NE, $n = 4$ in wild types and $n = 5$ in MAOA mutants. *, $P < 0.05$; **, $P < 0.01$ (t test).

required to elicit an eyeblink/head turn response between MAOA mutant and wild-type mice. Although they initially started out at comparable intensities, the MAOA-deficient mice needed increasingly higher voltages than the wild types to elicit the same unconditioned response over the course of training sessions. This finding suggests that MAOA mutants may have an elevated pain threshold. It is conceivable that the alteration in pain sensitivity is due to the elevated 5-HT level. For example, decreasing brain 5-HT increases sensitivity to electric shock in rats, whereas increasing brain 5-HT decreases pain sensitivity (29). It is also possible that the MAOA mutants exhibit stronger conditioned analgesia (due to enhance fear conditioning associated with periorbital shock US) and therefore subsequently require stronger US intensities. Conditioned fear is known to decrease pain sensitivity via activating an endogenous analgesic system (30). This may explain why MAOA-deficient and wild-type mice did not differ in US intensities prior to undergoing eyeblink conditioning. Thus, the MAOA mutants might have demonstrated impaired eyeblink conditioning if a constant US intensity had been used (rather than variable US intensities adjusted to each animal). Regardless, the enhanced fear learning (i.e., conditioned freezing and step-down avoidance) observed in

the MAOA mutant mice is unlikely to be due to an increase in pain sensitivity since they appear to be less sensitive to (periorbital) electric shock.

As mentioned in the Introduction, the men of a Dutch family with deficient MAOA activity manifest impulsive aggression as well as a borderline mental retardation (11). The MAOA mutant mice similarly exhibit enhanced aggressive behavior (8), and as indicated by the present results, also show a selective enhancement in the performance of emotional (fear), but not motor (eyeblink conditioning), tasks. [It is not known if fear conditioning is modified in humans with MAOA deficiency. It is also possible (but not yet tested) that more complex behavioral tasks like spatial memory may be impaired in these mice.] Although the enhanced performance in fear tasks shown by MAOA-deficient mice might be due to an alteration of the fear memory process *per se* as mentioned above (e.g., the elevated NE levels modulating memory consolidation process), it cannot be ruled out that there may be a general alteration of emotional reactivity to threatening (learned or unlearned) stimuli in the MAOA-deficient mice. Since MAOA mutants lack barrelfields in their somatosensory cortex (8, 9), it is possible that their exploratory behavior is altered to favor freezing and step-down avoidance. Indeed, there was a trend toward MAOA-deficient mice taking a longer latency to step-down than the wild types prior to experiencing the footshock. However, the preshock baseline latency did not correlate with postshock test latencies, indicating that a longer latency to step-down prior to the footshock does not necessarily lead to enhanced step-down inhibitory avoidance learning. Likewise, in the fear conditioning experiment, the MAOA mutants exhibited less cage crossover behavior than the wild types during the 3-min preshock baseline (data not shown). Again, the crossover behavior and the conditioned freezing response did not correlate, suggesting that the limited crossover behavior is not responsible for the augmented conditioned freezing. Pharmacological manipulations, such as infusions of various monoaminergic drugs (e.g., β-adrenergic receptor antagonist propranolol) into various brain structures (e.g., the amygdala) prior to training and testing, may provide the means to separate this learning and performance issue in MAOA-deficient mice.

Acknowledgments

We thank Michael Davis and James L. McGaugh for comments on this manuscript and Mi Jeong Shin for assistance. This work was supported by grants from the National Institute of Mental Health (1F32MN10521-01 BNR) to J.J.K., from the National Institute of Mental Health (R37 MH39085, MERIT Award, K05 MH00795 RSAward, ROMH37020) and Welin Professorship Award to J.C.S., and from the National Science Foundation (BNS-8718300), the National Institutes of Health (AG05142), and Sankyo to R.F.T.

References

1. Feldman, R. S. & Quenzer, L. F. (1984) *Fundamentals of Neuropsychopharmacology* (Sinauer, Sunderland, MA).

2. Snyder, S. H. (1974) *Science* 184, 1243–1253.

3. Palmer, A. M. & DeKosky, S. T. (1993) *J. Neural Transm. Gen. Sect.* 91, 135–159.

4. Schildkraut, J. J. (1965) *Am. J. Psychiatry* 122, 509–522.

5. Hornykiewicz, O. (1974) *Life Sci.* 15, 1249–1259.

6. Elliott, G. R., Edelman, A. M., Renson, J. F. & Berger, P. A. (1977) in *Psychopharmacology: From Theory to Practice*, eds. Barchas, J. D., Berger, P. A., Cicaranello, R. D. & Elliott, G. R. (Oxford Univ. Press, New York), pp. 33–50.

7. Shih, J. C. (1990) *Neuropsychopharmacology* 4, 1–7.

8. Cases, O., Seif, I., Grimsby, J., Gaspar, P., Chen, K., Pournin, S., Muller, U., Aguet, M., Babinet, C., Shih, J. C. & De Maeyer, E. (1995) *Science* 268, 1763–1766.

9. Cases, O., Vitalis, T., Seif, I., De Maeyer, E., Sotelo, C. & Gaspar, P. (1996) *Neuron* 16, 297–307.

10. Freeman, H. (1993) *Lancet* 342, 1528–1532.

11. Brunner, H. G., Nelen, M., Breakefield, X. O., Ropers, H. H. & van Oost, B. A. (1993) *Science* 262, 578–580.

12. Goldman-Rakic, P. S. (1992) *Sci. Am.* 267, 110–117.

13. Squire, L. R. & Zola-Morgan, S. (1991) *Science* 253, 1380–1386.

14. Thompson, R. F. (1986) *Science* 233, 941–947.

15. Kim, J. J. & Fanselow, M. S. (1992) *Science* 256, 675–677.

16. Chen, L., Bao, S., Lockard, J. M., Kim, J. J. & Thompson, R. F. (1996) *J. Neurosci.* 16, 2829–2838.

17. Kalivas, P. W. (1985) *J. Pharmacol. Exp. Ther.* 235, 544–550.

18. Lowry, O. H., Rosebrough, N. J., Farr, A. L. & Randall, R. J. (1951) *J. Biol. Chem.* 193, 265–275.

19. Haycock, J. W., van Buskirk, R. & McGaugh, J. L. (1977) *Behav. Biol.* 20, 281–310.

20. Stein, L., Belluzzi, J. D. & Wise, C. D. (1975) *Brain Res.* 84, 329–335.

21. Davis, M. (1992) *Annu. Rev. Neurosci.* 15, 353–375.

22. Lavond, D. G., Kim, J. J. & Thompson, R. F. (1993) *Annu. Rev. Psychol.* 44, 317–342.

23. LeDoux, J. E. (1994) *Sci. Am.* 270, 50–57.

24. McGaugh, J. L. (1989) *Annu. Rev. Neurosci.* 12, 255–287.

25. McGaugh, J. L., Introini-Collison, I. B., Naga-hara, A. H. & Cahill, L. (1990) *Neurosci. Biobehav. Rev.* 14, 425–431.

26. Liang, K. C., McGaugh, J. L. & Yao, H. Y. (1990) *Brain Res.* 508, 225–233.

27. Ito, M. (1984) *The Cerebellum and Neural Control* (Raven, New York).

28. Freedman, R., Hoffer, B. J., Woodward, D. J. & Puro, D. (1977) *Exp. Neurol.* 55, 269–288.

29. Seiden, L. S. & Dykstra, L. A. (1977) *Psycho-pharmacology: A Biochemical and Behavioral Approach* (Van Nostrand Reinhold, New York).

30. Fanselow, M. S. (1984) *Trends Neurosci.* 7, 460–462.

36 The Mind of an Addicted Brain: Neural Sensitization of Wanting versus Liking

Kent C. Berridge and Terry E. Robinson

What compels an addict to take a drug like cocaine, heroin, or amphetamine? That is the most important question to be answered about addiction. It is different from "What motivates a person to try a drug in the first place?" or "Why might a nonaddict continue to take drugs occasionally for recreation?" The defining features of addiction are its compulsive nature and persisting susceptibility to relapse. Those are the features we have sought to explain in our biopsychological theory of addiction.[1]

Most expert explanations of addiction parallel the explanations likely to be given by the lay public: Addicts take drugs for the pleasure they produce, and to avoid the unpleasant consequences of withdrawal.[2] But critical examination shows that these explanations are not sufficient to explain addiction.[1,3] The truth is that addicts continue to seek drugs even when no pleasure can be obtained, and even when no withdrawal exists. For instance, addicts seek drugs when they know those available will be insufficient for pleasure.[1,3] Further, addicts crave drugs again even before withdrawal begins: Craving is often highest immediately after taking a drug.[1,3] And addicts continue to crave drugs long after withdrawal is finished: Relapse remains a potent danger when the addict has reentered normal life, after detoxification and recovery from withdrawal.[1,3] Of course, this is not to say that pleasure and withdrawal play no role in the use of drugs. But after one has accounted for all instances of drug use by addicts motivated by pleasure or withdrawal, a vast amount of compulsive drug use still remains to be explained.

We have offered the incentive-sensitization theory of addiction[1] to explain why addictive drug seeking extends beyond pleasure and withdrawal. The theory has four major tenets:

1. Compulsive drug seeking is the result of a progressive and extremely persistent hypersensitivity of specific neural systems (neural sensitization) induced in susceptible individuals by intermittent drug use. Neural sensitization refers to the persistent increased ability of a drug to elicit an effect from particular neurobehavioral systems, and is produced after the systems have received repeated and intermittent exposure to the drug.[1,4] Neural sensitization can more than double the original effect of the drug on the system. This phenomenon stands in contrast to drug tolerance, or reduced responsiveness. Neural sensitization is more than a simple pharmacological effect. Associative learning exerts a powerful role over neural sensitization, and the expression of sensitized drug effects is controlled by conditioned stimuli (stimuli that have previously signaled administration of the drug, and so may predict its future occurrence).[1,4]

2. The neural systems that are most sensitized by drugs normally mediate a specific motivational process we call "wanting" or, more formally, attribution of incentive salience.[1] This psychological process is not "liking" or pleasure, nor is it directly experienced in conscious awareness. Nonetheless, it causes the perception or representation of an event to become attractive, sought after, and capable of riveting attention. This process normally establishes the motivational value of ordinary incentives. But in addicts, the associative pairing of particular acts and drug stimuli with pharmacological consequences that overactivate the system causes excessive wanting to become focused specifically on drug use. (Note that we have placed "wanting" and "liking" in quotation marks to emphasize that our meaning is different from the conscious, subjective awareness that is often meant by these words. We use the words to denote preconscious psychological processes that can cause conscious desire or pleasure but are not identical to them. Additional cognitive processes are required to transform

preconscious "wanting" and "liking" into subjective desire or pleasure. For the remainder of this review, we omit the quotation marks but continue to use wanting and liking to mean the underlying processes.)

3. Repeated drug use sensitizes the neural substrates of wanting but not of liking. With the development of sensitization, addicts come to want drugs more and more even if they like them less and less. In other words, the process of addiction leads to an increasing dissociation between wanting and liking.

4. Finally, as we have alluded to, people do not have direct conscious awareness of either wanting or liking. Rather, activation of the neural substrates of wanting or liking must be translated into subjective awareness by cognitive mechanisms, as are other complex perceptions. Because the basic processes that mediate wanting and liking are not directly accessible to consciousness, people may find themselves wanting particular things without knowing why. Under some circumstances, people may not even know that they want them.

Neural Sensitization and Drug Use

Many addictive drugs, when taken repeatedly and intermittently (as a developing addict would take them), cause certain neurobehavioral systems to become more and more responsive, or sensitized.[1] In particular, dramatic sensitization effects have been observed in mesotelencephalic dopamine systems.[1,4] The neurons of these systems release dopamine as a neurotransmitter. They originate in the midbrain and project to the neostriatum, nucleus accumbens, amygdala, neocortex, and other areas of the forebrain. Mesotelencephalic dopamine systems show robust sensitization after repeated exposure to drugs such as amphetamine, cocaine, or heroin.[1,4]

Once induced, neural sensitization is extremely persistent. In rats, behavioral effects of sensitiza-

tion, such as exaggerated hyperactivity to amphetamine, may persist undiminished for more than a year, and perhaps for life.[1] At the very least, sensitization persists much longer than do unconditioned physiological withdrawal symptoms, which decay within weeks after the cessation of drug use.

A crucial point for our hypothesis is that the development and expression of sensitization are powerfully controlled by associative learning, particularly by processes of classical or Pavlovian conditioning that help to establish conditioned reinforcers.[1,3–5] Sensitization effects can be markedly enhanced by stimuli that were previously associated with drug administration. Whether the consequences of sensitization are expressed at a particular place or time is determined to a large extent by whether such conditioned stimuli (including contextual stimuli) are present.[1,3,4] The reason why addicts focus excessive wanting specifically on drug use is primarily this interaction of neural sensitization with associative learning.[1]

Neural Systems of Wanting Are Sensitized by Drugs

The same mesotelencephalic dopamine systems that show prominent sensitization have long been recognized as crucial to incentive motivation. They have commonly been viewed as a major substrate for drug pleasure and for addiction.[1–3,5] But what precisely do dopamine systems contribute to reward? In particular, does their role in wanting a reward differ from their role in liking it? Most existing evidence fails to provide a clear answer, because most evidence has come primarily from animal studies that confound wanting and liking. For measures of instrumental behavior (i.e., work or effort directed at obtaining a reward), preference, goal-directed strategies, and voluntary consumption, changes in wanting look like changes in liking. Instrumental measures most directly reflect the degree to which a reward is wanted. Based on the assumption that rewards are wanted to the degree they are liked, a change in liking or pleasure after dopamine manipulations has often been inferred from altered instrumental performance.[5] It is important to note, however, that in studies of the role of dopamine in reward, there has never been independent evidence for the assumption that changes in performance reflect changes in liking as opposed to changes in wanting alone.

Recent experiments on food reward have examined the relation of liking to wanting directly. The results indicate that instrumental performance does not necessarily reflect liking, at least under certain circumstances.[1,6] A chief line of evidence against the assumption has come from studies in our laboratory.[6] Facial reactions elicited by sweet or bitter tastes can be used to assess the liking (hedonic or aversive affect) elicited by a taste, and are not instrumental in nature.[6] Several studies have shown that dopamine-related manipulations that appear to change the potency of food reward (according to instrumental or voluntary consumption measures of wanting) fail to change the palatability of the same food (as measured by facial reactions).[6] Unlike normal appetite, satiety, or a variety of neural manipulations that increase or decrease the potency of food reward—all of which alter the degree of wanting and liking together—manipulations of dopamine systems appear to change wanting alone.[6] For example, drugs that suppress or activate dopamine systems that alter instrumental measures of food reward failed to change hedonic patterns to sugar. Massive depletion of forebrain dopamine by lesions that destroyed only dopamine-containing neurons eliminated appetite but failed to decrease hedonic reactions to sweet tastes or to increase aversive reactions to bitter tastes. And elicitation of feeding by electrical stimulation of the lateral hypothalamus, which acts in part via activation of dopamine systems and which has been argued to enhance the potency of food reward, failed to

increase hedonic reactions or to decrease aversive reactions. Taken together, these observations indicate that dopamine manipulations alter appetite, or wanting, for food rewards but do not alter liking.

Recent neurophysiological evidence also supports the hypothesis that dopamine systems mediate wanting in particular, and not liking. For example, in studies of the neuronal activity of dopamine systems during reward, Schultz and colleagues have shown that monkeys that expected to receive a tasty reward showed maximum electrophysiological activation of dopamine neurons at the moment a conditioned stimulus signaled the reward was about to occur—a moment most relevant to wanting[1]—not at the moment the food was actually received or tasted.[7]

The combination of neurobiological and affective behavioral evidence has led us to suggest that mesotelencephalic dopamine-related systems mediate reward by a psychological process that is separable from sensory pleasure. The process we posit is the attribution of incentive salience to the brain's representations of stimuli and events.[1,6] Incentive salience transforms the representation to which it is attributed, making the event attractive and able to grab attention. Once its representation has been transformed into a salient incentive, an event can elicit approach, instrumental action, goal-directed strategies of cognition, and the conscious experience of desire. Such a transformation by itself is wanting alone—no pleasure need necessarily accompany it.[1,6] Indeed, when a powerful incentive is much desired but not obtainable, as in the myth of Tantalus, the experience becomes unpleasant: To be tantalized but never gratified can be a form of torture.

Incentive salience, or wanting, must be actively attributed to a percept or representation. The active nature of the attribution is critical to understanding the neural bases of motivation and addiction. Although the mesotelencephalic dopamine systems that we suggest mediate the attribution of incentive salience are not primary sensory systems, they nonetheless modulate the brain's responsiveness to sensory stimuli. This modulatory role results from the embedment of mesotelencephalic dopamine systems within larger corticostriatal neural systems that receive extensive high-level, highly processed sensory inputs.

Only Wanting—Not Liking—Is Sensitized by Drugs

Addiction is due to sensitized wanting—not to liking. Normally, liking—the pleasure engendered by an encounter with a new incentive—serves as the trigger to activate and direct wanting (via associative learning[1,6]). The degree to which an ordinary incentive becomes wanted depends essentially on the degree to which it is liked. But in drug addiction, because of neural sensitization of wanting, these two processes become decoupled.

The precise locus of neural sensitization is not known, but changes in mesotelencephalic dopaminergic neurons or the inputs and outputs of these neurons seem to be involved.[1,4] A consequence is that drug wanting increases markedly while liking for a given dose may fade. Because the attribution of incentive salience to particular targets is guided by associative learning, sensitized incentive salience for addicts becomes targeted on drug-associated stimuli and mental representations of drug taking. The act of drug taking and associated stimuli, such as drug paraphernalia, become salient incentives themselves. Crack cocaine addicts who have run out of drug, for example, may compulsively and repeatedly examine every small particle they can find that bears any resemblance to a piece of crack, such as a pebble, bit of plaster, or food crumb, even though they know the search for crack is useless; this phenomenon is sometimes described as chasing ghosts.[8] The generation of incentive salience may sometimes be irrational, but it is no less powerful for that.

People Are Not Directly Aware of Wanting and Liking

Addicts who give up their drug often experience intense subjective craving. But addicts who have unimpeded access to their drug may take it routinely, arranging their lives so they can do so without fail, yet habitually and as a matter of course, without intense conscious craving of any kind. To reconcile such craving-free drug use with our hypothesis of sensitized wanting in addiction, it is important to note that subjective experience can sometimes be a misleading guide to underlying liking and wanting. An important postulate of our hypothesis is that conscious awareness has only indirect access to attributions of incentive salience.

It may seem strange to assert that people are not directly aware of their own likes and wants. After all, whether or not people know much about anything else, don't they know what they like? And wouldn't they know if wanting and liking weren't the same? Perhaps nothing strikes a person with greater immediacy than intense pleasure or pain; nothing seizes the mind more completely than an intense craving. But the intensity of these experiences no more implies that people are directly aware of the activation of the elementary processes that have engendered these emotions than the visual experience of the sun as an extremely intense brightness implies that people are directly aware of the neural or computational processes that mediate visual perception.

Visual perception is perhaps the most telling example to illustrate this point. For instance, in the psychological phenomenon known as blindsight, which occurs after damage to the primary visual cortex, people may retain the ability to report the location, brightness, orientation, and even shape of simple visual stimuli in forced-choice tests—yet be completely unaware of what they are looking at or that they are reporting correctly.[9] The brain of a blindsighted person retains many aspects of visual processing, but the subjective mind is not aware of those visual processes.

Regarding addiction, a consequence of the separation of elementary psychological processes from conscious awareness is that it is not nonsensical to speak of unconscious wanting or of unconscious pleasure, just as it is not nonsensical to speak of implicit knowledge or unconscious perception. People are not directly aware of their own elementary processes of either wanting or liking. These go on independently of consciousness. The transformation of elementary visual processes into conscious visual perception is primarily a change of consciousness, not a change of the fundamental visual processes themselves. Many basic visual processes go on equally in the brains of normal and blindsighted people. Analogously, the translation of incentive salience into conscious craving is primarily a change of consciousness, not of the processes of wanting or liking themselves.

Although this point may be controversial, a variety of examples show that people's conscious awareness of what they want can be dissociated from underlying processes of wanting and liking:

1. Choosing what one most dislikes. In a study by Kahneman et al., people freely chose between two procedures that produced pain by prolonged immersion of the hand in ice-cold water.[10] Subjects often chose the experience that they liked less (in the sense that they said it hurt more) because this procedure entailed a small decrement in pain at the end of the trial.

2. Liking induced by events that one does not perceive consciously. Murphy and Zajonc asked people to rate how much they liked a neutral visual stimulus, such as the sight of an unfamiliar Chinese ideograph. These affective ratings were increased if the ideograph was preceded by a too-brief-to-be-perceived tachistoscopic presentation of a smiling face—even though the subjects never consciously detected the face.[11] In this case, liking was elicited by an unconscious perception,

and then was integrated—inappropriately—into the conscious rating of the ideograph.

3. Liking distorted by excessive introspection. Even slow, considered judgments of pleasure can be distorted by the very factor—painstaking introspection—that might be expected to improve the accuracy of affective evaluation. When ordinary people were asked by Wilson and Schooler to judge the taste pleasure of several strawberry jams, the subjects' immediate judgments roughly paralleled the judgments of experts.[12] However, if subjects were asked to analyze their reasons, their pleasure ratings were different and diverged more strongly from the experts' ratings. In other words, rather than revealing the subtleties of underlying affect to conscious awareness, prolonged introspection buried them deeper under additional layers of cognitive interpretation.

4. Wanting without awareness of liking. Finally, people may want without being aware either that they like or want the object they demonstrably seek. Several studies of addiction itself provide the most compelling demonstrations of this fact. For example, Lamb et al. provided "recovered" heroin addicts the opportunity to press a lever to earn an injection that contained either morphine or saline.[13] The addicts were subsequently asked to rate subjectively how much they liked each injection, how much drug they thought it contained, and how much it would cost on the street. The addicts rated saline as worthless and empty, and after several trials chose not to work for it. Conversely, the intermediate to high doses of morphine were rated as pleasant and drug rich, and the addicts worked at high rates to obtain them. Most important, a remarkable dissociation occurred for the lowest dose of morphine. Every addict rated this injection as empty and worthless, identical to saline in its subjective consequences. But despite their subjective evaluation of the low dose as worthless, four out of five addicts worked for the injection at rates as high as those they showed for the higher morphine doses.

Similar dissociations between subjective evaluation and behavioral indices of wanting have been reported for cocaine. For example, Fischman and colleagues offered recovered addicts the opportunity to earn intravenous infusions of cocaine or saline by pressing either of two levers, after they had received desipramine (which blocks the reuptake of dopamine at synapses).[14] In addition, the subjects were asked to rate their subjective evaluations of the drug they chose. Desipramine significantly suppressed the addicts' subjective craving, measured by agreement with the statement "I want cocaine." Also, desipramine administered with cocaine induced unpleasant subjective states assessed by scales of confusion and anger. But desipramine did not at all reduce the behavioral self-administration of cocaine, measured by lever presses for infusions, despite its marked suppression of the subjective experience of drug craving. Desipramine, by our interpretation, disrupted the translation of sensitized incentive salience into conscious awareness, thus reducing subjective craving, but did not disrupt wanting itself.

Such dissociations between the underlying affective processes that drive behavioral seeking and conscious awareness are inexplicable by the conventional assumption that people seek things because they consciously like them. But these dissociations stand as testimony that people can fail to know the relation between their own wanting and liking. Under some conditions, wanting can powerfully direct human behavior while the person's conscious mind remains unaware of wanting or of the motivated behavior. Because of the inability of cognitive introspection to access underlying wanting or liking processes directly, wanting is sometimes best measured by observing what people actually do.

In order to rise to conscious awareness, a salient incentive, like other events, must be translated into subjective experience by processes of cognitive interpretation. Those processes leave room for significant error about what has tran-

spired, even for highly noticeable events.[15] Questionnaires that purport to measure drug craving by addicts must be interpreted with this in mind. It is quite possible that questions intended to measure drug wanting will in many instances fail to do so because of the accidental masking of these processes by cognitive factors. The occurrence of drug self-administration in the absence of reported subjective craving has led some researchers to suggest that persistent drug use becomes automatic or decoupled from conscious volitional control as a consequence of habitual repetition.[16] We would add that the compulsive quality of automatic habits of drug seeking arises from sensitized incentive salience, acquired through associative pairing of neural hyperactivity with the act of drug use, and not the mere repetition of the act itself.

Pharmacotherapies for Addiction?

Finally, the incentive-sensitization theory makes a unique prediction for what any as-yet-to-be-discovered medication must do if it is to cure addiction. The theory predicts that the only pharmacotherapy able to constitute a cure will be one that reverses associatively controlled processes of neural sensitization. Medications that simply prevent sensitization will not work. Addicts would not willingly take them until after they became addicted—when it would be too late. Nor will a cure be found in medications that simply suppress the function of dopaminergic or related neural systems. At low doses of such medications, drug-associated stimuli are still relatively strong incentives. The higher doses that would be needed to suppress all incentive salience are incapacitating. Still other medications, which suppress drug liking, focus on the wrong component of reward, and can at best be only partly successful. Only reversal of neural sensitization would transform the brain and mind of an addict back into the brain and mind of a nonaddict. As yet, a pharmacological cure for addiction does not exist. But the incentive-sensitization theory tells in advance how to recognize a cure: It will reverse the physiological changes that constitute neural sensitization.

Acknowledgments

We thank Barry Everitt, Randy Gallistel, Jane Stewart, Frederick Toates, and Robert Zajonc for their helpful comments on an earlier version of this manuscript.

Notes

1. T. E. Robinson and K. C. Berridge, The neural basis of drug craving: An incentive-sensitization theory of addiction, *Brain Research Reviews*, 18, 247–291 (1993).
2. For example, "Drug craving is characterized by both the desire to experience the hedonic effects of the drug ... and the desire to avoid aversive withdrawal symptoms"; A. Markou, F. Weiss, L. H. Gold, S. Barak Caine, G. Schulteis, and G. F. Koob, Animal models of drug craving, *Psychopharmacology*, 112, 163–182 (1993), p. 176.
3. J. Stewart, H. de Wit, and R. Eikelboom, Role of unconditioned and conditioned drug effects in the self-administration of opiates and stimulants, *Psychological Review*, 91, 251–268 (1984); R. A. Wise and M. A. Bozarth, A psychomotor stimulant theory of addiction, *Psychological Review*, 94, 469–492 (1987).
4. T. E. Robinson and J. B. Becker, Enduring changes in brain and behavior produced by chronic amphetamine administration: A review and evaluation of animal models of amphetamine psychosis, *Brain Research Reviews*, 11, 157–198 (1986); P. W. Kalivas and J. Stewart, Dopamine transmission in the initiation and expression of drug- and stress-induced sensitization of motor activity, *Brain Research Reviews*, 16, 223–244 (1991).
5. D. Bindra, How adaptive behavior is produced: A perceptual-motivation alternative to response reinforcement, *Behavioral and Brain Sciences*, 1, 41–91 (1978); F. Toates, *Motivational Systems* (Cambridge University Press, Cambridge, England, 1986); R. A. Wise, Neuroleptics and operant behavior: The anhedonia hypothesis, *Behavioral and Brain Sciences*, 5,

39–87 (1982); T. W. Robbins and J. J. Everitt, Functions of dopamine in the dorsal and ventral striatum, *Seminars in the Neurosciences*, 4, 119–127 (1992).
6. K. C. Berridge, I. L. Venier, and T. E. Robinson, Taste reactivity analysis of 6-hydroxydopamine-induced aphagia: Implications for arousal and anhedonia hypotheses of dopamine function, *Behavioral Neuroscience*, 103, 36–45 (1989); K. C. Berridge and E. S. Valenstein, What psychological process mediates feeding evoked by electrical stimulation of the lateral hypothalamus? *Behavioral Neuroscience*, 105, 3–14 (1991); D. Treit and K. C. Berridge, A comparison of benzodiazepine, serotonin, and dopamine agents in the taste-reactivity paradigm, *Pharmacology, Biochemistry and Behavior*, 37, 451–456 (1990); K. C. Berridge, Wanting and liking in food reward: A taste reactivity analysis of process and brain substrates, *Neuroscience and Biobehavioral Reviews* (in press).
7. W. Schultz and R. Romo, Dopamine neurons of the monkey midbrain: Contingencies of responses to stimuli eliciting immediate behavioral reactions, *Journal of Neurophysiology*, 63, 607–624 (1990); W. Schultz, Activity of dopamine neurons in the behaving primate, *Seminars in Neuroscience*, 4, 129–138 (1992). For further review, see pp. 262–267 in Robinson and Berridge, note 1.
8. R. B. Rosse, M. Fay-McCarthy, J. Collins, Jr., D. Risher-Flowers, T. N. Alim, and S. I. Deutsch, Transient compulsive foraging behavior associated with crack cocaine use, *American Journal of Psychiatry*, 150, 155–156 (1993).
9. L. Weiskrantz, *Blindsight: A Case Study and Implications* (Oxford University Press, Oxford, England, 1986); M. S. Gazzaniga, R. Fendrich, and C. M. Wessinger, Blindsight reconsidered, *Current Directions in Psychological Science*, 3, 93–96 (1994).
10. D. Kahneman, B. L. Fredrickson, C. A. Schreiber, and D. A. Redelmeier, When more pain is preferred to less: Adding a better end, *Psychological Science*, 4, 401–405 (1993).
11. S. T. Murphy and R. B. Zajonc, Affect, cognition, and awareness: Affective priming with optimal and suboptimal stimulus exposures, *Journal of Personality and Social Psychology*, 64, 723–739 (1993).
12. T. D. Wilson and J. W. Schooler, Thinking too much: Introspection can reduce the quality of preferences and decisions, *Journal of Personality and Social Psychology*, 60, 181–192 (1991).

13. R. J. Lamb, K. L. Preston, C. W. Schindler, R. A. Meisch, F. Davis, J. L. Katz, J. E. Henningfield, and S. R. Goldberg, The reinforcing and subjective effects of morphine in post-addicts: A dose-response study, *Journal of Pharmacology and Experimental Therapeutics,* 259, 1165–1173 (1991).

14. M. W. Fischman and R. W. Foltin, Self-administration of cocaine by humans: A laboratory perspective, in *Cocaine: Scientific and Social Dimensions,* Ciba Foundation Symposium Vol. 166, G. R. Bock and J. Whelan, Eds. (Wiley, Chichester, England, 1992).

15. R. E. Nisbett and T. D. Wilson, Telling more than we can know: Verbal reports on mental processes, *Psychological Review,* 84, 231–259 (1977).

16. S. T. Tiffany, A cognitive model of drug urges and drug-use behavior: Role of automatic and non-automatic processes, *Psychological Review,* 97, 147–168 (1990).

IV SOCIAL NEUROSCIENCE OF MOTIVATION, EMOTION, AND ATTITUDES

B. Social Applications

ii. Attitudes and Preferences

37

Negative Information Weighs More Heavily on the Brain: The Negativity Bias in Evaluative Categorizations

Tiffany A. Ito, Jeff T. Larsen, N. Kyle Smith, and John T. Cacioppo

A growing catalog of errors, biases, and asymmetries points to the conclusion that negative information more strongly influences people's evaluations than comparably extreme positive information (Kanouse & Hansen, 1971; Peeters & Czapinski, 1990; Skowronski & Carlston, 1989). Impression formation is one area in which this is especially evident. In an illustrative study, Anderson (1965) found that evaluations of people described by multiple positive traits of differing extremity followed an averaging rule. The evaluation of such a person was similar to the average of the evaluations that had been given to people possessing each of the positive traits in isolation. By contrast, the evaluation of a person described by multiple negative traits of differing extremity was less favorable than expected from an averaging model. This suggests that negative traits are given greater weight in overall evaluations than are positive traits (see also Birnbaum, 1972; Feldman, 1966; Fiske, 1980; Hodges, 1974). A greater weighting for negative information than positive information can also be seen in risk-taking research, where the axiom that losses loom larger than gains often holds. The distress that people report in association with the loss of a given quantity of money typically exceeds the amount of pleasure associated with gain of that same amount (e.g., Kahneman & Tversky, 1984). More generally, Taylor (1991) has noted a tendency for negative events to result in a greater mobilization of an organism's physiological, cognitive, emotional, and social responses.

These disparate instances of greater sensitivity to negative information represent the operation of what has been termed a *negativity bias*. Cacioppo and colleagues have incorporated the negativity bias into a more general model of evaluative space in which positive and negative evaluative processes are assumed to result from the operation of separable positive and negative motivational substrates, respectively (Cacioppo & Berntson, 1994; Cacioppo, Gardner, & Berntson, 1997; Ito & Cacioppo, in press). Positivity and negativity are further posited as having partially separable neurophysiological substrates that have functional outputs best viewed within a multidimensional bivariate space as opposed to a single bipolar continuum.

An important advantage of the model of evaluative space is that it incorporates instances in which positivity and negativity are activated in a reciprocal (i.e., bipolar) manner and instances in which positivity and negativity vary in other combinations. Research by Goldstein and Strube (1994) demonstrated that positive and negative evaluations do not always operate reciprocally by revealing independence in the positive and negative reactions students reported at the beginning and end of three consecutive class periods. Specifically, the intensity of positivity and negativity within each class period was uncorrelated, and the two valent reactions were differentially affected by exam feedback. Cacioppo and colleagues referred to instances in which the positive and negative motivational systems operate independently as uncoupled activation (Cacioppo & Berntson, 1994; Cacioppo et al., 1997).

Multiple modes of evaluative activation were also observed by Ito, Cacioppo, and Lang (1998), who assessed the relation between positive and negative evaluations of nearly 500 color pictures from the International Affective Picture System (IAPS; Center for the Study of Emotion and Attention, 1995). For many of the pictures, positivity and negativity were negatively correlated, suggesting a reciprocal relation between the two motivational systems. However, positivity and negativity were uncorrelated for other pictures, revealing uncoupled activation. Uncoupled activation can occur as singular activation of either the positive or the negative motivational system, both of which were observed by Ito et al.

Finally, the model of evaluative space proposes a nonreciprocal mode of activation in which both valent systems are coactivated or coinhibited, resulting in a positive correlation between positivity and negativity ratings. Racial prejudice is one area in which coactivation has been observed such that White participants sometimes report both strong positive attitudes and strong negative attitudes toward African Americans (Hass, Katz, Rizzo, Bailey, & Eisenstadt, 1991).

Certainly, the model of evaluative space is not the first model to note the separability of positive and negative evaluative processes (for a review, see Cacioppo & Gardner, in press). This notion has a long tradition, for example, within the attitude and judgment literature. Although bipolar measures of attitudes are used widely and attitudes are often conceptualized as the net difference between the positive and negative valent processes aroused by a stimulus, many attitude theorists have nevertheless grappled with the separability of positive and negative evaluations (e.g., Edwards, 1946; Kaplan, 1972; Priester & Petty, 1996; Scott, 1968; Thompson, Zanna, & Griffin, 1995). The bivariate structure of evaluations was noted by Scott (1968) in his review of attitude measurement:

The conception of favorable and unfavorable as "opposites" implies that persons will not be found with attitudes simultaneously at both ends of the dimensions. Yet an alternative formulation might treat degree of favorableness and degree of unfavorableness as conceptually distinct (although no doubt empirically correlated) components, on which persons may make, simultaneously, a variety of position combinations. In other words, it is only by convention that direction of an attitude is conceptualized as a single bipolar continuum. (p. 206)

For our present purposes, the most important implication of conceptualizing positivity and negativity as separable is the ability to stipulate different currency or activation functions for the two systems. Activation functions can be thought of as a means of expressing the value of separate

and multifarious appetitive and aversive inputs on a common scale of positivity and negativity, respectively. In the model of evaluative space (Cacioppo & Berntson, 1994; Cacioppo et al., 1997), the negative motivation system is characterized by a negativity bias. This refers to a tendency for the negative motivational system to respond more intensely than the positive motivational system to comparable amounts of activation. That is, the gradient for the currency function for negativity is steeper than the one for positivity (see also Lewin, 1935; Peeters & Czapinski, 1990).

The steeper gradient for the negative motivational system was evident in the evaluations of IAPS stimuli reported by Ito et al. (1998). To assess the negativity bias, Ito et al. performed a regression analysis, in which mean negativity scores were regressed onto mean arousal ratings used as a proxy for motivational activation, for the 212 slides in the set that participants found more negative than positive. They similarly regressed mean positivity scores onto arousal ratings for the subset of 258 slides that participants found more positive than negative. As predicted, the slope of the regression line for negativity was steeper than the regression line for positivity. Similar results were obtained using bipolar valence scores as the measures of evaluative activation, in which the dataset was dichotomized at the scale median.

To assess the generalizability of this effect across stimulus items, we have replicated this analysis on data for the English Affective Lexicon (Bradley, Lang, & Cuthbert, 1997). This stimulus set currently contains 620 verbs (e.g., *activate*), nouns (e.g., *lion*), adverbs (e.g., *leisurely*), and adjectives (e.g., *quiet*) for which normative ratings of bipolar valence, arousal, and dominance are available. Prior to the analyses, the data were dichotomized at the median of the mean valence ratings. This median split yielded two subsets of words that elicited either predominantly positive or predominantly negative evaluations. Separate regression analyses in which valence ratings were predicted from arousal ratings for the two subsets of words were then performed. As in Ito et al. (1998), arousal ratings were used as a proxy for motivational activation. Consistent with the regression analyses in Ito et al., a negativity bias was found such that the regression line relating arousal to valence among evaluatively negative words was steeper than the line relating arousal to valence among evaluatively positive words.[1]

Although the extant research clearly reveals evidence of the negativity bias (e.g., see Skowronski & Carlston, 1989), much less is known about the stage at which this bias operates. Observable expressions of an evaluation represent the output of at least two stages—evaluative categorization and response output—and the negativity bias could operate at either stage. A negativity bias may be produced through processes occurring at the response-output stage by response priming, for example. This could occur if negative stimuli are more likely to prime or activate a fight-or-flight response, thereby producing more extreme reactions to (including more extreme ratings of) negative stimuli than positive stimuli (Cannon, 1929). Although not denying the possibility of response priming, the model of evaluative space views the negativity bias as an inherent characteristic of the underlying motivational substrate. This led to the prediction that the negativity bias will manifest at the initial evaluative categorization stage of information processing (Cacioppo & Berntson, 1994; Cacioppo et al., 1997). In the present research, we report two experiments designed to test this hypothesis.

This research makes use of event-related brain potentials (ERPs) as measures of the evaluative categorization stage (Cacioppo, Crites, Berntson, & Coles, 1993). ERPs are changes in electrocortical activity that occur in response to discrete stimuli. Time-locked topographical features of the ERP are referred to as *components* and are typically identified by the peaks in and the spatial distributions of the waveforms (for reviews,

see Coles, Gratton, & Fabiani, 1990; Coles, Gratton, Kramer, & Miller, 1986). An ERP component is assumed to reflect one or more information-processing operations, and the amplitude of the component is thought to reflect the extent to which an information-processing operation is engaged (Donchin & Coles, 1988; Gehring, Gratton, Coles, & Donchin, 1992).

The paradigm we use is a modification of the oddball paradigm frequently used to study the P300 component of the ERP. In the standard oddball paradigm, simple stimuli representing two distinct categories (e.g., low- and high-pitched tones) are presented with differing probabilities to participants. On average, the low-probability stimulus (also called the *oddball* or *target stimulus*) evokes a larger positive-going potential, called the *P300*, as compared with the high-probability stimulus. The P300 has a maximal amplitude over central and parietal scalp areas, and manifests from approximately 300 to 900 ms following stimulus onset (Donchin, 1981).

To study evaluative processes, we have presented stimuli that are either positive, negative, or neutral in valence, with stimuli from one evaluative category occurring more frequently than the others (e.g., Cacioppo et al., 1993; Crites, Cacioppo, Gardner, & Berntson, 1995).[2] We refer to the frequently presented stimuli in each sequence as the *context* and those from the less probable categories as *targets*. Evaluative inconsistency between the target and context (e.g., a negative target stimulus embedded within a sequence of positive-context stimuli) results in an enhancement of a late positive potential (LPP) of the ERP, which shares many of the signature characteristics of the P300: (a) The LPP is typically largest over the parietal scalp area, intermediate over the central scalp area, and smallest over the frontal scalp area; (b) larger amplitude LPPs are elicited by the (evaluatively) inconsistent stimuli than by (evaluatively) consistent stimuli, particularly over central-parietal regions; (c) the average latency of the LPP falls within the

300 to 900 ms latency window typical of the P300; and (d) the amplitude of the LPP elicited over the central-parietal region varies as a function of the evaluative distance of the target from the context even when targets are equally probable (Cacioppo, Crites, Gardner, & Berntson, 1994; Crites & Cacioppo, 1996; Crites et al., 1995; Gardner, Cacioppo, Berntson, & Crites, in press). Furthermore, these LPP variations are found when individuals perform evaluative categorizations of the stimuli but not when they perform various nonevaluative categorizations (Cacioppo, Crites, & Gardner, 1996; Crites & Cacioppo, 1996).

As we have noted, we conceptualize evaluative categorization as separate from response selection and execution (or output; Cacioppo & Berntson, 1994; Cacioppo et al., 1993), which raises the issue of whether greater responsivity to negative cues is a function of processes operating at either the evaluative-categorization stage or response selection–execution stage. ERPs provide a means of assessing the evaluative-categorization stage independent of response selection and execution processes. This was demonstrated by Crites et al. (1995), who recorded LPPs to positive, negative, and neutral stimuli embedded within sequences of positive-context stimuli. On some trials participants accurately reported their evaluations, whereas on others they were instructed to misreport their evaluations of either negative or neutral items as being positive. The misreport instructions had the intended effect on overt responses. However, the LPPs to evaluatively inconsistent stimuli, as compared with consistent stimuli, were enhanced, regardless of the accuracy of the overt evaluative report. These results were also replicated in a negative evaluative context in which participants either accurately reported their evaluations or misreported their neutral or positive evaluations (Crites et al., 1995; see also Gardner et al., in press). Therefore, ERPs provide an especially sensitive probe of the evaluative-categorization stage, allowing us to assess whether the underly-

ing negative motivational system responds more intensely than does the positive system to comparable amounts of activation.

To test the hypothesis that the negativity bias operates at the evaluative-categorization stage, we performed two experiments in which ERPs were recorded while participants evaluated positive, negative, and neutral pictorial stimuli. Neutral pictures served as the most frequently presented contextual stimuli. The positive and negative pictures were equated for (a) probability of occurrence, (b) evaluative extremity relative to the neutral pictures, and (c) level of arousal, resulting in a design in which the positive and negative pictures differed primarily in terms of whether they activated the positive or negative motivational system. If the negativity bias operates at the evaluative-categorization stage, it should manifest itself as larger LPPs to evaluatively negative pictures as compared with positive pictures.

Experiment 1

Method

Participants
Thirty-three Ohio State University (OSU) undergraduates (24 men) participated in the experiment for partial class credit. All were right-handed and had right-handed parents. Data from 8 participants were removed because of equipment malfunction ($n = 5$), voluntary withdrawal from the study ($n = 2$), or excessive artifact in the electroencephalograph (EEG) from vertical eye movement ($n = 1$). Analyses were conducted on the data obtained from the remaining 25 participants.

Materials
Thirty-six affectively neutral, two positive, and two negative pictures were selected from Sets 1–8 of the IAPS (Center for the Study of Emotion and Attention—National Institute of Mental Health, 1995). Because neutral pictures were

shown much more frequently than positive or negative pictures, the inclusion of a greater number of neutral pictures ensured that exemplars from all three categories were presented an equal number of times.[3] Using normative data collected from OSU undergraduates in a previous term (Ito et al., 1998), we selected neutral pictures that had (a) bipolar valence ratings near the midpoint (5.0) and median (5.19) of the scale ($M = 5.10$ on a 1–9 scale; range = 4.21–6.15); (b) low levels of positive activation as measured by a unipolar positivity scale ($M = 2.10$ on a 5-point scale, where lower values indicate less positivity); (c) low levels of negative activation as measured by a unipolar negativity scale ($M = 1.48$ on a 5-point scale, where lower values indicate less negativity); and (d) low levels of arousal ($M = 2.75$, as measured on a 9-point bipolar scale where lower values indicate greater calmness). The 36 neutral pictures were divided into two equal-sized groups with comparable normative ratings: (a) bipolar valence $M = 5.10, 5.10$; (b) unipolar positivity $M = 2.12, 2.08$; (c) unipolar negativity $M = 1.49, 1.47$; and (d) arousal $M = 2.74, 2.75$. Examples of neutral pictures include a plate, hair dryer, and an electrical outlet.

The two positive and two negative pictures were selected to have high valence and arousal ratings that were equally extreme from the mean values for the neutral pictures. The positive pictures, which depicted a red Ferrari and people enjoying a roller coaster, had the following normative ratings: (a) bipolar valence $M = 8.31$, (b) unipolar positivity $M = 4.19$, (c) unipolar negativity $M = 1.23$, and (d) arousal $M = 7.43$. The negative pictures, which depicted a mutilated face and a handgun aimed at the camera, had the following normative ratings: (a) bipolar valence $M = 1.89$, (b) unipolar positivity $M = 1.16$, (c) unipolar negativity $M = 4.07$, and (d) arousal $M = 7.34$.[4]

Procedure

Potential participants were informed that the purpose of the study was to measure electrical activity occurring in the brain when people view pictures. Once they arrived for the experimental session, they received a brief overview of the procedures, then read and signed an informed consent form. Participants then had the electrodes attached and received more detailed task instructions.

Participants were seated in a comfortable reclining chair in a sound-attenuated, electrically shielded room. Following procedures used in prior research on evaluative categorization (Gardner et al., in press), pictures were shown to participants in sequences of five on a color computer monitor located approximately 76 cm in front of the chair.

LPPs are affected by surrounding contextual stimuli as well as by the stimuli currently being processed. As a result, LPPs observed in prior research (in which targets were embedded in positive or negative stimulus sequences) may have varied with the valence of the context stimuli as well as the target stimulus. To examine the negativity bias in the present experiment, we therefore established a neutral evaluative context and recorded ERP responses to pictures that were either evaluatively consistent (i.e., neutral) or inconsistent (i.e., positive or negative) with that context. To accomplish this, all participants were exposed to 120 sequences of five pictures. These sequences were divided into two 60-sequence blocks. Both blocks contained primarily neutral pictures but differed in whether positive or negative pictures were also embedded in some of the sequences (see Table 37.1). Specifically, in half of the sequences in each block, a single positive or negative target (depending on the block) was embedded in the neutral context. In the remaining sequences in each block, all pictures within the sequences were neutral, and one of these neutral pictures was designated as the target picture. In all sequence types, targets randomly appeared in either the third, fourth, or fifth position in a sequence, thereby ensuring that targets were always preceded by at least two neutral pictures and that participants could not easily

Table 37.1

Types of five-picture sequences used in experiment 1

	Stimulus position				
Sequence type	1	2	3	4	5
Block with positive targets					
1. Neutral in neutral	ϕ	ϕ	**ϕ**	ϕ	ϕ
2. Neutral in neutral	ϕ	ϕ	ϕ	**ϕ**	ϕ
3. Neutral in neutral	ϕ	ϕ	ϕ	ϕ	**ϕ**
4. Positive in neutral	ϕ	ϕ	**P**	ϕ	ϕ
5. Positive in neutral	ϕ	ϕ	ϕ	**P**	ϕ
6. Positive in neutral	ϕ	ϕ	ϕ	ϕ	**P**
Block with negative targets					
7. Neutral in neutral	ϕ	ϕ	**ϕ**	ϕ	ϕ
8. Neutral in neutral	ϕ	ϕ	ϕ	**ϕ**	ϕ
9. Neutral in neutral	ϕ	ϕ	ϕ	ϕ	**ϕ**
10. Negative in neutral	ϕ	ϕ	**N**	ϕ	ϕ
11. Negative in neutral	ϕ	ϕ	ϕ	**N**	ϕ
12. Negative in neutral	ϕ	ϕ	ϕ	ϕ	**N**

Note. Within each sequence type, psychophysiological data were recorded to an evaluatively consistent or inconsistent target located in either the third, fourth, or fifth stimulus position; these stimuli are designated by boldface characters. ϕ = a stimulus position in which neutral targets were presented; P = a stimulus position in which positive targets were presented; N = a stimulus position in which negative targets were presented.

predict when a positive or negative picture might appear. This resulted in 12 trial types (see Table 37.1). Types 1–6 were shown to each participant an equal number of times within one of the blocks, and Types 7–12 were shown an equal number of times within the other block. Order of the trial types was randomized within each block for each participant. Participants were not informed of the distinction between context and target pictures and evaluated all pictures in a similar fashion. Psychophysiological data were recorded during the presentation of the single target picture in each sequence.

Half of the participants saw the block with embedded positive targets first, and the remaining participants saw the block with embedded negative targets first. Moreover, a different set of 18 neutral pictures was presented in each block. This was intended to prevent attenuation of LPP amplitude to the neutral pictures in the second block because of repeated presentations of specific neutral pictures. Prior to viewing the second block, participants took a short (<5 min) break and read a brief history of OSU. The passage was intended to induce a neutral mood and mitigate potential carryover effects.

Each picture in a sequence was presented for 1,000 ms. Participants were instructed to look at the picture for its entire presentation and to think about whether it showed something they found to be positive (or negative, depending on the block) or neutral. After stimulus offset, participants registered their evaluation by pressing one of two labeled keys on a computer keypad. Either the left (or right, counterbalanced) key indicated *neutral*. The other key indicated *positive* or *negative*, depending on which block was being presented. Participants used the left and right thumbs to press the left and right keys, respectively. After a 1,000 ms interstimulus interval, the next picture was shown. We stressed to participants that there were no right or wrong answers in evaluating the pictures and that we were interested in their first impressions. After the fifth picture in a sequence, the word *pause* was shown on the screen. Participants were instructed to use either thumb to press a third button on the keypad when they were ready to initiate the next sequence of five pictures.

To summarize, data were recorded from both target (positive and negative) and context (neutral) pictures. The design, therefore, featured two within-subject variables: picture category (valenced or context) and target valence (positive or negative). There were also three between-subject variables, representing the hand used to register a neutral evaluation (left or right), block order (positive or negative block first), and set of neutral pictures shown in the first block (Subset

A or B). An additional within-subject factor, sagittal scalp site, is described below.

Psychophysiological Data Collection and Reduction

EEG data were recorded at sites over midline frontal (Fz), central (Cz), and parietal (Pz) scalp areas using tin electrodes sewn into an elastic cap (Electro-Cap International, Eaton, OH).[5] An additional site at the top of the forehead served as an electrical ground. Miniature tin electrodes were also placed over the left and right mastoids. Active scalp sites were referenced on-line to the left mastoid. Additional miniature tin electrodes were placed above and below the left eye and on the outer canthus of each eye to monitor vertical and horizontal eye movements, respectively. Electrode impedances were below 5 KΩ at all sites. EEG and electrooculogram (EOG) recordings were amplified by NeuroScan Synamps amplifiers with a bandpass of 0.1–30 Hz (12-dB roll-off) and digitized at 1,000 Hz. For all targets, EEG and EOG data recording began 128 ms before picture onset and continued throughout the 1,000 ms picture presentation.

Off-line, the data were rereferenced to a computed average of the left and right mastoids.[6] EEG data were next corrected to the mean voltage of the 128-ms prestimulus recording period before applying a regression procedure to remove the effects of vertical eye movements from the EEG, which can distort measurements from scalp sites (Semlitsch, Anderer, Schuster, & Presslich, 1986). The regression correction was applied to 14 of the participants' data. The remaining 11 participants did not blink enough during the EEG recording period for the regression procedure to reliably estimate eye activity from the vertical EOG channel. For these participants, we visually inspected the EEG data and deleted any trials on which ocular or other artifact occurred (e.g., because of movement). We similarly inspected the EEG data from those participants for whom the regression procedure was applied for remaining ocular or other arti-

fact. For all participants, if artifact was detected at any of the three scalp sites, data from all sites for that trial were eliminated from further analysis. A 9-Hz low-pass digital filter was then applied to the remaining data.

We next constructed ensemble averages to extract the LPP component from the EEG signal (Coles et al., 1990). For each participant's data, we computed four averaged waveforms. These waveforms aggregated the electrical activity associated with the evaluation of positive targets, neutral targets in the positive block, negative targets, and neutral targets in the negative block. We calculated separate ensemble-averaged ERP waveforms for each scalp site for each participant. The amplitude of the LPP of the ERP was quantified by locating within each ERP waveform the largest positive-going potential at Pz between 400–900 ms after stimulus onset. The amplitude of the LPP in the other two sites was defined as the largest positive-going potential occurring within ±100 ms of the LPP at Pz.

Results

We first examined whether we replicated prior research on evaluative categorizations showing that the LPP amplitude has a central-parietal scalp distribution and varies as a function of evaluative inconsistency. To do this, we subjected the LPP amplitudes to a 2 (picture category: context, valenced) × 2 (target valence: positive, negative) × 3 (sagittal scalp site: frontal, central, parietal) × 2 (hand for *neutral* response) × 2 (block order: positive first, negative first) × 2 (set of neutral pictures paired with positive targets: Subset A, Subset B) multivariate analysis of variance (MANOVA). All F tests reported represent the Wilks's lambda approximation. Our results confirmed both prior effects. First, we obtained a main effect of sagittal scalp site, $F(2, 16) = 22.15$, $p < .0001$. Two sets of planned contrasts were conducted to test specifically for the central-parietal scalp distribution. The first contrast compared the mean of the LPP amplitudes at Cz and Pz with the mean at Fz, revealing significantly larger LPPs at the combined Cz–Pz areas (combined Cz–Pz $M = 7.42\ \mu V$) than at Fz ($M = 3.28\ \mu V$), $F(1, 17) = 34.46$, $p < .0001$. The second planned contrast compared LPP amplitudes at Pz and Cz, revealing larger LPPs at Pz ($M = 8.49\ \mu V$) than at Cz ($M = 6.35\ \mu V$), $F(1, 17) = 9.84$, $p < .01$. Second, the MANOVA revealed main effects of picture category, $F(1, 17) = 59.98$, $p < .0001$, and target valence, $F(1, 17) = 8.79$, $p < .01$, which were qualified by a significant Picture Category × Target valence interaction, $F(1, 17) = 19.45$, $p < .01$. Both positive and negative targets ($M_{positive} = 7.43\ \mu V$, $M_{negative} = 10.90\ \mu V$) were associated with larger LPPs than their corresponding context pictures ($M = 2.95\ \mu V$ and $M = 2.89\ \mu V$, respectively), $F(1, 17) = 27.08$, $p < .001$, and $F(1, 17) = 52.66$, $p < .001$, respectively. Across both blocks, then, LPPs were larger for evaluatively inconsistent pictures than consistent pictures.

It is important to note that this interaction also revealed the predicted negativity bias at the evaluative categorization stage. Negative targets resulted in larger LPPs than positive targets, $F(1, 24) = 15.51$, $p < .001$, whereas LPP amplitudes to neutral pictures in the two blocks did not differ (see Figure 37.1). Thus, the evaluative categorization of negative stimuli was associated with a larger amplitude LPP than was the evaluative categorization of equally probable, equally evaluatively extreme, and equally arousing positive stimuli.

A Picture Category × Sagittal Scalp Site interaction was also obtained, $F(2, 16) = 16.38$, $p < .0001$. For the target pictures, follow-up comparisons revealed larger amplitude LPPs at the central-parietal area (combined Cz–Pz $M = 10.78\ \mu V$) as compared to Fz ($M = 4.55\ \mu V$), $F(1, 24) = 74.30$, $p < .0001$. LPPs at Pz ($M = 12.54\ \mu V$) were also significantly larger than those at Cz ($M = 9.01\ \mu V$) for the target pictures, $F(1, 24) = 23.92$, $p < .0001$. For the neutral pictures, follow-up comparisons revealed

larger amplitude LPPs at the central-parietal area (combined Cz–Pz $M = 3.55\ \mu V$) as compared to Fz ($M = 1.48\ \mu V$), $F(1, 24) = 9.89$, $p < .005$; LPP amplitudes at Pz and Cz did not differ for the context pictures.

More interesting from a theoretical perspective, we obtained a Picture Category × Target Valence × Sagittal Scalp Site interaction, $F(2, 16) = 6.73$, $p < .01$. The mean amplitudes as a function of picture category, target valence, and sagittal scalp site are shown in Table 37.2, and the stimulus-aligned averaged waveforms at Pz are shown in Figure 37.1. LPP amplitudes were larger to negative than positive targets at Pz, Cz, and Fz, all $ps < .05$. The interaction was attributable to a greater sensitivity to evaluative inconsistency at central and parietal areas. When participants were viewing negative target pictures, the target pictures resulted in larger LPP amplitudes than the neutral pictures did at all sites, all $ps < .01$. When participants were viewing positive target pictures, the target pictures resulted in larger LPP amplitudes than neutral pictures did at Pz and Cz, $ps < .005$, a difference that was not significant at Fz, $p < .06$.[7]

Discussion

The results of Experiment 1 reveal three important findings. First, the present results replicate prior research results, revealing both the scalp distribution of the LPP and the LPP's sensitivity to evaluative inconsistency (e.g., Cacioppo et al., 1993; Cacioppo et al., 1994; Crites & Cacioppo, 1996; Crites et al., 1995). Specifically, the LPP was largest over central-parietal regions, and its amplitude was enhanced for the evaluatively inconsistent positive and negative pictures as compared with the neutral-context pictures. Moreover, the LPP was maximally sensitive to evaluative inconsistency effects at Pz and Cz.

Second, the sensitivity of the LPP to evaluative inconsistency in the present experiment builds upon prior research by using an evaluatively neutral context. In prior research, LPP

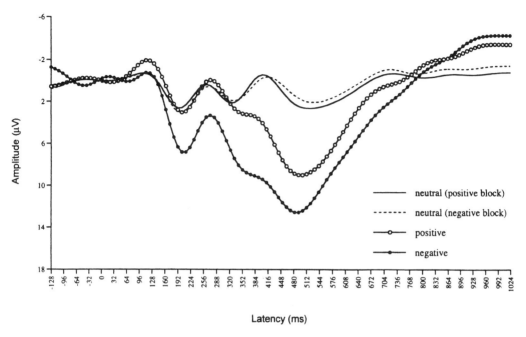

Figure 37.1

Averaged event-related brain potential waveforms at the midline parietal electrode (Pz) to neutral and positive targets in the block of trials containing neutral (frequent) and positive (rare) targets and to neutral and negative targets in the block of trials containing neutral (frequent) and negative (rare) targets. The amplitude of the late positive potential is not only larger to the rare (positive and negative) targets than the frequent (neutral) targets, but it is larger to the negative targets than the positive targets. These results were obtained even though the positive and negative targets were equally extreme, arousing, rare, and task relevant. These results, therefore, are consistent with the operation of a negativity bias at the evaluative categorization stage of information processing.

enhancement to evaluative inconsistency was obtained across a range of evaluative context–target combinations, including positive contexts with negative targets (Cacioppo et al., 1993; Cacioppo et al., 1994; Crites et al., 1995; Crites & Cacioppo, 1996) and neutral targets (Crites et al., 1995), as well as negative contexts with positive targets (Cacioppo et al., 1993; Crites et al., 1995) and neutral targets (Crites et al., 1995). Note that the context in these prior studies was always either positive or negative. The present research demonstrates that LPP enhancement to evaluative inconsistency also occurs with positive

and negative targets in a neutral context. As predicted, LPPs for the positive and negative targets were larger than LPPs for the neutral context. When added to the cumulative research, the present results demonstrate that the effects of evaluative inconsistency are not dependent on the valences of the contextual stimuli.

More important, larger LPPs were obtained in response to negative target pictures as compared with positive target pictures, suggesting the operation of a negativity bias as early as the eval-uative-categorization stage. This occurred even though the positive and negative pictures were

Table 37.2
Mean LPP amplitude (and SEM) as a function of picture category, target valence, and sagittal scalp site in experiment 1

Site	Target									
	Negative		Positive		Neutral (negative block)		Neutral (positive block)			
	M	*SEM*	*M*	*SEM*	*M*	*SEM*	*M*	*SEM*	*M*	*SEM*
Pz	14.99	1.22	10.87	1.04	3.67	0.59	4.44	0.82	8.49	0.72
Cz	11.51	1.20	7.38	1.03	3.26	0.64	3.26	0.87	6.35	0.68
Fz	6.20	1.16	4.04	1.07	1.57	0.78	1.14	0.93	3.28	0.77
M	10.90	1.09	7.43	0.87	2.89	0.43	2.95	0.73		

Note. All values are in µV. LPP = late positive potential; Pz = midline parietal electrode; Cz = midline central electrode; Fz = midline frontal electrode.

equally improbable in the stimulus sequences and equally discrepant from the neutral pictures in terms of mean valence and arousal ratings. The stimuli in Experiment 1 were chosen based on the normative responses from a separate sample of OSU undergraduates. Examination of the behavioral responses in Experiment 1 indicated that 10 of the 25 participants consistently categorized at least one of the four normatively valenced targets as neutral. Therefore, we conducted two ancillary analyses to determine whether the ERP evidence for evaluative inconsistency or negativity bias effects could reflect the operation of a possible confounding variable. Neither analysis provided any evidence for this possibility. First, analyses of the 15 participants whose behavioral responses matched the normative classifications revealed the same evaluative inconsistency and negativity bias effects as were obtained in the full sample. Second, among those participants who tended to misclassify one of the positive or negative targets, the LPP amplitude for the misclassified target did not differ from the amplitude for the target of the same valence that was correctly classified. For instance, the amplitude of the misclassified positive target did not differ from the correctly classified positive target. Further, LPP amplitude for the misclassified

positive or negative target was uncorrelated with LPP amplitude for the neutral pictures from the relevant block. At the electrocortical level, then, evidence shows that positive and negative targets were perceived as evaluatively inconsistent from the neutral context, even when the participants pressed the *neutral* rather than normatively consistent *positive* or *negative* button on the keypad.

Experiment 2

Although the ancillary analyses suggest that the results of Experiment 1 were not qualified by normatively inconsistent classifications, we were nevertheless concerned about the occurrence of these responses. The normative data on which stimulus selection was based were collected in sessions in which roughly equal numbers of positive, negative, and neutral pictures were shown (Ito et al., 1998). The judgments of pictures in Experiment 1, in contrast, were made in a context of primarily neutral pictures. The numerous presentations of neutral pictures may have affected participants' subjective evaluative criterion by expanding the range of neutral classifications. In essence, this would have produced an assimilation of valent stimuli to the neutral category.

To counter this possibility, we replicated Experiment 1 but preceded the experimental trials with a picture preview period in which positive, negative, and neutral pictures were shown to participants. We reasoned that participants would be less likely to expand their subjective range of neutral stimuli if they had recently been exposed to anchors of relatively extreme positivity and negativity.

In addition, we intermixed positive and negative targets in a single block in Experiment 2 to increase external validity. Whereas the valence of the target differed by blocks in Experiment 1, people more typically encounter positive and negative events in close proximity in everyday settings. A situation in which the activation and deactivation of the positive and negative motivational systems occur in a random sequence may therefore more closely mimic the evaluative situations typically faced in everyday life. Moreover, whereas participants in Experiment 1 were presented with only two response options (i.e., positive and neutral in the positive target block and negative and neutral in the negative target block), participants in Experiment 2 were presented with all three options for every picture. When people naturally evaluate objects in their environment, it is more likely that they choose from the full range of evaluative responses, which includes positivity, negativity, and neutrality. Thus, the presence of all three options may also more closely correspond to people's everyday evaluative experiences than did the situation in Experiment 1. Finally, to increase the generalizability of the effects obtained in Experiment 1, we used different positive and negative pictures in Experiment 2.

Method

Participants

Twenty-one OSU undergraduates (11 men) participated in the experiment for partial class credit. Data from 7 participants were unusable because of equipment failure ($n = 1$) or excessive artifact

($n = 6$). Analyses were conducted on the data obtained from the remaining 14 participants.

Materials

Twenty-six affectively neutral, two positive, and two negative pictures were used in the experiment. Eighteen of the neutral pictures and all of the positive and negative pictures were selected from Sets 1–8 of the IAPS using normative data from Ito et al. (1998). Some of the neutral pictures (but none of the positive or negative pictures) used in Experiment 1 were also used in Experiment 2.[8]

The 18 neutral IAPS pictures had the following characteristics: (a) bipolar valence ratings near the midpoint of the scale ($M = 5.00$), (b) bipolar valence ratings not greater than 1 scale point away from the midpoint (range = 4.60–5.40), (c) low levels of positive activation as measured by unipolar positivity scale ($M = 1.91$), (d) low levels of negative activation as measured by unipolar negativity scale ($M = 1.47$), and (e) low levels of arousal ($M = 2.64$). The two positive and two negative pictures were selected to have high and equally extreme affect and arousal ratings. The positive pictures, which showed a pizza and a bowl of chocolate ice cream, had the following normative ratings: (a) bipolar valence = 7.81, (b) unipolar positivity = 3.65, (c) unipolar negativity = 1.42, and (d) arousal = 6.17. The negative pictures, which showed a dead cat and a dead and decomposing cow, had the following normative ratings: (a) bipolar valence = 2.10, (b) unipolar positivity = 1.09, (c) unipolar negativity = 4.08, and (d) arousal = 6.22. Eighteen pictures in the IAPS met our criteria for neutral pictures. To ensure equal rates of presentation of each individual picture, we included eight additional neutral pictures from the PC Paintbrush Photo-Library CD (1994).[9]

Procedure

Experiment 2 followed the same procedure as Experiment 1, with the following exceptions. First, participants were exposed to 90 sequences

Table 37.3
Types of five-picture sequences used in experiment 2

	Stimulus position				
Sequence type	1	2	3	4	5
1. Neutral in neutral	φ	φ	**φ**	φ	φ
2. Neutral in neutral	φ	φ	φ	**φ**	φ
3. Neutral in neutral	φ	φ	φ	φ	**φ**
4. Positive in neutral	φ	φ	**P**	φ	φ
5. Positive in neutral	φ	φ	φ	**P**	φ
6. Positive in neutral	φ	φ	φ	φ	**P**
7. Negative in neutral	φ	φ	**N**	φ	φ
8. Negative in neutral	φ	φ	φ	**N**	φ
9. Negative in neutral	φ	φ	φ	φ	**N**

Note. Within each sequence type, psychophysiological data were recorded to an evaluatively consistent or inconsistent target located in either the third, fourth, or fifth stimulus position; these stimuli are designated by boldface characters. φ = a stimulus position in which neutral targets were presented; P = a stimulus position in which positive targets were presented; N = a stimulus position in which negative targets were presented.

of five stimuli, and each of the 9 possible sequences in Table 37.3 was shown 10 times in a different random order for each participant. Second, just prior to the presentation of experimental trials, participants were preexposed to 30 positive, 30 negative, and 30 neutral pictures. To provide anchors of extreme positivity and negativity, all participants viewed the neutral preview pictures last. Half of the participants were randomly assigned to view the positive pictures first, and the remaining participants viewed the negative pictures first. Six pictures were shown at a time on the screen, and participants paced themselves through the preview screens. The 26 neutral, 2 positive, and 2 negative pictures selected for use in the experiment were among those shown during the preview period. These were augmented with 4 additional neutral pictures from the PC Paintbrush PhotoLibrary CD (1994), 28 positive pictures from the IAPS, and

28 negative pictures from the IAPS. Participants were told that the pictures were shown so they could preview some of the pictures they would see in the experiment.

As in Experiment 1, participants were instructed to make evaluative categorizations of what was depicted in the pictures. Unlike Experiment 1, participants were exposed to positive, neutral, and negative stimuli across the 90 sequences. Therefore, participants were instructed to determine whether each picture showed something they found positive, negative, or neutral. They indicated their evaluation by pressing one of three appropriately labeled keys on a computer keypad once the picture was removed from the screen. The middle key was always labeled *neutral*. For half of the participants, keys labeled *positive* and *negative* were located to the right and left, respectively. The order of these keys was reversed for the remaining participants. The right thumb was used to respond to the rightmost key and the left thumb for the leftmost key. Either thumb could be used for the middle key. The screen remained blank for 1,200 ms after participants responded, then the next picture appeared. Participants pushed a fourth key to initiate the next picture sequence following the word *pause*.

Psychophysiological Data Collection and Reduction
Experiment 2 used the same data-collection and reduction procedures as Experiment 1. We computed separately for each participant an ensemble-averaged ERP for positive targets, negative targets, and neutral targets. This was done separately at all sites, producing nine separate ERP waveforms for each participant. LPP amplitude was quantified in the same manner as in Experiment 1.

Results

As in Experiment 1, we tested for the expected scalp distribution and the effects of evaluative

Table 37.4
Mean LPP amplitude (and SEM) as a function of target variance and sagittal scalp site in experiment 2

Site	Target Negative		Positive		Neutral			
	M	*SEM*	*M*	*SEM*	*M*	*SEM*	*M*	*SEM*
Pz	17.01	0.85	13.01	1.34	5.20	0.62	11.95	0.65
Cz	9.03	0.91	8.73	1.13	2.29	0.91	6.68	0.68
Fz	3.14	0.90	4.44	1.08	1.01	1.45	2.87	0.93
M	9.73	0.65	8.94	0.98	2.83	0.88		

Note. All values are in µV. LPP = late positive potential; Pz = midline parietal electrode; Cz = midline central electrode; Fz = midline frontal electrode.

inconsistency before testing for the posited negativity bias. All F tests reported represent the Wilks's lambda approximation. A 3 (target valence: neutral, positive, negative) × 3 (sagittal scalp location: frontal, central, parietal) × 2 (hand for *positive* response: left, right) × 2 (valence of first preview pictures: positive, negative) MANOVA revealed the expected main effect of sagittal scalp site, $F(2, 9) = 37.47$, $p < .0001$. As in Experiment 1, we performed two planned contrasts, the first of which compared the mean of the LPP amplitudes at Cz and Pz to those at Fz, and the second of which compared LPP amplitudes at Pz to those at Cz. As in prior research and in Experiment 1, LPPs were larger at the combined central-parietal area (combined Cz–Pz $M = 9.53$ µV) than at Fz ($M = 2.87$ µV), $F(1, 10) = 40.64$, $p < .0001$, and LPP amplitudes at Pz ($M = 11.95$ µV) were larger than those at Cz ($M = 6.68$ µV), $F(1, 10) = 83.13$, $p < .0001$. Thus, the scalp distribution of the LPP conformed to the expected central-parietal maximum.

In addition, the main effect of target valence confirmed that the LPP was sensitive to evaluative inconsistency, $F(2, 9) = 20.94$, $p < .0001$. A planned contrast revealed that across all sites, LPPs were larger for the evaluatively inconsistent positive and negative pictures (combined positive–negative $M = 9.45$ µV) than

for the neutral-context pictures ($M = 2.83$ µV), $F(1, 10) = 45.95$, $p < .0001$. We also obtained a significant Target Valence × Sagittal Scalp Site interaction, $F(4, 7) = 15.86$, $p < .001$. Follow-up contrasts revealed evaluative inconsistency effects at each scalp site: LPPs for the evaluatively inconsistent positive and negative pictures exceeded those for neutral pictures at Pz, $F(1, 13) = 74.40$, $p < .0001$, Cz, $F(1, 13) = 26.60$, $p < .0001$, and Fz, $F(1, 13) = 5.10$, $p < .05$.

The Target Valence × Sagittal Scalp Site interaction also revealed evidence of the operation of the posited negativity bias at the evaluative-categorization stage of information processing. The mean LPP amplitudes as a function of target valence and sagittal scalp site are shown in Table 37.4, and the stimulus-aligned averaged waveforms for each valence at Pz are shown in Figure 37.2. Follow-up contrasts comparing LPP amplitude for negative pictures to LPP amplitude for positive pictures at all sites revealed the negativity bias at Pz, where LPP amplitude was larger for negative targets ($M = 17.01$ µV) than for positive targets ($M = 13.01$ µV), $F(1, 13) = 5.29$, $p < .05$.[10]

Discussion

In Experiment 1, we noted unexpectedly high rates of normatively inconsistent categoriza-

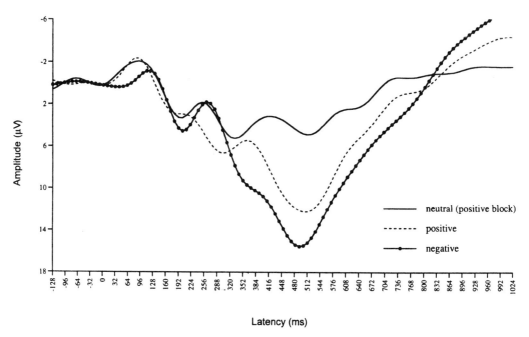

Figure 37.2

Averaged event-related brain potential waveforms at the midline parietal electrode (Pz) to neutral (frequent), positive (rare), and negative (rare) targets. The amplitude of the late positive potential is not only larger to the rare
(positive and negative) targets than the frequent (neutral) targets, but it is larger to the negative targets than the
positive targets. These results were obtained even though the positive and negative targets were equally extreme,
arousing, rare, and task relevant. These results, therefore, are consistent with the operation of a negativity bias at
the evaluative-categorization stage of information processing.

tions of the valenced targets. Although ancillary
analyses discounted the possibility that non-
normative responses produced the evaluative
inconsistency and negativity bias effects in Experiment 1, we nevertheless hoped to decrease
the rate of normatively inconsistent responses
in Experiment 2. Examination of the behavioral
responses from participants in Experiment 2
suggests we were successful in doing so in that
only three of the participants in Experiment 2
displayed normatively inconsistent classifications
of valent stimuli.[11]

Several design changes in Experiment 2 may
have increased participants' agreement with the

normative classifications. First, we introduced the
picture preview period in which positive, negative, and neutral pictures were shown to participants before the experimental trials. Presenting
such a large number of neutral pictures may
have assimilated valent stimuli into the neutral
category in Experiment 1. To counteract this in
Experiment 2, we provided participants with relatively extreme anchors of positivity and negativity before the experimental trials by presenting
the positive and negative preview pictures before
the neutral ones. Experiment 2 also used different exemplars of positive and negative stimuli
and had a partially nonoverlapping set of neutral

stimuli, raising the possibility that the particular exemplars chosen in Experiment 1 resulted in fewer consensual classifications than the exemplars in Experiment 2 did. This seems unlikely, however, because the variability in the normative ratings of stimuli in Experiments 1 and 2 was comparable. Another difference between the two experiments was the presence of two (Experiment 1) as opposed to three (Experiment 2) response options. If anything, the presence of an additional response option would increase response variability, leading one to expect more normatively inconsistent classifications in Experiment 2.

Although changes in the specific exemplars used and in the number of response options presented to participants were unlikely to have affected the rate of normatively inconsistent classifications, those design changes were implemented to increase the external validity of Experiment 2. In real-world evaluative situations, evaluatively positive and negative events and objects are often encountered in close proximity, and when we evaluate such events and objects, we most likely think in terms of both positivity and negativity as well as neutrality, as opposed to choosing between positivity or negativity and neutrality, as was the task in Experiment 1. Despite these methodological variations, the results of Experiment 2 replicate those of Experiment 1 in revealing a negative bias as early as the evaluative-categorization stage.

General Discussion

Experiments 1 and 2 replicate prior research showing that evaluatively inconsistent stimuli are associated with larger amplitude late positive brain potentials than evaluatively consistent stimuli (Cacioppo et al., 1993, 1994, 1996; Crites & Cacioppo, 1996; Crites et al., 1995; Gardner et al., in press). Furthermore, and as in prior research, variations in evaluative categorizations were more apparent over parietal regions

(Cacioppo et al., 1993; see, also, Coles et al., 1990). The present research is also the first to demonstrate the LPP's sensitivity to evaluative inconsistencies within a neutral context. Prior research has used either positive or negative contexts. Because the LPP is sensitive to both the valence of the target and of the contextual stimuli in which it is embedded, the neutral context of the present experiments provides a clearer depiction of positive and negative categorization processes per se. The results of both experiments showed clearly that the evaluative categorization of negative stimuli was associated with a larger amplitude LPP than was the evaluative categorization of equally probable, equally evaluatively extreme, and equally arousing positive stimuli.

Locating the Negativity Bias

Cacioppo et al. (1997) describe the negativity bias as the tendency for a unit of activation to result in a greater change in output in the negative motivational system as compared with the positive motivational system. As a consequence of the negativity bias, attitudinal and behavioral expressions should be more strongly influenced by negative input than positive input (Cacioppo & Berntson, 1994). Ample evidence demonstrates greater responsivity to negative stimuli than positive stimuli, as reviewed in the introduction. What is not clear from prior research is the stage at which the negativity bias operates. As we noted, Cannon's (1929) notion that threatening stimuli are more likely to elicit general and diffuse sympathetic activation as part of an adaptive fight-or-flight response emphasizes the relative impact of negative information on action tendencies. Such an analysis may suggest that the negativity bias is introduced at the response output stage through some form of response priming. The model of evaluative space, although not denying the possibility of response priming, treats the negativity bias as an inherent characteristic of the negative motivational system in the central nervous system (Cacioppo et al.,

1997; Cacioppo & Berntson, 1994), leading to the prediction that the negativity bias operates automatically at the evaluative-categorization stage.

Assuming that the negativity bias operates at the evaluative-categorization stage, one question that can be asked is whether the negativity bias will always operate at this stage. Although greater responsivity to comparable activation is viewed in the model of evaluative space as an inherent characteristic of the negative motivation system, the negativity bias does not imply that the intensity of observed or reported negative evaluations will always exceed positive evaluations because of the associated axiom of a positivity offset (Cacioppo & Berntson, 1994; Cacioppo et al., 1997). The positivity offset refers to a tendency toward greater output from the positive motivational system than negative motivational system when motivational activation is low.

Operation of the positivity offset was seen in the activation functions reported by Ito et al. (1998). As we noted in the introduction, regression analyses relating ratings of positivity and negativity to ratings of arousal (used as a proxy for motivational activation) revealed a steeper slope for the activation function of negativity. In addition to demonstrating the negativity bias, these analyses also revealed a positivity offset in the form of a higher intercept value for the regression line of positivity than for negativity (see Ito et al., 1998, Figure 9).[12] That is, when motivational activation is low, the motivation to approach exceeds the motivation to withdraw. The positivity offset is likely responsible for a wide range of effects, such as the tendency to rate new acquaintances more positively than negatively, even when little is known about them (e.g., Kaplan, 1972; Gardner, 1996).

The steeper slope for the activation function of negativity suggests that the negative motivational system is structured to respond more intensely than the positive motivational system to comparable levels of motivational activation, but

whether these differences in responsivity manifest themselves as more extreme negative evaluations depends on how much motivational activation is present. At the lowest levels, the higher intercept value for positivity results in more extreme positive evaluations than negative evaluations. As motivational activation increases, the steeper slope for the activation function of negativity leads the two activation functions to cross. After this intersection, output from the negative motivational system is greater than output from the positive motivational system (given equal motivational input to both systems), resulting in more extreme negative evaluations than positive evaluations. In sum, the underlying motivational system for negativity is predicted to always respond more intensely per unit of activation than the positive motivational system, but whether these differences manifest themselves as more extreme negative evaluations than positive evaluations will depend on the activation levels of each and whether relatively weak or strong input is present. In the present experiments, relatively intense positive and negative stimuli were used, leading us to predict LPP amplitude differences as a function of picture valence.

Another relevant question is why the negativity bias operates as early as the evaluative-categorization stage. If the negativity bias operated only at response stages, it would be difficult to redirect attention immediately, seamlessly, and effortlessly to potentially threatening events. Indeed, the adaptive advantage that the negativity bias confers to affective processing led us to suggest its operation at the earliest stages of evaluative processing (Cacioppo & Berntson, 1994; Cacioppo et al., 1997; see also Peeters & Czapinski, 1990). The notion that the negativity bias reflects a rapid, automatic feature of evaluative (i.e., affective) processing is further suggested by the correspondence between the experimental conditions and the conditions required for what Bargh (1989) has referred to as an *unintended, goal-dependent automaticity*. As Bargh notes, all automaticities are to some extent conditional, in that they depend on the occurrence of some minimal set of circumstances. In the case of an unintended goal-dependent automaticity, the individual must be aware of the instigating stimulus and have a specific processing goal in mind, but intention for the effect to occur and conscious guidance of the process to completion are not required. The operationalizations in the present experiments appear to have met the conditions for unintended goal-dependent automaticity. The experimental stimuli were presented above sensory thresholds, and participants were given the processing goal of performing evaluative categorizations. At the same time, no mention of the negativity bias was made prior to the experimental trials, and there is no reason to expect that participants intended to display a negativity bias or that they consciously guided the negative and positive motivational systems to respond in ways that produced the observed differences in LPP amplitudes.

We do not assume that evaluative categorizations in general or the operation of the negativity bias in particular are necessarily goal-dependent, however. To the contrary, numerous studies have shown that the activation of evaluations stored in memory is a relatively unconditional phenomenon that can be triggered by the mere presence of an attitude object in the environment (Bargh, Chaiken, Govender, & Pratto, 1992; Fazio, Sanbonmatsu, Powell, & Kardes, 1986). Similarly, evidence consistent with the negativity bias has been obtained in paradigms in which an explicit evaluative task was not given (Pratto & John, 1991). This specific ability to operate automatically may increase the adaptive utility of the negativity bias by allowing organisms to avoid harm even when they are not explicitly sensitized to do so.

Implications of Other Models

As we have noted, the present results suggest that the negativity bias operates as an automatic feature of the underlying negative motivational system. Alternatively, the negativity bias has been explained in terms of differential diagnosticity for negative information as compared with positive information within the impression-formation domain (Reeder & Brewer, 1979; Skowronski & Carlston, 1989). According to this view, behaviors differ in how diagnostic they are of membership in a particular category, with negative behaviors often carrying more diagnostic information than positive ones.

Whereas impressions can covary as a function of diagnosticity, several lines of research suggest that the operation of a negativity bias in the underlying negative motivational system has more explanatory power than a diagnosticity-based explanation for negativity bias effects. The negativity bias has been observed in impression-formation tasks, even when negative behaviors are not the most diagnostic (Ganzach, 1995; Gardner, 1996; Rowe, 1989), and in domains in which trait diagnosticity is not relevant (e.g., Ito et al., 1998; Miller, 1959). An explanation that makes reference to the underlying motivational system rather than diagnosticity also has the power to generalize to a greater number of situations. The diagnosticity explanation addresses information integration (i.e., how an impression of a person is formed from knowledge of that individual's different traits and behaviors) and has dealt with the attribution of traits to an individual (i.e., determining how moral a person is). In addition, diagnosticity effects may depend on learning, occurring only after the organism learns which behaviors are diagnostic for a particular domain. In contrast, the negativity bias as we have conceptualized it functions as a property of the underlying negative motivational system alone. As such, it is expected to manifest itself in domains other than trait attribution and impression formation and to operate independent of learning. At the same time, although we believe that differences in the activation functions of negativity and positivity are sufficient to result in greater responsivity to negative information, we do not doubt that differences in diagnosticity can affect evaluations. The latter effects, however, may be more limited in scope.

It is also possible that the effects observed in the present experiments were due not to the activation function of the negative motivational system but to differences in the ease with which negative and positive stimuli could be classified; that is, negative stimuli may have contained greater informational value than positive stimuli, and this may have resulted in larger LPPs to negative stimuli. Although it seems clear that stimuli can differ in the extent to which they convey their evaluative meaning, there is no evidence that ease of classification varied systematically with stimulus valence in the present experiments. If stimuli of one valence were more easily classified, then we might expect faster classifications for those items. When latencies of the LPPs were examined, however, no differences in stimulus valence were found. LPP latency is relevant to this issue because it is thought to reflect relative stimulus evaluation time (Donchin, 1979) so that latencies increase as the categorization task becomes more difficult (Kutas, McCarthy, & Donchin, 1977). If negative stimuli were more easily classified than positive stimuli, shorter LPP latencies should have been found for negative pictures as compared with positive pictures. Instead, LPP latencies were equivalent for negative, positive, and neutral stimuli (see Figures 37.1 and 37.2), suggesting equal ease of classification across stimulus valence.

A final alternative explanation for the larger LPPs for negative pictures is that they may have been more surprising or novel than positive pictures. This possibility stems from an assumed greater base rate of positive occurrences than negative occurrences in everyday life. Although we did not obtain direct measures of surprise or novelty in the present experiments, extant research indicates that there have been no systematic differences in the novelty of positive and negative stimuli within an experimental setting. Prior research involving similar stimuli reveals that positive and negative stimuli are (a) viewed for an equivalent duration in free-viewing periods (and for a longer duration than are neutral stimuli; Bradley, Cuthbert, & Lang, 1990, 1991; Lang, Greenwald, Bradley, & Hamm, 1993); (b) recalled with equal frequency and at a higher rate than neutral items (Bradley, Cuthbert, & Lang, 1996; Bradley, Greenwald, Petry, & Lang, 1992); and (c) rated as more interesting than neutral stimuli. In fact, positive pictures are rated as more interesting than the negative ones (Bradley et al., 1990, 1991; Lang, Greenwald, Bradley, & Hamm, 1993). If the negative pictures were more novel or surprising, then we might expect them to have been viewed longer than positive or neutral pictures, to have been more memorable, or to have received higher interest ratings (e.g., Fisk & Schneider, 1984; Pratto & John, 1991). As can be seen, this has not been the case.

Specific features of our experimental paradigm also argue against a novelty explanation. The preexposure period in Experiment 2, in which participants paced themselves through sets of positive, negative, and neutral pictures from which the experimental stimuli were drawn, would have helped to diminish any possible global novelty differences between the classes of stimuli. The negativity bias effect was seen both when preexposure occurred (Experiment 2) and when it did not (Experiment 1). The stimuli were also specifically presented in a way that would minimize global novelty effects. This was accomplished by establishing a local context in which positive and negative stimuli were equally unlikely. From the perspective of a participant in Experiment 1, for example, the structuring of the sequences resulted in 540 presentations of neutral pictures but in only 30 each of positive and negative pictures. The local context of the experiment was therefore very potent in establishing equally low local base-rate expectations for positive and negative pictures. Research on the conceptually similar P300-ERP component reveals that its amplitude is more sensitive to the local (as opposed to global) context (Squires, Wickens, Squires, & Donchin, 1976). Extant research and specific features of the present experiments suggest that a confound between valence and novelty is unlikely to have produced the LPP results obtained.

Whereas novelty effects were unlikely to have produced the present results, Pratto and John (1991) argued that humans possess a mechanism effortlessly directing attention to negative stimuli. Participants in their study performed a modified Stroop task in which they named the ink color used to print various desirable and undesirable traits. Color-naming latencies were longer for the undesirable traits, suggesting that the negatively valenced stimuli attracted more attention from the primary task (ink-color naming) than the positively valenced stimuli. Although potential differences in arousal between the words in the two valence categories could also produce attentional differences (Lang et al., 1993), greater attention to negative stimuli is a plausible adaptive behavior. It is important to note that in Pratto and John's research, participants were not explicitly instructed to attend to stimulus valence, whereas an explicit evaluative task was performed in the present experiments. Taken together, Pratto and John's results suggest that negative stimuli may attract attention through an automatic vigilance mechanism, and the present results suggest that once attended, negative information has a greater impact than equally extreme positive information.

Acknowledgments

Preparation of this article was supported by National Science Foundation Grant SBR-9512459 and National Institute of Mental Health Grant P50MH52384-01A1. We thank Allyson Holbrook for assistance with statistical analyses.

Notes

1. In fact, Cacioppo and Berntson (1994) proposed that the activation functions for positivity and nega-

tivity were nonlinear with exponents less than 1. Therefore, nonlinear regression analyses were also performed on the IAPS ratings in Ito et al. (1998). These analyses used the equation $E = A^X + b$, where E is either unipolar negativity ratings or positivity ratings, A is arousal ratings, X is the exponent that represents both the slope of the line and the rate of deceleration in the impact of increasing activation of the valent system of interest, and b represents the intercept value. To model activation of the negative motivational system, we computed the above equation using data from the 212 slides that participants found to be more negative than positive, with unipolar negativity ratings serving as E. To model activation of the positive motivational system, we computed the above equation using data from the 258 slides that participants found more positive than negative, with unipolar positivity ratings serving as E. As predicted by the negativity bias, the exponent was larger in the model estimating activation of the negative motivational system as compared with the model estimating activation of the positive motivational system. Similar results were obtained when bipolar valence ratings were used as E, dichotomizing the dataset at the scale median. Comparable analyses were also performed for stimuli in the English Affective Lexicon. Results again revealed a larger exponent in the model estimating activation of the negative motivational system.

2. In the traditional oddball paradigm, stimuli are presented in long sequences (e.g., 200 stimuli). Evaluative categorization of long sequences of affectively valenced stimuli proved difficult for participants to perform (see Cacioppo et al., 1993, Note 1). As a result, we present stimuli in short sequences of 5 or 6 stimuli in our modified paradigm. The shorter sequences reduce variability in the ERP by presumably increasing participants' attention to and discrimination of the stimuli.

3. Although we intended to present each picture 15 times, an error in the stimulus randomization program, which was detected after data collection, resulted in one exemplar from each valent category being presented 20 times, whereas the other exemplar from the same valent category was presented 10 times. Thus, for each participant the probability of seeing a given valent picture was either .033 or .067 instead of being equiprobable. This difference in probability of presentation between exemplars of the same valent category was crossed, not confounded, with experimental variables, however, and had no effect on LPP amplitude.

Therefore, we collapsed across this factor in all subsequent analyses.

4. The IAPS pictures in Neutral Subset A were 1910, 2190, 4100, 5500, 5800, 6150, 7002, 7025, 7035, 7040, 7080, 7090, 7140, 7217, 7224, 7285, 7550, and 7820. Those in Neutral Subset B were 2230, 2840, 5900, 7000, 7006, 7009, 7010, 7030, 7050, 7100, 7130, 7150, 7170, 7190, 7233, 7235, 7284, and 9210. The IAPS pictures in the positive category were 8490 and 8510; those in the negative category were 3030 and 6230.

5. Data were also recorded from 25 additional scalp sites (F3, F4, F7, F8, FT7, FT8, FC3, FC4, T3, T4, TP7, TP8, C3, C4, CP3, CP4, T5, T6, P3, P4, O1, O2, and OZ) for initial exploratory analyses of dipole sources. Thus, they are not relevant to the present psychological hypotheses.

6. The off-line referencing of EEG data to a combined left and right mastoid reference eliminates bias in asymmetry measures that can be introduced from even slight differences in impedances between the two mastoids (R. J. Davidson, personal communication, September 21, 1995). Other referencing schemes have been used to eliminate the biasing effects of differential impedances, such as common referencing (referencing each site to an average of all the sites), but the method used here results in more precise and less biased measures of ERP amplitudes.

7. The MANOVA also revealed two higher order interactions that did not bear on theoretical issues: (a) Picture Category × Block Order × Set of Neutral Pictures Paired with Positive Targets, $F(1, 17) = 11.23$, $p < .01$; (b) Picture Category × Hand for *Neutral* Response × Block Order × Set of Neutral Pictures Paired with Positive Targets, $F(1, 17) = 7.31$, $p < .01$. None of these interactions were theoretically interesting, nor did they qualify the effects reported in the text.

8. The IAPS pictures in the neutral category were 6150, 7006, 7009, 7010, 7025, 7030, 7035, 7040, 7080, 7090, 7100, 7150, 7170, 7190, 7233, 7235, 7820, and 7830. Picture 7830 was the only neutral IAPS picture used in Experiment 2 but not in Experiment 1. The IAPS pictures in the positive category were 7340 and 7350, and those in the negative category were 9140 and 9571.

9. The PhotoLibrary CD images used had the file names 5740081, 9320065, 9430083, 14060015, 14070024, 14070035, 20110049, and 2040092.

10. Of less theoretical interest was a main effect of hand for *positive* response, $F(1, 10) = 7.84$, $p < .05$. LPPs were larger for participants who used their left thumb to indicate a positive evaluation ($M = 8.70$ µV) as opposed to those who used their right thumb ($M = 5.64$ µV).

11. It is important to note that the evaluative inconsistency and negativity bias effects obtained in the full sample in Experiment 2 were replicated in the subsample of participants whose categorizations of the valenced targets matched the normative classifications.

12. The positivity offset, in the form of a higher intercept value for the gradient relating positive evaluations and motivational activation, was also seen in the regression analyses on stimuli from the English Affective Lexicon (Bradley et al., 1997). In addition, all nonlinear regression analyses discussed in note 1 also contained a higher intercept value for the positive gradient.

References

Anderson, N. H. (1965). Averaging versus adding as a stimulus-combination rule in impression formation. *Journal of Personality and Social Psychology, 2*, 1–9.

Bargh, J. A. (1989). Conditional automaticity: Varieties of automatic influence in social perception and cognition. In J. S. Uleman & J. A. Bargh (Eds.), *Unintended thought* (pp. 3–51). New York: Guilford Press.

Bargh, J. A., Chaiken, S., Govender, T., & Pratto, F. (1992). The generality of the automatic attitude activation effect. *Journal of Personality and Social Psychology, 62*, 893–912.

Birnbaum, M. (1972). Morality judgements: Tests of an averaging model. *Journal of Experimental Psychology, 93*, 35–42.

Bradley, M. M., Cuthbert, B. N., & Lang, P. J. (1990). Startle reflex modification: Emotion or attention? *Psychophysiology, 27*, 513–522.

Bradley, M. M., Cuthbert, B. N., & Lang, P. J. (1991). Startle and emotion: Lateral acoustic probes and the bilateral blink. *Psychophysiology, 28*, 285–295.

Bradley, M. M., Cuthbert, B. N., & Lang, P. J. (1996). Picture media and emotion: Effects of a sustained affective context. *Psychophysiology, 33*, 662–670.

Bradley, M. M., Greenwald, M. K., Petry, M., & Lang, P. J. (1992). Remembering pictures: Pleasure and arousal in memory. *Journal of Experimental Psychology: Learning, Memory, and Cognition,* 18, 379–390.

Bradley, M. M., Lang, P. J., & Cuthbert, B. N. (1997). *Affective norms for English words.* Gainesville: Center for the Study of Emotion and Attention—National Institute of Mental Health (CSEA–NIMH), University of Florida.

Cacioppo, J. T., & Berntson, G. G. (1994). Relationship between attitudes and evaluative space: A critical review, with emphasis on the separability of positive and negative substrates. *Psychological Bulletin,* 115, 401–423.

Cacioppo, J. T., Crites, S. L., Jr., Berntson, G. G., & Coles, M. G. H. (1993). If attitudes affect how stimuli are processed, should they not affect the event-related brain potential? *Psychological Science,* 4, 108–112.

Cacioppo, J. T., Crites, S. L., Jr., & Gardner, W. L. (1996). Attitudes to the right: Evaluative processing is associated with lateralized late positive event-related brain potentials. *Personality and Social Psychology Bulletin,* 22, 1205–1219.

Cacioppo, J. T., Crites, S. L., Jr., Gardner, W. L., & Berntson, G. G. (1994). Bioelectrical echoes from evaluative categorizations: I. A late positive brain potential that varies as a function of trait negativity and extremity. *Journal of Personality and Social Psychology,* 67, 115–125.

Cacioppo, J. T., & Gardner, W. L. (in press). Emotion. *Annual Review of Psychology,* 50.

Cacioppo, J. T., Gardner, W. L., & Berntson, G. G. (1997). Beyond bipolar conceptualizations and measures: The case of attitudes and evaluative space. *Personality and Social Psychology Review,* 1, 3–25.

Cannon, W. B. (1929). *Bodily changes in pain, hunger, fear, and rage* (2nd ed.). New York: Appleton-Century-Crofts.

Center for the Study of Emotion and Attention—National Institute of Mental Health (CSEA–NIMH). (1995). *The international affective picture system: Digitized photographs.* Gainesville: The Center for Research in Psychophysiology, University of Florida.

Coles, M. G. H., Gratton, G., & Fabiani, M. (1990). Event-related brain potentials. In J. T. Cacioppo & L. G. Tassinary (Eds.), *Principles of psychophysiology:*

Physical, social, and inferential elements (pp. 413–455). Cambridge, England: Cambridge University Press.

Coles, M. G. H., Gratton, G., Kramer, A. F., & Miller, G. A. (1986). Principles of signal acquisition and analysis. In M. G. H. Coles, E. Donchin, & S. W. Porges (Eds.), *Psychophysiology: Systems, processes, and applications* (pp. 183–226). New York: Guilford Press.

Crites, S. L., Jr., & Cacioppo, J. T. (1996). Electrocortical differentiation of evaluative and nonevaluative categorizations. *Psychological Science,* 7, 318–321.

Crites, S. L., Jr., Cacioppo, J. T., Gardner, W. L., & Berntson, G. G. (1995). Bioelectrical echoes from evaluative categorizations: II. A late positive brain potential that varies as a function of attitude registration rather than attitude report. *Journal of Personality and Social Psychology,* 68, 997–1013.

Donchin, E. (1979). Event-related potentials: A tool in the study of human information processing. In H. Begleiter (Ed.), *Evoked potentials and behavior* (pp. 13–75). New York: Plenum.

Donchin, E. (1981). Suprise!... Surprise? *Psychophysiology,* 18, 493–513.

Donchin, E., & Coles, M. G. H. (1988). Is the P300 component a manifestation of context updating? *Behavioral and Brain Sciences,* 11, 357–374.

Edwards, A. L. (1946). A critique of "neutral" items in attitude scales constructed by the method of equally appearing intervals. *Psychological Review,* 53, 159–169.

Fazio, R. H., Sanbonmatsu, D. M., Powell, M. C., & Kardes, F. R. (1986). On the automatic activation of attitudes. *Journal of Personality and Social Psychology,* 50, 229–238.

Feldman, S. (1966). Motivational aspects of attitudinal elements and their place in cognitive interaction. In S. Feldman (Ed.), *Cognitive consistency* (pp. 76–114). San Diego, CA: Academic Press.

Fisk, A. D., & Schneider, W. (1984). Memory as a function of attention, level of processing, and automatization. *Journal of Experimental Psychology: Learning, Memory, and Cognition,* 38, 889–906.

Ganzach, Y. (1995). Negativity (and positivity) in performance evaluation: Three field studies. *Journal of Applied Psychology,* 80, 491–499.

Gardner, W. L. (1996). *Biases in impression formation: A demonstration of a bivariate model of evaluation (positivity, negativity)*. Unpublished doctoral dissertation, Ohio State University, Columbus.

Gardner, W. L., Cacioppo, J. T., Berntson, G. G., & Crites, S. L., Jr. (in press). Distinguishing hostile from hospitable events: Individual differences in evaluative categorizations as indexed by a late positive brain potential. *Social Cognition*.

Gehring, W. J., Gratton, G., Coles, M. G. H., & Donchin, E. (1992). Probability effects on stimulus evaluation and response processes. *Journal of Experimental Psychology: Human Perception and Performance, 18, 198–216.*

Goldstein, M. D., & Strube, M. J. (1994). Independence revisited: The relation between positive and negative affect in a naturalistic setting. *Personality and Social Psychology Bulletin, 20, 57–64.*

Hass, R. G., Katz, I., Rizzo, N., Bailey, J., & Eisenstadt, D. (1991). Cross-racial appraisal as related to attitude ambivalence and cognitive complexity. *Personality and Social Psychology Bulletin, 17, 83–92.*

Hodges, B. H. (1974). Effect of valence on relative weighting in impression formation. *Journal of Personality and Social Psychology, 30, 378–381.*

Ito, T. A., & Cacioppo, J. T. (in press). The psychophysiology of utility appraisals. In D. Kahneman, E. Diener, & N. Schwartz (Eds.), *Understanding quality of life: Scientific perspectives on enjoyment and suffering.* New York: Russell Sage Foundation.

Ito, T. A., Cacioppo, J. T., & Lang, P. J. (1998). Eliciting affect using the International Affective Picture System: Bivariate evaluation and ambivalence. *Personality and Social Psychology Bulletin, 24, 855–879.*

Kahneman, D., & Tversky, A. (1984). Choices, values, and frames. *American Psychologist, 39, 341–350.*

Kanouse, D. E., & Hansen, L. R., Jr. (1971). Negativity in evaluations. In E. E. Jones, D. E. Kanouse, H. H. Kelley, R. E. Nisbett, S. Valin, & B. Weiner (Eds.), *Attribution: Perceiving the causes of behavior* (pp. 47–62). Morristown, NJ: General Learning Press.

Kaplan, K. J. (1972). On the ambivalence–indifference problem in attitude theory and measurement: A suggested modification of the semantic differential technique. *Psychological Bulletin, 77, 361–372.*

Kutas, M., McCarthy, G., & Donchin, E. (1977). Augmenting mental chronometry: The P300 as a measure of stimulus evaluation time. *Science, 197, 792–795.*

Lang, P. J., Greenwald, M. K., Bradley, M. M., & Hamm, A. O. (1993). Looking at pictures: Affective, facial, visceral, and behavioral reactions. *Psychophysiology, 30, 261–273.*

Lewin, K. (1935). *A dynamic theory of personality.* New York: McGraw-Hill.

Miller, N. E. (1959). Liberalization of the basic S–R concepts: Extensions to conflict behavior, motivation, and social learning. In S. Kock (Ed.), *Psychology: A study of a science* (pp. 198–292). New York: McGraw-Hill.

PC Paintbrush PhotoLibrary [Computer software]. (1994). Cambridge, MA: Softkey International.

Peeters, G., & Czapinski, J. (1990). Positive–negative asymmetry in evaluations: The distinction between affective and informational negativity effects. In W. Stroebe & M. Hewstone (Eds.), *European review of social psychology* (Vol. 1, pp. 33–60). Chichester, England: Wiley.

Pratto, F., & John, O. P. (1991). Automatic vigilance: The attention-grabbing power of negative social information. *Journal of Personality and Social Psychology, 61, 380–391.*

Priester, J. R., & Petty, R. E. (1996). The gradual threshold model of ambivalence: Relating the positive and negative bases of attitudes to subjective ambivalence. *Journal of Personality and Social Psychology, 71, 442–447.*

Reeder, G. D., & Brewer, M. B. (1979). A schematic model of dispositional attribution in interpersonal perception. *Psychological Review, 86, 61–79.*

Rowe, P. M. (1989). Unfavorable information and interview decisions. In R. W. Eder & G. R. Ferris (Eds.), *The employment interview: Theory, research, and practice* (pp. 77–89). Newbury Park, CA: Sage.

Scott, W. A. (1968). Attitude measurement. In G. Lindzey & E. Aronson (Eds.), *Handbook of social psychology* (Vol. 2, pp. 204–273). Reading, MA: Addison-Wesley.

Semlitsch, H. V., Anderer, P., Schuster, P., & Presslich, O. (1986). A solution for reliable and valid reduction of ocular artifacts, applied to the P300 ERP. *Psychophysiology, 23, 695–703.*

Skowronski, J. J., & Carlston, D. E. (1989). Negativity and extremity biases in impression formation: A review of explanations. *Psychological Bulletin, 105, 131–142.*

Squires, K. C., Wickens, C., Squires, N. K., & Donchin, E. (1976). The effect of stimulus sequence on the waveform of the cortical event-related potential. *Science,* 193, 1142–1146.

Taylor, S. E. (1991). Asymmetrical effects of positive and negative events: The mobilization-minimization hypothesis. *Psychological Bulletin,* 110, 67–85.

Thompson, M. M., Zanna, M. P., & Griffin, D. W. (1995). Let's not be indifferent about (attitudinal) ambivalence. In R. E. Petty & J. A. Krosnick (Eds.), *Attitude strength: Antecedents and consequences* (pp. 361–386). Mahwah, NJ: Erlbaum.

38 Face-Elicited ERPs and Affective Attitude: Brain Electric Microstate and Tomography Analyses

D. Pizzagalli, D. Lehmann, T. Koenig, M. Regard, and R. D. Pascual-Marqui

1 Introduction

Neuroscientific investigations of face processing identified the occipito-temporal pathway (or "ventral stream") as crucially involved in face identification. Functional magnetic resonance imaging (fMRI; Puce et al., 1995; Kanwisher et al., 1997, 1999; Aguirre et al., 1999), positron emission tomography (PET; Sergent et al., 1992; Haxby et al., 1994) and intracerebral recordings (Allison et al., 1994; Halgren et al., 1994) demonstrated that maximal activation within this pathway is task-dependent and hierarchically organized from posterior to anterior regions. Whereas structural encoding typically activates posterior regions (e.g. posterior fusiform gyrus), identification of specific faces or retrieval of semantic knowledge about individuals is associated with activation of more anterior regions (e.g. midfusiform, parahippocampal, and mid-temporal gyrus).

Ethologically, faces are crucial channels of social cognition because they have high emotional value, and they permit deciphering the intentions of others (Brothers, 1990). Face recognition may thus indirectly reflect encoding and storage of social acts (Brothers, 1990). As expected, brain electric or magnetic signatures of face recognition occur quickly, 50–200 ms post-stimulus (Allison et al., 1994; Halgren et al., 1994; Bötzel et al., 1995; Jeffreys, 1996; Sams et al., 1997; Seeck et al., 1997; Debruille et al., 1998; Swithenby et al., 1998; Eimer and Mc-Carthy, 1999).

In behavioral studies, processing bias while perceiving emotional information (including faces) was demonstrated in induced or pathological affective states. Depressed subjects displayed processing bias towards emotionally negative information (George et al., 1998); induced emotions (e.g. happiness, sadness) influenced information processing accordingly (Halberstadt and Niedenthal, 1997). However, no studies have investigated brain mechanisms during face perception as a function of affect-related personality features of the perceiver.

Combining the 3 issues discussed above, the present study investigates the influence of personal affective attitude (subjects' affective reactivity or style; Goldsmith, 1993; Davidson, 1995) on brain electric field data during face processing. Brain electric field analysis can identify the occurrence times of different brain processes. As physical phenomena, different brain field configurations (map landscapes) must have been caused by different active neuronal populations (Fender, 1987), and in terms of physiology it is reasonable to assume that different active neural populations implement different functions. When examining the temporal development of sequences of momentary maps of potential distributions (landscapes of potentials) on the head surface, a recurrent observation is that these sequences consist of brief epochs of quasi-stable map configurations (landscapes), called microstates, that are concatenated by rapid transitions (e.g. Lehmann and Skrandies, 1984; Lehmann, 1987; Koenig and Lehmann, 1996; Koenig et al., 1998). Thus, brain electric field characteristics change in a stepwise manner rather than steadily, although each step or microstate must consist of the activity of many parallel neuronal processes. The microstates were suggested to be the building blocks of a stepwise information processing in the brain; this was supported by several studies (e.g. Lehmann et al., 1998).

In the present study, temporal brain microstate segmentation (Koenig and Lehmann, 1996; Koenig et al., 1998; Lehmann et al., 1998) together with a new brain electric tomography approach: low resolution electromagnetic tomography (LORETA; Pascual-Marqui et al., 1994, 1999) allowed the assessment of the timing and cortical localization of personality-modulated, face-elicited processes, issues not covered in a previous analysis (Pizzagalli et al., 1998). The present study analyzed 27 channel event-related potential (ERP) fields recorded while subjects (dichotomized for their affective, approaching vs. withdrawing attitude towards faces) passively observed face images without tasks, i.e. during unrequested, automatic, emotional evaluation of faces.

2 Materials and Methods

2.1 Subjects

Eighteen healthy subjects (7 female; mean age: 29.4; range 22–37) with no history of neurological or psychiatric disorders and with normal or corrected-to-normal vision participated after informed, written consent to the study (approved by the Ethics Committee). All subjects were right-handed (Oldfield, 1971).

2.2 EEG Recordings

Twenty-seven channel ERPs were recorded during passive observation of face images in a sound, light and electrically shielded room with an intercom system. ERPs were recorded from 27 electrodes (Fpz as recording reference, Fp1/2, Fz, F3/4, F7/8, FC1/2, Cz, C3/4, T7/8, CP1/2, Pz, P3/4, P7/8, PO3/4, Oz and O1/O2) of the 10/10 system (American Electroencephalographic Society, 1991; filter: 0.3–70 Hz; sampling: 256 Hz; electrode impedances < 5 kΩ). Eye movements were recorded from outer left canthus vs. Fpz.

2.3 Face Images and Presentation

Face images were 32 black and white photographic portraits of psychiatric patients ("Szondi-portraits"), particularly suited to evoke emotional decisions (Regard and Landis, 1986). Subjects were naïve to the images to minimize

post-perceptual semantic processing, and were instructed to look passively at the face images. The size-, contrast- and brightness-adjusted faces (size: 8×11 cm) were presented binocularly, centered in a continually visible frame (size: 18.8×12.5 cm) on light gray background on a computer screen (exposure: 450 ms at intervals of 2000 ms; distance: 100 cm). The presentation of the 32 faces was repeated 20 times in newly randomized sequence (1 min intervals).

2.4 Affective Face Ratings and Subject Group Dichotomization

After recording, subjects rated each face image for its affective appeal (liking or disliking) on a vertical 10 cm scale, whose upper and lower ends were labeled "liked face" and "disliked face," respectively, or vice versa (constant for given faces). Each face, together with a vertical scale, was presented on an individual hard-copy. Order of rating presentation was randomized over subjects. For each subject, affective attitude was operationalized as mean affective rating of all face images. Subjects were dichotomized into two groups: the 9 subjects with the lowest mean ratings ("general negative affective attitude"; mean = 3.89, SD = 0.89, range: 1.68–4.59), and the 9 subjects with the highest mean ratings ("general positive affective attitude"; mean = 5.34, SD = 0.36, range: 4.72–5.83). The groups did not differ in age, sex, and laterality index (Oldfield, 1971).

2.5 Data and Statistical Analyses

Off-line, all data epochs were reviewed for eye, body movement or other artifacts. After artifact rejection, the ERP map series covering 1024 ms post-stimulus were averaged for each subject using all 32 stimuli and all 20 sequence repetitions, and subsequently recomputed off-line to average reference (digital 1.5–30 Hz temporal bandpass). A grand mean ERP map series was computed across all subjects.

2.5.1 Microstate Analysis

In order to identify the start and end time points of the brain electric microstates, relevant changes of the landscape of the momentary potential maps must be detected in the sequence of maps. In the present approach, the map landscapes are assessed by the locations of map descriptors, e.g. the locations of the centroids of the areas of positive and negative potential in the map (Wackermann et al., 1993). In the first map of a sequence, spatial windows are erected around the descriptors. If in a subsequent map a descriptor falls outside of a window, a microstate end is recognized, and a new one starts; the spatial windows are shifted to accommodate the next map's descriptors. Originally, predetermined window sizes were used (Lehmann and Skrandies, 1984; Lehmann, 1987). In the present study, a data-driven approach is used so that window size preselection is avoided (Koenig and Lehmann, 1996; Koenig et al., 1998). This approach involves three basic steps. First, increasing window sizes in steps of 0.01 electrode distance are applied to the map sequence until no more microstate end points are found. Second, the total number of end points across all window sizes is determined for each moment in time, resulting in a probability function of microstate end points. Third, a cut-off level for this function is determined that equally satisfies two goals, stability (i.e. assignment of a maximal number of maps to a given microstate; operationalized as the number of time points where microstate end probability function is smaller than cut-off), and discrimination (i.e. detection of a maximal number of different microstates; operationalized as number of peaks of the end probability function above cut-off). Time points with an end probability above cut-off are accepted as moments of relevant change of map landscape (i.e. as microstate start/end time points). This procedure was applied to the grand mean ERP map series.

For each subject, landscapes were averaged between the identified microstate start and end

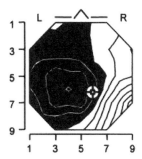

Figure 38.1

Spatial feature extraction from a momentary scalp field map. Numbers correspond to the electrode positions of the international 10-10 system as columns (horizontal, left (L) = 1, center = Cz = 5, right (R) = 9) and rows (vertical, anterior = 1, center = Cz = 5, posterior = 9). The head is seen from above, nose up, left ear left. The cross shows the location of the electric gravity center (point of gravity of the absolute map voltages), indicating the orthogonally underlying location of the mean of all momentarily active processes that produced the measured scalp potential map. Equipotential lines are linearly interpolated in steps of 1 μV (black = negative areas, white = positive areas vs. average reference).

times; the landscape of each microstate was then reduced to the location of the point of gravity of all absolute voltages (Pizzagalli et al., 1998). As displayed in Fig. 38.1, this electric gravity center is a conservative estimate of the mean localization of all active, brain electric sources projected orthogonally onto the scalp surface. For each microstate, a global test using a two-dimensional vector analysis approach assessed group differences between gravity centers. This approach treats differences of electric gravity center location between subject groups as two-dimensional vectors, and consists of 3 steps. First, the electric gravity center location of the two subject groups was separately averaged; then the mean difference vector between the two groups was calculated. Finally, the electric gravity center of each subject was projected onto the difference vector, and these positions were compared between attitudes using an unpaired t test. Post hoc unpaired t tests assessed group differences along the left-right and anterior–posterior brain axis. Overall, two-tailed P values are reported.

Only microstates showing significant attitude-dependent differences were further analyzed.

To assess the variance of microstate timing across subjects, microstate start and end times were determined for each subject by computing spatial correlations between the individual map at each time frame and the averaged ("model") microstate maps from the grand mean ERP map series (Brandeis et al., 1992). This individual microstate time recognition used time windows larger than the conventional durations of given components. For example, to assess the individual start and end times for microstate #2, a time window including microstates #1–#4 was used; for microstate #3, microstates #2–#5 were included. For microstate #2, four correlations were computed for each time frame, i.e. between the individual map at that time frame and the model map of microstate #1–#4. The highest correlation assigned each individual map to a specific microstate; the start and end times of the assignments defined the individual microstate start and end times for each subject.

It was further explored whether these assignments were statistically supported, i.e. whether the highest correlations were also significantly different from the other three. For each subject, the averaged map between the individual microstate start and end time was computed; then, 3 t values were computed between the highest correlation and the other three using the formula described by Steiger (1980). This procedure allows to test whether the correlation between A (i.e. a specific individual map) and B (i.e. the model map of microstate B) is significantly different from the correlation between A and C (the model map of microstate C), presupposing that the correlation between B and C is also known. Bonferroni corrected P values are reported ($P < 0.017$).

2.5.2 Brain Electric Tomography

For the relevant microstates, LORETA (Pascual-Marqui et al., 1994, 1999) computed the three-dimensional intracerebral distributions of current density. The method does not assume a specific number of sources, but solves the inverse problem by computing the "smoothest" of all possible activity distributions (i.e. assuming related orientations and strengths of neighboring neuronal sources). The assumption of simultaneous and synchronous activation of neighboring neurons is supported by animal single unit recordings (Llinas, 1988; Kreiter and Singer, 1992; Haalman and Vaadia, 1997). At each voxel, LORETA computes current density as the linear, weighted sum of the scalp electric potentials. Previous studies employing LORETA showed that the method is able to provide physiologically meaningful results, e.g. during basic visual and auditory tasks (Pascual-Marqui et al., 1994), epileptic discharges (Lantz et al., 1997), as well as cognitive tasks known to engage specific brain regions as assessed with other imaging techniques (Brandeis et al., 1998; Strik et al., 1998).

The utilized LORETA version (Pascual-Marqui et al., 1999) was registered to the Talairach brain atlas (Talairach and Tournoux, 1988), and computations were restricted to cortical gray matter and hippocampus (using the digitized Talairach and probability atlases of the Brain Imaging Centre, Montreal Neurologic Institute). The solution space consisted of 2394 voxels with a spatial resolution of 7 mm. For microstates with significant differences between groups, two average LORETA images were constructed across subjects: the brain electric activity during the microstates, and the voxel-by-voxel t test differences between groups. The Structure-Probability Maps atlas (Lancaster et al., 1997) was used to assess which brain regions were involved in personality-modulated microstate as well as in differences between the subject groups: Brodmann area(s) and brain regions closest to the observed locations identified by the Talairach coordinates are reported.

2.6 Test–retest Reliability of Affective Attitude as Trait

The 18 subjects were asked by mail 14 months (on the average) after the ERP experiment to rate the same face images again; 14 replied.

3 Results

3.1 Microstate Analysis

In the present data, 9 microstates with different mean topographies (see Table 38.1, third column) were identified. For each of the 9 grand mean microstates and both subject groups, Table 38.1 lists the location of the electric gravity center and the vector tested for group differences. The gravity centers differed significantly between groups in microstates #2 (132–196 ms; $t = 3.46$, d.f. $= 16$; $P < 0.003$) and #3 (196–272 ms; $t = 2.38$, d.f. $= 16$; $P < 0.03$). Post hoc testing revealed that the electric gravity center for subjects with negative affective attitude was significantly more to the right than for subjects with positive attitude in both microstates (both $t = 2.38$, d.f. $= 16$; $P < 0.03$). Anterior–posterior differences were not significant.

As shown in Table 38.1, microstate #2 had a posterior negative landscape, #3 a posterior positive landscape, both with strongest gradients over occipital areas. Beyond polarity, and across subjects, the landscape of microstates #2 and #3 assessed by the electric gravity center differed in a global test (vector analysis approach) at $P < 0.028$ ($t = 2.41$, d.f. $= 16$); post hoc testing showed that microstate #2's electric gravity center was more posterior ($t = 2.16$, d.f. $= 16$; $P < 0.046$).

Fig. 38.2 displays the locations of the electric gravity centers for the two subject groups for all 9 microstates. This allows following how the activity generally developed as well as how the group differences changed in time. Fig. 38.2A,B shows the locations for the microstates before and after offset of the stimulus presentation

(occurring at 450 ms), respectively. Generally, the subject groups clearly differed during stimulus presentation but not after stimulus offset. Moreover, both after stimulus onset and again after stimulus offset, the gravity center was located most posteriorly, and for the subsequent microstates it moved more anterior (microstate #5 was an exception but its posteriorization is most probably related to the stimulus offset occurring during its time duration).

The start and end times of microstates #2 and #3 were successfully identified with small variance in all subjects. (The time window, where the spatial correlations were computed, was 80–332 ms for microstate #2 and 132–576 ms for microstate #3). Across subjects, the means of the individual start and end times were 134.2 ± 8.7 and 190.7 ± 8.7 ms for microstate #2 (grand mean ERP map series: 132–196 ms), and 195.3 ± 8.3 and 275.6 ± 28.2 ms for microstate #3 (grand mean ERP map series: 196–272 ms). Two additional results were of relevance. First, for each subject, the sequence of the assignments for both microstates was always uninterrupted (i.e. the occurrence of a new assignment unambiguously started the occurrence of the next microstate). Second, the assignments were not only unambiguous but also very robust, as assessed by testing the differences between dependent correlations (Steiger, 1980). Considering the individual microstate start and end times related to microstate #2, all 18 subjects displayed significantly higher correlations for the model map of microstate #2 than of microstates #1, #3 and #4 (all P values < 0.017). Similarly, for microstate #3, 17 of 18 subjects (binomial $P(17/18) < 0.0001$) displayed significantly higher correlations for the model map of microstate #3 than of microstates #2, #4 and #5 (all P values < 0.017).

3.2 LORETA Tomography

The results of the microstate analysis demonstrated that significantly different neural

Table 38.1
Mean locations (and SD) of the electric gravity centers on the left-right (L-R) and anterior-posterior (A-P) axes of the head in the 9 identified microstates, for subjects with negative ($n = 9$) and with positive ($n = 9$) affective attitude

No.	Timing (ms)	Topography		Negative	Positive	Difference	Vector	*P* value
	Microstate			Affective attitude				
#1	80–132		L-R	5.14 (0.14)	5.01 (0.20)	0.126		
			A-P	5.92 (0.15)	5.93 (0.18)	−0.010	0.126	0.138
#2	132–196		L-R	5.16 (0.11)	5.04 (0.10)	0.120		
			A-P	5.83 (0.19)	5.77 (0.18)	0.059	0.134	0.003
#3	196–272		L-R	5.24 (0.13)	5.03 (0.22)	0.204		
			A-P	5.72 (0.18)	5.63 (0.31)	0.092	0.224	0.030
#4	272–332		L-R	5.18 (0.20)	5.02 (0.25)	0.156		
			A-P	5.56 (0.39)	5.32 (0.26)	0.237	0.284	0.096
#5	332–576		L-R	5.19 (0.22)	5.12 (0.13)	0.066		
			A-P	5.58 (0.11)	5.52 (0.32)	0.064	0.092	0.318
#6	576–616		L-R	5.09 (0.19)	5.07 (0.23)	0.022		
			A-P	5.95 (0.43)	5.89 (0.32)	0.061	0.065	0.724
#7	616–668		L-R	5.09 (0.13)	5.11 (0.24)	−0.020		
			A-P	5.60 (0.16)	5.47 (0.29)	0.130	0.131	0.280
#8	668–876		L-R	5.09 (0.25)	5.07 (0.11)	0.019		
			A-P	5.39 (0.20)	5.44 (0.33)	−0.055	0.058	0.661
#9	876–948		L-R	5.20 (0.35)	5.13 (0.25)	0.073		
			A-P	5.46 (0.46)	5.38 (0.31)	0.083	0.111	0.516

The locations are the electrode positions as in Fig. 38.1. Equipotential lines are linearly interpolated in steps of 1 μV (vertical hatching = negative areas, white = positive areas vs. average reference). Group differences were assessed as two-dimensional vectors. Two-tailed *P* values are reported.

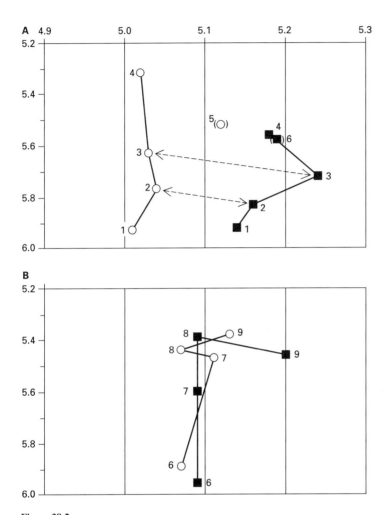

Figure 38.2
Mean locations of the brain's electric gravity centers of the nine identified microstates for subjects with negative ($n = 9$; ■) and for subjects with positive ($n = 9$; ○) affective attitude. The frames (head seen from above, anterior is up) display an area near the vertex, around the sagittal midline (heavy vertical line at 5.0), extending from electrode position 4.9 to 5.3 on the left-right axis (x axis) and from position 5.2–6.0 on the anterior-posterior axis (y axis), using the position numbering of Fig. 38.1. Dashed arrows display significant group differences. (A) Locations of the electric gravity centers for the microstates #1–#5. (B) Locations of the electric gravity centers for the microstates #6–#9. The location of microstate #5 (332–576 ms) is in brackets because it straddled the end of the stimulus exposure, which occurred at 450 ms.

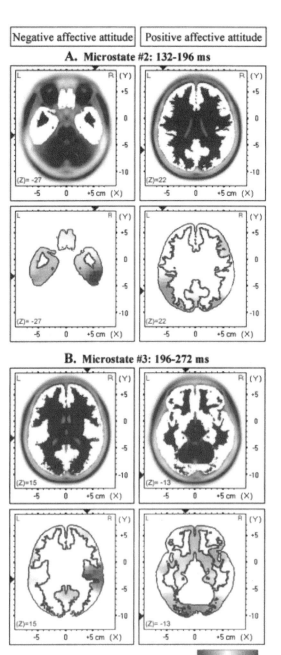

Negative affective attitude | Positive affective attitude

A. Microstate #2: 132-196 ms

B. Microstate #3: 196-272 ms

$t = -4.26$ 0 4.26

populations were active in the two subject groups during microstates #2 and #3. The LORETA analysis showed that microstates #2 and #3 were characterized by a bilateral occipito-temporal activation, involving the lingual and fusiform gyri, and extending to the inferior temporal gyri (Brodmann areas 18, 19, 37, 39). Difference tests (Fig. 38.3 and Table 38.2) comparing activity between subject groups showed, for subjects with negative attitude, the strongest activity excess in both microstates in right temporal areas (for microstate #2 more inferior than for #3), whereas for subjects with positive attitude, the strongest activity excess occurred in microstate #2 in left temporo-parietal areas and in microstate #3 in left occipital areas.

Besides the voxels with maximal t values, other voxels showed group differences with a P value < 0.05 (uncorrected for multiple testing). As listed in Table 38.2, for microstate #2, subjects with negative attitude had stronger activity in the right middle temporal gyrus, right post-

Figure 38.3
Images of voxel-by-voxel LORETA t-statistics of brain electric activity comparing subjects with negative ($n = 9$) and positive ($n = 9$) affective attitude during the microstate #2 (132–196 ms; A) and #3 (196–272 ms; B). Axial brain slices (head seen from above, nose up, L = left, R = right) are shown at the level (indicated as Z-axis values at the lower left corners) of the extreme t values. In (A) and (B), the upper images show LORETA's cortical solution areas in white; the lower images display the t values as gray shades (see calibration) in these areas. Locations of extreme t values (values, see table 38.2) are indicated by black triangles. Left images show relative hyperactivity for subjects with negative affective attitude; right images show relative hyperactivity for subjects with positive affective attitude. Coordinates in mm after Talairach and Tournoux (1988); origin at anterior commissure; (X) = left (−) to right (+); (Y) = posterior (−) to anterior (+); (Z) = inferior (−) to superior (+). Note that paired upper and lower images are at the same Z-level.

Table 38.2
Results of the voxel-by-voxels LORETA t statistics comparing subjects with negative ($n = 9$) and positive ($n = 9$) affective attitude for microstate #2 (132–196 ms) and #3 (196–272 ms)

Micro-state	Affective attitude	X	Y	Z	t value	BA	Region	Side
#2	Negative	53	−32	−27	4.26[a]	BA 20	Fusiform gyrus	Right
		60	−25	−6	3.79[b]	BA 21	Middle temporal gyrus	Right
		67	−11	22	2.82[b]	BA 43	Postcentral gyrus	Right
		11	24	36	2.41[b]	BA 32	Cingulate gyrus	Right
		−3	24	36	2.38[b]	BA 32	Cingulate gyrus	Left
		46	−25	43	2.15[b]	BA 2	Postcentral gyrus	Right
	Positive	−59	−60	22	−1.84[a]	BA 44	Superior temporal gyrus	Left
#3	Negative	39	−32	15	3.39[a]	BA 29	Superior temporal gyrus	Right
		60	−32	15	2.99[b]	BA 42	Superior temporal gyrus	Right
		67	−11	29	2.75[b]	BA 6	Precentral gyrus	Right
		60	−25	−27	2.67[b]	BA 20	Inferior temporal gyrus	Right
		60	−39	−27	2.54[b]	BA 20	Fusiform gyrus	Right
		39	−53	43	2.51[b]	BA 40	Inferior parietal lobule	Right
	Positive	−17	−102	−13	−2.48[a]	BA 17	Lingual gyrus	Left

Coordinates in mm after Talairach and Tournoux (1988); origin at anterior commisure; X = left (−) to right (+); Y = posterior (−) to anterior (+); Z = inferior (−) to superior (+). Brodmann areas (BA) and anatomical regions of the extreme t values[a] and t values associated with P values < 0.05 ([b]; uncorrected for multiple testing) are reported (d.f. = 16). Positive t values indicate relative hyperactivity, negative values relative hypoactivity in subjects with negative affective attitude.

central gyrus, and bilateral cingulate gyri. For microstate #3, subjects with negative attitude had stronger activity in the precentral, inferior temporal and fusiform gyrus as well as in the inferior parietal lobule, all in the right hemisphere.

3.3 ERP Waveform Analysis

In order to compare the present results with those obtained with conventional ERP waveform analyses, average amplitudes were computed (vs. technical zero baseline) for every subject using the individual microstate start and end times of microstates #2 and #3. These values were subjected to analyses of variance (ANOVA) separately for midline (Fpz, Fz, Cz, Pz, Oz), anterior (Fp1/2, F3/4, F7/8, FC1/2), central (C3/4, T7/8, CP1/2) and posterior (P3/4, P7/8, PO3/4, O1/2) electrodes using *Group*, *Electrode* and *Hemisphere* (when appropriate) as factors. Figure 38.4 displays the ERP waveshapes separately averaged for subjects with positive and for those with negative affective attitude.

For microstate #2, the only effect approaching significance was a *Group × Electrode × Hemisphere* interaction for posterior electrodes ($F(3, 48) = 2.46$; $P < 0.074$). Follow-up analyses showed that this triple interaction was caused by more negative amplitudes at P7 for subjects with positive affective attitude but a reversed pattern at P8 and O2. These results fit well with the left-right group differences demonstrated in the microstate analysis. However, no group differences emerged at single electrodes in the conventional waveshape analysis. The microstate analysis was therefore more sensitive in assessing group differences.

For microstate #3, a significant $Group \times Electrode$ interaction emerged ($F(4, 64) = 3.30$; $P < 0.016$) in the ANOVA analysis with midline electrodes: negative affective attitude was associated with more negative amplitude at Fz ($t = 2.47$, d.f. $= 16$; $P < 0.025$) but more positive amplitudes at Oz ($t = 2.75$, d.f. $= 16$; $P < 0.014$). For anterior electrodes, a $Group \times Electrode \times Hemisphere$ interaction was found ($F(3, 48) = 3.17$; $P < 0.032$). Follow-up analyses demonstrated group differences at F4 ($t = 2.44$, d.f. $= 16$; $P < 0.027$), F8 ($t = 2.32$, d.f. $= 16$; $P < 0.034$), F3 ($t = 2.23$, d.f. $= 16$; $P < 0.041$), and FC1 ($t = 2.26$, d.f. $= 16$; $P < 0.038$) with larger (more negative) amplitudes for subjects with negative affective. The main effect of $Group$ approached significance ($F(1, 16) = 3.67$; $P < 0.073$). For posterior electrodes, a main effect of $Group$ was demonstrated ($F(1, 16) = 4.59$; $P < 0.048$): again, subjects with negative affective attitude had generally higher amplitudes. Significant $Group \times Hemisphere$ ($F(1, 16) = 4.98$; $P < 0.040$) and $Group \times Electrode \times Hemisphere$ ($F(3, 48) = 6.33$; $P < 0.001$) interactions modulated this effect. Follow-up analyses for the $Group \times Hemisphere$ interaction showed that subjects with negative affective attitude had larger amplitudes at electrodes over the right than left hemisphere (2.38 ± 0.77 vs. 1.91 ± 0.63; $t = 1.93$, d.f. $= 8$; $P < 0.089$), and differed from subjects with positive affective attitude only at electrodes over the right hemisphere (2.38 ± 0.77 vs. 1.66 ± 0.67; $t = 2.11$, d.f. $= 16$; $P < 0.05$). Group differences were only found at P8 ($t = 2.07$, d.f. $= 16$; $P < 0.055$), O2 ($t = 2.67$, d.f. $= 16$; $P < 0.017$) and PO4 ($t = 2.15$, d.f. $= 16$; $P < 0.048$). For central electrodes, no significant effects emerged.

3.4 Test–retest Reliability of Affective Attitude as Trait

Re-rating of the face images by the same subjects showed that repeat (on the average 416 days after the experiment) and original affective attitudes correlated with Spearman's $\rho = 0.61$ ($n = 14$, $P < 0.02$).

4 Discussion

4.1 Temporal Aspects of the Personality-Modulated, Face-Elicited ERP Microstates

The space-oriented microstate analysis employed in the present study allowed the discrimination of sequential brain microstates as basic elements of brain information processing (Koenig and Lehmann, 1996; Koenig et al., 1998; Lehmann et al., 1998). The two microstates at 132–196 ms and at 196–272 ms after stimulus onset were systematically influenced by the subjects' affective attitude towards the face images (assessed after the experiment). The timing of these microstates was consistent over subjects (i.e. identifiable unambiguously and reliably in all subjects). During both microstates, the electric gravity center for subjects with negative affective attitude was located more to the right compared to subjects with positive affective attitude. Evidently, different, attitude-dependent neuronal populations were active in the two microstates between 132 and 272 ms after stimulus onset during the passive, task-free observation of faces.

4.2 Spatial Aspects of the Personality-Modulated, Face-Elicited ERP Microstates

During the two personality-modulated microstates, the 3 dimensional distribution of neuronal electrical activity in the brain as computed with LORETA tomography (Pascual-Marqui et al., 1994, 1999) showed maximal differences between groups as follows: stronger activity at right tem-

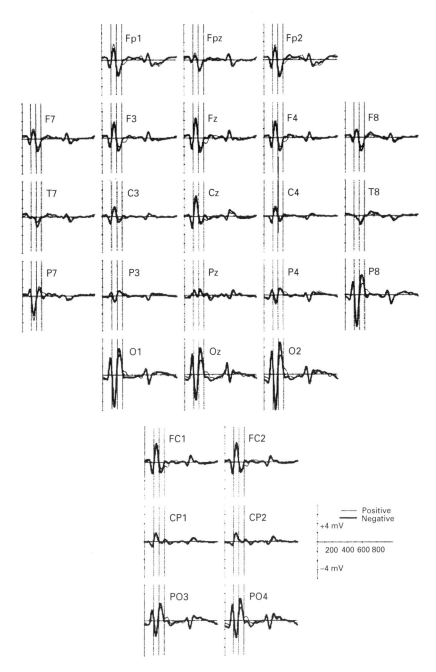

Figure 38.4

Mean ERP waveshapes (vs. average reference) separately averaged for subjects with negative affective attitude ($n = 9$; heavy lines) and for subjects with positive affective attitude ($n = 9$; thin lines). The vertical dashed lines illustrate the start and end times for the microstates showing significant group differences in the microstate analysis (microstate #2: 132–196 ms; microstate #3: 196–272 ms). Note that plotting of ERPs at different electrode positions cannot be easily interpreted in terms of the spatial configuration of a momentary field map. Electrode nomenclature according to the international 10-10 system.

poral regions for negative affective attitude in both microstates (however, clearly more inferior in microstate #2 than #3), and stronger activity at left temporo-parietal (in microstate #2) or left occipital (in microstate #3) regions for positive attitude. The relative right temporal hyperactivity associated with negative affective attitude agrees with other studies demonstrating involvement of this region in negative, withdrawal-related emotions, such as disgust (Davidson et al., 1990), aversive conditioning (Hugdahl et al., 1995), anticipatory anxiety and predisposition to panic attack (Reiman, 1997) and processing of negatively loaded films (Lane et al., 1997). The relative left temporo-parietal hyperactivity associated with positive affective attitude parallels recent reports of left-sided activation during positive emotion (fronto-temporal junction during assessment of face attractiveness: Nakamura et al., 1998) as well as left-sided inhibition during negative emotion (left temporo-occipital junction during aversive conditioning: Hugdahl et al., 1995). Taken together, the group differences at the scalp (in both the space-oriented and conventional ERP waveform analysis) and in the brain agree with differential hemispheric involvement in emotions (Regard and Landis, 1986; Canli et al., 1998; see Silberman and Weingartner, 1986; Davidson, 1995 for reviews), i.e. with relatively greater involvement of the right (left) hemisphere during negative (positive) emotions. Thus, the automatically generated, differential geometry of brain activity in the present subjects would account for their varying, affective posthoc rating of the face pictures. These phasic responses may well arise, however, from a background of tonic differences between the subject groups. Indeed, subjects with the (highest) positive and negative affective attitude were found to differ already in their baseline EEG activity (i.e. recorded before any stimulus exposure; Pizzagalli et al., 1999). Relevant to the present results, a negative attitude was associated with a right-lateralized intracerebral model source for the EEG beta frequency band.

4.3   Functional Significance of the Personality-modulated Microstates

The first microstate (132–196 ms) with group differences had maximal activity at 160 ms, which parallels latencies of face-sensitive brain activity measured with scalp ERP's (Bötzel et al., 1995; Jeffreys, 1996; Eimer and McCarthy, 1999), depth ERP's (Allison et al., 1994; Halgren et al., 1994) and magnetoencephalogram (Sams et al., 1997; Swithenby et al., 1998). These studies consistently found an automatic, stimulus-related stage of face processing (configuration extraction) between 120 and 200 ms post-stimulus. It is intriguing that the personality-modulated brain electric responses to face stimuli differed already at such early configuration extraction stages ("structural encoding stages," see Bruce and Young, 1986). The LORETA analysis supported this by demonstrating an inferior, bilateral occipito-temporal activation, in an area reportedly associated with the structural encoding stage of face processing (see Section 1).

PET and fMRI studies using visual stimuli demonstrated activation of primary and secondary visual areas during emotional processing (Lane et al., 1997; Lang et al., 1998; Morris et al., 1998; Nakamura et al., 1998). This was accounted for by reentrant processes from more anterior structures (e.g. cingulate, amygdala) associated with attention and/or motivation, indexing adaptive significance (Lang et al., 1998). A direct test of this hypothesis confirmed a modulatory role of the amygdala for brain activity in the extrastriate cortex (Morris et al., 1998). Similar reentrant processing linked to affect-related personality features might have been active in the present paradigm. At least in microstate #2, the relative hyperactivity in the right inferior temporal area was suggestively close to limbic structures. In terms of individual differences in emotional reactivity, a close relationship ($r = 0.75$) between activity in the right amygdala and electrodermal responses during extinction of fear conditioning was recently reported (Furmark et al., 1997).

4.4 Possible Influences of the Imposed Task on Face-elicited ERPs

Several ERP studies investigating face processing while engaging the subjects in more demanding, cognitive tasks (e.g. semantic matching tasks, or tasks with long-term memory requirements) demonstrated considerably later face-elicited potentials (300–600 ms; Smith and Halgren, 1987; Sommer et al., 1991; Bobes et al., 1994). However, the subjects in the present study had no prior experience with the face images and they were engaged in a passive viewing condition, where possible influences of explicit identification or memory searches were minimized or absent. Therefore, the latency differences between studies investigating unconstrained, automatic vs. cognitively demanding face processing may be accounted for by the fact that the brain regions implementing "more cognitive" operations are probably activated in later (i.e. more anteriorly located) stages of the face processing flow (Sergent et al., 1992; Halgren et al., 1994). Although not directly tested, this assumption receives partial support from the present findings of a continuous and systematic anteriorization of the brain electric activity after stimulus onset (and offset).

Summarizing, it has been suggested that a face "… is immediately and obligatorily transformed into the representation of a person (with dispositions and intentions) before having access to consciousness" (Brothers, 1990, p. 35). The present results demonstrate that not only the salience (i.e. its behavioral appetitive or aversive significance) or the perceptual features of a face, but also the disposition of the perceiving subject modulate this immediate and obligatory encoding within a sufficiently brief time for the decision to be interactively useful. This is, to our knowledge, the first demonstration that specific, trait-like, affect-related personality features in-

fluence face-elicited brain processes, and it raises the intriguing issue of experience-dependent brain plasticity not only in sensory and motor functions but also in higher brain functions such as face perception, emotional processing, and personality.

Acknowledgements

We thank Drs. B. Heider and C. Röhrenbach for the digitized Szondi face images, Drs. A. C. Evans and P. Neelin for providing the Talairach MRI and probability atlases, Dr. V. L. Towle for useful information about electrode coordinates in realistic head geometry, and Dr. R. J. Davidson for helpful comments on the manuscript. This study was partially supported by grants from the Swiss National Science Foundation (81ZH-52864) and "Holderbank"-Stiftung zur Förderung der wissenschaftlichen Fortbildung to D.P.

References

Aguirre GK, Singh R, D'Esposito M. Stimulus inversion and the responses of face and object-sensitive cortical areas. NeuroReport 1999; 10:189–194.

Allison T, Ginter H, McCarthy G, Norbe A, Puce A, Luby M, Spencer D. Face recognition in human extrastriate cortex. J Neurophysiol 1994; 71:821–825.

American Electroencephalographic Society Guidelines for Standard Electrode Position Nomenclature. J Clin Neurophysiol 1991; 8:200–202.

Bobes MA, Valdés-Sosa M, Olivares E. An ERP study of expectancy violation in face perception. Brain Cogn 1994; 26:1–22.

Bötzel K, Schulze S, Stodieck SRG. Scalp topography and analysis of intracerebral sources of face-evoked potentials. Exp Brain Res 1995; 104:135–143.

Brandeis D, Naylor H, Halliday R, Callaway E, Yano L. Scopolamine effects on visual information processing, attention, and event-related potential map latencies. Psychophysiology 1992; 29:315–336.

Brandeis D, van Leeuwen TH, Rubia K, Vitacco D, Steger J, Pascual-Marqui RD, Steinhausen HC. Neuroelectric mapping reveals precursor of stop failures in children with attention deficits. Behav Brain Res 1998; 94:111–125.

Brothers L. The social brain: a project for integrating primate behavior and neurophysiology in a new domain. Concepts Neurosci 1990; 1:27–51.

Bruce V, Young A. Understanding face recognition. Br J Psychol 1986; 77:305–327.

Canli T, Desmond JE, Zhao Z, Clover G, Gabrieli JDE. Hemispheric asymmetry for emotional stimuli detected with fMRI. NeuroReport 1998; 9:3233–3239.

Davidson RJ. Cerebral asymmetry, emotion, and affective style. In: Davidson RJ, Hugdahl K, editors. Brain asymmetry, Cambridge: MIT Press, 1995. pp. 361–387.

Davidson RJ, Ekman P, Saron CD, Senulis JA, Friesen WV. Approach/withdrawal and cerebral asymmetry: I. Emotional expression and brain physiology. J Pers Soc Psychol 1990; 58:330–341.

Debruille JB, Guillem F, Renault B. ERPs and chronometry of face recognition: following-up Seek et al. and George et al. NeuroReport 1998; 9:3349–3353.

Eimer M, McCarthy RA. Prosopagnosia and structural encoding of faces: evidence from event-related potentials. NeuroReport 1999; 10:255–259.

Fender DH. Source localization of brain electric activity. In: Gevins AS, Remond A, editors. Handbook of electroencephalography and clinical neurophysiology: methods of analysis of brain electrical and magnetic signals, revised series, vol. 1, Amsterdam: Elsevier, 1987. pp. 355–403.

Furmark T, Fischer H, Wik G, Larsson M, Fredrikson M. The amygdala and individual differences in human fear conditioning. NeuroReport 1997; 8:3957–3960.

George MS, Huggins T, McDermut W, Parekh PI, Rubinow D, Post RM. Abnormal facial emotion recognition in depression: serial testing in an ultra-rapid-cycling patient. Behav Modif 1998; 22:192–204.

Goldsmith HH. Temperament: variability in developing emotion systems. In: Lewis M, Haviland JM, editors. Handbook of emotions, New York: Guilford Press, 1993. pp. 353–364.

Haalman I, Vaadia E. Dynamics of neuronal interactions: relation to behavior, firing rates, and distance between neurons. Human Brain Map 1997; 5:249–253.

Halberstadt JB, Niedenthal PM. Emotional state and the use of stimulus dimensions in judgment. J Pers Soc Psychol 1997; 72:1017–1033.

Halgren E, Baudena P, Heit G, Clarke M, Marinkovic K. Spatio-temporal stages in face and word processing: I. Depth recorded potentials in the human occipital and parietal lobes. J Physiol (Lond) 1994; 88:1–50.

Haxby JV, Horwitz B, Ungerleider LG, Maisog JM, Pietrini P, Grady CL. The functional organization of human extrastriate cortex: a PET-rCBF study of selective attention to faces and locations. J Neurosci 1994; 14:6336–6353.

Hugdahl K, Berardi A, Thompson WL, Kosslyin SM, Macy R, Baker DP, Alpert NM, LeDoux JE. Brain mechanisms in human classical conditioning: a PET blood flow study. NeuroReport 1995; 6:1723–1728.

Jeffreys DA. Evoked potential studies of face and object processing. Vis Cogn 1996; 3:1–38.

Kanwisher N, McDermott J, Chun MM. The fusiform face area: a module in human extrastriate cortex specialized for face perception. J Neurosci 1997; 17:4302–4311.

Kanwisher N, Stanley D, Harris A. The fusiform face area is selective for faces not animals. NeuroReport 1999; 10:183–187.

Koenig T, Lehmann D. Microstates in language-related brain potential maps show noun-verb differences. Brain Lang 1996; 53:169–182.

Koenig T, Kochi K, Lehmann D. Event-related electric microstates of the brain differ between words with visual and abstract meaning. Electroenceph clin Neurophysiol 1998; 106:535–546.

Kreiter AK, Singer W. Oscillatory neuronal responses in the visual cortex of the awaque macaque monqui. Eur J Neurosci 1992; 4:369–375.

Lancaster JL, Rainey LH, Summerlin JL, Freitas CS, Fox PT, Evans AC, Toga AW, Mazziotta JC. Automated labeling of the human brain—a preliminary report on the development and evaluation of a forward-transform method. Human Brain Map 1997; 5:238–242.

Lane RD, Reiman EM, Ahern GL, Schwartz GE, Davidson RJ. Neuroanatomical correlates of happiness, sadness, and disgust. Am J Psychiatry 1997; 154:926–933.

Lang PJ, Bradley MM, Fitzsimmons JR, Cuthbert BN, Scott JD, Moulder B, Nangia V. Emotional arousal and activation of the visual cortex: an fMRI analysis. Psychophysiology 1998; 35:199–210.

Lantz G, Michel CM, Pascual-Marqui RD, Spinelli L, Seeck M, Seri S, Landis T, Rosen I. Extracranial localization of intracranial interictal epileptiform activity using LORETA (low resolution electromagnetic tomography). Electroenceph clin Neurophysiol 1997; 102:414–422.

Lehmann D. Principles of spatial analysis. In: Gevins AS, Remond A, editors. Handbook of electroencephalography and clinical neurophysiology: methods of analysis of brain electrical and magnetic signals, revised series, vol. 1, Amsterdam: Elsevier, 1987. pp. 309–354.

Lehmann D, Skrandies W. Spatial analysis of evoked potentials in man. A review. Progr Neurobiol 1984; 23:227–250.

Lehmann D, Strik WK, Henggeler B, Koenig T, Koukkou M. Brain electric microstates and momentary conscious mind states as building blocks of spontaneous thinking: I. Visual imagery and abstract thoughts. Int J Psychophysiol 1998; 29:1–11.

Llinas RR. The intrinsic electrophysiological properties of mammalian neurons: insights into central nervous system function. Science 1988; 242:1654–1664.

Morris JS, Friston KJ, Büchel C, Frith CD, Young AW, Calder AJ, Dolan RJ. A neuromodulatory role for the amygdala in processing emotional facial expressions. Brain 1998; 121:47–57.

Nakamura K, Kawashina R, Nagumo S, Ito K, Sugiura M, Kato T, Nakamura A, Hatano K, Kubota K, Fukuda H, Kojima S. Neuroanatomical correlates of the assessment of facial attractiveness. NeuroReport 1998; 9:753–757.

Oldfield RC. The assessment and analysis of handedness: the Edinburgh inventory. Neuropsychologia 1971; 9:97–113.

Pascual-Marqui RD, Michel CM, Lehmann D. Low resolution electromagnetic tomography: a new method for localizing electrical activity in the brain. Int J Psychophysiol 1994; 7:49–65.

Pascual-Marqui RD, Lehmann D, Koenig T, Kochi K, Merlo MCG, Hell D, Koukkou M. Functional imaging in acute, neuroleptic-naive, first-episode, productive schizophrenia. Psychiatry Res. Neuroimag 1999; 90: 169–179.

Pizzagalli D, Koenig T, Regard M, Lehmann D. Faces and emotions: brain electric field sources during covert emotional processing. Neuropsychologia 1998; 36:323–332.

Pizzagalli D, Koenig T, Regard M, Lehmann D. Affective attitudes to face images associated with intracerebral EEG source location before face viewing. Cogn Brain Res 1999; 7:371–377.

Puce A, Allison T, Gore JC, McCarthy G. Face-sensitive regions in human extrastriate cortex studied by functional MRI. J Neurophysiol 1995; 74:1192–1199.

Regard M, Landis T. Affective and cognitive decisions on faces in normals. In: Ellis HD, Jeeves MA, Newcombe F, Young A, editors. Aspects of face processing, Dordrecht: NATO ASI Series, Martinus Nijhoff, 1986. pp. 363–369.

Reiman EM. The application of positron emission tomography to the study of normal and pathologic emotions. J Clin Psychiatry 1997; 58:4–12.

Sams M, Hietanen JK, Hari R, Ilmoniemi RJ, Lounasmaa OV. Face-specific responses from the human inferior occipito-temporal cortex. Neuroscience 1997; 77:49–55.

Seeck M, Michel CM, Mainwaring N, Cosgrove R, Blume H, Ives J, Landis T, Schomer DL. Evidence for rapid face recognition from human scalp and intracranial electrodes. NeuroReport 1997; 8:2749–2754.

Sergent J, Ohta S, MacDonald B. Functional neuroanatomy of face and object processing. Brain 1992; 115:15–36.

Silberman EK, Weingartner H. Hemispheric lateralization of functions related to emotion. Brain Cogn 1986; 5:322–353.

Smith ME, Halgren E. Event-related potentials elicited by familiar and unfamiliar faces. In: Johnson Jr. R, Rohrbaugh JW, Parasuram R, editors. Current trends in event-related potential research (EEG Supplement, 40), Amsterdam: Elsevier, 1987. pp. 422–426.

Sommer W, Schweinberger SR, Matt J. Human brain potential correlates of face encoding into memory. Electroenceph clin Neurophysiol 1991; 79:457–463.

Steiger JH. Tests for comparing elements of a correlation matrix. Psychol Bull 1980; 87:245–251.

Strik WK, Fallgatter AJ, Brandeis D, Pascual-Marqui RD. Three-dimensional tomography of event-related potentials during response inhibition: evidence for phasic frontal lobe activation. Electroenceph clin Neurophysiol 1998; 108:406–413.

Swithenby SJ, Bailey AJ, Bräutigam S, Josephs OE, Jousmäki V, Tesche CD. Neural processing of human faces: a magnetoencephalographic study. Exp Brain Res 1998; 118:501–510.

Talairach J, Tournoux P. Co-planar stereotaxic atlas of the human brain, Stuttgart: Thième, 1988.

Wackermann J, Lehmann D, Michel CM, Strik WK. Adaptive segmentation of spontaneous EEG map series into spatially defined microstates. Int J Psychophysiol 1993; 14:269–283.

39

Performance on Indirect Measures of Race Evaluation Predicts Amygdala Activation

Elizabeth A. Phelps, Kevin J. O'Connor, William A. Cunningham, E. Sumie Funayama, J. Christopher Gatenby, John C. Gore, and Mahzarin R. Banaji

Introduction

Over the last several decades, research has shown that expressions of prejudicial attitudes toward Black and White social groups, as measured by self-report, have declined steadily (Biernat & Crandall, 1999; Schuman, Steeh, & Bobo, 1997). In spite of this decline, robust evidence of negative evaluations has been observed on indirect measures that bypass access to conscious awareness and conscious control (Banaji, in press; Cunningham, Nezlek, & Banaji, 2000; Nosek, Cunningham, Banaji, & Greenwald, 2000; Bargh & Chen, 1997; Dovidio, Kawakami, Johnson, Johnson, & Howard, 1997; Fazio, Jackson, Dunton, & Williams, 1995; Devine, 1989). Studies such as these have shown, time and again, negative indirect (automatic) evaluations of and behavior toward Black compared with White Americans. Understanding the nature of these unconscious evaluations of social groups is regarded to be a primary achievement of the field of social cognition. The present investigation expands research on social evaluation by measuring brain activity, in addition to behavior, with two primary goals: (1) to examine the neural correlates of responses to racial groups, and (2) to examine the relation between individual variability in conscious and unconscious social evaluation and brain activity.

Although the neural systems involved in the evaluation of social groups are likely to be extensive and complex, in the present study, we chose to focus on the amygdala, a subcortical structure known to be involved in emotional learning, memory, and evaluation. The amygdala is critically involved in emotional learning as measured by fear conditioning, a task in which a neutral stimulus comes to acquire emotional properties through direct association with an aversive stimulus (Davis, 1997; LeDoux, 1996; Kapp, Pascoe,

& Bixler, 1984). In humans, the amygdala's role extends beyond fear conditioning to the expression of learned emotional responses that have been acquired without direct aversive experience (Funayama, Grillon, Davis, & Phelps, in press; Phelps, LaBar, et al., 1998). The amygdala has also been shown to play a role in the evaluation of social stimuli in both humans and nonhumans (Adolphs, 1998; Adolphs et al., 1999; Kling & Brothers, 1992). In addition, patients with amygdala damage show deficits in the evaluation of fearful faces, suggesting that it is necessary for learning responses to social and emotional signals (Phelps & Anderson, 1997). In normal adults, the amygdala's involvement in perceiving emotional faces is demonstrated by its preferential response to fearful faces as measured by fMRI (Breiter et al., 1996), even if such faces are presented subliminally (Whalen, 1998).

The amygdala has been shown to be important in numerous forms of emotional learning and evaluation. In humans, however, its role is often limited to the indirect expression of the learned emotional response (Bechara et al., 1995). For example, a classic finding is that the startle reflex response is enhanced or potentiated in the presence of negative stimuli (Grillon, Ameli, Woods, Merikangus, & Davis, 1991; Lang, Bradley, & Cuthbert, 1990). The startle potentiation is used to indirectly indicate the emotional evaluation of the stimulus. Patients with amygdala damage, in contrast to controls, do not exhibit this startle potentiation in the presence of negative stimuli (Angrilli et al., 1996). Interestingly, these patients explicitly rate these stimuli as equally arousing and negative as control subjects (Funayama et al., in press). Given the amygdala's involvement in the indirect expression of learned emotional responses coupled with the importance of learning and memory in social evaluation (see Eagly & Chaiken, 1993) suggests that the amygdala is an obvious starting point to investigate the neural systems underlying the indirect evaluation of social groups.

Using fMRI, we investigated amygdala activity in White American subjects in response to Black and White male faces with neutral expressions. In Experiment 1, the faces presented belonged to individuals who were unfamiliar to the subjects. In Experiment 2, the faces belonged to famous and positively regarded Black and White individuals. In each experiment, we also measured conscious and unconscious evaluations of racial groups. Previous research using behavioral measures with White American samples have shown stronger unconscious negative reactions to Black compared to White social groups (Dasgupta, McGhee, Greenwald, & Banaji, in press; Greenwald, McGhee, & Schwartz, 1998). To the extent that Black faces evoke greater negative emotional evaluations, we should observe greater activity in the amygdala. In particular, we measured the correlation between amygdala activity and measures of unconscious and conscious evaluation.

Results

Experiment 1

White American subjects first participated in the fMRI portion of the experiment that was described as a study about memory for faces. During image acquisition, subjects viewed pictures of Black and White unfamiliar male faces with neutral expressions taken from a college yearbook. For each face, subjects indicated if the face was the same or different than the one immediately preceding it, using a button press. After scanning, we obtained three behavioral responses, one of which was a direct (i.e., conscious) measure of racial evaluation and two of which were indirect (i.e., unconscious) measures of racial evaluation.

First, subjects took a version of the Implicit Association Test (IAT) (Greenwald et al., 1998)

to indirectly measure race bias. The term "bias" in this context refers to the presence of an indirect or noncontrollable behavioral response that exhibits preference for one group over another. It is distinguished from the colloquial use of the term "racial bias" that often implies a purposeful and conscious action of discrimination. The IAT measures the degree to which social groups (e.g., Black vs. White, old vs. young) are automatically associated with positive and negative evaluations (for a demonstration of selected IAT procedures visit www.yale.edu/implicit). Subjects categorized the same faces viewed during imaging as "Black" or "White," while simultaneously categorizing words as "good" (joy, love, peace) or "bad" (cancer, bomb, devil). The difference in response latencies to the Black + good/White + bad pairing compared to the Black + bad/White + good pairing provided the indirect measure of group evaluation. Several studies have now robustly shown negative evaluation among White Americans in the form of faster responding in the Black + bad/White + good pairings (Banaji, in press; Dasgupta et al., in press; Cunningham, Preacher, & Banaji, 2000; Greenwald et al., 1998). The IAT was followed by the Modern Racism Scale, a commonly used measure of conscious, self-reported beliefs, and attitudes toward Black Americans (McConahay, 1986).

Approximately 1 week after the IAT and Modern Racism assessments, we measured the magnitude of the eyeblink startle response to the same Black and White faces as another measure of indirect racial bias. Previous studies examining the startle response suggest that it is potentiated in the presence of negative or fearful stimuli (Lang et al., 1990) and this potentiation has been shown to be related to amygdala function (Davis, 1992; Funayama et al., in press; Angrilli et al., 1996).

Results

Performance on the IAT revealed significantly slower responses to Black + good/White + bad pairings compared to Black + bad/White +

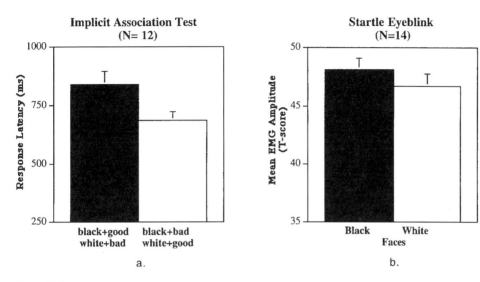

Figure 39.1
(a) Mean IAT response latency to black+good/white+bad and black+bad/white+good. (b) Mean startle eyeblink respnse (EMG amplitude) to Black and White faces.

good, $t(11) = 7.26$, $p < .001$ (see Figure 39.1a). This result is consistent with previous studies using White subjects and suggests an unconscious negative anti-Black or pro-White evaluation (Banaji, in press; Dasgupta et al., 2000; Mc-Conahay, 1986). There was a trend toward greater or potentiated startle eyeblink when viewing Black compared to White faces, $t(13) = 1.33$, $p = .10$, one-tailed (see Figure 39.1b). This pro-White race bias on the indirect measures (IAT and eyeblink startle) was in contrast to responses on the Modern Racism Scale where subjects consciously expressed pro-Black beliefs and attitudes. The average score for subjects was 1.89 (with 6 being strongly anti-Black and 1 strongly pro-Black) with a standard deviation of .66 and an effect size of -2.44 (Cohen's d).

With the imaging data, we were primarily interested in activity of the amygdala and limited our image acquisition to slices covering this region. Several previous studies assessing amygdala activity using fMRI in human subjects

(Buchel, Morris, Dolan, & Friston, 1998; LaBar, Gatenby, Gore, & Phelps, 1998; Phelps, O'Connor, et al., 1998; Whalen et al., 1998; Breiter et al., 1996) and electrophysiology in nonhuman animals (Quirk, Armony, & LeDoux, 1997; Maeda, Morimoto, & Yanagimoto, 1993; Pascoe & Kapp, 1985) have found that this region responds maximally to the onset and early presentations of a stimulus with emotional significance, including emotional faces. In light of these results, we compared early responses of the amygdala to Black and White faces. To localize responses in the amygdala we used a region-of-interest (ROI) analysis. With this ROI analysis, we assessed the strength of amygdala activity for each individual subject. This ROI analysis revealed that the majority of White subjects showed greater amygdala activation when viewing unfamiliar Black compared to White faces. These data also showed that the extent of amygdala activation to Black-versus-White faces varied across subjects. Eight subjects showed

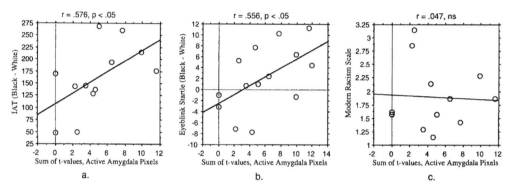

Figure 39.2
Correlations between the magnitude of amygdala activation to Black-versus-White faces as measured by the sum of the *t*-values for active amygdala pixels and behavioral measures: (a) IAT response latency for Black–White. (b) Difference in eyeblink startle response to Black-White faces, and (c) Score on the Modern Racism Scale. Similar results were obtained when magnitude of amygdala activation was assessed by counting the number of active amygdala pixels: IAT, $r = .52$, $p < .08$; startle eyeblink, $r = .54$, $p < .07$. Modern Racism Scale, ns.

greater amygdala activation in the Black-versus-White comparison than the White-versus-Black comparison. An additional four subjects showed some evidence of significant amygdala activation in the Black-versus-White comparison. As a result of this variability, a group composite analysis did not show significant amygdala activity.

We were particularly interested in this variability because it offered an opportunity to assess the relationship between activity in the amygdala and behavioral measures of race bias. There was a significant correlation between bias in response time on the IAT and strength of the amygdala activation to Black-versus-White faces (see Figure 39.2a). There was also a significant correlation between amygdala activity and the potentiation of the eyeblink startle response to Black faces (see Figure 39.2b). There was no correlation between amygdala activity and the conscious measure of racial attitudes assessed with the Modern Racism Scale (see Figure 39.2c). In addition, we correlated all three behavioral measures with the strength of amygdala activation in the White-versus-Black comparison and no tests reached statistical significance.

In order to determine the precise brain regions whose activity were most strongly related to performance on indirect measures of racial bias, composite correlation maps were generated. This technique, of generating composite images portraying regions where variability in brain activity is correlated with variability on a behavioral measure, has been previously used in PET (Hamann, Ely, Grafton, & Clinton, 1999; Cahill et al., 1996) and is conceptually similar to the selection of event types based on behavior used in event-related fMRI studies (Brewer, Zhao, Desmond, Glover, & Gabrieli, 1998; Wagner et al., 1998). On the composite image, individual subjects' activation in a region was correlated with (1) the magnitude of the IAT effect, (2) the magnitude of the startle eyeblink potentiation to Black-versus-White faces, and (3) the score on the Modern Racism Scale. The resulting correlation values (*r*) are plotted on the composite anatomical image, displaying regions where the strength of activation to Black-versus-White faces is correlated with the magnitude of the behavioral response.

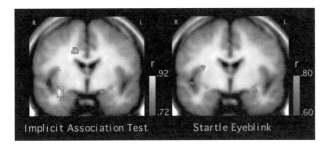

Figure 39.3
Composite correlation maps displaying regions where magnitude of activation to Black-versus-White faces is correlated with indirect behavioral measures. (left) IAT response latency Black-White, regions of significant correlation include: left superior amygdala (Talairach and Tournoux coordinates: −17.6, −5, −10.8), right amygdala extending to the inferior insula (31.7, −5, 12.2), and right anterior cingulate (14.1, −5, 36.1). (right) Eyeblink startle difference Black–White, regions of significant correlation include: left superior amygdala (−22.1, −5, −11.7) and two small regions in the right insular cortex (31.8, −5, 17.1; 41.4, −5, −2.4).

As can be seen in Figure 39.3, activation in the left amygdala is correlated with both the IAT reaction-time bias (Figure 39.3 left) and the startle eyeblink potentiation bias (Figure 39.3 right, see figure caption for all Talairach & Tournoux, 1998 coordinates). Consistent with the results from the ROI analysis, there was no region within the amygdala where activation was correlated with performance on the Modern Racism Scale. As can be seen in Figure 39.3a, there are two additional regions that were correlated with IAT reaction time bias. There was a large region of activation that extends from the right amygdala to the inferior insular cortex. The insular cortex has numerous reciprocal connections with the amygdala and is often active in tasks assessing emotional responses (Shi & Davis, 1999; Ploghaus et al., 1999). In addition, a region in the anterior cingulate was correlated with IAT performance. The anterior cingulate is thought to play a role in attentional processes and is often active in tasks where there is response competition, such as the Stroop task (Pardo, Pardo, Janer, & Raichle, 1990). As seen in Figure 39.3b, there were also two small regions within the more superior region of the insular cortex that were correlated with the magnitude of eyeblink startle potentiation to Black faces. However, the only common region of activity on the two correlation maps examining both indirect behavioral measures of racial bias was the left-superior amygdala.

Discussion
These data show for the first time that representations of social groups that differ in race evoke differential amygdala activity and that such activation is related to unconscious social evaluation. Notably, variability in amygdala activation among White subjects is correlated with negative indirect responses to Black compared to White faces on behavioral measures. Additionally, this relationship between amygdala activity and indirect measures of racial bias is in contrast to the lack of such a relationship with the direct or conscious measure of racial attitudes.

For both indirect measures, the region in the amygdala most strongly correlated with negative evaluation was the left-superior amygdala. This is of interest because this region is also known to be activated when viewing (supraliminally presented) faces with fearful versus neutral expressions (Breiter et al., 1996).

Experiment 2

We propose that the variability in the response of the amygdala to Black compared with White faces in Experiment 1 is likely to be a reflection of culturally acquired knowledge about social groups filtered through individual experience. We expected that the greater amygdala activity in response to unfamiliar Black faces is the result of a general learned negative evaluation of Black Americans (Adolphs, 1998; Fiske, 1998). If the results of Experiment 1 reflect a learned negative evaluation of the group, the pattern of results from Experiment 1 should disappear when presenting exemplars of Black Americans who are as familiar and well liked as White Americans.

To demonstrate a boundary condition on the results obtained in Experiment 1, we conducted a similar fMRI study and used the same behavioral measures with an independent group of White American subjects. However, the faces in both categorization tasks (scanning and IAT) belonged to famous and positively regarded Black and White males. The Black and White individuals portrayed were roughly equivalent in degree of fame, age, and domain of achievement.

Results

The data analysis for Experiment 2 was identical to Experiment 1. Consistent with Experiment 1, subjects consciously expressed pro-Black attitudes on the Modern Racism Scale. The average score was 1.92 with a standard deviation of .67 and an effect size of -2.35 (Cohen's d). However, unlike Experiment 1, the two indirect measures yielded different patterns of results. The IAT continued to show positive evaluation of famous White compared to famous Black faces, $t(12) = 3.61$, $p < .01$, although there was a reduction compared to Experiment 1 in the mean difference in response time between the Black + good/White + bad and Black + bad/White + good conditions. In contrast, there was no evidence of eyeblink startle potentiation to the

Black famous faces. In fact, the mean eyeblink startle response was slightly greater to the White famous faces. The continued observation of race bias on the IAT is likely to be a result of the emphasis that task places on attention to Black and White group labels in categorization, unlike the other behavioral tasks that did not require identification of the race of the face stimuli. It is clear from other research using the IAT that the particular labels that are used are critical in the evaluative effect that is produced (Mitchell, Nosek, & Banaji, 2000). By using labels that allow categorization on dimensions other than race, it is possible to elicit positive evaluations of familiar and positively regarded Black individuals. If such a task were used in the present study, we would expect no differences in evaluation of White and Black faces.

The imaging data revealed no consistent pattern of amygdala activity when White subjects viewed well-known Black and White faces. Although some subjects showed evidence of amygdala activation, this was observed equally often in the Black-versus-White and White-versus-Black comparisons. More importantly, there were no significant correlations between the indirect or direct measures of racial bias and the strength of amygdala activation for either the Black-versus-White or White-versus-Black comparisons.

Discussion

These results suggest that the amygdala's response to Black faces in White subjects is not observed when they are familiar and positively regarded. With this data, however, we cannot distinguish responses due purely to familiarity from those due to positive evaluation, independent of familiarity. In fact, these two factors may be difficult to untangle because of the documented role of familiarity in producing positive evaluation (Kunst-Wilson & Zajonc, 1980). However, there is evidence to suggest that race bias cannot be explained merely in terms of familiarity. After controlling for the effects of familiarity on the IAT test, a preference for White over Black still remains (Dasgupta et al., 2000; Ottaway, Hayden, & Oakes, in press). In addition, studies examining responses to familiar emotional scenes suggest that the presentation of familiar, negative stimuli will result in the potentiation of the startle response (Funayama et al., in press; Angrilli et al., 1996). Although we cannot rule out a role for familiarity in the differences observed between Experiments 1 and 2, previous behavioral studies suggest that the positive evaluation of the famous individuals is also a significant factor. Finally, we express caution in interpreting this null result, especially as it stands in comparison to the significant findings of Experiment 1. These were, after all, independent experiments and future research ought to test the main variable of interest in a single study.

General Discussion

These studies have shown for the first time that members of Black and White social groups can evoke differential amygdala activity and that this activity is related to unconscious social evaluation. In Experiment 1, the strength of amygdala activation to Black-versus-White faces was correlated with two indirect (unconscious) measures of race evaluation (IAT and potentiated startle), but not with the direct (conscious) expression of race attitudes. In Experiment 2, these patterns were not obtained when the faces observed belonged to familiar and positively regarded Black and White individuals. Together, these results suggest that the amygdala response to Black-versus-White faces in White subjects is a function of culturally acquired information about social groups, modified by individual knowledge and experience.

Although the present studies found that activity in the amygdala to unfamiliar Black-versus-White faces is related to indirect measures of

race bias, these results do not specify a particular behavioral function for the observed amygdala activation. The neural systems underlying racial evaluation are most likely extensive and expand beyond the amygdala. Results from previous studies showing that the amygdala is not necessary for conscious learning about the emotional nature of stimuli (Phelps, LaBar, et al., 1998; Bechara et al., 1995; LaBar, Ledoux, Spencer, & Phelps, 1995) suggest that it is not likely to play a role in the formation of conscious attitudes toward social groups. Our results indicate that the amygdala may be specifically involved in indirect or nonconscious responses to racial groups. One possible mechanism by which the amygdala may affect racial responses is suggested by studies showing its involvement in nonconsciously signaling the presence of stimuli that have acquired an emotional significance based on previous experience (Whalen, 1998; Whalen et al., 1998).

Because the combination of procedures used in these studies are novel, several caveats are in order. It is important to reaffirm that although we have obtained significant correlations between amygdala activity and indirect behavioral measures of racial bias, these data cannot speak to the issue of causality. Our own interpretation is that both amygdala activation as well as behavioral responses of race bias are reflections of social learning within a specific culture at a particular moment in the history of relations between social groups. Specifically, the influences that predict such responses (both brain and behavior) may include knowledge of cultural evaluations of social groups, personal experience with social group members, and one's own group membership.

An obvious question regarding one's own group membership as a determinant of race bias concerns the likely performance of Black subjects in these studies. Although we have yet to collect such data, we do offer a speculation. From preliminary IAT data it appears that Black Americans show more favorable evaluations of

Blacks than do White Americans. However, they do not show as strong an in-group preference as White subjects. We take this finding to show that Black American's own indirect evaluations may be determined in part by the larger culture's negative evaluation of their group (Banaji, in press). Based on the results of the present study, we expect to see less amygdala activation for Black subjects in response to Black-versus-White faces. Importantly, we expect the correlations in the data of Black subjects to mimic the data observed here. That is, the extent to which individual Black subjects show overall greater favorability toward their own group on the IAT, we expect greater relative amygdala activity to unfamiliar White compared to Black faces.

For a century, psychologists have measured attitudes toward social groups as if they existed solely in conscious form. Recent research in social cognition has shown that unconscious social evaluations, however dissociated they may be from their conscious counterparts, are robust and reliable (Fiske, 1998; Greenwald & Banaji, 1995). Unless one is socially isolated, it is not possible to avoid acquiring evaluations of social groups, just as it is not possible to avoid learning other types of general world knowledge. Having acquired such knowledge, however, does not require its conscious endorsement. Yet such evaluations can affect behavior in subtle and often unintentional ways (see Bargh & Chen, 1997; Fazio et al., 1995).

In the present studies, we have for the first time related indirect behavioral measures of social evaluation to neuronal activity. Understanding the mechanisms underlying these indirect responses can initiate discovery of the means by which they are learned and modulated. Besides the finding itself of a relationship between brain activity and behavioral race bias, such data have the potential to shift orthodox thinking about the separation of social, mental, and physical spheres. They start to reveal how social learning and evaluation are rooted in the ordinary mechanics of mind and brain.

Method

Experiment 1

Subjects
Fourteen subjects (seven female, seven male) were submitted for final analysis. A total of 20 subjects were run. All subjects gave informed consent. Six subjects were excluded because center of mass motion during scan exceeded our criterion of 0.33 pixels in any direction. There were no systematic differences observed between male and female subjects.

Stimuli
Subjects were presented photographs of nine Black and nine White male faces, with neutral facial expressions. The photographs were taken from college yearbooks. All photographs were in black and white and depicted men with short hair, no facial hair, and no distinctive clothing.

FMRI: Procedure and Parameters
Prior to image acquisition, the anterior and posterior commissures (AC and PC, respectively) were localized for slice orientation. Whole-brain sagittal T1-weighted anatomical images were acquired using a spin echo pulse sequence (5 mm contiguous slices, TE = 12 msec, TR = 600 msec, matrix size = 256 × 192, in-plane resolution = 1.56 × 1.56 mm, and FOV = 40 × 40 cm). Five 6-mm coronal slices (slice skip = 2 mm) were then prescribed perpendicular to the AC–PC line, with the middle slice centered on the amygdala. Amygdala localization was accomplished by placing the middle (third) slice 4–5 mm posterior to the AC in the midsagittal view and assessing the position of the amygdala in the subsequent coronal sections using anatomical landmarks and a standardized atlas (Talairach & Tournoux, 1998). During the study, echoplanar functional images were acquired using an asymmetric spin echo pulse sequence (TE = 30 msec, echo offset = 30 msec, TR = 1.5 sec, in-plane

resolution $= 3.125 \times 3.125$ mm, matrix size $= 128 \times 64$, and FOV $= 40 \times 20$ cm). The experimental paradigm was a standard block design consisting of six blocks of each stimulus condition, Black and White, resulting in 12 trials. During image acquisition subjects were presented pictures of nine Black and nine White unfamiliar male faces. The pictures were presented as six blocks each of Black and White faces. Each face was presented for 2 sec and each block lasted 18 sec. The face presented on any given trial was randomly selected from among the set of nine for that racial group. For each face, subjects indicated with a button press if the face was the same or different than the one immediately preceding it. During each trial, 12 images were acquired over 18 sec (TR $= 1.5$ sec). In the described analysis, subjects' functional activation was averaged across the first six images of the first three trials of each condition.

FMRI Analysis

A t test analysis was conducted on the individual subject data. Resultant t maps were generated by subtraction to reveal differential activation between conditions. Pixels showing significant differential activation ($p < .05$, uncorrected) were used in subsequent ROI and correlation analyses. For each subject, ROI analyses were performed on the amygdala. This region was first outlined on anatomical images. The functional maps of Black versus White were then superimposed on the anatomical images to identify active pixels within these regions. To determine if an individual subject showed greater amygdala activation to Black-versus-White faces, a count of significantly active amygdala pixels was conducted (t value, $p < .05$, cluster value $= 1$) for the Black-versus-White and the White-versus-Black comparisons. To calculate the correlation between a behavioral response and activation, the behavioral measure of interest was regressed on the magnitude of amygdala activity. The magnitude of amygdala activity was calculated using the sum of t values for significantly active pixels

within each ROI and also counting the number of significantly active pixels (t value, $p < .05$, cluster value $= 0$, see Constable et al., 1998 for more details). Each measure of amygdala activity was used in separate regression analyses and virtually identical results were obtained. Additional regression analyses were performed examining the White-versus-Black activation and no significant correlations were obtained.

Two types of group analyses were conducted. The first examined the overall group effect for the Black-minus-White comparison. Activation maps were generated by in-plane transformation of the individual subjects' statistical parametric maps (SPMs) and the anatomic images into a proportional three-dimensional grid defined by Talairach and Tournoux (1998). The individual activation maps were smoothed using a Gaussian filter (FWHM $= 5.2$ mm). In order to obtain p values for significantly active pixels across subjects, a contrast composite map was generated using a randomization test to create a distribution of task-related t values for each pixel (Bullmore et al., 1998), from which p values were calculated. The p value for each pixel was overlaid upon a mean anatomic image.

The second group analysis generated composite correlation maps designed to determine the pixels for which Black–White activation magnitude was correlated with behavioral performance. The SPMs and the anatomic images for the 12 individual subjects who had valid IAT results were transformed by in-plane transformation into a proportional three-dimensional grid defined by Talairach and Tournoux (1998). The individual activation maps were smoothed using a Gaussian filter (FWHM $= 5.2$ mm). For each pixel, the subjects' Black-minus-White t values were correlated with the (1) difference in response latency on the IAT, (2) eyeblink startle difference to Black-versus-White faces, and (3) score on the Modern Racism Scale. The r value for each pixel was overlaid upon a mean anatomic image. Only significantly correlated pixels are displayed.

IAT

Subjects were asked to categorize the same faces they viewed during imaging as Black or White, while simultaneously categorizing words as good (joy, love, peace) or bad (cancer, bomb, devil). For half of the trials, subjects were asked to press a right button if the stimulus was either a White face or a good word and a left button if the stimulus was either a Black face or a bad word. For the remaining half of the trials, the pairings were reversed. The two conditions were counterbalanced. The difference in speed to respond to the Black + good/White + bad pairing compared to the Black + bad/White + good pairing provided the indirect measure of group evaluation. Some subjects were given the IAT immediately after scanning and others were given the test a week later. There was no difference in IAT performance related to the timing of the test. Two subjects were dropped from the IAT analyses; the first because of an unusually high error rate in categorization (28%), the second because of an error in the IAT program that resulted in the subject receiving only stimuli corresponding to the left key in the second half of the Black + good categorization condition.

Eyeblink Startle

The startle response is a defensive reflex, one component of which is an eyeblink response (Lang et al., 1990; Knorkski, 1967). Using electromyogram (EMG) to measure responses of the muscles below the eye, we assessed the magnitude of the eyeblink response as an indication of startle in the presence of the Black and White faces. The startle stimulus was a 50-msec burst of 100-dB white noise that was delivered through headphones. There were six habituation trials to the startle stimulus alone. All 18 faces were presented for 6 sec each. Startle eyeblink was assessed during the presentation of six White and six Black faces. The startle probes occurred 2 to 4 sec following stimulus onset. The eyeblink component of subjects' startle response was measured by EMG (BioPac Systems) and stored off-

line for later analysis. Two Ag–AgCl electrodes were placed on the skin over the orbicularis oculi muscle under subjects' left eye. A reference electrode was placed behind subjects' left ear. Prior to analysis, the raw EMG signal was fully rectified, followed by a 10-Hz, two-pole, low-pass filter. The signal was fully integrated and a running value of the area under the curve was calculated. An eyeblink was defined as the difference between the preblink baseline, taken as the mean EMG activity in the 50-msec prior to the startle probe, and the peak amplitude occurring 120 msec following the startle probe. Subjects' EMG amplitudes were standardized (t scores = $z(10) +$ 50) before analysis due to large between-subject differences in baseline eyeblink amplitude.

Modern Racism Scale

The Modern Racism Scale is a commonly used measure of conscious, self-reported beliefs and attitudes toward Black Americans. Examples of items are: "Discrimination against Blacks is no longer a problem in the United States"; "It is easy to understand the anger of Black people in America." Scores on a six-point scale asking for agreement or disagreement with items were computed, with lower scores representing pro-Black and larger scores representing anti-Black beliefs and attitudes. This scale is a standard measure of attitudes and beliefs about the current status and rights of Black Americans and does not tap purely evaluative responses toward the group.

Experiment 2

Subjects

Thirteen subjects (six female, seven male) were submitted to final analysis. A total of 26 subjects were run. All subjects gave informed consent. Thirteen subjects were excluded because center of mass motion during scanning exceeded our criterion of 0.33 pixels in any direction. There were no systematic differences observed between the male and female subjects and these data were combined.

Stimuli

The Black individuals whose faces were portrayed were Muhammad Ali, Arsenio Hall, Bill Cosby, Magic Johnson, Michael Jordan, Martin Luther King Jr., Colin Powell, Will Smith, and Denzel Washington. The White individuals were Larry Bird, Conan O'Brian, Tom Cruise, Harrison Ford, John F. Kennedy, Mark McGwire, Joe Namath, Norman Schwartzkopf, and Jerry Seinfeld. The photographs were taken from published books and the Internet. All photos were in black and white. All of the photographs were of the face and neck only with a frontal view and neutral facial expressions.

Procedures

The procedures and analysis were identical to Experiment 1.

Acknowledgments

We thank David Armor, R. Bhaskar, John Bargh, Siri Carpenter, Geoffrey Cohen, Michael Davis, Thierry Devos, Anthony Greenwald, Richard Hackman, Kristin Lane, Kristi Lemm, Joseph LeDoux, Jeansok Kim, Kevin LaBar, Matthew Lieberman, Brian Nosek, Kevin Ochsner, and Scott Yancey for helpful comments. We especially thank Adam Anderson for suggesting the fMRI composite analysis technique and Pawel Skudlarski for developing the techniques. This research was supported by grants from the McDonnell Foundation (97-26 to EAP), the National Science Foundation (SBR 97099324 to MRB), the National Institute of Mental Health (MH57672 to MRB), and National Institute of Health (NS3332 to JCG).

References

Adolphs, R. A. (1998). The human amygdala in social judgment. *Nature,* 393, 470–474.

Adolphs, R., Tranel, D., Hamann, S., Young, A. W., Calder, A. J., Phelps, E. A., Anderson, A., Lee, G. P., & Damasio, A. R. (1999). Recognition of facial emotion in nine individuals with bilateral amygdala damage. *Neuropsychologia,* 37, 1111–1117.

Angrilli, A., Mauri, A., Palomba, D., Flor, H., Birbaumer, N., Sartori, G., & di Paola, F. (1996). Startle reflex and emotion modulation impairment after a right amygdala lesion. *Brain,* 119, 1991–2000.

Banaji, M. R. (in press). Implicit attitudes can be measured. In H. L. Roediger, III, J. S. Nairne, I. Neath, & A. Surprenant (Eds.), *The nature of remembering: Essays in honor of Robert G. Crowder.* Washington, DC: American Psychological Association.

Bargh, J. A., & Chen, M. (1997). Nonconscious behavioral confirmation processes: The self-fulfilling consequences of automatic stereotype activation. *Journal of Experimental Social Psychology,* 33, 541–560.

Bechara, A., Tranel, D., Damasio, H., Adolphs, R., Rockland, C., & Damasio, A. R. (1995). Double dissociation of conditioning and declarative knowledge relative to the amygdala and hippocampus in humans. *Science,* 269, 1115–1118.

Biernat, M., & Crandall, C. S. (1999). Racial attitudes. In J. P. Robinson, P. H. Shaver, & L. S. Wrightsman (Eds.), *Measures of political attitudes* (pp. 291–412). San Diego: Academic Press.

Breiter, H. C., Etcoff, N. L., Whalen, P. J., Kennedy, W. A., Rauch, S. L., Buckner, R. L., Strauss, M. M., Hyman, S., & Rosen, B. (1996). Response and habituation of the human amygdala during visual processing of facial expression. *Neuron,* 17, 875–887.

Brewer, J. B., Zhao, Z., Desmond, J. E., Glover, G. H., & Gabrieli, J. D. E. (1998). Marking memories: Brain activity that predicts how well visual experience will be remembered. *Science,* 281, 1185–1187.

Buchel, C., Morris, J., Dolan, R. J., & Friston, K. J. (1998). Brain systems mediating aversive conditioning: An event-related fMRI study. *Neuron,* 20, 947–957.

Bullmore, E., Brammer, M., Williams, S. C., Rabe-Hesketh, S., Janot, N., David, A., Mellers, J., Howard, R., & Sham, P. (1998). Statistical methods of estimation and interference for functional MR image analysis. *Magnetic Resonance in Medicine,* 35, 261–277.

Cahill, L., Haier, R. J., Fallon, J., Alkire, M. T., Tang, C., Keator, D., Wu, J., & McGaugh, J. L. (1996). Amygdala activity at encoding correlated with long-term, free recall of emotional information. *Proceedings* of the National Academy of Sciences, U.S.A., 93, 8016–8021.

Constable, R. T., Skudlarski, P., Mencl, E., Pugh, K. R., Fulbright, R. K., Lacadie, C., Shaywitz, S. E., & Shaywitz, B. A. (1998). Quantifying and comparing region-of-interest activation patterns in functional brain imaging: Methodology considerations. *Magnetic Resonance Imaging*, 16, 289–300.

Cunningham, W. A., Nezlek, J. B., & Banaji, M. R. (2000). *Conscious and unconscious ethnocentrism: Revisting the ideologies of prejudice*. Unpublished manuscript: Yale University.

Cunningham, W. A., Preacher, K. J., & Banaji, M. R. (2000). *Psychometric properties of implicit attitude measures: Inter-item consistency, stability, and convergent validity*. Unpublished manuscript: Yale University.

Dasgupta, N., McGhee, D. E., Greenwald, A. G., & Banaji, M. R. (2000). Automatic preference for White-Americans: Eliminating the familiarity explanation. *Journal of Experimental Social Psychology*, 36, 316–328.

Davis, M. (1992). The role of the amygdala in conditioned fear. In J. P. Aggleton (Ed.), *The amygdala: Neurobiological aspects of emotion, memory, and mental dysfunction* (255–306). New York: Wiley.

Davis, M. (1997). Neurobiology of fear responses: The role of the amygdala. *Journal of Neuropsychiatry and Clinical Neurology*, 9, 382–402.

Devine, P. G. (1989). Stereotypes and prejudice: Their automatic and controlled components. *Journal of Personality and Social Psychology*, 56, 680–690.

Dovidio, J. F., Kawakami, K., Johnson, C., Johnson, B., & Howard, A. (1997). On the nature of prejudice: Automatic and controlled processes. *Journal of Experimental Social Psychology*, 33, 510–540.

Eagly, A. H., & Chaiken, S. (1993). *The psychology of attitudes*. Fort Worth, TX: Harcourt.

Fazio, R. H., Jackson, J. R., Dunton, B. C., & Williams, C. J. (1995). Variability in automatic activation as an unobtrusive measure of racial attitudes: A bona fide pipeline? *Journal of Personality and Social Psychology*, 69, 1013–1027.

Fiske, S. T. (1998). Stereotyping, prejudice, and discrimination. In D. T. Gilbert, S. T. Fiske, & G. Lindzey (Eds.), *The handbook of social psychology* (vol. 2, pp. 357–411). New York: Oxford University Press.

Fiske, S. T., & Taylor, S. E. (1991). *Social Cognition* (2nd ed.). New York: McGraw-Hill.

Funayama, E. S., Grillon, C. G., Davis, M., & Phelps, E. A. (in press). A double dissociation in the affective modulation of startle in humans: Effects of unilateral temporal lobectomy. *Journal of Cognitive Neuroscience*.

Greenwald, A. G., & Banaji, M. R. (1995). Implicit social cognition: Attitudes, self-esteem, and stereotypes. *Psychological Review*, 102, 4–27.

Greenwald, A. G., McGhee, J. L., & Schwartz, J. L. (1998). Measuring individual differences in social cognition: The Implicit Association Test. *Journal of Personality and Social Psychology*, 74, 1464–1480.

Grillon, C., Ameli, R., Woods, S. W., Merikangus, K., & Davis, M. (1991). Fear-potentiated startle in humans: Effects of anticipatory anxiety on the acoustic blink reflex. *Pscyhophysiology*, 28, 588–595.

Hamann, S. B., Ely, T. D., Grafton, S. T., & Clinton, D. K. (1999). Amygdala activity related of enhanced memory for pleasant and aversive stimuli. *Nature Neuroscience*, 2, 289–293.

Kapp, B. S., Pascoe, J. P., & Bixler, M. A. (1984). The amygdala: A neuroanatomical systems approach to its contribution to aversive conditioning. In N. Butters & L. S. Squire (Eds.), *The neuropsychology of memory* (473–488). New York: Guilford Press.

Kling, A. S., & Brothers, L. A. (1992). The amygdala and social behavior. In J. P. Aggleton (Ed.), *The amygdala: Neurobiological aspects of emotion, memory, and mental dysfunction* (pp. 255–306). New York: Wiley.

Knorkski, J. (1967). *Integrative activity of the brain: An interdisciplinary approach*. Chicago: University of Chicago Press.

Kunst-Wilson, W. R., & Zajonc, R. B. (1980). Affective discrimination of stimuli that cannot be recognized. *Science*, 207, 557–558.

LaBar, K. S., Gatenby, C., Gore, J. C., LeDoux, J. E., & Phelps, E. A. (1998). Amygdolo-cortical activation during conditioned fear acquisition and extinction: A mixed trial fMRI study. *Neuron*, 20, 937–945.

LaBar, K. S., LeDoux, J. E., Spencer, D. D., & Phelps, E. A. (1995). Impaired fear conditioning following unilateral temporal lobectomy in humans. *Journal of Neuroscience*, 15, 6846–6855.

Lang, P. J., Bradley, M. M., & Cuthbert, B. N. (1990). Emotion, attention, and the startle reflex. *Psychological Review, 97,* 377–395.

LeDoux, J. E. (1996). *The emotional brain.* New York: Simon & Schuster.

Maeda, H., Morimoto, H., & Yanagimoto, K. (1993). Response charactersitics of amygdaloid neurons provoked by emotionally significant environmental stimuli in cats, with special reference to response durations. *Canadian Journal of Physiology and Pharmacology, 7,* 374–378.

McConahay, J. P. (1986). Modern racism, ambivalence, and the Modern Racism Scale. In J. F. Dovidio & S. L. Gaertner (Eds.), *Prejudice, discrimintion, and racism* (pp. 91–125). Orlando: Academic Press.

Mitchell, J., Nosek, B. A., & Banaji, M. R. (2000). *Category salience determines implicit attitudes toward black females and white male targets.* Nashville, TN: Society of Personality and Social Psychology.

Nosek, B. A., Cunningham, W. A., Banaji, M. R., & Greenwald, A. G. (2000). *Measuring implicit attitudes on the Internet.* Nashville, TN: Society for Personality and Social Psychology.

Ottaway, S. A., Hayden, D. C., & Oakes, M. A. (in press). Implicit attitudes and racism: The effects of word familiarity and frequency in the Implicit Association Test. *Social Cognition.*

Pardo, J. V., Pardo, P. J., Janer, K. W., & Raichle, M. E. (1990). The anterior cingulate cortex mediates processing selection in the Stroop attentional conflict paradigm. *Proccedings of the National Academy of Sciences, U.S.A., 87,* 256–259.

Pascoe, J. P., & Kapp, B. S. (1985). Electrophysiological characteristics of amygdaloid central nucleus neurons during Pavlovian conditioning in the rabbit. *Behavioral Brain Research, 16,* 117–133.

Phelps, E. A., & Anderson, A. K. (1997). Emotional memory: What does the amygdala do? *Current Biology, 7,* 311–314.

Phelps, E. A., LaBar, K. S., Anderson, A. K., O'Connor, K. J., Fulbright, R. K., & Spencer, D. S. (1998). Specifying the contributions of the human amygdala to emotional memory: A case study. *Neurocase, 4,* 527–540.

Phelps, E. A., O'Connor, K. J., Gatenby, J. C., Anderson, A. K., Grillon, C., Davis, M., & Gore, J. C. (1998). Activation of the human amygdala by a cogni-

tive representation of fear. *Society for Neuroscience Abstracts, 24,* 1524.

Ploghaus, A., Tracey, I., Gati, J. S., Clare, S., Menon, R. S., Matthews, P. M., Rawlins, J., & Nicholas, P. (1999). Dissociating pain from its anticipation in the human brain. *Science, 284,* 1979–1981.

Quirk, G. J., Armony, J. L., & LeDoux, J. E. (1997). Fear conditioning enhances different temporal components of tone evodek spike trains in auditory cortex and lateral amygdala. *Neuron, 19,* 1029–1039.

Schuman, H., Steeh, C., & Bobo, L. (1997). *Racial attitudes in America: Trends and interpretations.* Cambridge: Harvard University Press.

Shi, C. J., & Davis, M. (1999). Pain pathways involved in fear conditioning measured with fear-potentiated startle: Lesion studies. *Journal of Neuroscience, 19,* 420–430.

Talairach, J., & Tournoux, P. (1998). *Co-planar stereotaxic atlas of the human brain: 3-dimensional proportional system: An approach to cerebral imaging.* New York: Thieme.

Wagner, A. D., Schacter, D. L., Rotte, N., Koutstaal, W., Maril, A., Dale, A. M., Rosen, B. R., & Buckner, R. L. (1998). Building memories: Remembering and forgetting of verbal experiences as predicted by brain activity. *Science, 281,* 1188–1191.

Whalen, P. J. (1998). Fear, vigilance, and ambiguity: Initial neuroimaging studies of the human amygdala. *Current Directions in Psychological Science, 7,* 177–188.

Whalen, P. J., Rauch, S. L., Etcoff, N. L., McInerney, S. C., Lee, M. B., & Jenike, M. A. (1998). Masked presentations of emotional facial expressions modulate amygdala activity without explicit knowledge. *Journal of Neuroscience, 18,* 411–418.

40

Deciding Advantageously before Knowing the Advantageous Strategy

Antoine Bechara, Hanna Damasio, Daniel Tranel, and Antonio R. Damasio

In a gambling task that simulates real-life decision-making in the way it factors uncertainty, rewards, and penalties, the players are given four decks of cards, a loan of $2000 facsimile U.S. bills, and asked to play so that they can lose the least amount of money and win the most (1). Turning each card carries an immediate reward ($100 in decks A and B and $50 in decks C and D). Unpredictably, however, the turning of some cards also carries a penalty (which is large in decks A and B and small in decks C and D). Playing mostly from the disadvantageous decks (A and B) leads to an overall loss. Playing from the advantageous decks (C and D) leads to an overall gain. The players have no way of predicting when a penalty will arise in a given deck, no way to calculate with precision the net gain or loss from each deck, and no knowledge of how many cards they must turn to end the game (the game is stopped after 100 card selections). After encountering a few losses, normal participants begin to generate SCRs before selecting a card from the bad decks (2) and also begin to avoid the decks with large losses (1). Patients with bilateral damage to the ventromedial prefrontal cortices do neither (1, 2).

To investigate whether subjects choose correctly only after or before conceptualizing the nature of the game and reasoning over the pertinent knowledge, we continuously assessed, during their performance of the task, three lines of processing in 10 normal participants and in 6 patients (3) with bilateral damage of the ventromedial sector of the prefrontal cortex and decision-making defects. These included (i) behavioral performance, that is, the number of cards selected from the good decks versus the bad decks; (ii) SCRs generated before the selection of each card (2); and (iii) the subject's account of how they conceptualized the game and of the strategy they were using. The latter was assessed by interrupting the game briefly after

each subject had made 20 card turns and had already encountered penalties, and asking the subject two questions: (i) "Tell me all you know about what is going on in this game." (ii) "Tell me how you feel about this game." The questions were repeated at 10-card intervals and the responses audiotaped.

After sampling all four decks, and before encountering any losses, subjects preferred decks A and B and did not generate significant anticipatory SCRs. We called this period pre-punishment. After encountering a few losses in decks A or B (usually by card 10), normal participants began to generate anticipatory SCRs to decks A and B. Yet by card 20, all indicated that they did not have a clue about what was going on. We called this period pre-hunch (Fig. 40.1). By about card 50, all normal participants began to express a "hunch" that decks A and B were riskier and all generated anticipatory SCRs whenever they pondered a choice from deck A or B. We called this period hunch. None of the patients generated anticipatory SCRs or expressed a "hunch" (Fig. 40.1). By card 80, many normal participants expressed knowledge about why, in the long run, decks A and B were bad and decks C and D were good. We called this period conceptual. Seven of the 10 normal participants reached the conceptual period, during which they continued to avoid the bad decks, and continued to generate SCRs whenever they considered sampling again from the bad decks. Remarkably, the three normal participants who did not reach the conceptual period still made advantageous choices (4). Just as remarkably, the three patients with prefrontal damage who reached the conceptual period and correctly described which were the bad and good decks chose disadvantageously. None of the patients generated anticipatory SCRs (Fig. 40.1). Thus, despite an accurate account of the task and of the correct strategy, these patients failed to generate autonomic responses and

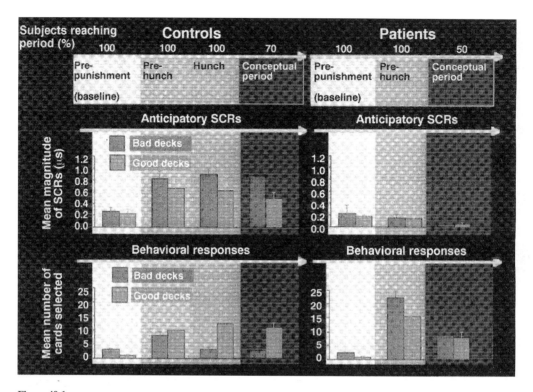

Figure 40.1
Presentation of the four periods in terms of average numbers of cards selected from the bad decks (A and B) versus the good decks (C and D), and the mean magnitudes of anticipatory SCRs associated with the same cards. The pre-punishment period covered the start of the game when subjects sampled the decks and before they encountered the first loss (that is, up to about the 10th card selection). The pre-hunch period consisted of the next series of cards when subjects continued to choose cards from various decks, but professed no notion of what was happening in the game (on average, between the 10th (range: 7–13) and 50th card (range: 30–60) in normals, or between the 9th (3–10) and 80th (60–90) in patients. The hunch period (never reached in patients) corresponded to the period when subjects reported "liking" or "disliking" certain decks, and "guessed" which decks were risky or safe, but were not sure of their answers [on average, between the 50th (30–60) and 80th card (60–90) in normals]. The conceptual period corresponded to the period when subjects were able to articulate accurately the nature of the task and tell for certain which were the good and bad decks, and why they were good or bad [on average, after the 80th card (60–90) in both normals and patients]. (Top panels) Bars represent means ($\pm$ SEM) of the mean magnitude of anticipatory SCRs generated before the selection of cards from the bad decks versus the good decks. Anticipatory SCRs are generated in the time window before turning a card from any given deck, that is, during the time the subject ponders from which deck to choose (2). SCRs in association with the good and bad decks from normal controls or patients were not significantly different during the pre-punishment (baseline) period. However, there was a significant increase in the magnitude of these SCRs during the pre-hunch period, but only for normal controls. During the next two periods, SCR activity in normal subjects was sustained in the case of the bad decks, but it began to subside in the case of the good decks (8). (Bottom panels) Bars in the "Behavioral responses" plots represent means ($\pm$ SEM) of the mean number of cards selected from the bad decks versus those selected from the good decks. Normal controls selected more cards from the good decks during the pre-hunch, hunch, and conceptual periods. In contrast, prefrontal patients selected more cards from the bad decks during these periods (9).

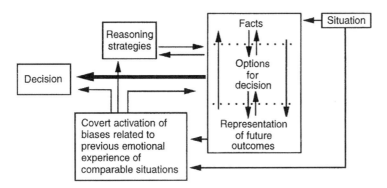

Figure 40.2
Diagram of the proposed steps involved in decision-making.

continued to select cards from the bad decks. The patients failed to act according to their correct conceptual knowledge.

On the basis of these results, we suggest that the sensory representation of a situation that requires a decision leads to two largely parallel but interacting chains of events (Fig. 40.2). In one, either the sensory representation of the situation or of the facts evoked by it activate neural systems that hold nondeclarative dispositional knowledge related to the individual's previous emotional experience of similar situations (5). The ventromedial frontal cortices are among the structures that we suspect hold such dispositional knowledge, the activation of which, in turn, activates autonomic and neurotransmitter nuclei (such as those that deliver dopamine to selected cortical and subcortical forebrain regions), among other regions. The ensuing nonconscious signals then act as covert biases on the circuits that support processes of cognitive evaluation and reasoning (6). In the other chain of events, the representation of the situation generates (i) the overt recall of pertinent facts, for example, various response options and future outcomes pertaining to a given course of action; and (ii) the application of reasoning strategies to facts and options. Our experiment indicates that in normal participants, the activation of covert

biases preceded overt reasoning on the available facts. Subsequently, the covert biases may have assisted the reasoning process in cooperative manner, that is, biases would not decide per se, but rather facilitate the efficient processing of knowledge and logic necessary for conscious decisions (7). We suspect that the autonomic responses we detected are evidence for a complex process of nonconscious signaling, which reflects access to records of previous individual experience—specifically, of records shaped by reward, punishment, and the emotional state that attends them. In this light, damage to ventromedial cortices acts by precluding access to a particular kind of record of previous and related individual experience.

References and Notes

1. A. Bechara, A. R. Damasio, H. Damasio, S. W. Anderson, *Cognition* 50, 7 (1994).

2. A. Bechara, D. Tranel, H. Damasio, A. R. Damasio, *Cereb. Cortex* 6, 215 (1996).

3. The patients who participated in the experiment were drawn from the Division of Cognitive Neuroscience's Patient Registry and have been described previously (1, 2). Three are female (ages 53, 63, and 64), and three are male (ages 51, 52, and 65). All have stable focal lesions. Years of education: 13 ± 2

(mean ± SEM); verbal IQ: 111 ± 8 (mean ± SEM); performance IQ: 102 ± 8 (mean ± SEM).

4. The results in this group of normal participants are similar to the results described previously in other normal participants (2).

5. A. R. Damasio, *Descartes' Error: Emotion, Reason, and the Human Brain* (Grosset/Putnam, New York, 1994).

6. We envision these biases to act as markers or qualifiers in the manner suggested by A. Damasio [in (5), chap. 8] and by A. R. Damasio, D. Tranel, and H. Damasio [in *Frontal Lobe Function and Dysfunction*, H. S. Levin, H. M. Eisenberg, A. L. Benton, Eds. (Oxford Univ. Press, New York, 1991), pp. 217]. See also P. R. Montague, P. Dayan, C. Person, T. J. Sejnowski, *Nature* 377, 725 (1995). This action might occur both at the cortical level and in subcortical structures such as basal ganglia.

7. On the basis of a series of related studies [A. Bechara, D. Tranel, H. Damasio, S. W. Anderson, A. R. Damasio, *Soc. Neurosci. Abstr.* 21, 1210 (1995); D. Tranel, A. Bechara, H. Damasio, A. R. Damasio, *ibid.* 22, 1108 (1996)], we believe that the bias mechanism identified here is distinct from other neural mechanisms whose integrity is crucial for decision-making. Such mechanisms include response inhibition [J. M. Fuster, *The Prefrontal Cortex: Anatomy, Physiology, and Neuropsychology of the Frontal Lobe* (Raven, New York, ed. 3, 1996); R. Dias, T. W. Robbins, A. C. Roberts, *Nature* 380, 69 (1996); A. Diamond, in *The Development and Neural Bases of Higher Cognitive Functions*, A. Diamond, Ed. (New York Academy of Sciences, New York, 1990), vol. 608, pp. 637–669], working memory [P. S. Goldman-Rakic, in *Handbook of Physiology; The Nervous System*, F. Plum, Ed. (American Physiological Society, Bethesda, MD, 1987), vol. 5, pp. 373–401], and selective attention [M. I. Posner and S. Dehaene, *Trends Neurosci.* 17, 75 (1994)]. In other words, we propose an addition to mechanisms already recognized as necessary for proper reasoning rather than an alternative to those mechanisms.

8. A three-way analysis of variance (ANOVA) on the anticipatory SCRs generated by normal participants and patients (between group), during the pre-punishment and pre-hunch periods (within group), and in association with the bad and good decks (within group) revealed, most importantly, a significant two-way interaction of group with period [$F(1, 14) = 16.24$, $P < 0.001$]. Subsequent Newman-Keuls tests on these SCRs revealed that, during the pre-punishment (baseline) period, the SCRs associated with the good or bad decks of normals or patients were not significantly different. However, there was a significant increase in the magnitude of these SCRs during the pre-hunch period, relative to the pre-punishment period, but only for normals ($P < 0.01$). The SCRs from normals during pre-hunch were also significantly higher than the SCRs of patients during both pre-punishment and pre-hunch ($P < 0.01$). Because all normals generated anticipatory SCRs, whereas all patients did not, Fisher's exact test, based on the hypergeometric distribution, yielded a one-sided $P < 0.001$. SCRs from normals who selected cards from the bad decks during the hunch period were compared to the SCRs associated with sampling the good decks. The same comparisons of SCRs were done for the conceptual period. Although SCRs from the bad decks during the hunch or the conceptual period were generally higher than those from the good decks, the difference did not reach statistical significance. However, Newman-Keuls tests comparing SCRs from the hunch or the conceptual period to those from the pre-punishment period revealed significant differences in the case of the bad decks ($P < 0.01$) but not the good decks. This suggests that SCR activity was sustained in the case of the bad decks, but may have been subsiding in the case of the good decks.

9. A similar ANOVA in which mean number of cards selected was used instead of SCRs revealed, most importantly, a significant three-way interaction of group with period with decks [$F(1, 14) = 6.9$, $P < 0.02$]. With subsequent Newman-Keuls tests, the most relevant comparison was that patients selected significantly more cards from the bad decks relative to the good decks during the pre-hunch period ($P < 0.01$). By contrast, controls selected more from the good decks relative to the bad decks (the difference was not statistically significant). During the hunch and conceptual periods, controls selected significantly more cards from the good decks relative to the bad decks ($P < 0.01$). By contrast, patients still selected more cards from the bad decks relative to the good decks during the conceptual period (the difference was not statistically significant).

Supported by the National Institute of Neurological Diseases and Stroke grant PO1 NS19632.

41

Do Amnesics Exhibit Cognitive Dissonance Reduction? The Role of Explicit Memory and Attention in Attitude Change

Matthew D. Lieberman, Kevin N. Ochsner, Daniel T. Gilbert, and Daniel L. Schacter

A fox saw some ripe black grapes hanging from a trellised vine. He resorted to all his tricks to get at them, but wearied himself in vain, for he could not reach them. At last he turned away, hiding his disappointment and saying: "The grapes are sour, and not ripe as I thought."
—Aesop (trans. 1961, p. 100)

When a person responds to disappointments in the same fashion as Aesop's fox, revising his or her attitudes to fit with the current circumstances, other people may doubt the sincerity of the person's new beliefs and may be tempted to think of this change as rationalization or self-deception. If the grapes were suddenly available, the fox might not pass over them for being sour. The research we report here, however, suggests that such conventional wisdom may be wrong, that the grapes may indeed continue to be unappealing even if the memory that they were once unobtainable is completely removed. In this chapter, we present two experiments suggesting that the incongruency between one's attitudes and behaviors can automatically result in real changes in those attitudes. Such behavior-induced attitude changes may require minimal conscious effort and may endure without memory for the behavior that induced them.

Although rhetoricians since Aristotle have been interested in how and why people change their minds, scientific research on attitude change began in earnest only after the Second World War (Asch, 1956; Hovland, Janis, & Kelley, 1953; see Jones, 1998). Although much was learned about the conditions that elicit attitude change, only in the past two decades have psychologists become invested in understanding the information processing mechanisms that underlie it (Chaiken, Liberman, & Eagly, 1989; Petty & Cacioppo, 1986).

In the current analysis, we focus on the role of conscious reasoning in behavior-induced attitude change (i.e., changing an attitude to fit with recent behavior). We consider conscious reasoning to be composed largely of the attentional operations of working memory and the contents of explicit memory (O'Reilly, Braver, & Cohen, 1997). In two experiments, we examined the role of these two components by severely degrading their contributions to the process of attitude change.

Conscious Content: The Role of Explicit Memory

Explicit memory refers to one's ability to consciously recollect past events, behaviors, and experiences (Schacter, Chiu, & Ochsner, 1993) and thus is a central component of most social abilities. Indeed, people's memory for the identities and actions of other people and themselves forms the adhesive that gives them a continuing sense of place in their social world. Revising personal attitudes and beliefs in response to a counterattitudinal behavior naturally seems to depend on retrospective capacities. If Aesop's forlorn lover of grapes could not remember that the grapes were out of reach, he would have no reason to persuade himself of their reduced quality.

Current Models of Attitude Change

Explicit memory plays an important role in the dominant models of behavior-induced attitude change. Festinger's (1957) theory of cognitive dissonance posits that when a person's actions and attitudes are discrepant, physiological arousal results, leading to psychological discomfort, which in turn motivates the person to restore harmony between his or her attitudes and behavior by altering the attitudes to fit the behavior. For example, in Brehm's (1956) free-choice paradigm, women were asked to rate how much they liked a set of eight appliances.

The experimenter then asked each participant to choose which of two appliances she preferred to take home as compensation for participation. After making a difficult choice between two appliances that they had rated nearly equally, participants were asked to rate the eight items again. In the final ratings, participants rated the chosen item higher, and the rejected item lower, than they had in their original ratings. In essence, participants spread the difference in desirability between the chosen and rejected items.

Dissonance theory explains attitude change in the free-choice paradigm in terms of the arousal caused by making a decision that does not logically follow from the participant's initial ratings. Presumably, this arousal leads to increasing psychological discomfort, which draws attention. Once noticed, the discomfort is attributed back to the discrepancy between the counterattitudinal behavior and the initial attitude. Motivated reasoning ensues and alters the participant's attitudes toward the chosen and rejected items so that the attitudes and behavior become consonant. Explicit memory is implicated in this account at the point when an attribution of the psychological discomfort to the counterattitudinal behavior occurs. In short, the behavior must be remembered in order for it to be an attributional target.

The major alternative to dissonance theory, Bem's (1965) self-perception theory, also relies on explicit memory. According to self-perception theory, people infer their own attitudes the same way they infer the attitudes of others, namely, by observing their own behavior. Asked to report their attitudes toward the appliances, Brehm's participants presumably constructed new attitudes based on the most accessible information, their recent behavior. In order to do this, they needed to have explicit memory for that behavior.

Anterograde Amnesia

A strong test of whether explicit memory is involved in behavior-induced attitude change would require that individuals perform a counterattitudinal behavior and then completely forget it soon afterward. Patients with anterograde amnesia constitute a neuropsychological population that is likely to do exactly that. This form of amnesia results from either hippocampal or diencephalic damage, and greatly reduces or even eliminates the ability to form new memories that can be consciously retrieved (Squire, 1992). Any information currently held in mind is lost quickly upon distraction. Amnesic patients should not exhibit behavior-induced attitude change if explicit memory is required for it to occur.

Experiment 1

We tested 12 amnesic patients and 12 age-matched adults using Gerard and White's (1983) modified version of Brehm's (1956) free-choice paradigm. All tasks were completed in a single testing session that was divided into four phases. In Phase 1, participants examined two sets of 15 art prints and ranked each set, from most liked to least liked. In Phase 2, participants were shown six groups of two pairs of prints, and indicated for each group which pair they would prefer to hang in their home. For one of the groups, one pair comprised the 4th- and 10th-ranked prints from one of the sets used in Phase 1, and the other pair comprised the 6th- and 12th-ranked prints from the same set. In Phase 3, participants were required to rerank the two sets of prints from Phase 1 to reflect their current liking of them. In Phase 4, participants were shown the prints and asked to identify the 4 prints that constituted the two critical pairs that were used in Phase 2. The participants were then asked to identify each of the 4 prints as having been chosen or rejected in Phase 2.

The primary measures were (a) the average change in ranks of the selected and rejected pairs between Phases 1 and 3 and (b) in Phase 4, how accurately participants could identify the prints they had chosen in Phase 2.

Table 41.1
Patient characteristics

Patient group	Age	WAIS-R IQ	WMS-R score				
			Attention	Verbal	Visual	General	Delayed
Medial							
Temporal							
AB	59	105	92	72	96	76	50
PD	61	109	89	72	73	65	61
RL	69	103	93	70	75	68	66
JM	49	89	95	84	56	70	52
PS	40	95	115	89	95	90	<50
SS	71	126	114	104	100	102	<50
Korsakoff's							
PB	72	87	93	77	94	82	60
RD	68	83	99	75	75	82	50
RG	80	94	104	58	82	61	66
WR	70	88	96	78	85	76	53
WK	57	94	93	63	78	59	57
RM	78	112	95	88	100	90	68
Mean	64.5	98.8	98.2	77.5	84.0	76.8	59.4

Note. WAIS-R = Wechsler Adult Intelligence Scale, Revised; WMS-R = Wechsler Memory Scale, Revised. The WAIS-R and the five WMS-R indices yield a mean of 100 and a standard deviation of 15 in the normal population. The WMS-R does not provide numerical scores for participants who score below 50. Therefore, such values were scored as 50 for computing means.

Method

Participants

Participants were 12 amnesic patients (9 men and 3 women; for patients' characteristics, see Table 41.1) and 12 control participants (8 men and 4 women). They were matched for age (for control participants, $M = 61.7$, range: 43–73; for amnesics, $M = 64.5$, range: 40–80) and years of education (for control participants, $M = 12.9$ years, range: 8–17; for amnesics, $M = 14.2$ years, range: 7–20).

Procedure

When participants entered the testing room, they were informed that they would be completing some tasks that would allow the experimenter to assess their verbal skills and their aesthetic preferences. In Phase 1, they were given a stack of 15 art prints measuring 3 in. by 5 in. and were asked to rank them in order of preference. A sorting board was placed in front of each participant to help him or her in sorting the cards while making the rankings. Participants sorted a set of 15 cards that reproduced paintings by Claude Monet and a second set of 15 cards that reproduced paintings by unknown Aboriginal artists. The order in which they sorted these two sets was counterbalanced across participants, and the second set was always designated as the *critical set*. After finishing their rankings, participants completed a filler verbal task called the "city generation task," which required them to generate the names of 15 U.S. cities from single-letter cues. While they performed the filler task, the experimenter removed two pairs of prints from the critical set. These were designated as the *critical pairs*. One consisted of the 4th- and 10th-ranked prints (referred to as the 4–10 pair), and the other consisted of the 6th- and 12th-ranked prints (referred to as the 6–12 pair). Thus, each critical pair was composed of a relatively liked and a relatively disliked print.

After 3 min of the filler task, the second phase of the study began. Participants were told that they were now going to complete another aesthetic task, and this time they were going to indicate which of two pairs of art prints they would prefer to hang in their home if they could have full-size reproductions of that pair to take with them. Participants made six such choices, five involving novel pairs of prints and one involving the critical pairs. For each choice, two pairs of prints were placed on the table in front of the participant, with one pair on the left and one pair on the right. The participant pointed to the pair that he or she preferred. This pair was designated the *selected* pair, and the other pair was designated the *rejected* pair. As soon as a choice was made, the next pairs of prints were placed before the participant. The pairs of prints used for the participant's fourth choice were the two critical pairs. The sides of the table on which the 4–10 pair and 6–12 pair were placed were counterbalanced across participants.

The third phase began after participants completed another iteration of the city-generation task, with a slightly different instruction to generate only the names of foreign cities. Phase 3 was similar to Phase 1, with a minor change in instructions. Participants were told that preferences can sometimes fluctuate over time, and that they were to rank each set of prints again, in order of their preference, but that they should do so according to how they felt about them "right now." It was emphasized that this was not a memory test, and that they need not

try to recollect how they had ranked the items initially. The critical set was always presented second.

The fourth phase began immediately upon completion of Phase 3. Participants were shown the 15 prints from the critical set (either the Monet set or the Aboriginal set) and asked to identify the 4 prints that had appeared in Phase 2. As a test of memory for their choice, participants were also asked to indicate which pair they had selected and which pair they had rejected during Phase 2.

Results and Discussion

Attitude Change

The age-matched control participants showed the typical behavior-induced attitude change. That is, there was a greater difference between the mean ranks of the selected and rejected pairs in Phase 3 than in Phase 1, $t(10) = 3.07$, $p < .02$, $r = .68$.[1] Amnesic patients also showed attitude change, $t(9) = 2.52$, $p < .03$, $r = .62$. Table 41.2 shows the average change in rank for the two groups, as well as the spread (increase in rank for the selected prints minus decrease in rank for the rejected prints). A comparison of the attitude change shown by the amnesic patients and age-matched control participants revealed no difference, $t(21) = 0.10$, $p > .3$. Participants also ranked and reranked another set of prints for which no choices were made. Prints with initial ranks equivalent to the ranks of the selected and rejected prints from the critical set provided baseline levels of attitude change in the absence of choice. As shown in Table 41.2, amnesic patients and control participants showed no significant attitude change in the noncritical set, $t(9) = 0.10$, $p > .3$, and $t(10) = 0.12$, $p > .3$, respectively.

Explicit Memory

All participants had great difficulty identifying the 4 critical prints from the set of 15. Both amnesic patients (25% correct) and control partic-

Table 41.2
Attitude change and explicit memory in experiment 1

	Amnesic	Controls
Rank change for choice prints		
Selected pair	+1.13	+0.86
Rejected pair	−1.20	−1.12
Spread (selected-rejected)	+2.33	+1.98
Rank change for non-choice prints [a]		
Selected pair	−0.15	−0.21
Rejected pair	0.00	−0.29
Spread (selected-rejected)	+0.15	+0.08
Identification of choice prints	25%	33%
Categorization of choice prints	44%	91%

a. Non-choice prints are prints from the non-critical set that were ranked and re-ranked without an intervening choice. Prints with the equivalent rank as those a participant selected and rejected in the critical set were designated as selected and rejected in the non-critical set for comparison purposes.

ipants (33% correct) performed at or near the level of accuracy expected by chance alone (27%). Not surprisingly, these low levels of performance did not differ significantly between the two groups, $t(21) = 0.86$, $p < .2$, $r = .25$. The poor performance is probably attributable to the requirement that participants remember when or how often during the experiment they had encountered the critical pairs. Remembering such contextual information constitutes a type of source memory judgment, which is impaired in both amnesic patients (e.g., Schacter, Harbluk, & McLachlan, 1984) and elderly adults (e.g., Schacter, Osowiecki, Kaszniak, Kihlstrom, & Valdiserri, 1994). Our control group consisted of primarily elderly adults.

More important, however, amnesic patients and control participants did differ with regard to their memory for which critical prints were chosen and which were rejected, a type of memory that specifically references the counter-attitudinal behavior. Of the cards correctly identified as critical prints, the age-matched control participants categorized nearly all of the prints correctly as chosen or rejected (91%), and outperformed amnesic patients (44%), $t(21) = 3.00$, $p < .02$, $r = .67$, who performed at chance (50%). In short, control participants remembered their counterattitudinal behavior, whereas amnesics did not, but the two groups showed identical amounts of attitude change.

Perhaps the most important measure bearing on our hypothesis that explicit memory does not necessarily play a role in behavior-induced attitude change is the correlation between attitude change and explicit memory. Although amnesic patients showed generally poor memory for the prints, it is still possible that whatever memory they did possess could be related to the amount of attitude change they exhibited. If anything, however, it appears the opposite is more likely true: For both amnesic patients, $r = −.41$, $p = .25$, and control participants, $r = −.63$, $p < .04$, greater attitude change was observed when fewer prints were accurately identified. In addition, the ability to correctly categorize prints as selected or rejected was not significantly correlated with amount of attitude change for either group, both ps > .3.

Conclusion
The amnesic patients in this experiment showed just as much behavior-induced attitude change as did matched control participants despite the fact that they had no explicit memory for which prints they had chosen and no explicit memory for which prints were involved in the choice. Furthermore, for both groups, the degree of explicit memory for the prints involved in the choice was negatively correlated with the amount of attitude change. These results suggest that explicit memory for one's counterattitudinal behavior is not a necessary component of behavior-induced attitude change, and might even disrupt the process.

Of course, the data from this experiment do not rule out the possibility that attitude change occurred right at the moment of choice, while the behavioral information was still accessible in working memory, even for amnesic patients. If this is the case, the current data suggest that if behavior-induced attitude change is a consciously controlled process, it is happening on a much smaller time scale than previously imagined (Festinger, 1964; Steele, Spencer, & Lynch, 1993). In our second experiment, we incorporated a cognitive-load manipulation to provide a more traditional test of the involvement of controlled processing in behavior-induced attitude change.

Conscious Processes: The Role of Attention and Working Memory

If only to live up to its name, rationalization seems to require a good deal of effortful thinking. It seems scarcely metaphorical to say that a friend "on the short end of the stick" of a romantic breakup appears to be working hard to reconceptualize the extinguished relationship as expendable. Attention seems to be deliberately focused on those elements of the relationship that were undesirable from the start or were ambiguous enough that they can now be reinterpreted in a negative light.

Conscious attention to the counterattitudinal behavior and conscious work in the service of attitude revision are both unspecified, but implied, components of cognitive dissonance theory. Language alluding to the use of consciously controlled processing in attitude change is often used by dissonance researchers: Across four decades of research, there have been references to the need to "engage in cognitive work" (Petty & Wegener, 1998, p. 336), statements that dissonance research is "primarily concerned with processes which are conscious and capable of verbalization" (Hovland & Rosenberg, 1960,

p. 202) and that attitude change requires "awareness of . . . his [the participant's] discrepant commitment" (Brehm & Cohen, 1962, p. 168), and mention of the "phenomenological experience of cognitive dissonance" (Elliot & Devine, 1994, p. 391). Most significant, Festinger (1964) concluded that "dissonance reduction does, indeed, require that time be spent in thinking about the characteristics of the alternative" (p. 59). Given these references and prior research on implicit attitude change more generally (Kunst-Wilson & Zajonc, 1980; Wilson, Lindsey, & Schooler, 2000), it is somewhat surprising that the necessity of conscious attention and effort for behavior-induced attitude change seldom has been investigated (Brock & Grant, 1963; Nisbett & Wilson, 1977).

On the basis of our results from Experiment 1, we hypothesized that the attentional resources associated with working memory are not a necessary component of behavior-induced attitude change. To test this hypothesis, we ran normal participants through the free-choice paradigm under normal or cognitive-load conditions. Cognitive load (e.g., counting the occurrences of a tone) severely reduces the resources available for attentional and cognitive processing (Baddeley, 1986), and processes unimpaired by cognitive load are considered to be relatively automatic (Gilbert, Pelham, & Krull, 1988; Wegner & Bargh, 1998). We predicted that participants under cognitive load would show as much attitude change in the free-choice paradigm as participants under no load.

Experiment 2

Method

Participants

Sixteen male and 16 female undergraduate students at Harvard University received $10 each for their voluntary participation. All participants were right-handed and between 17 and 21 years of age.

Procedure

The procedure was identical to the procedure used in Experiment 1 with the exception that for half the participants, the two phases during which attitude change might occur (i.e., the choice and reranking phases) were performed under cognitive load. Participants in the cognitive-load condition heard a series of tones, each at one of three pitches, and were required to keep track of the number of tones at the lowest pitch (Gilbert & Silvera, 1996; Lieberman, Gilbert, & Jarcho, 2000). In the no-load condition, participants were told to ignore the tones.

Results and Discussion

Attitude Change

No-load participants showed the standard behavior-induced attitude change; there was a greater difference between the mean rank of the selected and rejected pairs in Phase 3 than there was in Phase 1, $t(14) = 2.23$, $p < .05$, $r = .51$. Our prediction that participants under a cognitive load would also show attitude change was supported, $t(14) = 2.64$, $p < .02$, $r = .58$. As shown in Table 41.3, nearly identical levels of attitude change were evidenced by participants in the two conditions in response to the counterattitudinal behavior. A comparison between the two groups revealed no differences, $t(28) = 0.71$, $p > .2$, $r = .10$. As in Experiment 1, there was no attitude change in the noncritical set; this was true for participants in both the no-load and the cognitive-load conditions, $t(14) = 0.21$, $p > .3$, and $t(14) = 0.12$, $p > .3$, respectively (see Table 41.3).

Explicit Memory

The cognitive-load manipulation did not attenuate attitude change, but did it affect other kinds of processing? To answer this question, we exam-

Table 41.3
Attitude change and explicit memory in experiment 2

	Load	No load
Rank change for choice prints		
Selected pair	+0.44	+0.94
Rejected pair	−0.91	−0.38
Spread (selected-rejected)	+1.35	+1.32
Rank change for non-choice prints [a]		
Selected pair	−0.41	−0.41
Rejected pair	−0.47	−0.25
Spread (selected-rejected)	+0.06	−0.16
Identification of choice prints	35%	67%
Categorization of choice prints	67%	73%

a. Non-choice prints are prints from the non-critical set that were ranked and re-ranked without an intervening choice. Prints with the equivalent rank as those a participant selected and rejected in the critical set were designated as selected and rejected in the noncritical set for comparison purposes.

ined participants' ability to identify which of the 15 prints were presented in the choice phase. Because cognitive load impairs encoding (e.g., Fletcher, Shallice, & Dolan, 1998), we expected that load would impair memory for the counterattitudinal behavior. This is exactly what we found: Subjects under cognitive load were able to identify only half as many prints (35%) as their no-load counterparts (67%), $t(30) = 4.89$, $p < .001$, $r = .67$. Though participants under load were near chance in their identification accuracy, they correctly categorized as chosen or rejected those prints that they accurately identified as often as did the no-load participants (67% vs. 73%, respectively), $t(30) = 0.03$, $p > .2$, $r = .01$. In short, even though cognitive load impaired participants' ability to think about their behavior, they showed the same amount of attitude change as participants not under cognitive load.

As in Experiment 1, we assessed the extent to which degree of attitude change correlated with explicit memory measures. For both the cognitive-load and the no-load participants, there were no significant correlations between attitude change and either memory measure, all $ps > .3$.

Conclusion

Regardless of cognitive-load condition, participants showed substantial attitude change in response to their counterattitudinal behavior. Attitudes changed despite the fact that participants under a cognitive load were significantly impaired in their recall of which prints were involved in the choice phase of the experiment.

These data, combined with the results of Experiment 1, suggest that the process of behavior-induced attitude change is a relatively automatic one (cf. Zanna & Aziza, 1976). It is possible that attitude change requires some minimal amount of attention, conscious awareness, or mental effort, but it is fair to claim that unaltered performance under cognitive load indicates that this attitude-change process is toward the automatic end of the automatic-controlled continuum (Bargh & Tota, 1988; Gilbert, 1989; Wegner, 1994).

General Discussion

The current experiments provide strong evidence that behavior-induced attitude change requires minimal ability to encode and retrieve new explicit memories and minimal ability to engage in consciously controlled processing. In fact, if one compares the performance of the amnesic patients in Experiment 1 and the no-load participants in Experiment 2, it appears that intact explicit memory may actually attenuate the magnitude of behavior-induced attitude change (cf. Snyder & Ebbesen, 1972). This hypothesis is bolstered by the negative correlations between degree of attitude change and explicit memory in Experiment 1.

The possibility that behavior-induced attitude change can take place automatically and without conscious processing casts new light on the role of motivation in rationalization. People tend to look unfavorably on individuals who change their attitudes to justify their behaviors because these individuals should be able to see that they are "just rationalizing" and thus realize that their new attitudes are glaringly inauthentic. Our results suggest, however, that the behavior-induced attitude-change process may not be consciously experienced. Because the results of automatic attitude processes are often experienced as given by the environment rather than constructed by the mind, what looks like disingenuous rationalization from without may feel genuine from within (Bargh, 1989).

Automatically changed attitudes can be especially hardy inasmuch as their maintenance does not require the individual to remember the reason why the attitude was changed in the first place. In the fable that opened this chapter, it appears that the fox continued to believe the grapes were undesirable only because they continued to be unobtainable. The new attitude toward grapes seems to serve as the continuing justification for not ruminating over the loss. The results from Experiment 1, however, indicate that this teleological interpretation of attitude change may be unnecessary, because the amnesics did not remember that there was a prior conflict that they would prefer to keep avoiding. Not revisiting the conflict may be a by-product of the new attitude's presence, but it is not the case that the new attitude is sustained because of a need to avoid the conflict.

The current data also place new constraints on the change processes posited by any theory of behavior-induced attitude change. Self-perception theory and cognitive dissonance theory have depended on both explicit memory and conscious processing to differing degrees in their explanations of attitude change. Although the current data do not address either theory's general viability, they do suggest that the processing components of these theories need clearer specification. Future research integrating the methods of neuroscience into social cognition should yield clearer specification of these processes (Lieberman, 2000; Ochsner & Lieberman, 2000).

Acknowledgments

It is a pleasure to thank Paula Koseff, Michelle Woodbury, and Annapurna Duleep for their contributions. This research was supported in part by McDonnell-Pew grants to Matthew Lieberman (JSMF 99-25 CN-QUA.05) and Kevin Ochsner (JSMF 98-23 CM-QUA.04), National Institute of Mental Health Grant No. RO1-MH56075 to Daniel Gilbert, and National Institute of Neurological Disorders and Stroke Center Grant No. NS26985 awarded to Boston University.

Notes

1. The amnesic patients and elderly control participants in Experiment 1 chose the 4–10 pair 64% of the time. Gerard and White (1983) reported that 75% of their participants chose the higher-ranked pair in a choice that was objectively easier than the one we used. The difference between their result and ours is non-significant, $[chi]^2(1) = 0.99$, $p > .3$, one-tailed. Gerard and White also reported that eliminating the data of those participants who selected the lower-ranked pair did not change their results. Given the constraints on our sample size, we chose to include data from participants who selected the lower-ranked pair. In Experiment 2, participants chose the 4–10 pair more than 75% of the time.

References

Aesop. (1961). *Aesop without morals: The famous fables and a life of Aesop* (L. W. Daly, ed. & trans.). New York: Barnes and Co.

Asch, S. E. (1956). Studies of independence and conformity: A minority of one against a unanimous majority. *Psychological Monographs, 7*(9, Whole No. 416).

Baddeley, A. (1986). *Working memory.* New York: Oxford University Press.

Bargh, J. A. (1989). Conditional automaticity: Varieties of automatic influence in social perception and cognition. In J. S. Uleman & J. A. Bargh (Eds.), *Unintended thought* (pp. 3–51). New York: Guilford Press.

Bargh, J. A., & Tota, M. E. (1988). Context-dependent automatic processing in depression: Accessibility of negative constructs with regard to self but not others. *Journal of Personality and Social Psychology, 54,* 925–939.

Bem, D. J. (1965). An experimental analysis of self-persuasion. *Journal of Experimental Social Psychology, 1,* 199–218.

Brehm, J. W. (1956). Post-decision changes in the desirability of alternatives. *Journal of Abnormal and Social Psychology, 52,* 384–389.

Brehm, J. W., & Cohen, A. R. (1962). *Explorations in cognitive dissonance.* New York: Wiley.

Brock, T. C., & Grant, L. D. (1963). Dissonance, awareness and motivation. *Journal of Abnormal and Social Psychology, 67,* 53–60.

Chaiken, S., Liberman, A., & Eagly, A. H. (1989). Heuristic and systematic information processing within and beyond the persuasion context. In J. S. Uleman & J. A. Bargh (Eds.), *Unintended thought* (pp. 212–252). New York: Guilford Press.

Elliot, A. J., & Devine, P. G. (1994). On the motivational nature of cognitive dissonance: Dissonance as psychological discomfort. *Journal of Personality and Social Psychology, 67,* 382–394.

Festinger, L. (1957). *A theory of cognitive dissonance.* Evanston, IL: Row, Peterson.

Festinger, L. (1964). *Conflict, decision, and dissonance.* Stanford, CA: Stanford University Press.

Fletcher, P. C., Shallice, T., & Dolan, R. J. (1998). The functional roles of prefrontal cortex in episodic memory: I. Encoding. *Brain, 121,* 1239–1248.

Gerard, H. B., & White, G. L. (1983). Post-decisional reevaluation of choice alternatives. *Personality and Social Psychology Bulletin, 9,* 365–369.

Gilbert, D. T. (1989). Thinking lightly about others. In J. S. Uleman & J. A. Bargh (Eds.), *Unintended thought* (pp. 189–211). New York: Guilford Press.

Gilbert, D. T., Pelham, B. W., & Krull, D. S. (1988). On cognitive busyness: When person perceivers meet persons perceived. *Journal of Personality and Social Psychology,* 54, 733–740.

Gilbert, D. T., & Silvera, D. S. (1996). Overhelping. *Journal of Personality and Social Psychology,* 70, 678–690.

Hovland, C. I., Janis, I. L., & Kelley, H. H. (1953). *Communication and persuasion.* New Haven, CT: Yale University Press.

Hovland, C. I., & Rosenberg, M. J. (1960). Summary and further theoretical issues. In M. J. Rosenberg, C. I. Hovland, W. J. McGuire, R. P. Abelson, & J. W. Brehm (Eds.), *Attitude organization and change: An analysis of consistency among attitude components* (pp. 198–232). New Haven, CT: Yale University Press.

Jones, E. E. (1998). Major developments in five decades of social psychology. In D. T. Gilbert, S. T. Fiske, & G. Lindzey (Eds.), *The handbook of social psychology* (4th ed., pp. 3–57). New York: Oxford University Press.

Kunst-Wilson, W. R., & Zajonc, R. B. (1980). Affective discrimination of stimuli that cannot be recognized. *Science,* 207, 557–558.

Lieberman, M. D. (2000). Intuition: A social cognitive neuroscience approach. *Psychological Bulletin,* 126, 109–137.

Lieberman, M. D., Gilbert, D. T., & Jarcho, J. (2000). *Automatic and controlled attribution processes across cultures.* Unpublished manuscript, University of California, Los Angeles.

Nisbett, R. E., & Wilson, T. D. (1977). Telling more than we can know: Verbal reports on mental processes. *Psychological Review,* 84, 231–259.

Ochsner, K. N., & Lieberman, M. D. (2000). *The social cognitive neuroscience approach.* Manuscript submitted for publication.

O'Reilly, R., Braver, T. S., & Cohen, J. D. (1997). A biologically-based computational model of working memory. In A. Maykae & P. Shah (Eds.), *Models of working memory* (pp. 375–411). New York: Oxford University Press.

Petty, R. E., & Cacioppo, J. T. (1986). The elaboration likelihood model of persuasion. In L. Berkowitz (Ed.), *Advances in experimental social psychology* (Vol. 19, pp. 123–205). New York: Academic Press.

Petty, R. E., & Wegener, D. T. (1998). Attitude change: Multiple roles for persuasion variables. In D. T. Gilbert, S. T. Fiske, & G. Lindzey (Eds.), *The handbook of social psychology* (4th ed., pp. 323–390). New York: Oxford University Press.

Schacter, D. L., Chiu, C. Y. P., & Ochsner, K. N. (1993). Implicit memory: A selective review. *Annual Review of Neuroscience,* 16, 159–182.

Schacter, D. L., Harbluk, J. L., & McLachlan, D. R. (1984). Retrieval without recollection: An experimental analysis of source amnesia. *Journal of Verbal Learning and Verbal Behavior,* 23, 593–611.

Schacter, D. L., Osowiecki, D., Kaszniak, A., Kihlstrom, J., & Valdiserri, M. (1994). Source memory: Extending the boundaries of age-related deficits. *Psychology and Aging,* 9, 81–89.

Snyder, M., & Ebbesen, E. B. (1972). Dissonance awareness: A test of dissonance theory versus self-perception theory. *Journal of Experimental Social Psychology,* 8, 502–517.

Squire, L. R. (1992). Declarative and nondeclarative memory: Multiple brain systems supporting learning and memory. *Journal of Cognitive Neuroscience,* 4, 232–243.

Steele, C., Spencer, S., & Lynch, M. (1993). Self-image resilience and dissonance: The role of affirmational resources. *Journal of Personality and Social Psychology,* 64, 885–896.

Wechsler, D. (1981). *Manual for the Wechsler Adult Intelligence Scale-Revised.* New York: Psychological Corp.

Wechsler, D. (1987). *Manual for the Wechsler Memory Scale-Revised.* San Antonio, TX: Psychological Corp.

Wegner, D. M. (1994). Ironic processes of mental control. *Psychological Review,* 101, 34–52.

Wegner, D. M., & Bargh, J. A. (1998). Control and automaticity in social life. In D. T. Gilbert, S. T. Fiske, & G. Lindzey (Ed.), *The handbook of social psychology* (4th ed., pp. 446–496). New York: Oxford University Press.

Wilson, T. D., Lindsey, S., & Schooler, T. Y. (2000). A model of dual attitudes. *Psychological Review,* 107, 101–126.

Zanna, M. P., & Aziza, C. (1976). On the interaction of repression-sensitization and attention in resolving cognitive dissonance. *Journal of Personality,* 44, 577–593.

42 Impaired Preference Conditioning after Anterior Temporal Lobe Resection in Humans

Ingrid S. Johnsrude, Adrian M. Owen, Norman M. White, W. Vivienne Zhao, and Veronique Bohbot

An extensive body of research on animals has linked structures within the amygdaloid nuclear complex (ANC) to emotional associative learning. Much of this work has focussed on aversive phenomena such as fear conditioning (Gallagher and Chiba, 1996; Killcross et al., 1997; Rogan et al., 1997; Walker and Davis, 1997; Davis, 1998; LeDoux, 1998; Fanselow and LeDoux, 1999; Fendt and Fanselow, 1999). Studies of fear and aversive conditioning in humans have produced results consistent with the animal literature: patients with bilateral (Bechara et al., 1995) and even unilateral (LaBar et al., 1995) ANC lesions do not show normal fear conditioning responses. Functional neuroimaging studies also suggest a role for the ANC in fear conditioning in humans (Büchel et al., 1998; LaBar et al., 1998; Morris et al., 1998).

It has long been recognized in the animal literature that selective amygdala lesions can affect the ability of animals to associate stimuli with reward value (Weiskrantz, 1956; Jones and Mishkin, 1972; Speigler and Mishkin, 1981; Gaffan and Harrison, 1987; Cador et al., 1989; Robbins et al., 1989; Gallagher et al., 1990; Everitt et al., 1991; Hiroi and White, 1991; White and McDonald, 1993) (for review, see Aggleton, 1993; McDonald and White, 1993; Gallagher and Holland, 1994; Ono et al., 1995; Hatfield et al., 1996; Gallagher and Chiba, 1996; Robbins and Everitt, 1996; Hitchcott et al., 1997; Hitchcott and Phillips, 1998; Everitt et al., 1999; Holland and Gallagher, 1999). Place-preference conditioning is one of the most common procedures for assessing conditioned reward associations (Carr et al., 1989; Schechter and Calcagnetti, 1993; Tzschentke, 1998). In this paradigm, a particular set of environmental cues is first paired with reward, and then an animal's tendency to approach and spend time in that environment, compared to a neutral one, is assessed. Place-preference conditioning procedures can be considered a special case of a more general conditioning paradigm (stimulus–reward association learning) in which biologically relevant stimuli (which normally elicit approach responses due to their rewarding affective significance) become associated with neutral stimuli that subsequently elicit approach on their own.

Conditioned preferences have been demonstrated previously in healthy human participants (Razran, 1954; Staats and Staats, 1957, 1958; Levey and Martin, 1975, 1983; Martin and Levey, 1978; Kirk-Smith et al., 1983; Bierley et al., 1985; Rozin and Zellner, 1985; Stuart et al., 1987, 1991; Allen and Janiszewski, 1989; Niedenthal, 1990; Baeyens et al., 1993, 1995; Todrank et al., 1995), but the underlying anatomical substrates have not been examined in any detail. A few studies have investigated mechanisms of preference formation in brain-damaged populations, but these have focussed on the effects of exposure alone, rather than evaluating the effects of associative learning (Redington et al., 1984; Johnson et al., 1985).

In a recent study (Johnsrude et al., 1999), conditioned preferences for novel, abstract, monochrome patterns were induced in young, normal volunteer participants using a method based on cue, or place, preference procedures originally developed for use with rats (Carr et al., 1989). Care was taken to minimize the subjects' awareness of the experimental contingencies and of the goal of the study by presenting the abstract patterns in the context of a cognitively demanding working memory task. Participants subsequently preferred the pattern paired most often with reward to that paired least often with reward. Importantly, participants did not attribute their preferences to the conditioning procedure, but instead attributed them to the physical characteristics of the patterns themselves, indicating

Table 42.1
Demographic information on participants in each group

Group	N	Sex M	Sex F	Handedness R	Handedness L	Testing language English	Testing language French	Age Mean	Age Range	Years of education Mean	Years of education Range	Time since surgery Median	Time since surgery Range
LA	15	12	3	15	0	13	2	36	23–48	13	9–18	4 years	3 months–27 years
RA	18	7	11	15	3	8	10	38	22–55	12	6–18	1 year	3 months–16 years
FNTL	13	7	6	9	4	10	3	30	16–39	14	9–20	1 year	3 months–10 years
NC	21	10	11	20	1	15	6	37	23–58	13	11–18		

that they were largely unaware of the effects of the conditioning procedure on their subsequent behavior.

In the present study, we used this procedure to assess preference conditioning in a group of neurosurgical patients with known damage to the amygdaloid region. In the majority of these patients, surgery was used to control pharmacologically intractable epilepsy. The resection always included the ANC and immediately surrounding tissue, as well as a variable amount of hippocampus, parahippocampal gyrus, and lateral neocortex in one hemisphere. The documented neuropsychological deficits after unilateral lesions of this type depend on the extent of the removal, but are generally mild and do not preclude the patient having a normal and productive life (Hermann et al., 1991; Eliashiv et al., 1997). We tested a matched group of normal volunteers and a group of patients with surgical lesions confined unilaterally to frontal cortex to evaluate the anatomical specificity of any resulting deficit.

Materials and Methods

Participants

Thirty-three patients with unilateral anterior temporal lobe resections (15 left; 18 right) who had undergone surgery at the Montreal Neuro-

logical Institute for the relief of intractable epilepsy or for the removal of benign tumors were included in this study. In all of these patients, the lesion included the ANC and periamygdalar cortices, as described below. The study was approved by the Research and Ethics Committee of the Montreal Neurological Institute and Hospital, and all participants gave written consent. Patients with brain damage outside of the operated zone were excluded, and so were those who exhibited no improvement in their seizure frequency or intensity after surgery. All patients were either right-handed, or were left-hemisphere dominant for speech as determined by a preoperative sodium amobarbital test (Milner, 1997), and had full-scale intelligence quotient (IQ) ratings over 80 on the Wechsler Adult Intelligence Scale-Revised (WAIS-R).

Table 42.1 presents demographic information on participants in the four groups. The 15 patients with left ANC removals (LA) included one case of cortical dysplasia and one low-grade ganglioglioma. The pathology in the rest of the patients in this group was focal gliosis and sclerosis. Three of these patients were tested 3–4 months after surgery, two were tested 5 months to a year after surgery, three were tested between 1 and 5 years after surgery, and the rest were tested >10 years after surgery. Two of the 18 patients with removals of the right ANC (RA) were operated for neuroepithelial tumors, and one for a low-grade oligodendroglioma. The pathology in the rest of the group was gliosis and sclerosis. Seven of these patients were tested 3–4 months after surgery, two were tested 5 months to a year after surgery, two were tested between 1 and 5 years after surgery, another two were tested between 5 and 10 years after surgery, and the rest were tested more than 10 years after surgery. A group of 13 surgical patients with lesions confined unilaterally to frontal cortex (FNTL; seven patients with left-sided removals, six patients with right-sided removals) were also tested. Pathology reports cited low-grade gliomas in five cases (two left, three right) a cavernous hemangioma in one left-sided case, an aneurysm and hematoma in another left-sided patient, an arteriovenous malformation (AVM) in a right-sided patient, and cortical dysplasia, gliosis, and/or sclerosis in the other five patients. The resection did not encroach on temporal lobe structures in any of these patients. Two of these patients were tested 3–4 months postoperatively, five were tested 5 months to a year after surgery, three were tested between 1 and 5 years after surgery, two others were tested 5–10 years after surgery, and one was tested more than 10 years after surgery. Twenty-one neurologically normal volunteers (NC) who were matched to the patients with respect to age and years of education were also tested. One-way ANOVAs demonstrated no difference in age or years of education among the four groups. Nonparametric (Kruskal–Wallis) ANOVAs did not reveal any significant differences in the distributions of handedness, sex, or testing language (English or French) across the four groups.

Imaging in Patients with Temporal Lobe Resections

For conclusions about functional specialization within the medial temporal lobe to be drawn, it was important to confirm the site and extent of the resections in the patients with temporal lobe resections, and quantify the degree of overlap. The resections were labeled on postoperative

T1-weighted magnetic resonance (MR) images, acquired on each subject (Philips Gyroscan; 1.5 T). These images were linearly transformed into standardized stereotaxic space (Talairach and Tournoux, 1988), using DISPLAY, an interactive three-dimensional imaging software package (MacDonald et al., 1994; McConnell Brain Imaging Center, Montreal Neurological Institute). Postoperative MR images were not available for two patients in the LA group. The surgical reports for these two patients describe left anterior temporal lobe resections that include the amygdala and uncus, the pes of the hippocampus in one case, 3 cm of hippocampus in the other, and lateral neocortical resections in both extending to ~4.5 cm along the Sylvian fissure and along the base of the temporal lobe, measured from the temporal pole. A postoperative MR image was not available for one patient in the RA group. The surgical report for this patient describes a right anterior temporal lobe resection including the amygdala and uncus, 3 cm of the hippocampus, and a lateral neocortical resection extending to 4 cm along the Sylvian fissure and 6 cm along the base of the temporal lobe. The label volumes resulting from analysis of the 13 postoperative MRs in the LA group and the 17 MRs in the RA group were coregistered and averaged to produce probability volumes of lesion location, as shown in Figure 42.1. The area of maximal overlap in resection site (100%, resected in all patients) in each group is centered on the ANC (Talairach coordinates: LA, −24, −15, −18; RA, 24, −15, −19).

Materials and Procedure

A computerized touch-screen task based on place-preference procedures used with rats was used. This task has been described in detail elsewhere (Johnsrude et al., 1999). Participants chose between raisins and fruit-flavored candy pellets (Dweebs; The Willy Wonka Candy Factory, Nestle, York, UK) before the start of the procedure, and they were always rewarded with that

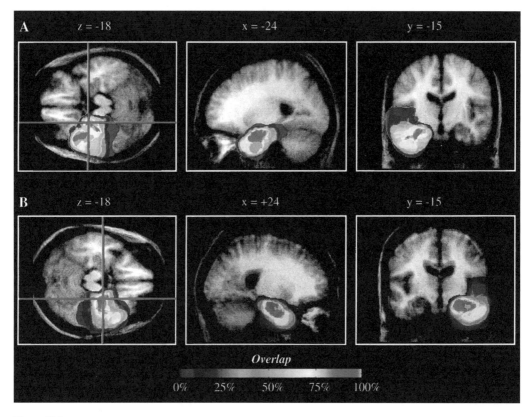

Figure 42.1
Overlap of lesions in patients with left (LA) or right (RA) anterior temporal lobe resection, as indexed by the color scale, superimposed on the averaged MR image for each group. (A) $n = 13$ LA patients. (B) $n = 17$ RA patients. In both LA and RA groups, the area of maximal overlap in lesion location includes the region of the amygdala.

type of food. Raisins were chosen by 16 of 21 participants in the NC group, 12 of 15 patients in the LA group, 16 of 18 in the RA group, and 8 of 13 in the FNTL group. The rest chose candy pellets. These proportions are not significantly different across groups, as tested using χ^2 tests.

There were three phases to the experimental procedure: formation of conditioned preferences, a test of preference expression, and an assessment of preference attribution. These are shown schematically in Fig. 42.2.

At the beginning of the formation phase, participants were presented with three black squares on the screen and were given the following instructions:

"You see three boxes on the screen. At any time, one of the boxes is hiding a red ball, and the other two are hiding black balls. What you have to do is guess where the red ball is. I would like you to find as many red balls as you can. You can choose a box by lightly touching the screen. Once you have touched a box, it will

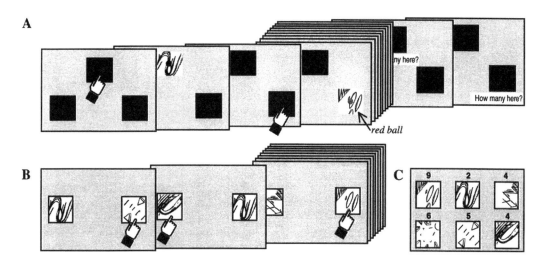

Figure 42.2
The three phases of the experimental procedure. (A) Schematic drawing of a block of trials in the formation phase. On the first trial, the subject picked the top box and heard a buzzer at the same time as the pattern and black ball appeared. On the second trial, the subject selected the rightmost box and heard a melodic flourish at the same time as the pattern and the red ball appeared. After seeing the red ball, they took the chosen food reward (one candy or raisin) from the bowl beside the monitor. At the end of each block of trials the subject was asked to remember how many times they had found the red ball in each of the three boxes. (B) Expression test. The subject saw successive pairs of patterns and was told to "touch the pattern you prefer." The six patterns used in this phase included the three used in the formation phase and three novel ones. (C) In the final phase, the subject was shown the six patterns used in the preference expression test together with a number representing the number of times that pattern had been chosen (of 10). For the three patterns most frequently chosen, the subject was asked, "Why do you like this pattern?" to assess whether participants attributed their preferences to their experience during the formation phase.

open up and show you which ball was hidden underneath. Every so often, you will be asked how many times you have found the red ball in a particular box. Thus, while you are choosing boxes you have also to try and remember how many times you have found a red ball in each of the three boxes. I would like you to eat one candy/raisin every time you find a red ball."

The participants then proceeded to guess where the red "ball" was hidden by touching one of the three black "boxes." After each guess, the selected box would "open" revealing one of three abstract black-and-white line drawings or patterns, and either a red or a black circle (or ball) superimposed on the center of that pattern (Fig. 42.2A). If the circle was red, the participants heard a melodic flourish and picked the chosen type of food reward (one candy or one raisin) from a bowl placed beside the computer screen. If the circle was black, they heard a buzzer and were not permitted to take a food reward. After 3 sec, the selected box returned to black, and the subject was required to make the next guess. This interval ensured that participants had sufficient time to taste the food in the presence of the stimulus patterns on the rewarded trials. Unknown to the subjects, the stimulus pattern and circle color were predetermined for each trial, regardless of the location chosen.

A total of 180 trials were presented over six blocks. In total, each of the stimulus patterns was presented 60 times, together with either a red ball or a black ball according to the contingency relationship for that pattern (see below). At the end of each block, the participants were asked how many times they had found the red circle in each of the three boxes during the previous block of trials; this was the working memory task.

Three versions of the formation procedure were prepared. Each subject was tested using one of the three different versions, chosen pseudorandomly, in such a way that the distribution of the versions across the sexes and across the reward types (candy or raisins) was approximately equal. In each version, a different set of pattern–outcome contingency pairings was used. Thus, in one version, pattern A was accompanied by reward (red circle, melodic flourish, and food reward) on 90% of trials in which it appeared (i.e., 54 trials) and by nonreward (black circle, buzzer sound and no food) on 10% of those trials (i.e., six trials). Pattern B was accompanied by reward on 50% of trials in which it appeared and by nonreward on the other 50%. Pattern C was accompanied by reward on 10% of trials and by nonreward on the other 90%. In the second version of the task the ratios were: Pattern A, 10:90; Pattern B, 90:10; Pattern C, 50:50, whereas in the third version, the corresponding ratios were: 50:50; 10:90, and 90:10.

The trial order was pseudorandom and fixed. The rarest combinations were always presented just before or just after the more frequent combinations (e.g., for the first version described above, Pattern A paired with a black circle was presented just after Pattern A paired with a red circle). In addition, an identical pattern/outcome pair could not occur more than twice in a row. These provisions served to break up runs of similar trials that might otherwise have alerted the participants to the different outcome contingencies. In addition, each block of trials contained an equal number of red and black circles,

and at least one occurrence of each of the six possible combinations of circles and patterns.

Immediately after the conditioning procedure, preferences were assessed. Six different patterns were used in this part of the study: three of the patterns were those used in the conditioning procedure, whereas three others were novel. On each trial, a pair of patterns was presented, one on each side of the screen, as shown in Figure 42.2B. The participants were told to choose the pattern they preferred, by touching it. They were told not to think too hard about it, but to go with their first impression. There were a total of 30 trials, and each pattern was presented 10 times: five times on the left, and five times on the right, twice with each of the other five patterns.

After the preference assessment all six patterns were presented simultaneously on the screen for the preference attribution test. A number on top of each pattern indicated the number of times (out of 10) the subject had chosen each one (Fig. 42.2C). To assess the participants' perceptions of their preferences, they were asked, "Why did you like this pattern?" for their three most frequently chosen patterns. At the end of this phase, each participant was informed of the nature of the study.

Data Scoring

The dependent variables analyzed included the preference scores for each pattern (the number of times, out of a possible ten, that it was chosen in the preference assessment phase), and counting error in the working memory component of the formation procedure. This variable was calculated by computing, for each of the boxes (left, top, and right) in each block of trials, the absolute discrepancy between the observed number of red balls (how many the subject actually saw) and the estimated number (how many the subject reported). These discrepancy values were summed across boxes and across blocks of trials to determine the overall discrepancy score. The discrepancy values were also categorized as

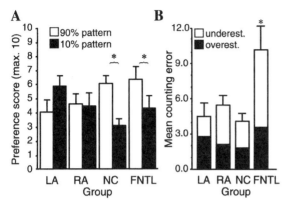

Figure 42.3

(A) The mean preference scores (maximum = 10) and SEs for the 90 and 10% patterns in patients with left or right temporal lobe damage, including the amygdaloid body (LA, RA), normal control participants (NC), and patients with unilateral frontal lobe lesions (FNTL). Error bars indicate SEM. LA and RA participants fail to show a preference effect; see Results. (B) Mean discrepancy scores on the working memory task in normal control participants (NC) and in patients with left (LA) or right (RA) anterior temporal lobe resection and frontal lobe resections (FNTL). The patients with frontal lobe lesions are impaired relative to all other groups. Error bars indicate SEM for the overall discrepancy scores. When the errors are categorized as overestimations or underestimations, the FNTL group is shown to produce significantly more underestimations relative to the other three groups; see Results.

underestimations or overestimations, and the values were summed separately to determine the total amount of each type of error for each subject. One LA subject had a total discrepancy score > 3 SDs away from the mean for this group: his data were not included in the analysis.

Results

It was decided, a priori, to exclude from the analysis data from those participants who demonstrated any spontaneous knowledge of the relationship between their experience with the patterns and their preferences. In fact, none of the participants related their preferences to the previous stage of the task during the preference attribution test or debriefing. Instead, they attributed their preferences to the physical characteristics of the patterns themselves. Sample responses (from normal participants and patients

with frontal lobe damage) to the question, "Why did you like this pattern?" included "looks like the sun," "reminds me of pizza," "has more of a design, is a little more complicated," "is symmetrical," "I liked the lines and curves," and "was an interesting sort of pattern, and caught my eye."

When the preference scores for the 90 and 10% patterns were compared across groups using a two-way ANOVA, a significant group-by-pattern interaction was obtained ($F_{(3, 63)} = 4.09$; $p < 0.01$). Planned comparisons between the two preference scores in each group demonstrated that participants in the NC and FNTL groups preferred the 90% pattern to the 10% pattern (NC: $t_{(20)} = 4.0$, $p < 0.0005$; FNTL: $t_{(12)} = 1.92$, $p < 0.05$, one-tailed), whereas LA and RA participants did not (Fig. 42.3A). The LA group tended to prefer the 10% pattern to the 90% pattern, but not to a significant degree, $t_{(14)} = 1.35$, $p = 0.1$.

Preference scores for the 50% pattern and for the novel patterns were intermediate between those for the 10 and the 90% patterns (range of mean preference scores on 50% pattern, 3.9–5.7; novel patterns, 4.9–5.4). These patterns were included for reasons of experimental design, and we did not expect or observe any differences among the groups in preference scores for these patterns (as tested using one-way ANOVAs). Furthermore, the value 5, which is the value expected if participants were choosing at random during the preference assessment phase, was within 1 SD of the cell mean preference scores for these patterns.

One-way ANOVA on the overall discrepancy scores revealed that NC, LA, and RA participants were equally able to keep track of the number of times they had found the red ball in each of the three boxes, whereas patients with frontal lobe damage were significantly impaired [Tukey's honestly significant difference (HSD) tests: main effect, $F_{(3, 62)} = 5.22$; $p < 0.005$]. When the discrepancy values were categorized as overestimations and underestimations, it was apparent that patients with frontal lobe damage significantly underestimated the number of times they had found the red ball in each location (Tukey's HSD tests after one-way ANOVA: $F_{(3, 62)} = 7.92$; $p < 0.0005$). There were no differences among the groups in overestimation (one-way ANOVA: $F_{(3, 62)} = 1.35$; p, ns). This is shown in Figure 42.3B. Total discrepancy, overestimation, and underestimation scores for patients with left frontal ($n = 7$) and right frontal ($n = 6$) excisions were then examined separately to look for hemisphere effects. Mann–Whitney U tests were used to compare these two subgroups with normal participants and with each other. Both frontal groups differed significantly from normals on total discrepancy scores and underestimation scores (p values < 0.05), but not on overestimation scores, consistent with the F tests. Left frontal and right frontal groups did not differ on any measure.

Discussion

In a previous experiment, a task based on place-preference conditioning procedures was used to induce conditioned reward associations in normal human volunteers (Johnsrude et al., 1999). The same task was used in the present study to investigate whether the ANC might be critically involved in conditioned reward learning in humans, as it is in other animals. Compared to normal control subjects and patients with unilateral frontal cortex excisions, patients with unilateral anterior temporal lobe resections that included the amygdaloid complex showed severely impaired preference conditioning. In contrast, patients with anterior temporal lobe resections performed normally on the counting task, whereas patients with frontal cortex damage were severely impaired. This task, which required that subjects monitor the frequency of occurrence of red balls in each of the three boxes, places significant demands on aspects of working memory that are known to depend on the integrity of the prefrontal cortex rather than the medial temporal lobe structures (Petrides and Milner, 1982; Smith and Milner, 1988; Owen et al., 1990, 1996; Jonides et al., 1993; Smith, 1996; Owen, 1997). This double dissociation provides clear evidence that, in humans as in other animals, reward-related learning (conditioned reward) critically depends on a circuit involving inferotemporal cortex and the ANC.

Several features of the experimental design were included to minimize the participants' awareness of the conditioning procedure and the goals of the experiment. The subjects' attention was not explicitly drawn to the stimuli to be conditioned before or during conditioning, and these stimuli were irrelevant to performance of the counting task. Furthermore, the counting task was made quite demanding to minimize the subjects' opportunity to attend to anything but that task and the occurrence of reward or non-reward. The three patterns were paired with reward on 90, 50, and 10% of the trials in which they occurred. By avoiding the absolutes of 100 and 0%, and by including a pattern paired on equal number of trials with reward and non-reward, the experimental contingencies were made more difficult to discern. Participants were also asked, at the end of the study, why they showed the preferences they did, to determine whether preferences would be attributed to previous experience with the patterns. Without exception, participants attributed their preferences to the characteristics of the pattern itself. Because the patterns were randomly assigned to the different reward contingencies for each subject, these responses may be subjective rationalizations of a conditioned preference. This suggests that participants were largely unaware of the effect of their previous experience on their behavior. The patients with temporal lobe removals also attributed their preferences to the characteristics of the patterns themselves. They did show preferences, but their preferences were not consistently related to the frequency with which patterns were associated with reward in the conditioning procedure. They did not "learn to like," as the normal subjects and those with frontal lobe damage did.

All patients in the LA and RA groups had extensive damage to the amygdaloid region, including the perirhinal and entorhinal cortices, as well as white matter tracts passing through this area (Fig. 42.1). Both groups, particularly the LA group, also had significant damage to anterior temporal neocortex. Work in monkeys indicates that bilateral lesions of either the anterior part of inferior temporal cortex or the ANC (but not the posterior part of inferior temporal cortex or the hippocampus) produce impairments in object–reward association learning (Jones and Mishkin, 1972; Speigler and Mishkin, 1981; Gaffan and Harrison, 1987). The impairments seen in many of these studies may not be attributable to damage to the ANC per se, but may be caused by entorhinal and/or perirhinal cortex damage, or to damage to white matter tracts passing

through the amygdalar region that normally connect rhinal and more lateral temporal cortex with ventral frontal cortex and medial thalamus (see, for example, Málková et al., 1997). However, considerable evidence from experiments with rats does implicate the ANC, particularly the lateral and basolateral nuclei to the exclusion of other surrounding tissue, in conditioned reward (Peinado-Manzano, 1987, 1988; Cador et al., 1989; Everitt et al., 1989, 1991; Everitt, 1990; McDonald and White, 1993; White and Hiroi, 1993). The lesions in the patients we tested encompassed the amygdala and surrounding tissue and so we are unable to draw conclusions about functional specialization of structures within this region. A notable difference between the present study and the existing animal literature is that the amygdala is typically lesioned or inactivated bilaterally in animal studies of reward-related learning (Coleman-Mesches et al., 1996). The LA and RA participants tested in the present study had predominantly unilateral damage, although undiagnosed dysfunction in some structures contralateral to the site of the excised epileptic focus may have contributed to the impairment (Incisa della Rocchetta et al., 1995). LaBar et al. (1995) found significant impairments in fear conditioning in unilateral temporal lobectomy patients, also with no effect of side of excision.

The findings presented here of impaired preference conditioning in patients with even unilateral lesions of the medial temporal area contrast with those of Tranel and Damasio (1993), who found evidence for preserved learning of affective associations in Boswell, a patient with bilateral medial-temporal damage (including the ANC). In that study, three previously novel people were instructed to act toward Boswell in either a positive (e.g., giving compliments and treats), negative (e.g., requiring him to participate in tedious experiments), or neutral way, over a 5 d period. Boswell was subsequently unable to identify the stimulus persons, but when asked to "choose the person that you would go to for a treat" he consistently chose the positive stimulus person, suggesting that he was able to learn to associate faces with reward outcomes. However, Tranel and Damasio (1993) speculate that Boswell's preserved learning might reflect the action of another learning system, that for reinforced stimulus–response associations. This type of learning appears to be mediated by a neural system that includes the dorsal striatum (e.g., Mishkin et al., 1985; McDonald and White, 1993), which is intact in Boswell. This learning system would also be expected to be intact in our patients with more restricted lesions. The apparent discrepancy in the results of the two studies therefore probably reflects the different requirements of the two tasks.

Because the anterior temporal lobe is considered to be the final stage in the cortical visual system, our results accord well with the idea that visual stimuli acquire affective significance through an interaction between high-level visual areas and the ANC. Temporal lobe excisions do not generally result in marked visual perceptual impairments, although patients with right temporal lobe lesions can show subtle deficits when normal stimulus redundancy has been reduced, by presenting items tachistoscopically, for example (Milner, 1990). The stimuli used in the present study were not degraded in any way, and all patients in both temporal lobe groups appeared able to discriminate them, judging from their physical descriptions of the patterns during the last phase.

The findings of the present study are also consistent with a body of literature demonstrating that aspects of working memory may be dependent on the integrity of the prefrontal cortex (Petrides and Milner, 1982; Funahashi et al., 1989; Owen et al., 1990, 1996; Jonides et al., 1993; Petrides et al., 1993; Wilson et al., 1993; Cohen et al., 1994; Courtney et al., 1996; Rao et al., 1997) (for review, see Owen, 1997; Rushworth and Owen, 1998). Thus, unlike the anterior temporal lobe group, the patients with excisions of the frontal lobe were unable to maintain an ongoing record of how many red balls had been found in each location, a requirement that undoubtedly placed demands on aspects of working memory.

Smith and Milner (1988) and Smith (1996) presented series of words and abstract designs to normal volunteers and patients with unilateral frontal or temporal lobe excisions. The words and designs differed in the number of times that they were repeated within a series. Whereas normal participants and patients with anterior temporal lobe resections were equally able to estimate frequency of occurrence, patients with frontal lobe excisions, particularly the right frontal group, significantly underestimated the frequency of occurrence of either words or designs. Furthermore, Smith noticed a trend toward material-specificity in this deficit: patients with left frontal-lobe lesions were more impaired than patients with right frontal-lobe lesions at estimating the frequency of occurrence of words, and the reverse pattern was observed for designs. No effect of side of excision was seen in the present study: patients with right- and left-frontal-lobe resections appeared equally impaired. The lack of hemispheric asymmetry may be owing to the nature of the stimuli to be monitored in the present study: participants were required to monitor the conjunction of a particular event (red ball) with three distinct locations (left, top, or right). This is qualitatively different from monitoring the occurrence of words or abstract designs that are all presented in the same spatial position.

In conclusion, the results of this study suggest that working memory and stimulus–reward association learning are doubly dissociable in humans. Patients with unilateral frontal lesions were impaired at the working memory component of the task, but did show preference conditioning. Conversely, patients with anterior temporal lobe resections performed normally on the working memory component, but did not acquire stimulus–reward associations. To date, the work on mediation of emotional learning by the ANC in humans has focussed on negative affect, such as fear (Bechara et al., 1995; LaBar et al., 1995, 1998; Büchel et al., 1998; Morris et al., 1998; but see, Hamann et al., 1999). The results presented in this chapter demonstrate that, in humans as in other species, structures in the region of the amygdala are required for cues to acquire affective significance through their association with rewarding events.

Acknowledgments

This work was supported by the Medical Research Council of Canada through a Career Investigatorship awarded to B. A. Milner. We gratefully acknowledge her assistance. I.S.J. was funded by the Wellcome Trust during the preparation of this manuscript. This work was conducted in the Neuropsychology/Cognitive Neuroscience Unit, Montreal Neurological Institute, McGill University, while I.S.J. and A.M.O. were working there. We thank the participants, the neurosurgeons A. Olivier, W. Feindel, and R. Leblanc, and numerous colleagues for helpful discussions.

References

Aggleton JP (1993) The contribution of the amygdala to normal and abnormal emotional states. Trends Neurosci 16:328–333.

Allen CT, Janiszewski CA (1989) Assessing the role of contingency awareness in attitudinal conditioning with implications for advertising research. J Marketing Res 26:30–43.

Baeyens F, Hermans D, Eelen P (1993) The role of CS-US contingency in human evaluative conditioning. Behav Res Ther 31:731–737.

Baeyens F, Eelen P, Crombez G (1995) Pavlovian associations are forever: on classical conditioning and extinction. J Psychophysiol 9:127–141.

Bechara A, Tranel D, Damasio H, Adolphs R, Rockland C, Damasio AR (1995) Double dissociation of conditioning and declarative knowledge relative to the amygdala and hippocampus in humans. Science 269:1115–1118.

Bierley C, McSweeney FK, Vannieuwkerk R (1985) Classical conditioning of preferences for stimuli. J Consumer Res 12:316–323.

Büchel C, Morris J, Dolan RJ, Friston KJ (1998) Brain systems mediating aversive conditioning: An event-related fMRI study. Neuron 20:947–957.

Cador M, Robbins TW, Everitt BJ (1989) Involvement of the amygdala in stimulus–reward associations: interaction with the ventral striatum. Neuroscience 30:77–86.

Carr GD, Fibiger HC, Phillips AG (1989) Conditioned place preference as a measure of drug reward. In: The neuropharmacological basis of reward (Leibman JM, Cooper SJ, eds), pp 264–319. Oxford: Oxford UP.

Cohen JD, Forman SD, Braver TS, Casey BJ, Servan-Schreiber D, Noll DC (1994) Activation of prefrontal cortex in a non-spatial working memory task with functional MRI. Hum Brain Mapp 1:293–304.

Coleman-Mesches K, Salinas JA, McGaugh JL (1996) Unilateral amygdala inactivation after training attenuates memory for reduced reward. Behav Brain Res 77:175–180.

Courtney SM, Ungerlieder LG, Keil K, Haxby JV (1996) Object and spatial visual working memory activate separate neural systems in human cortex. Cereb Cortex 6:39–49.

Davis M (1998) Anatomic and physiologic substrates of emotion in an animal model. J Clin Neurophysiol 15:378–387.

Eliashiv SD, Dewar S, Wainwright I, Engel J Jr, Fried I (1997) Long-term follow-up after temporal lobe resection for lesions associated with chronic seizures. Neurology 48:1383–1388.

Everitt BJ (1990) Sexual motivation: A neural and behavioural analysis of the mechanisms underlying appetitive and copulatory responses of male rats. Neurosci Biobehav Rev 14:217–232.

Everitt BJ, Cador M, Robbins TW (1989) Interactions between the amygdala and ventral striatum in stimulus–reward associations: studies using a second-order schedule of sexual reinforcement. Neuroscience 30:63–75.

Everitt BJ, Morris KA, O'Brien A, Robbins TW (1991) The basolateral amygdala-ventral striatal system and conditioned place preference: further evidence of limbic-striatal interactions underlying reward-related processes. Neuroscience 42:1–18.

Everitt BJ, Parkinson JA, Olmstead MC, Arroyo M, Robledo P, Robbins TW (1999) Associative processes in addition and reward. The role of amygdala-ventral striatal subsystems. Ann N Y Acad Sci 877:412–438.

Fanselow M, LeDoux J (1999) Why we think plasticity underlying Pavlovian fear conditioning occurs in the basolateral amygdala. Neuron 23:229–232.

Fendt M, Fanselow MS (1999) The neuroanatomical and neurochemical basis of conditioned fear. Neurosci Biobehav Rev 23:743–760.

Funahashi S, Bruce CJ, Goldman-Rakic PS (1989) Mnemonic coding of visual space in the monkey's dorsolateral prefrontal cortex. J Neurophysiol 61:1–19.

Gaffan D, Harrison S (1987) Amygdalectomy and disconnection in visual learning for auditory secondary reinforcement by monkeys. J Neurosci 7:2285–2292.

Gallagher M, Chiba AA (1996) The amygdala and emotion. Curr Opin Neurobiol 6:221–227.

Gallagher M, Holland PC (1994) The amygdala complex: multiple roles in associative learning. Proc Natl Acad Sci USA 91:11771–11776.

Gallagher M, Graham PW, Holland PC (1990) The amygdala central nucleus and appetitive Pavlovian conditioning: lesions impair one class of conditioned behavior. J Neurosci 10:1906–1911.

Hamann SB, Ely TD, Grafton ST, Kilts CD (1999) Amygdala activity related to enhanced memory for pleasant and aversive stimuli. Nat Neurosci 2:289–294.

Hatfield T, Han J-S, Conley M, Gallagher M, Holland P (1996) Neurotoxic lesions of basolateral, but not central, amygdala interfere with Pavlovian second-order conditioning and reinforcer devaluation effects. J Neurosci 16:5256–5265.

Hermann BP, Wyler AR, Somes G (1991) Preoperative psychological adjustment and surgical outcome are determinants of psychosocial status after anterior temporal lobectomy. J Neurol Neurosurg Psychiatry 55:491–496.

Hiroi N, White NM (1991) The lateral nucleus of the amygdala mediates expression of the amphetamine-produced conditioned place preference. J Neurosci 11:2107–2116.

Hitchcott PK, Phillips GD (1998) Double dissociation of the behavioural effects of R(+) 7-OH-DPAT infusions in the central and basolateral amygdala nuclei upon Pavlovian and instrumental conditioned appetitive behaviours. Psychopharmacology 140:458–469.

Hitchcott PK, Bonardi CM, Phillips GD (1997) Enhanced stimulus–reward learning by intra-amygdala administration of a D3 dopamine receptor agonist. Psychopharmacology 133:240–248.

Holland PC, Gallagher M (1999) Amygdala circuitry in attention and representational processes. Trends Cognit Sci 3:65–73.

Incisa della Rocchetta A, Gadian DG, Connelly A, Polkey CE, Jackson GD, Watkins KE, Johnson CL, Mishkin M, Vargha-Khadem F (1995) Verbal memory impairment after right temporal lobe surgery: role of contralateral damage as revealed by 1H magnetic resonance spectroscopy and T2 relaxometry. Neurology 45:797–802.

Johnson MK, Kim JK, Risse G (1985) Do alcoholic Korsakoff's syndrome patients acquire affective reactions? J Exp Psychol: Learn Mem Cog 11:22–36.

Johnsrude IS, Owen AM, Zhao WV, White NM (1999) Conditioned preference in humans: a novel experimental approach. Learn Motiv 30:250–264.

Jones B, Mishkin M (1972) Limbic lesions and the problem of stimulus-reinforcement associations. Exp Neurol 36:362–377.

Jonides J, Smith EE, Koeppe RA, Awh E, Minoshima S, Mintun MA (1993) Spatial working memory in humans as revealed by PET. Nature 363:623–625.

Killcross S, Robbins TW, Everitt BJ (1997) Different types of fear-conditioned behaviour mediated by separate nuclei within the amygdala. Nature 388: 377–380.

Kirk-Smith MD, van Toller C, Dodd GH (1983) Unconscious odour conditioning in human subjects. Biol Psychol 17:221–231.

LaBar KS, LeDoux JE, Spencer DO, Phelps EA (1995) Impaired fear conditioning following unilateral temporal lobectomy in humans. J Neurosci 15:6846–6855.

LaBar KS, Gatenby JC, Gore JC, LeDoux JE, Phelps EA (1998) Human amygdala activation during conditioned fear acquisition and extinction: A mixed-trial fMRI study. Neuron 20:937–945.

LeDoux JE (1998) Fear and the brain: where have we been, and where are we going? Biol Psychiatry 44:1229–1238.

Levey AB, Martin I (1975) Classical conditioning of human "evaluative" responses. Behav Res Ther 13:221–226.

Levey AB, Martin I (1983) Part I. Cognitions, evaluations and conditioning: rules of sequence and rules of consequence. Adv Behav Res Ther 4:181–195.

MacDonald JD, Avis D, Evans AC (1994) Multiple surface identification and matching in magnetic resonance images. Proc Soc Vis Biomed Comput 2359: 160–169.

Málková L, Gaffan D, Murray EA (1997) Excitotoxic lesions of the amygdala fail to produce impairment in visual learning for auditory secondary reinforcement but interfere with reinforcer devaluation effects in rhesus monkeys. J Neurosci 17:6011–6020.

Martin I, Levey AB (1978) Evaluative conditioning. Adv Behav Res Ther 1:57–102.

McDonald RJ, White NM (1993) A triple dissociation of memory systems: hippocampus, amygdala, and dorsal striatum. Behav Neurosci 107:3–22.

Milner B (1990) Right temporal-lobe contribution to visual perception and visual memory. In: Vision, temporal lobe and memory (Iwai E, ed), pp 43–53. New York: Elsevier.

Milner B (1997) Amobarbital memory testing: Some personal reflections. Brain Cogn 33:14–17.

Mishkin M, Malamut B, Bachevalier J (1985) Memories and habits: two neural systems. In: Neurobiology of learning and memory (Lynch G, McGaugh JL, Weinberger NM, eds) New York: Guilford.

Morris JS, Öhman A, Dolan RJ (1998) Conscious and unconscious emotional learning in the human amygdala. Nature 393:467–470.

Niedenthal PM (1990) Implicit perception of affective information. J Exp Social Psychol 26:505–527.

Ono T, Nishijo H, Uwano T (1995) Amygdala role in conditioned associative learning. Prog Neurobiol 46:401–422.

Owen AM (1997) The functional organization of working memory processes within human lateral frontal cortex: the contribution of functional neuroimaging. Eur J Neurosci 9:1329–1339.

Owen AM, Downes JJ, Sahakian BJ, Polkey CE, Robbins TW (1990) Planning and spatial working memory following frontal lobe lesions in man. Neuropsychologia 28:1021–1034.

Owen AM, Morris RG, Sahakian BJ, Polkey CE, Robbins TW (1996) Double dissociations of memory and executive functions in working memory tasks following frontal lobe excisions, temporal lobe exci-

sions or amygdalo-hippocampectomy in man. Brain 119:1597–1615.

Peinado-Manzano MA (1987) Role of the lateral nucleus of the amygdala in successive conditional visual discrimination learning in rats. Med Sci Res 15:383–384.

Peinado-Manzano MA (1988) Effects of bilateral lesions of the central and lateral amygdala on free operant successive discrimination. Behav Brain Res 29:61–72.

Petrides M, Milner BA (1982) Deficits on subject-ordered tasks after frontal- and temporal-lobe lesions in man. Neuropsychologia 20:249–262.

Petrides M, Alivisatos B, Evans AC, Meyer E (1993) Dissociation of human mid-dorsolateral from posterior dorsolateral frontal cortex in memory processing. Proc Natl Acad Sci USA 90:873–877.

Rao SC, Rainer G, Miller EK (1997) Integration of what and where in the primate prefrontal cortex. Science 276:821–824.

Razran GHS (1954) The conditioned evocation of attitudes (cognitive conditioning?). J Exp Psychol 48:278–282.

Redington K, Volpe BT, Gazzaniga MS (1984) Failure of preference formation in amnesia. Neurology 34: 536–538.

Robbins TW, Everitt BJ (1996) Neurobehavioural mechanisms of reward and motivation. Curr Opin Neurobiol 6:228–236.

Robbins TW, Cador M, Taylor JR, Everitt BJ (1989) Limbic-striatal interactions in reward-related processes. Neurosci Biobehav Rev 13:155–162.

Rogan MT, Staubli UV, LeDoux JE (1997) Fear conditioning induces associative long-term potentiation in the amygdala. Nature 390:604–607.

Rozin P, Zellner D (1985) The role of Pavlovian conditioning in the acquisition of food likes and dislikes. In: Experimental assessments and clinical applications of conditioned food aversions (Braveman NS, Bronstein P, eds), pp 189–202. New York: N Y Acad Sci.

Rushworth MFS, Owen AM (1998) The functional organization of the lateral frontal cortex: conjecture or conjuncture in the electrophysiology literature. Trends Cognit Sci 2:46–53.

Schechter MD, Calcagnetti DJ (1993) Trends in place preference conditioning with a cross-indexed bibliography: 1957–1991. Neurosci Biobehav Rev 17:21–41.

Smith ML (1996) Recall of frequency of occurrence of self-generated and examiner-provided words after frontal or temporal lobectomy. Neuropsychologia 34:553–563.

Smith ML, Milner B (1988) Estimation of frequency of occurrence of abstract designs after frontal or temporal lobectomy. Neuropsychologia 26:297–306.

Speigler BJ, Mishkin M (1981) Evidence for the sequential participation of inferior temporal cortex and amygdala in the acquisition of stimulus–reward associations. Behav Brain Res 3:303–317.

Staats AW, Staats CK (1958) Attitudes established by classical conditioning. J Abnorm Psychol 57:37–40.

Staats CK, Staats AW (1957) Meaning established by classical conditioning. J Exp Psychol 54:74–80.

Stuart EW, Shimp TA, Engle RW (1987) Classical conditioning of consumer attitudes: four experiments in an advertising context. J Consumer Res 14:334–349.

Stuart EW, Shimp TA, Engle RW (1991) A program of classical conditioning experiments testing variations in the conditioned stimulus and context. J Consumer Res 18:1–12.

Talairach J, Tournoux P (1988) Co-planar stereotaxic atlas of the human brain: 3-dimensional proportional system: an approach to cerebral imaging. Stuttgart, Germany: Thieme.

Todrank J, Byrnes D, Wrzesniewski A, Rozin P (1995) Odors can change preferences for people in photographs: a cross-modal evaluative conditioning study with olfactory USs and visual CSs. Learn Motiv 26:116–140.

Tranel D, Damasio AR (1993) The covert learning of affective valence does not require structures in hippocampal system or amygdala. J Cogn Neurosci 5:79–88.

Tzschentke TM (1998) Measuring reward with the conditioned pace preference paradigm: a comprehensive review of drug effects, recent progress and new issues. Prog Neurobiol 56:613–672.

Walker DL, Davis M (1997) Double dissociation between the involvement of the bed nucleus of the stria terminalis and the central nucleus of the amygdala in startle increases produced by conditioned versus unconditioned fear. J Neurosci 17:9375–9383.

White NM, Hiroi N (1993) Amphetamine conditioned cue preference and the neurobiology of drug seeking. Semin Neurosci 5:329–336.

White NM, McDonald RJ (1993) Acquisition of a spatial conditioned place preference is impaired by amygdala lesions and improved by fornix lesions. Behav Brain Res 55:269–281.

Wilson FA, O Scalaidhe SP, Goldman-Rakic PS (1993) Dissociations of object and spatial processing domains in primate prefrontal cortex. Science 260:1955–1958.

Weiskrantz L (1956) Behavioural changes associated with ablation of the amygdaloid complex in monkeys. J Comp Physiol Psychol 9:381–391.

V BIOLOGY OF SOCIAL RELATIONSHIPS AND INTERPERSONAL PROCESSES

A. Basic Processes

43 Biobehavioral Responses to Stress in Females: Tend-and-Befriend, Not Fight-or-Flight

Shelley E. Taylor, Laura Cousino Klein, Brian P. Lewis, Tara L. Gruenewald, Regan A. R. Gurung, and John A. Updegraff

Survival depends on the ability to mount a successful response to threat. The human stress response has been characterized as fight-or-flight (Cannon, 1932) and has been represented as an essential mechanism in the survival process. We propose that human female responses to stress (as well as those of some animal species) are not well characterized by fight-or-flight, as research has implicitly assumed, but rather are more typically characterized by a pattern we term "tend-and-befriend." Specifically, we suggest that, by virtue of differential parental investment, female stress responses have selectively evolved to maximize the survival of self and offspring. We suggest that females respond to stress by nurturing offspring, exhibiting behaviors that protect them from harm and reduce neuroendocrine responses that may compromise offspring health (the tending pattern), and by befriending; namely, affiliating with social groups to reduce risk. We hypothesize and consider evidence from humans and other species to suggest that females create, maintain, and utilize these social groups, especially relations with other females, to manage stressful conditions. We suggest that female responses to stress may build on attachment–caregiving processes that downregulate sympathetic and hypothalamic-pituitary-adrenocortical (HPA) responses to stress. In support of this biobehavioral theory, we consider a large animal and human literature on neuroendocrine responses to stress, suggesting that the tend-and-befriend pattern may be oxytocin mediated and moderated by sex hormones and endogenous opioid peptide mechanisms.

Background

The fight-or-flight response is generally regarded as the prototypic human response to stress. First described by Walter Cannon in 1932, the fight-or-flight response is characterized physiologically by sympathetic nervous system activation that innervates the adrenal medulla, producing a hormonal cascade that results in the secretion of catecholamines, especially norepinephrine and epinephrine, into the bloodstream. In addition to its physiological concomitants, fight-or-flight has been adopted as a metaphor for human behavioral responses to stress, and whether a human (or an animal) fights or flees in response to sympathetic arousal is thought to depend on the nature of the stressor. If the organism sizes up a threat or predator and determines that it has a realistic chance of overcoming the predator, then attack is likely. In circumstances in which the threat is perceived to be more formidable, flight is more probable.

A coordinated biobehavioral stress response is believed to be at the core of reactions to threats of all kinds, including attacks by predators; assaults by members of the same species; dangerous conditions such as fire, earthquake, tornado, or flooding; and other threatening events. As such, an appropriate and modulated stress response is at the core of survival. Through principles of natural selection, an organism whose response to stress was successful would likely pass that response on to subsequent generations, and the fight-or-flight response is thought to be such an evolved response.

A little-known fact about the fight-or-flight response is that the preponderance of research exploring its parameters has been conducted on males, especially on male rats. Until recently, the gender distribution in the human literature was inequitable as well. Prior to 1995, women constituted about 17% of participants in laboratory studies of physiological and neuroendocrine responses to stress. In the past 5 years, the gender balance has been somewhat redressed. We identified 200 studies of physiological and neuroendocrine responses to an acute experimental stressor conducted between 1985 and the present, utilizing 14,548 participants, 66% of whom were male, and 34% of whom were female. Despite movement toward parity, the inclusion of women in human stress studies remains heavily dependent on the specific topic under investigation. For example, women are overrepresented in studies of affiliative responses to stress, and men are overrepresented in studies of neuroendocrine responses to physical and mental challenges (Gruenewald, Taylor, Klein, & Seeman, 1999).

Why have stress studies been so heavily based on data from males? The justification for this bias is similar to the rationale for the exclusion, until recently, of females from many clinical trials of drugs, from research on treatments for major chronic diseases, and from animal research on illness vulnerabilities. The rationale has been that, because females have greater cyclical variation in neuroendocrine responses (due to the reproductive cycle), their data present a confusing and often uninterpretable pattern of results. The fight-or-flight response may also be affected by female cycling, and, as a result, evidence concerning a fight-or-flight response in females has been inconsistent. However, what if the equivocal nature of the female data is not due solely to neuroendocrine variation but also to the fact that the female stress response is not exclusively, nor even predominantly, fight-or-flight?

Theoretical Model

An empirical gap such as the identified gender bias in stress studies provides a striking opportunity to build theory. From a metatheoretical perspective, we reasoned that a viable theoretical framework for understanding female responses to stress may be derived by making a few conservative evolutionary assumptions and then building parallel and mutually constraining biological and behavioral models.

We propose, first, that successful responses to stress have been passed on to subsequent generations through principles of natural selection: Those without successful responses to threat are disproportionately unlikely to reach an age when reproduction is possible. An additional assumption is that, because females have typically borne a greater role in the care of young offspring, responses to threat that were successfully passed on would have been those that protected offspring as well as the self. The female of the species makes a greater investment initially in pregnancy and nursing and typically plays the primary role in activities designed to bring the offspring to maturity. High maternal investment should lead to selection for female stress responses that do not jeopardize the health of the mother and her offspring and that maximize the likelihood that they will survive.[1] "Tending," that is, quieting and caring for offspring and blending into the environment, may be effective for addressing a broad array of threats. In contrast, fight responses on the part of females may put themselves and their offspring in jeopardy, and flight behavior on the part of females may be compromised by pregnancy or the need to care for immature offspring. Thus, alternative behavioral responses are likely to have evolved in females.

The protection of self and offspring is a complex and difficult task in many threatening circumstances, and those who made effective use of the social group would have been more successful against many threats than those who did not. This assumption leads to the prediction that females may selectively affiliate in response to stress, which maximizes the likelihood that multiple group members will protect both them and their offspring. Accordingly, we suggest that the female stress response of tending to offspring and affiliating with a social group is facilitated by the process of "befriending," which is the creation of networks of associations that provide resources and protection for the female and her offspring under conditions of stress.

We propose that the biobehavorial mechanism underlying the tend-and-befriend pattern is the attachment–caregiving system, a stress-related system that has been previously explored largely for its role in maternal bonding and child development. In certain respects, the female tending response under stressful conditions may represent the counterpart of the infant attachment mechanism that appears to be so critical for the development of normal biological regulatory systems in offspring (Hofer, 1995). Numerous investigations have explored the effects of the mother–infant bond on infants' emotional, social, and biological development, but less literature has explored the counterpart maternal mechanism, that is, what evokes tending behavior in the mother. We attempt to redress that balance here. In addition, we suggest that the befriending pattern may have piggybacked onto the attachment–caregiving system and thus may be at least partially regulated by the same biobehavioral systems that regulate tending. From this analysis, it follows that neuroendocrine mechanisms would have evolved to regulate these responses to stress, much as sympathetic activation is thought to provide the physiological basis for the fight-or-flight response. We propose that the neurobiological underpinnings of the attachment–caregiving system (e.g., Panksepp, 1998) provide a foundation for this stress regulatory system. Specifically, oxytocin and endogenous opioid mechanisms may be at the core of the tend-and-befriend response.

In essence, then, we are proposing the existence of an endogenous stress regulatory system that has heretofore been largely ignored in the biological and behavioral literatures on stress, especially in humans. Accordingly, the empirical evaluation of the viability of this theoretical position requires us to address several questions: Is there neuroendocrine and behavioral evidence for our contention that fight-or-flight is less characteristic of female than male responses to stress? Is there a neuroendocrinological basis for and behavioral evidence for tending under stress in

females, that is, nurturing and caring for offspring under conditions of threat? Is there evidence of differential affiliation by females under stress and a neuroendocrine mechanism that may underlie it?

To evaluate these hypotheses, we draw on several sources of scientific evidence. We begin with evidence for gender divergences in biological and behavioral responses to stress and examine substantial neuroendocrine data from animal studies that may account for these divergences. We use the animal literature not to draw direct connections to human behavior but because animal studies enable researchers to test neuroendocrine mechanisms directly, whereas such evidence is typically more indirect in human studies. We then consider whether there are neuroendocrine and behavioral parallels in the literature on human and nonhuman primate responses to stress. Clearly, there are risks in combining evidence from multiple sources that include behavioral studies with humans and nonhuman primates and neuroendocrine research from animal studies. However, any effort to understand stress responses that ignores one or more of these lines of evidence is potentially risky because a comprehensive biobehavioral account of stress response requires integration across multiple sources of evidence. We suggest appropriate caveats in generalizing from one line of work to another when they are warranted.

Females and the Fight-or-Flight Response

The basic neuroendocrine core of stress responses does not seem to vary substantially between human males and females.[2] Both sexes experience a cascade of hormonal responses to threat that appears to begin with the rapid release of oxytocin, vasopressin, corticotropin-releasing factor (CRF), and possibly other hormones produced in the paraventricular nucleus of the hypothalamus.[3] Direct neural activation of the adrenal medulla triggers release of the catecholamines, norepinephrine and epinephrine, and concomitant sympathetic responses, as noted. Hypothalamic release of CRF and other hormones stimulate the release of adrenocorticotropin hormone (ACTH) from the anterior pituitary, which, in turn, stimulates the adrenal cortex to release corticosteroids, especially cortisol or corticosterone, depending on the species (Jezova, Skultetyova, Tokarev, Bakos, & Vigas, 1995; Sapolsky, 1992b). As such, both males and females are mobilized to meet the short-term demands presented by stress.

As already noted, however, a stress response geared toward aggressing or fleeing may be somewhat adaptive for males but it may not address the different challenges faced by females, especially those challenges that arise from maternal investment in offspring. The demands of pregnancy, nursing, and infant care render females extremely vulnerable to external threats. Should a threat present itself during this time, a mother's attack on a predator or flight could render offspring fatally unprotected. Instead, behaviors that involve getting offspring out of the way, retrieving them from threatening circumstances, calming them down and quieting them, protecting them from further threat, and anticipating protective measures against stressors that are imminent may increase the likelihood of survival of offspring. Given the adaptiveness of such behaviors for females, neuroendocrine mechanisms may have evolved to facilitate these behaviors and inhibit behavioral tendencies to fight or flee.

Neuroendocrine Perspective on Fight

Consistent with the above analysis, neuroendocrine differences between the sexes suggest that females are unlikely to show a physical "fight" response to threat. Females largely lack androgens, which, in many species, act to develop the male brain for aggression either pre- or postnatally and then activate aggressive behavior in specific threatening contexts (such as responses to territorial establishment and defense).[4] In humans, gonadal hormones appear to influence the development of both rough-and-tumble play and tendencies toward aggression, both of which show moderate to large sex differences (Collaer & Hines, 1995).

Although the exact role of testosterone in male attack behaviors remains controversial, testosterone has been associated with hostility and aggressive behavior in both human (e.g., Bergman & Brismar, 1994; Olweus, Mattson, Schalling, & Low, 1980) and animal studies (Lumia, Thorner, & McGinnis, 1994). In humans, testosterone has been shown to increase with acute stress, including high-intensity exercise (e.g., Cumming, Brunsting, Strich, Ries, & Rebar, 1986; Mathur, Toriola, & Dada, 1986; Wheeler et al., 1994) and psychological stress (although the effects vary by the nature of the stressor and by individual differences; Christensen, Knussmann, & Couwenbergs, 1985; Hellhammer, Hubert, & Schurmeyer, 1985; Williams et al., 1982). Girdler, Jamner, and Shapiro (1997) found that, in men, testosterone increased significantly with acute stress and testosterone reactivity to acute stressors was significantly associated with level of hostility. Although human male aggression is generally regarded as being under greater cortical control than is true for lower order animals, a small but consistently positive relation between self-reported hostility and testosterone has been found in meta-analyses of aggression, as has a consistent relationship between testosterone levels and assessments of aggression made by others (Archer, 1990). Studies of captive human male populations, including incarcerated felons and psychiatric patients, also show positive relations between testosterone and ratings of aggressive behavior (Benton, 1992). Thus testosterone may be a link by which sympathetic arousal is channeled into hostility and interpersonal attack behavior among males.

The androgens, especially testosterone, are also implicated in the development of rough-and-tumble play (Beatty, 1984; Collaer & Hines,

1995). From an early age, one male acts as an evocative stimulus for another male, inducing aggressive behavior (Maccoby & Jacklin, 1974). In the human male, rough-and-tumble play is believed to be organized prenatally by testosterone and androgens, but because it occurs before puberty, it may not be dependent on testosterone for activation (see Beatty, 1984; Collaer & Hines, 1995, for reviews).

Human female aggressive responses are not organized by testosterone or androgens either pre- or postnatally, and the typical low levels of those hormones in juvenile and adult females means that predominantly male hormones are unlikely to be the organizing factors that evoke a female fight response as they do in males. The presence of either another male or another female does not typically act as an evocative stimulus for human female attack behavior, and human females do not engage in rough-and-tumble play at the levels observed in males (Maccoby & Jacklin, 1974).[5] In human males, there appears to be a link between sympathetic reactivity and hostility, whereas hostility in females is not reliably linked to sympathetic arousal, suggesting that it is not a necessary component of a fight-or-flight response (Girdler et al., 1997).

Female aggression is well documented. Our argument is not that female aggression fails to occur but that it is not mediated by the sympathetic arousal–testosterone links that appear to be implicated in fight responses for men. Extensive reviews of the human aggression literature suggest that males may not be inherently more aggressive than females, but that the patterns of aggression between males and females differ (see Bjorkqvist & Niemela, 1992, for a review). Males are more likely to use physical aggression in struggles for power within a hierarchy or to defend territory against external enemies. Females reliably show less physical aggression than males but they display as much or more indirect aggression (Holmstrom, 1992), that is, aggression in the form of gossip, rumor-spreading, and enlisting the cooperation of a third party in un-

dermining an acquaintance. However, human females still show lower levels of verbal aggression than males, although this sex difference is smaller than that for physical aggression (Eagly & Steffen, 1986). Overall, female aggressive responses appear to be tied less to sympathetic arousal than male aggression and are instead more cerebral in nature. For example, female aggressive behavior may be more moderated by social norms and learning and by cultural, situational, and individual differences (Bjorkqvist & Niemela, 1992; Eagly & Steffen, 1986).

The physical fight response is the most robust area of aggression that shows higher levels for males than females, and these differences are found in rodents, primates, and humans (Archer, 1990; Eagly & Steffen, 1986; Hyde, 1984). When female attack behavior is observed, it appears to be confined to particular circumstances. For example, female adult rats are aggressive toward intruder (i.e., unfamiliar) males and females, primarily when they are pregnant or nursing, behaviors that fall off rapidly as pups mature (Adams, 1992). In addition, maternal attack behavior toward potential predators that threaten offspring has been well documented (Adams, 1992; Brain, Haug, & Parmigiani, 1992; Sandnabba, 1992). In summary, female physical aggression appears to be confined to situations requiring defense, rather than to the broader array of threats that is found in males.[6]

Neuroendocrine Perspective on Flight

Although flight may appear to be the more probable first line of defense of females to stressful events or threatening circumstances, this response, too, may not be dominant in the hierarchy of stress responses of females. Females who are pregnant, nursing, or otherwise responsible for offspring may be unable to flee without jeopardizing the health and safety of their offspring. Although flight behavior among females is well documented in species whose offspring have the capability to flee within hours after birth (e.g., ungulates such as deer or antelope), in species whose offspring remain immature for long periods of time, flight by the female can require abandonment of offspring. Females of most species spend a substantial proportion of their fertile lives either pregnant, nursing, or raising young children, and until recently, this was largely true of human females as well. Given the very central role that these activities play in the perpetuation of the species, stress responses that enabled the female to protect simultaneously herself and her offspring are likely to have resulted in more surviving offspring.

If flight behavior in response to stress is indeed inhibited in females, may there be a neuroendocrine basis for this inhibition? McCarthy (1995) alluded to such a mechanism in her animal studies of the behavioral effects of oxytocin and its modulation by estrogen. In particular, she argued that animals in the natural environment face a constant barrage of stress and a continuous stress response can have deleterious physiological effects. Consequently, reactions that control stress responses have physiological advantages. Oxytocin release may be such a reaction. Oxytocin is a posterior pituitary hormone that is released to a broad array of stressors by both males and females. It is associated with parasympathetic (vagal) functioning, suggesting a counterregulatory role in fear responses to stress (Dreifuss, Dubois-Dauphin, Widmer, & Raggenbass, 1992; Sawchenko & Swanson, 1982; Swanson & Sawchenko, 1980). In experimental studies of the effects of exogenously administered oxytocin with rodents, oxytocin has been found to enhance sedation and relaxation, reduce fearfulness, and decrease sympathetic activity, patterns of responses that are antithetical to the fight-or-flight response (Uvnas-Moberg, 1997). These effects appear to be substantially more pronounced in female rats than in males for several reasons. First, oxytocin release in response to stress appears to be greater in females than in males (Jezova, Jurankova, Mosnarova, Kriska, & Skultetyova, 1996). Second, androgens have

been shown to inhibit oxytocin release under conditions of stress (Jezova et al., 1996). Third, the effects of oxytocin are strongly modulated by estrogen (McCarthy, 1995).

The estrogen-enhanced anxiolytic properties of oxytocin (e.g., Windle, Shanks, Lightman, & Ingram, 1997) may explain the consistent sex differences found in stress-related behavior among rats. For example, in response to acute stress, female laboratory rats show fewer behavioral indications of fear (e.g., freezing) than males (e.g., Klein, Popke, & Grunberg, 1998), slower withdrawal latencies to heat and mechanical stimuli, a longer tail-flick response (Uvnas-Moberg, 1997), higher ambulation scores in openfield tests, faster time to emerge from familiar into novel territory, and a greater amount of exploration of novel territory (Gray's studies, as cited in Gray & Lalljee, 1974). The exogenous administration of oxytocin in rats results in decreased blood pressure (effects that last longer in females), decreased pain sensitivity, and decreased corticosteroid levels, among other findings also suggestive of a reduced stress response (Uvnas-Moberg, 1997). Oxytocin is also known to promote maternal and other forms of affiliative behavior, which, McCarthy (1995) argued, may be functional under stress, representing more adaptive responses than extreme fear. Although McCarthy's oxytocin-based argument did not address flight behavior per se, its emphasis on fear reduction for moderating the typical behavioral responses to fear suggests that oxytocin may be implicated in the processes by which fear in the rat is reduced, flight is avoided, and maternal and other forms of affiliative behavior are increased under conditions of threat (see McCarthy, 1995). These effects may be conditional on the development of a maternal bond between mother and infant: Among mother–infant pairs where attachment bonds have been formed, abandonment of infants under stress is rarely, if ever, found (Keverne, Nevison, & Martel, 1999; Mendoza & Mason, 1999).

Whether and exactly how McCarthy's argument can be applied to the human situation remains to be seen. For example, although female rats show fewer behavioral signs of anxiety than males, that pattern may be reversed in nonhuman primates and humans, although the data are ambiguous (Gray's studies, as cited in Gray & Lalljee, 1974).[7] Nonetheless, as we describe below, oxytocin in human females has been found to have similar effects on anxiety, affiliation, and maternal behavior (e.g., Uvnas-Moberg, 1997), and estrogen is associated with reduced anxiety in human females (Gray, 1971). In humans, oxytocin inhibits the release of glucocorticoids, also suggesting an anxiolytic effect (Chiodera et al., 1991). Consequently, the role of oxytocin in the inhibition of flight responses merits continued cross-species investigations.

In summary, we suggest that the flight response to stress may be inhibited in females and that such inhibition favors the survival of the female and her offspring under conditions of stress. The neuroendocrine underpinnings of this response may be oxytocin mediated.

Tending under Stress

Tending

As we previously stated, the basic neuroendocrine core of stress responses does not seem to vary substantially between human males and females. In both sexes, threat triggers sympathetic-adrenal-medullary (SAM) and hypothalamic-pituitary-adrenal (HPA) activation, as well as the release of other neuroendocrine responses that operate to prepare the organism to respond to the stressor. How would a female responding to stress with sympathetic arousal nonetheless quiet and calm down offspring? We propose that the biobehavioral mechanism for the tending process builds on the attachment-caregiving system. We explore the hypothesis that the neuroendocrine mechanisms that may act to modulate sympathetic arousal and HPA activation also act to encourage tending to offspring under conditions of threat.

Attachment was originally conceived as a stress-related biobehavioral system that is the mainstay of maternal bonding and of child socialization (Bowlby, 1988). This largely innate caregiving system is thought to be especially activated in response to threat and to signs of offspring distress (such as "distress vocalization"). The caregiving system has been heavily explored through animal studies, with parallels in human developmental investigations. A paradigm researchers frequently adopt for empirical investigations of mother–infant attachment–caregiving processes involves separation, and under these circumstances, in a number of species, both mothers and offspring show distress at separation. For example, in a study of squirrel monkeys (*Saimiri sciureus*), a 30- to 60-min separation of mother and infant led to signs of distress and increased plasma cortisol in both mothers and infants (Coe, Mendoza, Smotherman, & Levine, 1978); however, on being reunited, the stress responses of both mother and infant declined (Mendoza, Coe, Smotherman, Kaplan, & Levine, 1980). Meaney and colleagues (e.g., Francis, Diorio, Liu, & Meaney, 1999; Liu et al., in press; Liu et al., 1997) explicitly link tending responses to stress and demonstrate consequent effects on the development of stress regulatory systems. In one of Meaney and colleagues' paradigms, infant rats are removed from the nest, handled by a human experimenter, and then returned to the nest. The immediate response of the mother is intense licking and grooming and arched-back nursing, which provides the pup with immediate stimulation that nurtures and soothes it. Over the long term, this maternal behavior results in better regulation of somatic growth and neural development, especially enhancing hippocampal synaptic development and consequent spatial learning and memory in offspring. In certain respects, the female tending response under stressful conditions may represent the counterpart of the infant attachment and separation distress signaling system (Hofer, 1995). Although considerable research has explored the effects of the mother–infant bond on infants' development, less literature has explored the counterpart mechanism in the mother. We attempt here to outline elements of that response.

Oxytocin and endogenous opioid mechanisms may be at the core of the tending response (Panksepp, Nelson, & Bekkedal, 1999). Evidence from a broad array of animal studies involving rats, prairie voles, monkeys, and sheep show that central administration of oxytocin reduces anxiety and has mildly sedative properties in both males and females (e.g., Carter, Williams, Witt, & Insel, 1992; Drago, Pederson, Caldwell, & Prange, 1986; Fahrbach, Morrell, & Pfaff, 1985; McCarthy, Chung, Ogawa, Kow, & Pfaff, 1991; McCarthy, McDonald, Brooks, & Goldman, 1996; Uvnas-Moberg, 1997; Witt, Carter, & Walton, 1990). As noted, this response appears to be stronger in females than in males, and oxytocin may play two roles with regard to the female stress response. It may serve both to calm the female who is physiologically aroused by a stressor and also to promote affiliative behaviors, including maternal behavior toward offspring. For example, studies of ewes (*Ovis*) have found that intracerebroventricular administration of oxytocin stimulates maternal behavior (Kendrick, Keverne, & Baldwin, 1987; see also Kendrick et al., 1997). The resulting grooming and touching that occurs in mother–infant contact may help quiet infants. These effects appear to be bidirectional, inasmuch as oxytocin enhances affiliative and affectionate contact, which, in turn, enhances the flow of oxytocin (Uvnas-Moberg, 1999).[8] As noted above, endogenous opioid mechanisms are also implicated in maternal attachment processes. In rhesus monkeys (*Macaca mulatta*), administration of naloxone (an opioid antagonist) is associated with less caregiving and protective behavior toward infants (Martel, Nevison, Rayment, Simpson, & Keverne, 1993). Similarly, administration of naltrexone, another opioid antagonist, inhibits maternal behavior in sheep under experimental conditions (Kendrick & Keverne, 1989). In rat studies, administration of oxytocin antagonists diminishes the attractive qualities of conditioned maternal cues and blocks behavioral indices of infant–mother attachment (Panksepp et al., 1999).

A large number of animal studies suggest that this maternal contact under stressful conditions has a wide array of immediate benefits for offspring. Maternal touching among rats reduces HPA alterations indicative of a stress response in pups (Liu et al., 1997; Pihoker, Owens, Kuhn, Schanberg, & Nemeroff, 1993; Wang, Bartolome, & Schanberg, 1996). Separation from the mother increases corticosterone secretion in rat pups, which is reduced when the mother returns (Kuhn, Pauk, & Schanberg, 1990; Stanton, Gutierrez, & Levine, 1988). Studies of rhesus monkeys have found that ventral contact between offspring and mother following a threatening event promotes rapid decreases in HPA activity and sympathetic nervous system arousal (Gunnar, Gonzalez, Goodlin, & Levine, 1981; Mendoza, Smotherman, Miner, Kaplan, & Levine, 1978; Reite, Short, Seiler, & Pauley, 1981).

The estrogen-enhanced oxytocin responses documented in rats and now explored in humans appear to be very strong. McCarthy (1995), for example, referred to the effects of estrogen on oxytocin as among the strongest known effects of estrogen. Uvnas-Moberg (1997) found that, in rats, oxytocin-induced calming may last for several weeks, suggesting that it is not continuously maintained by oxytocin flow but, instead, is maintained by secondary changes induced by the peptide. Moreover, these effects are not easily blocked by oxytocin antagonists. The surprisingly robust, long duration of these oxytocin-mediated effects suggests that they may be exerted at the level of the genome (Uvnas-Moberg, 1997). Thus, the oxytocin effect in females is potent, long-lasting, and maintained by secondary changes, suggesting centrality and importance, at least in animal studies.

Although studies with humans are less able to provide evidence of underlying mechanisms, mother–infant attachment processes have been found to have much the same benefits on human infants, and, as has been true in animal studies, oxytocin and endogenous opioid mechanisms are thought to be at their core. Some of the human evidence on the behavioral concomitants of oxytocin has involved studies of nursing mothers, because oxytocin levels are known to be high at this time. As in animal studies, nursing is soothing to both mothers and infants. Blass (1997) reported that consuming milk significantly reduced crying in human infants, and sucking on a nipple is known to have a physiologically calming effect in infants and can also reduce crying (Field & Goldson, 1984). Lower levels of sympathetic arousal have also been found in lactating versus nonlactating women (Wiesenfeld, Malatesta, Whitman, Grannose, & Vile, 1985). Women who are breastfeeding are calmer and more social than matched-age women who are not breastfeeding or pregnant, as determined by personality inventories (Uvnas-Moberg, 1996); moreover, the levels of oxytocin in these breast-feeding women correlated strongly with the level of calm reported, and oxytocin pulsatility was significantly correlated with self-reported sociability (Uvnas-Moberg, 1996). Similar findings are reported by Adler, Cook, Davidson, West, and Bancroft (1986). Altemus, Deuster, Galliven, Carter, and Gold (1995) found that lactating women showed suppressed HPA responses to stress, which is consistent with the animal literature showing reduced HPA activity in response to oxytocin (see also Chiodera et al., 1991; Lightman & Young, 1989). Dunn and Richards (1977) also reported higher levels of maternal behavior among lactating versus nonlactating mothers.

Until recently, it was difficult to examine the relation of oxytocin to human social behavior except during lactation, in part because of ethical issues involved with manipulating oxytocin levels and in part because there were no commercially available assays to measure oxytocin at the levels suspected to be implicated in stress responses. Emerging evidence suggests that oxytocin is associated with relaxation and interpersonal outcomes in nonlactating women as well. For example, in a sample of nulliparous women, Turner, Altemus, Enos, Cooper, and McGuinness (1999) found that oxytocin levels increased in response to relaxation massage and decreased in response to sad emotions. Women who reported fewer interpersonal problems of intrusiveness showed greater increases in oxytocin in response to these sources of stimulation. Data showed that maintaining oxytocin levels during sadness was associated with lower anxiety in close relationships, and high basal levels of oxytocin were associated with greater interpersonal distress. In an experimental study with older women, Taylor, Klein, Greendale, and Seeman (1999) found that higher levels of oxytocin were associated with reduced cortisol responses to stress and with faster HPA recovery following an acute stress laboratory challenge.

As is true in animal studies, human studies show that nurturing behaviors under conditions of stress benefit both mother and offspring. Field and colleagues have shown that touching an infant and carrying an infant close to the mother's chest can soothe and calm the infant (Field, Malphurs, Carraway, & Pelaez-Nogueras, 1996; Field, Schanberg, Davalos, & Malphurs, 1996). High levels of physical affection and warmth between mother and child during stressful circumstances have been tied to normal HPA activation profiles in response to stress in offspring (e.g., Chorpita & Barlow, 1998; Flinn & England, 1997; Hertsgaard, Gunnar, Erickson, & Nachmias, 1995). In humans (as well as in nonhuman primates), these processes appear to be mediated by mother–infant attachment, with securely attached offspring less likely to show elevated cortisol in response to challenging circumstances (e.g., Gunnar, Brodersen, Krueger, & Rigatuso, 1996; Gunnar, Brodersen, Nachmias, Buss, & Rigatuso, 1996; Nachmias, Gunnar, Mangelsdorf, Parritz, & Buss, 1996).

Nurturing behavior under stressful conditions may not only quiet and soothe offspring but it may also have discernible effects on health-related outcomes, directly affecting the likelihood that offspring will survive and mature properly.[9] For example, in humans, inadequate physical maternal care has been tied to growth retardation, social withdrawal, and poor interpersonal relatedness, among other complications (e.g., Harlow, 1986; Shaffer & Campbell, 1994). Premature human infants given a pacifier or massage grow better, become calmer, and become more tolerant to pain (Bernbaum, Pereira, Watkins, & Peckham, 1983; Field & Goldson, 1984; Scafidi, Field, & Schanberg, 1993; Uvnas-Moberg, Marchini, & Winberg, 1993). In experimental investigations with humans, touch and massage have been found to increase immune system function, decrease pain, reduce subjective reports of stress, and maintain normal growth in infants (Field, 1995, 1996; Ironson et al., 1996; Scafidi & Field, 1996).[10]

If mothers in particular exhibit nurturing behavior under conditions of stress, it should also be possible to see behavioral evidence for this prediction in parenting behaviors. Such evidence is provided by Repetti's (Repetti, 1989, 1997) studies of the effects of stressful workdays on parenting behavior. Repetti gave questionnaires to both fathers and mothers about their workdays and their behaviors at home on those days and to children regarding their experiences with their parents on those days. She found that fathers who had experienced an interpersonally conflictual day at work were more likely to be interpersonally conflictual in the home after work. Fathers who had highly stressful workdays, but not involving interpersonal conflict, were more likely to withdraw from their families (Repetti, 1989). A very different pattern was found for mothers. Specifically, women were more nurturant and caring toward their children on their stressful work days. In particular, on days when women reported that their stress levels at work had been the highest, their children

reported that their mothers had shown them more love and nurturance (Repetti, 1997). A second study replicated these differences in mothers' and fathers' responses to offspring under stress (Repetti, 2000).[11]

The underpinnings of the tending response appear to be oxytocin based initially, at least in rodent and animal species and possibly also in human females;[12] prolactin, endogenous opioids, and social learning may be more important for sustaining the tending response, once the behavior pattern has developed (Panksepp, 1998). The extent to which the tending response is hormonally regulated over the long term is unclear, however. Rat studies show that tending responses under stress (e.g., pup retrieval) lose their complete dependence on hormonal regulation relatively quickly and are thought to be socially maintained instead in response to distress vocalizations (DeVries & Villalba, 1999). Tending responses in human females also appear to depend, in part, on characteristics of human infant cries, and such qualities as pitch and tone convey often quite subtle information to mothers about the urgency and nature of the infants' needs (Bates, Freeland, & Lounsbury, 1979; Crowe & Zeskind, 1992; Zeskind, 1980, 1987; Zeskind & Collins, 1987; Zeskind, Sale, Maio, Huntington, & Weiseman, 1985). The human female not only brings the possibility of social evocation by offspring to stressful situations but a large neocortex as well, and so tending behavior in human females may be oxytocin based, socially mediated, mediated by higher-order brain functions, or some combination of these three processes.

In summary, whereas male responses to stress may be tied to sympathetic arousal and to a fight-or-flight pattern that is, at least in part, organized and activated by androgens, female stress responses do not show these androgen links and, instead, may be tied, at least in part, to the release of oxytocin and its biobehavioral links to caregiving behavior. Oxytocin is believed not only to underlie attachment processes between mothers and offspring but it may also be implicated in other close social bonds. We extend this analysis in the next section by arguing that female responses to stress are also characterized by affiliation with social groups because group living provides special benefits for females.

Befriending among Females

Group living is generally regarded as an evolutionary adaptation among many species that benefits both males and females (Caporeal, 1997). Groups provide more eyes for the detection of predators, and most predators are reluctant to attack potential prey if they believe there are others who may come to that prey's rescue (Janson, 1992; Rubenstein, 1978). Moreover, groups can create confusion in a predator. If a predator charges a large group, the group may disband in many directions, which may confuse the predator long enough to reduce the likelihood that any one member of the group can be taken down. Group life, then, is fundamental to primate existence, making it an important evolutionary strategy by which primates have survived (Caporeal, 1997; Dunbar, 1996). As we have noted, female stress responses have likely evolved in ways that not only protect the female herself but also protect her offspring. As such, group life is likely to have been an especially important adaptation for females and offspring, because of the limitations of fight-or-flight as a female response to stress. Like human males, human females once required successful defense against external predators, such as tigers, leopards, hyenas, packs of hunting dogs, and other primates. In addition, human females have much to fear from human males, including rape, assault, homicide, and abuse of offspring.[13] The pairing of human females with human males may be, in part, an evolutionary adaptation that protects females and offspring against random assault by males. However, under some conditions, human females also have reason to fear their own male partners. In North America, estimates of the percentage of women who have been assaulted by their partners range from 20% to 50% (Bray, 1994; Goodman, Koss, Fitzgerald, Russo, & Keita, 1993; Koss et al., 1994; Malamuth, 1998; Straus & Gelles, 1986), and statistical analyses of assault and homicide data reveal that human females are most likely to be assaulted or killed by their own partners (see Daly & Wilson, 1988; Daly, Wilson, & Weghorst, 1982). There is no reason to believe that this is a particularly modern phenomenon. Thus, evolved mechanisms of female survival likely protected against a broad array of threats, including those from males of her own species.

If the above reasoning is true, one would predict a strong tendency among females to affiliate under conditions of stress. There is animal data consistent with this analysis. Crowding has been found to stress male rodents but to calm female rodents, as assessed by corticosteroid levels (specifically, spatial crowding is problematic for males, whereas the number of other animals present is positively related to calming in females; Brown, 1995; Brown & Grunberg, 1995). McClintock (personal communication, May 6, 1998) has reported that female rats housed together in five-female groupings live 40% longer than females housed in isolation.[14] Research on prairie voles (*Microtus ochrogaster*), a preferred species for studying behavioral concomitants of oxytocin, has found that, under conditions of stress, female prairie voles show selective preference for their same-sex cage companions (DeVries & Carter, unpublished raw data, as cited in Carter, 1998).

Human Evidence for Affiliation under Stress

Research on human males and females shows that, under conditions of stress, the desire to affiliate with others is substantially more marked among females than among males. In fact, it is one of the most robust gender differences in adult human behavior, other than those directly tied to pregnancy and lactation, and it is the primary gender difference in adult human behavioral responses to stress (Belle, 1987; Luckow, Reifman, & McIntosh, 1998). In their analysis of gender differences in coping, Luckow et al. (1998) found that the largest difference arose on seeking and using social support, and the combined significance of their effect was significant beyond the $p < .0000001$ level. Of the 26 studies that tested for gender differences, one study showed no differences, and 25 favored women. There were no reversals (Luckow et al., 1998). Indeed, so reliable is this effect that, following the early studies on affiliation in response to stress by Schachter (1959), most subsequent research on affiliation under stress used only female participants.[15]

Nonetheless, some research has compared males' and females' responses to stress. Bull et al. (1972) found that exposure to noise stress led to decreased liking among male participants but greater liking by females toward familiar others. Bell and Barnard (1977) found that males prefer less social interaction in response to heat or noise stress, whereas females preferred closer interpersonal distance. Affiliation under stress, however, is not random (Bull et al., 1972; Kenrick & Johnson, 1979; Schachter, 1959). Women's affiliative tendencies under stress are heavily to affiliate with other women (Schachter, 1959). When given a choice to affiliate with an unfamiliar male versus alone prior to a stressful experience, women choose to wait alone (Lewis & Linder, 2000). In summary, then, women are more likely than men to choose to affiliate in response to a laboratory challenge, but affiliation appears to be selectively with similar others, especially with other women.

Across the entire life cycle, females are more likely to mobilize social support, especially from other females, in times of stress. They seek it out more, they receive more support, and they are more satisfied with the support they receive. Adolescent girls report more informal sources of support than do boys, and they are more likely to turn to their same-sex peers for support than are boys (e.g., Copeland & Hess, 1995; see Belle,

1987, for a review). Female college students report more available helpers and report receiving more support than do males (e.g., Ptacek, Smith, & Zanas, 1992; see Belle, 1987, for a review). Adult women maintain more same-sex close relationships than do men, they mobilize more social support in times of stress than do men, they rely less heavily than do men on their spouses for social support, they turn to female friends more often, they report more benefits from contact with their female friends and relatives (although they are also more vulnerable to network events as a cause of psychological distress), and they provide more frequent and more effective social support to others than do men (Belle, 1987; McDonald & Korabik, 1991; Ogus, Greenglass, & Burke, 1990). Although females give help to both males and females in their support networks, they are more likely to seek help and social support from other female relatives and female friends than from males (Belle, 1987; Wethington, McLeod, & Kessler, 1987).[16]

Women are also more engaged in their social networks than are men. They are significantly better at reporting most types of social network events than men, such as major illnesses of children, and they are more likely to report being involved if there is a crisis event in the network (Wethington et al., 1987). In an extensive study of social networks, Veroff, Kulka, and Douvan (1981) reported that women were 30% more likely than men to have provided some type of support in response to network stressors, including economic and work-related difficulties, interpersonal problems, death, and negative health events. So consistent and strong are these findings that theorists have argued for basic gender differences in orientation toward others, with women maintaining a collectivist orientation (Markus & Kitayama, 1991) or connectedness (Clancy & Dollinger, 1993; Kashima, Yamaguchi, Choi, Gelfand, & Yuki, 1995; Niedenthal & Beike, 1997) and males, a more individualistic orientation (Cross & Madson, 1997). These findings appear to have some cross-cultural generalizability: In their study of six cultures, Whiting and Whiting (1975) found that women and girls seek more help from others and give more help to others than men and boys do. Edwards (1993) found similar sex differences across 12 cultures.

In stressful circumstances where resources are scarce, female networks for child care and exchange of resources often emerge and become very well developed. Large kin networks among disadvantaged African Americans, as well as the fictive kin networks that often evolve when real kin are not available, are well documented (Stack, 1975). Newman (1999) described the all-female economic networks that impoverished Dominican women develop, so as to protect themselves and their children when male breadwinners are unemployed or leave the family. Studies of Black families, White working class families, White ethnic families, and low-income families of all races reveal the importance of the instrumental assistance and emotional support shared among female kin, friends, and neighbors, especially around the tasks of childrearing (Belle, 1987).[17]

The preceding analysis is not intended to suggest that males are not benefited by social group living or that they do not form social groups in response to external threats or stress. However, anthropological accounts, as well as survey literature, suggest that the functions of the groups that men and women form and turn to under stress are somewhat different. In a broad array of cultures, men have been observed to form groups for purposes of defense, aggression, and war (Tiger, 1970). They tend toward larger social groups than is true of women (Baumeister & Sommer, 1997), and these groups are often organized around well-defined purposes or tasks. Although men orient toward and invest in a large number of social relationships, many of these relationships emphasize hierarchies of status and power rather than intimate bonding (Baumeister & Sommer, 1997; Spain, 1992). Female groupings tend to be smaller, often consisting of dyads or a few women, and although

some such groups are focused around tasks (such as food preparation, sewing, or collective child care), these groups often have the establishment and maintenance of socioemotional bonds at their core, a characteristic less true of male groupings (Cross & Madson, 1997). Women in women's social groups show more affiliative behaviors, including smiling, disclosure, attention to others, and ingratiation (Baumeister & Sommer, 1997; Pearson, 1981), and they interact at closer physical distances than do men's groups (Patterson & Schaeffer, 1977).

A Neuroendocrine Perspective on Affiliation under Stress

Studies of affiliative behaviors in animal studies suggest a mechanism whereby enhanced social activity of females may occur under conditions of stress. In particular, they suggest that oxytocin reduces stress and enhances affiliation. For example, social contact is enhanced and aggression diminished following central oxytocin treatment in estrogen-treated female prairie voles (Witt et al., 1990), and the exogenous administration of oxytocin in rats causes an increase in social contact and in grooming (Argiolas & Gessa, 1991; Carter, DeVries, & Getz, 1995; Witt, Winslow, & Insel, 1992). With reference to humans, Carter (1998) suggested that oxytocin may be at the core of many forms of social attachment, including not only mother–infant attachments but also adult pair bonds and friendships (Drago et al., 1986; Fahrbach et al., 1985; Panksepp, 1998). Keverne et al. (1999) suggested that female-to-female bonding may have piggybacked onto maternal–infant bonding attachment processes. Consistent with Keverne et al.'s (1999) hypothesis, research has reported that animals prefer to spend time with animals in whose presence they have experienced high brain oxytocin and endogenous opioid activities in the past (Panksepp, 1998), suggesting that friendships may be mediated by the same neurochemical systems that mediate maternal urges. As is true of the maternal–infant caregiving system, contact with a friend or a supportive other person during stressful events down-regulates sympathetic and neuroendocrine responses to stress and facilitates recovery from the physiological effects of acute stress (Christenfeld et al., 1997; Fontana, Diegnan, Villeneuve, & Lepore, 1999; Gerin, Milner, Chawla, & Pickering, 1995; Gerin, Pieper, Levy, & Pickering, 1992; Glynn, Christenfeld, & Gerin, 1999; Kamarck, Manuck, & Jennings, 1990; Kirschbaum et al., 1995; Kors, Linden, & Gerin, 1997; Lepore, Allen, & Evans, 1993; Roy, Steptoe, & Kirschbaum, 1998; Sheffield & Carroll, 1994; Thorsteinsson, James, & Gregg, 1998). Both men and women experience these stress-regulatory benefits of social support, but women disproportionately seek such contact, and the stress-reducing benefits are more consistent when the support provider is female rather than male (e.g., Gerin et al., 1995).

The enhanced desire for social contact that females demonstrate under conditions of stress, relative to males, may also be modulated by endogenous opioid mechanisms. Endogenous opioid peptides are released during stress and are believed to influence social interaction (Benton, 1988; Jalowiec, Calcagnetti, & Fanselow, 1989). Animal studies suggest that higher levels of endogenous opioids are associated with higher levels of social interaction and maternal behavior. For example, Martel et al. (1993) found that administration of naloxone (an opioid antagonist) in female rhesus monkeys reduced both maternal behavior as well as social grooming of other females. Further support for this hypothesis and for its possible differential relevance for females is provided by an experimental investigation of the effects of opioids on affiliative behavior in humans. Jamner, Alberts, Leigh, and Klein (1998) found that administration of naltrexone (a long-acting opioid antagonist) increased the amount of time women spent alone, reduced the amount of time that they spent with friends, and reduced the pleasantness of women's social interactions, as compared with men. In

addition, women who were given naltrexone initiated fewer social interactions than when they received a placebo. Thus, endogenous opioids appear to play a role in regulating social interactions, especially for women. Endogenous opioids also moderate the release of other peptides in the limbic system (e.g., oxytocin, vasopressin), as well as other "stress-related" neurohormones, such as norepinephrine (Keverne et al., 1999), and cortisol (Klein, Alberts, et al., 1998), which may contribute to the sex differences observed in social behavior under conditions of stress.

Advantages of Affiliation under Stress

What are the advantages of social affiliation under stress, and why do females seek to do it more? Why does female affiliation under stress appear to be at least somewhat selectively with other females? We reasoned that an examination of evidence from humans' closest relatives, namely Old World nonhuman primates, may provide some insights into the patterns and functions of female affiliative responses to stress.[18]

Female–female networks of associations are common in nonhuman primate societies. Among many Old World primates, female coalitions, and networks are formed early and are in place when they are needed (Dunbar, 1996; Wallen & Tannenbaum, 1997). For example, in Gelada baboons (*Theropithecus gelada*), a mother and her two daughters, or a sister, mother, and daughter may form an alliance to provide support against threat. These long-term commitments are solidified through grooming behavior, which may take up as much as 10% to 20% of an animal's time (Dunbar, 1996). Intrasexual aggression within these matrilineal groupings is reported to be low among females (although high among males), whereas the reverse is true of affiliative behavior, with females exhibiting more affiliative behaviors than males. These findings appear to be similar across several species of monkeys and other primates (Burbank, 1987;

Glazer, 1992; Keverne et al., 1999). Although these bonds and their functions appear to be stronger when kin relationships are involved (Silk, 2000), unrelated females in several primate species form similar bonds. Wallen and Tannenbaum (1997) found that rhesus monkeys establish social bonds with female peers, which provide security and promote the maintenance of a matrilineal social system. Squirrel monkeys typically associate with females of roughly the same age and spend considerable time in close association (Baldwin, 1985; Mason & Epple, 1969). In captive situations, female squirrel monkeys show signs of distress in response to being separated from their cagemates. In an experimental investigation, when female squirrel monkeys were introduced to a novel environment, they showed more distress when alone than when they experienced the new environment in the company of their same-sex cagemates (Hennessy, Mendoza, & Kaplan, 1982). These adverse reactions were stronger for lactating mothers with infants than for nonlactating females (Jordan, Hennessy, Gonzalez, & Levine, 1985).

The so-called harem structure that characterizes the breeding patterns of many primates also suggests what some of the protective functions of female groups may be (Wrangham, 1980). The harem structure typically consists of a dominant male and several females and their offspring. Primatologists have tended to emphasize the benefits that the harem structure has for males, enabling them to have all their eggs in one basket, so to speak, and have somewhat overlooked the functions that the harem may afford to females and offspring. Evidence suggests that the female harem may provide protection for females. With reference to the Gelada baboons, Dunbar (1996) noted that daughters mature into a harem grouping of females to join their mothers, older sisters, aunts, and female cousins in a "coalition of great intensity and loyalty . . . these alliances are formed at birth, the product of being born to a particular mother" (p. 20). Mother–daughter, sister–sister, and female friend grooming are all widely docu-

mented and are described by Dunbar as "the cement that holds alliances together" (p. 20). Although males rarely groom each other, adult females will often groom their close female relations and friends in this fashion. Grooming does not occur at random but rather takes place within the context of clearly defined social relationships, most of which involve matrilineal relatives or special friends (see also De Waal, 1996; Wrangham, 1980).

Grooming can be an indication of status as well as a form of hygiene and an expression of friendship. The frequency with which a female is groomed by others predicts how likely it is that those others will come to her aid if she is attacked by members of another harem, the male in her own harem, or an outside predator (Dunbar, 1996; Wrangham, 1980). In his studies of rhesus monkeys, S. Datta (cited in Dunbar, 1996, p. 25) noted that whether a particular female is attacked may depend on such factors as whether that female's mother or other females with whom that female has formed alliances are nearby. The probability of attack is reduced if the targeted female is of high status or if her mother is of high status, because there is greater potential to enlist the support of other females to drive off a potential attacker. Grooming behavior appears to be enhanced by oxytocin and may be moderated by endogenous opioid mechanisms. For example, among monkeys, naxolone has been found to reduce mothers' grooming behavior toward their infants and toward other group members (Martel et al., 1993).

These female groups may also provide protection for females from their own males. On the one hand, the harem itself may be protected by a dominant male who attempts to keep the females in line, in particular, preventing them from breeding with other males. On the other hand, if he is overly aggressive or threatening to a particular female, the chances that her female relatives will come to her aid and threaten the male as a group is very high. Dunbar (1996) described an example of this protection:

The harem male's attempts to ride herd on his females when they stray too far from him often backfire. The luckless victim's grooming partners invariably come to her aid. Standing shoulder-to-shoulder, they outface the male with outraged threats and furious barks of their own. The male will usually back off, and walk huffily away, endeavoring to maintain an air of ruffled dignity. However, occasionally, the male will persist, feeling, perhaps, unusually sensitive about his honor and security. This only leads to more of the group's females racing in to support their embattled sisters. The male invariably ends up being chased 'round the mountainside by his irate females in an impressive display of sisterly solidarity. (pp. 20–21)[19]

Similar accounts are found in De Waal (1996).

Female bonded groups also appear to be important for the control of resources related to food (Silk, 2000; Wrangham, 1980). Wrangham (1980) suggested that female bonded groups may have evolved, in part, because of the competition that exists for high quality food patches under conditions of limited feeding sites. Cooperative relationships among females may provide for the sharing of information about food sites and also help supplant others from preferred food patches (Silk, 2000; Wrangham, 1980). Matrilocal primate groupings also provide opportunities for the exchange of caretaking responsibilities under some circumstances (Wrangham, 1980), and examples of one female taking care of the offspring of another female appear commonly throughout the primate literature (e.g., De Waal, 1996).

Studies of primates suggest that these groups of females and their offspring may also constitute a critical mechanism by which juvenile females gain experience in the tending of infants, enabling them to observe the behaviors of other mothers. For example, studies with rhesus macaque monkeys have reported that females who have not yet given birth frequently help care for younger siblings (Keverne et al., 1999). Research data from monkeys that have been deprived of maternal or social contact during the first 8 months of their lives reveal significant adverse effects on subsequent maternal care, including infanticide and abuse. Social contact and opportunities to provide maternal care subsequently improves maternal care, but that care does not approach that of feral mothers (e.g., Ruppenthal, Harlow, Eisele, Harlow, & Suomi, 1974). When mothers and infants are given opportunities to form bonds with each other, abandonment of infants is rarely observed (Keverne et al., 1999; Mendoza & Mason, 1999), but in captive-reared animals and other circumstances when mother–infant bonds have not formed, mothering behavior can be inadequate. Researchers believe this maternal behavior is mediated, in part, by endogenous opioid mechanisms. Related findings appear in studies of human affiliative behavior (Jamner et al., 1998).

Although oxytocin and endogenous opioid mechanisms may be important in affiliative and maternal behavior in primates and humans, the important role of higher brain functioning must also be noted. As Keverne et al. (1999) pointed out, the development of a large neocortex in primates has allowed affiliative behavior and maternal caregiving to take place without the hormonal regulation prompted by pregnancy and parturition that elicits similar behaviors in rats. Freeing behavior from exclusive neuroendocrine control enables females to engage in affiliation and infant caregiving through learning by modeling other females. These points suggest an important socialization role for these all-female social groupings. Indeed, Keverne et al. (1999) argued that, through such learning, females provide social stability and group cohesion, with their affiliative processes helping to maintain the continuity of the group over successive generations.

Two caveats regarding the research on female networks in primate groups are warranted. First, there are more than 130 different primate species, and there is substantial variability in the specifics of female networks. For example, female associations are based on kin in some primate social groupings but on nonkin dominance hierarchies in others. In most primate species, networks of females are responsible for rearing offspring, but in titi monkeys (*Callicebus*), fathers are responsible for the rearing of offspring, and titi females actually show aversion to being left alone with their offspring (Mendoza & Mason, 1999). Although it would be unwise to draw direct links from primate behavior to humans, it would be foolish to claim that there is nothing to be learned from primate behavior merely because there is variability among primate species. Thus, although these primate examples should be interpreted with caution, they provide illustrations of the befriending patterns common to many primates, including human females.

Second, the preceding analysis runs the risk of romanticizing the networks that females create. It must be noted that these networks are by no means stress-free, particularly nonkin female networks (e.g., Silk, 2000). Studies of primates reveal how females who are more dominant in a hierarchy may harass less dominant females, a behavior that can have many adverse effects, including the suppression of fertility (Abbott, Saltzman, Schultz-Darken, & Smith, 1999; Shively, Laber-Laird, & Anton, 1997). A more extreme response has been reported by Fossey (1983) in gorillas and by Goodall (1986) in chimpanzees. The researchers found that, in both species, dominant females, together with their oldest female offspring occasionally cannibalized the young of less dominant females. In humans, interpersonal strain, conflict, and the potential for misunderstanding and mistreatment are common in social groups, and all-female groups are no exception. The networks that women help create and may become enmeshed in are themselves sources of stress, and women report that interpersonal stressors are the most common and stressful types of stressors they experience (Davis, Matthews, & Twamley, 1999). Nonetheless, on the whole, these female networks may confer more benefits than harm.

Conclusions, Implications, and Limitations

We propose a theory of female responses to stress characterized by a pattern termed "tend-and-befriend." Specifically, we propose that women's responses to stress are characterized by patterns that involve caring for offspring under stressful circumstances, joining social groups to reduce vulnerability, and contributing to the development of social groupings, especially those involving female networks, for the exchange of resources and responsibilities. We maintain that aspects of these responses, both maternal and affiliative, may have built on the biobehavioral attachment–caregiving system that depends, in part, on oxytocin, estrogen, and endogenous opioid mechanisms, among other neuroendocrine underpinnings. We suggest that these patterns may have evolved according to principles of natural selection and by virtue of differential parental investment. We propose this theory as a biobehavioral alternative to the fight-or-flight response (Cannon, 1932), which has dominated stress research of the past 5 decades and has been disproportionately based on studies of males.

To evaluate our theory, we examined several empirical literatures that provide convergent support. A neuroendocrine literature on stress hormones and their relation to behavior derived largely from studies with male rats and, to a lesser extent, on nonhuman primates, suggests that the fight-or-flight response may be heavily tied to androgenic pre- or postnatal organization of an aggressive response to threat that is activated, in part, by testosterone. A substantial neuroendocrine literature from animal studies with females suggests, in contrast, that sympathetic and HPA responses may be downregulated by oxytocin under stressful circumstances and that oxytocin, coupled with endogenous opioid mechanisms and other sex-linked hormones, may foster maternal and affiliative behavior in response to stress. The neuroendocrine model links to a literature on humans, suggesting that oxytocin and endogenous opioid mechanisms may have similar maternal and affiliative concomitants. Finally, literatures on both human and nonhuman primates point to differential maternal and affiliative activities among females, compared with males and provides evidence of a substantial female preference to affiliate under stress. The tend-and-befriend pattern may be maintained not only by sex-linked neuroendocrine responses to stress but by social and cultural roles as well.

Theoretical and Empirical Limitations

There are limitations in our analysis. We have combined observations from stress literatures on rats, primates, and humans in a manner that requires considerable leaps, both empirically and inferentially. As noted, the reason for this unusual mode of argumentation is because the neuroendocrine mechanisms are addressed heavily by one literature (rodent) and the behavioral responses to stress are addressed by two others (primate, human). It is impossible to build a coherent and informed biobehavioral model that covers what is known about female stress responses without drawing on these diverse and largely unintegrated sources of evidence. This need does not diminish the risks that such an analytic strategy entails, however.

Some of the points in the preceding argument remain conjectural. In particular, we have suggested that oxytocin and endogenous opioids may play important roles in female responses to stress, and it remains to be seen if these are as significant players as we have suggested. It should be noted that the present argument does not posit that oxytocin and endogenous opioids are either necessary or sufficient bases for the behavioral responses identified: We have argued that the tending response is consistent with maternal investment in offspring and maternal behavior under stressful conditions is socially responsive to distress vocalizations by offspring and is likely to be mediated by cortical processes as well. The befriending pattern is one of the

most robust sex differences reported in the literature on adult human behavior under stress (e.g., Belle, 1987; Luckow et al., 1998), and it, too, may depend heavily on social and cortical processes. At present, the potential roles of oxytocin and endogenous opioids in mediating these patterns are sufficient to be considered credible hypotheses but they are not definitively established.

Our analysis has included little consideration of the nature of the stressor in moderating stress responses. Neuroendocrine responses under stress are not uniform but depend on the stress stimulus involved and other environmental conditions such as predictability and chronicity of a stressor (e.g., Glass & Singer, 1972; Sapolsky, 1992a; Staub, Tursky, & Schwartz, 1971). Under certain stressful circumstances, we might find the tend-and-befriend pattern to be quite descriptive of female responses to stress and, in other cases, not descriptive (Jezova et al., 1996). In addition, because different stressors elicit different patterns of stress hormones, oxytocin may be involved in some kinds of stressful events but not others (cf. Kalin, Gibbs, Barksdale, Shelton, & Carnes, 1985; Sapolsky, 1992b).

Another limitation is that, at present, the model largely ignores the very reason why stress responses in females have been so understudied: cyclical variation. If the hypothesized neuroendocrine underpinnings of female stress responses are correct, then we might expect to see cyclical variation in these responses, as well as a degree of dependence on critical reproductive-related events in a woman's life, including onset of puberty, pregnancy, lactation, and menopause. For example, if estrogen is involved in the modulation of oxytocin-related affiliative or maternal responses, the so-called tending–befriending pattern may be stronger during the late luteal phase of cycle, as opposed to the follicular phase, and diminished in postmenopausal women. Consistent with these suggestions, in rhesus monkeys, females are most social around the time of ovulation or when they are treated with estrogen (Wallen & Tannenbaum, 1997), and oxytocin, in interaction with estrogen, has been suggested as the mechanism by which this sociability occurs (Carter, 1998). At present, however, more evidence is needed to assess the validity of these hypotheses.

Social and Political Implications

The issue arises as to whether sex differences in human behavior would be better understood as differences in social roles rather than as evolved biobehavioral responses (Eagly & Wood, 1999). For example, given substantial human behavioral flexibility, one can question whether maternal investment in offspring continues to be higher than that of fathers.[20] In response, we note that current differences between men and women in parental investment do not matter as much as differential parental investment during the period of time that stress responses evolved. An evolutionary biobehavioral argument does not constrain current human behavior but neither is it necessarily challenged by current human behavioral flexibility. We also note that, although human social roles vary substantially across cultures and may, in some cases, prescribe behavioral patterns for women similar to the tend-and-befriend pattern, social roles alone are unlikely to account for it. A social role position neither addresses the cross-species similarities we have identified nor accounts for the underlying biological evidence for our position. Nonetheless, it will be important for future research to detail the parts of our biobehavioral model that are sensitive to environmental input.

An analysis that posits biological bases for gender differences in behavior raises important political concerns as well. Many women feel, with some justification, that such models can be used to justify patterns of discrimination and social oppression. To head off any such effort, we emphatically point out that our analysis makes no prescriptive assumptions about the social roles that women occupy. Our analysis should

not be construed to imply that women should be mothers, will be good mothers, or will be better parents than men by virtue of these mechanisms. Similarly, this analysis should not be construed as evidence that women are naturally more social than men or that they should shoulder disproportionate responsibility for the ties and activities that create and maintain the social fabric.

Other political concerns, however, may be based on false assumptions about what biological underpinnings signify. Biological analyses of human behavior are sometimes misconstrued by social scientists as implying inflexibility or inevitability in human behavior or as reductionist efforts that posit behavioral uniformity. These perceptions constitute unwarranted concerns about biological bases of behavior. Biology is not so much destiny as it is a central tendency, but a central tendency that influences and interacts with social, cultural, cognitive, and emotional factors, resulting in substantial behavioral flexibility (Crawford & Anderson, 1989; Tooby & Cosmides, 1992). The last few decades of biological research have shown that, just as biology affects behavior, so behavior affects biology, in ways ranging from genetic expression to acute responses to stressful circumstances. Rather than viewing social roles and biology as alternative accounts of human behavior, a more productive theoretical and empirical strategy will be to recognize how biology and social roles are inextricably interwoven to account for the remarkable flexibility of human behavior.

Implications for Future Research

The present analysis suggests several areas of research for future investigation. We have presented a relatively primitive neuroendocrine model, ascribing a heavy role to oxytocin, endogenous opioid mechanisms, and estrogen. However, other neurohormones such as serotonin (e.g., Bagdy & Arato, 1998; Insel & Winslow, 1998; Knutson et al., 1998), prolactin

(Insel, 1997; Panksepp et al., 1999), vasopressin (Panksepp et al., 1999), dopamine (Berridge & Robinson, 1998; Kreek & Koob, 1998), and norepinephrine (Kraemer, 1992; Panksepp et al., 1999) may also be implicated in these pathways, as well, in ways not yet fully identified. Examination of the patterning of these neuroendocrine responses in subsequent studies of both lower animals and humans may help to clarify the neuroendocrine model further. Additional behavioral sequelae of these patterns merit investigation, such as suppression of sexual behavior in females under stress; the role of stress responses in moderating gender differences in negative affect, especially high levels of depression and anxiety in females (Craske & Glover, in press; Frasch, Zetzsche, Steiger, & Jirikowski 1995; Levine, Lyons, & Schatzberg, 1999); and the neuroendocrine and behavioral underpinnings of eating behavior, social withdrawal, and substance abuse under conditions of stress.

The range of female responses to stress, as outlined in this article, go beyond the acute fight-or-flight response that has been argued to be the foundation of stress responses. Our analysis suggests, instead, that aspects of a coordinated stress response are structurally in place, which are then activated under conditions of stress. This is not a particularly novel observation, inasmuch as group living is precisely such a structural adaptation. The interplay of such structural adaptations with acute stress conditions suggests how primate and human stress responses may have assumed increasingly complex forms as nonhuman primates and humans encountered an ever more diverse array of stressors. Indeed, it suggests a layering and patterning of means for responding to stress that may provide quite a flexible set of reactions to a broad array of situations and, as such, may be suited to managing chronic stress, as well as acutely stressful conditions.

In this context, there may be value in thinking about the fight-or-flight response as only part of a range of equally flexible male responses. Fight-or-flight may have garnered disproportionate attention in the scientific literature because of the potent behavioral responses it produces, such as aggression, and from the risks it may create for men's health, such as the early development of cardiovascular disease (CVD). Other male responses to stress may be meritorious of investigation. For example, some aspects of the tend-and-befriend model may characterize male responses to stress under some conditions as well. A more complete model would also consider a broader range of male behavioral responses to stress, such as affiliative behavior, protective behavior, and social withdrawal; a broader array of stress-related disorders, including substance abuse, accident rates, homicide and suicide, and a broader range of neuroendocrine responses, such as the roles of serotonin, oxytocin, vasopressin, and endogenous opioid mechanisms in mediating or moderating male responses to stress. For example, some intriguing effects of vasopressin in male prairie voles include guarding of territory, self defense, and guarding of females in response to stress, and studies of the effects of oxytocin in male rodents reveal effects on pair-bonding and affiliation (see Carter, 1998, for a review). In short, much remains to be discovered about men's responses to stress as well.

Although our analysis has focused on human stress responses, the present analysis may apply to some other mammalian species as well. Under what circumstances should we see tending-and-befriending responses to stress in females? Evidence of female tending under conditions of stress may be especially pronounced under conditions where there are long gestational periods of offspring; when females spend a high proportion of their life in activities related to pregnancy, nursing, and the rearing of offspring; and in any species in which offspring remain biologically immature for a long period of time. The befriending response may be especially prevalent under conditions of resource scarcity, in any species where females are smaller and less powerful than males, when males are unavailable, when there is a high differential mortality between the sexes, when there is a high rate of rape or attack of females, and when males commonly abandon their partners or where monogamous associations are otherwise unlikely or unstable.

The present analysis is suggestive of health implications for females. If a downregulated stress response in females produces relaxation and affiliation, this may help to explain the $7\frac{1}{2}$ nonspecific years that women live longer than men. That is, a stress response moderated by a counter-regulatory system such as the tend-and-befriend pattern proposed here may reduce women's vulnerability to a broad array of stress-related disorders, including episodes of violence, such as homicide and suicide; dependence on stress-reducing substances, such as alcohol or drugs; stress-related accidents and injuries; and patterns of cardiovascular reactivity that represent risk factors for CVD.

The analysis also suggests important implications for social support processes. It is now well established that both animals and humans show health benefits from social contact (e.g., House, Umberson, & Landis, 1988). Positive physical contact in the form of touching, hugging, cuddling, and the like is known to release oxytocin, which, in turn, has antistress properties. The present analysis suggests some mechanisms whereby social support may provide health protection, in particular, by engaging a counterveiling anabolic response to stress characterized by decreased sympathoadrenal activity, decreased HPA, and increased parasympathetic activity and accompanying relaxation. As such, oxytocin may confer health benefits (cf. Ryff & Singer, 1998).

Finally, the present analysis underscores the importance of studying both sexes in investigations of stress and stress responses. We have contended that the disproportionate representation of males in studies of stress has obscured significant influences on and patterns of responses to stress in females. Similarly, virtually all of the studies on affiliation under stress have been conducted on women; the absence of male data makes interpretation of these patterns difficult. Strenuous arguments against the inclusion of single-sex samples for understanding the pathology and treatment of health and mental health disorders (with the exception of sex-linked disorders) have prompted major changes in requirements for clinical trials and treatment evaluation. The threat that single-sex investigations pose to basic research endeavors is no less significant, both because the knowledge that is gained is skewed in favor of one sex's life experiences and because basic knowledge often becomes the basis for subsequent clinical intervention.

Acknowledgments

Support for preparation of this article was provided by National Science Foundation Grant SBR 9905157, National Institute of Mental Health Grant MH 056880, and the MacArthur Foundation's SES and Health Network. All of the authors except Shelley E. Taylor were supported by a National Institute of Mental Health Training Grant MH 15750 in health psychology at various points throughout the preparation of this chapter. We are grateful to Nancy Adler, David A. Armor, Lisa Aspinwall, John Cacioppo, Elissa Epel, Alan Fiske, Gregg Gold, Melissa Hines, Margaret Kemeny, Jennifer Lerner, Sonja Lyubomirsky, Karen Matthews, Bruce McEwen, L. Anne Peplau, Lien Pham, Inna Rivkin, Joan Silk, Robert Trivers, and Rosemary Veniegas for their comments on previous versions of this article.

Notes

1. We note here that the term *parental investment* is a technical term from evolutionary theory, referring to time and effort devoted to offspring and not a judgmental evaluation suggesting that women care more about children than men do, or a proscriptive term suggesting that women are or must be the only parents who can take appropriate care of offspring.

2. Both sexes show sympathetic arousal in response to the perception of threat, with men showing somewhat stronger vascular responses and women somewhat stronger heart rate responses (Allen, Stoney, Owens, & Matthews, 1993; Matthews & Stoney, 1988; Stoney, Davis, & Matthews, 1987; Stoney, Matthews, McDonald, & Johnson, 1988).

3. Different combinations of these hormones may be released in response to different types of stressors. Vasopressin secretion, for example, is not stimulated by a variety of stressors, although oxytocin release appears to be a more consistent, though not universal, component of the neuroendocrine response to stress (Jezova et al., 1995; Kalin et al., 1985).

4. The exact role that testosterone plays in aggression varies by species, particularly whether it has organizational effects, activational effects, or both (Archer, 1990; Beatty, 1984). In rodent species, for example, aggression is organized perinatally by testosterone and requires androgen for the activation of aggression in adulthood. Researchers believe aggression in primates is organized by testosterone prenatally but is not necessarily dependent on androgens for later activation.

5. Female rhesus monkeys exposed to testosterone in utero show intermediate levels of rough-and-tumble play (greater than normal for females and less than normal for males), underscoring the organizational effect that testosterone appears to play prenatally for physical aggression in at least some primates (Goy, 1966, 1978; Phoenix, 1974a, 1974b, 1974c; Phoenix, Goy, & Resko, 1968). There is also some evidence that aggression in extremely aggressive women is associated with testosterone (Benton, 1992).

6. When female attack behavior is documented in rats, primates, or human females, it is much more likely to be female–female aggression than female-to-male aggression (Burbank, 1987; Fry, 1992; except when threats to offspring are involved). This female-to-female aggression appears to be directed primarily against outsiders, such as intruder females in the rat and females outside one's immediate social grouping in primates and humans.

7. Women report more psychological distress in response to stressful events than do men, but these self-reports do not necessarily parallel physiological processes (e.g., Collins & Frankenhaeuser, 1978; Frankenhaeuser, Dunne, & Lundberg, 1976).

8. Relevant to this point is a study of gender differences in responsivity to touch in humans in response to the stress of hospitalization (Whitcher & Fisher, 1979). Results revealed that, under stress, touch produced more favorable affective, behavioral, and physiological (especially cardiovascular) effects in females than was true for males, and touch was actually experienced as aversive by males.

9. Bowlby's (1988) theory of attachment maintains that the formation of an attachment bond between infant and mother (or a suitable substitute) is essential for adequate socialization. For example, human play behavior and exploration in early ages is heavily dependent on physical proximity to a caregiver with whom that infant has formed a strong bond (see Hazan & Shaver, 1994).

10. It should be noted that touch (Panksepp et al., 1999) and smell (Kendrick, Levy, & Keverne, 1992) have been implicated in animal studies of mother–infant attachment, and these same behaviors may be implicated in human mother–infant attachment processes to some degree as well (e.g., Fleming, Steiner, & Corter, 1997).

11. There appears to be an upper limit on this phenomenon, inasmuch as chronically stressed or distressed mothers are somewhat more likely to show withdrawal behavior on especially stressed days rather than increases in affection (Repetti & Wood, 1997).

12. Oxytocin may have important effects on social learning and social memory (de Wied, 1997; Popik, Vetulani, & Van Ree, 1992). For example, low doses of oxytocin strengthen social memories, and, as such, oxytocin may play a role in learning and memory for social bonds, infant caregiving, and friendships.

13. Although abuse of children does not differ significantly by gender of perpetrator (U.S. Department of Health & Human Services, 1999), correcting for time spent with children yields considerably higher rates for men than women. Stepfather status is a particularly potent predictor of abuse, with much higher rates of abuse of stepchildren by stepfathers than abuse of children by their biological fathers (Daly & Wilson, 1996).

14. No males were included in this particular study.

15. The late Stanley Schachter maintained, in several contexts, that he had not found affiliative behavior in men under stress and, consequently, conducted his subsequent studies on affiliation using females only.

16. It should be noted that, although men are less likely to seek and give social support than women, they are often recipients of social support, and such support, especially from a female partner, close relative, or close female friend, appears to be successful in reducing physiological arousal in response to stress (e.g., Kirschbaum, Klauer, Filipp, & Hellhammer, 1995). Similar findings emerge in the primate literature. Sapolsky (1994) reported that males who are the recipients of grooming efforts by females have better physiological functioning.

17. Studies of human female networks suggest that matrilineal and matrilocal societies are typically characterized by peaceful interfemale relations (Glazer, 1992). When generations of related women and girls live together all their lives and participate in cooperative work groups, interfemale aggression is reported to be low (Benedict, 1934; Glazer, 1992; Murphy & Murphy, 1974). Reliably, however, when women join patriarchal extended families, interfemale aggression is considerably higher, especially between in-laws. These findings are true both for human social groupings and for primate social groupings (Glazer, 1992; Keverne et al., 1999).

An intriguing study of hunting among women of the Agta Negrito of Luzon (the Philippines) underscores the functions of networks of female kin. Women's hunting has largely been regarded as biologically impractical because hunting is assumed to be incompatible with the obligations of maternal care of offspring (Dahlberg, 1981; Hiatt, 1970; Lee, 1979). Specifically, hunting forays are thought to impair women's abilities to nurse, care for, and carry children, and female odor itself may constitute a handicap to effective hunting. However, studies of cultures where the females do hunt suggest exceptions that prove the rule. Agta women participate actively in hunting precisely because others are available to provide child care responsibilities (Goodman, Griffin, Estioko-Griffin, & Grove, 1985). When women were observed to hunt, they either brought nursing children with them or gave the children to their mothers or oldest female siblings for care. Whereas men typically hunted alone, women almost always hunted with dogs and/or in groups, often with other females, especially sisters. Thus, proximity to hunting grounds, use of dogs, hunting in groups, and cooperation in child care appear to be the key factors that make it possible for Agta female hunters to be successful.

18. Old World primates include bonobos (*Pan paniscus*), gorillas (*Gorilla gorilla*), orangutans (*Pongo pygmaeus*), and chimpanzees (*Pan troglodytes*; chimpanzees are believed to be the closest relations of humans), as well as certain monkeys, including baboons (*Papio*) and macaques (*Macaca*). New World monkeys include the capuchin (*Cebus*), spider (*Ateles*), squirrel (*Saimin*), and other subfamilies.

19. We are not suggesting that the female kin network evolved primarily or even significantly to protect females against their own partners. It is, however, likely that females have evolved mechanisms that protect them and their offspring against jealous and suspicious partners, and female kin networks may constitute one basis for doing so.

20. Survey data (Burden & Googins, 1987; Ferber, O'Farrell, & Allen, 1991; Staines & Pleck, 1983), interview data (Hochschild, 1989), and analyses of time-use diaries (Robinson & Godbey, 1997) indicate that women continue to bear the major responsibility for childcare, whether or not they work for pay. These estimates suggest that mothers' childcare exceed fathers' childcare by a factor of approximately three to one, on average.

References

Abbott, D. H., Saltzman, W., Schultz-Darken, N. J., & Smith, T. E. (1999). Specific neuroendocrine mechanisms not involving generalized stress mediate social regulation of female reproduction in cooperatively breeding marmoset monkeys. In C. S. Carter, I. I. Lederhendler, & B. Kirkpatrick (Eds.), *The integrative neurobiology of affiliation* (pp. 199–220). Cambridge, MA: MIT Press.

Adams, D. (1992). Biology does not make men more aggressive than women. In K. Bjorkqvist & P. Niemela (Eds.), *Of mice and women: Aspects of female aggression* (pp. 17–26). San Diego, CA: Academic Press.

Alder, E. M., Cook, A. Davidson, D., West, C., & Bancroft, J. (1986). Hormones, mood and sexuality in lactating women. *British Journal of Psychiatry, 148,* 74–79.

Allen, M. T., Stoney, C. M., Owens, J. F., & Matthews, K. A. (1993). Hemodynamic adjustments to laboratory stress: The influence of gender and personality. *Psychosomatic Medicine, 55,* 505–517.

Altemus, M. P., Deuster, A., Galliven, E., Carter, C. S., & Gold, P. W. (1995). Suppression of hypothalamic-pituitary-adrenal axis response to stress in lactating women. *Journal of Clinical Endocrinology and Metabolism, 80,* 2954–2959.

Archer, J. (1990). The influence of testosterone on human aggression. *British Journal of Psychology, 82,* 1–28.

Argiolas, A., & Gessa, G. L. (1991). Central functions of oxytocin. *Neuroscience and Biobehavioral Reviews, 15,* 217–231.

Bagdy, G., & Arato, M. (1998). Gender-dependent dissociation between oxytocin but not ACTH, cortisol or TSH responses to *m*-chlorophenylpiperazine in healthy subjects. *Psychopharmacology, 136,* 342–348.

Baldwin, J. D. (1985). The behavior of squirrel monkeys (*Saimiri*) in natural environments. In L. A. Rosenblum & C. L. Coe (Eds.), *Handbook of squirrel monkey research* (pp. 35–53). New York: Plenum.

Bates, J. E., Freeland, C. A. B., & Lounsbury, M. L. (1979). Measurement of infant difficulties. *Child Development, 50,* 794–802.

Baumeister, R. F., & Sommer, K. L. (1997). What do men want? Gender differences and two spheres of belongingness: Comment on Cross and Madson (1997). *Psychological Bulletin, 122,* 38–44.

Beatty, W. W. (1984). Hormonal organization of sex differences in play fighting and spatial behavior. In G. J. De Vries, J. P. C. De Bruin, H. B. M. Uylings, & M. A. Corner (Eds.), *Progress in brain research* (Vol. 61, pp. 315–330). Amsterdam: Elsevier.

Bell, P. A., & Barnard, S. W. (1977, May). *Sex differences in the effects of heat and noise stress on personal space permeability.* Paper presented at the annual meetings of the Rocky Mountain Psychological Society, Albuquerque, NM.

Belle, D. (1987). Gender differences in the social moderators of stress. In R. C. Barnett, L. Biener, & G. K. Baruch (Eds.), *Gender and stress* (pp. 257–277). New York: Free Press.

Benedict, R. (1934). *Patterns of culture.* New York: Mentor.

Benton, D. (1988). The role of opiate mechanisms in social relationships. In M. Lader (Ed.), *The psychopharmacology of addiction.* (British Association for Psychopharmacology Monography, 10, pp. 115–140). London: Oxford University Press.

Benton, D. (1992). Hormones and human aggression. In K. Bjorkqvist & P. Niemela (Eds.), *Of mice and women: Aspects of female aggression* (pp. 37–50). San Diego, CA: Academic Press.

Bergman, B., & Brismar, B. (1994). Hormone levels and personality traits in abusive and suicidal male alcoholics. *Alcoholism: Clinical and Experimental Research, 18,* 311–316.

Bernbaum, J. C., Pereira, G., Watkins, J., & Peckham, G. (1983). Nonnutritive sucking during gavage feeding enhances growth and maturation in premature infants. *Pediatrics, 71,* 41–45.

Berridge, K. C., & Robinson, T. E. (1998). What is the role of dopamine in reward: Hedonic impact, reward learning, or incentive salience? *Brain Research Reviews, 28,* 309–369.

Bjorkqvist, K., & Niemela, P. (1992). New trends in the study of female aggression. In K. Bjorkqvist & P. Niemela (Eds.), *Of mice and women: Aspects of female aggression* (pp. 3–16). San Diego, CA: Academic Press.

Blass, E. M. (1997). Infant formula quiets crying human newborns. *Journal of Developmental and Behavioral Pediatrics, 18,* 162–165.

Bowlby, J. (1988). *A secure base: Parent–child attachment and healthy human development.* New York: Basic Books.

Brain, P. F., Haug, M., & Parmigiani, S. (1992). The aggressive female rodent: Redressing a "scientific" bias. In K. Bjorkqvist & P. Niemela (Eds.), *Of mice and women: Aspects of female aggression* (pp. 27–36). San Diego, CA: Academic Press.

Bray, R. L. (1994, September/October). Remember the children, *Ms. Magazine, 5,* 38–43.

Brown, K. J. (1995). *Effects of housing conditions on stress responses, feeding, and drinking in male and female rats.* Unpublished master's thesis, Uniformed Services University of the Health Sciences, Bethesda, MD.

Brown, K. J., & Grunberg, N. E. (1995). Effects of housing on male and female rats: Crowding stresses males but calms females. *Physiology and Behavior, 58,* 1085–1089.

Bull, A. J., Burbage, S. E., Crandall, J. E., Fletcher, C. I. Lloyd, J. T., Ravenberg, R. L., & Rockett, S. L. (1972). Effects of noise and intolerance of ambiguity upon attraction for similar and dissimilar others. *Journal of Social Psychology, 88,* 151–152.

Burbank, V. K. (1987). Female aggression in cross-cultural perspective. *Behavior Science Research,* 21, 70–100.

Burden, D. S., & Googins, B. (1987). *Balancing job and homelife study: Managing work and family stress in corporations.* Boston: Boston University School of Social Work.

Cannon, W. B. (1932). *The wisdom of the body.* New York: Norton.

Caporeal, L. R. (1997). The evolution of truly social cognition: The core configuration model. *Personality and Social Psychology Review,* 1, 276–298.

Carter, C. S. (1998). Neuroendocrine perspectives on social attachment and love. *Psychoneuroendocrinology,* 23, 779–818.

Carter, C. S., DeVries, A. C., & Getz, L. L. (1995). Physiological substrates of mammalian monogamy: The prairie vole model. *Neuroscience and Biobehavioral Reviews,* 19, 303–314.

Carter, C. S., Williams, J. R., Witt, D. M., & Insel, T. R. (1992). Oxytocin and social bonding. In C. A. Pedersen, G. F. Jirikowski, J. D. Caldwell, & T. R. Insel (Eds.), Oxytocin in maternal sexual and social behaviors. *Annals of the New York Academy of Science,* 652, 204–211.

Chiodera, P., Salvarani, C., Bacchi-Modena, A., Spailanzani, R., Cigarini, C., Alboni, A., Gardini, E., & Coiro, V. (1991). Relationship between plasma profiles of oxytocin and adrenocorticotropic hormone during sucking or breast stimulation in women. *Hormone Research,* 35, 119–123.

Chorpita, B. F., & Barlow, D. H. (1998). The development of anxiety: The role of control in the early environment. *Psychological Bulletin,* 124, 3–21.

Christenfeld, N., Gerin, W., Lindon, W., Sanders, M., Mathur, J., Deich, J. D., & Pickering, T. G. (1997). Social support effects on cardiovascular reactivity: Is a stranger as effective as a friend? *Psychosomatic Medicine,* 59, 388–398.

Christensen, K., Knussman, R., & Couwenbergs, C. (1985). Sex hormones and stress in the human male. *Hormones and Behavior,* 19, 426–440.

Clancy, S. M., & Dollinger, S. J. (1993). Photographic description of the self: Gender and age differences in social connectedness. *Sex Roles,* 29, 477–495.

Coe, C. L., Mendoza, S. P., Smotherman, W. P., & Levine, S. (1978). Mother–infant attachment in the squirrel monkey: Adrenal response to separation. *Behavior and Biology,* 22, 256–263.

Collaer, M. L., & Hines, M. (1995). Human behavioral sex differences: A role for gonadal hormones during early development? *Psychological Bulletin,* 118, 55–107.

Collins, A., & Frankenhaeuser, M. (1978). Stress responses in male and female engineering students. *Journal of Human Stress,* 4, 43–48.

Copeland, E. P., & Hess, R. S. (1995). Differences in young adolescents' coping strategies based on gender and ethnicity. *Journal of Early Adolescence,* 15, 203–219.

Craske, M. G., & Glover, D. A. (in press). Anxiety disorder. In E. M. Palance (Ed.), *Women's health: A behavioral medicine approach.* New York: Oxford University Press.

Crawford, C. B., & Anderson, J. L. (1989). Sociobiology: An environmentalist discipline? *American Psychologist,* 44, 1449–59.

Cross, S. E., & Madson, L. (1997). Models of the self: Self-construals and gender. *Psychological Bulletin,* 122, 5–37.

Crowe, J. J. P., & Zeskind, P. S. (1992). Psychophysiological and perceptual responses to infant cries varying in pitch: Comparison of adults with low and high scores on the child abuse potential inventory. *Child Abuse and Neglect,* 16, 19–29.

Cumming, D. C., Brunsting, L. A., Strich, G., Ries, A. L., & Rebar, R. W. (1986). Reproductive hormone increases in response to acute exercise in men. *Medical Science in Sports and Exercise,* 18, 369–373.

Dahlberg, F. (Ed.) (1981). *Woman the gatherer.* New Haven, CT: Yale University Press.

Daly, M., & Wilson, M. (1988). *Homicide.* New York: Aldine de Gruyter.

Daly, M., & Wilson, M. (1996). Violence against stepchildren. *Current Directions in Psychological Science,* 5, 77–81.

Daly, M., Wilson, M., & Weghorst, S. J. (1982). Male sexual jealousy. *Ethology and Sociobiology,* 3, 11–27.

Davis, M. C., Matthews, K. A., & Twamley, E. W. (1999). Is life more difficult on Mars or Venus? A meta-analytic review of sex differences in major and minor life events. *Annals of Behavioral Medicine,* 21, 83–97.

DeVries, G. J., & Villalba, C. (1999). Brain sexual dimorphism and sex differences in parental and other social behaviors. In C. S. Carter, I. I. Lederhendler, & B. Kirkpatrick (Eds.), *The integrative neurobiology of affiliation* (pp. 155–168). Cambridge, MA: MIT Press.

De Waal, F. (1996). *Good natured: The origins of right and wrong in humans and other animals.* Cambridge, MA: Harvard University Press.

De Wied, D. (1997). Neuropeptides in learning and memory process. *Behavioural Brain Research,* 83, 83–90.

Drago, F., Pederson, C. A., Caldwell, J. D., & Prange, A. J., Jr. (1986). Oxytocin potently enhances novelty-induced grooming behavior in the rat. *Brain Research,* 368, 287–295.

Dreifuss, J. J., Dubois-Dauphin, M., Widmer, H., & Raggenbass, M. (1992). Electrophysiology of oxytocin actions on central neurons. *Annals of the New York Academy of Science,* 652, 46–57.

Dunbar, R. (1996). *Grooming, gossip, and the evolution of language.* Cambridge, MA: Harvard University Press.

Dunn, J. B., & Richards, M. P. (1977). Observations on the developing relationship between mother and baby in the neonatal period. In H. R. Scaefer (Ed.), *Studies in mother–infant interaction* (pp. 427–455). New York: Academic Press.

Eagly, A. H., & Steffen, V. J. (1986). Gender and aggressive behavior: A meta-analytic review of the social psychological literature. *Psychological Bulletin,* 100, 309–330.

Eagly, A. H., & Wood, W. (1999). The origins of sex differences in human behavior. *American Psychologist,* 54, 408–423.

Edwards, C. P. (1993). Behavioral sex differences in children of diverse cultures: The case of nurturance to infants. In M. E. Pereira & L. A. Fairbanks (Eds.), *Juvenile primates: Life history, development, and behavior* (pp. 327–338). New York: Oxford University Press.

Fahrbach, S. E., Morrell, J. I., & Pfaff, D. W. (1985). Possible role for endogenous oxytocin in estrogen-facilitated maternal behavior in rats. *Neuroendocrinology,* 40, 526–532.

Ferber, M. A., O'Farrell, B., & Allen, L. R. (1991). *Work and families: Policies for a changing work force.* Washington, DC: National Academy Press.

Field, T. M. (1995). Massage therapy for infants and children. *Journal of Developmental & Behavioral Pediatrics,* 16, 105–111.

Field, T. M. (1996). Touch therapies for pain management and stress reduction. In R. J. Resnick & H. R. Ronald (Eds.), *Health psychology through the life span: Practice and research opportunities* (pp. 313–321). Washington, DC: American Psychological Association.

Field, T., & Goldson, E. (1984). Pacifying effects of nonnutritive sucking on term and preterm neonates during heelstick procedures. *Pediatrics,* 74, 1012–1015.

Field, T. M., Malphurs, J., Carraway, K., & Pelaez-Nogueras, M. (1996). Carrying position influences infant behavior. *Early Child Development & Care,* 121, 49–54.

Field, T. M., Schanberg, S., Davalos, M., & Malphurs, J. (1996). Massage with oil has more positive effects on normal infants. *Pre- & Peri-Natal Psychology Journal,* 11, 75–80.

Fleming, A. S., Steiner, M., & Corter, C. (1997). Cortisol, hedonics, and maternal responsiveness in human mothers. *Hormones and Behavior,* 32, 85–98.

Flinn, M. V., & England, B. G. (1997). Social economics of childhood gluticosteroid stress responses and health. *American Journal of Physical Anthropology,* 102, 33–53.

Fontana, A. M., Diegnan, T., Villeneuve, A., & Lepore, S. J. (1999). Nonevaluative social support reduces cardiovascular reactivity in young women during acutely stressful performance situations. *Journal of Behavioral Medicine,* 22, 75–91.

Fossey, D. (1983). *Gorillas in the mist.* Boston: Houghton Mifflin.

Francis, D., Diorio, J., Liu, D., & Meaney, M. J. (1999, November). Nongenomic transmission across generations of maternal behavior and stress responses in the rat. *Science,* 286, 1155–1158.

Frankenhaeuser, M., Dunne, E., & Lundberg, U. (1976). Sex differences in sympathetic-adrenal medullary reactions induced by different stressors. *Psychopharmacology,* 47, 1–5.

Frasch, A., Zetzsche, T., Steiger, A., & Jirikowski, G. F. (1995). Reduction of plasma oxytocin levels in patients suffering from major depression. In R. Ivell & J. Russell (Eds.), *Oxytocin: Cellular and molecular approaches in medicine and research* (pp. 257–258). New York: Plenum Press.

Fry, D. P. (1992). Female aggression among the Zapotec of Oaxaca, Mexico. In K. Bjorkqvist & P. Niemela (Eds.), *Of mice and women: Aspects of female aggression* (pp. 187–200). San Diego, CA: Academic Press.

Gerin, W., Milner, D., Chawla, S., & Pickering, T. G. (1995). Social support as a moderator of cardiovascular reactivity: A test of the direct effects and buffering hypothesis. *Psychosomatic Medicine, 57,* 16–22.

Gerin, W., Pieper, C., Levy, R., & Pickering, T. G. (1992). Social support in social interaction: A moderator of cardiovascular reactivity. *Psychosomatic Medicine, 54,* 324–336.

Girdler, S. S., Jamner, L. D., & Shapiro, D. (1997). Hostility, testosterone, and vascular reactivity to stress: Effects of sex. *International Journal of Behavioral Medicine, 4,* 242–263.

Glass, D., & Singer, J. (1972). *Urban stress.* New York: Academic Press.

Glazer, I. M. (1992). Interfemale aggression and resource scarcity in a cross-cultural perspective. In K. Bjorkqvist & P. Niemela (Eds.), *Of mice and women: Aspects of female aggression* (pp. 163–172). San Diego, CA: Academic Press.

Glynn, L. M., Christenfeld, N., & Gerin, W. (1999). Gender, social support, and cardiovascular responses to stress. *Psychosomatic Medicine, 61,* 234–242.

Goodall, J. (1986). *The chimpanzees of Gombe: Patterns of behavior.* Cambridge, MA: Belknap Press of Harvard University Press.

Goodman, L. A., Koss, M. P., Fitzgerald, L. F., Russo, N. F., & Keita, G. P. (1993). Male violence against women: Current research and future directions. *American Psychologist, 48,* 1054–1058.

Goodman, M. J., Griffin, P. B., Estioko-Griffin, A. A., & Grove, J. S. (1985). The compatibility of hunting and mothering among the Agta hunter–gatherers of the Philippines. *Sex Roles, 12,* 1199–1209.

Goy, R. W. (1966). Role of androgens in the establishment and regulation of behavioral sex differences in mammals. *Journal of Animal Science, 25*(Suppl.), 21–35.

Goy, R. W. (1978). Development of play and mounting behavior in female rhesus virilized prenatally with esters of testosterone or dihydrotestosterone. In D. J. Chivers & J. Herbert (Eds.), *Recent advances in primatology* (Vol. 1, pp. 449–462). London: Academic Press.

Gray, J. A. (1971). Sex differences in emotional behaviour in mammals including Man: Endocrine bases. *Acta Psychologica, 35,* 29–46.

Gray, J. A., & Lalljee, B. (1974). Sex differences in emotional behaviour in the rat: Correlation between open-field defecation and active avoidance. *Animal Behaviour, 22,* 856–861.

Gruenewald, T. L., Taylor, S. E., Klein, L. C., & Seeman, T. E. (1999). Gender disparities in acute stress research [Abstract]. *Proceedings of the Society of Behavioral Medicine's 20th Annual Meeting: Annals of Behavioral Medicine, 21*(Suppl.), S141.

Gunnar, M. R., Brodersen, L., Krueger, K., & Rigatuso, J. (1996). Dampening of adrenocortical responses during infancy: Normative changes and individual differences. *Child Development, 67,* 877–889.

Gunnar, M. R., Brodersen, L., Nachmias, M., Buss, K., & Rigatuso, J. (1996). Stress reactivity and attachment security. *Developmental Psychology, 29,* 191–204.

Gunnar, M. R., Gonzalez, C. A., Goodlin, B. L., & Levine, S. (1981). Behavioral and pituitary-adrenal responses during a prolonged separation period in rhesus monkeys. *Psychoneuroimmunology, 6,* 65–75.

Harlow, C. M. (Ed.) (1986). *Learning to love: The selected papers of H. F. Harlow.* New York: Praeger.

Hazan, C., & Shaver, P. R. (1994). Attachment as an organizational framework for research on close relationships. *Psychological Inquiry, 5,* 1–22.

Hellhammer, D. H., Hubert, W., & Schurmeyer, T. (1985). Changes in saliva testosterone after psychological stimulation in men. *Psychoneuroendocrinology, 10,* 77–81.

Hennessy, M. B., Mendoza, S. P., & Kaplan, J. N. (1982). Behavior and plasma cortisol following brief peer separation in juvenile squirrel monkeys. *American Journal of Primatology, 3,* 143–151.

Hertsgaard, L. G., Gunnar, M. R., Erickson, M. R., & Nachmias, M. (1995). Adrenocortical responses to the strange situation in infants with disorganized/disoriented attachment relationships. *Child Development, 66,* 1100–1106.

Hiatt, B. (1970). Woman the gatherer. In F. Gale (Ed.), *Woman's role in aboriginal society, Australian aboriginal studies.* Canberra, Australian Capital Territory, Australia: Australian Institute of Aboriginal Studies.

Hochschild, A. (1989). *The second shift: Working parents and the revolution at home.* New York: Viking Penguin.

Hofer, M. A. (1995). Hidden regulators: Implications for a new understanding of attachment, separation, and loss. In S. Goldberg, R. Muir, & J. Kerr (Eds.), *Attachment theory: Social, developmental, and clinical perspectives* (pp. 203–230). Hillsdale, NJ: Analytic Press.

Holmstrom, R. (1992). Female aggression among the great apes: A psychoanalytic perspective. In K. Bjorkqvist & P. Niemela (Eds.), *Of mice and women: Aspects of female aggression* (pp. 295–306). San Diego, CA: Academic Press.

House, J. S., Umberson, D., & Landis, K. R. (1988). Structures and processes of social support. *American Review of Sociology, 14,* 293–318.

Hyde, J. S. (1984). How large are gender differences in aggression? A developmental meta-analysis. *Developmental Psychology, 20,* 722–736.

Insel, T. R. (1997). A neurobiological basis of social attachment. *American Journal of Psychiatry, 154,* 726–735.

Insel, T. R., & Winslow, J. T. (1998). Serotonin and neuropeptides in affiliative behaviors. *Biological Psychiatry, 44,* 207–219.

Ironson, G., Field, T., Scafidi, F., Hashimoto, M., Kumar, M., Kumar, A., Price, A., Goncalves, A., Burman, I., Tetenman, C., Patarca, R., & Fletcher, M. A. (1996). Massage therapy is associated with enhancement of the immune system's cytotoxic capacity. *International Journal of Neuroscience, 84,* 205–217.

Jalowiec, J. E., Calcagnetti, D. J., & Fanselow, M. S. (1989). Suppression of juvenile social behavior requires antagonism of central opioid systems. *Pharmacology Biochemistry and Behavior, 33,* 697–700.

Jamner, L. D., Alberts, J., Leigh, H., & Klein, L. C. (1998, March). *Affiliative need and endogenous opioids.* Paper presented at the annual meetings of the Society of Behavioral Medicine, New Orleans, LA.

Janson, C. H. (1992). Evolutionary ecology of primate structure. In E. A. Smith & B. Winterhalder (Eds.), *Evolutionary ecology and human behavior* (pp. 95–130). New York: Aldine.

Jezova, D., Jurankova, E., Mosnarova, A., Kriska, M., & Skultetyova, I. (1996). Neuroendocrine response during stress with relation to gender differences. *Acta Neurobiologae Experimentalis, 56,* 779–785.

Jazova, D., Skultetyova, I., Tokarev, D. I., Bakos, P., & Vigas, M. (1995). Vasopressin and oxytocin in stress. In G. P. Chrousos, R. McCarty, K. Pacak, G. Cizza, E. Sternberg, P. W. Gold, & R. Kvetnansky (Eds.), *Stress: Basic mechanisms and clinical implications* (Vol. 771, pp. 192–203). New York, NY: Annals of the New York Academy of Sciences.

Jordan, T. C., Hennessy, M. B., Gonzalez, C. A., & Levine, S. (1985). Social and environmental factors influencing mother–infant separation–reunion in squirrel monkeys. *Physiology and Behavior, 34,* 489–493.

Kalin, N. H., Gibbs, D. M., Barksdale, C. M., Shelton, C. E., & Carnes, M. (1985). Behavioral stress decreases plasma oxytocin concentrations in primates. *Life Science, 36,* 1275–1280.

Kamarck, T. W., Manuck, S. B., & Jennings, J. R. (1990). Social support reduces cardiovascular reactivity to psychological challenge: A laboratory model. *Psychosomatic Medicine, 52,* 42–58.

Kashima, Y., Yamaguchi, S. K., Choi, S., Gelfand, M. J., & Yuki, M. (1995). Culture, gender, and self: A perspective from the individualism–collectivism research. *Journal of Personality and Social Psychology, 69,* 925–937.

Kendrick, K. M., Da Costa, A. P., Broad, K. D., Ohkura, S., Guevara, R., Levy, F., & Keverne, E. B. (1997). Neural control of maternal behavior and olfactory recognition of offspring. *Brain Research Bulletin, 44,* 383–395.

Kendrick, K. M., & Keverne, E. B. (1989). Effects of intracerebroventricular infusions of naltrexone and phentolamine on central and peripheral oxytocin release and on maternal behaviour induced by vaginocervical stimulation in the ewe. *Brain Research, 505,* 329–332.

Kendrick, K. M., Keverne, E. B., & Baldwin, B. A. (1987). Intracerebroventricular oxytocin stimulates maternal behaviour in the sheep. *Neuroendocrinology, 46,* 56–61.

Kendrick, K. M., Levy, F., & Keverne, E. B. (1992, May 8). Changes in the sensory processing of olfactory signals induced by birth in sheep. *Science, 256,* 833–836.

Kenrick, D. T., & Johnson, G. A. (1979). Interpersonal attraction in aversive environments: A problem for the classical conditioning paradigm? *Journal of Personality and Social Psychology, 37,* 572–579.

Keverne, E. B., Nevison, C. M., & Martel, F. L. (1999). Early learning and the social bond. In C. S.

Carter, I. I. Lederhendler, & B. Kirkpatrick (Eds.), *The integrative neurobiology of affiliation* (pp. 263–274). Cambridge, MA: MIT Press.

Kirschbaum, C., Klauer, T., Filipp, S., & Hellhammer, D. H. (1995). Sex-specific effects of social support on cortisol and subjective responses to acute psychological stress. *Psychosomatic Medicine, 57*, 23–31.

Klein, L. C., Alberts, J., Jamner, J. D., Leigh, H., Levine, L. J., & Orenstein, M. D. (1998). Naltrexone administration increases salivary cortisol units in women but not men. *Psychophysiology, 35*, S49.

Klein, L. C., Popke, E. J., & Grunberg, N. E. (1998). Sex differences in effects of opioid blockade on stress-induced freezing behavior. *Pharmacology Biochemistry and Behavior, 61*, 413–417.

Knutson, B., Wolkowitz, O. M., Cole, S. W., Chan, T., Moore, E. A., Johnson, R. C., Terpstra, J., Turner, R. A., & Reus, V. I. (1998). Selective alteration of personality and social behavior by serotonergic intervention. *American Journal of Psychiatry, 155*, 373–379.

Kors, D., Linden, W., & Gerin, W. (1997). Evaluation interferes with social support: Effects on cardiovascular stress reactivity. *Journal of Social and Clinical Psychology, 16*, 1–23.

Koss, M. P., Goodman, L. A., Browne, A., Fitzgerald, L. F., Keita, L. F., & Russo, N. F. (1994). *No safe haven: Male violence against women at home, at work, and in the community.* Washington, DC: American Psychological Association.

Kraemer, G. W. (1992). A psychobiological theory of attachment. *Behavior and Brain Science, 15*, 493–541.

Kreek, M. J., & Koob, G. F. (1998). Drug dependence: Stress and dysregulation of brain reward pathways. *Drug and Alcohol Pathways, 51*, 23–47.

Kuhn, C. M., Pauk, J., & Schanberg, S. M. (1990). Endocrine responses to mother–infant separation in developing rats. *Developmental Psychobiology, 23*, 395–410.

Lee, R. B. (1979). *The Kung San: Man, women and work in a foraging society.* New York: Cambridge University Press.

Lepore, S. J., Allen, K. A. M., & Evans, G. W. (1993). Social support lowers cardiovascular reactivity to an acute stress. *Psychosomatic Medicine, 55*, 518–524.

Levine, S., Lyons, D. M., & Schatzberg, A. F. (1999). Psychobiological consequences of social relationships. In C. S. Carter, I. I. Lederhendler, & B. Kirkpatrick

(Eds.), *The integrative neurobiology of affiliation* (pp. 83–92). Cambridge, MA: MIT Press.

Lewis, B. P., & Linder, D. E. (2000). *Fear and affiliation: Replication and extension of Schachter.* Manuscript in preparation.

Lightman, S. L., & Young, W. S., III. (1989). Lactation inhibits stress-mediated secretion of corticosterone and oxytocin and hypothalamic accumulation of corticotropin-releasing factor and enkephalin messenger ribonucleic acids. *Endocrinology, 124*, 2358–2364.

Liu, D., Diorio, J., Day, J. C., Francis, D. D., Mar, A., & Meaney, M. J. (in press). Maternal care, hippocampal synaptogenesis and cognitive development in the rat. *Science.*

Liu, D., Diorio, J., Tannenbaum, B., Caldji, C., Francis, D., Freedman, A., Sharma, S., Pearson, D., Plotsky, P. M., & Meaney, M. J. (1997, September 12). Maternal care, hippocampal glucocorticoid receptors, and hypothalamic-pituitary-adrenal responses to stress. *Science, 277*, 1659–1662.

Luckow, A., Reifman, A., & McIntosh, D. N. (1998, August). *Gender differences in coping: A meta-analysis.* Poster session presented at the 106th Annual Convention of the American Psychological Association, San Francisco, CA.

Lumia, A. R., Thorner, K. M., & McGinnis, M. Y. (1994). Effects of chronically high doses of anabolic androgenic steroid, testosterone, on intermale aggression and sexual behavior in male rats. *Physiology and Behavior, 55*, 331–335.

Maccoby, E. E., & Jacklin, C. H. (1974). *The psychology of sex differences.* Stanford, CA: Stanford University Press.

Malamuth, N. M. (1998). An evolutionary-based model integrating research on the characteristics of sexually coercive men. In J. G. Adair, D. Belanger, & K. L. Dion (Eds.), *Advances in psychological science* (Vol. 1, pp. 151–184). New York: Psychology Press.

Markus, H. R., & Kitayama, S. (1991). Culture and the self: Implications for cognition, emotion, and motivation. *Psychological Review, 98*, 224–253.

Martel, F. L., Nevison, C. M., Rayment, F. D., Simpson, M. J. A., & Keverne, E. B. (1993). Opioid receptor blockade reduces maternal affect and social grooming in rhesus monkeys. *Psychoneuroimmunology, 18*, 307–321.

Mason, W. A., & Epple, G. (1969). Social organization in experimental groups of *Saimiri* and *Callicebus*. *Proceedings of the Second International Congress of Primatology*, 1, 59–65.

Mathur, D. N., Toriola, A. L., & Dada, O. A. (1986). Serum cortisol and testosterone levels in conditioned male distance runners and non-athletes after maximal exercise. *Journal of Sports Medicine and Physical Fitness*, 26, 245–250.

Matthews, K. A., & Stoney, C. M. (1988). Influences of sex and age on cardiovascular responses during stress. *Psychosomatic Medicine*, 50, 46–56.

McCarthy, M. M. (1995). Estrogen modulation of oxytocin and its relation to behavior. In R. Ivell & J. Russell (Eds.), *Oxytocin: Cellular and molecular approaches in medicine and research* (pp. 235–242). New York: Plenum Press.

McCarthy, M. M., Chung, S. K. Ogawa, S., Kow, L., & Pfaff, D. W. (1991). Behavioral effects of oxytocin: Is there a unifying principle? In S. Jard & J. Ramison (Eds.), *Vasopressin* (pp. 195–212). Montrouge, France: John Libbey Eurotext.

McCarthy, M. M., McDonald, C. H., Brooks, P. J., & Goldman, D. (1996). An anxiolytic action of oxytocin is enhanced by estrogen in the mouse. *Physiology and Behavior*, 60, 1209–1215.

McDonald, L. M., & Korabik, K. (1991). Sources of stress and ways of coping among male and female managers. *Journal of Social Behavior and Personality*, 6, 185–198.

Mendoza, S. P., Coe, C. L., Smotherman, W. P., Kaplan, J., & Levine, S. (1980). Functional consequences of attachment: A comparison of two species. In R. W. Bell & W. P. Smotherman (Eds.), *Maternal influences and early behavior* (pp. 235–252). New York: Spectrum.

Mendoza, S. P., & Mason, W. A. (1999). Attachment relationships in New World primates. In C. S. Carter, I. I. Lederhendler, & B. Kirkpatrick (Eds.), *The integrative neurobiology of affiliation* (pp. 93–100). Cambridge, MA: MIT Press.

Mendoza, S. P., Smotherman, W. P., Miner, M., Kaplan, J., & Levine, S. (1978). Pituitary-adrenal response to separation in mother and infant squirrel monkeys. *Developmental Psychology*, 11, 169–175.

Murphy, Y., & Murphy, R. (1974). *Women of the forest.* New York: Columbia University Press.

Nachmias, M., Gunnar, M. R., Mangelsdorf, S., Parritz, R. H., & Buss, K. (1996). Behavioral inhibition and stress reactivity: The moderating role of attachment security. *Child Development*, 67, 508–522.

Newman, K. (1999). *No shame in my game: The working poor in the inner city.* New York: Alfred Knopf, with Russell Sage Foundation.

Niedenthal, P. M., & Beike, D. R. (1997). Interrelated and isolated self-concepts. *Personality and Social Psychology Review*, 1, 106–128.

Ogus, E. D., Greenglass, E. R., & Burke, R. J. (1990). Gender-role differences, work stress and depersonalization. *Journal of Social Behavior and Personality*, 5, 387–398.

Olweus, D., Mattson, A., Schalling, D., & Low, H. (1980). Testosterone, aggression, physical, and personality dimensions in normal adolescent males. *Psychosomatic Medicine*, 42, 352–369.

Panksepp, J. (1998). *Affective neuroscience.* London: Oxford University Press.

Panksepp, J., Nelson, E., & Bekkedal, M. (1999). Brain systems for the mediation of social separation distress and social-reward: Evolutionary antecedents and neuropeptide intermediaries. In C. S. Carter, I. I. Lederhendler, & B. Kirkpatrick (Eds.), *The integrative neurobiology of affiliation* (pp. 221–244). Cambridge, MA: MIT Press.

Patterson, M. L., & Schaeffer, R. E. (1977). Effects of size and sex composition on interaction distance, participation, and satisfaction in small groups. *Small Group Behavior*, 8, 433–442.

Pearson, J. C. (1981). The effects of setting and gender on self-disclosure. *Group and Organization Studies*, 6, 334–340.

Phoenix, C. H. (1974a). Effects of dihydrotestosterone on sexual behavior of castrated male rhesus monkeys. *Physiology and Behavior*, 12, 1045–1055.

Phoenix, C. H. (1974b). Prenatal testosterone in the nonhuman primate and its consequences for behavior. In R. C. Friedman, R. M. Richart, R. L. Vande Wiele, & L. O. Stern (Eds.), *Sex differences in behavior* (pp. 495–532). New York: Wiley.

Phoenix, C. H. (1974c). The role of androgens in the sexual behavior of adult male rhesus monkeys. In W. Montagna & W. A. Sadler (Eds.), *Reproductive behavior* (pp. 376–404). New York: Plenum.

Phoenix, C. H., Goy, R. W., & Resko, J. A. (1968). Psychosexual differentiation as a function of androgenic stimulation. In M. Diamond (Ed.), *Perspectives in reproduction and sexual behavior* (pp. 215–246). Bloomington: Indiana University Press.

Pihoker, C., Owens, M. J., Kuhn, C. M., Schanberg, S. M., & Nemeroff, C. B. (1993). Maternal separation in neonatal rats elicits activation of the hypothalamic-pituitary-adrenocortical axis: A putative role for corticotropin-releasing factor. *Psychoneuroendocrinology,* 18, 485–493.

Popik, P., Vetulani, J., & Van Ree, J. M. (1992). Low doses of oxytocin facilitate social recognition in rats. *Psychopharmacology,* 106, 71–74.

Ptacek, J. T., Smith, R. E., & Zanas, J. (1992). Gender, appraisal, and coping: A longitudinal analysis. *Journal of Personality,* 60, 747–770.

Reite, M., Short, T., Seiler, C., & Pauley, J. D. (1981). Attachment, loss, and depression. *Journal of Child Psychology and Psychiatry,* 22, 141–169.

Repetti, R. L. (1989). Effects of daily workload on subsequent behavior during marital interactions: The role of social withdrawal and spouse support. *Journal of Personality and Social Psychology,* 57, 651–659.

Repetti, R. L. (1997, April). *The effects of daily job stress on parent behavior with preadolescents.* Paper presented at the biennial meeting of the Society for Research in Child Development, Washington, DC.

Repetti, R. L. (2000). *The differential impact of chronic job stress on mothers' and fathers' behavior with children.* Manuscript in preparation.

Repetti, R. L., & Wood, J. (1997). Effects of daily stress at work on mothers' interactions with preschoolers. *Journal of Family Psychology,* 11, 90–108.

Robinson, J., & Godbey, G. (1997). *Time for life.* State College: Pennsylvania State University Press.

Roy, M. P., Steptoe, A., & Kirschbaum, C. (1998). Life events and social support as moderators of individual differences in cardiovascular and cortisol reactivity. *Journal of Personality and Social Psychology,* 75, 1273–1281.

Rubenstein, D. E. (1978). On predation, competition, and the advantages of group living. In P. P. G. Bateson & P. H. Klopfer (Eds.), *Perspectives in ethnology* (Vol. 3, pp. 205–31). New York: Plenum Press.

Ruppenthal, G. C., Harlow, M. K., Eisele, C. D., Harlow, H. F., & Suomi, S. F. (1974). Development of

peer interactions of monkeys reared in a nuclear family environment. *Child Development,* 45, 670–682.

Ryff, C. D., & Singer, B. (1998). The contours of positive human health. *Psychological Inquiry,* 9, 1–28.

Sandnabba, N. K. (1992). Aggressive behavior in female mice as a correlated characteristic in selection for aggressiveness in male mice. In K. Bjorkqvist & P. Niemela (Eds.), *Of mice and women: Aspects of female aggression* (pp. 367–381). San Diego, CA: Academic Press.

Sapolsky, R. M. (1992a). Cortisol concentrations and the social significance of rank instability among wild baboons. *Psychoneuroendocrinology,* 17, 701–709.

Sapolsky, R. M. (1992b). *Stress, the aging brain, and the mechanisms of neuron death.* Cambridge, MA: MIT Press.

Sapolsky, R. M. (1994). *Why zebras don't get ulcers.* New York: Friedman.

Sawchenko, P. E., & Swanson, L. W. (1982). Immunohistochemical identification of neurons in the paraventricular nucleus of the hypothalamus that project to the medulla or to the spinal cord in the rat. *Journal of Comparative Neurology,* 205, 260–272.

Scafidi, F., & Field, T. (1996). Massage therapy improves behavior in neonates born to HIV-positive mothers. *Journal of Pediatric Psychology,* 21, 889–897.

Scafidi, F. A., Field, T., & Schanberg, C. M. (1993). Factors that predict which preterm infants benefit most from massage therapy. *Journal of Developmental and Behavioral Pediatrics,* 14, 176–180.

Schachter, S. (1959). *The psychology of affiliation.* Stanford, CA: Stanford University Press.

Shaffer, D., & Campbell, M. (1994). Reactive attachment disorder of infancy or early childhood. In A. Frances, H. A. Pincus, & H. B. First (Eds.), *Diagnostic and statistical manual of mental disorders: DSM–IV* (4th ed., pp. 116–118). Washington, DC: American Psychiatric Association.

Sheffield, D., & Carroll, D. (1994). Social support and cardiovascular reactions to active laboratory stressors. *Psychology and Health,* 9, 305–316.

Shively, C. A., Laber-Laird, K., & Anton, R. F. (1997). Behavior and physiology of social stress and depression in female Cynomolgus monkeys. *Biological Psychiatry,* 41, 871–882.

Silk, J. B. (2000). Ties that bond: The role of kinship in primate societies. In L. Stone (Ed.), *New directions in anthropological kinship.* Boulder, CO: Rowman and Littlefield.

Spain, D. (1992). The spatial foundations of men's friendships and men's power. *Men's friendships, 246,* 59–73.

Stack, C. (1975). *All my kin.* New York: Harper and Row.

Staines, G. L., & Pleck, J. L. (1983). *The impact of work schedules on the family.* Ann Arbor: University of Michigan Survey Research Center, Institute for Social Research.

Stanton, M. E., Gutierrez, Y. R., & Levine, S. (1988). Maternal deprivation potentiates pituitary-adrenal stress responses in infant rats. *Behavioral Neuroscience, 102,* 692–700.

Staub, E., Tursky, B., & Schwartz, G. E. (1971). Self-control and predictability: Their effects on reactions to aversive stimuli. *Journal of Personality and Social Psychology, 18,* 157–162.

Stoney, C. M., Davis, M. C., & Matthews, K. A. (1987). Sex differences in physiological responses to stress and in coronary heart disease: A causal link? *Psychophysiology, 24,* 127–131.

Stoney, C. M., Matthews, K. A., McDonald, R. H., & Johnson, C. A. (1988). Sex differences in lipid, lipo-protein, cardiovascular, and neuroendocrine responses to acute stress. *Psychophysiology, 25,* 645–656.

Straus, M. A., & Gelles, R. J. (1986). Societal change and change in family violence from 1975 to 1985 as revealed by two national surveys. *Journal of Marriage and the Family, 48,* 465–479.

Swanson, L. W., & Sawchenko, P. E. (1980). Para-ventricular nucleus: A site for the integration of neuroendocrine and autonomic mechanisms. *Neuroendocrinology, 31,* 410–417.

Taylor, S. E., Klein, L. C., Greendale, G., & Seeman, T. E. (1999). *Oxytocin and HPA responses to acute stress in women with or without HRT.* Manuscript in preparation.

Thorsteinsson, E. B., James, J. E., & Gregg, M. E. (1998). Effects of video-relayed social support on hemodynmaic reactivity and salivary cortisol during laboratory-based behavioral challenge. *Health Psychology, 17,* 436–444.

Tiger, L. (1970). *Men in groups.* New York: Vintage Books.

Tooby, J., & Cosmides, L. (1992). Psychological foundations of culture. In J. Barkow, L. Cosmides, & J. Tooby (Eds.), *The adapted mind* (pp. 19–136). New York: Oxford University Press.

Turner, R. A., Altemus, M., Enos, T., Cooper, B., & McGuinness, T. (1999). Preliminary research on plasma oxytocin in healthy, normal cycling women investigating emotion and interpersonal distress. *Psychiatry, 62,* 97–113.

U.S. Department of Health and Human Services. (1999). *Child Maltreatment 1997: Reports from the States to the National Child Abuse and Neglect Data System.* Washington, DC: U.S. Government Printing Office.

Uvnas-Moberg, K. (1996). Neuroendocrinology of the mother–child interaction. *Trends in Endocrinology and Metabolism, 7,* 126–131.

Uvnas-Moberg, K. (1997). Oxytocin linked antistress effects—the relaxation and growth response. *Acta Psychologica Scandinavica, 640*(Suppl.), 38–42.

Uvnas-Moberg, K. (1999). Physiological and endocrine effects of social contact. In C. S. Carter, I. I. Lederhendler, & B. Kirkpatrick (Eds.), *The integrative neurobiology of affiliation* (pp. 245–262). Cambridge, MA: MIT Press.

Uvnas-Moberg, K., Marchini, G., & Winberg, J. (1993). Plasma cholecystokinin concentrations after breast feeding in healthy four-day-old infants. *Archives of Diseases in Childhood, 68,* 46–48.

Veroff, J., Kulka, R., & Douvan, E. (1981). *Mental health in America: Patterns of help-seeking from 1957 to 1976.* New York: Basic Books.

Wallen, K., & Tannenbaum, P. L. (1997). Hormonal modulation of sexual behavior and affiliation in rhesus monkeys. *Annals of the New York Academy of Science, 807,* 185–202.

Wang, S., Bartolome, J. V., & Schanberg, S. M. (1996). Neonatal deprivation of maternal touch may suppress ornithine decarboxylase via downregulation of the proto-oncogenes c- myc and max. *Journal of Neuroscience, 16,* 836–842.

Wethington, E., McLeod, J. D., & Kessler, R. C. (1987). The importance of life events for explaining sex differences in psychological distress. In R. C. Barnett, L. Biener, & G. K. Baruch (Eds.), *Gender and stress* (pp. 144–156). New York: Free Press.

Wheeler, G., Cumming, D., Burnham, R., Maclean, I., Sloley, B. D., Bhambhani, Y., & Steadward, R. D. (1994). Testosterone, cortisol and catecholamine responses to exercise stress and autonomic dysreflexia in elite quadiplegic athletes. *Paraplegia, 32*, 292–299.

Whitcher, S. J., & Fisher, J. D. (1979). Multidimensional reaction to therapeutic touch in a hospital setting. *Journal of Personality and Social Psychology, 37*, 87–96.

Whiting, B., & Whiting, J. (1975). *Children of six cultures.* Cambridge, MA: Harvard University Press.

Wiesenfeld, A. R., Malatesta, C. Z., Whitman, P. B., Grannose, C., & Vile, R. (1985). Psychophysiological response of breast- and bottle-feeding mothers to their infants' signals. *Psychophysiology, 22*, 79–86.

Williams, R. B., Lane, J. D., Kuhn, C. M., Melosh, W., White, A. D., & Schanberg, S. M. (1982, October 29). Type A behavior and elevated physiological and neuroendocrine responses to cognitive tasks. *Science, 218*, 483–485.

Windle, R. J., Shanks, N., Lightman, S. L., & Ingram, C. D. (1997). Central oxytocin administration reduces stress-induced corticosterone release and anxiety behavior in rats. *Endocrinology, 138*, 2829–2834.

Witt, D. M., Carter, C. S., & Walton, D. (1990). Central and peripheral effects of oxytocin administration in prairie voles (*Microtus ochrogaster*). *Pharmacology Biochemistry and Behavior, 37*, 63–69.

Witt, D. M., Winslow, J. T., & Insel, T. R. (1992). Enhanced social interactions in rats following chronic, centrally infused oxytocin. *Pharmacology Biochemistry and Behavior, 43*, 855–886.

Wrangham, R. W. (1980). An ecological model of female-bonded primate groups. *Behaviour, 75*, 262–300.

Zeskind, P. S. (1980). Adult responses to cries of low and high risk infants. *Infant Behavior and Development, 3*, 167–177.

Zeskind, P. S. (1987). Adult heart rate responses to infant cry sounds. *British Journal of Developmental Psychology, 5*, 73–79.

Zeskind, P. S. & Collins, V. (1987). The pitch of infant crying and caregiver responses in a natural setting. *Infant Behavior and Development, 10*, 501–504.

Zeskind, P. S., Sale, J., Maio, M. L., Huntington, L., & Weiseman, J. (1985). Adult perceptions of pain and hunger cries: A synchrony of arousal. *Child Development, 14*, 549–554.

Oxytocin, Vasopressin, and Autism: Is There a Connection?

Thomas R. Insel, Derek J. O'Brien, and James F. Leckman

Introduction

Autism remains one of the most challenging frontiers of psychopathology. Although the syndrome's incidence is generally reported at less than 0.1%, its emergence early in life, its profound impact on families, and its chronic, treatment-refractory course have resulted in enormous emotional and financial costs (Bristol et al. 1996). The absence of a specific, reliable medical treatment for autistic children has proven especially vexing. Over the past two decades successful new pharmacotherapies have been developed for most other major psychiatric illnesses, but for autism little significant medical progress has been made since the syndrome was first described by Kanner in 1943 (Bailey et al. 1996; Kanner 1943).

There is general agreement between DSM-IV and ICD-10 over the major diagnostic criteria for autism (American Psychiatric Association 1994; World Health Organization 1993). These criteria define autism as a disorder of early childhood with the following triad of behavioral signs: 1) social impairment (lack of social reciprocity, decreased eye contact, failure to recognize the uniqueness of others); 2) communication abnormalities (delayed or incomplete language acquisition, deficits in both prelinguistic and verbal expression, decreased play); and 3) stereotyped behaviors (unusual attachments to objects, rigid adherence to routines or rituals, simple motor mannerisms such as hand flapping).

Several aspects of this syndrome may prove especially important for investigating the neurobiology of autism. First, this is a developmental syndrome. The onset of autism is virtually always observed before 3 years of age, and often parents report abnormalities in social interest even in the first months of life (Lord 1995). Affected children show a range of cognitive deficits, with about 75% functioning at a retarded level (reviewed in Gillberg and Coleman 1992). As with many neu-rodevelopmental syndromes, boys are affected about 4–5 times more often than girls (Gillberg and Coleman 1992). Together these observations suggest that the relevant neurobiological events may occur relatively early in the course of central nervous system (CNS) development, involving a cascade of complex gene–environment interactions.

Second, autism has an important genetic component. Siblings have an incidence of 2.9–3.7% (Bolton et al. 1994; Jorde et al. 1990; Szatmari and Jones 1991), representing nearly a 100-fold increased risk relative to the general population. Twin studies have found a concordance of 36–91% in monozygotic twins compared to a <1% concordance rate in dizygotic twins (Bailey et al. 1995; Folstein and Rutter 1977; Steffenberg et al. 1989). After pooling the data from two British twin samples and using the sibling rate of non-twin probands to estimate the dizygotic rate, Bailey et al. calculated a heritability of 91–93% for autism (Bailey et al. 1995). In addition, autism or autistic behavior is associated with several specific genetic disorders, including fragile X disorder (Bailey et al. 1993; Gillberg and Wahlström 1985) and tuberous sclerosis (Gillberg et al. 1994; Hunt and Shepherd 1993; Smalley et al. 1992) as well as several rare chromosomal anomalies (reviewed in Gillberg and Coleman 1992). On the basis of the available evidence, Bailey et al. (1996) have concluded that "genetic influences predominate in the etiology of autism and, moreover, that this is likely to apply to the great majority of cases" (p 96). It should be noted, however, that the genetic component of etiology is likely to be complex, involving multiple genes that act additively or possibly act via genetic heterogeneity. In addition, the phenotype may extend beyond DSM-IV autism to include what Rutter has called the "lesser variant" (Rutter et al. 1993). It seems likely that the putative genes do not cause autism; they increase the probability of developing one or more of the features of this complex disorder.

Finally, in spite of broad recognition that autism is a neurodevelopmental syndrome, there is still no consistent neurochemical, neurophysiological, or neuroanatomical abnormality. Although several reports have noted hyperserotonemia in autism, there is little evidence for a specific abnormality of serotonin in the CNS, and treatments that target serotonin (e.g., fluvoxamine) have proven only modestly helpful (Gordon et al. 1993; McBride et al. 1996; McDougle et al. 1996). Brain opiates have been implicated in social behavior, but there are no data demonstrating that these peptides are involved in autism, nor is there a clear therapeutic effect of opiate agonists or antagonists (Gillberg and Coleman 1992). Several neuroanatomic abnormalities have been noted by magnetic resonance imaging and by postmortem examination, but the significance of these findings and their relationship to the symptom complex remain to be demonstrated (Bailey et al. 1996; Bauman 1991; Courchesne et al. 1994).

An etiologic theory of autism needs to account for the social, cognitive, and communication deficits, as well as the compulsive behavior of these children. In addition, this theory should address the early onset, predominance in boys, genetic loading, and subtle neuroanatomical anomalies observed in this disorder. In this chapter, we suggest that abnormalities in the neural pathways for either oxytocin or vasopressin could account for many of these aspects of autism. This suggestion, which is based on animal studies of oxytocin and vasopressin effects on social and cognitive function (see, for instance, Insel 1992; Panksepp 1992), is enhanced by recent molecular studies of these neuropeptide systems in humans.

Oxytocin and Vasopressin as Candidate Neuropeptides

Oxytocin (OT) and vasopressin (AVP), nine amino acid peptides synthesized in the hypo-

thalamus, are released into the bloodstream via axon terminals in the posterior pituitary or neurohypophysis (hence their designation as neurohypophyseal peptides). The peptides are closely related structurally, differing at only two amino acids. Both are part of a family of nine amino acid peptides (nonapeptides) that can be traced phylogenetically to invertebrates (Gainer and Wray 1994). Ancestral nonapeptides have been implicated in various forms of nonmammalian reproductive behaviors such as nest building. Oxytocin and vasopressin are unique among this family in that they are found exclusively in mammals, probably evolving from the ancestral peptide arginine vasotocin, from which oxytocin and vasopressin each differ in only a single amino acid (Archer 1974).

The traditional view of the neurohypophyseal peptides as endocrine hormones acting on peripheral organs has recently been revised to consider these peptides as neurotransmitters or neuromodulators, that is, peptides with central actions. Within the hypothalamus, oxytocin and vasopressin are synthesized in the paraventricular nucleus (PVN) and supraoptic nucleus (SON). Not only do PVN cells synthesizing oxytocin and vasopressin project to diverse sites within the brain and brainstem (Sofroniew and Weindl 1981), receptors for both peptides have been found throughout the limbic system in the forebrain and autonomic centers in the brainstem (Barberis and Tribollet 1996). Furthermore, both peptides are released within the brain following chemical depolarization of the appropriate neurons, and fibers have been demonstrated at the ultrastructural level to make synaptic contacts in the CNS (Buijs and van Heerikhuize 1982). Thus, the evidence is quite strong that the brain is a target organ for these peptides. As vasopressin can bind to oxytocin receptors, and expression of oxytocin and vasopressin genes appears linked (see below), the most conservative approach to understanding how these peptides function in the brain is to discuss them together, rather than focusing on either one in isolation.

Three aspects of the central pathways for oxytocin and vasopressin deserve special note. First, specific vasopressin pathways appear to be sexually dimorphic. In both rodents (De Vries and Buijs 1983) and primates (Wang et al. 1997), extrahypothalamic vasopressin cells (e.g., cells in the bed nucleus of the stria terminalis) and their projections (e.g., lateral septum) are androgen-dependent and markedly more abundant in males. Second, neurotransmission for both peptides appears to depend largely on an unusual variability in their respective receptor. Oxytocin receptors are remarkably plastic, induced severalfold after gonadal steroid administration (Johnson et al. 1990) and expressed in different brain regions even in closely related species (Insel and Shapiro 1992; Insel et al. 1994a). In the hypothalamus, vasopressin receptors are sexually dimorphic and dependent on both steroids and photoperiod (Dubois-Dauphin et al. 1991; Johnson et al. 1995). Finally, both oxytocin and vasopressin receptors are developmentally regulated and expressed more in the immature brain (Shapiro and Insel 1989; Tribollet et al. 1989, 1991), and both peptides have been shown to have effects on neural development (Boer 1991, 1993). Vasopressin can be detected by embryonic day 16 in the developing rat brain and increases to high levels prior to birth. Oxytocin is also found in the fetal brain, although in the rat it is not processed to its mature, amidated form until after birth (Whitnall et al. 1985). It has long been known that vasopressin has mitogenic effects on various cell lines and can alter neurite outgrowth (reviewed in Boer and Swaab 1985). Chronic perinatal administration of both vasopressin and oxytocin has been associated with altered adult brain weight, with the most significant and persistent changes observed in the cerebellum (Boer 1991).

More than three decades of research indicates that both peptides have important cognitive and behavioral effects (Argiolas and Gessa 1991; de Wied et al. 1993) (Table 44.1). In 1965, De Wied reported that rats trained to avoid one side of a shuttle box appeared to "forget" this training following removal of the posterior–intermediate lobes of the pituitary unless treated with a vasopressin analogue (de Wied 1965). Several subsequent studies have demonstrated that vasopressin and oxytocin modulate learning and memory processes (reviewed in Kovacs and Telegdy 1985). In general, vasopressin facilitates learning of both active and passive avoidance behavior in a dose-dependent fashion. The peptide appears to influence both the consolidation and retrieval phases of learning, possibly with different metabolites affecting consolidation and retrieval independently. Although many of the early studies were based on peripheral administration of vasopressin, it is now clear from studies using central administration of the peptide that vasopressin effects on learning are mediated by a central receptor, probably in the hippocampus (reviewed in de Wied et al. 1993). Oxytocin's effects on learning are also dose-dependent, but generally opposite to vasopressin, with an inhibition of extinction in both passive and active avoidance paradigms.

Although the majority of patients diagnosed with autism also show mental retardation, the nature of the cognitive deficit is complex and not simply a defect in consolidation or retrieval (Rutter 1983). Paradoxically, although vasopressin facilitates learning in adults, vasopressin given during gestation has been reported to confer long-term deficits in memory (in male subjects) (Tinius et al. 1987). The mechanism of these effects is unclear, as the increase in vasopressin undoubtedly alters maternal physiology with a number of potential effects on fetal perfusion and nutrition.

Social Behavior

One form of memory that may be especially relevant to autism is the recognition of a familiar conspecific. A rodent test of this form of recognition, termed "social memory" was developed by Thor and Holloway (1982) and has been used

Table 44.1
Central effects of oxytocin and vasopressin

Effects	OT	OTA	AVP	V1A
Social behaviors				
Initiate maternal care (rat)	+++	—	+	?
Paternal care (vole)	?	?	+++	—
Onset sexual receptivity (rat)	+++	—	—	+++
Male sexual behavior (rat)	+++	—	?	?
Female pair bonding (vole)	+++	—	0	0
Male pair bonding (vole)	0	0	+++	—
Aggression (vole, hamster)	0	0	+++	—
Decrease isolation calls (rat)	+++	0	+++	0
Cognition				
Active avoidance (rat)	—	0	+++	—
Passive avoidance (rat)	—	0	+++	—
Social memory (rat)	+++/—	?	+++	—
Pup's memory (rat)	+++	—	?	?
Stereotypies				
Grooming (rat, monkey)	+++	—	+++	0
Flank-marking (hamster)	?	?	+++	—

References are provided in text. OT, oxytocin; OTA, oxytocin antagonist; AVP, vasopressin; V1A, antagonist at V1a receptor. +++ indicates facilitation of behavior; — indicates inhibition of behavior or, in some cases, blockage of agonist effect; 0 indicates no effect; ? indicates no data available.

by Dantzer et al. (1987) as well as others (Popik et al. 1992) to determine the role of vasopressin and oxytocin. After a brief exposure to a novel juvenile, a male rat may recognize this juvenile after 60 min but not after a 120-min interval. Vasopressin appears to facilitate and a vasopressin (V1a) receptor antagonist inhibits the consolidation of a social memory (Dantzer et al. 1987). A rat treated with vasopressin after being briefly exposed to a novel juvenile appears to recognize this juvenile 120 min later, whereas treatment with a vasopressin antagonist leads to no evidence of recognition when tested 30 min postexposure. Vasopressin's effects on social memory have been described only in male rats and appear to be androgen-dependent (Bluthe et al. 1990). In contrast to vasopressin's effects

on avoidance behavior, which are believed to be mediated via the hippocampus, effects on social memory involve the lateral septum (Dantzer et al. 1988), which receives more vasopressinergic innervation in males. Oxytocin, although initially reported to inhibit social memory (Dantzer et al. 1987), has more recently been shown to facilitate social memory at low doses (Popik et al. 1992). Oxytocin knockout mice show a remarkable deficit in social memory, although performance on spatial memory and olfactory discrimination tasks is unimpaired (author's unpublished data). In a recent experiment with rat pups, oxytocin was shown to facilitate conditioning to olfactory cues associated with the mother (Nelson and Panksepp 1996). These results suggested that oxytocin may not be essential for recognizing the mother, but that the peptide was critical for learning about factors associated with the mother. Curiously, as with the selective social memory deficits of oxytocin knockout mice, other forms of learning in rat pups, such as conditioning to odors associated with nonsocial stimuli, did not appear to be oxytocin-dependent.

A growing body of evidence has implicated oxytocin and vasopressin in the central mediation of sociosexual behaviors (Carter 1992; Insel 1992; Witt 1995). Oxytocin, given chronically by ICV minipump, increases affiliation, as measured by the amount of time rats spend in side-by-side contact (Witt et al. 1992). Oxytocin has been demonstrated to facilitate both maternal and sexual behaviors in rats (and maternal behavior in sheep). Both rats and sheep shift from avoiding to approaching neonates just prior to parturition. Oxytocin appears to be important for this transition to maternal behavior, but is not essential once this behavior has been initiated (Insel 1990). Vasopressin can also facilitate the emergence of maternal behavior (Pedersen et al. 1982), but it appears weaker than oxytocin and its effects on female sexual behavior may be opposite to oxytocin (Södersten et al. 1983). Vasopressin has also been implicated in paternal behavior (Wang et al. 1993) and, consistent with nest-defense, appears to facilitate certain forms of aggression (Ferris 1992; Winslow et al. 1993a).

Perhaps most relevant to autism, both peptides have been implicated in the development of social attachments. In monogamous prairie voles that form pair bonds, oxytocin has been shown to be both necessary and sufficient for the normal development of a partner preference in females (Insel and Hulihan 1995). In this species, pair bonds normally develop as a consequence of mating. For females, central administration of an oxytocin antagonist prevents pair bonding without inhibiting mating, while central administration of oxytocin facilitates pair bonding even in the absence of mating. Vasopressin appears to influence an analogous process of pair bond formation in males (Winslow et al. 1993a).

Communication

As language is restricted to humans, there are obvious limitations to the study of linguistic abnormalities in nonhuman animals. Nevertheless, other species communicate using visual, olfactory, and audiovocal cues. Some of these species-typical forms of communication appear to be influenced by the nonapeptides. For instance, flank-marking, a form of social communication observed in golden hamsters, is used by a dominant male to mark his territory. Flank marking can be elicited by microinjection of vasopressin into the lateral hypothalamus and is inhibited by administration of a vasopressin (V1a) receptor antagonist (Ferris et al. 1984, 1988, 1993). Similar effects, including an increase in scent marking and auto-grooming, have been observed in squirrel monkeys but only when socially isolated (Winslow and Insel 1991a, 1991b).

In most infant mammals, social separation results in a high-frequency distress call. In the infant rat, these calls, which are ultrasonic, are a potent stimulus for maternal retrieval. Central administration of oxytocin and vasopressin reduces the isolation calls of infant rats in a dose-dependent fashion (Insel and Winslow 1991; Winslow and Insel 1993). This potent central effect of these peptides may be related to the transient, exuberant expression of oxytocin and vasopressin receptors in the developing cortex (especially in cingulate).

In adult male canaries, the related nonapeptide vasotocin induces singing behavior (Voorhuis et al. 1991). This effect is complex, as vasotocin's effects on singing depend on the season and apparently on the gonadal status of the male bird.

Rituals

Both peptides have been shown to induce stereotypic behaviors such as stretching, repetitive grooming, startle, and squeaking responses when administered ICV to mice (reviewed in Meisenberg and Simmons 1983). Grooming, particularly grooming of the genital regions, is consistently observed following ICV administration of oxytocin in rats (Drago et al. 1986; van Wimersma Greidanus et al. 1990). In chicks, oxytocin induces wing-flapping (Panksepp 1992). Repeated central administration of vasopressin induces seizures in rats, including so-called "barrel-rolling" seizures that may be fatal. Although seizures have been reported in 25% of patients with autism, there appear to be no distinctive features of these seizures that make them unique to autism (reviewed in Gillberg and Coleman 1992). Self-injurious behavior is also a common feature of autism. It is certainly possible that the increase in aggression and self-directed behaviors observed in rodents after central administration of vasopressin could be related to the self-injurious behavior, often stereotyped, observed in autistic children.

Summary

In summary, results from nonhuman animal studies suggest that these neuropeptide systems influence behaviors that are abnormal in autism, including deficits in social, cognitive, and communicative behaviors as well as motor stereotypies. In addition, the early abundance of oxytocin and vasopressin receptors is consistent with a developmental role, and the sexual dimorphism of vasopressin pathways might be related to the male preponderance of this disorder; however, there are problems extrapolating the animal data to autism. The direction of the effect is not always consistent; these peptides facilitate social behavior and learning (suggesting a nonapeptide deficit in autism) but also induce grooming and stereotypic behavior (suggesting an excess). Although vasopressin induces flank-marking, the neurobiological relationship of olfactory communication to human language is highly speculative. In addition, the developmental effects are confusing. Vasopressin administered during gestation has been reported to inhibit rather than

facilitate subsequent cognitive performance. Perhaps some resolution of these apparent contradictions resides in the transition from adult pharmacology (administering microgram quantities of peptide) to developmental pathophysiology (selective deficits rather than excesses through early development). If autism is a genetic disorder, then one might expect that some alteration in one of these two neuropeptide systems throughout development would contribute to this disorder. Over the past decade, we have gained a greater understanding of the molecular biology of both these peptides and their receptors, providing several potential genetic mechanisms for autism.

Potential Genetic Mechanisms

The search for a genetic mechanism involving oxytocin or vasopressin neurotransmission logically breaks down into studies of the genes for these peptides, genes for their receptors, and developmental genes that specify for oxytocin and vasopressin pathways (see Table 44.2).

Peptide Genes

The genes for oxytocin and vasopressin have been among the most intensively studied in neuroendocrinology. First cloned and sequenced in 1984, these genes were localized to chromosome 20 in the human genome, where they are arranged in antiparallel orientation with a long interspersed repeated DNA element (LINE) (reviewed in Gainer and Wray 1994). The genes for both peptides consist of three exons (and two introns) with little change in structure across species from mouse to human. Transgenic studies with the rat oxytocin gene demonstrate that oxytocin expression is dependent upon sequences within or near the vasopressin gene, as only transgenes containing both oxytocin and vasopressin direct cell-specific expression. This suggests that the genes are closely linked and that a

Table 44.2
Human genes for OT, AVP, and their receptors

Gene	Chromo-somal location	Poly-morphism	Comments
OT	20	?	OT knockout mice show social deficits
AVP	20	Yes	Brattleboro rats show cognitive deficits, brain anomalies
OTR	3p25–26	Yes	Receptor distribution associated with affiliative behavior
V1a	12	Yes	Receptor distribution associated with affiliative behavior
V1b	?	?	May be located in brain as well as pituitary
V2	Xq28	Yes	Mutations associated with nephrogenic diabetes insipidus

single critically placed mutation could influence expression of both oxytocin and vasopressin.

Rodents with mutations of oxytocin and vasopressin have been studied for behaviors relevant to autism. We have recently described a mouse with a null mutation of the oxytocin gene (i.e., an oxytocin knockout mouse) (Nishimori et al. 1996). Homozygous mice completely lack oxytocin and are unable to lactate. These mice show deficits in social behavior, including decreased social investigation, increased aggression, and decreased vocal response to social separation (author's unpublished data). As noted above, these mice also show selective deficits in social memory. The consequences of vasopressin deficiency have been studied in the Brattleboro rat, which fails to make vasopressin because of a point mutation leading to a frameshift in the vasopressin gene. In addition to diabetes insip-

idus, these rats show various cognitive deficits, including impaired extinction of avoidance behavior and decreased social memory (de Wied et al. 1988). Brattleboro rats also show a number of neurochemical and neuroanatomical abnormalities, including reduced catecholamine concentrations and smaller brain volume (Boer et al. 1982). Brattleboro rats have been reported to show increased oxytocin synthesis, suggesting that some of the observed abnormalities in these animals may not be a direct effect of the deficiency in vasopressin (Boer et al. 1988). Neither the oxytocin knockout mouse nor the Brattleboro rat is a convincing animal model of autism, but each exhibits key features of the syndrome.

There are no reported cases of human oxytocin gene mutations, although a family with multigenerational problems with lactation has been recently suggested for study (Hans Zingg, personal communication, August, 1997). A series of pedigrees with mutations of the human AVP gene have been recently described (Rittig et al. 1996). Although the affected individuals have diabetes insipidus, behavioral and cognitive abnormalities have not been assessed.

Receptor Genes

There are four known genes in the neurohypophyseal receptor family: oxytocin or OTR (uterus, mammary tissue, and brain), V1a (liver and brain), V1b or V3 (pituitary), and V2 (kidney). All of these have been cloned and sequenced in the past 5 years (reviewed in Barberis and Tribollet 1996; Zingg 1996). These genes are approximately equivalent in size, with 40–60% homology in their amino acid sequences. Each codes for a receptor that belongs to the seven transmembrane spanning domain, G-protein coupled receptor family. Large regions, particularly within the transmembrane domains and the second and third extracellular loops, are conserved across the four different OT/AVP receptors. In addition to ligand binding, coupling to G proteins differs across this group. The OTR,

V1a, and V1b receptors use Gq/11 to induce phosphoinositol hydrolysis and increase intracellular calcium. The V2 receptor is coupled to Gs to stimulate adenylate cyclase.

By far, the greatest attention has been focused on the V2 receptor gene. Over 40 mutations (mostly point mutations) in this gene have been shown to be associated with nephrogenic diabetes insipidus (Merendino et al. 1993; Rosenthal et al. 1992; Seibold et al. 1992). While it seems likely that the other genes in this family might reveal similar functional sequence variability, there has been only limited study of the OTR (Michelini et al. 1995) and V1a receptor genes (Thibonnier et al. 1994).

The human OTR gene is roughly 17 kb, with four exons and three introns (Inoue et al. 1994). In the human genome, the OTR gene is localized to chromosome 3p25–3p26 in a region near the loci for Von Hippel–Lindau disease and renal cell carcinoma (Kimura et al. 1994; Michelini et al. 1995). The promoter sequence for this gene includes several cytokine-responsive elements. A polymorphic tandem repeat sequence in the 3′ flanking region of this gene has been described, but not yet characterized functionally (Michelini et al. 1995). This area, downstream from the coding sequence, shows sequence variability in an area where the nucleotides cytosine and adenine (CA) are repeated 30 times in most subjects but 28 times in others. As this is not in a regulatory or coding region of the gene, this variability may be entirely insignificant. In other species, this gene has shown remarkable sequence variability, particularly in the promoter region around a tandem repeat sequence 100–400 bp upstream from the start site. Although the OTR complementary DNA, which encodes a 388 amino acid polypeptide shows relatively little difference across species, the sequence variability in the promoter region may account for the profound differences in this receptor's regional expression in the brains of different mammals (Young et al. 1996). For instance, monogamous prairie voles and nonmonogamous montane voles show markedly different patterns of oxytocin receptor distribution in brain (Insel and Shapiro 1992) and as a consequence, respond differently to exogenous peptide (Winslow et al. 1993b). A similar variation in the human OTR promoter might lead to changes in the distribution or the developmental regulation of the receptor protein in brain. As a result, a different set of targets would be influenced within the brain, and attachment behavior or cognitive function could be impaired even in the presence of normal oxytocin concentrations.

The V1a receptor gene has also been sequenced in several species, including humans (Thibonnier et al. 1994). The human V1a receptor gene encodes a 394 amino acid protein and has been studied extensively by transfection into CHO cells (Thibonnier et al. 1994). Polymorphisms for the human V1a receptor have been detected in the second intron, and three tandem repeat microsatellites have been found in the 5′ flanking region (Thibonnier, personal communication, December, 1996). As with the oxytocin receptor, the V1a receptor also shows marked species variability in the promoter region across species (Young et al. unpublished) and even more striking species differences in regional expression (Insel et al. 1994b). For instance, the V1a receptor is most heavily expressed in the lateral septum, bed nucleus of the stria terminalis, lateral hypothalamus, and ventral thalamus within the rat brain, yet shows a broad cortical distribution in the primate brain with most intense expression in both cortical and subcortical regions important for memory, such as entorhinal cortex, mammillary bodies, insula, and cingulate cortex (Toloczko et al. 1997). Curiously, although there is only a modest homology between neurohypophyseal peptide receptor subtypes, point mutation experiments have shown that changing only a single amino acid residue within the agonist binding domain in the transmembrane part of the V1a receptor results in a shift of binding specificity toward the oxytocin subtype (Chini et al. 1995). Therefore, one might expect that a mutation in this region would confer significant functional consequences, just as a change in the promoter sequence appears to be associated with important differences in regional distribution.

Developmental Genes

It is also worth considering that developmentally regulated genes involved in cell lineage determination of the PVN or functionally related areas may be altered in autism. A fundamental aspect of neurogenesis is the requirement for precise spatial and temporal coordination of sequential events that underlie the appearance of mature cellular phenotypes. Some of the genes active in the formation of the hypothalamus have been characterized. Many of these genes code for transcription factors that are likely to regulate the expression of downstream effector genes. Some of the most intriguing hypothalamic transcription factors that have been identified thus far are in a family of recently discovered proteins called POU proteins. Genes coding for proteins in this family, including Brn-1, Brn-2, and Brn-4, are expressed in magnocellular neurons of the PVN and SON (Rosenfeld et al. 1996) and are capable of binding to the distal 5′ flanking region of the oxytocin gene, meaning that they may influence transcription. In a remarkable experiment, mice engineered to lack the Brn-2 gene fail to develop a mature PVN and SON (Schonemann et al. 1995). Other less well-characterized homeobox-containing genes (i.e., genes with homeobox sequences that may be important for determining polarity or orientation in the developing neuraxis) including dbx and otp are also expressed in the anterior hypothalamus, as well as other regions that receive oxytocin and vasopressin projections (Lu et al. 1992, 1994; Simeone et al. 1994). Alterations in these genes may have the potential to disrupt the normal genetic program, leading to dysfunctional outcomes in anatomically discrete circuits.

In summary, if an alteration in oxytocin or vasopressin neurotransmission accounts for the pathophysiology of autism, and autism is a genetic disease, one might expect to find an associated allele in either the oxytocin or vasopressin genes or the genes for their neural receptors (OTR and V1a). Animals with mutations of either the oxytocin or vasopressin genes exhibit some of the features of autism (social deficits in the oxytocin knockout mouse, memory deficits in the vasopressin-deficient rat), but also demonstrate abnormalities not observed in autism (e.g., diabetes insipidus in the Brattleboro rat). Experience with the V2 receptor (localized in kidney) demonstrates that at least one member of this family is subject to functional mutations. What would be the result of a similar alteration in the receptors expressed in brain? We do not yet have animals with null mutations for the OTR or V1a receptors, but comparative studies demonstrate marked species differences in both the promoter regions of these receptor genes and the patterns of expression of these receptors in brain. As species with different patterns of receptor distribution also differ in patterns of social affiliation, we have previously suggested that either the OTR or V1a receptor may represent a molecular basis for the capacity to form selective, enduring social attachments, as seen in monogamous mammals (Insel et al. 1996). Given the profound species differences in OTR and V1a receptor distribution, even among primates (Toloczko et al. 1997), one might expect to find within-species variability in the expression of one or both receptors in the human brain, with associated changes in social behavior.

Oxytocin and Vasopressin in Human Psychopathology

Several of the results from animal studies suggest that human diseases involving abnormal social attachments could be due to abnormalities of oxytocin or vasopressin pathways. Although there has been remarkably little research on oxytocin or vasopressin in autism (see below), there

Table 44.3
Oxytocin and vasopressin in neuropsychiatric disorders

Disorder	Finding	Reference
Schizophrenia	Decreased NPI (AVP), increased NPII (OT)	(Linkowski et al. 1984)
	Increased CSF OT	(Beckmann et al. 1985)
	No change in CSF OT	(Glovinsky et al. 1994)
	Altered neurophysin profiles	(Mai et al. 1993)
Affective disorders	CSF NPI (AVP) decreased UP, increased BP	(Linkowski et al. 1984)
	CSF NPII (OT) no change UP, increased BP	(Linkowski et al. 1984)
	Decreased CSF AVP	(Gjerris et al. 1985)
	No change in CSF AVP or OT with medication	(Pitts et al. 1995)
	56% increase of AVP and 23% increase of OT in PVN	(Purba et al. 1996)
OCD	Increased CSF OT, normal CSF AVP (nontic group)	(Leckman et al. 1994)
	Increased CSF AVP	(Altemus et al. 1992)
	Negative correlation of CSF AVP and severity	(Swedo et al. 1992)
	Positive correlation of CSF OT and depression	(Swedo et al. 1992)
Prader–Willi	Decreased OT cells, no change in AVP	(Swaab et al. 1995)
AIDS	Decreased OT cells, no change in AVP	(Purba et al. 1993)
Alzheimer's	No change in OT or AVP cells	(Van der Woude et al. 1995)

NP, neurophysin; AVP, vasopressin; OT, oxytocin; CSF, cerebrospinal fluid; UP, unipolar; BP, bipolar; PVN, paraventricular nucleus of hypothalamus.

are several studies that have reported abnormalities of central oxytocin or vasopressin in neuropsychiatric populations (Table 44.3).

The evidence for abnormality in cerebrospinal fluid (CSF) oxytocin or vasopressin in schizophrenia is not compelling (Beckmann et al. 1985; Glovinsky et al. 1994; Linkowski et al. 1984), but a recent postmortem study by Mai et al. has described abnormal morphometric profiles of neurophysin-stained cell bodies and terminals in untreated schizophrenics. It is not clear if these abnormalities are specific to schizophrenia or restricted to either oxytocin or vasopressin pathways (Mai et al. 1993).

Similarly, results from measuring CSF oxytocin or vasopressin concentrations in either untreated (Gjerris et al. 1985; Linkowski et al. 1984) or treated (Pitts et al. 1995) affectively ill patients have not been consistent across studies.

More intriguing results emerged in a recent postmortem study that found a 56% increase in vasopressin-positive cells and a 23% increase in oxytocin-positive cells in the hypothalamus of depressed subjects (Purba et al. 1996). This study used stereologic techniques to quantify immunoreactive cells in the PVN for 8 depressed patients (all medicated) and 8 age-matched controls (age 23–88 years). As this same group previously reported no change in the number of vasopressin cells in the PVN or SON with Alzheimer's disease (Van der Woude et al. 1995), a 40% decrease in the number of oxytocin cells but no change in the number of vasopressin cells in AIDS (Purba et al. 1993), and a 42% decrease in the number of oxytocin cells in Prader–Willi syndrome (Swaab et al. 1995), the findings in depression appear relatively selective.

Perhaps the most surprising clinical data suggest that obsessive–compulsive disorder (OCD) patients may have increased oxytocin concentrations in CSF, although this finding appears to be limited to OCD subjects without tics (Leckman et al. 1994). One other study including a broad spectrum of OCD subjects found a difference in CSF vasopressin levels relative to normals (Altemus et al. 1992), and another found CSF vasopressin to be negatively correlated with OCD symptoms while CSF oxytocin concentrations were correlated with severity of depressive symptoms in this disorder (Swedo et al. 1992). It is not immediately clear how these evolving findings with OCD relate to an abnormality with social attachments, but the evidence that these neuropeptides may stimulate grooming behavior and may influence the extinction of avoidance behaviors could provide a link between oxytocin or vasopressin and OCD. A controlled trial of intranasal oxytocin in 12 OCD patients found no significant effects on obsessions or compulsions (Den Boer and Westenberg 1992).

Oxytocin and Vasopressin in Autism

Analogous data are not yet available for autism. A recent study reported that the plasma concentration of oxytocin in autistic children is about half that observed in healthy age-matched control subjects, and that autistic children failed to show the normal developmental increase of plasma oxytocin with age or interpersonal skills (Modahl et al. 1998), consistent with a genetic deficiency of oxytocin. Although there is little relationship of blood oxytocin to CSF concentrations, a genetic defect in oxytocin synthesis might be expected to lower both pools. To date, CSF data on oxytocin and vasopressin in autism have not been reported. Systemic administration of synthetic oxytocin to autistic children reportedly increases social interaction (Hollander, oral communication, December, 1996), which could also support the notion of an oxytocin

deficit in autism. It is not clear, however, that systemic peptide crosses into the brain. In short, there is no current compelling clinical evidence that central pathways for either oxytocin or vasopressin are important for this disorder.

Nevertheless, the available results from preclinical research suggest that these pathways are critical for normal social behavior and memory, and that these pathways are a reasonable place to look for abnormalities in autism. Specifically, we hypothesize that abnormalities in either the OTR or V1a receptor genes, or in developmental genes active in the specification of oxytocin or vasopressin pathways, are involved in the etiology of some forms of autism. This hypothesis is supported by the results of comparative research, the discovery of polymorphisms in both receptor genes, and the anatomical localization of these receptors in the primate brain to sites important for social behavior and cognition.

Although the animal studies may prove important in guiding the search for what to look for and where to look in humans with impaired attachment behavior, the tests of this hypothesis remain to be done in people with autism. Traditional studies of plasma or CSF concentrations will be important if there is a mutation in either the peptide genes or developmental genes critical for hypothalamic differentiation. Normal concentrations of oxytocin or vasopressin will not preclude a mutation of the receptor genes. As the changes in very discrete clusters of receptors appear important for regulating social behaviors in animal studies, it seems likely that measures of CSF or plasma hormone concentrations will not be definitive in human neuropsychiatric illness.

Three techniques will be important.

• First, the study of candidate genes should allow the detection of sequence variations in the OTR and V1a receptor genes in DNA from autistic patients. As both OTR and V1a receptors can be expressed in cell lines, the functional significance of any variation in sequence can be determined. Association studies will be necessary to determine if functional alleles are relevant to some subset of patients with autism (Risch and Merikangas 1996). If sequence variations in the OTR and V1a receptor genes are not associated with autism, then the candidate gene search should be extended to the peptide genes and the family of developmental genes that specify for differentiation of the endocrine hypothalamus.

• Second, pharmacologic techniques can be used to assess the responsiveness of OTR and V1a receptors in brain. Although systemically and intranasally administered peptides are unlikely to cross the blood–brain barrier, the recent development of nonpeptide ligands for both receptors provides an opportunity for assessing central receptors after peripheral administration (Evans et al. 1993; Imaizumi et al. 1992).

• Finally, neuroanatomical studies should prove informative. We know that both receptors are highly variable in their regional expression. Localization of these receptors, either in vivo with positron-emission tomography imaging or in vitro with receptor autoradiography, will be an important test of the hypothesis. It may also be useful to complete postmortem studies of the PVN in autism and compare both messenger-RNA and protein levels to previous reports in depression, AIDS, and Prader–Willi syndrome.

Although the discovery of an etiology for autism would be an important advance, the development of a treatment of a genetic defect of oxytocin or vasopressin neurotransmission may prove an even greater challenge. Thus far, we have been successful in developing nonpeptide analogues to antagonists but not to agonists (Manning et al. 1995), so replacement therapy remains a problem. If the receptor is either not responsive or expressed in an abnormal pattern, replacement therapy will not suffice. We have recently described a transgenic mouse with an altered promoter sequence capable of guiding OTR expression to specific brain sites (Young et al. 1997). Using a similar gene therapy strategy, it may soon be possible to induce receptor expression in a predictable pattern based on the construction of a normal receptor gene.

In summary, molecular, cellular, and behavioral studies demonstrate a role for oxytocin and vasopressin neural pathways in species-typical social behavior, cognition, communication, and motor stereotypies. We hypothesize that these neural systems are involved in autism. Experience with the structurally related V2 receptor that is found in the kidney demonstrates that this family of receptor genes is prone to functional mutations. We predict that similar mutations in the OTR and V1a receptors, or in relevant developmental genes expressed in the brain, will be found in autism. We now have the tools with which to test this prediction. If this prediction is borne out, even in a subset of patients with autism, a strategy for treatment can be devised to increase either oxytocin or vasopressin neurotransmission.

References

Altemus M, Pigott T, Kalogeras KT, Demitrack M, Dubbert B, Murphy DL, et al. (1992): Abnormalities in the regulation of vasopressin and corticotropin releasing factor secretion in obsessive-compulsive disorder. *Arch Gen Psychiatry* 49:9–20.

American Psychiatric Association (1994): *The Diagnostic and Statistical Manual of Mental Disorders,* 4th ed. Washington, DC: American Psychiatric Press.

Archer R (1974): Chemistry of the neurohypophyseal hormones: An example of molecular evolution. In: Knobil E, Sawyer W, editors. *Handbook of Physiology,* vol 4. Washington, DC: American Physiological Society: pp 119–130.

Argiolas A, Gessa GL (1991): Central functions of oxytocin. *Neurosci Biobehav Rev* 15:217–231.

Bailey AJ, Bolton P, Butler L, LeCouteur A, Murphy M, Scott S, et al. (1993): Prevalence of the fragile X anomaly amongst autistic twins and singletons. *J Child Psychol Psychiatry* 34:673–688.

Bailey A, LeCouteur A, Gottesman I, Bolton P, Simonoff E, Yuzda E, et al. (1995): Autism as a strongly genetic disorder: Evidence from a British twin study. *Psychol Med* 25:63–78.

Bailey A, Phillips W, Rutter M (1996): Autism: Towards an integration of clinical, genetic, neuropsychological, and neurobiological perspectives. *J Child Psychol Psychiatry* 37:89–126.

Barberis C, Tribollet E (1996): Vasopressin and oxytocin receptors in the central nervous system. *Crit Rev Neurobiol* 10:119–154.

Bauman M (1991): Microscopic neuroanatomic abnormalities in autism. *Pediatrics* 87(suppl):791–796.

Beckmann H, Lang RE, Gattaz WF (1985): Vasopressin: Oxytocin in cerebrospinal fluid of schizophrenic patients and normal controls. *Psychoneuroendocrinology* 10:187–191.

Bluthe R-M, Schoenen J, Dantzer R (1990): Androgen-dependent vasopressinergic neurons are involved in social recognition in rats. *Brain Res* 519:150–157.

Boer GJ (1991): Neuropeptides: A new class of transmitters, a new class of functional teratogens. In: Fujii T, Boer GJ, editors. *Functional Neuroteratology of Short-Term Exposure to Drugs.* Teikyo University Press, Teikyo, Japan, pp 73–84.

Boer GJ (1993): Chronic oxytocin treatment during late gestation and lactation impairs development of rat offspring. *Neurotoxicol Teratol* 15:383–389.

Boer GJ, Swaab DF (1985): Neuropeptide effects on brain development to be expected from behavioral teratology. *Peptides* 6:21–28.

Boer GJ, Van Rheenen-Verberg CMF, Uylings HBM (1982): Impaired brain development of the diabetes insipidus Brattleboro rat. *Dev Brain Res* 3:557–575.

Boer GJ, Van Heerikhuize J, Van der Woude TP (1988): Elevated serum oxytocin of the vasopressin-deficient Brattleboro rat is present throughout life and is not sensitive to treatment with vasopressin. *Acta Endocrinol (Copenh)* 117: 442–450.

Bolton P, Macdonald H, Pickles A, Rios P, Goode S, Crowson M, et al. (1994): A case-control family history study of autism. *J Child Psychol Psychiatry* 35:877–900.

Bristol MM, Cohen DJ, Costello EJ, Denckla M, Eckberg TJ, Kallen R, et al. (1996): State of the science in autism: Report to the national institutes of health. *J Autism Dev Disord* 26:121–154.

Buijs RM, van Heerikhuize JJ (1982): Vasopressin and oxytocin release in the brain—A synaptic event. *Brain Res* 252:71–76.

Carter CS (1992): Oxytocin and sexual behavior. *Neurosci Biobehav Rev* 16:131–144.

Chini B, Mouillac B, Ala Y, Balestre M, Trumpp-Kallmeyer S, Hoflack J, et al. (1995): Tyr 115 is the key residue for determining agonist selectivity in the V1a vasopressin receptor. *EMBO J* 14:2176–2182.

Courchesne E, Townsend J, Saitoh O (1994): The brain in infantile autism: Posterior fossa structures are abnormal. *Neurology* 44:214–223.

Dantzer R, Bluthe R, Koob G, Le Moal M (1987): Modulation of social memory in male rats by neurohypophyseal peptides. *Psychopharmacology (Berl)* 91:363–368.

Dantzer R, Koob G, Bluthe R, Le Moal M (1988): Septal vasopressin modulates social memory in male rats. *Brain Res* 457:143–147.

Den Boer JA, Westenberg HGM (1992): Oxytocin in obsessive compulsive disorders. *Peptides* 13:1083–1085.

De Vries G, Buijs R (1983): The origin of vasopressinergic and oxytocinergic innervation of the rat brain with special reference to the lateral septum. *Brain Res* 273:307–317.

de Wied D (1965): The influence of the posterior and intermediate lobes of the pituitary and pituitary peptides on the maintenance of a conditioned avoidance response in rats. *Int J Neuropharmacol* 4:157–167.

de Wied D, Joëls M, Burbach JPH (1988): Vasopressin effects on the central nervous system. In: Conn PM, Negro Villar A, editors. *Peptide Hormones: Effects of Mechanisms of Action.* Boca Raton, FL: CRC Press, pp 97–140.

Drago F, Pedersen CA, Caldwell JD, Prange AJ Jr (1986): Oxytocin potently enhances novelty-induced grooming behavior in the rat. *Brain Res* 368:287–295.

Dubois-Dauphin M, Theler J-M, Zaganidis N, Dominik W, Tribollet E, Pevet P, et al. (1991): Expression of vasopressin receptors in hamster hypothalamus is sexually dimorphic and dependent on photoperiod. *Proc Natl Acad Sci (USA)* 88: 11163–11167.

Evans BE, Lundell GF, Gilbert KF, Bock MG, Kenneth ER, Carroll LA, et al. (1993): Nanomolar-affinity, non-peptide oxytocin receptor antagonists. *J Med Chem* 36:3994–4005.

Ferris C (1992): Role of vasopressin in aggressive and dominant/subordinate behaviors. In: Pedersen C, Caldwell J, Jirikowski G, Insel T, editors. *Oxytocin in*

Maternal, Sexual, and Social Behaviors, vol 652. New York: New York Academy of Sciences Press, pp 212–227.

Ferris C, Albers H, Wesolowski S, Goldman B, Leeman S (1984): Vasopressin injected into the hypothalamus triggers a stereotypic behavior in golden hamsters. *Science* 224:521–523.

Ferris C, Singer E, Meenan D, Albers H (1988): Inhibition of vasopressin-stimulated flank marking behavior by V1-receptor antagonists. *Eur J Pharmacol* 154: 153–159.

Ferris C, Delville Y, Grzonka Z, Insel T (1993): An iodinated vasopressin (V1) antagonist blocks flank marking and selectively labels neural binding sites in golden hamsters. *Physiol Behav* 54:737–747.

Folstein S, Rutter M (1977): Infantile autism: A genetic study of 21 twin pairs. *J Child Psychol Psychiatry* 18:297–321.

Gainer H, Wray S (1994): Cellular and molecular biology of oxytocin and vasopressin. In: Knobil E, Neill J, editors. *The Physiology of Reproduction,* 2 ed. vol 1. New York: Raven Press, pp 1099–1130.

Gillberg C, Coleman M (1992): *The Biology of the Autistic Syndromes,* 2nd ed. London: MacKeith Press.

Gillberg C, Wahlström J (1985): Chromosome abnormalities in infantile autism and other childhood psychoses: A population study of 66 cases. *Dev Med Child Neurol* 27:293–304.

Gillberg IC, Gillberg C, Ahlsén G (1994): Autistic behaviour and attention deficits in tuberous sclerosis: A population-based study. *Dev Med Child Neurol* 36:50–56.

Gjerris A, Hummer M, Vendsborg P, Christiensen N, Rafaelson D (1985): Cerebrospinal fluid vasopressin changes in depression. *Br J Psychiatry* 147:696–701.

Glovinsky D, Kalogeras KT, Kirch DG, Suddath R, Wyatt RJ (1994): Cerebrospinal fluid oxytocin concentration in schizophrenic patients does not differ from control subjects and is not changed by neuroleptic medication. *Schizophr Res* 11:273–276.

Gordon C, State R, Nelson J, Hamburger S, Rapoport J (1993): A double-blind comparison of clomipramine, desipramine, and placebo in the treatment of autistic disorder. *Arch Gen Psychiatry* 50:441–447.

Hunt A, Shepherd C (1993): A prevalence study of autism in tuberous sclerosis. *J Autism Dev Disord* 23:329–339.

Imaizumi T, Harada S, Hirooka Y, Masaki H, Momohara M, Takeshita A (1992): Effects of OPC-21268, an orally effective vasopressin V1 receptor antagonist in humans. *Hypertension* 20:53–58.

Inoue T, Kimura T, Azuma C, Inazawa J, Takemura M, Kikuchi T, et al. (1994): Structural organization of the human oxytocin receptor gene. *J Biol Chem* 269:32451–32456.

Insel TR (1990): Oxytocin and maternal behavior. In: Krasnegor N, Bridges R, editors. *Mammalian Parenting: Biochemical, Neurobiological, and Behavioral Determinants.* New York: Oxford University Press, pp 260–280.

Insel TR (1992): Oxytocin: A neuropeptide for affiliation—Evidence from behavioral, receptor autoradiographic, and comparative studies. *Psychoneuroendocrinology* 17:3–33.

Insel TR, Hulihan TJ (1995): A gender specific mechanism for pair bonding: Oxytocin and partner preference formation in monogamous voles. *Behav Neurosci* 109:782–789.

Insel TR, Shapiro LE (1992): Oxytocin receptor distribution reflects social organization in monogamous and polygamous voles. *Proc Natl Acad Sci USA* 89:5981–5985.

Insel TR, Winslow JT (1991): Central oxytocin administration reduces rat pup isolation calls. *Eur J Pharmacol* 203:149–152.

Insel TR, Wang Z, Ferris CF (1994a): Patterns of brain vasopressin receptor distribution associated with social organization in microtine rodents. *J Neurosci* 14:5381–5392.

Insel TR, Wang Z, Ferris CF (1994b): Patterns of vasopressin receptor distribution associated with social organization in monogamous and non-monogamous microtine rodents. *J Neurosci* 14:5381–5392.

Insel TR, Winslow JT, Wang Z-X, Young L, Hulihan TJ (1996): Oxytocin and the molecular basis of monogamy. *Adv Exp Med Biol* 395:227–234.

Johnson AE, Barberis C, Albers HE (1995): Castration reduces vasopressin receptor binding in the hamster hypothalamus. *Brain Res* 674:153–158.

Johnson AE, Coirini H, Insel TR, McEwen BS (1990): The regulation of oxytocin receptor binding in the ventromedial hypothalamic nucleus by testosterone and its metabolites. *Endocrinology* 128:891–896.

Jorde LB, Mason-Brothers A, Waldman R, Ritvo ER, Freeman BJ, Pingree C, et al. (1990): The UCLA-

University of Utah epidemiologic survey of autism: Genealogical analysis of familiar aggregation. *Am J Med Genet* 36:85–88.

Kanner L (1943): Autistic disturbances of affective contact. *Nervous Child* 2:217–250.

Kimura T, Makino Y, Saji F, Takemura M, Inoue T, Kikuchi T, et al. (1994): Molecular characterization of a cloned human oxytocin receptor. *Eur J Endocrinol* 131:385–390.

Kovacs GL, Telegdy G (1985): Role of oxytocin in memory, amnesia, and reinforcement. In: Amico J, Robinson AG, editors. *Oxytocin: Clinical and Laboratory Studies*. New York: Elsevier, pp 359–371.

Leckman J, Goodman W, North W, Chappell P, Price L, Pauls D, et al. (1994): Elevated cerebrospinal fluid levels of oxytocin in obsessive compulsive disorder. Comparison with Tourette's syndrome and healthy controls. *Arch Gen Psychiatry* 51:782–792.

Linkowski P, Genen V, Kerkhofs M, Mendlewicz J, Legros J (1984): Cerebrospinal fluid neurophysins in affective illness and schizophrenia. *Eur Arch Psychiatry Neurol Sci* 234:162–165.

Lord C (1995): Follow-up of two-year-olds referred for possible autism. *J Child Psychol Psychiatry* 36:1365–1382.

Lu S, Bogarad LD, Murtha MT, Ruddle FH (1992): Expression pattern of the murine homeobox gene, Dbx, displays extreme spatial restriction in embryonic forebrain and spinal cord. *Proc Natl Acad Sci (USA)* 89:8053–8057.

Lu S, Wise TL, Ruddle FH (1994): Mouse homeobox gene Dbx: Sequence, gene structure and expression pattern during midgestation. *Mech Dev* 47:187–195.

Mai JK, Berger K, Sofroniew MV (1993): Morphometric evaluation of neurophysin-immunoreactivity in the human brain: Pronounced inter-individual variability and evidence for altered staining patterns in schizophrenia. *J Hirnforschung* 34:133–154.

Manning M, Cheng LL, Klis WA, Stoev S, Przybylski J, Bankowski K, et al. (1995): Advances in the design of selective antagonists, potential tocolytics, and radioiodinated ligands for oxytocin receptors. In: Ivell R, Russell JA, editors. *Oxytocin: Cellular and Molecular Approaches in Medicine and Research*. New York: Plenum Press, pp 559–583.

McBride P, Anderson G, Shapiro T (1996): Autism research: Bringing together approaches to pull apart the disorder. *Arch Gen Psychiatry* 53:980–982.

McDougle C, Naylor S, Cohen D, Volkmar F, Heninger G, Price L (1996): A double-blind placebo-controlled study of fluvoxamine in adults with autistic disorder. *Arch Gen Psychiatry* 53:1001–1008.

Meisenberg G, Simmons W (1983): Centrally mediated effects of neurohypophyseal hormones. *Neurosci Biobehav Rev* 7:263–280.

Merendino JJ, Spiegel AM, Crawford JD, A-M OC, Brownstein MJ, Lolait SJ (1993): A mutation in the V2 vasopressin receptor gene in a kindred with X-linked nephrogenic diabetes insipidus. *N Engl J Med* 328:1538–1541.

Michelini S, Urbanek M, Dean M, Goldman D (1995): Polymorphism and genetic mapping of the human oxytocin receptor gene on chromosome 3. *Am J Med Gen* 60:183–187.

Modahl C, Green LA, Fein D, Morris M, Waterhouse L, Feinstein C, et al. (1998): Plasma oxytocin levels in autistic children. *Biol Psychiatry* 43:270–277.

Nelson E, Panksepp J (1996): Oxytocin and infant-mother bonding in rats. *Behav Neurosci* 100:583–592.

Nishimori K, Young L, Guo Q, Wang Z, Insel T, Matzuk M (1996): Oxytocin is required for nursing but is not essential for parturition or reproductive behavior. *Proc Natl Acad Sci USA* 93:777–783.

Panksepp J (1992): Oxytocin effects on emotional processes: Separation distress, social bonding, and relationships to psychiatric disorders. In: Pedersen C, Caldwell J, Jirikowski G, Insel T, editors. *Oxytocin in Maternal, Sexual, and Social Processes*, vol 652. New York: New York Academy of Sciences, pp 243–252.

Pedersen CA, Ascher JA, Monroe YL, Prange AJ Jr (1982): Oxytocin induces maternal behavior in virgin female rats. *Science* 216:648–649.

Pitts A, Samuelson S, Meller W, Bissette G, Nemeroff C, Kathol R (1995): Cerebrospinal fluid corticotropin releasing factor, vasopressin, and oxytocin concentrations in treated patients with major depression and controls. *Biol Psychiatry* 38:330–335.

Popik P, Vos P, van Ree J (1992): Neurohypophyseal hormone receptors in the septum are implicated in social recognition in the rat. *Behav Pharmacol* 3:351–358.

Purba JS, Hoogendijk W, Hofman M, Swaab D (1996): Increased number of vasopressin- and oxytocin-expressing neurons in the paraventricular nucleus of the hypothalamus in depression. *Arch Gen Psychiatry* 53:137–143.

Purba JS, Hofman MA, Portegies P, Troost D, Swaab DF (1993): Decreased number of oxytocin neurons in the paraventricular nucleus of the human hypothalamus in AIDS. *Brain* 116:795–809.

Risch N, Merikangas K (1996): The future of genetic studies of complex human disease. *Science* 273:1516–1517.

Rittig S, Robertson GL, Siggaard C, Kovács L, Gregersen N, Nyborg J, et al. (1996): Identification of 13 new mutations in the vasopressin-neurophysin II gene in 17 kindreds with familial autosomal dominant neurohypophyseal diabetes insipidus. *Am J Hum Genet* 58:107–117.

Rosenthal W, Siebold A, Antaramian A (1992): Molecular identification of the gene responsible for nephrogenic congenital diabetes insipidus. *Nature* 359:233–235.

Rosenfeld MG, Bach I, Erkman L, Li P, Lin C, Lin S, et al. (1996): Transcriptional control of cell phenotypes in the neuroendocrine system. *Recent Prog Horm Res* 51:217–239.

Rutter M (1983): Cognitive deficits in the pathogenesis of autism. *J Child Psychol Psychiatry* 24:513–531.

Rutter M, Bailey A, Bolton P, LeCouteur A (1993): Autism: Syndrome definition and possible genetic mechanisms. In: McClearn PR, McClearn GE, editors. *Nature, Nurture, and Psychology.* Washington, DC: APA Books, pp 269–284.

Schonemann MD, Ryan AK, McEvilly RJ, O'Connell SM, Arias CA, Kalla KA, et al. (1995): Development and survival of the endocrine hypothalamus and posterior pituitary gland requires the neuronal POU domain factor Brn-2. *Genes Dev* 9:3122–3135.

Seibold A, Brabet P, Rosenthal W, Birnbaumer M (1992): Structure and chromosomal localization of the human antidiuretic hormone receptor gene. *Am J Hum Genet* 51:1078–1083.

Shapiro LE, Insel TR (1989): Ontogeny of oxytocin receptors in rat forebrain: A quantitative study. *Synapse* 4:259–266.

Simeone A, D'Apice MR, Nigro V, Casanova J, Graziani F, Acampora D, et al. (1994): Orthopedia, a novel homeobox-containing gene expressed in the developing CNS of both mouse and *Drosophila. Neuron* 13:83–101.

Smalley SL, Tanguay PE, Smith M, Gutierrez G (1992): Autism and tuberous sclerosis. *J Autism Dev Disord* 22:339–355.

Södersten P, Henning M, Melin P, Ludin S (1983): Vasopressin alters female sexual behaviour by acting on the brain independently of alterations in blood pressure. *Nature* 301:608–610.

Sofroniew MV, Weindl A (1981): Central nervous system distribution of vasopressin, oxytocin, and neurophysin. In: Martinez JL, Jensen RA, Mesing RB, Rigter H, McGaugh JL, editors. *Endogenous Peptides and Learning and Memory Processes.* New York: Academic Press, pp 327–369.

Steffenberg S, Gillberg C, Helgren L, Anderson L, Gillberg L, Jakobsson G, et al. (1989): A twin study of autism in Denmark, Finland, Iceland, Norway, and Sweden. *J Child Psychol Psychiatry* 30:405–416.

Swaab DF, Purba JS, Hofman MA (1995): Alterations in the hypothalamic paraventricular nucleus and its oxytocin neurons (putative satiety cells) in Prader-Willi syndrome: A study of five cases. *J Clin Endocrinol Metab* 80:573–579.

Swedo SE, Leonard HL, Kruesi MJP, Rettew DC, Listwak SJ, Berrettini W, et al. (1992): Cerebrospinal fluid neurochemistry in children and adolescents with obsessive-compulsive disorder. *Arch Gen Psychiatry* 49:29–36.

Szatmari P, Jones MB (1991): IQ and the genetics of autism. *J Child Psychol Psychiatry* 35:215–229.

Thibonnier M, Auzan C, Madhun Z, Wilkins P, Berti-Mattera L, Clauser E (1994): Molecular cloning, sequencing, and functional expression of a cDNA encoding the human V_{1a} vasopressin receptor. *Journal Biol Chem* 269:3304–3310.

Thor DH, Holloway WR (1982): Social memory of the male laboratory rat. *J Comp Physiol Psychol* 96:1000–1006.

Tinius T, Beckwith B, Preussler D (1987): Prenatal administration of arginine vasopressin impairs memory retrieval in adult rats. *Peptides* 8:1–7.

Toloczko DM, Young L, Insel TR (1997): Are there oxytocin receptors in the primate brain? In: Carter CS, Lederhendler II, Kirkpatrick B, editors. *The Integrative Neurobiology of Affiliation.* New York: The New York Academy of Sciences, pp 506–509.

Tribollet E, Charpak S, Schmidt A, Dubois-Dauphin M, Dreifuss JJ (1989): Appearance and transient expression of oxytocin receptors in fetal, infant, and peripubertal rat brain studied by autoradiography and electrophysiology. *J Neurosci* 9:1764–1773.

Tribollet E, Goumaz M, Raggenbass M, Dubois-Dauphin M, Dreifuss JJ (1991): Early appearance and transient expression of vasopressin receptors in the brain of the rat fetus and infant. An autoradiographical and electrophysiological study. *Dev Brain Res* 58:13–24.

Van der Woude P, Goudsmit E, Wierda M, Purba J, Hofman M, Swaab D (1995): No vasopressin cell loss in the human paraventricular or supraoptic nucleus during aging and in Alzheimer's disease. *Neurobiol Aging* 16:11–18.

van Wimersma Greidanus TB, Kroodsma JM, Pot MLH, Stevens M, Maigret C (1990): Neurohypophyseal hormones and excessive grooming behavior. *Eur J Pharmacol* 187:1–8.

Voorhuis TAM, De Kloet ER, De Wied D (1991): Effect of a vasotocin analogue on singing behavior in the canary. *Horm Behav* 25:549–559.

Wang ZX, Ferris CF, De Vries GJ (1993): The role of septal vasopressin innervation in paternal behavior in prairie voles (*Microtus ochrogaster*). *Proc Natl Acad Sci USA* 91:400–404.

Wang Z, Moody K, Newman JD, Insel TR (1997): Vasopressin and oxytocin immunoreactive neurons and fibers in the forebrain of male and female common marmosets (*Callithrix jacchus*). *Synapse* 27:14–25.

Whitnall MH, Key S, Ben-Barak Y, Ozato K, Gainer H (1985): Neurophysin in the hypothalamo-neurohypophyseal system. II. Immunocytochemical studies on the ontogeny of oxytocinergic and vasopressinergic neurons. *J Neurosci* 5:98–109.

Winslow JT, Insel TR (1991a): Social status in pairs of male squirrel monkeys determines response to central oxytocin administration. *J Neurosci* 11:2032–2038.

Winslow JT, Insel TR (1991b): Vasopressin modulates male squirrel monkeys' behavior during social separation. *Eur J Pharmacol* 200:95–101.

Winslow JT, Insel TR (1993): Effects of central vasopressin administration to infant rats. *Eur J Pharmacol* 233:101–107.

Winslow JT, Hastings N, Carter CS, Harbaugh CR, Insel TR (1993a): A role for central vasopressin in pair bonding in monogamous prairie voles. *Nature* 365:545–548.

Winslow JT, Shapiro LE, Carter CS, Insel TR (1993b): Oxytocin and complex social behaviors: Species comparisons. *Psychopharmacol Bull* 29:409–414.

Witt DM (1995): Oxytocin and rodent sociosexual responses: From behavior to gene expression. *Neurosci Biobehav Rev* 19:315–324.

Witt DM, Winslow JT, Insel TR (1992): Enhanced social interactions in rats following chronic, centrally infused oxytocin. *Pharmacol Biochem Behav* 43:855–861.

World Health Organization (1993): *International Classification of Diseases (ICD-10)*. Geneva: World Health Organization.

Young LJ, Huot B, Nilsen R, Wang Z, Insel TR (1996): Species differences in central oxytocin receptor gene expression: Comparative analysis of promoter sequences. *J Neuroendocrinol* 8:777–783.

Young LJ, Winslow JT, Wang Z, Gingrich B, Guo Q, Matzuk MM, et al. (1997): Gene targeting approaches to neuroendocrinology: Oxytocin, maternal behavior, and affiliation. *Horm Behav* 31:221–231.

Zingg HH (1996): Vasopressin and oxytocin receptors. In: *Baillière's Clinical Endocrinology and Metabolism*, vol 10. Baillière Tindall, Paris, pp 75–96.

45 Tryptophan Depletion, Executive Functions, and Disinhibition in Aggressive, Adolescent Males

David G. LeMarquand, Robert O. Pihl, Simon N. Young, Richard E. Tremblay, Jean R. Séguin, Roberta M. Palmour, and Chawki Benkelfat

Serotonin (5-HT) has been linked to aggressive behavior in animals (Pucilowski and Kostowski 1980) and humans (Kavoussi et al. 1997), although the evidence supporting this relationship has been debated (Berman et al. 1997; Tuinier et al. 1995). Dietary depletion of tryptophan, a method known to lower brain 5-HT synthesis in humans (Nishizawa et al. 1997), increases human aggression in the laboratory (Cleare and Bond 1995; Moeller et al. 1996; Pihl et al. 1995), although the effect is relatively small. Other studies have found no such effect (Salomon et al. 1994; Smith et al. 1987). In clinical samples, studies with adults (Brown et al. 1982) and children (Kruesi et al. 1990) suggest that reduced baseline functioning of the central 5-HT system is associated with aggressive/violent behavior in general, and more specifically with *impulsive* violent behavior (Linnoila et al. 1983; Virkkunen et al. 1994). Thus, at a more fundamental level, 5-HT may be controlling the inhibition of behavior (Soubrié 1986).

Studies investigating the role of 5-HT in impulsive aggression have primarily utilized self-report measures of impulsivity. The first goal of the present study was to test the hypothesis that lowered 5-HT synthesis (and presumably function) might transiently increase behavioral disinhibition measured objectively in the laboratory in a sample of stable aggressive young men who were part of a larger cohort followed longitudinally since the age of five. Disinhibition was defined as behavior committed in the presence of stimuli previously associated with punishment or loss of potential reward, conceptually representing one component of impulsivity. Commission errors on a go/no-go passive avoidance learning task assessed disinhibition; this measure discriminates disinhibited groups from controls (Iaboni et al. 1995; Newman et al. 1985).

The second goal of the present study was to assess the relationship between disinhibition and cognitive functioning in this sample. Cognitive-neuropsychological processes have been implicated in the regulation of aggressive behavior (Pennington and Ozonoff 1996). Specifically, selective deficits in executive functions have been correlated with physical aggression (Séguin et al. 1995). Executive functions subsume the capacities for initiation and maintenance of goal attainment (Lezak 1985). These include the planning of motor skills, modulation of behavior in light of expected future consequences, learning of contingencies, ability to use feedback, abstract reasoning, problem solving, and sustained attention and concentration (Séguin et al. 1995). Given the association between aggression and impulsivity, it was predicted that decreased executive functioning would be associated with increased disinhibition. (In addition to executive functioning, measures of conventional memory processes were also included to account for possible confounds).

Methods and Materials

Participants

Participants were selected from a sample of 1,037 17-year-old boys followed since kindergarten (Mâsse and Tremblay 1997). They were classified according to their percentile scores on the teacher-rated physical aggression subscale of the Social Behavior Questionnaire (Tremblay et al. 1991) assessed at ages 6, 10, 11, and 12. Those boys scoring >70th percentile on the aggression subscale at age 6 and at least two of the three additional assessment points were classified as Stable Aggressive (SA). Those scoring <65th percentile were classified as Nonaggressive (NA). A list of 92 potential participants was generated, of which 38 participated in the study (18 SA, 20 NA).

Procedure and Instruments

Demographic Variables

IQ was estimated according to Sattler (1988) using the Vocabulary and Block Design subtests of
Wechsler Intelligence Scale for Children-Revised
(Wechsler 1974) administered at age 15. Self-
reported number of years in school, assessed
in 1995, was included. Teacher-rated aggression
and anxiety represent the average of participants' ratings at ages 6, 10, 11, and 12 on the
fighting and anxiety subscales of the Social Behavior Questionnaire (Tremblay et al. 1991). A
family adversity index (Tremblay et al. 1991)
was constructed using parental age at the birth
of the first child, parental education, parental
occupational status (Blishen et al. 1987), and
family structure, all assessed when the participant was in kindergarten. Participant-reported
fathers' and mothers' occupational status (average of 1994 and 1995 assessments) (Blishen et al.
1987) and total family revenue (in 1993) provided a more recent assessment of the participants' family socioeconomic status.

Cognitive/Neuropsychological Variables

At ages 13 and 14 (1991/92), participants were
administered a neuropsychological test battery,
described previously (Séguin et al. 1995). These
tests results were factor analyzed in a larger
sample ($n = 177$) (Séguin et al. 1995). Four factors accounting for 58% of the variance were
found, including Verbal Learning (composed of
the Semantic and Letter Fluency [Lezak 1983],
Paired Associates and Digit Span [Wechsler
1987] tests), Incidental Spatial Learning (composed of the Spatial Memory subtests, see Smith
and Milner 1981, 1989), and Executive Function
(composed of the Nonspatial Conditional Association [Petrides 1990], Number Randomization
[Wiegersma et al. 1990], Self-Ordered Pointing
[Milner et al. 1985], and Strategic Problem Solving [Becker et al. 1986] tests). Participants' scores
on these three factors were used in the present
study to assess cognitive-neuropsychological correlates of disinhibition on the go/no-go task.

Verbal and spatial learning were included to
assess conventional memory processes (Séguin
et al. 1995).

Acute Tryptophan Depletion

Prospective participants were mailed an information sheet outlining the study, and parental
and participant consent forms. Those boys interested in participating were asked to sign the consent form and to obtain parental consent. They
were scheduled for the first lab test day, and
asked to avoid consumption of certain foods
high in protein (e.g., meats), abstain from alcohol and/or recreational drug use the day before
each lab session, and refrain from eating breakfast on test days.

A 2 (group; SA, NA) × 2 (amino acid administration; tryptophan depletion [T-] and balanced
amino acid mixture [B]) between-/within-subjects
design was employed. Each participant was
tested on 2 days, separated by at least 1 week.
On each day, participants consumed an amino
acid mixture administered double-blind. Assignment to order of amino acid administration (T-
and B, or B and T-) was counterbalanced within
groups. Research assistants who administered
the amino acid mixtures, tests, questionnaires,
and other procedures were blind to the young
mens' behavior ratings.

One or two participants were scheduled per
test day. Early in the morning, the boys were
transported by car from their homes to the laboratory. Testing commenced at approximately
9:00 A.M. Upon arrival at the lab, adherence to
the previous day's specified menu and the pro-
hibitions against recreational drug/alcohol use
and breakfast consumption were assessed (by
means of self-report). Next, 10 milliliters (ml) of
venous blood was drawn from each participant
to obtain a measure of pretreatment plasma total
and free (nonalbumin-bound) tryptophan levels.

Amino Acid Administration

The T- amino acid mixture was the same as that
employed by Benkelfat et al. (1994). The B mixture contained the same amino acids plus 2.3 g

L-tryptophan. The amino acids were combined with 150 ml orange juice and 0.8 g artificial sweetener (sodium cyclamate) to improve taste. An alternate combination consisting of 150 ml water and 40 ml chocolate syrup (in lieu of the orange juice) was offered to guard against the development of a conditioned taste aversion. Participants were additionally required to swallow 12 capsules containing three amino acids (4.9 g L-arginine, 2.7 g L-cysteine, and 3.0 g L-methionine) not included in the mixture because of their bitter taste. They were allowed water ad libitum to accomplish this. Chewing gum was provided to participants to remove the aftertaste.

Immediately following amino acid administration, on the first test day only, paper-and-pencil questionnaires measuring various personality dimensions were administered. Participants were weighted. A 5 hour wait period was implemented following the completion of amino acid consumption. This time period has been shown to result in significant declines in plasma free and total tryptophan (Benkelfat et al. 1994) and brain serotonin synthesis (Nishizawa et al. 1997), as well as in behavioral changes (Benkelfat et al. 1994; LeMarquand et al. 1997). During the waiting period, participants were allowed to read or watch one or two movies. They were prohibited from sleeping. Five hours after amino acid administration, a second 10 ml blood sample was drawn from each participant for analysis of the effects of the amino acid mixtures on plasma tryptophan levels.

Assessment of Disinhibition: The Go/No-Go Task

Participants were required to learn, by trial-and-error, to respond (press a button) to "active" stimuli (two-digit numbers paired with reward) and withhold responses to "passive" stimuli (two-digit numbers paired with punishment). For the first session, eight numbers (four active, four passive) were repeated 10 times in different, randomized orders for a total of 80 trials. For the second session, 10 different numbers (five active, five passive) were repeated eight times in

randomized orders, again for a total of 80 trials. Four different sets of stimuli were employed per session, one for each condition. Additional characteristics of the stimuli have been presented elsewhere (Newman and Kosson 1986).

Visual, auditory, and monetary feedback followed each response. Correct responses were rewarded with a high-pitched tone, presentation of the word "CORRECT" on the computer screen, and the addition of 10 cents to a running tally of the participant's earnings presented on screen. Incorrect responses were punished by a low-pitched tone, the word "WRONG," and subtraction of 10 cents from the participant's earnings. Each participant did four conditions of the go/no-go task. In the reward–punishment (Rew–Pun) condition, participants started with one dollar. Responses to active stimuli were rewarded, and responses to passive stimuli punished. In the punishment-only (Pun–Pun) condition, participants began with four dollars and had no opportunity to win more money. Responses to passive stimuli and failures to respond to active stimuli were punished. In the reward-only (Rew–Rew) condition, participants began with no money and could not lose money. Responses to active stimuli and withholding responses to passive stimuli were rewarded. In the final punishment–reward (Pun–Rew) condition, participants started with one dollar; failures to respond to active stimuli were punished, and nonresponses to passive stimuli were rewarded. Each condition was preceded by a reward pretreatment (12 [first session] or 15 [second session] trials presented in the format described above with the frequency of active and passive stimuli in the ratio of 2:1) before the standard 80 trials of the condition. This pretreatment served to establish a dominant response set for reward (Newman et al. 1990).

Participants received instructions concerning the nature of go/no-go task, the reinforcement contingencies, and the process of trial-and-error learning. In the presence of the experimenter, they received eight practice trials involving four presentations of each of two practice stimuli

(01 as an active stimulus; 02 as a passive stimulus). The experimenter answered any questions the participant had, but was not present during actual testing. Participants were randomly assigned to one of the 24 possible orders of presentation of the four conditions. At the conclusion of each condition, the experimenter re-entered the room to explain the demands of the next condition. Dependent measures for this task included commission errors (failures to inhibit responses to passive stimuli) and omission errors (failures to respond to active stimuli) for each condition.

Tryptophan Repletion

Following completion of the go/no-go task, participants were provided with a high-protein snack and a 1 g L-tryptophan tablet to normalize plasma tryptophan levels if the individual was tryptophan-depleted, or to maintain the double-blind status of the study if the individual received the B amino acid mixture. The tryptophan preparation used (Tryptan) is available by prescription in Canada and has not been associated with any cases of eosinophilia-myalgia syndrome (Wilkins 1990). One hour following the start of meal consumption, a final 10 ml blood sample was drawn to measure plasma tryptophan concentrations following repletion. Plasma-free tryptophan was measured in all blood samples. This procedure has been fully detailed previously (Benkelfat et al. 1994). The participants were remunerated for their time and given their winnings on the go/no-go task. After completing both amino acid administrations, participants were debriefed. They were provided with an information sheet outlining the basic goals of the study, and any questions were answered.

Data Analysis

Variables were initially inspected by group for normality, homogeneity of variance, and outliers. Appropriate transformations or treatment of outliers were applied to correct for viola-

tions of these assumptions (Tabachnick and Fidell 1989), and, where employed, are specified. Demographic characteristics of SA and NA participants were compared using t-tests for continuous variables or Fisher's Exact Test (two-tailed) for frequencies. Plasma-free tryptophan levels were analyzed using a 2 (group; SA, NA) $\times$ 2 (treatment; T-, B) $\times$ 3 (time; pre-, 5 hours post-amino acid consumption, 1 hour postrepletion) between–within analysis of variance (ANOVA). For the go/no-go discrimination task, separate 2 (group) $\times$ 2 (treatment) $\times$ 4 (condition; Rew–Pun, Pun–Pun, Rew–Rew, Pun–Rew) mixed-model ANOVAs were performed on omission and commission errors. Statistically significant interactions were further analyzed using simple interaction effects tests followed by pairwise comparisons using the Newman–Keuls procedure. Geisser–Greenhouse corrections were used for all main effects and interactions involving repeated measures. Relationships between cognitive/neuropsychological functioning and disinhibition on the go/no-go were explored using multiple regression.

Ethical Approval

All participants involved in this study, as well as their parents, gave written informed consent. The study was approved by the Research Ethics Board of the Department of Psychiatry, McGill University.

Results

Six participants (three SA, three NA) completed only one of the two amino acid test days. Go/no-go data for the missing test day for these participants was estimated using group means. Additionally, three participants (one SA, two NA), who completed both amino acid test days, came for cognitive testing at age 13 but not at age 14. Missing test scores on two factors (verbal learning and executive function) were estimated using multiple regression to predict missing test data within each factor, then multiplying the predicted test scores by the factor weights to estimate the factor scores. All analyses reported below were rerun omitting participants with missing data; the results were not different.

Three NA and two SA participants vomited during one of the test days, were retained for testing on that day, and subsequently completed the entire experiment. In four cases, emesis occurred during the T- amino acid session. The analyses below were rerun omitting the participants who vomited during the T- session; again the results were not different.

Demographic Data

Demographic characteristics of the study sample are presented in Table 45.1. SA participants had lower estimated IQs [$t(23.14) = -2.90$, $p = .008$], fewer years of education [$t(17) = -3.42$, $p = .003$], lower family revenues in 1993 [$t(36) = -2.17$, $p = .037$], and higher (square root) teacher-rated averaged aggression [$t(36) = 19.62$, $p < .001$] and averaged anxiety [$t(36) = 2.94$, $p = .006$].

Comparisons between those SA participants tested ($n = 38$) versus those not tested ($n = 54$) revealed that those tested were higher in teacher-rated aggression ($p = .10$) and anxiety [$t(35.39) = -2.24$, $p = .03$] than those not tested. In the NA group, those tested were no different in aggression or anxiety compared to those not tested.

Serum Free and Total Tryptophan Levels

Plasma free tryptophan concentrations were square root transformed to correct for positive skewness and violations of the homogeneity of variance assumption. Analysis of plasma free tryptophan concentrations revealed a highly significant treatment by time interaction [Geisser–Greenhouse F $(1.11, 39.80) = 28.47$, $p < .001$].

Table 45.1
Demographic characteristics of stable aggressive (SA) and nonaggressive (NA) participants[1]

Measure (year of assessment)	SA	NA
Number	18	20
Age, years	17.2 ± 0.4	17.0 ± 0.6
Weight, lb	158 ± 36.9	147 ± 17.1
IQ, (WISC—R short form)[2]	93 ± 14.9	104 ± 6.7[4]
Education, years (1995)	10.3 ± 0.9	11.0 ± 0.0[4]
Teacher-rated aggression	2.9 ± 0.9	0.1 ± 0.1[4]
Teacher-rated anxiety	4.8 ± 1.7	2.9 ± 2.1[4]
Family adversity (1984)	0.4 ± 0.2	0.4 ± 0.2
Family revenue (1993)	5.8 ± 2.7	8.0 ± 3.4[3]
Mother's occupational prestige (1994–95)	34.1 ± 6.9	38.1 ± 11.6
Father's occupational prestige (1994–95)	40.9 ± 10.2	46.2 ± 11.3

1. Values represent raw data and are expressed as mean ± standard deviation.
2. WISC—R, Wechsler Intelligence Scale for Children—Revised.
3. $p < .05$.
4. $p < .01$.

The T- amino acid mixture significantly decreased; whereas the B mixture significantly increased, plasma free tryptophan levels 5 hours postconsumption across groups. The T- mixture led to a decline in plasma free tryptophan of 81% across groups; whereas the B mixture led to, on average, a 95% increase in plasma free tryptophan concentration. In those four individuals (1 SA, 3 NA) who vomited in the T- session and were retained for testing, plasma total and free tryptophan dropped 64.8 and 48.2%, respectively.

Consumption of the snack and the 1 g tryptophan supplement led to a 353% increase in plasma free tryptophan in the B condition and a 269% increase in the T- condition relative to pre-amino acid administration levels (see Table 45.2). Levels of total and free tryptophan were significantly lower in those who received the

Table 45.2
Total and free plasma tryptophan levels (mean $\pm$ SD) at baseline and 5 h following the ingestion of a balanced (B) and tryptophan-depleted (T-) amino acid load, and following tryptophan repletion, in SA (stable aggressive) and NA (nonaggressive) participants

Time of blood draw	SA ($n = 18$)		NA ($n = 20$)	
	B mixture	T- mixture	B mixture	T- mixture
Total tryptophan baseline, µg/ml	10.8 $\pm$ 2.3	11.1 $\pm$ 2.9	11.6 $\pm$ 2.1	11.6 $\pm$ 2.4
5 h Post amino acid mixture, µg/ml	15.6 $\pm$ 6.8 (+42.4%)	1.4 $\pm$ 0.5 (−87.0%)	18.9 $\pm$ 3.1 (+65.8%)	2.0 $\pm$ 1.5 (−82.1%)
Repletion, µg/ml	25.9 $\pm$ 10.9 (+147%)	18.7 $\pm$ 13.9 (+78%)	35.3 $\pm$ 11.7 (+206%)	26.2 $\pm$ 16.3 (+136%)
Free tryptophan baseline, µg/ml	1.3 $\pm$ 0.3	1.5 $\pm$ 0.3	1.5 $\pm$ 0.4	1.5 $\pm$ 0.3
5 h Post amino acid mixture, µg/ml	2.3 $\pm$ 1.0 (+76.9%)	0.2 $\pm$ 0.1 (−85.3%)	3.0 $\pm$ 0.8 (+114%)	0.3 $\pm$ 0.3 (−76.9%)
Repletion, µg/ml	5.1 $\pm$ 3.0 (+279%)	4.6 $\pm$ 3.6 (+220%)	7.3 $\pm$ 3.2 (+428%)	5.7 $\pm$ 4.7 (+317%)

T- mixture as compared to the B mixture following repletion.

Go/No-Go Task

Errors (omission and commission) were summed separately across the 80 trials within each condition. Square root transformations were applied to normalize the positively skewed distributions of the omission and commission errors. Analysis of square root commission errors revealed significant group [$F(1, 36) = 8.96$, $p = .005$] and condition [Geisser–Greenhouse $F(2.67, 96.07) = 5.07$, $p < .01$] main effects. SA participants made more (square root) commission errors as compared to NA participants, and all participants made fewer (square root) commission errors in the Rew–Pun condition relative to the Pun–Rew condition. No main effects or interactions involving treatment were significant, indicating that tryptophan depletion had no effect on square root commission errors by group or condition (see Figure 45.1).

Analysis of square root omission errors revealed a significant group $\times$ treatment $\times$ condition interaction [Geisser–Greenhouse $F(2.81, 101.15) = 3.51$, $p = .02$] (see Figure 45.1). Further analysis revealed a significant group $\times$ treatment interaction in the Rew–Pun condition [$F(1, 36) = 5.66$, $p < .03$]; however, post-hoc testing revealed no significant differences between the means.

Square root omission and commission errors were reanalyzed (separately) using estimated IQ, years of education, family revenue, and average teacher-rated anxiety as covariates in separate analyses of covariance (ANCOVAs). In the analyses of square root omission errors, none of the covariates altered the significant group $\times$ treatment $\times$ condition interaction. In the analyses of square root commission errors, estimated IQ was a marginally significant covariate [$F(1, 35) = 4.04$, $p = .052$], reducing the group main effect to a trend [$F(1, 35) = 3.56$, $p = .068$]. Average teacher-rated anxiety was a significant covariate [$F(1, 35) = 6.22$, $p = .02$], similarly reducing the group main effect to a trend [$F(1, 35) = 3.16$, $p = .08$]. Years of education and family revenue were not significant covariates and did not affect the group difference in commission errors.

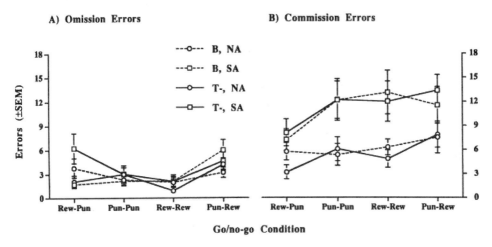

A) Omission Errors

B) Commission Errors

Go/no-go Condition

Figure 45.1

Mean ($\pm$ SE) omission and commission errors by condition in each of the two groups following consumption of the two amino acid loads. Rew–Pun indicates the reward-punishment go/no-go condition; Pun–Pun, punishment-punishment; Rew–Rew, reward-reward; Pun–Rew, punishment-reward. T- indicates tryptophan-depleted amino acid mixture; B, balanced amino acid mixture; SA, stable aggressive participants; NA, nonaggressive participants.

Go/No-Go and Cognitive Variables: Interrelationships

To explore relationships between disinhibition on the go/no-go task and cognitive functioning, square root omission and commission errors were averaged (separately) across conditions, then treatments, and used as dependent variables in separate multiple regression analyses. Estimated IQ was employed as a measure of general intellectual ability, and the factor scores for the verbal learning, incidental spatial learning, and executive function factors were used as indicators of cognitive functioning. These variables were entered on separate steps, in that order, to test whether executive function was associated with disinhibition over and above IQ, spatial memory, and verbal abilities, the latter two assessing conventional memory processes. Group membership (stable aggressive versus nonaggressive) was added on the last step to see if aggres-

sive status was related to disinhibition over and above cognitive functioning. Executive function significantly predicted average square root commission errors [B (unstandardized) $= -0.50$, $t = -3.07$, $p = .004$] over and above IQ, spatial memory, and verbal skill. Aggressive group status did not predict (square root) commission errors [B $= 0.34$, $t = -1.08$, $p = .29$] over and above cognitive functioning. The final equation accounted for 39% of the variance [adjusted R^2; $F(5, 32) = 5.72$, $p = .0007$]. Addition of the executive function factor accounted for 21% of the variance in (square root) commission errors over and above the 18% accounted for by estimated IQ and the spatial and verbal factors. Figure 45.2 shows the relationship between commission errors (by group, averaged across conditions and treatments) and executive function factor scores. None of the cognitive variables, nor group membership, predicted average square root omission errors.

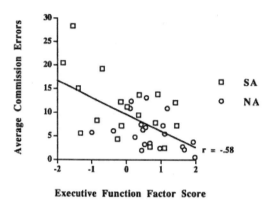

Figure 45.2
Correlation between commission errors on the go/no-go (averaged across conditions and treatments) and executive function factor scores. SA indicates stable aggressive participants; NA, nonaggressive participants.

Discussion

The effect of tryptophan depletion on disinhibition (commission errors), and the relationship between executive functions and disinhibition, were investigated in this sample of stable aggressive and nonaggressive adolescent males, a subsample of a larger, well-defined, longitudinal cohort followed for 12 years. First, SA participants made more commission errors than NA participants across go/no-go and amino acid conditions. This finding was robust after controlling for group differences in years of education or family revenue. IQ and teacher-rated anxiety, although significantly related to commission errors, only reduced the group difference marginally. This difference was also not caused by group differences in mood (in general, there were few group or amino acid treatment effects on mood measures [data not shown]).

The group difference in commission errors is congruent with previous work demonstrating increased commission errors (but similar omission errors) in incarcerated psychopaths, extraverts, and juvenile delinquents (Newman and Kosson 1986; Newman et al. 1985, 1990; Patter-

son et al. 1987) and children with attention deficit hyperactivity disorder (Iaboni et al. 1995). Increased commission errors in psychopaths, extraverts, and juvenile delinquents were found in the reward–punishment condition only (not in the reward–reward or punishment–punishment conditions), leading to the hypothesis that, in situations with competing reward and response cost, a dominant response set for reward is formed making response inhibition difficult when confronted with stimuli associated with response cost (Newman and Wallace 1993). In the present study, commission errors were increased across go/no-go conditions in SA participants (as in attention deficit and hyperactivity disorder children; Iaboni et al.), suggesting a more global impairment in behavioral inhibition in SA young men. Taken together, these studies suggest that disinhibition is an important characteristic of individuals with a history of aggressive behavior.

Two caveats concerning this finding must be noted. First, recent drug use was not formally assessed; the effects of recent drug intoxication and/or withdrawal could have had an impact on passive avoidance learning. Second, participants in the present study and in Iaboni et al. (1995)

did all four conditions of the go/no-go; whereas, in other studies (Newman and Wallace 1993), go/no-go conditions were administered between subjects. This procedural change may have an effect on the pattern of results across go/no-go conditions.

The second important finding of the present study is the association between executive functions and commission errors. This association was robust even after controlling for IQ and conventional memory processes, and it accounted for the difference in commission errors between the SA and NA participants, because group membership was no longer associated with commission errors after controlling for executive functions. These results suggest that behavioral disinhibition and reduced executive functioning are correlated and underlie aggressive behavior. Aggressive individuals may have deficits in any combination of abilities tapped by tests of executive function, including learning contingencies or modulating behavior in light of expected future consequences.

Current research supports associations between these variables. Executive functions have been related to aggressive behavior in the laboratory (Giancola and Zeichner 1994; Lau et al. 1995). Neuroimaging studies implicate the dorsolateral prefrontal cortex in the performance of tests measuring executive functions (Petrides et al. 1993a, b). Furthermore, neuropsychological tests associated with areas 9 and 46 of the dorsolateral prefrontal cortex are most associated with physical aggression after controlling for attention deficit hyperactivity disorder and IQ. A recent positron emission tomography (PET) study found that no-go responses (inhibition of thumb flexing) were associated with activation in the right prefrontal cortex (approximately area 46) in healthy males (Kawashima et al. 1996). Future investigation might focus on which specific executive functions and which neuroanatomical areas in the frontal cortex are most highly correlated with commission errors on the go/no-go task.

Tryptophan depletion had no effect on disinhibition on the go/no-go task in aggressive, disruptive young men, in contrast to an earlier study in which tryptophan depletion increased commission errors in young men with family histories of alcoholism (LeMarquand et al. 1997). Although the absence of a tryptophan depletion effect on disinhibition seems to go against the original hypothesis, alternative interpretations should be considered. This result may have been caused by ceiling effects: SA participants made more commission errors as compared to NA participants in the B amino acid condition as well as the T- condition. This suggests that the SA group was disinhibited at baseline (i.e., after the B amino acid mixture), washing out a potential T- effect. Alternatively, the SA group was higher in anxiety compared to: (1) the NA group; and (2) those SA individuals not tested. The presence of anxiety in the SA participants may have mitigated against finding an effect of tryptophan depletion.

Reduced baseline serotonin functioning in aggressive children and adolescents has been suggested in a number of studies (Halperin et al. 1994, 1997; Kruesi et al. 1990, 1992). SA and NA participants did not differ on one possible factor influencing serotonin synthesis—baseline plasma tryptophan levels prior to amino acid administration. Following tryptophan depletion and subsequent repletion, however, plasma tryptophan levels in SA participants were somewhat lower than those of NA participants, possibly suggesting a lag in the availability of tryptophan for 5-HT synthesis in some circumstances. If aggressive young men do have somewhat lower baseline serotonergic functioning, augmenting baseline serotonin function could decrease disinhibition (Coccaro and Kavoussi 1997).

In summary, stable aggressive adolescent males were more disinhibited (i.e., made more commission errors) as compared to nonaggressive young men on a go/no-go task. Moreover, executive functions accounted for a significant proportion of the variance in commission errors in the entire sample, over and above IQ, memory abilities, and group membership (stable aggressive vs. nonaggressive). Tryptophan depletion had no effect on disinhibition in stable aggressive young men, possibly because of a ceiling effect.

Acknowledgments

We thank Molly Fortin, Fabienne Gauthier, and Claudine Morin for assistance with blood draws; Carole Blanchet, Dorothy Opatowski, Isabelle Tremblay, Jolène Gauthier, Richard Legros, and Jennifer Weiner for assistance in testing; Mark Gross and Franceen Lenoff for technical assistance; and Judi Young and Liz Rusnak for secretarial assistance. This research was conducted by David LeMarquand in partial fulfillment of the requirements for the Ph.D. degree from the Department of Psychology, McGill University. This work was supported by grants from the Medical Research Council of Canada, Ottawa, Ontario (Drs. Pihl, Young, and Benkelfat), and doctoral and dissertation fellowships to D. LeMarquand from the Fonds pour la Formation de Chercheurs et L'Aide à la Recherche (FCAR), and the Guggenheim Foundation, New York. Portions of this research were presented at the Society for Biological Psychiatry, New York, May 1996; the Canadian College of Neuropsychopharmacology, Toronto, Canada, June 1996; and the NATO Advanced Study Institute on the Biosocial Bases of Violence: Theory and Research, Rhodes, Greece, May 1996.

References

Becker JT, Butters N, Rivoira P, Miliotis P (1986): Asking the right questions: Problem solving in male alcoholics and male alcoholics with Korsakoff's Syndrome. Alcohol Clin Exp Res 10:641–646.

Benkelfat C, Ellenbogen M, Dean P, Palmour R, Young SN (1994): Mood-lowering effect of tryptophan depletion: Enhanced susceptibility in young men at genetic risk for major affective disorders. Arch Gen Psychiat 51:687–697.

Berman ME, Tracy JI, Coccaro EF (1997): The serotonin hypothesis of aggression revisited. Clin Psychol Rev 17:651–665.

Blishen BR, Carroll WK, Moore C (1987): The 1981 socioeconomic index for occupations in Canada. Can Rev Sociol Anthropol 24:465–488.

Brown GL, Ebert MH, Goyer PF, Jimerson DC, Klein WJ, Bunney WE, Goodwin FK (1982): Aggression, suicide, and serotonin: Relationships to CSF amine metabolites. Am J Psychiat 139:741–746.

Cleare AJ, Bond AJ (1995): The effect of tryptophan depletion and enhancement on subjective and behavioural aggression in normal male subjects. Psychopharmacology 118:72–81.

Coccaro EF, Kavoussi RJ (1997): Fluoxetine and impulsive aggressive behavior in personality-disordered subjects. Arch Gen Psychiat 54:1081–1088.

Giancola PR, Zeichner A (1994): Neuropsychological performance on tests of frontal-lobe functioning and aggressive behavior in men. J Abnorm Psychol 103:832–835.

Halperin JM, Sharma V, Siever LJ, Schwartz ST, Matier K, Wornell G, Newcorn JH (1994): Serotonergic function in aggressive and nonaggressive boys with attention deficit hyperactivity disorder. Am J Psychiat 151:243–248.

Halperin JM, Newcorn JH, Schwartz ST, Sharma V, Siever LJ, Koda VH, Gabriel S (1997): Age-related changes in the association between serotonergic function and aggression in boys with ADHD. Biol Psychiatry 41:682–689.

Iaboni F, Douglas VI, Baker AG (1995): Effects of reward and response costs on inhibition in ADHD children. J Abnorm Psychol 104:232–240.

Kavoussi R, Armstead P, Coccaro EF (1997): The neurobiology of impulsive aggression. Psychiat Clin North Am 20:395–403.

Kawashima R, Satoh K, Itoh H, Ono S, Furumoto S, Gotoh R, Koyama M, Yoshioka S, Takahashi T, Takahashi K, Yanagisawa T, Fukuda H (1996): Functional anatomy of GO/NO-GO discrimination and response selection—A PET study in man. Brain Res 728:79–89.

Kruesi MJ, Rapoport JL, Hamburger S, Hibbs E, Potter WZ, Lenane M, Brown GL (1990): Cerebrospinal fluid monoamine metabolites, aggression, and impulsivity in disruptive behavior disorders of children and adolescents. Arch Gen Psychiat 47:419–426.

Kruesi MJP, Hibbs ED, Zahn TP, Keysor CS, Hamburger SD, Bartko JJ, Rapoport JL (1992): A 2-year prospective follow-up study of children and adolescents with disruptive behavior disorders. Arch Gen Psychiat 49:429–435.

Lau MA, Pihl RO, Peterson JB (1995): Provocation, acute alcohol intoxication, cognitive performance, and aggression. J Abnorm Psychol 104:150–155.

LeMarquand DG, Pihl RO, Young SN, Tremblay RE, Palmour RM, Benkelfat C (1997): Tryptophan depletion and behavioral disinhibition in men at risk for alcoholism and antisocial behavior. In Raine A, Brennan PA, Farrington DP, Mednick SA (eds), Biosocial Bases of Violence. New York, Plenum, pp 337–339.

Lezak M (1983): Neuropsychological Assessment. New York, Wiley.

Lezak MD (1985): Neuropsychological assessment. In Frederiks JAM (ed), Handbook of clinical neurology: Vol. 1. Clinical neuropsychology. New York, Elsevier, pp 515–530.

Linnoila M, Virkkunen M, Scheinin M, Nuutila A, Rimon R, Goodwin FK (1983): Low cerebrospinal fluid 5-hydroxyindoleacetic acid concentration differentiates impulsive from nonimpulsive violent behavior. Life Sci 33:2609–2614.

Mâsse LC, Tremblay RE (1997): Behavior of boys in kindergarten and the onset of substance use during adolescence. Arch Gen Psychiat 54:62–68.

Milner B, Petrides M, Smith ML (1985): Frontal lobes and the temporal organization of memory. Human Neurobiol 4:137–142.

Moeller FG, Dougherty DM, Swann AC, Collins D, Davis CM, Cherek DR (1996): Tryptophan depletion and aggressive responding in healthy males. Psychopharmacology 126:97–103.

Newman JP, Widom CS, Nathan S (1985): Passive avoidance in syndromes of disinhibition: Psychopathy and extraversion. J Pers Soc Psychol 48:1316–1327.

Newman JP, Kosson DS (1986): Passive avoidance learning in psychopathic and nonpsychopathic offenders. J Abnorm Psychol 95:252–256.

Newman JP, Patterson CM, Howland EW, Nichols SL (1990): Passive avoidance in psychopaths: The effects of reward. Person Individ Diff 11:1101–1114.

Newman JP, Wallace JF (1993): Diverse pathways to deficient self-regulation: Implications for disinhibitory psychopathology in children. Clin Psychol Rev 13:699–720.

Nishizawa S, Benkelfat C, Young SN, Leyton M, Mzengeza S, de Montigny C, Blier P, Diksic M (1997): Differences between males and females in rates of serotonin synthesis in human brain. Proc Natl Acad Sci USA 94:5308–5313.

Patterson CM, Kosson DS, Newman JP (1987): Reaction to punishment, reflectivity, and passive avoidance learning in extraverts. J Pers Soc Psychol 52:565–575.

Pennington BF, Ozonoff S (1996): Executive functions and developmental psychopathology. J Child Psychol Psychiat 37:51–87.

Petrides M (1990): Nonspatial conditional learning impaired in patients with unilateral frontal but not unilateral temporal lobe excisions. Neuropsychologia 28:137–149.

Petrides M, Alivisatos B, Evans AC, Meyer E (1993a): Dissociation of human mid-dorsolateral from posterior dorsolateral frontal cortex in memory processing. Proc Natl Acad Sci USA 90:873–877.

Petrides M, Alivisatos B, Meyer E, Evans AC (1993b): Functional activation of the human frontal cortex during the performance of verbal working memory tasks. Proc Natl Acad Sci USA 90:878–882.

Pihl RO, Young SN, Harden P, Plotnick S, Chamberlain B, Ervin FR (1995): Acute effect of altered tryptophan levels and alcohol on aggression in normal human males. Psychopharmacology 119:353–360.

Pucilowski O, Kostowski J (1980): Aggressive behavior and the central serotonergic system. Behav Brain Res 9:33–48.

Salomon RM, Mazure CM, Delgado PL, Mendia P, Charney DS (1994): Serotonin function in aggression: The effects of acute plasma tryptophan depletion in aggressive patients. Biol Psychiatry 35:570–572.

Sattler JM (1988): Assessment of Children. San Diego, CA, JM Sattler (Publisher).

Séguin JR, Harden PW, Pihl RO, Tremblay RE, Boulerice B (1995): Cognitive and neuropsychological characteristics of physically aggressive boys. J Abnorm Psychol 104:614–624.

Smith ML, Milner B (1981): The role of right hippocampus in the recall of spatial location. Neuropsychologia 19:781–793.

Smith ML, Milner B (1989): Right hippocampal impairment in the recall of spatial location: Encoding deficit or rapid forgetting? Neuropsychologia 27:71–81.

Smith SE, Pihl RO, Young SN, Ervin FR (1987): Elevation and reduction of plasma tryptophan and their effects on aggression and perceptual sensitivity in normal males. Aggress Behav 12:393–407.

Soubrié P (1986): Reconciling the role of central serotonin neurons in human and animal behavior. Behav Brain Sci 9:319–364.

Tabachnick BG, Fidell LS (1989): Using Multivariate Statistics. New York, HarperCollins.

Tremblay RE, Loeber R, Gagnon C, Charlebois P, Larivée S, LeBlanc M (1991): Disruptive boys with stable and unstable high fighting behavior patterns during junior elementary school. J Abnorm Child Psychol 19:285–300.

Tuinier S, Verhoeven WMA, van Praag HM (1995): Cerebrospinal fluid 5-hydroxyindoleacetic acid and aggression: A critical reappraisal of the clinical data. Int Clin Psychopharmacol 10:147–156.

Virkkunen M, Rawlings R, Tokola R, Poland RE, Guidotti A, Nemeroff C, Bissette G, Kalogeras K, Karonen S-L, Linnoila M (1994): CSF biochemistries, glucose metabolism, and diurnal activity rhythms in alcoholic, violent offenders, fire setters, and healthy volunteers. Arch Gen Psychiat 51:20–27.

Wechsler D (1974): Manual for the Wechsler Intelligence Scale for Children—Revised. New York, Psychological Corporation.

Wechsler D (1987): Wechsler Memory Scale—Revised. New York, Psychological Corporation.

Wiegersma S, van der Scheer E, Hijman R (1990): Subjective ordering, short-term memory, and the frontal lobes. Neuropsychologia 28:95–98.

Wilkins K (1990): Eosinophilia-myalgia syndrome. Can Med Ass J 142:1265–1266.

46 Nature over Nurture: Temperament, Personality, and Life Span Development

Robert R. McCrae, Paul T. Costa Jr., Fritz Ostendorf, Alois Angleitner, Martina Hřebíčková, Maria D. Avia, Jesús Sanz, Maria L. Sánchez-Bernardos, M. Ersin Kusdil, Ruth Woodfield, Peter R. Saunders, and Peter B. Smith

There are both empirical and conceptual links between child temperaments and adult personality traits. The empirical associations are modest, but the conceptual relations are profound. Explaining how this is so requires a complicated chain of arguments and evidence. For example, we report cross-sectional data showing (among other things) that adolescents are lower in Conscientiousness than are middle-aged and older adults in Germany, the United Kingdom, Spain, the Czech Republic, and Turkey. The relevance of such data may not be immediately obvious, but in fact they speak to the transcontextual nature of personality traits and thus to the fundamental issue of nature versus nurture.

The gist of our argument is easily stated: Personality traits, like temperaments, are endogenous dispositions that follow intrinsic paths of development essentially independent of environmental influences. That idea is simple, but it is so foreign to the thinking of most psychologists that it requires a detailed exposition and defense. Once grasped, however, it offers a new and fruitful perspective on personality and its development.

A Theoretical Perspective on Temperament

There is no hard and fast distinction between temperament and personality. *The American Heritage Dictionary of the English Language* defines *temperament* as "the manner of thinking, behaving, or reacting characteristic of a specific individual" (Morris, 1976, p. 1324), a definition which might serve equally well for *personality trait*. One of the first omnibus personality inventories, measuring such traits as ascendance, emotional stability, and thoughtfulness, was designated by J. P. Guilford and his colleagues (Guilford, Zimmerman, & Guilford, 1976) as a

"temperament survey." In some respects, then, there is a long tradition of equating these two sets of individual differences variables.

There is also a long tradition of distinguishing them. Temperament is frequently regarded as a constitutional predisposition, observable in preverbal infants and animals, and tied, at least theoretically, to basic psychological processes. Personality traits, in contrast, are often assumed to be acquired patterns of thought and behavior that might be found only in organisms with sophisticated cognitive systems. Constructs like authoritarianism, self-monitoring, and narcissism do not appear to be directly applicable to chimpanzees or human infants.

Some theorists divide personality traits into two categories, corresponding to innate and acquired characteristics. For example, Cloninger and his colleagues (Cloninger, Przybeck, Svrakic, & Wetzel, 1994) classified Novelty Seeking, Harm Avoidance, Reward Dependence, and Persistence as temperaments, and Self-Directedness, Cooperativeness, and Self-Transcendence as aspects of character. Other theorists assume that temperament provides the starting place for personality development, a tabula that is not quite rasa. All those personality theorists who nod to "constitutional factors" (e.g., Kluckhohn & Murray, 1953) adopt some such position. An appealing version of this constitutional perspective would distinguish between broad factors, like Extraversion, that might correspond to basic temperamental influences, and specific traits, like sociability or dominance, that might be interpreted as acquired personality traits.

There is, however, a completely different way to conceptualize these important distinctions. McAdams (1996) has offered a formulation of the personality system as a whole in terms of three levels. Personality traits are assigned to

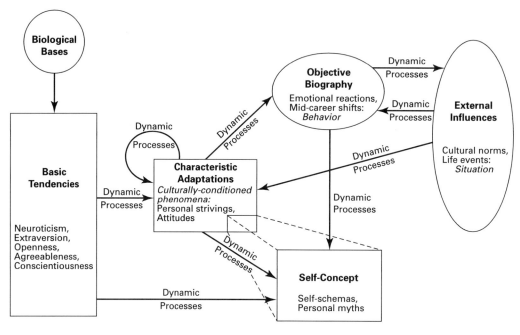

Figure 46.1

A model of the personality system according to five-factor theory, with examples of specific content in each category and arrows indicating paths of causal influence. (Adapted from "A Five-Factor Theory of Personality," by R. R. McCrae and P. T. Costa, Jr., 1999, in *Handbook of Personality*, second ed., p. 142, edited by L. Pervin and O. P. John, New York: Guilford Press.)

Level 1 in McAdams's scheme, whereas "constructs that are contextualized in time, place or role" (p. 301), such as coping strategies, skills, and values, occupy Level 2. (Level 3 includes life narratives that give unity and purpose to the self.) A related system has been proposed by McCrae and Costa (1996, 1999) in a five-factor theory (FFT) of personality. As shown schematically in Figure 46.1, the FFT highlights the distinction between biologically based *basic tendencies* and culturally conditioned *characteristic adaptations* (which include the important subcategory of self-concepts). Basic tendencies comprise abstract potentials and dispositions (including the traits in McAdams's Level 1), whereas characteristic adaptations include ac-

quired skills, habits, beliefs, roles, and relationships (constructs from McAdams's Level 2).

In the terminology of FFT, Cloninger and colleagues (Cloninger et al., 1994) would presumably place Novelty Seeking and Harm Avoidance in the category of basic tendencies, and Self-Directedness and Cooperativeness in the category of characteristic adaptations. The alternative, constitutional view would perhaps hold that the temperamental basis of personality—including the five factors listed in Figure 46.1—is a part of basic tendencies, whereas personality traits like sociability and dominance are characteristic adaptations.

According to FFT, however, both broad personality factors and the specific traits that define them are best understood not as characteristic adaptations, but rather as endogenous basic tendencies. FFT has returned, as it were, to Guilford's (Guilford et al., 1976) view that the attributes measured by personality questionnaires can be identified as temperaments (Costa & McCrae, in press).

Some readers will be surprised by the claim that the whole range of personality traits can be subsumed by temperament. In support of that claim, most of the findings summarized in this article are taken from research on the five-factor model of personality, which is intended to provide a comprehensive taxomomy of traits (Goldberg, 1993). It should be noted, however, that the basic ideas are likely to be applicable to many alternative models as well. For example, there is evidence of cross-cultural invariance for three- and seven-factor models (Benet-Martínez & Waller, 1997; S. B. G. Eysenck, 1983), and the pattern of adult age differences reported here can also be seen in California Psychological Inventory scales (Gough, 1987; Labouvie-Vief, Diehl, Tarnowski, & Shen, in press; Yang, McCrae, & Costa, 1998).

Most readers will probably be startled by the conspicuous absence in Figure 46.1 of an arrow from *external influences* to *basic tendencies*. This is not an oversight; FFT deliberately asserts that personality traits are endogenous dispositions, influenced not at all by the environment. That assertion is, of course, an oversimplification, but we believe it is a heuristically valuable one and a useful corrective to what Asendorpf and Wilpers (1998) recently called "the naive environmentalism that has for a long time dominated the literature on personality development" (p. 1543). In this chapter we hope to show that FFT provides a useful framework for understanding child temperament and adult personality development.

The Roles of the Environment

First, however, we must reassure the reader that environmental influences play crucial roles in the

functioning of the personality system in several different respects: They define the conditions under which human personality evolved; they shape a vast array of skills, values, attitudes, and identities; they provide the concrete forms in which personality traits are expressed; and they supply the trait indicators from which personality traits are inferred and trait levels are assessed.

At one level, all psychological characteristics must be understood as end results of evolutionary processes by which organisms have adapted to their environment (D. M. Buss, 1991). Evolutionary principles are most easily applied to explain characteristics that distinguish different species, and their application to the explanation of individual differences within species is controversial (D. M. Buss & Greiling, 1999). Indeed, Tooby and Cosmides (1990) argued that differences among human beings in personality traits are best regarded as noise of no evolutionary significance. At a minimum, however, that implies that personality variations are compatible with the usual human environment: We know from their continued presence among us that both introverts and extraverts can survive in the human world.

The environment also operates at a much more direct level. A recent book on the limited influences of parenting (Harris, 1998) was greeted with alarm by many psychologists, who interpreted it to imply that the way parents treat their children does not matter (Begley, 1998). In contrast, FFT explicitly recognizes that

The influence of parents on their children is surely incalculable: they nourish and protect them, teach them to walk and talk, instill habits, aversions, and values, and provide some of the earliest models for social interaction and emotional regulation (McCrae & Costa, 1994, p. 107).

In short, parenting has important long-term consequences for the development of characteristic adaptations, including, of course, the lifelong relationship between parent and child. Many other aspects of the environment are also significant influences on characteristic adaptations, including peers (Harris, 1998), the media, educational systems, and so on. Vocational interests, religious beliefs, food preferences, tactics of interpersonal manipulation, and group loyalties are some of the products of these influences, and it is possible to view and study psychological development as the creation and integration of these characteristic adaptations. This approach may be particularly appealing in collectivistic cultures, in which the individual's evolving place in social networks is of more concern than are autonomous features of the individual (Kagitçibaşi, 1996). But important as this form of development may be, FFT asserts that it is not what personality psychologists get at when they administer personality questionnaires to assess such characteristics as assertiveness, curiosity, or shyness.

However, the environment also has a direct relation to personality traits, because characteristic adaptations are always involved in their expression. To take a simple example, interpersonal traits are most often inferred from communication with others, and that normally requires a common acquired language such as English, Shona, or Hindi. At what is perhaps a more psychologically meaningful level, trait manifestations must fit within a cultural context. An expression of sympathy for the deceased could be insulting in a culture in which the dead are never mentioned by name; thus, an agreeable person must learn how to be polite in terms of the culture's rules of etiquette. Even apparently direct manifestations of personality, such as the chronic anxiety of an individual high in Neuroticism, are usually contextualized: Anxious Americans worry about computer viruses and the future of Social Security; anxious Navahos—at least when they were studied by Clyde Kluckhohn (1944)—worried about ghosts and witches (cf. Kitayama & Markus, 1994).

According to FFT, traits cannot be directly observed, but rather must be inferred from patterns of behavior and experience that are known to be valid trait indicators (Tellegen, 1988). Personality scales rely on these indicators and need to be sensitive to variations introduced by culture, age, and other contexts. But although they may ask respondents about their values, habits, or concerns, personality inventories are designed to allow the inference of deeper psychological constructs.

Personality Traits as Endogenous Basic Tendencies

If the environment has such obvious and pervasive effects on characteristic adaptations and the expression of personality traits, why not presume that it also affects traits themselves? According to FFT, personality is biologically based, but it is well established that perceptual and learning experiences can reshape the developing brain (Kolb & Whishaw, 1998), and recent studies suggest that traumatic stress may contribute to atrophy in the hippocampus (Bremner, 1998). Thus, life experience might affect personality through its effects on the brain (Nelson, 1999). There is cross-sectional evidence that the experience of acculturation can change personality profiles (McCrae, Yik, Trapnell, Bond, & Paulhus, 1998), and some longitudinal research has shown that personality change is associated with life events (Agronick & Duncan, 1998).

All of these findings are useful reminders that the theoretical generalizations represented in Figure 46.1 certainly have exceptions. However, the generalization that personality traits are more or less immune to environmental influences is supported by multiple, converging lines of empirical evidence that significant variations in life experience have little or no effect on measured personality traits. Any one of these lines of evidence is subject to many alternative interpretations, but taken together, they make a strong case for regarding personality traits as fundamentally temperament-like. That assumption makes sense of many findings that would remain puzzling from the perspective of naive environmentalism. In the following section, we review some research consistent with this premise of FFT.

Heritability of Personality

The study of behavior genetics has flourished in the past 20 years, and the results of many twin and adoption studies have shown remarkable unanimity (Loehlin, 1992): Personality traits have a substantial genetic component, little or no component that can be attributed to shared environmental effects (e.g., attending the same school or having the same parents), and a residual component about which little is yet known. Heritability is virtually a sine qua non of biologically based theories of personality, so it is crucial to note that it is not limited to Neuroticism and Extraversion, which are often conceded to be temperamental traits (H. J. Eysenck, 1990). All five factors are heritable; in fact, some estimates find the strongest evidence of heritability for Openness to Experience (Loehlin, 1992).

Further, people inherit more than the global dispositions summarized by the five major personality factors; specific traits such as self-consciousness, gregariousness, and openness to ideas are also specifically heritable (Jang, Mc-Crae, Angleitner, Riemann, & Livesley, 1998), and in this regard can better be considered basic tendencies than characteristic adaptations.

But behavior–genetic studies also speak to the importance of environmental effects, although what they say is subject to different interpretations. The sheer weight of evidence has by now convinced most psychologists familiar with that literature that environmental influences shared by children in the same family have little or no effect on adult personality (Plomin & Daniels, 1987). If the environment is to have any effect, it must be through what is typically labeled the *nonshared environment,* the set of experiences unique to different children in the same family (e.g., having different first-grade teachers or being a parent's favorite). However, this term is not measured directly, but rather it is calculated as

a residual, and as such it includes far more than experience; in particular, it includes both random error of measurement and systematic method bias. When Riemann, Angleitner, and Strelau (1997) reduced method variance by combining self-reports and observer ratings from two peers, their heritability estimates for the five factors, ranging from .66 to .79, were considerably higher than the .50 usually cited. The remaining 21% to 34% of the variance might include nonshared influences from the psychological environment, such as peer groups, but it might instead reflect wholly biological sources, such as the prenatal hormonal environment (Resnick, Gottesman, & McGue, 1993), minor brain damage or infection, or simply the imperfect operation of genetic mechanisms. Behavior–genetic studies still allow for the possibility of some kinds of environmental influences on traits, but they do not as yet offer a compelling reason to modify Figure 46.1.

Studies of Parental Influences

Behavior–genetic designs infer effects indirectly from the phenotypic similarity of people with different kinds and degrees of relatedness; they do not directly measure any putative cause of personality traits. There are, however, studies that have linked child-rearing behaviors or parent–child relations to adult personality traits (e.g., Rapee, 1997). Most of these studies were retrospective, and many found some association. McCrae and Costa (1988), for example, previously reported that men and women who recalled their parents as being especially loving described themselves as being better adjusted and more agreeable. Although this appears to provide direct support for parental influences on personality, there are many alternative interpretations. Perhaps parents had been more loving because these adjusted and agreeable children had been more lovable. Perhaps the same genes that made the parents loving made the children adjusted. Perhaps retrospective bias made kind children recall their childhood with exaggerated fondness. Despite the possible operation of all these artifacts, the observed correlations were only in the range from .10 to .30, accounting for at most 10% of the variance in adult personality traits (cf. Rapee, 1997).

It is possible that the effects of parenting are more focused, affecting specific personality traits rather than broad factors. But when the 30 facet scales of the Revised NEO Personality Inventory (NEO-PI-R; Costa & McCrae, 1992a) were correlated with Loving/Rejecting, Casual/Demanding, and Attention scales for father and for mother, none of the 180 correlations reached .30 ($Mdn |r| = .08$; McCrae & Costa, 1994).

The results of the rare prospective-longitudinal studies are more informative. In one of the first and best of these, Kagan and Moss (1962) examined maternal characteristics during three age periods from infancy to age 10 and assessed the child's personality at ages 19–29. Of 552 relevant correlations, only 35 (6%) reached statistical significance at the $p < .05$ level. If parenting has an effect on personality, it is subtle indeed (Harris, 1998).

All these findings are consistent with the results of adoption studies (e.g., Plomin, Corley, Caspi, Fulker, & DeFries, 1998), which showed that children bear little resemblance to either their adoptive parents or their adoptive siblings. Neither parental role modeling nor the parenting practices that would affect all children in a family seem to have much influence on personality traits.

Cross-cultural Studies of Personality Structure

It is possible that environmental influences relevant to personality development lie outside the family, in the broader institutions that are collectively called *culture*. As a biologically based phenomenon common to the human species, the fundamental structure of infant and child temperament ought to transcend culture, and there is some evidence that it does (Ahadi, Rothbart, & Ye, 1993). But over time, many psychologists would find it reasonable to argue that the pervasive forces of culture can arbitrarily redefine the parameters of personality—indeed, that was a central premise of the school of culture and personality that flourished in the first half of this century (Singer, 1961). Some contemporary social scientists still find this a plausible argument. Juni (1996) challenged the idea that the five-factor model would apply cross-culturally: "Different cultures and different languages should give rise to other models that have little chance of being five in number nor of having any of the factors resemble those . . . of middle-class Americans" (p. 864).

However, studies using the Personality Research Form (Paunonen, Jackson, Trzebinski, & Forsterling, 1992; Stumpf, 1993) and the NEO-PI-R (e.g., Martin et al., 1997; McCrae & Costa, 1997; McCrae, Costa, del Pilar, Rolland, & Parker, 1998) have reported clear and detailed replication of the five-factor model in cultures ranging from Malaysia to Estonia. The traits that define the five factors in American samples define the same factors around the world. In this respect, the structure of individual differences appears to be a universal feature of human groups, relatively impervious to cultural variation.

Some authors have argued that there are additional personality factors, such as Chinese Tradition (Cheung et al., 1996) and (Filipino) Temperamentalness (Church, Katigbak, & Reyes, 1998) that are indigenous to specific cultures. Such culture-based factors would constitute evidence against a purely endogenous theory of the origins of personality. As yet, however, we know too little about indigenous factors to understand how to evaluate this evidence. Perhaps they are measurement artifacts or social attitudes that should be distinguished from personality traits per se; perhaps they really are universal factors that have so far gone unnoticed in other cultures. Because of their importance in the nature–nurture controversy, such proposed factors merit intensive longitudinal, cross-observer, and behavior–genetic research.

Comparative Studies

The five-factor model may be found in every culture because it is a product of human biology; recent research on animals suggests that at least some of the five factors may also be shared by nonhuman species. Gosling and John (1998) asked cat and dog owners to describe their pets, with terms taken from the five-factor model or from a list intended to describe temperament in animals. In both instruments and in both species, they found four factors: three corresponding to Neuroticism, Extraversion, and Agreeableness, and the fourth combining features of Openness to Experience and Conscientiousness in a kind of animal Intellect factor. King and Figueredo (1997) analyzed zookeeper ratings of chimpanzees and found six factors, which corresponded to the five-factor model plus a large dominance factor.

It has been known for many years that the five-factor structure of personality can be approximated even in ratings of strangers (Passini & Norman, 1966), so it might be suspected that these ratings of animals were merely projections of implicit personality theory. But Gosling and John (1998) could not replicate a five-factor structure of personality in cats or dogs, even when they used Procrustes rotation, suggesting that something other than sheer implicit personality theory was at work. King and Figueredo (1997) demonstrated substantial agreement between observers on chimpanzee personality ratings—the same kind of evidence that Norman and Goldberg (1966) had used to rebut the claim that personality ratings of humans were mere cognitive fictions.

The use of personality ratings in the description of nonhuman species may seem odd—is it meaningful to assess a dog's efficiency, harshness, or creativity?—but there is by now substantial scientific literature on the topic (A. H. Buss, 1997; Gosling, 1998). It seems much less odd to speak about temperament in animals; if traits are temperaments, then the literature on individual differences in animals can be more easily understood.

Temporal Stability of Adult Personality

Beginning in the 1970s, several independent longitudinal studies (e.g., Block, 1981; Siegler, George, & Okun, 1979) began to address the stability of individual differences in personality traits. Results, with researchers using a variety of samples, instruments, and methods of measurement, showed a consistent pattern of stability. Retest correlations over 6, 12, or 20 years were not much smaller than short-term retest reliabilities; personality in 70-year-olds could be predicted with remarkable accuracy from assessments made 30 years earlier (Costa & McCrae, 1992b; Finn, 1986).

On the one hand, these findings pointed to the existence of something in the individual that endured over long periods of time—a key piece of evidence for the reality of personality traits. On the other hand, it cast into doubt the influence of intervening events. Over the course of a 30-year study, many participants would have had major life changes in occupation, marital status, family stage, physical health, and place of residence. They would have shared their cohort's experience of assassinations, wars, and recessions; read dozens of books; watched thousands of hours of television. But the cumulative force of all these external influences on personality test scores is barely detectable.

Again, it is possible that life events and experiences affect some specific traits even if they do not have a major impact on broad factors. However, in a study of 2,274 men and women traced from about age 40 to age 50, retest correlations for the 30 eight-item NEO-PI-R facet scales were uniformly high, ranging from .64 for Vulnerability to .80 for Assertiveness and Openness to Aesthetics (Siegler & Costa, 1999).

The Intrinsic Maturation of Personality

Studies of heritability, limited parental influence, structural invariance across cultures and species, and temporal stability all point to the notion that personality traits are more expressions of human biology than products of life experience. Another more recent line of evidence concerns maturation and personality change. Here we present the latest findings from a series of studies that have examined age differences in the mean levels of personality traits across cultures. The basic argument is straightforward: If personality development reflects environmental influences, then groups whose histories have led them through different environments should show different developmental outcomes. Conversely, if personality development proceeds independently of life experiences, then similar trends should be seen everywhere.

The data reviewed above on the temporal stability of personality traits were retest correlations that reflect the consistency of rank order across two occasions. High stability of individual differences does not mean that personality trait scores are unchanging, only that people retain their relative standing across any changes that occur. If the trait score of every individual in a sample increased by exactly the same amount over an interval, the retest correlation would be 1.0, no matter how large or small the increase. The personality changes of interest here must be examined by comparing mean levels.

Initial work in studies of adults conducted in the United States found very modest mean level effects after age 30. For example, in a large and representative sample of men and women between ages 35 and 84, the correlations of age with Neuroticism, Extraversion, and Openness to Experience were $-.12$, $-.16$, and $-.19$, respectively (Costa et al., 1986). Later comparisons of college students with older adults showed larger effects, albeit in the same direction: Students scored about one-half standard deviation higher than adults on Neuroticism, Extraversion, and Openness to Experience (Costa & McCrae, 1994). They also scored consistently lower than adults on Agreeableness and Conscientiousness.

In themselves, these data are powerfully ambiguous. Perhaps they represent the effects of intrinsic maturation, but there are many other possibilities as well. This pattern of maturation may be purely American, a response to an educational and economic system that encourages an extended adolescence. Or it may reflect cohort differences, the effects of coming of age at specific times in history. Perhaps present-day adolescents are less conscientious than their grandparents are because they have grown up in an era of affluence, or of easily available drugs, or of rock music.

The usual suggestion for a research design to help untangle such confounds is the longitudinal study. Because comparisons are made between the same individuals tested on two (or more) occasions, birth cohort effects are controlled in longitudinal designs. If increases in Conscientiousness were documented in a group of college students as they grew into middle adulthood, that would provide more direct evidence of a true maturational effect. In fact, some studies have reported just such longitudinal changes in variables related to Conscientiousness (Jessor, 1983; McGue, Bacon, & Lykken, 1993).

Longitudinal studies take time to conduct, however, and longitudinal studies of Americans tell us nothing directly about age changes in different cultural and historical contexts. Cross-sectional studies of age differences conducted in other cultures, however, provide a simple way to circumvent some limitations of both cohort and culture, because different cultures have usually had differing recent histories.

Consider Turkey and the Czech Republic. Turkey is an Islamic country, and its citizens speak an Altaic language. Following the disintegration of the Ottoman Empire at the end of World War I, a new and radically secular society was established, modeled on the West. Institutions from the alphabet to style of dress were reformed; most significantly, women were given unprecedented opportunities for education and occupations outside the home. Turkey was not directly involved in World War II and has progressed slowly toward multiparty democracy.

Throughout the century it has grown in prosperity and urbanization, with a concomitant decline in strong kinship systems.

The Czech Republic, a traditionally Christian nation whose citizens speak a language from the Slavic branch of the Indo-European family, began the century as part of the Austro-Hungarian Empire. Between world wars it functioned as a democracy with a highly industrialized economy. In 1938, Germany began an occupation of Czechoslovakia that was ended by Soviet troops in 1945; Soviet dominance continued thereafter, with nationalization of industry and collectivization of agriculture. Attempted reform in 1968 led to a military response from the Warsaw Pact, and political repression continued until the collapse of Communist control in 1989.

The life experiences of Turks and Czechs have thus been radically different in this century, and both have differed from those of Americans. If experiences shape personality, then cohorts born at the same time in these three countries would presumably differ in mean levels. Czech adolescents, for example, who have spent much of their lives in a democratic society, might be better adjusted than their politically traumatized parents and grandparents. In contrast, American adolescents are known to be higher in Neuroticism than their parents' generation (Costa & McCrae, 1994).

Two previous studies have compared age differences on NEO-PI-R scale scores across cultures (Costa et al., in press; McCrae et al., 1999). In each, data were standardized within culture (to eliminate translation effects) and means were calculated for the age groups of 18–21, 22–29, 30–49, and 50+. Data were available for secondary analysis from Germany, Italy, Portugal, Croatia, South Korea, Russia, Estonia, and Japan. In four of the cultures (Italy, Croatia, Russia, and Estonia), there were no significant age effects for Neuroticism. In the other four cultures, Neuroticism was higher in younger respondents—just as it had been in American studies. Results for the remaining factors are

easily summarized: In every culture, the American pattern was replicated. Extraversion and Openness to Experience declined and Agreeableness and Conscientiousness increased with age in Germany, Italy, Portugal, Croatia, South Korea, Russia, Estonia, and Japan.

Xiu, Wu, Wu, and Shui (1996) examined age differences on a Chinese version of the short form of the NEO-PI-R, the NEO Five-Factor Inventory (NEO-FFI; Costa & McCrae, 1992a). In a sample of 593 men and women between ages 20 and 84, small but significant age effects were found for Neuroticism and Openness to Experience, which declined with age, and Agreeableness, which increased with age. Thus, this study offers a partial replication of American effects (see also Yang, McCrae, & Costa, 1998).

New Data from Five Cultures

In this chapter we report analyses of the NEO-FFI administered in Germany, the United Kingdom, Spain, the Czech Republic, and Turkey. The American version was adapted for use in the U.K., and translations were made into the other languages and checked by review of a back-translation. Internal consistency for the five 12-item scales ranged from .48 (for Agreeableness in the Turkish sample) to .85, with a median of .76; in every sample, internal consistency was lowest for the Agreeableness and Openness to Experience scales, suggesting that results with these two scales should be viewed with some caution.

Previous cross-cultural studies using the NEO-PI-R have examined only adult development, in part because American normative data have been published only for college-age and older adults. The present chapter includes data from adolescents between ages 14 and 17 from four of the samples. The NEO-FFI has demonstrated validity when used in samples of intellectually gifted American sixth graders (Parker & Stumpf, 1998); internal consistencies in the four adoles-

Table 46.1
Composition of the samples by age group and gender

| | Age group (in years) | | | | | | | | | |
| | 14–17 | | 18–21 | | 22–29 | | 30–49 | | 50+ | |
Sample	M	W	M	W	M	W	M	W	M	W
German	42	149	85	252	215	515	182	615	73	230
British	41	39	135	135	28	29	40	72	12	9
Spanish			49	74	145	116	117	143	67	53
Czech	147	263	117	116	26	25	78	76	40	24
Turkish	157	112	16	7			84	108	21	6

Note. None of the Spanish respondents was under 18 years old; none of the Turkish students or their parents was between ages 22 and 29. M = men; W = women.

cent subsamples studied here ranged from .57 to .86, with a median of .75, values which are comparable to those seen in adults.

Data were originally collected for a variety of purposes, and as Table 46.1 shows, the distribution by age group is not optimal in several instances. Nevertheless, there appear to be sufficient cases in most age groups to make secondary analyses worthwhile. The German sample consists of mono- and dizygotic twins, on whom both self-reports and mean peer ratings of personality are available (Riemann et al., 1997). These respondents are part of a large German sample whose full NEO-PI-R scale scores were previously analyzed (McCrae et al., 1999). They are included here not as an independent replication, but rather as a check on the consistency of results from the long and short versions of the NEO-PI-R.

Data from the U.K. were obtained in three studies that involved adolescent school children, their parents, and university students. An effort was made to include respondents from all occupational groups; most respondents were from the southern part of the U.K. The Turkish sample consisted of adolescents from many regions in Turkey that attended a summer camp, and families in the city of Bursa, a major industrial cen-

ter. The Spanish and Czech samples were both recruited by undergraduate psychology students who invited friends, relatives, and partners to join the study. None of these samples is either random or nationally representative, but it seems unlikely that they share any systematic sampling bias that might explain common age trends.

As in previous studies, T scores were computed within each culture using means and standard deviations from the adults over age 21 (following the American convention). The only meaningful comparisons are thus among age groups within each culture. Analyses of variance (ANOVAs) with age group and gender as classifying variables showed generally similar patterns in men and women: Of the 25 ANOVAs, only 5 showed significant interaction terms, with no pattern replicated across cultures. Four of the interactions were quite small, accounting for less than 2% of the variance. A somewhat larger effect was seen for Openness to Experience in the Turkish sample, in which age differences were found only in women.

Results for the total sample are summarized in Figures 46.2–46.6. The ANOVAs confirm that there are significant cross-sectional declines in Neuroticism and Extraversion and increases in Conscientiousness in all five samples. There

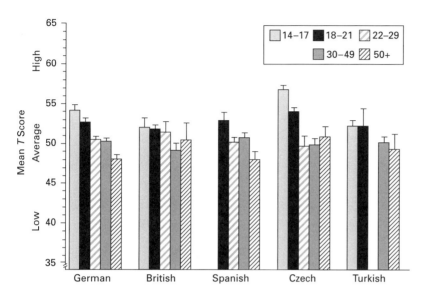

Figure 46.2
Mean levels of Neuroticism in five cultures. *T* scores are based on the mean and standard deviation of all respondents over age 21 within each culture. Error bars: SEM.

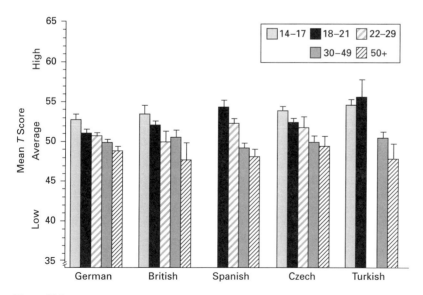

Figure 46.3
Mean levels of Extraversion in five cultures. *T* scores are based on the mean and standard deviation of all respondents over age 21 within each culture. Error bars: SEM.

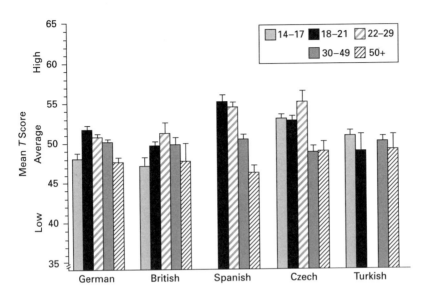

Figure 46.4
Mean levels of Openness to Experience in five cultures. *T* scores are based on the mean and standard deviation of all respondents over age 21 within each culture. Error bars: SEM.

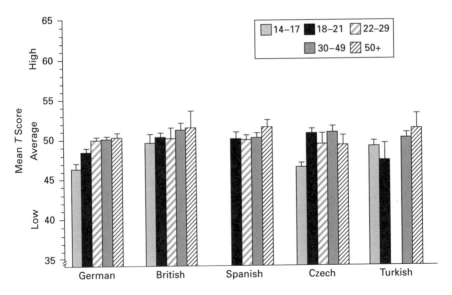

Figure 46.5
Mean levels of Agreeableness in five cultures. *T* scores are based on the mean and standard deviation of all respondents over age 21 within each culture. Age groups do not differ significantly in the British and Spanish samples. Error bars: SEM.

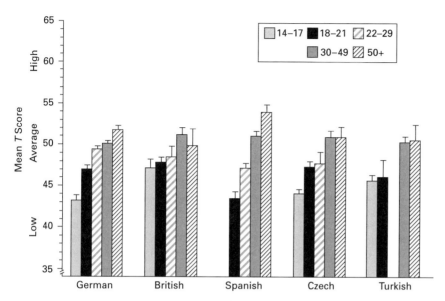

Figure 46.6
Mean levels of Conscientiousness in five cultures. *T* scores are based on the mean and standard deviation of all respondents over age 21 within each culture. Error bars: SEM.

are significant increases in Agreeableness in the German, Czech, and Turkish samples, but these trends do not reach significance in the British and Spanish samples. The hypothesized decline in Openness to Experience is seen clearly in the Spanish sample, and is significant in the Czech and Turkish samples. In contrast, German and British samples show significantly lower levels of Openness to Experience in the youngest group than in the group of 18- to 21-year-olds. (The same pattern was seen when mean peer ratings were examined in the German sample.) It is not clear whether this reflects a true developmental trend, a sampling bias, or some culture-specific phenomenon.

Although the pattern of results across these samples conforms very closely to hypotheses, it is important to recall that most of the effects are quite small in magnitude. Across cultures, the median correlations of age with Neuroticism,

Extraversion, Openness to Experience, Agreeableness, and Conscientiousness scales are $-.17$, $-.21$, $-.08$, .09, and .23, respectively. Thus, previous reviews of the literature that concluded that mean levels of personality traits are generally stable in adulthood (McCrae & Costa, 1990) are only modestly qualified by the present findings.

To date, most information on adult age differences in personality has been based on analyses of self-reports. Comparison of peer ratings of college-age men (Costa, McCrae, & Dembroski, 1989) with older adult men (see Costa & McCrae, 1989) on the original NEO Personality Inventory showed significant effects in the expected direction for all five domains, which were substantial in magnitude (greater than one-half standard deviation) for Neuroticism and Conscientiousness. However, in the German sample examined here, mean peer ratings showed significant correlations with age only for Neuroticism

(−.05), Agreeableness (.06), and Conscientious-ness (.21). Research using the full NEO-PI-R in other cultures would be helpful in clarifying the nature and extent of age differences and changes in observer-rated personality traits.

The NEO-FFI used in the present study does not assess specific facets of the five factors. Earlier research, however, has shown that individual facet scales of the NEO-PI-R show distinctive age trends across cultures. For example, the Excitement-Seeking facet of Extraversion declined markedly in nine out of nine cultures, whereas the Assertiveness facet showed significant (and small) declines in only four of them. Additional analyses on the specific variance in facet scales (net of the five factors) also showed generalizable, albeit very small, effects (Costa et al., in press).

Intrinsic Maturation and Adult Temperament

The data in Figures 46.2–46.6 are largely consistent with earlier observations that the same pattern of age differences in personality traits can be seen across different cultures with different recent histories. There appear to be three possible explanations for this phenomenon. The first is that age differences are cohort effects, reflecting the influence of historical forces common to all these cultures, such as the rise of the mass media or the near-universal improvement in health care. Although this possibility cannot be excluded, it would seem to be a remarkable coincidence that common historical forces affect all five factors, whereas historical experiences unique to each culture affect none of the factors enough to reverse the usual pattern.

One way to test this hypothesis would be to assess the effect within cultures of variables that might plausibly account for common cohort differences. For example, higher levels of Openness to Experience in younger cohorts might be due to increasing levels of formal education over the course of this century in most cultures. If so, covarying years of education would reduce or

eliminate age differences in Openness to Experience. We tested that hypothesis in the Spanish, German, and Turkish samples, in which data on education were available, but found that significant age differences in Openness to Experience remained.

A second possibility is that societies everywhere (or perhaps modern industrial societies everywhere) spontaneously develop parallel institutions that encourage the same trends in personality development. Adult responsibilities may make adults more responsible; caring for children may make them more caring. This possibility cannot be easily dismissed, but it is not yet proven. Even if there is an association between age-role demands and personality traits, it is possible that the causal order is reversed, and that social norms have been crafted to accommodate intrinsic maturational trends in personality. This is quite clear in the case of laws defining a minimum age for driving, voting, and drinking.

A third possibility is that there are natural progressions of personality development that occur without regard to cultural and historical context. Just as children learn to talk, count, and reason in a fixed order and time course, so too may adults become more agreeable and less extraverted as a natural consequence of aging. This notion of intrinsic maturation is consistent with the other lines of evidence—heritability, stability, and cross-cultural universality—that point to the interpretation of traits as endogenous basic tendencies.

It is also supported more directly by behavior–genetic and comparative evidence on age changes in personality. Changes in personality traits between adolescence and young adulthood have been shown to be modestly to moderately heritable (McGue et al., 1993), and developmental trends in chimpanzees (King, Landau, & Guggenheim, 1998) and rhesus monkeys (Suomi, Novak, & Well, 1996) have shown some intriguing parallels to adult human development.

Whether age grading in the social structure shapes personality development or vice-versa—

or whether both processes are at work—cannot be determined from available data. Future research might test these alternative hypotheses in third-world nations where adult responsibilities are assumed at an earlier age or among people with different relevant life experiences, such as parenting. But viewing personality as temperament at least has the virtue of making intrinsic maturation a plausible hypothesis that merits testing.

Linking Child Temperament and Adult Personality

The intent of the whole preceding argument was to demonstrate that if by temperament we mean biologically based psychological tendencies with intrinsic paths of development, then standard personality inventories assess temperament, and traits such as aesthetic sensitivity, achievement striving, and modesty are as much temperaments as are activity level and behavioral inhibition. From this perspective it is perhaps not surprising that when Angleitner and Ostendorf (1994) factored adult temperament measures (A. H. Buss & Plomin, 1975; Strelau, Angleitner, Bantelmann, & Ruch, 1990) along with other markers they found the familiar structure of the five-factor model.

But if the individual differences identified by temperament researchers and personality trait psychologists are much the same, the goals and methods of these two research traditions are not. Researchers within the temperament tradition often emphasize basic processes and mechanisms. Ahadi and Rothbart (1994), for example, have examined psychological systems such as Approach and Effortful Control, and Strelau and colleagues (Strelau et al., 1990) have developed a set of constructs based on hypothesized Pavlovian properties of the central nervous system. In contrast, trait psychologists more often focus on outcomes and other correlates of traits. For example, Barrick and Mount (1991) showed

that Conscientiousness is associated with superior job performance. By identifying personality traits with temperaments, researchers may begin to integrate these different emphases on causes and effects and come to a better understanding of both the origins and the expressions of basic tendencies (Costa & McCrae, in press).

The Structure and Stability of Individual Differences

It cannot be assumed that the adult structure of temperament will appear in analyses of temperament variables in children, but there is evidence that something similar to the five factors can be found in adult ratings of school children (Digman & Shmelyov, 1996; Kohnstamm, Halverson, Mervielde, & Havill, 1998) and in self-reports from children as young as 5 years old (Measelle & John, 1997). Ahadi and Rothbart (1994) have offered conceptual analyses that link child temperament constructs to adult personality factors: Approach to Extraversion, Anxiety to Neuroticism, and Effortful Control to Conscientiousness and Agreeableness. Classic efforts at understanding infant temperament (Thomas, Chess, & Birch, 1968) were not informed by the five-factor model; if investigators looked for these factors, they might find them even in neonates, just as they have been found in nonhuman animals (King & Figueredo, 1997).

Even if identical factors were found in infants and adults, it would not imply that infant temperament is a good predictor of adult personality. Reviews of the longitudinal literature have reported that temperament variables in fact show limited stability across relatively short intervals, especially among infants (e.g., Lemery, Goldsmith, Klinnert, & Mrazek, 1999), and very modest prediction of adult traits (Wachs, 1994). Block (1993), for example, examined retest correlations for ego undercontrol and ego resiliency at age 3 and age 23 in boys and girls; only one of these four correlations reached significance (although all were positive). In a recent review of the longitudinal attachment literature, Fraley (1998) reported an average correlation of .19 between attachment at age 1 and age 19. Kagan and Zentner (1996) found only modest associations between characteristics of early childhood and adult psychopathology.

Even modest associations can be meaningful if the outcomes are socially significant. Caspi and colleagues (Caspi, Elder, & Herbener, 1990) have shown that childhood personality traits (including shyness and ill-temperedness) can predict important life outcomes such as delayed marriage and downward mobility. Undercontrol at age 3 predicts health-risk behaviors in young adults through the mediation of personality traits in adolescence (Caspi et al., 1997).

With shorter intervals and older children, stronger associations are found. For example, ego control showed a retest correlation of .70 between age 3 and age 4, and .67 between age 14 and age 23 (Block, 1993). Siegler and colleagues (Siegler et al., 1990) estimated that half of the variance in personality dimensions is stable from late adolescence to middle adulthood, and Helson and Moane (1987) reported greater stability between age 27 and age 43 (a 16-year interval) than between age 21 and age 27 (a 6-year interval). When adults initially over age 30 are studied, uncorrected retest coefficients near .70 are not uncommon over 30-year periods (Costa & McCrae, 1992b).

One very general principle of life span personality development thus appears to be that the stability of individual differences over a fixed time interval increases steadily from infancy up to at least age 30. Environmentalists might assume that this phenomenon is attributable to the accumulation of life experiences: Any single new experience should affect more change when it occurs in the context of the limited experience of early life than when it competes with a lifetime of other experiences.

In contrast, FFT suggests another answer: Endogenous dispositions develop over time in ways that redistribute rank orderings. The func-

tioning of genes, after all, is not fixed at birth; they switch on and off across the life span and contribute to individual patterns of aging. The brain itself continues to grow and develop until at least the mid-20s (Pujol, Vendrell, Junqué, Martí-Vilalta, & Capdevila, 1993), so it is hardly surprising that personality traits would also change in this period.

Developmental Trends for Five Factors

At the aggregate level, it is possible to describe general developmental trends for the five factors (and the specific traits that define them; see McCrae et al., 1999). From age 18 to age 30 there are declines in Neuroticism, Extraversion, and Openness to Experience, and increases in Agreeableness and Conscientiousness; after age 30 the same trends are found, although the rate of change seems to decrease.

In this chapter we presented some of the first data tracing the five factors backward from age 18, with German, British, Czech, and Turkish samples. For the most part, high-school-age boys and girls appeared to continue the same trends: They were even higher in Neuroticism and Extraversion and lower in Agreeableness and Conscientiousness than were college-age students. No clear trend could be discerned for Openness to Experience, as lower instead of higher scores were found in the German and British samples.

The present data do support the use of instruments like the NEO-FFI in younger adolescents, and it would be a relatively simple matter to conduct cross-sectional studies on representative samples of this age group. Research with even younger samples is possible, but would require new instruments. Measelle and John (1997), for example, used a puppet interview to assess personality in young children and reported increases in Conscientiousness between ages 5 and 7. Calibrating puppet interviews and NEO-FFIs would be difficult, so it is likely that developmental trends will have to be pieced together from studies of overlapping segments of childhood.

What could account for these developmental trends? Evolutionary arguments might be offered. High levels of Extraversion and Openness to Experience might be useful in finding a mate, whereas higher Agreeableness and Conscientiousness might be more important for raising a family. Comparative studies of personality development in other primates (King et al., 1998) with different patterns of mating and child rearing might be used to test such evolutionary hypotheses.

The Development of Characteristic Adaptations

Finally, it is worth recalling that FFT postulates developments on two separate tracks: Basic tendencies follow a pattern of intrinsic maturation, whereas characteristic adaptations respond to the opportunities and incentives of the social environment. To the extent that the theory is correct, psychologists, educators, and parents will have relatively little impact on the long-term development of personality traits, but they can have an influence on characteristic adaptations (cf. Harkness & Lilienfeld, 1997). Traits can be channeled even if they cannot be changed. What kinds of habits, skills, beliefs, and social networks are optimal for shy or ill-tempered children? These are likely to be the most productive questions for those concerned about shaping human development.

References

Agronick, G. S., & Duncan, L. E. (1998). Personality and social change: Individual differences, life path, and importance attributed to the women's movement. *Journal of Personality and Social Psychology, 74,* 1545–1555.

Ahadi, S. A., & Rothbart, M. K. (1994). Temperament, development, and the Big Five. In C. F. Halverson, Jr., G. A. Kohnstamm, & R. P. Martin (Eds.), *The developing structure of temperament and personality from infancy to adulthood* (pp. 189–207). Hillsdale, NJ: Erlbaum.

Ahadi, S. A., Rothbart, M. K., & Ye, R. (1993). Children's temperament in the US and China: Similarities and differences. *European Journal of Personality, 7,* 359–377.

Angleitner, A., & Ostendorf, F. (1994). Temperament and the Big Five factors of personality. In C. F. Halverson, G. A. Kohnstamm, & R. P. Martin (Eds.), *The developing structure of temperament and personality from infancy to adulthood* (pp. 69–90). Hillsdale, NJ: Erlbaum.

Asendorpf, J. B., & Wilpers, S. (1998). Personality effects on social relationships. *Journal of Personality and Social Psychology, 74,* 1531–1544.

Barrick, M. R., & Mount, M. K. (1991). The Big Five personality dimensions and job performance: A meta-analysis. *Personnel Psychology, 44,* 1–26.

Begley, S. (1998, September 7). The parent trap. *Newsweek,* 52–59.

Benet-Martínez, V., & Waller, N. G. (1997). Further evidence for the cross-cultural generality of the Big Seven Factor model: Indigenous and imported Spanish personality constructs. *Journal of Personality, 65,* 567–598.

Block, J. (1981). Some enduring and consequential structures of personality. In A. I. Rabin, J. Aronoff, A. M. Barclay, & R. A. Zucker (Eds.), *Further explorations in personality* (pp. 27–43). New York: Wiley-Interscience.

Block, J. (1993). Studying personality the long way. In D. C. Funder, R. D. Parke, C. Tomlinson-Keasey, & K. Widaman (Eds.), *Studying lives through time: Personality and development* (pp. 9–41). Washington, DC: American Psychological Association.

Bremner, J. D. (1998). Neuroimaging of posttraumatic stress disorder. *Psychiatric Annals, 28,* 445–450.

Buss, A. H. (1997). Evolutionary perspectives on personality traits. In R. Hogan, J. Johnson, & S. R. Briggs (Eds.), *Handbook of personality psychology* (pp. 345–366). San Diego, CA: Academic Press.

Buss, A. H., & Plomin, R. (1975). *A temperament theory of personality development.* New York: Wiley.

Buss, D. M. (1991). Evolutionary personality psychology. *Annual Review of Psychology, 42,* 459–491.

Buss, D. M., & Greiling, H. (1999). Adaptive individual differences. *Journal of Personality, 67,* 209–243.

Caspi, A., Begg, D., Dickson, N., Harrington, H. L., Langley, J., Moffitt, T. E., & Silva, P. A. (1997). Personality differences predict health-risk behaviors in young adulthood: Evidence from a longitudinal study. *Journal of Personality and Social Psychology, 73,* 1052–1063.

Caspi, A., Elder, G. H., Jr., & Herbener, E. S. (1990). Childhood personality and the prediction of life-course patterns. In L. N. Robins & M. Rutter (Eds.), *Straight and devious pathways from childhood to adulthood* (pp. 13–35). New York: Cambridge University Press.

Cheung, F. M., Leung, K., Fan, R. M., Song, W. Z., Zhang, J. X., & Zhang, J. P. (1996). Development of the Chinese Personality Assessment Inventory. *Journal of Cross-Cultural Psychology, 27,* 181–199.

Church, A. T., Katigbak, M. S., & Reyes, J. A. S. (1998). Further exploration of Filipino personality structure using the lexical approach: Do the Big-Five or Big-Seven dimensions emerge? *European Journal of Personality, 12,* 249–270.

Cloninger, C. R., Przybeck, T. R., Svrakic, D. M., & Wetzel, R. D. (1994). *The Temperament and Character Inventory (TCI): A guide to its development and use.* St. Louis, MO: Washington University, Center for Psychobiology of Personality.

Costa, P. T., Jr., & McCrae, R. R. (1989). *The NEO-PI/NEO-FFI manual supplement.* Odessa, FL: Psychological Assessment Resources.

Costa, P. T., Jr., & McCrae, R. R. (1992a). *Revised NEO Personality Inventory (NEO-PI-R) and NEO Five-Factor Inventory (NEO-FFI) professional manual.* Odessa, FL: Psychological Assessment Resources.

Costa, P. T., Jr., & McCrae, R. R. (1992b). Trait psychology comes of age. In T. B. Sonderegger (Ed.), *Nebraska Symposium on Motivation: Psychology and aging* (pp. 169–204). Lincoln: University of Nebraska Press.

Costa, P. T., Jr., & McCrae, R. R. (1994). Stability and change in personality from adolescence through adulthood. In C. F. Halverson, G. A. Kohnstamm, & R. P. Martin (Eds.), *The developing structure of temperament and personality from infancy to adulthood* (pp. 139–150). Hillsdale, NJ: Erlbaum.

Costa, P. T., Jr., & McCrae, R. R. (in press). A theoretical context for adult temperament. In T. D. Wachs & G. A. Kohnstamm (Eds.), *Temperament in context.* Hillsdale, NJ: Erlbaum.

Costa, P. T., Jr., McCrae, R. R., & Dembroski, T. M. (1989). Agreeableness vs. antagonism: Explication of a potential risk factor for CHD. In A. Siegman & T. M. Dembroski (Eds.), *In search of coronary-prone behavior: Beyond Type A* (pp. 41–63). Hillsdale, NJ: Erlbaum.

Costa, P. T., Jr., McCrae, R. R., Martin, T. A., Oryol, V. E., Senin, I. G., Rukavishnikov, A. A., Shimonaka, Y., Nakazato, K., Gondo, Y., Takayama, M., Allik, J., Kallasmaa, T., & Realo, A. (in press). Personality development from adolescence through adulthood: Further cross-cultural comparisons of age differences. In V. J. Molfese & D. Molfese (Eds.), *Temperament and personality development across the life span.* Hillsdale, NJ: Erlbaum.

Costa, P. T., Jr., McCrae, R. R., Zonderman, A. B., Barbano, H. E., Lebowitz, B., & Larson, D. M. (1986). Cross-sectional studies of personality in a national sample: 2. Stability in neuroticism, extraversion, and openness. *Psychology and Aging, 1,* 144–149.

Digman, J. M., & Shmelyov, A. G. (1996). The structure of temperament and personality in Russian children. *Journal of Personality and Social Psychology, 71,* 341–351.

Eysenck, H. J. (1990). Genetic and environmental contributions to individual differences: The three major dimensions of personality. *Journal of Personality, 58,* 245–262.

Eysenck, S. B. G. (1983). One approach to cross-cultural studies of personality. *Australian Journal of Psychology, 35,* 383–390.

Finn, S. E. (1986). Stability of personality self-ratings over 30 years: Evidence for an age/cohort interaction. *Journal of Personality and Social Psychology, 50,* 813–818.

Fraley, R. C. (1998). *Attachment continuity from infancy to adulthood: Meta-analysis and dynamic modeling of developmental mechanisms.* Unpublished manuscript, University of California, Davis.

Goldberg, L. R. (1993). The structure of phenotypic personality traits. *American Psychologist, 48,* 26–34.

Gosling, S. D. (1998). *From mice to men: What can animal research tell us about human personality?* Unpublished manuscript, University of California, Berkeley.

Gosling, S. D., & John, O. P. (1998, May). Personality dimensions in dogs, cats, and hyenas. In S. D. Gosling

& S. Suomi (Chairs), *From mice to men: Bridging the gap between personality and animal researchers.* Symposium conducted at the 10th Annual Convention of the American Psychological Society, Washington, DC.

Gough, H. G. (1987). *California Psychological Inventory administrator's guide.* Palo Alto, CA: Consulting Psychologists Press.

Guilford, J. S., Zimmerman, W. S., & Guilford, J. P. (1976). *The Guilford–Zimmerman Temperament Survey Handbook: Twenty-five years of research and application.* San Diego, CA: EdITS.

Harkness, A. R., & Lilienfeld, S. O. (1997). Individual differences science for treatment planning: Personality traits. *Psychological Assessment, 9,* 349–360.

Harris, J. R. (1998). *The nurture assumption: Why children turn out the way they do.* New York: Free Press.

Helson, R., & Moane, G. (1987). Personality change in women from college to midlife. *Journal of Personality and Social Psychology, 53,* 176–186.

Jang, K. L., McCrae, R. R., Angleitner, A., Riemann, R., & Livesley, W. J. (1998). Heritability of facet-level traits in a cross-cultural twin study: Support for a hierarchical model of personality. *Journal of Personality and Social Psychology, 74,* 1556–1565.

Jessor, R. (1983). The stability of change: Psychosocial development from adolescence to young adulthood. In D. Magnusson & V. L. Allen (Eds.), *Human development: An interactional perspective* (pp. 321–341). New York: Academic Press.

Juni, S. (1996). Review of the revised NEO Personality Inventory. In J. C. Conoley & J. C. Impara (Eds.), *12th Mental Measurements Yearbook* (pp. 863–868). Lincoln: University of Nebraska Press.

Kagan, J., & Moss, H. A. (1962). *From birth to maturity.* New York: Wiley.

Kagan, J., & Zentner, M. (1996). Early childhood predictors of adult psychopathology. *Harvard Review of Psychiatry, 3,* 341–350.

Kagitçibaşi, Ç. (1996). *Family and human development across cultures: A view from the other side.* Hillsdale, NJ: Erlbaum.

King, J. E., & Figueredo, A. J. (1997). The five-factor model plus dominance in chimpanzee personality. *Journal of Research in Personality, 31,* 257–271.

King, J. E., Landau, V. I., & Guggenheim, C. B. (1998, May). Age-related personality changes in chim-panzees. In S. D. Gosling & S. Suomi (Chairs), *From mice to men: Bridging the gap between personality and animal researchers.* Symposium conducted at the 10th Annual Convention of the American Psychological Society, Washington, DC.

Kitayama, S., & Markus, H. R. (Eds.). (1994). *Emotion and culture: Empirical studies of mutual influences.* Washington, DC: American Psychological Association.

Kluckhohn, C. (1944). Navaho witchcraft. *Papers of the Peabody Museum of American Archaeology and Ethnology* (Vol. 22, No. 3). Cambridge, MA: Harvard University.

Kluckhohn, C., & Murray, H. A. (1953). Personality formation: The determinants. In C. Kluckhohn, H. A. Murray, & D. M. Schneider (Eds.), *Personality in nature, society, and culture* (2nd ed., pp. 53–67). New York: Knopf.

Kohnstamm, G. A., Halverson, C. F., Jr., Mervielde, I., & Havill, V. L. (Eds.). (1998). *Parental descriptions of child personality: Developmental antecedents of the Big Five?* Hillsdale, NJ: Erlbaum.

Kolb, B., & Whishaw, I. Q. (1998). Brain plasticity and behavior. *Annual Review of Psychology, 49,* 43–64.

Labouvie-Vief, G., Diehl, M., Tarnowski, A., & Shen, J. (in press). Age differences in adult personality: Findings from the United States and China. *Journal of Gerontology: Psychological Sciences.*

Lemery, K. S., Goldsmith, H. H., Klinnert, M. D., & Mrazek, D. A. (1999). Developmental models of infant and childhood temperament. *Developmental Psychology, 35,* 189–204.

Loehlin, J. C. (1992). *Genes and environment in personality development.* Newbury Park, CA: Sage.

Martin, T. A., Draguns, J. G., Oryol, V. E., Senin, I. G., Rukavishnikov, A. A., & Klotz, M. L. (1997, August). *Development of a Russian-language NEO-PI-R.* Paper presented at the 105th Annual Convention of the American Psychological Association, Chicago, IL.

McAdams, D. P. (1996). Personality, modernity, and the storied self: A contemporary framework for studying persons. *Psychological Inquiry, 7,* 295–321.

McCrae, R. R., & Costa, P. T., Jr. (1988). Recalled parent–child relations and adult personality. *Journal of Personality, 56,* 417–434.

McCrae, R. R., & Costa, P. T., Jr. (1990). *Personality in adulthood.* New York: Guilford Press.

McCrae, R. R., & Costa, P. T., Jr. (1994). The para-dox of parental influence: Understanding retrospective studies of parent–child relations and adult personality. In C. Perris, W. A. Arrindell, & M. Eisemann (Eds.), *Parenting and psychopathology* (pp. 107–125). New York: Wiley.

McCrae, R. R., & Costa, P. T., Jr. (1996). Toward a new generation of personality theories: Theoretical contexts for the five-factor model. In J. S. Wiggins (Ed.), *The five-factor model of personality: Theoretical perspectives* (pp. 51–87). New York: Guilford Press.

McCrae, R. R., & Costa, P. T., Jr. (1997). Personality trait structure as a human universal. *American Psychologist, 52,* 509–516.

McCrae, R. R., & Costa, P. T., Jr. (1999). A five-factor theory of personality. In L. Pervin & O. P. John (Eds.), *Handbook of personality* (2nd ed., pp. 139–153). New York: Guilford Press.

McCrae, R. R., Costa, P. T., Jr., del Pilar, G. H., Rolland, J. P., & Parker, W. D. (1998). Cross-cultural assessment of the five-factor model: The Revised NEO Personality Inventory. *Journal of Cross-Cultural Psychology, 29,* 171–188.

McCrae, R. R., Costa, P. T., Jr., Lima, M. P., Simões, A., Ostendorf, F., Angleitner, A., Marušić, I., Bratko, D., Caprara, G. V., Barbaranelli, C., Chae, J. H., & Piedmont, R. L. (1999). Age differences in personality across the adult life span: Parallels in five cultures. *Developmental Psychology, 35,* 466–477.

McCrae, R. R., Yik, M. S. M., Trapnell, P. D., Bond, M. H., & Paulhus, D. L. (1998). Interpreting personality profiles across cultures: Bilingual, acculturation, and peer rating studies of Chinese undergraduates. *Journal of Personality and Social Psychology, 74,* 1041–1055.

McGue, M., Bacon, S., & Lykken, D. T. (1993). Personality stability and change in early adulthood: A behavioral genetic analysis. *Developmental Psychology, 29,* 96–109.

Measelle, J., & John, O. P. (1997, May). *Young children's self-perceptions on the Big Five: Consistency, stability, and school adaptation from age 5 to age 7.* Paper presented at the Biennial Meeting of the Society for Research in Child Development, Washington, DC.

Morris, W. (1976). *The American heritage dictionary of the English language.* Boston: Houghton Mifflin.

Nelson, C. A. (1999). Neural plasticity and human development. *Current Directions in Psychological Science, 8,* 42–45.

Norman, W. T., & Goldberg, L. R. (1966). Raters, ratees, and randomness in personality structure. *Journal of Personality and Social Psychology, 4,* 681–691.

Parker, W. D., & Stumpf, H. (1998). A validation of the five-factor model of personality in academically-talented youth across observers and instruments. *Personality and Individual Differences, 25,* 1005–1025.

Passini, F. T., & Norman, W. T. (1966). A universal conception of personality structure? *Journal of Personality and Social Psychology, 4,* 44–49.

Paunonen, S. V., Jackson, D. N., Trzebinski, J., & Forsterling, F. (1992). Personality structure across cultures: A multimethod evaluation. *Journal of Personality and Social Psychology, 62,* 447–456.

Plomin, R., Corley, R., Caspi, A., Fulker, D. W., & DeFries, J. (1998). Adoption results for self-reported personality: Evidence for nonadditive genetic effects? *Journal of Personality and Social Psychology, 75,* 211–218.

Plomin, R., & Daniels, D. (1987). Why are children in the same family so different from one another? *Behavioral and Brain Sciences, 10,* 1–16.

Pujol, J., Vendrell, P., Junqué, C., Martí-Vilalta, J. L., & Capdevila, A. (1993). When does human brain development end? Evidence of corpus callosum growth up to adulthood. *Annals of Neurology, 34,* 71–75.

Rapee, R. M. (1997). Potential role of childrearing practices in the development of anxiety and depression. *Clinical Psychology Review, 17,* 47–67.

Resnick, S. M., Gottesman, I. I., & McGue, M. (1993). Sensation seeking in opposite-sex twins: An effect of prenatal hormones? *Behavior Genetics, 23,* 323–329.

Riemann, R., Angleitner, A., & Strelau, J. (1997). Genetic and environmental influences on personality: A study of twins reared together using the self- and peer-report NEO-FFI scales. *Journal of Personality, 65,* 449–475.

Siegler, I. C., & Costa, P. T., Jr. (1999, August). *Personality continuity and change in midlife men and women.* Symposium presented at the 107th Annual Convention of the American Psychological Association, Boston, MA.

Siegler, I. C., George, L. K., & Okun, M. A. (1979). Cross-sequential analysis of adult personality. *Developmental Psychology, 15,* 350–351.

Siegler, I. C., Zonderman, A. B., Barefoot, J. C., Williams, R. B., Jr., Costa, P. T., Jr., & McCrae, R. R. (1990). Predicting personality in adulthood from college MMPI scores: Implications for follow-up studies in psychosomatic medicine. *Psychosomatic Medicine, 52,* 644–652.

Singer, M. (1961). A survey of culture and personality theory and research. In B. Kaplan (Ed.), *Studying personality cross-culturally* (pp. 9–90). Evanston, IL: Row, Peterson.

Strelau, J., Angleitner, A., Bantelmann, J., & Ruch, W. (1990). The Strelau Temperament Inventory—Revised (STI-R): Theoretical considerations and scale development. *European Journal of Personality, 4,* 209–235.

Stumpf, H. (1993). The factor structure of the Personality Research Form: A cross-national evaluation. *Journal of Personality, 61,* 27–48.

Suomi, S. J., Novak, M. A., & Well, A. (1996). Aging in rhesus monkeys: Different windows on behavioral continuity and change. *Developmental Psychology, 32,* 1116–1128.

Tellegen, A. (1988). The analysis of consistency in personality assessment. *Journal of Personality, 56,* 621–663.

Thomas, A., Chess, S., & Birch, H. G. (1968). *Temperament and behavior disorders in children.* New York: New York University Press.

Tooby, J., & Cosmides, L. (1990). On the universality of human nature and the uniqueness of the individual: The role of genetics and adaptation. *Journal of Personality, 58,* 17–68.

Wachs, T. D. (1994). Fit, context, and the transition between temperament and personality. In C. F. Halverson, Jr., G. A. Kohnstamm, & R. P. Martin (Eds.), *The developing structure of temperament and personality from infancy to adulthood* (pp. 209–220). Hillsdale, NJ: Erlbaum.

Xiu, S., Wu, Z., Wu, Z., & Shui, C. (1996). Study of age differences on personality features of adults. *Psychological Science, 19,* 1–5. [in Chinese]

Yang, J., McCrae, R. R., & Costa, P. T., Jr. (1998). Adult age differences in personality traits in the United States and the People's Republic of China. *Journal of Gerontology: Psychological Sciences, 53B,* P375–P383.

V BIOLOGY OF SOCIAL RELATIONSHIPS AND INTERPERSONAL PROCESSES

B. Social Applications

i. Attachment

Dario Maestripieri

In 1969, Bowlby published the first volume of his trilogy on *Attachment and Loss*. In it, he laid out the basic principles of a new theory aimed at explaining the nature of the social bond between infants and their caregivers, most notably their mothers. After 30 years of research focused on the processes associated with the formation, maintenance, and breaking of infants' bonds with their caregivers, psychologists are now turning their attention to attachment from the caregiver's perspective (George & Solomon, 1999).

Maternal attachment can be viewed as a set of behaviors whose function is to maintain proximity and interaction with the infant. As the early conceptualizations and empirical studies of infant attachment were informed by research with nonhuman primates (hereafter, primates), so the recent research on maternal attachment has been informed by primate studies. For example, both primate and human studies have recently investigated whether motivation for caregiving changes across pregnancy in relation to hormonal changes, whether the first few postpartum days are a sensitive period for this motivation, and whether hormonal variables predict differences in caregiving motivation and behavior among individuals. In this chapter, I review some recent findings in these three areas of research and discuss similarities and differences between primate and human data.

Changes in Caregiving Motivation during Pregnancy

In group-living macaques, caregiving motivation during pregnancy can be measured by the frequency with which females touch, hold, groom, or carry other females' newborn infants. Interactions with young infants are by no means limited to pregnant females. Macaque females of all ages and reproductive stages show some interest

in young infants and attempt to interact with them. This suggests that in primates, just as in humans and other mammals, pregnancy hormones (such as estradiol and progesterone) are not necessary for the expression of caregiving motivation. The question addressed by recent primate studies, however, is not whether hormones are necessary for caregiving motivation but whether the hormonal changes underlying pregnancy enhance caregiving motivation.

A recent study of pigtail macaques reported that the frequency of interaction with infants increased during late pregnancy and peaked the week before birth (Maestripieri & Zehr, 1998). The increase in caregiving motivation during late pregnancy was correlated with an increase in the concentrations of estradiol in the blood and in the estradiol to progesterone ratio. This correlational evidence that hormones can affect caregiving motivation was corroborated by experimental manipulations. Rhesus macaque females whose ovaries had been removed increased significantly their frequency of interactions with other females' infants after receiving estradiol in doses similar to those of middle-late pregnancy (Maestripieri & Zehr, 1998). Furthermore, nonpregnant marmoset females treated with estrogen and progesterone in concentrations similar to those of late pregnancy showed a significantly higher motivation to interact with infants than nontreated females (Pryce, Döbeli, & Martin, 1993).

Human pregnancy is characterized by hormonal changes very similar to those occurring in primates and other mammals. Both longitudinal and cross-sectional studies of women in their first pregnancy have shown that, in most cases, women experience increased maternal feelings toward their own fetus at about 20 to 24 weeks of gestation (Corter & Fleming, 1995). Changes in maternal feelings during pregnancy do not appear to be correlated with changes in concentrations of hormones such as estradiol, progesterone, prolactin, or cortisol (Corter & Fleming, 1995). However, it is possible that if changes in maternal attachment during pregnancy were assessed with behavioral and psychophysiological measures (e.g., heart rate responses to infant cries) instead of women's self-reports on their feelings of attachment, an association between changes in caregiving motivation and hormones would become apparent.

Is There a Postpartum Sensitive Period for Caregiving Motivation?

Klaus and Kennell (1976) hypothesized that there may be a sensitive period shortly after birth during which it is necessary for mothers to be in close contact with their infants for later child development to be optimal. Many subsequent studies of bonding concluded that the evidence for such a sensitive period was at best equivocal and, consequently, research on bonding was abandoned. Although the concept of mother-infant bonding was extrapolated from animal research, what most human studies attempted to demonstrate (i.e., that slight differences in time spent in contact during the postpartum period would have long-lasting consequences for the parent-child relationship) has never been demonstrated in animals either. In fact, a recent reanalysis of the primate data has provided some evidence that the postpartum period may be a sensitive period for caregiving motivation, but not necessarily for infant attachment or development (Maestripieri, in press).

Naturalistic observations of macaques have shown that a mother whose infant died shortly after birth may kidnap a newborn from another new mother and adopt it. Occasionally, a new mother with a live infant may adopt another newborn and raise both infants as if they were twins. Interestingly, although infant mortality is by no means limited to the early postpartum period, all cases of newborn adoption have been reported to occur within the first 2 postpartum weeks, suggesting that the potential for adoption is highest during this period.

Experimental studies in which infants have been swapped between mothers also suggest that there is a postpartum sensitive period for caregiving motivation (Maestripieri, in press). In particular, the evidence suggests that (a) when mother and infant are separated during the sensitive period, the mother is likely to accept her own infant or an alien infant with similar characteristics if reunion occurs before the end of the sensitive period; (b) when mother and infant are separated during the sensitive period, the mother is likely to reject her own infant and any other infant if reunion occurs after the end of the sensitive period; and (c) when mother and infant are separated after the sensitive period and later reunited, the mother is likely to accept her own infant but reject any other infant. These findings are unlikely to be accounted for by learning processes related to recognition of offspring. Rather, they suggest that the physiological changes associated with childbirth and early lactation may be associated with a period of heightened responsiveness to infant stimuli and motivation for caregiving behavior.

Whether humans also have a postpartum sensitive period for caregiving motivation is not clear. Even if such a sensitive period were discovered, its implications for later parenting and child development would remain to be established. It is obvious that human adoption is the product of deliberate choice and that foster parents can provide excellent care. Nevertheless, the fact remains that if hormones and other biological variables have some effects on caregiving motivation, however small these effects might be, psychologists can no longer afford to overlook them.

Individual Differences in Caregiving Motivation and Behavior

Investigating whether differences in caregiving motivation or behavior among individuals are, at least in part, accounted for by hormonal or other biological variables is probably the greatest challenge for research on maternal attachment. This is because, in both primates and humans individual differences in motivation and behavior are affected to a great extent by previous experience and the surrounding environment. Therefore, a full understanding of the causes of individual differences in caregiving would require knowledge of the complex interactions among biological, cognitive, and social processes.

Some of the most obvious individual differences in behavior are related to sex. In most mammalian species, there is a clear sex difference in caregiving motivation and behavior, with females being far more involved in caregiving than males. In only a few species of primates do males participate in caregiving, and these cases appear to reflect special reproductive and ecological circumstances. For example, in New World monkeys such as marmosets and tamarins, females give birth to twins and fathers share the energetic costs of infant carrying with mothers. In rhesus macaques, the sex difference in interest in infants appears in the 1st year of life and persists through adulthood. A rhesus macaque female begins handling newborn infants when she is only a few months old and barely big and strong enough to lift them off the ground. In contrast, males of the same age show little or no interest in interacting with infants. A similar sex difference in interaction with infants has been reported for human children and adolescents in a number of cultures. In humans, such difference may, at least in part, be the product of socialization, and in particular the different expectations that parents in most cultures have for their sons and daughters in terms of child-care roles. In macaques, however, the sex difference in behavior toward infants is unlikely to be the product of socialization because there are no consistent differences in the way mothers, or other group members, interact with males and females during their first year of life (Fairbanks, 1996).

An alternative explanation has to do with prenatal hormones. In rhesus macaques, prenatal exposure to male hormones (androgens) is known to affect sex differences in play later in life, so that juvenile females prenatally exposed to excess androgens engage in the rough-and-tumble play that is typical of males (Goy & Phoenix, 1971). Unfortunately, no primate studies to date have investigated the relation between prenatal hormones and caregiving motivation. In a study with humans, however, girls affected by congenital adrenal hyperplasia (a common inherited syndrome in which the adrenal gland overproduces androgens) played less frequently with dolls than unaffected girls, suggesting that prenatal exposure to excess androgens may play a role in the development of sex differences in caregiving motivation (Geary, 1998).

Primate studies investigating differences in caregiving motivation or behavior among adult females have produced conflicting evidence. In a laboratory study of red-bellied tamarins, mothers that had poor parenting skills and whose infants did not survive had lower urinary concentrations of estradiol in the last week of pregnancy than mothers that had good parenting skills and whose infants survived (Pryce, Abbott, Hodges, & Martin, 1988). This difference, however, was found only in females without previous caregiving experience, not in experienced mothers. In macaques, not all pregnant females are more interested in infants than nonpregnant females, and individual differences in behavior toward infants are not necessarily related to differences in hormone levels. Rhesus macaque mothers who physically abuse their infants interact more frequently with other females' infants than nonabusive mothers during both pregnancy and lactation. However, the hormonal profiles of abusive and nonabusive mothers are generally similar. Moreover, individual differences in parenting styles during early lactation are largely unrelated to the levels of estradiol and progesterone circulating in the blood of both abusive and nonabusive mothers (Maestripieri & Megna, in press).

In recent studies of humans, mothers who maintained high levels of estradiol before and after childbirth had higher feelings of attachment to their own infants in the early postpartum days than women whose levels of estradiol were lower (Fleming, Ruble, Krieger, & Wong, 1997). Interestingly, the hormone that was most closely related to maternal behavior in the early postpartum period was not estradiol but the stress hormone cortisol. Higher salivary concentrations of cortisol were associated with more intense caregiving behavior in both first-time and experienced mothers (Fleming, Steiner, & Corter, 1997). Mothers with higher salivary concentrations of cortisol on the 1st day after childbirth were also more attracted to their own infants' body odor and better able to recognize their infants' odor than mothers with lower cortisol concentrations. Mothers' attraction to infant odors was also affected by previous experience with infants, and experience, rather than cortisol, was the best predictor of individual differences in maternal responsiveness assessed with a questionnaire.

Conclusions

Taken together, these recent studies of primates and humans suggest that the study of hormonal correlates of individual differences in caregiving, and more generally of biological influences on maternal attachment, is an enterprise that is worth pursuing. Understanding the complex interaction among biological, cognitive, and social variables in the expression of caregiving behavior will not be an easy task. However, we already possess sophisticated theoretical models integrating multiple factors that may affect caregiving motivation and variability in caregiving across the life span and different individuals (e.g., Corter & Fleming, 1995; Pryce, 1995). Such models, along with comparative studies of animal parenting, can stimulate and inform future research on maternal attachment. There are

still many important questions that remain to be addressed. Is there an interaction between prenatal hormonal influences and early postnatal experiences in the development of caregiving behavior? Are the influences of biological variables on caregiving mostly limited to first-time parents, or can these influences still be detected in reproductively experienced individuals? What are the specific similarities and differences between the processes affecting maternal and paternal attachment? Are there any biological correlates of neglectful or abusive parenting? Answering these questions will have important implications for understanding the normative processes underlying maternal attachment, as well as its pathologies.

Recommended Reading

Corter, C., & Fleming, A. S. (1995). (See References)

Maestripieri, D. (1999). The biology of human parenting: Insights from nonhuman primates. *Neuroscience & Biobehavioral Reviews, 23,* 411–422.

Acknowledgments

This work was supported by National Institute of Mental Health Awards R01-MH57249 and R01-MH62577. I thank Martha McClintock for helpful comments on this manuscript.

References

Bowlby, J. (1969). *Attachment and loss: 1. Attachment.* New York: Basic Books.

Corter, C., & Fleming, A. S. (1995). Psychobiology of maternal behavior in human beings. In M. Bornstein (Ed.), *Handbook of parenting* (pp. 87–116). Hillsdale, NJ: Erlbaum.

Fairbanks, L. A. (1996). Individual differences in maternal styles: Causes and consequences for mothers and offspring. *Advances in the Study of Behavior, 25,* 579–611.

Fleming, A. S., Ruble, D., Krieger, H., & Wong, P. Y. (1997). Hormonal and experiential correlates of maternal responsiveness during pregnancy and the puerperium in human mothers. *Hormones and Behavior, 31*, 145–158.

Fleming, A. S., Steiner, M., & Corter, C. (1997). Cortisol, hedonics, and maternal responsiveness in human mothers. *Hormones and Behavior, 32*, 85–98.

Geary D. C. (1998). *Male, female: The evolution of human sex differences.* Washington, DC: American Psychological Association.

George, C., & Solomon, J. (1999). Attachment and caregiving: The caregiving behavioral system. In J. Cassidy & P. R. Shaver (Eds.), *Handbook of attachment* (pp. 649–670). New York: Guilford Press.

Goy, R. W., & Phoenix, C. H. (1971). The effects of testosterone propionate administered before birth on the development of behaviour in genetic female rhesus monkeys. In C. H. Sawyer & R. A. Gorski (Eds.), *Steroid hormones and brain function* (pp. 193–201). Berkeley: University of California Press.

Klaus, M. H., & Kennell, J. H. (1976). *Maternal-infant bonding.* St. Louis, MO: Mosby.

Maestripieri, D. (in press). Is there mother-infant bonding in primates? *Developmental Review.*

Maestripieri, D., & Megna, N. L. (in press). Hormones and behavior in rhesus macaque abusive and non-abusive mothers: 2. Mother-infant interactions. *Physiology and Behavior.*

Maestripieri, D., & Zehr, J. L. (1998). Maternal responsiveness increases during pregnancy and after estrogen treatment in macaques. *Hormones and Behavior, 34*, 223–230.

Pryce, C. R. (1995). Determinants of motherhood in human and nonhuman primates. A biosocial model. In C. R. Pryce, R. D. Martin, & D. Skuse (Eds.), *Motherhood in human and nonhuman primates: Biosocial determinants* (pp. 1–15). Basel, Switzerland: Karger.

Pryce, C. R., Abbott, D. H., Hodges, J. H., & Martin, R. D. (1988). Maternal behavior is related to prepartum urinary estradiol levels in red-bellied tamarin monkeys. *Physiology and Behavior, 44*, 717–726.

Pryce, C. R., Döbeli, M., & Martin, R. D. (1993). Effects of sex steroids on maternal motivation in the common marmoset (*Callithrix jacchus*): Development and application of an operant system with maternal reinforcement. *Journal of Comparative Psychology, 107*, 99–115.

48 Maternal Care, Hippocampal Glucocorticoid Receptors, and Hypothalamic–Pituitary–Adrenal Responses to Stress

Dong Liu, Josie Diorio, Beth Tannenbaum, Christian Caldji, Darlene Francis, Alison Freedman,
Shakti Sharma, Deborah Pearson, Paul M. Plotsky, and Michael J. Meaney

Several years ago Levine, Denenberg, and others (1) showed that the development of hypothalamic-pituitary-adrenal (HPA) responses to stress is modified by early environmental events, including infantile stimulation [or handling (2)]. As adults, animals exposed to brief periods of handling daily for the first weeks of life show reduced pituitary adrenocorticotropic hormone (ACTH) and adrenal corticosterone (the principal glucocorticoid in the rat) responses to stress compared with nonhandled animals (3). These differences are apparent as late as 24 to 26 months of age (4), indicating that the handling effect on HPA function persists throughout life.

Glucocorticoids act at a number of neural sites to exert an inhibitory, negative-feedback effect over the synthesis of hypothalamic releasing-factors for ACTH, notably corticotropin-releasing hormone (CRH) and arginine vasopressin (AVP) (5). Postnatally handled animals show enhanced glucocorticoid negative-feedback sensitivity compared with nonhandled rats (6) and therefore decreased hypothalamic CRH and AVP mRNA expression, as well as lower levels of both CRH and AVP immuno-reactivity (7). The handling effect on feedback sensitivity is mediated by an increase in gluco-corticoid receptor (GR) expression in the hippo-campus (8, 9), a region that has been strongly implicated in glucocorticoid negative-feedback regulation (10). The increased hippocampal GR gene expression is therefore a central feature of the handling effect on HPA responsivity to stress, resulting in increased feedback inhibition of CRH and AVP synthesis and reduced pituitary ACTH release during stress.

A number of authors (11) have proposed that the effects of postnatal handling are mediated by changes in mother-pup interactions and that the handling manipulation itself might map onto naturally occurring individual differences in ma-ternal care. Specifically, Levine proposed that handling of the pups altered the behavior of the mother and that these differences in mother-pup interactions then mediate the effect of handling on the development of endocrine and behav-ioral responses to stress. The question, then, is how this maternal mediation might occur and whether such factors might contribute to natu-rally occurring individual differences in HPA responses to stress.

In the Norway rat, mother-pup contact oc-curs primarily within the context of a nest-bout, which begins when the mother approaches the litter and gathers the pups under her; she then nurses her offspring, intermittently licking and grooming the pups (12, 13). Handling results in changes in mother-pup interactions (14). Mothers of handled pups spend the same amount of time with their litters as mothers of nonhandled pups; however, mothers of handled litters had shorter, but more frequent, nest-bouts (15).

We examined the behavior of mothers of han-dled or nonhandled litters over the first 10 days of life, a "critical" period for the handling effect on HPA development (16). Mothers of handled pups showed increased levels of licking and grooming of pups and arched-back nursing (LG-ABN) compared with mothers of nonhandled pups (Table 48.1). The frequency of these two behaviors was highly correlated ($r = +0.91$); over 90% of the instances of licking and groom-ing occurred while the mother was nursing her pups in the arched-back posture. Mothers of nonhandled pups nursed no less frequently than those of handled pups (17), but tended to more frequently adopt a "blanket" or passive posture when nursing, lying over or beside the pups. These differences in licking and grooming (and the accompanying arched-back nursing posture) were the only behaviors that served to reliably

Table 48.1

Mean (± SEM) number of observations (from a total of 1200) of licking and grooming in the mothers of handled or nonhandled litters (Handling study) or high– or low–LG-ABN mothers (Maternal behavior study)

Group	Licking and grooming
Handling study	
Handled	155 ± 21*
Nonhandled	78 ± 25
Maternal behavior study	
High LG-ABN	136 ± 22*
Low LG-ABN	72 ± 8

Differences in maternal behavior were stable over the 10-day period of observation. In neither study were there group differences in the frequency with which dams nursed pups or in pup contact (16).
* $P < 0.01$.

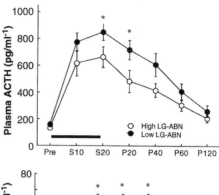

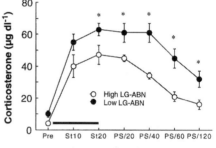

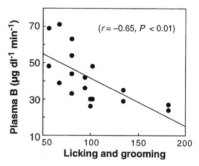

distinguish mothers of handled from those of nonhandled pups.

To determine whether the increased maternal licking and grooming affects the development of HPA responses to stress, we examined the relation between naturally occurring individual differences in maternal care and HPA development (18). We detected pronounced and stable individual differences in maternal licking and grooming (which again was highly correlated with arched-back nursing; $r = +0.94$). The variability among the dams in licking and grooming was substantial and of sufficient range to meaningfully study the relation between variations in postnatal maternal care and the development of adult responses to stress (19).

As adults, the offspring of high–LG-ABN mothers that showed significantly reduced plasma ACTH and corticosterone responses to restraint stress (20) compared with the offspring of low–LG-ABN mothers (Fig. 48.1). There were no differences in basal hormone levels (Fig. 48.1). These findings parallel those observed in

Figure 48.1

Mean (± SEM) plasma ACTH (top) and corticosterone (middle) responses to a 20-min period of restraint stress (solid bar) in the offspring of high- versus low-licking and grooming and arched-back nursing (LG-ABN) mothers. (*) Significantly different at $P < 0.05$. Two animals from each of the nine litters were randomly chosen for testing, that is, $n = 8$ to 10 per group. (Bottom) Scattergram for the correlation between the frequency of maternal licking and grooming during the first 10 days of life and the integrated plasma corticosterone response to stress (calculated by use of the trapezoidal rule).

handled versus nonhandled rats, which differ in stress-induced, but not basal HPA, activity (3). Moreover, the frequency of maternal licking and grooming was significantly correlated with the magnitude of the plasma ACTH ($r = -0.66$, $P < 0.01$) and corticosterone ($r = -0.65$, $P < 0.01$) responses to stress in the adult offspring. Thus, the greater the frequency of maternal licking and grooming during infancy, the lower the HPA response to stress in adulthood.

We then examined glucocorticoid feedback sensitivity in the high– and low–LG-ABN offspring by administering a bolus injection of corticosterone 3 hours before acute restraint stress (21). Corticosterone treatment suppressed plasma ACTH responses to restraint stress to a significantly greater extent in the high–LG-ABN offspring compared with their low–LG-ABN counterparts (75 ± 5 versus $37 \pm 12\%$, respectively; $P < 0.01$). These findings suggest that the offspring of the high–LG-ABN mothers, like the handled animals, show increased sensitivity to the inhibitory effects of glucocorticoids on stress-induced HPA activity.

Glucocorticoid inhibition of hypothalamic CRH gene expression represents a critical feature of feedback action (5). Thus, we examined CRH mRNA expression (22) in parvocellular neurons of the paraventricular nucleus of the hypothalamus (PVNh), which send projections to the median eminence and provide the neural signal for the stimulation of ACTH release (23). CRH mRNA expression in the PVNh was significantly decreased in the offspring of high–LG-ABN mothers compared with those of low–LG-ABN mothers (Fig. 48.2). Moreover, CRH mRNA expression in the PVNh was significantly correlated with the frequency of maternal licking and grooming during the first 10 days of life (Fig. 48.2).

Considering the importance of the hippocampal GR system for negative-feedback regulation of HPA activity (10), we examined GR mRNA expression in the hippocampus of the offspring of high– and low–LG-ABN mothers

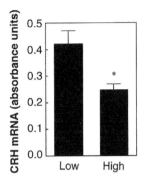

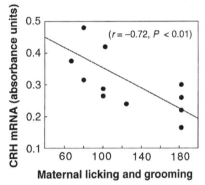

Figure 48.2
(Top) Mean ($\pm$ SEM) levels of CRH mRNA in the PVNh in the adult offspring of high- ($n = 5$) versus low-LG-ABN mothers ($n = 7$) from in situ hybridization studies of corticotropin-releasing hormone mRNA levels. CRH mRNA levels are expressed as arbitrary absorbance units. *$P < 0.001$. (Bottom) Scattergram of the correlation between the frequency of maternal licking and grooming during the first 10 days of life and CRH mRNA expression in PVNh neurons in adulthood.

(24). Across each of the hippocampal cell fields there was increased GR mRNA expression in the offspring of the high– compared to low–LG-ABN mothers (Fig. 48.3). Again, GR mRNA levels in each cell field of the hippocampus were significantly correlated with the frequency of maternal licking and grooming ($r = +0.76$, $P < 0.002$ for the dentate gyrus; $r = +0.64$,

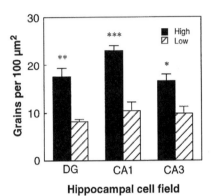

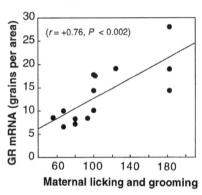

Figure 48.3
(Top) Mean ($\pm$ SEM) grains over individual cells (as a function of cell area) in dentate gyrus (DG), CA1, and CA3 cell fields of the hippocampus in adult offspring of high- ($n = 8$) versus low-LG-ABN mothers ($n = 6$) from in situ hybridization studies of GR mRNA levels. $* P < 0.01$; $** P < 0.001$; $*** P < 0.0001$. (Bottom) Scattergram of the correlation between the frequency of maternal licking and grooming during the first 10 days of life and GR mRNA expression in dentate gyrus neurons in adulthood.

$P < 0.02$ for the CA1 region; $r = +0.79$, $P < 0.001$ for the CA3 region) (Fig. 48.3).

These findings reveal a marked similarity between the HPA responses to stress in the offspring of high–LG-ABN mothers and those of handled animals. The offspring of high–LG-ABN mothers, like handled animals, show

dampened plasma ACTH and corticosterone responses to stress, increased hippocampal GR expression, enhanced glucocorticoid feedback sensitivity, and decreased hypothalamic CRH expression. There is considerable evidence for the importance of the hippocampus as a critical site for glucocorticoid feedback inhibition over hypothalamic CRH synthesis (10). Indeed, hippocampal GR levels have been directly correlated with CRH concentrations in the portal system of the anterior pituitary as well as with pituitary-adrenal activity (25). The offspring of the high–LG-ABN mothers showed increased glucocorticoid feedback sensitivity coupled with decreased hypothalamic CRH mRNA expression and, as in the handled animals, the increased hippocampal GR expression appears likely to mediate these effects.

The magnitude of the HPA response to stress in adult animals was strongly correlated with maternal licking and grooming (Figs. 48.1 to 48.3). These findings support the hypothesis of Levine that the effect of postnatal handling on HPA development is mediated by effects on mother-pup interactions. Thus, handling increases the frequency of licking and grooming (Table 48.1) and these maternal behaviors are, in turn, associated with dampened HPA responsivity to stress (Figs. 48.1 to 48.3). Tactile stimulation derived from maternal licking and grooming regulates pup physiology and affects central nervous system (CNS) development (26). Variation among dams in this form of maternal behavior appears also to be associated with the development of individual differences in neuroendocrine responses to stress.

The results of the handling study suggest that the frequency of maternal licking and grooming can be regulated by stimuli associated with the pup. Thus, handling pups consistently increased maternal licking and grooming (Table 48.1), effectively ensuring a consistently high level of licking and grooming by the dam. This is consistent with earlier studies showing that handling increases ultrasonic vocalizations in pups which, in turn, serve to increase maternal care, including licking and grooming (14). However, it remains possible that the differences in maternal behavior observed here are associated with factors intrinsic to the mother—such as emotionality—in which case the data presented here may, in part, offer an example of a nongenomic mode of inheritance between parent and offspring.

We believe that the effects of early environment on the development of HPA responses to stress reflect a naturally occurring plasticity whereby factors such as maternal care are able to program rudimentary, biological responses to threatening stimuli. Like humans, the Norway rat inhabits a great variety of ecological niches, each with varied sets of environmental demands. Such plasticity could allow animals to adapt defensive systems to the unique demands of the environment. Since most mammals usually spend their adult life in an environment that is either the same as or similar to the one in which they were born, developmental "programming" of CNS responses to stress in early life is likely to be of adaptive value to the adult (12, 27). Such programming affords the animal an appropriate HPA response, minimizing the need for a long and perhaps unaffordable period of adaptation in adult life. Our results suggest that this neonatal programming occurs via the differentiation of the GR system in forebrain neurons that govern HPA activity in response to variations in maternal behavior.

References and Notes

1. S. Levine, *Science* 126, 405 (1957); *ibid.* 135, 795 (1962); ———, G. C. Haltmeyer, G. G. Karas, V. H. Denenberg, *Physiol. Behav.* 2, 55 (1967); M. X. Zarrow, P. S. Campbell, V. H. Denenberg, *Proc. Soc. Exp. Biol. Med.* 356, 141 (1972).

2. The handling procedure involves removing the mother and then rat pups from their cage, placing the pups together in a small container, and returning the animals 15 min later to their cage and their moth-

ers. The manipulation is generally performed daily for the first 21 days of life. Handling does not represent a period of maternal deprivation, because over the course of the day mothers are routinely off their nests and away from pups for periods of 20 to 25 min. At the same time, the artificial and nonspecific nature of the handling paradigm is unsettling [M. Daly, *Br. J. Psychol.* 64, 435 (1972)]. Normal development in a rat pup most often occurs in the rather dark, tranquil confines of a burrow where the major source of stimulation is the mother and littermates.

3. S. Bhatnagar, N. Shanks, M. J. Meaney, *J. Neuroendocrinol.* 7, 107 (1995); J. L. Hess, V. H. Denenberg, M. X. Zarrow, W. D. Pfeifer, *Physiol. Behav.* 4, 109 (1969); M. Vallée et al., *J. Neurosci.* 17, 2626 (1997).

4. M. J. Meaney, D. H. Aitken, S. Bhatnagar, Ch. Van Berkel, R. M. Sapolsky, *Science* 238, 766 (1988); M. J. Meaney, D. H. Aitken, S. Bhatnagar, R. M. Sapolsky, *Neurobiol. Aging* 12, 31 (1991).

5. T. Imaki, J.-L. Nahan, C. Rivier, P. E. Sawchenko, W. Vale, *J. Neurosci.* 11, 585 (1991); P. M. Plotsky and P. E. Sawchenko, *Endocrinology* 120, 1361 (1987); P. M. Plotsky, S. Otto, R. M. Sapolsky, *ibid.* 119, 1126 (1986); P. E. Sawchenko, *J. Neurosci.* 7, 1093 (1987).

6. M. J. Meaney, D. H. Aitken, S. Sharma, V. Viau, A. Sarrieau, *Neuroendocrinology* 50, 597 (1989); V. Viau, S. Sharma, P. M. Plotsky, M. J. Meaney, *J. Neurosci.* 13, 1097 (1993).

7. P. M. Plotsky and M. J. Meaney, *Mol. Brain Res.* 18, 195 (1993); D. Francis, S. Sharma, P. M. Plotsky, M. J. Meaney, *Ann. N.Y. Acad. Sci.* 794, 136 (1996).

8. M. J. Meaney et al., *Behav. Neurosci.* 99, 760 (1985); A. Sarrieau, S. Sharma, M. J. Meaney, *Dev. Brain Res.* 43, 158 (1988).

9. D. O'Donnell, S. Larocque, J. R. Seckl, M. J. Meaney, *Mol. Brain Res.* 26, 242 (1994).

10. E. R. de Kloet, *Front. Neuroendocrinol.* 12, 95 (1991); L. Jacobson and R. M. Sapolsky, *Endocr. Rev.* 12, 118 (1991).

11. S. A. Barnett and J. Burn, *Nature* 213, 150 (1967); S. Levine, in *Society, Stress and Disease*, L. Levi, Ed. (Oxford Univ. Press, London, 1975), pp. 43–50; W. P. Smotherman and R. W. Bell, in *Maternal Influences and Early Behavior*, R. W. Bell and W. P. Smotherman, Eds. (Spectrum, New York, 1980), pp. 201–210.

12. J. R. Alberts and C. P. Cramer, in *Handbook of Behavioral Neurobiology,* E. M. Blass, Ed. (Plenum, New York, 1989), vol. 9, pp. 1–39.

13. A. Fleming and J. S. Rosenblatt, *Behav. Neurosci.* 86, 221 (1974); J. E. Jans and B. C. Woodside, *Dev. Psychobiol.* 23, 519 (1990); M. Leon, P. G. Croskerry, G. K. Smith, *Physiol. Behav.* 21, 793 (1978).

14. R. W. Bell, W. Nitschke, T. H. Gorry, T. Zachma, *Dev. Psychobiol.* 4, 181 (1971); M. H. S. Lee and D. I. Williams, *Anim. Behav.* 22, 679 (1974).

15. B. C. Woodside, M. J. Meaney, J. E. Jans, unpublished data.

16. S. Levine and G. W. Lewis, *Science* 129, 42 (1959); M. J. Meaney and D. H. Aitken, *Dev. Brain Res.* 22, 301 (1985). The animals used in all studies were Long-Evans hooded rats obtained from Charles River Labs. (St. Constant, Québec, Canada) and housed in 46 cm by 18 cm by 30 cm Plexiglas cages that permitted a clear view of all activity within the cage. Food and water were provided ad libidum. The colony was maintained on a 12:12 light:dark (L:D) schedule with lights on at 0800. All procedures were done in accordance with guidelines developed by the Canadian Council on Animal Care and protocol approved by the McGill University Animal Care Committee. Handling was done as described (2). Nonhandled animals were completely undisturbed until day 12 of life at which time normal cage maintenance was initiated. The behavior of each dam was observed [M. M. Myers, S. A. Brunelli, H. N. Shair, J. M. Squire, M. A. Hofer, *Dev. Psychobiol.* 22, 55 (1989)] for eight 60-min observation periods daily for the first 10 days after birth with six periods during the light phase and two periods during the dark phase of the L:D cycle. The distribution of the observations was based on the finding that nursing in rats occurs more frequently during the light phase of the cycle. Handling occurred each day at 1100, and an observation was scheduled at 1130 to correspond to the reunion of the mothers and pups. Within each observation period the behavior of each mother was scored every 4 min (15 observations per period × 8 periods per day = 120 observations per mother per day) for mother off pups, mother licking and grooming any pup, or mother nursing pups in either an arched-back posture, a "blanket" posture in which the mother lies over the pups, or a passive posture in which the mother lies either on her back or side while the pups nurse. Behavioral categories are not mutually exclusive.

17. D. Liu et al., data not shown.

18. Nine Long-Evans female rats were mated in our animal facility and housed and observed as described (16). The animals underwent routine cage maintenance beginning on day 12 but were otherwise not manipulated. At the time of weaning on day 22 of life, the male offspring were housed in same-sex, same-litter groups. Testing of offspring occurred no earlier than 100 days of age.

19. We then rank-ordered the dams on licking and grooming, identifying those mothers whose scores fell above the mean, and as a group these dams were classified as high LG-ABN. The remaining dams were classified as low LG-ABN. The offspring were tested beginning at 100 days of age.

20. For restraint stress (20 min) testing (6), two animals from each of the nine litters were randomly selected for testing. Blood samples were collected from indwelling right jugular vein catheters (6), implanted 4 days before restraint stress testing, and replaced with an equal volume of normal saline (0.9%) via the same route. We have found that by 72 hours after surgery, basal ACTH and corticosterone levels have returned to normal (6). Plasma corticosterone was measured by radioimmunoassay [L. C. Krey et al., *Endocrinology* 96, 1088 (1975)]. Plasma (25 μl) ACTH was measured by radioimmunoassay as described [C.-D. Walker, S. F. Akana, C. S. Cascio, M. F. Dallman, *ibid.* 127, 832 (1990); V. Viau and M. J. Meaney, *ibid.* 129, 2503 (1991)]. All samples were run within a single assay. In our lab the intra- and interassay coefficients of variation are 7 and 10%, respectively, for corticosterone and 8 and 11% for ACTH. The data were analyzed by two-way analyses of variance (ANOVA) with one between (group) and one within (sample) measure. Post hoc analysis was performed by Tukey test.

21. We used a delayed negative-feedback paradigm [M. Keller-Wood and M. F. Dallman, *Endocr. Rev.* 5, 1 (1984)] in which animals are steroid-treated 2 to 4 hours before acute stress. The animals used in this study were the same animals prepared with jugular catheters for acute restraint testing. The animals were tested 4 days after restraint stress, and all but one of the catheters remained patent during this interval. The critical measure here is the ability of the steroid to inhibit subsequent HPA responses to stress. Animals were injected subcutaneously with either vehicle alone or a low to moderate dose of corticosterone (1 mg/kg

in ethanol:saline/1:9) on the basis of earlier studies (6) showing that this dose discriminates feedback sensitivity in handled versus nonhandled rats. Restraint stress was done as described above and plasma samples were obtained from jugular catheters immediately before and at the end of the 20-min period of restraint, a time point that corresponds to the peak plasma ACTH level (6). The percentage suppression of plasma ACTH responses to stress for the high– versus low–LG-ABN groups was derived by comparing Δ(peak stress level— basal level) for each of the corticosterone-treated animals in both groups with that of the mean for the respective control groups (vehicle-treated high– or low– LG-ABN animals). Percentage suppression scores were used to accommodate for the groups differences in plasma ACTH responses to acute stress. The results were examined statistically by Mann-Whitney U test on the basis of percentage scores.

22. CRH mRNA in situ hybridization was done with a 48–base pair (bp) oligonucleotide sequence (CAGTT-TCCTGTTGCTGTGAGCTTGCTGAGCTAACTG-CTCTGCCCTGGC) (Perkin-Elmer, Warrington, UK) and a modified version of the procedure previously described [N. Shanks, S. Larocque, M. J. Meaney, *J. Neurosci.* 15, 376 (1995)] with brain sections obtained from animals rapidly killed under resting-state conditions. After hybridization, sections were apposed to Hyperfilm (Amersham) for 21 days along with sections of ^{35}S-labeled standards prepared with known amounts of radiolabeled ^{35}S in a brain paste. The hybridization signal within the parvocellular subregion of the PVNh was quantified by densitometry with an MCID image analysis system (Imaging Research, St. Catherine's, Ontario, Canada). The data are presented as arbitrary absorbance units after correction for background. These data were analyzed by *t* test for unpaired groups.

23. P. M. Plotsky, *J. Neuroendocrinol.* 3, 1 (1991); W. H. Whitnall, *Prog. Neurobiol.* 40, 573 (1993).

24. GR in situ hybridization was done as described [(9); J. R. Seckl, K. L. Dickson, G. Fink, *J. Neuroendocrinol.* 2, 911 (1990)] with [^{35}S]UTP-labeled cRNA antisense probes transcribed with T7 RNA polymerase from a 674-bp Pst I–Eco RI fragment of the rat GR cDNA linearized with Ava I. After hybridization, sections were dehydrated, dried, and dipped in photographic emulsion (NTB-2, Kodak), and then stored at 4°C for 21 days before development and counterstaining with Cresyl Violet. The hybridization signal within dorsal hippocampal subregions was quantified by grain counting within high-power microscopic fields under brightfield illumination. Grain counting was performed by an individual unaware of the group from which the slide was derived. For each cell field, grains over ~40 to 50 individual neurons per section were counted, on three sections per animal (9). After subtraction of background (grains over neuropil), mean values were derived for each hippocampal cell field for each animal. Background ranged between 10 and 15% of values found over hippocampal cells. Grain counts are presented as a function of cell area to account for possible morphological differences [J. T. McCabe, R. A. Desharnais, D. W. Pfaff, *Methods Enzymol.* 168, 822 (1989)]. These data were analyzed by two-way ANOVA with one between measures (group) and one repeated measure (hippocampal sub-field) by Tukey post hoc test.

25. R. M. Sapolsky, L. C. Krey, B. S. McEwen, *Proc. Natl. Acad. Sci. U.S.A.* 81, 6174 (1984); R. M. Sapolsky, M. P. Armanini, D. R. Packan, S. W. Sutton, P. M. Plotsky, *Neuroendocrinology* 51, 328 (1990); J. L. W. Yau, T. Olsson, R. G. M. Morris, M. J. Meaney, J. R. Seckl, *Neuroscience* 66, 571 (1995).

26. C. M. Kuhn, G. E. Evoniuk, S. M. Schanberg, *Science* 204, 1034 (1978); S. R. Butler, M. R. Suskind, S. M. Schanberg, *ibid.* 199, 445 (1978); S. Levine, *Ann. N.Y. Acad. Sci.* 746, 260 (1994); C. L. Moore, *Dev. Psychobiol.* 17, 347 (1984); M. M. Myers, H. N. Shair, M. A. Hofer, *Experentia* 48, 322 (1992); S. M. Schanberg and T. M. Field, *Child Dev.* 58, 1431 (1987).

27. M. A. Hofer, in L. A. Rosenblum and H. Moltz, Eds., *Symbiosis in Parent-Offspring Interactions* (Plenum, New York, 1983), pp. 61–75.

We thank R. Meisfield (Univ. of Arizona) for rat GR cDNA and H. Anisman and M. Hofer for comments on an earlier version of this manuscript. Supported by grants from the Medical Research Council of Canada (MRCC) (M.J.M.) and the National Institute of Mental Health (P.M.P. and M.J.M.). M.J.M. is the recipient of an MRCC Scientist award. D.L. is a graduate fellow of the MRCC.

49 Maternal Care and the Development of Stress Responses

Darlene D. Francis and Michael J. Meaney

Introduction

Stress is a risk factor for a variety of illnesses, ranging from auto-immune disorders to mental illness. The pathways through which stressful events can promote the development of such divergent forms of illness involve the same hormones that ensure survival during a period of stress [1**]. Stress-induced increases in adrenal release of catecholamines (adrenaline and noradrenaline) and glucocorticoids orchestrate an increase in catabolism, involving lipolysis and the mobilization of glucose reserves (see Table 49.1; [2, 3*]). These actions serve to increase the availability and distribution of energy substrates. There are also emotional and cognitive responses to stressors [4*]. During periods of stress, feelings of apprehension and fear predominate, and individuals become hypervigilant. The level of attention directed to the surrounding environment is increased at the expense of our ability to concentrate on tasks not related to the stressor. Glucocorticoids act on brain structures such as the hippocampus and amygdala, to disrupt episodic memory [5*]. At the same time, glucocorticoids and catecholamines act on areas of the brain, such as the amygdala, to enhance learning and memory for emotional stimuli (see [6–8]). Even though these responses are highly adaptive, chronic activation of these systems can promote the development of hyperlipidemia, hypertension, chronic immunosuppression and decreased viral resistance, states of anxiety and dysphoria, and sleep disorders [1**, 2, 9].

We will discuss the implications of altered maternal behavior early in an organism's life on its subsequent vulnerability to stress later in adulthood.

Corticotropin-releasing Hormone

Behavioral and endocrine responses to stress are largely governed by two central corticotropin-releasing factor (CRF) neuronal populations (see [10–12]). One population of CRF neurons is in the parvocellular region of the paraventricular nucleus of the hypothalamus (PVNh), which project to the hypophysial-portal system of the anterior pituitary [10]. In responses to stressors, CRF, as well as co-secretagogues such as arginine vasopressin, are released from PVNh neurons into the portal blood supply of the anterior pituitary, where it provokes the synthesis and release of adrenocorticotropin hormone (ACTH; see [10]). Pituitary ACTH, in turn, causes the release of glucocorticoids from the adrenal gland. CRF neurons in the PVNh also activate adrenomedullary catecholamine release [10]. The second population of CRF neurons is in the central nucleus of the amygdala (CnAmy) and projects to the locus coeruleus (LC). They increase the firing rate of LC neurons, resulting in increased noradrenaline release in the vast terminal fields of this ascending noradrenergic system (see [13, 14]).

The CRF neurons of the PVNh are an important noradrenergic target. Noradrenaline is the primary stimulus of CRF release from PVNh neurons during stress [10]. The amygdaloid CRF projection to the LC [13, 14] is also critical for the expression of behavioral responses to stress (see [8, 14, 15]). Hence, the CRF neurons in the PVNh and the CnAmy serve as important mediators of both behavioral and endocrine responses to stress.

These findings have provided a basis for understanding how stress can influence health. Yet, the influence of stress on health can only be fully appreciated when the individual's response to stress is taken into consideration. One hypothesis

Table 49.1
Summary of major metabolic/cardiovascular effects of stress-induced increases in catecholamines and glucocorticoids*

Target organ/tissue	Effect	Function
Liver	Increase gluconeogenesis	Maintain stable blood sugar level
Selected macromolecular storage sites	Increase glycogenolysis and lipolysis	Increase available energy substrates
Heart, circulatory system	Increase heart rate and blood pressure	Increase blood flow
GH target tissue	Decrease sensitivity to GH	Dampen anabolic processes

* Generated from [1**, 2, 9]. GH, growth hormone.

Table 49.2
A summary of the effects of postnatal handling or maternal separation on neural mediators of behavioral and HPA responses to stress in the rat*

Target	Postnatal handling	Maternal separation
CRF mRNA (PVNh)	↓	↑
CRF mRNA (CnAmy)	↓	↑
CRFir (locus coeruleus)	↓	↑
CRF receptor binding (locus coeruleus, raphé)	↓	↑
GR mRNA (hippocampus)	↑	↓
GR mRNA (PVNh)	No effect	↓
GC feedback inhibition of CRF	↑	↓
GABA_A receptor	↑	↓
CBZ receptor/γ2 mRNA† (amygdala, locus coeruleus, nucleus tractus solitarius)	↑	↓

* Generated from [16, 19, 21, 27]. † The γ2 subunit of the GABA_A receptor complex is thought to encode for the CBZ receptor site. CRFir, immunoreactive CRF; GC, glucocorticoid.

that guides research on the development of psychopathology focuses on the role of early life events in determining individual differences in vulnerability to stress [16–18]. This hypothesis is derived from the finding that chronic activation of central and endocrine stress responses can promote illness (see references cited above). Thus, early life events that increase stress reactivity result in a greater exposure to "stress hormones" and thus greater vulnerability for stress-induced illness over the lifespan. Support for this hypothesis has emerged from studies examining the influence of early life events on the development of neural systems that regulate the expression stress responses.

Environmental Regulation of the Hypothalamic–pituitary–adrenal Axis and Behavioral Responses to Stress

One of the strongest models for environmental regulation of the development of responses to stress is the postnatal handling research with

rodents. Handling involves a brief (i.e. 3–15 min) daily period of separation of the pup from the mother. In the rat and mouse, postnatal handling decreases the magnitude of behavioral and endocrine responses to stress in adulthood (see [19] for a review). In contrast, longer periods (i.e. 3–6 h) of daily separation from the mother increase behavioral and endocrine responses to stress [20*, 21]. These effects persist throughout the life of the animal (see e.g. [22]) and are associated with differences in health outcomes under conditions of stress [22–24].

The central CRF systems are critical targets for these environmental effects (see Table 49.2). Postnatal handling decreases, and maternal separation increases, CRF gene expression in the PVNh and the CnAmy. Moreover, there are potent effects on systems known to regulate CRF gene expression in the PVNh and the CnAmy.

Glucocorticoid receptor systems are modulated, which then serve to inhibit CRF synthesis and release in PVNh neurons [2, 3*]. GABAergic/central benzodiazepine (CBZ) systems, which regulate both amygdaloid CRF activity and noradrenergic neurons of the LC [12], are also affected. Predictably, stress-induced activation of ascending noradrenergic systems in adult animals is increased by maternal separation and decreased by handling in early life [25]. Thus, environmental manipulations can alter the expression of behavioral and endocrine responses to stress by altering the development of central CRF systems, as well as systems that regulate CRF activity.

In addition, maternal separation in early life alters the development of ascending serotonergic systems in both monkeys (see [26]) and rats [27]. Repeated periods of maternal separation in early life increase cerebrospinal fluid measures of central noradrenaline and serotonin responses to stress in the rhesus monkey [28]. Considering the importance of the ascending noradrenergic and serotonergic systems in depression, these findings suggest a mechanism whereby early life events might predispose an individual to depression in later life (see [17]).

Thus, long periods of maternal separation during infancy may have long-term effects on stress-mediating pathways. It is not clear, however, whether maternal care actively contributes to the normal development of the neural systems that mediate stress responses or whether it is simply the absence of the mother that is so disruptive to the development of these systems. If maternal care is important, then what are the relevant features of mother–infant interactions and how do they influence neural development?

What Are the Critical Features of Environmental Manipulations?

Handling, although a brief interlude in the routine of mother–pup interactions, does alter the behavior of the mother towards its offspring [29]. Mothers of handled pups spend the same amount of time with their litters as mothers of nonhandled pups; however, mothers of handled litters spend significantly more time licking/grooming their pups [30*]. The question, then, is whether this altered pattern of maternal behavior serves as a critical stimulus for the environmental effects on the development of endocrine and behavioral responses to stress.

Interestingly, there are substantial, naturally occurring variations in maternal licking/grooming in rat dams. Maternal licking/grooming of pups occurs most frequently while the mother nurses in the arched-back position; the frequency of the two behaviors are closely correlated (r = +0.91) across mothers [30*]. In a series of studies, mothers were divided into two groups: those that spent a large amount of time licking/grooming and arched-back nursing (LG-ABN) and those that spent little time performing these behaviors. Note, there were no differences between these groups in relation to the overall amount of time the mother was in contact with her pups [31*]. If handling-induced differences in licking/grooming or arched-back nursing are relevant for effects on HPA development, then the offspring of high LG-ABN mothers should resemble the handled animals. This is exactly what was found [30*]. As adults, the offspring of high LG-ABN mothers showed reduced plasma ACTH and corticosterone responses to restraint stress. In the adult rat, glucocorticoids act at specific receptor sites within selected brain regions, such as the hippocampus, to decrease CRF synthesis in PVNh neurons (see [3*]). The high LG-ABN animals also showed significantly increased hippocampal glucocorticoid receptor mRNA expression, enhanced glucocorticoid negative feedback sensitivity and decreased hypothalamic CRF mRNA levels. Moreover, the magnitude of the corticosterone response to acute stress was significantly correlated with the frequency of both maternal licking/grooming (r = −0.61) and arched-back nursing (r = −0.64) during the first

10 days of life, as were the levels of hippocampal glucocorticoid receptor mRNA and hypothalamic CRF mRNA expression (all correlation values > 0.70) [30•]. These studies suggest that the critical feature for the handling effect on HPA development involves an increase in maternal licking/grooming.

The offspring of the high and low LG-ABN mothers also differed in their behavioral responses to novelty [31•]. As adults, the offspring of the low LG-ABN mothers showed increased startle responses, decreased open-field exploration, and longer latencies to eat food provided in a novel environment, reflecting a greater fear of novelty. These animals also showed increased CRF receptor levels in the locus coeruleus and decreased CBZ receptor levels in the basolateral and central nucleus of the amygdala, as well as in the LC, and increased CRF mRNA expression in the CnAmy (DD Francis, J Diorio, MJ Meaney, unpublished data). These differences map perfectly onto the differences between handled and nonhandled animals, and provide support for the idea that the effects of handling are mediated by changes in maternal behavior.

It may be surprising that rather subtle variations in maternal behavior have such a profound impact on development. However, for a rat pup, the first weeks of life do not hold a great deal of stimulus diversity. Stability is the theme of the burrow, and the social environment in the first days of life is defined by the mother and littermates. The mother serves as a primary link between the environment and the developing animal. It seems reasonable that variations in the mother–pup interaction would serve to carry so much importance for development.

These findings are consistent with the results of studies using the cross-fostering technique as a test for the maternal-mediation hypotheses. For example, the spontaneously hypertensive rat (SHR) is a strain bred for hypertension. Even though the selective breeding suggests a genetic background, the expression of hypertension is also influenced by epigenetic factors (see [32]).

SHR pups reared by wild-type (Wistar–Kyoto [WKY]) mothers do not exhibit hypertension to the extent of kin reared by SHR dams. When borderline hypertensive rats (BHRs), a hybrid formed by SHR–WKY matings, are reared by WKY mothers, they do not express the hypertensive phenotype.

The influence of maternal behavior on the development of behavioral and endocrine responses to stress is also apparent in studies with BALBc mice, a strain that normally is very fearful and shows elevated HPA responses to stress. BALBc mice cross-fostered to C57 mothers are significantly less fearful and have reduced HPA responses to stress [33]. Importantly, C57 mothers normally lick and groom their pups about twice as frequently as BALBc mothers. C57 pups cross-fostered to BALBc mothers are more fearful, but not to the same level as non–cross-fostered BALBc mice. Comparable findings have emerged from studies of rat strains: for example, Fischer 344 rats, by comparison to Long-Evans rats, are more responsive to novelty and have increased HPA responses to acute stress. Interestingly, Long-Evans dams lick/groom their offspring significantly more often than do Fischer 344 mothers [34].

Under normal circumstances, of course, BALBc mice are reared by BALBc mothers. The genetic and environmental factors conspire to produce an excessively fearful animal. This is the essence of nature and nurture: genetic and environmental factors work in concert, and are often correlated (see [35]). Because parents provide both genes and environment for their biological offspring, the offspring's environment is correlated with their genes. The environment the parent provides commonly serves to enhance the genetic differences—they are redundant mechanisms. The knowledge of an animal's BALBc pedigree is sufficient to predict a high level of timidity in adulthood. Additional information on maternal care would statistically add little to the predictability—the two factors work in the same direction. But this is clearly different from concluding that maternal care is not relevant, and the results of cross-fostering studies attest to the importance of such epigenetic influences. The value of this process is that it can provide for variation. If a genetically determined trajectory is not adaptive for the animal, then development that can move in the direction of the current environmental signal would be of adaptive value. Hence, environmental events may alter the path of developmental trajectories in favor of more adaptive outcomes.

The Transmission of Individual Differences in Maternal Care to the Offspring

Individual differences in behavioral and neuroendocrine responses to stress are, in part, derived from variations in maternal care. Such effects might serve as a mechanism by which selected traits could be transmitted from one generation to the next. This includes individual differences in maternal behavior. Adult, female offspring of high LG-ABN mothers show significantly more LG-ABN than female offspring of low LG-ABN mothers (DD Francis et al., *Soc Neurosci Abstr* 1998, 24:452). Moreover, handling of female pups in early life causes them to become high LG-ABN mothers, regardless of parentage, which suggests that the mode of transmission is indeed behavioral.

The intergenerational transmission of parental behavior has also been reported in primates. In rhesus monkeys, for example, there is evidence for family lineages expressing abuse of infants [36]. Fairbanks [37] found that daughters reared by mothers who consistently spent a large amount of time in physical contact with their offspring became mothers who were similarly more attentive to their offspring. Also, in rhesus monkeys, Berman [38] found that the rejection of infants by their mothers is correlated to whether their mothers were rejected as infants. In all cases, these findings were independent of the social rank of the mother. In humans, measures of

parental bonding between a mother and daughter were highly correlated with the same measures of bonding between the daughter and her child [39]. These findings suggest a common process of intergenerational transmission of maternal behavior.

Environmental Regulation of Maternal Behavior

In humans, social, emotional and socio-economic context are overriding determinants of the quality of the relationship between a parent and child [40]. Parental care is disturbed under conditions of chronic stress. Conditions that most commonly characterize abusive and neglectful homes involve economic hardship, marital strife and a lack of social and emotional support (see [40]). Such homes, in turn, breed neglectful and even abusive parents. More subtle variations in parental care also show continuity across generations. Scores on the parental bonding index, a measure of parent–child attachment, are highly correlated across generations of mothers and daughters (DD Francis et al., *Soc Neurosci Abstr* 1998, 24:452). So what are the mechanisms that underlie this apparent transmission of parental behavior from one generation to the next?

Individual differences in behavioral and endocrine responses to stress in the rat are associated with variations in maternal care during infancy [31•, 32]. Predictably, the stress responsivity of the offspring mirrors that of their mothers. Low LG-ABN mothers are more fearful than are high LG-ABN dams, and likewise, their offspring are more fearful and timid than are those of high LG-ABN mothers. This is a crucial point in understanding the basis for the transmission of individual differences in parental behavior.

In the rat, maternal behavior emerges as a resolution of an interesting conflict [41]. Female rats, unless they are in late pregnancy or lactating, generally show an aversion towards pups. The novelty of the pups is a source of aversion for females, which is typical of the generally neophobic adult rat. Amygdaloid lesions or specific hormonal regimens that dampen fearful reactions to novelty also increase maternal responsivity in nulliparous females [42, 43]. Importantly, intracerebroventricular infusion of CRF reduces maternal responsivity [44]. In humans, the mother's attitude towards her newborn is highly correlated with her level of anxiety [43]. Mothers who feel depressed and anxious are, unsurprisingly, less positive towards their baby (see also [45]). That is to say, more fearful, anxious mothers, such as low LG-ABN rat dams, appear to be less maternally responsive towards their offspring. Uvnas-Moberg [46] has proposed a neural basis for these effects that is based on the functionally antagonist effects of oxytocin and CRF. She suggests that oxytocin has anxiolytic effects and promotes parental care, whereas CRF is anxiogenic and apparently disruptive of maternal behavior.

Under natural conditions, and the sanctity of the burrow, rat pups have little direct experience with the environment. Instead, it is their mother —and thus maternal care—that is affected by conditions such as the scarcity of food, social instability and low dominance status. The effects of these environmental challenges on the development of the pups may then be mediated by alterations in maternal care (see Figure 49.1). Variations in maternal care could, in turn, serve to transduce an environmental signal to the pups and thus influence the development of neural systems that mediate behavioral and HPA responses to stress. Unfavorable environmental conditions produce animals that are more neophobic (see [19]) and lower in maternal responsivity to pups (i.e. low LG-ABN mothers). This pattern of maternal care could then result in offspring that are more fearful and, ultimately, become low LG-ABN mothers. Hence, these individual differences in the quality of maternal care may serve as the basis for comparable patterns of maternal behavior in the offspring (F1) and for the transmission of these traits to subse-

quent generations (see Figure 49.1). A key question here concerns the effects of early life events on the development of neural systems that mediate maternal behavior (see Figure 49.1 and [46]).

Perhaps the most compelling evidence demonstrating perturbations in the nature of maternal care emerges from the studies of Rosenblum and colleagues (see [47]). Bonnet macaque mother–infant dyads were maintained under one of three foraging conditions: low foraging demand (LFD), where food was readily available; high foraging demand (HFD), where ample food was available, but required long periods of searching; and variable foraging demand (VFD), a mixture of the two conditions on a schedule that did not allow for predictability. Exposure to these conditions over a period of months had a significant influence on mother–infant interactions. The VFD condition was clearly the most disruptive. Mother–infant conflict increased in the VFD condition. Infants of mothers housed under these conditions were significantly more timid and fearful. These infants also showed signs of depression commonly observed in maternally separated macaque infants. As adolescents, the infants reared in the VFD conditions were more fearful, submissive and showed less social play behavior.

More recent studies have demonstrated the effects of these conditions on the development of neurobiological systems that mediate the organism's behavioral and endocrine/metabolic response to stress [48, 49••] As adults, monkeys reared under VFD conditions showed increased cerebrospinal fluid levels of CRF. Increased central CRF drive would suggest altered noradrenergic and serotonergic responses to stress, and this is exactly what was seen in adolescent VFD-reared animals. These findings provide a mechanism for the increased fearfulness observed in the VFD-reared animals. We would predict that if the environmental conditions remained stable, these differences would, in turn, be transmitted to the offspring (see Figure 49.1).

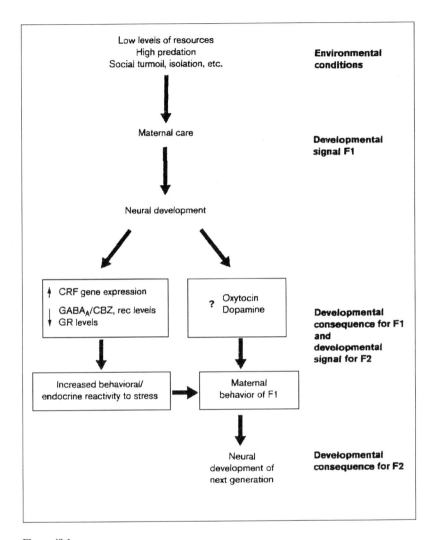

Figure 49.1

A schematic representing the potential outcomes of the proposed relationship between environmental adversity and infant care. The key feature of this formulation is the hypothesized relationship between fearfulness (i.e. reactivity to stress) and maternal behavior (see ref. 43 for a review). Thus, variations in maternal care affect the development of neural systems that mediate stress reactivity (see refs. 16, 19, 21, 27, 30*, 31*), which may then influence maternal behavior. These effects then serve to influence the development of the subsequent generation and thus provide a basis for the transmission of individual differences in stress reactivity from one generation to the next. F1, first generation; F2, second generation; rec, receptor.

Conclusions

The studies reviewed here underscore two critically important points. First, variations in maternal care that fall within the normal range of the species can still have a profound influence on development. One does not need to appeal to the more extreme conditions of abuse and neglect to see evidence for the importance of parental care. Second, environmental demands can alter parental care and thus infant development. Indeed, we hypothesize that environmentally induced alterations in maternal care mediate the effect of variations in the early postnatal environment on the development of specific neural systems that mediate the expression of fearfulness. Such individual differences in fearfulness, in turn, influence the parental care of the offspring, providing a neurobiological basis for the intergenerational transmission of specific behavioral traits. The key issue, and one with broad social implications, is understanding the neural mechanisms that underlie the relationship between environmental stressors and maternal care.

References and Recommended Reading

Papers of particular interest, published within the annual period of review, have been highlighted as:

• of special interest

•• of outstanding interest

•• 1. McEwen BS: Protective and damaging effects of stress mediators. *N Engl J Med* 1998, 338:171–179. This review outlines the importance of catecholamine and glucocorticoid action during a period of stress and the physiological costs associated with chronic activation of stress hormone release. The author summarizes our current understanding of the pathways through which elevated levels of corticosteroids and noradrenaline can promote various disease states. The article provides a physiological link between stress and illness.

2. Dallman MF, Akana SF, Strack AM, Hanson ES, Sebastian RJ: The neural network that regulates energy balance is responsive to glucocorticoids and insulin and also regulates HPA axis responsivity at a site proximal to CRF neurons. *Ann NY Acad Sci* 1995, 771:730–742.

• 3. De Kloet ER, Vregdenhil E, Oitzl MS, Joels M: Brain corticosteroid receptor balance in health and disease. *Endocr Rev* 1998, 19:269–301. This very timely review outlines the common actions of glucocorticoid and mineralocorticoid receptor activation on neurons, with a focus on the hippocampus, where GR and MR are co-expressed. The focus is on the role of these receptors in mediating negative feedback inhibition over HPA function. MR activation appears to mediate tonic inhibition over basal HPA activity, whereas GR activation regulates dynamic inhibition over stress-induced HPA activity. In addition, these steroid receptors regulate neuronal function in neocortical, limbic and midbrain regions. These actions appear to mediate the pronounced effects of corticosteroids on cognitive function.

• 4. Arnsten AF: The biology of being frazzled. *Science* 1998, 280:1711–1712. A very readable summary of the cognitive changes that occur during periods of acute stress with references to recent key studies.

• 5. Lupien S, Sharma S, Nair NPV, Hauger R, McEwen BS, de Leon M, Meaney MJ: Glucocorticoids and human brain aging. *Nat Neurosci* 1998, 1:69–73. This paper describes the relationship between individual differences in basal cortisol levels, hippocampal volume and episodic memory. Amongst elderly human subjects, cortisol levels were inversely correlated to hippocampal volume. In turn, hippocampal volume was correlated with episodic memory. These findings underscore the importance of individual differences in HPA activity for health over the lifespan.

6. Pitkanen A, Savander V, LeDoux JE: Organization of intra-amygdaloid circuitries in the rat: an emerging framework for understanding functions of the amygdala. *Trends Neurosci* 1998, 20:517–523.

7. Davis M, Walker DL, Lee Y: Amygdala and bed nucleus of the stria terminalis: different roles in fear and anxiety measured with the acoustic startle reflex. *Philos Trans R Soc Lond [Biol]* 1997, 352:1675–1687.

8. Quirarte GL, Roozendaal B, McGaugh JL: Glucocorticoid enhancement of memory storage involves noradrenergic activation in the basolateral amygdala. *Proc Natl Acad Sci USA* 1997, 94:14048–14053.

9. Rosmond R, Dallman MF, Bjorntorp P: Stress-related cortisol secretion in men: relationship with abdominal obesity and endocrine, metabolic and hemodynamic abnormalities. *J Clin Endocrinol Metabol* 1998, 83:1853–1859.

10. Plotsky PM: Pathways to the secretion of adreno-corticotropin: a view from the portal. *J Neuroendocrinol* 1991, 3:1–9.

11. Koob GF, Heinrichs SC, Menzaghi F, Pich EM, Britton KT: Corticotropin releasing factor, stress and behavior. *Semin Neurosci* 1994, 6:221–229.

12. Owens MJ, Nemeroff CB: Physiology and pharmacology of corticotropin-releasing factor. *Pharmacol Rev* 1991, 43:425–473.

13. Gray TS, Bingaman EW: The amygdala: cortico-tropin-releasing factor, steroids, and stress. *Crit Rev Neurobiol* 1996, 10:155–168.

14. Valentino RJ, Curtis AL, Page ME, Pavcovich LA, Florin-Lechner SM: Activation of the locus coeruleus brain noradrenergic system during stress: circuitry, consequences, and regulation. *Adv Pharmacol* 1998, 42:781–784.

15. Rosen JB, Schulkin J: From normal fear to pathological anxiety. *Psychol Rev* 1998, 105:325–350.

16. Caldji C, Francis D, Liu D, Plotsky PM, Meaney MJ: The role of early experience in the development of individual differences in behavioral and endocrine responses to stress. In *Handbook of Physiology: Coping with the Environment.* Edited by McEwen BS, Steller E. Oxford: Oxford University Press; in press.

17. Heim C, Owens MJ, Plotsky PM, Nemeroff CB: Persistent changes in corticotropin-releasing factor systems due to early life stress: relationship to the pathophysiology of major depression and post-traumatic stress disorder. *Psychopharmacol Bull* 1997, 33:185–192.

18. Seckl JR, Meaney MJ: Early life events and later development of ischaemic heart disease. *Lancet* 1994, 342:1236.

19. Meaney MJ, Diorio J, Widdowson J, LaPlante P, Caldji C, Seckl JR, Plotsky PM: Early environmental regulation of forebrain glucocorticoid receptor gene expression: implications for adrenocortical responses to stress. *Dev Neurosci* 1996, 18:49–72.

•20. van Oers HJ, de Kloet ER, Levine S: The ontogeny of glucocorticoid negative feedback: influence of maternal deprivation. *Endocrinology* 1998, 139:2838–2846. Maternal deprivation has immediate effects on neonatal physiology. Interestingly, these effects have revealed the importance of the mother in regulating the endocrine and metabolic responses to stress in the neonate. This paper is one of a series in which Levine and colleagues have described the role of the mother in maintaining a stable HPA environment during critical periods of neural development. In the absence of the mother, glucocorticoid feedback inhibition of HPA activity is reduced, permitting a greater HPA response to stress and exposure to elevated glucocorticoid levels. The importance of this research can be appreciated in terms of the well-established inhibitory effects of glucocorticoids on synaptic plasticity.

21. Plotsky PM, Meaney MJ: Early, postnatal experience alters hypothalamic corticotropin-releasing factor (CRF) mRNA, median eminence CRF content and stress-induced release in adult rats. *Mol Brain Res* 1993, 18:195–200.

22. Meaney MJ, Aitken DH, Bhatnagar S, Van Berkel CH, Sapolsky RM: Postnatal handling attenuates neuroendocrine, anatomical, and cognitive impairments related to the aged hippocampus. *Science* 1988, 238:766–768.

23. Bhatnagar S, Shanks N, Meaney MJ: Plaque-forming cell responses and antibody titers following injection of sheep-red blood cells in nonstressed, acute and/or chronically stressed handled and nonhandled animals. *Dev Psychobiol* 1996, 29:171–181.

24. Laban O, Markovic BM, Dimitrijevic M, Jankovic BD: Maternal deprivation and early weaning modulate experimental allergic encephalomyelitis in the rat. *Brain Behav Immunol* 1995, 9:9–19.

25. Liu D, Caldji C, Sharma S, Plotsky PM, Meaney MJ: The effects of early life events on *in vivo* release of norepinepherine in the paraventricular nucleus of the hypothalamus and hypothalamic-pituitary-adrenal responses during stress. *J Neuroendocrinol* 1999, in press.

26. Higley JD, Haser MF, Suomi SJ, Linnoila M: Nonhuman primate model of alcohol abuse: effects of early experience, personality and stress on alcohol consumption. *Proc Natl Acad Sci USA* 1991, 88:7261–7265.

27. Ladd CO, Owens MJ, Nemeroff CB: Persistent changes in corticotropin-releasing factor neuronal systems induced by maternal deprivation. *Endocrinology* 1996, 137:1212–1218.

28. Kraemer GW, Ebert MH, Schmidt DE, McKinney WT: A longitudinal study of the effect of different social rearing conditions on cerebrospinal fluid norepinephrine and biogenic amine metabolites in rhesus monkeys. *Neuropsychopharmacolgy* 1989, 2:175–189.

29. Smotherman WP, Bell RW: Maternal mediation of early experience. In *Maternal Influences and Early Behavior*. Edited by Bell RW, Smotherman WP. New York: Spectrum Publications; 1980:282–296.

•30. Liu D, Tannenbaum B, Caldji C, Francis D, Freedman A, Sharma S, Pearson D, Plotsky PM, Meaney MJ: Maternal care, hippocampal glucocorticoid receptor gene expression and hypothalamic–pituitary–adrenal responses to stress. *Science* 1997, 277:1659–1662. This report describes the differences in hypothalamic–pituitary–adrenal responses to stress in adults whose mothers showed naturally occurring variations in maternal behavior. The offspring of mothers who showed increased levels of pup licking/grooming and arched-back nursing during the first 10 days of postnatal life showed significantly reduced plasma adrenocorticotropin and corticosterone responses to stress. These effects appear to be mediated, in part, by changes in hippocampal glucocorticoid receptor gene expression.

•31. Caldji C, Tannenbaum B, Sharma S, Francis D, Plotsky PM, Meaney MJ: Maternal care during infancy regulates the development of neural systems mediating the expression of behavioral fearfulness in adulthood in the rat. *Proc Natl Acad Sci USA* 1998, 95:5335–5340. This is a follow-up to a previous study [30•], and it describes differences in the adult offspring of high or low LG-ABN mothers in behavioral responses to novelty as well as in potential neural mediators, including CRF, α2 adrenoreceptor, and central benzodiazepine/GABA_A receptor binding in locus coeruleus and amygdala.

32. McCarty R, Cierpial MA, Murphy CA, Lee JH: Maternal involvement in the development of cardiovascular phenotype. *Experientia* 1992, 48:315–322.

33. Anisman H, Zaharia MD, Meaney MJ, Merali Z: Do early life events permanently alter behavioral and hormonal responses to stressors? *Int J Dev Neurosci* 1998, 16:149–164.

34. Moore CL, Lux BA: Effects of lactation on sodium intake in Fischer-344 and Long-Evans rats. *Dev Psychobiol* 1998, 32:51–56.

35. Scarr S, McCartney K: How people make their own environments: a theory of genotype-environment effects. *Child Dev* 1983, 54:424–435.

36. Maestripieri D, Wallen K, Carroll KA: Genealogical and demographic influences on infant abuse and neglect in group-lining sooty mangabeys (Cerocebus atys). *Dev Psychobiol* 1997, 31:175–180.

37. Fairbanks LM: Individual differences in maternal style. *Adv Study Behav* 1996, 25:579–611.

38. Berman CM: Intergenerational transmission of maternal rejection rates among free-ranging rhesus monkeys on Cayo Santiago. *Anim Behav* 1990, 44:247–258.

39. Miller L, Kramer R, Warner V, Wickramaratne P, Weissman M: Intergenerational transmission of parental bonding among women. *J Am Acad Child Adolesc Psychiatry* 1997, 36:1134–1139.

40. Eisenberg L: The biosocial context of parenting in human families. In *Mammalian Parenting Biochemical, Neurobiological, and Behavioral Determinants*. Edited by Krasnegor NA, Bridges RS. New York: Oxford University Press; 1990:9–24.

41. Rosenblatt JS: Psychobiology of maternal behavior: contribution to the clinical understanding of maternal behavior among humans. *Acta Paediatr* 1994, 397(suppl):3–8.

42. Bridges RS: The role of lactogenic hormones in maternal behavior in female rats. *Acta Paediatr* 1994, 397(suppl):33–39.

43. Fleming AS: Factors influencing maternal responsiveness in humans: usefulness of an animal model. *Psychoneuroendocrinology* 1988, 13:189–212.

44. Pedersen CA, Caldwell JD, McGuire M, Evans DL: Corticotropin-releasing hormone inhibits maternal behavior and induces pup-killing. *Life Sci* 1991, 48:1537–1546.

45. Field T: Maternal depression effects on infants and early interventions. *Prev Med* 1998, 27:200–203.

46. Uvnas-Moberg K: The physiological and endocrine effects of social contact. *Ann NY Acad Sci* 1997, 807:146–163.

47. Rosenblum LA, Andrews MW: Influences of environmental demand on maternal behavior and infant development. *Acta Paediatr* 1994, 397(suppl):57–63.

48. Coplan JD, Andrews MW, Rosenblum LA, Owens MJ, Friedman S, Gorman JM, Nemeroff CB: Persistent elevations of cerebrospinal fluid concentrations of corticotropin-releasing factor in adult non-human primates exposed to early-life stressors: implications for psychopathology of mood and anxiety disorders. *Proc Natl Acad Sci USA* 1996, 93:1619–1623.

••49. Coplan JD, Trost RC, Owens MJ, Cooper TB, Gorman JM, Nemeroff CB, Rosenblum LA: Cerebrospinal fluid concentrations of somatostatin and biogenic amines in grown primates reared by mothers exposed to manipulated foraging conditions. *Arch Gen Psychiatry* 1998, 55:473–477. This paper represents a follow-up of an earlier study [48] documenting increased cerebrospinal levels of CRF in monkeys reared under conditions of variable (i.e. unpredictable) food (VF) resource availability. The VF rearing condition was associated with increased cerebrospinal levels of dopamine and serotonin metabolites, which, in turn, were correlated with CRF levels. The findings reflect the potential importance of the relationship between environmental stressors and mother–infant interactions for neural development and vulnerability to stress-induced pathology in later life.

50 Attachment in Rhesus Monkeys

Stephen J. Suomi

Attachment is not an exclusively human phenomenon. Although the theory that John Bowlby conceived and developed during the 1950s and 1960s reflected his clinical observations of infants and young children (even in the face of his psychoanalytic training), it also had a strong basis in his knowledge of (and near-constant interest in) ethological studies of developmental phenomena in animals, especially nonhuman primates. Indeed, it can be argued that Bowlby (1969/1982) tailored several essential features of his attachment theory specifically to account for clear-cut commonalities in the strong behavioral and emotional ties that infants inevitably develop with their mothers—not only across all of humanity, but also among our closest evolutionary relatives.

At about the time that Bowlby published, with James Robertson, his seminal studies of infant separation via hospitalization (Robertson & Bowlby, 1952), he became aware of the classic ethological studies of filial imprinting in precocial birds. During this period, he developed a close friendship with Robert Hinde, a world-class ethologist at Cambridge University, who was in the process of shifting his own basic research interests from song-learning in birds to mother–infant interactions in rhesus monkeys. Hinde soon had rhesus monkey mothers raising babies in small captive social groups (e.g., Hinde, Rowell, & Spencer-Booth, 1964), and Bowlby came to recognize patterns of behavior shown by the infant monkeys toward their mothers—but not toward other adult females in the group—that strikingly resembled recurrent response patterns of human infants and young children he had observed over years of clinical practice. These common patterns provided Bowlby with powerful evidence supporting his assumption that attachment has its basis in biology.

Indeed, virtually all of the basic features of human infant behavior that Bowlby's attachment theory specifically ascribed to our evolutionary history could be observed in the normative mother-directed behaviors of rhesus monkey infants described by Hinde and other primate researchers. For Bowlby (1958, 1969/1982), the fact that rhesus monkey infants and human babies share unique physical features, behavioral propensities, and emotional labilities linked to highly specific circumstances was consistent with the view that they also share significant parts of their respective evolutionary histories. He argued that these features, present in newborns of each species but often largely absent (or at least mostly hidden) in older individuals, represent successful adaptations to selective pressures over millions of years. To Bowlby, those characteristics common to human and monkey infants reflect evolutionary success stories and should be viewed as beneficial, if not essential, for survival of both the individual infant and the species.

What are those common characteristics—and what is their relevance for attachment theorizing? This chapter begins by describing how attachment relationships between rhesus monkey infants and their mothers are normally established and maintained throughout development. Next, those features that are unique to rhesus monkey infant–mother attachment relationships are examined, as is conflict within these relationships. Attachment relationships in rhesus monkeys and other primates are subject to influence from a variety of sources, and some of these influences are reviewed next. Some long-term biobehavioral consequences of different early attachment experiences are then examined in detail. Finally, the implications for attachment theory of recent findings regarding cross-generational transmission of specific attachment patterns in rhesus monkey families are discussed.

Normative Patterns of Infant–Mother Attachment in Rhesus Monkeys

The first detailed longitudinal studies of species-normative attachment relationships in rhesus monkeys were carried out over 30 years ago (e.g., Hansen, 1966; Harlow, Harlow, & Hansen, 1963; Hinde & Spencer-Booth, 1967). These seminal investigations provided descriptions of infant behavioral development and emerging social relationships that not only appear remarkably accurate even in today's light, but also have been repeatedly shown to generalize to other rhesus monkey infants growing up in a range of naturalistic settings, as well as to infants of other Old World monkey and ape species (see Higley & Suomi, 1986, for one of many comprehensive reviews). Virtually all infants in these species spend their initial days, weeks, and (for infant apes) months of life in near-continuous physical contact with their biological mothers, typically clinging to the mothers' ventral surface for most of their waking (and all of their sleeping) hours each day. Rhesus monkey neonates clearly and consistently display four of the five "component instinctual responses" that Bowlby (1958) listed as universal human attachment behaviors in his initial monograph on attachment: sucking, clinging, crying, and following (the fifth, smiling, is universally seen in chimpanzee but not monkey infants). All of these response patterns reflect efforts on the part of the infant to obtain and maintain physical contact with or proximity to its mother.

Rhesus monkey mothers, in turn, provide their newborns with essential nourishment; physical and psychological warmth (e.g., Harlow, 1958); and protection from the elements, potential predators, and even other members of the social group, including pesky older siblings. During this time a strong and enduring social bond inevitably develops between mother and infant—a bond that is unique in terms of its exclusivity, constituent behavioral features, and ultimate duration. The attachment bond that a rhesus monkey infant inevitably develops with its mother is like no other social relationship it will experience in its lifetime, except (in reciprocal form) for a female when she grows up to have infants of her own. Furthermore, for a male infant this bond will last at least until puberty, while for a female it will be maintained as long as mother and daughter are both alive (Suomi, 1995).

In their second month of life, most rhesus monkey infants start using their mothers as a "secure base" from which to begin exploring their immediate physical and social environment. At this age monkey infants are inherently curious (Harlow, 1953), and most attempt to leave their mothers' side for brief periods as soon as they become physically able. Mothers typically monitor these attempts quite closely, and they often physically restrain their infants' efforts— or retrieve them if they have wandered beyond arm's length—at the slightest sign of potential danger. Numerous studies (e.g., Hinde & White, 1974) have demonstrated that at this stage of infant development the mother is primarily responsible for maintaining mutual contact and/or proximity. With the emergence of social fear in the infant's emotional repertoire between 2 and 3 months of age (functionally and developmentally equivalent to human infant 9-month "stranger anxiety"; cf. Sackett, 1966; Suomi & Harlow, 1976), this pattern reverses; thereafter, the infant is primarily responsible for maintaining proximity and actual physical contact with its mother.

Once any rhesus monkey infant has become securely attached to its mother, it can then use her as an established base from which to make exploratory ventures toward stimuli that have caught its curiosity. The infant soon learns that if it becomes frightened or is otherwise threatened by the stimuli it has sought out, it can always run back to its mother, who can provide immediate safety and comfort via mutual ventral contact even if she has not already actively intervened on its behalf. Several studies have documented that initiation of ventral contact with the mother promotes rapid decreases in hypothalamic–pituitary–adrenal (HPA) activity (as indexed by lowered plasma cortisol concentrations) and in sympathetic nervous system arousal (as indexed by reductions in heart rate), along with other physiological changes commonly associated with soothing (e.g., Gunnar, Gonzalez, Goodlin, & Levine, 1981; Mendoza, Smotherman, Miner, Kaplan, & Levine, 1978; Reite, Short, Seiler, & Pauley, 1981).

As they grow older, most monkey infants voluntarily spend increasing amounts of time at increasing distances from their mothers, apparently confident that they can return to the mothers' protective care without interruption or delay should circumstances warrant it. Their mothers' presence as a secure base clearly promotes exploration of their ever-expanding physical and social world (Dienske & Metz, 1977; Harlow et al., 1963; Simpson, 1979). On the other hand, when rhesus monkey infants develop less than optimal attachment relationships with their mothers, their exploratory behavior is inevitably compromised (e.g., Arling & Harlow, 1967; Suomi, 1995); this is consistent with Bowlby's observations regarding human attachment relationships (e.g., Bowlby, 1969/1982, 1988), as will be discussed later.

At about 3 months of age, monkey infants begin to develop distinctive social relationships with other members of their social group. Increasingly, these come to involve other infants of like age and comparable physical, cognitive, and socioemotional capabilities. Following weaning (usually in the fourth and fifth months) and essentially until puberty (during the third or fourth year), play with peers represents the predominant social activity for young monkeys (Ruppenthal, Harlow, Eisele, Harlow, & Suomi, 1974). During this time the play interactions become increasingly gender-specific and sex-segregated (i.e., males tend to play more with males, and females with females; e.g., Harlow &

Lauersdorf, 1974). Peer play also becomes more and more behaviorally and socially complex, and by the third year the play bouts typically involve patterns of behavior that appear to simulate the full range of adult social activity (e.g., Suomi & Harlow, 1975). By the time they reach puberty, most rhesus monkey juveniles have had ample opportunity to develop, practice, and perfect behavioral routines that will be crucial for functioning as a normal adult, especially those patterns involved in reproduction and in dominance/aggressive interactions (Suomi, 1979a). Virtually all of them have also maintained close ties with their mothers (e.g., Berman, 1982).

The onset of puberty is associated with major life transitions for both male and female rhesus monkeys. Adolescence is associated not only with major hormonal alterations, pronounced growth spurts, and other obvious physical changes, but also with major social changes for both sexes (Suomi, Rasmussen, & Higley, 1992). Males experience the most dramatic and serious social disruptions: They sever all social ties not only with their mothers and other kin, but also with all others in their natal social troop. Virtually all of these adolescent males soon join all-male "gangs," and after several months most of them then attempt to enter a different established troop—typically one composed entirely of individuals of all ages and both genders, and largely unfamiliar to the adolescent males (Berard, 1989). Field data show that the process of natal group emigration represents an exceedingly dangerous transition for adolescent males. The mortality rate for these males from the time they leave their natal group until they become successfully integrated into another full-fledged group can be as high as 50%, depending on local circumstances (e.g., Dittus, 1979). Recent field studies have also identified and characterized substantial interindividual variability in both the timing of male emigration and the basic strategies followed in attempting to join other established social groups (Mehlman et al., 1995; Suomi et al., 1992).

Adolescent females, by contrast, never leave their maternal family or natal social group (Lindburg, 1971). Puberty for them is instead associated with increases in social activities directed toward maternal kin, typically at the expense of interactions with unrelated peers. Family interactions are heightened even more when these young females begin to have offspring of their own. Indeed, the birth of a new infant (especially to a new mother) often has the effect of "invigorating" the matriline—drawing its members closer both physically and socially, and, conversely, providing a buffer from external threats and stressors for mother and infant alike. Rhesus monkey females continue to be involved in family social affairs for the rest of their lives, even after they cease having infants of their own. Thus their experiences with specific attachment relationships tend to be lifelong (Suomi, 1998).

Unique Aspects of Rhesus Monkey Infant–Mother Attachment Relationships

Is infant–mother attachment different from any or all other social relationships a young rhesus monkey (or, for that matter, a human infant) will establish during its lifetime? Some aspects of the attachment relationship are clearly exclusive to the mother–infant dyad, because only the mother, and nobody else, provides an infant not only with all that passes through the placenta, but also with a prenatal environment uniquely attuned to her own circadian and other biological rhythms. In addition, there is increasing evidence of predictable fetal reactions that can be traced to specific activities (including vocalizations) of the mother, perhaps providing the basis for exclusive multimodal proto-communication between mother and fetus (e.g., Busnell & Granier-Deferre, 1981; DeCasper & Fifer, 1980; Fifer, 1987; Schneider, 1992). Such types of prenatal stimulation are, of course, routinely (and exclusively) provided by pregnant females of virtually all mammalian species, except perhaps for the egg-laying monotremes.

Some of these aspects of maternal support and stimulation are basically continued into an infant's initial postnatal months, including obviously the mother's status as the primary (if not sole) source of its nutrition. Mothers also keep sharing their own specific antibodies with their infants postnatally via the nursing process. Moreover, the essentially continuous contact or proximity between a mother and newborn provides the infant with extended exposure to its mother's odor, taste (of milk, at least), relative warmth, sound, and sight, representing a range and intensity of social stimulation seldom if ever provided by any other family or group members. In addition, rhesus monkey mothers continue to communicate their internal circadian and other biological rhythms to their offspring via extended ventral–ventral contact, and there is some evidence that their offspring typically develop synchronous parallel rhythms during their initial weeks of life (cf. Boyce, Champoux, Suomi, & Gunnar, 1995). As before, these maternally specific postnatal aspects of infant support and stimulation are not limited to the higher primates, but instead are characteristic of mothers of virtually all mammalian species (including the monotremes), at least up to the time of weaning (e.g., Hofer, 1995). But other aspects of a rhesus monkey mother's relationship with her infant are not shared by other mammalian mothers, not even by mothers of some other primate species.

What are these unique features of a rhesus monkey (and human) mother's relationship with her infant? It turns out that they are the very characteristics that Bowlby made the defining features of infant–mother attachment: (1) the mother's ability to reduce fear in her infant via direct social contact and other soothing behavior, and (2) the mother's capacity to provide a secure base to support her infant's exploration of the environment. Numerous longitudinal studies of rhesus monkey social ontogeny, carried out in both laboratory and field environments, have consistently found that mothers have a virtual monopoly on these capabilities—or at least the opportunity to express them with their infants (e.g., Berman, 1982; Harlow & Harlow, 1965). Thus, rhesus monkey infants rarely if ever use other group members (even close relatives) as secure bases, or even as reliable sources of ventral contact (Suomi, 1979b). Moreover, on those occasions when they "mistakenly" seek the company of someone other than their mothers, they are unlikely to experience decreases in physiological arousal comparable to those resulting from contact with their mothers; often, they experience increases in arousal instead.

The attachment relationship a rhesus monkey infant establishes with its mother differs in other fundamental ways from all other social relationships it will ever develop during its lifetime. Although numerous laboratory and field studies have shown that a rhesus monkey routinely develops a host of distinctive relationships with different siblings, peers, and adults of both sexes throughout development, each is strikingly different from the initial attachment to the mother in terms of primacy, constituent behaviors, reciprocity, and course of developmental change (Suomi, 1979b). Given these findings, perhaps Bowlby was not entirely correct when he argued that the infant's attachment to the mother provides the prototype for all subsequent social relationships (Bowlby, 1969/1982). On the other hand, Bowlby was absolutely correct (at least for rhesus monkeys) when he argued that the nature of the specific attachment relationship an infant develops with the mother can profoundly affect both concurrent and future relationships the infant may develop with others in its social sphere, as will be discussed in detail later.

A different issue regarding unique aspects of rhesus monkey attachment concerns not whether infant–mother attachment differs from other social relationships with conspecifics, but rather whether attachment as originally defined by Bowlby generalizes to other species, including other primates. As outlined above, Bowlby clearly believed that basic features of attachment phenomena are essentially homologous in rhesus

monkey infants and human babies—but are these characteristic features of attachment seen in other mammalian species as well? It all depends on how one defines "attachment," or such terms as "partner preference" and "imprinting."

Without question, infant preference for the mother (and vice versa) represents an exceedingly widespread phenomenon across most mammalian and avian species, as well as in numerous other taxa (Wilson, 1975). One specific (and, for Bowlby, a particularly relevant) form of partner preference involves "imprinting." According to Lorenz's (1937) classical definition, imprinting is restricted to those partner preferences that are (1) acquired during a critical (or "sensitive") period (or "phase"), (2) irreversible, (3) generally species-specific, and (4) typically established prior to any behavioral manifestation of the preference. According to this definition, imprinting-like phenomena can be observed in numerous insect, fish, avian, and mammalian species, including most if not all primates (Immelmann & Suomi, 1981).

On the other hand, it can be argued that infant–mother attachment as originally defined by Bowlby (1958, 1969/1982) represents a special case of imprinting that may itself be limited largely to Old World monkeys, apes, and humans (Suomi, 1995). To be sure, infants of all the other primate species (i.e., prosimians and New World monkeys) are initially at least as dependent on their mothers for survival, and spend at least as much time in physical contact with them, as rhesus monkey (and human) infants (Higley & Suomi, 1986). In these other primate species, however, the predominant form of mother–infant physical contact is usually different (dorsal–ventral vs. ventral–ventral); the frequency and diversity of mother–infant interactions are generally reduced; the patterns of developmental change differ dramatically; and, most importantly, the basic (indeed defining) features of attachment are largely absent.

Consider the case of capuchin monkeys (*Cebus apella*), a highly successful New World species whose natural habitat covers much of South America, including both Amazonian and Andean regions. These primates are remarkable in many respects, not the least of which is an amazing capability for manufacturing and using tools to manipulate their physical environment (Darwin, 1794; Visalberghi, 1990). In this respect they are clearly superior to rhesus monkeys—and, for that matter, all other primates except chimpanzees and humans. On the other hand, capuchin mother–infant relationships seem somewhat primitive by rhesus monkey standards.

A capuchin monkey spends virtually all of the first 3 months of life clinging to its mother's back, moving ventrally only during nursing bouts (Welker, Becker, Hohman, & Schafer-Witt, 1987). During this time there is very little visual, vocal, or grooming interaction between mother and infant, in marked contrast to a rhesus monkey infant, who by 3 months of age is already participating in extensive one-on-one interactions involving a wealth of visual, auditory, olfactory, tactile, and vestibular stimulation, and who typically has been using its mother as a secure base for exploration for over 2 months. When capuchin monkeys finally get off their mothers' backs in their fourth month, they seem surprisingly independent and can spend long periods away from the mothers without getting upset. If frightened, they are almost as likely to seek protective contact from other group members as from their mothers (Byrne & Suomi, 1995). At this age and thereafter, capuchin monkey youngsters spend only about one third as much time grooming their mothers as rhesus monkeys do, and their other activities with the mothers are not markedly different from their activities with siblings, peers, or unrelated adults (Byrne & Suomi, 1995; Welker, Becker, & Schafer-Witt, 1990), in sharp contrast to rhesus monkey of comparable age. All in all, capuchin monkey infants seem far less attached to their biological mothers in terms of the prominence of the relationship, the relative uniqueness of con-

stituent behaviors, and the nature and degree of secure-base-mediated exploration. One wonders how Bowlby's attachment theory might have looked if Hinde had been studying capuchin rather than rhesus monkeys!

Comparative studies of infant–mother relationships in other New World monkey and prosimian species have found that in most cases the relationships more closely resemble those of capuchin monkeys than those of rhesus monkeys (e.g., Fragaszy, Baer, & Adams-Curtis, 1991); in a few species (e.g., some marmosets and tamarins), the mother is not even an infant's primary caregiver (Higley & Suomi, 1986). To be sure, infants in all these primate species appear to be "imprinted" on their mothers, according to Lorenz's (1937) definition. However, attachment involves considerably more developmental complexity and reciprocity, especially with respect to secure-base phenomena, than do classical notions of imprinting. Indeed, it can be argued that, strictly speaking, attachment represents a special, *restricted case* of imprinting. Moreover, because infant–mother attachment is most apparent in humans and their closest phylogenetic kin, it also may well represent a relatively recent evolutionary adaptation among primates (Suomi, 1995).

Conflict in Rhesus Monkey Infant–Mother Relationships

The relationships that rhesus monkeys develop with their mothers over time involve many behavioral patterns that go beyond attachment phenomena per se (Hinde, 1976). Indeed, a rhesus monkey female is extensively involved in a wide variety of interactions with her mother virtually every day that both are alive (and a male is thus involved every day until adolescence). However, this does not mean that all of these interactions are uniformly positive and pleasant. To the contrary, conflicts between mothers and offspring are frequent and often predictable, if not inevitable, occurrences in everyday rhesus monkey social life.

Sociobiologists have long argued that although mothers and infants share many genes and (therefore) many long-term goals, their short-term interests are not always mutual, and hence periodic conflict is inevitable (Trivers, 1974). Regardless of the validity of this view, an obvious instance of parent–offspring conflict occurs for virtually every rhesus monkey infant at around 20 weeks of age, when its mother begins to wean it from her own milk to solid food. Whether this process begins because the mother "wants" her infant to cease nursing (so she can stop lactating, begin cycling, and be able to produce another offspring, as the sociobiologists propose); because she "knows" that she cannot continue to produce enough milk to sustain her infant's rapidly growing energy requirements; or because her infant's erupting teeth make nursing increasingly uncomfortable is certainly open to question. What *is* clear is that weaning is almost always associated with significant changes in the basic nature of the infant's relationship with its mother, and those changes are seldom placid (e.g., Hinde & White, 1974).

Mothers, for their part, make increasingly frequent efforts to deny their infants access to their nipples, albeit with considerable variation in the precise form, timing, and intensity of their weaning behavior, ranging from the exquisitely subtle to what borders on abuse. Infants, on the other hand, dramatically increase their efforts to obtain and maintain physical contact with their mothers, even when nipple contact is not attainable. As with mothers, there is substantial variation in the nature, intensity, and persistence of the infants' efforts to prevent or at least delay the weaning process (Berman, Rasmussen, & Suomi, 1993). In virtually all cases, an infant's newfound preoccupation with maintaining maternal contact clearly inhibits its exploratory behavior, and noticeably alters and diminishes its interactions with peers (and often other kin) as well. Indeed, it usually takes a month or more (if at all) before

those interaction patterns return to some semblance of normality (Hinde & White, 1974; Ruppenthal et al., 1974). Weaning therefore appears to undermine basic attachment security for the infant, perhaps permanently in some cases.

Postweaning "normality" for a young rhesus monkey seldom lasts for more than a few additional weeks before a second form of conflict with its mother typically arises. Most mothers return to reproductive receptivity at about the time their infants are 6–7 months old, at which point they begin actively soliciting selected adult males for the next 2 or 3 months (rhesus monkeys are seasonal breeders in nature). Throughout this period they may enter into consort relationships with several different males, typically lasting 1–3 days each. During this time a female and her chosen partner usually leave the main body of the monkey troop for most (if not all) of the time they are together, often seeking relative seclusion to avoid harassment or other interruptions from other troop members (Manson & Perry, 1993). At the same time, the offspring from the previous year's consort tends to be ignored, actively avoided, or even physically rejected by both the mother and her current mate (Berman, Rasmussen, & Suomi, 1994).

Not surprisingly, most rhesus monkey yearlings become quite upset in the face of such functional maternal separations; indeed, a few actually develop dramatic behavioral and physiological symptoms that parallel Bowlby's (1960, 1973) descriptions of separation-induced depression in human infants and young children (Suomi, 1995). Most of their cohorts likewise exhibit an initial period of intense protest following loss of access to their mothers, but soon begin directing their attention elsewhere. Interestingly, female offspring "left behind" by their mothers during consorts tend to seek out other family members during their mothers' absence, whereas young males are more likely to increase interactions with peers while their mothers are away (Berman et al., 1994). These gender differences in the prototypical response to maternal separation at 6–7 months of age thus appear to presage the much more dramatic gender differences in life course that emerge during adolescence and continue throughout adulthood.

It would seem that a rhesus monkey mother would always have the upper hand in conflicts with her offspring during both weaning and breeding periods, given her great size and strength advantage over even the most persistent 5- to 7-month-old infant. A number of research findings, however, suggest that infants bring resources of their own into these conflicts. For example, Simpson, Simpson, Hooley, and Zunz (1981) reported that infants who remained in physical contact with their mothers more and explored less during the preweaning months were more likely to delay the onset of weaning by several weeks, and in some cases even to preempt their mothers' cycling during the normal breeding season; this pattern was especially clear for male infants. More recently, Berman et al. (1993) found that infants who achieved the most frequent nipple contacts with their mothers during the breeding season had mothers who were least likely to conceive, even if they entered into relationships with multiple consorts during that period. The end result in both cases was that these infants could, by their own actions, "postpone" their mothers' next pregnancy for another year, thus gaining additional opportunities for unfetered access to her not shared by agemates whose mothers had become pregnant during the same period. In the process, such an infant was also able to postpone by at least a year the appearance of a new source of conflict—that of "rivalry" with the mother's next infant.

The birth of a new sibling has major consequences for a yearling rhesus monkey. From that moment on, the yearling's relationship with the mother is altered dramatically, especially with respect to attachment-related activities. No longer is a yearling the primary focus of its mother's attention. Instead, many of its attempts to use her as a source of security and comfort are often ignored or rebuffed, especially when its newborn sibling is nursing or merely clinging to the mother's ventrum (Suomi, 1982). Moreover, whenever the yearling tries to push its younger sibling off the mother, to obstruct its access to her, or to disrupt its activity when it moves away from her, the mother's most likely response is to physically punish the yearling quickly, without warning, and often with considerable severity. In contrast, the mother seldom if ever punishes the younger sibling when it interrupts the yearling's attempts to interact with her or otherwise disrupts the yearling's activities (Berman, 1992).

Thus the arrival of a younger sibling inevitably alters the yearling's attachment relationship with its mother. This relationship generally continues to wane (i.e., proximity seeking and secure-base exploratory behavior both diminish) throughout the rest of the childhood years, especially after the birth of each succeeding sibling. For males, the waning process continues into puberty, eventually culminating with their natal troop emigration, which effectively terminates any remnant of their relationship with their mothers. Although attachment-related activities likewise decline throughout childhood for females, the daughters tend to increase other forms of affiliative interaction with their mothers (e.g., mutual grooming bouts), most notably after they start having offspring of their own. Coincidentally, episodes involving obvious conflict with their mothers become increasingly frequent for both male and female offspring as they approach puberty; thereafter, any semblance of attachment-like behavior directed toward mothers is infrequent at best among daughters and, of course, impossible for sons once they have left their natal troop (Suomi, 1998).

Factors Influencing Attachment Relationships in Rhesus Monkeys

Although Bowlby (1969/1982) believed that attachment has a strong biological basis and represents the product of evolutionary processes, he also observed that there is substantial variation among mother–infant dyads in fundamental aspects of their attachment relationships, and he recognized the potential developmental significance of such variation. Indeed, he lived to see his research associate Mary Ainsworth's strange situation assessment paradigm become almost reified in its identification and characterization of different "types" (viz., A, B, C, and [more recently] D) and even "subtypes" (e.g., A1, A2, B3, or B4) of human infant–mother attachment relationships (e.g., Goldberg, 1995). Perhaps not surprisingly, there appears to be comparable variation in the attachment relationships formed by different rhesus monkey mother–infant dyads. Indeed, there exist compelling parallels in rhesus monkey attachment relationships to each of the major human attachment types, and at least arguable similarities for most of the classical subtypes (e.g., Higley & Suomi, 1989). Moreover, an increasing body of research has identified numerous factors that clearly can influence the nature and ultimate developmental trajectory of these different attachment relationships. Some of these influences derive from characteristics of the infant, some from characteristics of the mother, and still others to factors external to the mother–infant dyad.

Rhesus monkey infants are born with distinctive physical and physiognomic features, relatively mature sensory systems with preestablished preferences and biases, and behavioral propensities that serve to promote essential contact with their mothers. These include not only the above-mentioned "component instinctual responses" identified by Bowlby (1958), but also the full range of items on the Brazelton Neonatal Assessment Scale (Brazelton, 1973), as adapted for monkeys with surprisingly minimal modification (e.g., Schneider & Suomi, 1992). To the extent that any of these species-normative features, preferences, or propensities might be compromised in individual monkeys as a result of genetic defects, fetal insults, and/or perinatal complications, one might expect some degree of

disruption in their emerging relationships with their mothers. Indeed, the literature generally bears this out, although there are compelling anecdotal reports of mothers (and others in the social group) who make compensatory adjustments in long-term support of offspring who are clearly developmentally disabled (e.g., Fedigan & Fedigan, 1977). On the other hand, cases of severe infant developmental disability in which the affected individual survives beyond infancy are relatively rare in the wild. A more common source of infant variance in rhesus monkey attachment relationships comes from differences among infant monkeys in their temperamental characteristics and the physiological processes that underlie their behavioral expression.

Researchers studying rhesus and other monkey species in both laboratory and field settings have long recognized developmentally stable individual differences along certain temperamental dimensions. Perhaps the most thoroughly studied area of monkey temperamental research to date has focused on individual differences in prototypical biobehavioral response to environmental novelty and/or challenge. Several sets of investigators have identified a subgroup of "high-reactive" monkeys, constituting perhaps 15–20% of both wild and captive populations studied to date, who consistently respond to such mildly stressful situations with obvious behavioral expressions of fear and anxiety, as well as significant (and often prolonged) cortisol elevations, unusually high and stable heart rates, and dramatic increases in central nervous system metabolism of the neurotransmitter norepinepherine (e.g., Capitanio, Rasmussen, Snyder, Laudenslager, & Reite, 1986; Clarke & Boinski, 1995; Suomi, 1981, 1983, 1991; Suomi, Kraemer, Baysinger, & Delizio, 1981).

High-reactive monkeys can be readily identified in their first few weeks of life. Most begin leaving their mothers later, and explore their physical and social environments less, than the other monkeys in their birth cohort. High-reactive infants also tend to be shy and withdrawn in their initial encounters with peers. Laboratory studies have shown that they exhibit higher and more stable heart rates and greater cortisol output in such interactions than do their less reactive agemates (Suomi, 1991). These distinctive behavioral and physiological features appear early in infancy, they show remarkable interindividual stability throughout development, and there is increasing evidence that they are highly heritable (cf. Higley et al., 1993).

One consequence of such biobehavioral tendencies is that high-reactive infants tend to spend more time with their mothers and less time with peers during their initial weeks and months of life. Their attachment relationships with their mothers tend disproportionately to be "C"-like (ambivalent), especially in the face of such challenges as brief separations from their mothers. High-reactive young monkeys are also far more likely to exhibit depressive-like reactions to functional maternal separations during the breeding season, as described above, than the rest of their birth cohort (cf. Berman et al., 1994; Suomi, 1995). On the other hand, a high-reactive infant may ultimately be more "successful" than others in its peer group in postponing its mother's next pregnancy and, eventually, a new sibling rival for her attention (Berman et al., 1993; Simpson et al., 1981; Suomi, 1998). These and other findings provide impressive evidence that temperamental reactivity on the part of the infant can influence, if not alter substantially, fundamental aspects of its relationship with its mother throughout development.

Rhesus monkey infants in a second subgroup, constituting approximately 5–10% of populations studied to date, consistently exhibit response styles that are perhaps best described as highly impulsive in nature, especially in social settings (where such behavior often leads to aggressive exchanges). This temperamental pattern is most readily apparent in peer play interactions. Impulsive males in particular seem unable to moderate their behavioral responses to rough-and-tumble play initiations from peers,

instead escalating initially benign play bouts into full-blown, tissue-damaging aggressive exchanges, disproportionately at their own expense (Higley, Suomi, & Linnoila, 1996). Prospective longitudinal studies have shown that individuals who develop such response patterns typically exhibit poor state control and significant deficits in visual orienting capabilities during their first month of life (Champoux, Suomi, & Schneider, 1994). They also tend to exhibit chronically low rates of brain metabolism of serotonin, a prominent inhibitory neurotransmitter implicated in ubiquitous aspects of metabolic, regulatory, and emotional functioning (cf. Coccaro & Murphy, 1990). In particular, impulsive monkeys consistently have lower cerebrospinal fluid (CSF) concentrations of the primary central serotonin metabolite, 5-hydroxyindoleacetic acid (5-HIAA), than their peers throughout development (e.g., Champoux, Higley, & Suomi, 1997; Higley & Suomi, 1996; Higley, King et al., 1996; Mehlman et al., 1994). As is the case for high reactivity, these behavioral and neurochemical characteristics of impulsive aggression are remarkably stable throughout development, and they also appear to be highly heritable (cf. Higley et al., 1993; Higley & Suomi, 1996).

Highly impulsive rhesus monkeys typically develop difficult attachment relationships with their mothers. They seem to be unusually fussy in their initial weeks (reflecting their generally poor state control; cf. Champoux et al., 1994), and their conflicts with their mother intensify substantially during and shortly after the time of weaning (Suomi, in press). In Ainsworth's strange situation terminology, these infants tend to form "A"-like (avoidant) and "D"-like (disorganized) attachment relationships. As they grow older, highly impulsive youngsters usually continue to exhibit difficulties in their social interactions with their mothers, with peers, and with others in their social group, and these social problems generally carry over into adolescence and adulthood (cf. Higley & Suomi, 1996; Suomi, in press).

Thus, certain infant temperamental character-istics seem to have a strong influence on the nature and long-term course of mother–infant attachment relationships in rhesus monkeys. Numerous other studies have shown that differ-ences among monkey mothers in their charac-teristic maternal "style" can also affect the type of attachment relationships they develop with their offspring. Although a comprehensive re-view of the relevant literature is beyond the scope of this chapter, it is worth noting that most primate females tend to be remarkably consistent in the specific manner in which they rear their infants, at least after their initial pregnancy (cf. Higley & Suomi, 1986; Suomi, 1987). It is also worth noting that some of the differences one can observe among monkey mothers in their re-spective maternal styles can be related to specific temperamental characteristics they displayed as infants, as well as the nature of the attachment relationship they formed with their own mothers (e.g., Champoux, Byrne, Delizio, & Suomi, 1992; Suomi, 1995, in press; Suomi & Ripp, 1983), as will be discussed later.

Factors other than infant temperament or ma-ternal "style" per se can also influence emerging infant–mother attachment relationships in mon-keys. For example, numerous studies carried out over the past 30 years have demonstrated that most rhesus monkey mothers, no matter what their characteristic maternal style might be, are usually highly sensitive to those aspects of their immediate physical and social environment that pose a potential threat to their infants' well-being, and they appear to adjust their maternal behav-ior accordingly (Berman, Rasmussen, & Suomi, 1997). Both laboratory and field studies have consistently shown that low-ranking mothers typically are much more restrictive of their infants' exploratory efforts than are high-ranking mothers, whose maternal style tends to be more "laissez-faire." The standard interpretation of these findings has been that low-ranking mothers risk reprisal from others if they try to intervene whenever their infants are threatened, so they

minimize such risk by restricting their infants' exploration. High-ranking mothers usually have no such problem and hence can afford to let their infants explore as they please (cf. Suomi, 1998).

Other studies have found that mothers gener-ally become more restrictive and increase their levels of infant monitoring when their immediate social environment becomes less stable, such as when major changes in dominance hierarchies take place or when a new male tries to join the social group. Changes in various aspects of the physical environment, such as the food supply's becoming less predictable, have also been asso-ciated with increases in maternal restriction of early infant exploration (e.g., Andrews & Rosen-blum, 1991). For those infants whose oppor-tunities to explore are chronically limited during their first few months of life, their ability to de-velop species-normative relationships with others in their social group (especially peers) can be compromised, often with long-term consequences for both the infants and the troop (cf. Suomi, 1998).

Effects of Differential Attachment Relationships on Long-term Developmental Trajectories for Rhesus Monkeys

Although considerable evidence from both field and laboratory studies has shown that individual differences among rhesus monkeys in certain temperamental characteristics tend to be quite stable from infancy to adulthood and are at least in part heritable, this does not mean that these behavioral and physiological features are neces-sarily fixed at birth or are immune to subsequent environmental influence. On the contrary, an increasing body of evidence from laboratory studies demonstrates that prototypical bio-behavioral response patterns can be modified substantially by certain early experiences. In this respect, individual differences among monkeys in their early attachment relationships are espe-cially relevant.

One set of studies has focused on rhesus monkey infants raised with peers instead of their biological mothers. Those infants were permanently separated from their biological mothers at birth; hand-reared in a neonatal nursery for their first month of life; housed with same-age, like-reared peers for the rest of their first 6 months; and then moved into larger social groups containing both peer-reared and mother-reared age-mates. During their initial months, these infants readily developed strong social attachment bonds to each other, much as mother-reared infants develop attachments to their own mothers (Harlow, 1969). However, because peers are not nearly as effective as typical monkey mothers in reducing fear in the face of novelty, or in providing a "secure base" for exploration, the attachment relationships that these peer-reared infants developed were almost always "anxious" in nature (Suomi, 1995). As a result, while peer-reared monkeys showed completely normal physical and motor development, their early exploratory behavior was somewhat limited. They seemed reluctant to approach novel objects, and they tended to be shy in initial encounters with unfamiliar peers (Suomi, in press).

Even when peer-reared youngsters interacted with their same-age cagemates in familiar settings, their emerging social play repertoires were usually retarded in both frequency and complexity. One possible explanation for their relatively poor play performance is that their cagemates had to serve both as attachment figures and play-mates—a dual role that neither mothers nor mother-reared peers have to fulfill. Another is that they faced difficulties in developing sophisticated play repertoires with basically incompetent play partners. Perhaps as a result of either or both these factors, peer-reared youngsters typically dropped to the bottom of their respective dominance hierarchies when they were grouped with mother-reared monkeys their own age (Higley, King, et al., 1996).

Several prospective longitudinal studies have found that peer-reared monkeys consistently ex-

hibit more extreme behavioral, adrenocortical, and noradrenergic reactions to social separations than do their mother-reared cohorts, even after they have been living in the same social groups for extended periods (Higley & Suomi, 1989). Such differences in prototypical biobehavioral reactions to separation persist from infancy to adolescence, if not beyond. Interestingly, the general nature of the separation reactions of peer-reared monkeys seems to mirror that of "naturally occurring" high-reactive mother-reared subjects. In this sense, early rearing by peers appears to have the effect of making rhesus monkey infants generally more high-reactive than they might have been if reared by their biological mothers (Suomi, 1997).

Early rearing with peers has another long-term developmental consequence for rhesus monkeys: It tends to make them more impulsive, especially if they are males. Like the previously described impulsive monkeys growing up in the wild, peer-reared males initially exhibit aggressive tendencies in the context of juvenile play; as they approach puberty, the frequency and severity of their aggressive episodes typically exceed those of mother-reared group members of similar age. Peer-reared females tend to groom (and be groomed by) others in their social group less frequently and for shorter durations than their mother-reared counterparts, and, as noted above, they usually stay at the bottom of their respective dominance hierarchies. These differences between peer-reared and mother-reared agemates in aggression, grooming, and dominance remain relatively robust throughout the preadolescent and adolescent years (Higley, Suomi, & Linnoila, 1996). Peer-reared monkeys also consistently show lower CSF concentrations of 5-HIAA than their mother-reared counterparts. These group differences in 5-HIAA concentrations appear well before 6 months of age, and they remain stable at least throughout adolescence and into early adulthood (Higley & Suomi, 1996). Thus peer-reared monkeys as a group resemble the impulsive subgroup of wild-living (and mother-reared) monkeys, not only behaviorally but also in terms of decreased serotonergic functioning (Suomi, 1997).

Other laboratory studies utilizing peer-reared monkeys have disclosed additional differences from their mother-reared counterparts—differences that are not readily apparent in free-ranging populations of rhesus monkeys. For example, peer-reared adolescent and adult males require larger doses of the anesthetic ketamine to reach a comparable state of sedation. They also exhibit significantly higher rates of whole-brain glucose metabolism under mild isoflurane anesthesia, as determined by positron emission tomography (PET) imaging, than mother-reared controls (Doudet et al., 1995). Finally, peer-reared adolescent monkeys consistently consume larger amounts of alcohol under comparable *ad libitum* conditions than their mother-reared agemates (Higley, Hasert, Suomi, & Linnoila, 1991). Recent follow-up studies have demonstrated that the peer-reared subjects quickly develop a greater tolerance for alcohol; this can be predicted by their central nervous system serotonin turnover rates (Higley et al., in press), which in turn appear to be associated with differential serotonin transporter availability (Heinz et al., 1998).

This association between serotonin turnover rate and serotonin transporter availability has led to a collaboration with Lesch and his colleagues, who have recently identified and characterized the serotonin transporter gene (5-HTT)—a candidate gene for impaired serotonergic function, in that it mediates serotonin neurotransmission and is a target both for antidepressant compounds such as Prozac and for certain drugs of abuse (Lesch et al., 1996). They have shown that length variation of the 5-HTT gene-linked polymorphic region (5-HTT-LPR) results in allelic variation in 5-HTT expression, such that the "short" allele of the 5-HTT-LPR confers low transcriptional efficiency to the 5-HTT gene promoter (relative to the "long" allele), suggesting that the low 5-HTT expression

may result in decreased serotonergic function (Heils et al., 1998). Although this genetic polymorphism was first detected in humans, it also appears in rhesus monkeys; in fact, it is found uniquely among simian primates and humans (Lesch et al., 1997).

We have recently been able to apply polymerase-chain-reaction-based genotype analysis to most of the rhesus monkeys in our laboratory at the National Institutes of Health, in order to determine the relative frequencies of the "short" and "long" alleles of the 5-HTT gene. Some of these genotyped monkeys were peer-reared, while others were reared by their biological mothers since birth. We found that the relative frequency of subjects possessing the "short" 5-HTT allele did not differ significantly between the two rearing groups; this was not overly surprising, given that these monkeys had been more or less randomly preassigned to their respective rearing conditions at birth. Because we had collected CSF samples from these monkeys during their second and fourth years of life under comparable experimental conditions (and while they were all living in comparable social groups), it was possible to determine whether their 5-HIAA concentrations differed as a function of their 5-HTT polymorphic status, as might be expected from the extant literature. Interestingly, we did find such a predictive relationship, with individuals possessing the "short" allele having significantly lower 5-HIAA concentrations—*but only among peer-reared subjects*. For mother-reared subjects, 5-HIAA concentrations were essentially identical for monkeys with either allele (Bennett et al., 1998).

Thus there appears to be a significant genotype–environment *interaction* in the brain metabolism of serotonin, wherein the ultimate effect of a polymorphism in a specific gene for a given individual is, in fact, highly dependent on the specific early attachment experience of that individual. We are currently carrying out additional analyses involving other behavioral and physiological measures that have already been collected on those mother- and peer-reared monkeys whose 5-HTT polymorphic status has been individually specified. For example, we are now trying to determine whether rearing-condition differences in the incidence of impulsive aggressiveness per se can be traced to potentially different consequences of possessing the "short" allele as a function of peer vs. mother rearing, as appears to be the case for rearing-condition differences in 5-HIAA concentrations.

An additional risk that peer-reared females carry into adulthood concerns their maternal behavior. Peer-reared mothers are significantly more likely to exhibit neglectful and/or abusive treatment of their firstborn offspring than are their mother-reared counterparts, although their risk for inadequate maternal care is not nearly as great as is the case for females reared in social isolation; moreover, their care of subsequent offspring tends to improve dramatically (Ruppenthal, Arling, Harlow, Sackett, & Suomi, 1976). Nevertheless, most multiparous mothers who experienced early peer rearing continue to exhibit non-normative developmental changes in ventral contact with their offspring throughout the whole of their reproductive years (Champoux et al., 1992).

To summarize, early rearing by peers seems to make rhesus monkey infants both more highly reactive and more impulsive. Moreover, their resulting developmental trajectories not only resemble those of naturally occurring subgroups of rhesus monkeys growing up in the wild, but also persist in that vein long after their period of exclusive exposure to peers has been completed and they have been living in more species-typical social groups. Indeed, some effects of early peer rearing may well be passed on to the next generation via aberrant patterns of maternal care, as appears to be the case for both high-reactive and impulsive mothers rearing infants in their natural habitat (Suomi & Levine, 1998). As noted by Bowlby and other attachment theorists for the human case, the effects of inadequate early

social attachments may be both lifelong and cross-generational in nature.

What about the opposite situation? That is, are there any consequences, either short- or long-term, of *enhanced* early social attachment relationships for rhesus monkeys? We attempted to address this question by rearing rhesus monkey neonates selectively bred for differences in temperamental reactivity with foster mothers who differed in their characteristic maternal "style," as determined by their patterns of care of previous offspring. In this work, specific members of a captive breeding colony were selectively bred to produce offspring who, on the basis of their genetic pedigree, were either unusually high-reactive or within the normal range of reactivity. These selectively bred infants were then cross-fostered to unrelated multiparous females preselected to be either unusually nurturant with respect to attachment-related behavior or within the normal range of maternal care of previous offspring. The selectively bred infants were then reared by their respective foster mothers for their first 6 months of life, after which they were moved to larger social groups containing other cross-fostered agemates, as well as those reared by their biological mothers (Suomi, 1987).

During the period of cross-fostering, control infants (i.e., those whose pedigrees suggested normative patterns of reactivity) exhibited essentially normal patterns of biobehavioral development, independent of the relative nurturance of their foster mother. In contrast, dramatic differences emerged among genetically high-reactive infants as a function of their type of foster mother: Whereas high-reactive infants cross-fostered to control females exhibited expected deficits in early exploration and exaggerated responses to minor environmental perturbations, high-reactive infants cross-fostered to nurturant females actually appeared to be behaviorally precocious. They left their mothers earlier, explored their environment more, and displayed less behavioral disturbance during weaning than not only the high-reactive infants cross-fostered to control mothers, but even the control infants reared by either type of foster mother. Their attachment relationships with their nurturant foster mothers thus appeared to be unusually secure (Suomi, 1987).

When these monkeys were permanently separated from their foster mothers and moved into larger social groups at 6 months of age, additional temperament–rearing interaction effects appeared, marked by optimal outcomes for those high-reactive youngsters who had been reared by nurturant foster mothers. These individuals became especially adept at recruiting and retaining other group members as allies during agonistic encounters; perhaps as a consequence, most rose to and maintained top positions in their group's dominance hierarchy. In contrast, high-reactive youngsters who had been foster-reared by control females tended to drop to and remain at the bottom of the same hierarchies (Suomi, 1991).

Finally, some of the cross-fostered females from this study have since become mothers themselves, and their maternal behavior toward their firstborn offspring has been assessed. It appears that these young mothers have adopted the general maternal style of their foster mothers, independent of both their own original reactivity profile and the type of maternal style shown by their biological mothers. Thus the apparent benefits accrued by high-reactive females raised by nurturant foster mothers can seemingly be transmitted to the next generation of offspring, even though the mode of transmission is nongenetic in nature (Suomi & Levine, 1998). Clearly, high reactivity need not always be associated with adverse outcomes. Instead, following certain early experiences high-reactive infants appear to have relatively normal (if not actually optimal) long-term developmental trajectories, which in turn can be amenable to cross-generational transmission. Whether the same possibilities exist for genetically impulsive rhesus monkey infants is the focus of ongoing research.

These and other findings from studies with monkeys demonstrate that differential early social experiences can have major long-term influences on an individual's behavioral and physiological propensities, over and above any heritable predispositions. The nature of early attachment experiences appears to be especially relevant: Whereas insecure early attachments tend to make monkeys more reactive and impulsive, unusually secure early attachments seem to have essentially the opposite effect, at least for some individuals. In either case, the type of attachment relationship a rhesus monkey infant establishes with its mother (or mother substitute) can markedly affect its biobehavioral developmental trajectory, even long after its interactions with her have ceased (as is always the case for a male living in the wild).

Cross-Generational Consequences of Early Attachment Relationships: Implications for Human Attachment Theory

Among the most intriguing aspects of the long-term consequences of different early attachment experiences is the apparent transfer of specific features of maternal behavior across successive generations. Several studies of rhesus monkeys and other Old World monkey species have demonstrated strong continuities between the type of attachment relationship a female infant develops with her mother and the type of attachment relationship she develops with her own infant(s) when she becomes a mother herself. In particular, the pattern of ventral contact a female infant has with her mother (or mother substitute) during her initial months of life is a powerful predictor of the pattern of ventral contact she will have with her own infants during their first 6 months of life (Champoux et al., 1992; Fairbanks, 1989). This predictive cross-generational relationship is as strong in females who were foster-reared from birth by unrelated multiparous females as it is for females reared by their biological mothers, strongly suggesting that cross-generational transmission of at least one fundamental component of mother–infant attachment—patterning of mutual ventral contact—necessarily involves nongenetic mechanisms (Suomi & Levine, 1998). What those nongenetic mechanisms might be, and through what developmental processes they might act, are questions at the heart of ongoing investigations.

Contemporary attachment theorists considering the long-term consequences of differential early attachment relationships in humans have also been examining possible cross-generational continuities in attachment styles. Some authors have posited the likely existence of strong cross-generational continuities, such that mothers who experienced secure attachments when they were infants might tend to develop secure attachments with their own infants, while those who experienced avoidant or ambivalent attachments with their own mothers might tend to promote avoidant or ambivalent attachments as mothers themselves (e.g., Berlin & Cassidy, 1999; Main, 1995). Moreover, current attachment theorists attribute these postulated infancy-to-parenthood continuities in attachment type to "internal working models" initially based on early memories and periodically transformed by more recent experiences. Most of the empirical findings that have led to these hypotheses have come from comprehensive interviews of adults (e.g., the Adult Attachment Interview) retrospectively probing memories of events and experiences. On the other hand, the most powerful empirical support for apparently parallel long-term continuities in attachment behavior from the nonhuman primate literature comes from prospective longitudinal observations and physiological recordings, both in controlled experimental settings and in naturalistic habitats, as reviewed above.

One insight that the nonhuman primate data bring to discussions about long-term consequences of early experiences is that strong developmental continuities can unfold *in the absence of language or complex imagery*. It is difficult to argue that rhesus monkeys, for example, possess sufficient cognitive capabilities to develop "internal working models" requiring considerable self-reflection, given that they are probably not capable of "self-awareness" or "self-recognition" (e.g., Gallup, 1977; Povinelli, Parks, & Novak, 1992). What cognitive, emotional, and mnemonic processes might underlie these continuities—and do they have parallels in human nonverbal mental processes?

Alternatively, one might argue that working models are exclusively human constructions built upon a basic foundation that is essentially biological in nature and universal among the more advanced primate species. According to this view, cognitive constructions per se may not be necessary for long-term developmental or cross-generational continuities in attachment phenomena to transpire; that is, such continuities are essentially "programmed" to occur in the absence of major environmental disruption, and are in fact the product of strictly biological processes that reflect the natural evolutionary history of advanced primate species, human and nonhuman alike. If this is the case, then working models (or other comparable cognitive processes) might represent a "luxury" for humans that might enable individuals to cognitively "reinforce" the postulated underlying biological foundation, in which case the predicted developmental continuity might actually be strengthened.

On the other hand, the existence of a working model that has the potential to be *altered* by specific experiences (and/or insights) in late childhood, adolescence, or adulthood, might provide a basis for "breaking" an otherwise likely continuity between one's early attachment experiences and subsequent performance as a parent. These important issues deserve not only further theoretical consideration, but empirical investigation as well. As Bowlby (1988) himself said, "All of us, from cradle to the grave, are happiest when life is organized as a series of excursions, long or short, from the secure base provided by our attachment figure(s)'' (p. 62). Research with nonhuman primates has clearly provided compelling evidence in support of a strong biological foundation for attachment phenomena. Indeed, such a foundation may well serve as a "secure base" for future research excursions in the realm of attachment phenomena.

References

Andrews, M. W., & Rosenblum, L. A. (1991). Security of attachment in infants raised in variable- or low-demand environments. *Child Development, 62,* 686–693.

Arling, G. L., & Harlow, H. F. (1967). Effects of social deprivation on maternal behavior of rhesus monkeys. *Journal of Comparative and Physiological Psychology, 64,* 371–377.

Bennett, A. J., Lesch, K. P., Heils, A., Long, J., Lorenz, J., Shoaf, S. E., Suomi, S. J., Linnoila, M., & Higley, J. D. (1998). *Serotonin transporter gene variation, strain, and early rearing environment affect CSF 5-HIAA concentrations in rhesus monkeys (Macaca mulatta).* Manuscript submitted for publication.

Berard, J. (1989). Male life histories. *Puerto Rican Health Sciences Journal, 8,* 47–58.

Berlin, L. J., & Cassidy, J. (1999). Relations among relationships: Contributions from attachment theory and research. In J. Cassidy and P. Shaver (Eds.), *Handbook of attachment theory and research* (pp. 688–712). New York: Guilford.

Berman, C. M. (1982). The ontogeny of social relationships with group companions among free-ranging rhesus monkeys: I. Social networks and differentiation. *Animal Behavior, 30,* 149–162.

Berman, C. M. (1992). Immature siblings and mother–infant relationships among free-ranging rhesus monkeys on Cayo Santiago. *Animal Behavior, 44,* 247–258.

Berman, C. M., Rasmussen, K. L. R., & Suomi, S. J. (1993). Reproductive consequences of maternal care patterns during estrus among free-ranging rhesus monkeys. *Behavioral Ecology and Sociobiology, 32,* 391–399.

Berman, C. M., Rasmussen, K. L. R., & Suomi, S. J. (1994). Responses of free-ranging rhesus monkeys to a natural form of maternal separation: I. Parallels with mother–infant separation in captivity. *Child Development, 65,* 1028–1041.

Berman, C. M., Rasmussen, K. L. R., & Suomi, S. J. (1997). Group size, infant development, and social networks: A natural experiment with free-ranging rhesus monkeys. *Animal Behavior, 53,* 405–421.

Bowlby, J. (1958). The nature of the child's tie to his mother. *International Journal of Psycho-Analysis, 39,* 1–24.

Bowlby, J. (1960). Separation anxiety. *International Journal of Psycho-Analysis, 51,* 1–25.

Bowlby, J. (1969/1982). *Attachment and loss: Vol. 1.* New York: Basic Books.

Bowlby, J. (1973). *Attachment and loss: Vol. 2. Separation.* New York: Basic Books.

Bowlby, J. (1988). *A secure base.* New York: Basic Books.

Boyce, T. W., Champoux, M., Suomi, S. J., & Gunnar, M. R. (1995). Salivary cortisol in nursery-reared rhesus monkeys: Interindividual stability, reactions to peer interactions, and altered circadian rhythmicity. *Developmental Psychobiology, 28,* 257–267.

Brazelton, T. B. (1973). *Clinics in developmental medicine: No. 50. Neonatal Behavioral Assessment Scale.* London: Heinemann.

Busnell, M.-C., & Granier-Deferre, C. (1983). And what of fetal audition? In A. Oliverio & M. Zappella (Eds.), *The behavior of human infants* (pp. 93–126). New York: Plenum Press.

Byrne, G. D., & Suomi, S. J. (1995). Activity patterns, social interaction, and exploratory behavior in *Cebus apella* infants from birth to 1 year of age. *American Journal of Primatology, 35,* 255–270.

Capitanio, J. P., Rasmussen, K. L. R., Snyder, D. S., Laudenslager, M. L., & Reite, M. (1986). Long-term follow-up of previously separated pigtail macaques: Group and individual differences in response to unfamiliar situations. *Journal of Child Psychology and Psychiatry, 27,* 531–538.

Champoux, M., Byrne, E., Delizio, R. D., & Suomi, S. J. (1992). Motherless mothers revisited: Rhesus maternal behavior and rearing history. *Primates, 33,* 251–255.

Champoux, M., Higley, J. D., & Suomi, S. J. (1997). Behavioral and physiological characteristics of Indian and Chinese–Indian hybrid rhesus macaque infants. *Developmental Psychobiology, 31,* 49–63.

Champoux, M., Suomi, S. J., & Schneider, M. L. (1994). Temperamental differences between captive Indian and Chinese–Indian hybrid rhesus macaque infants. *Laboratory Animal Science, 44,* 351–357.

Clarke, A. S., & Boinski, S. (1995). Temperament in nonhuman primates. *American Journal of Primatology, 37,* 103–125.

Coccaro, E. F., & Murphy, D. L. (1990). *Serotonin in major psychiatric disorders.* Washington, DC: American Psychiatric Press.

Darwin, E. (1794). *Zoonomia, or the laws of organic life.* London: Johnson.

DeCasper, A. J., & Fifer, W. P. (1980). Of human bonding: Newborns prefer their mothers' voices. *Science, 208,* 1174–1176.

Dienske, H., & Metz, J. A. J. (1977). Mother–infant body contact in macaques: A time interval analysis. *Biology of Behaviour, 2,* 3–21.

Dittus, W. P. J. (1979). The evolution of behaviours regulating density and age-specific sex ratios in a primate population. *Behaviour, 69,* 265–302.

Doudet, D., Hommer, D., Higley, J. D., Andreason, P. J., Moneman, R., Suomi, S. J., & Linnoila, M. (1995). Cerebral glucose metabolism, CSF 5-HIAA, and aggressive behavior in rhesus monkeys. *American Journal of Psychiatry, 152,* 1782–1787.

Fairbanks, L. A. (1989). Early experience and cross-generational continuity of mother–infant contact in vervet monkeys. *Developmental Psychobiology, 22,* 669–681.

Fedigan, L. M., & Fedigan, L. (1977). The social development of a handicapped infant in a free-living troop of Japanese monkeys. In S. Chevalier-Skolnikoff & F. E. Poirier (Eds.), *Primate bio-social development: Biological, social and ecological determinants* (pp. 205–222). New York: Garland Press.

Fifer, W. P. (1987). Neonatal preference for mother's voice. In N. A. Krasnagor, E. M. Blass, M. A. Hofer, & W. P. Smotherman (Eds.), *Perinatal development: A psychobiological perspective* (pp. 39–60). New York: Academic Press.

Fragaszy, D. M., Baer, J., & Adams-Curtis, L. (1991). Behavioral development and maternal care in tufted capuchins (*Cebus apella*) and squirrel monkeys (*Saimiri sciureus*) from birth through seven months. *Developmental Psychobiology, 24,* 375–393.

Gallup, G. G. (1977). Self-recognition in primates: A comparative approach to the bidirectional properties of consciousness. *American Psychologist, 32,* 329–338.

Goldberg, S. (1995). Introduction. In S. Goldberg, R. Muir, & J. Kerr (Eds.), *Attachment theory: Social, developmental, and clinical perspectives* (pp. 1–15). Hillsdale, NJ: Analytic Press.

Gunnar, M. R., Gonzalez, C. A., Goodlin, B. L., & Levine, S. (1981). Behavioral and pituitary–adrenal responses during a prolonged separation period in rhesus monkeys. *Psychoneuroendocrinology, 6,* 65–75.

Hansen, E. W. (1966). The development of maternal and infant behaviour in the rhesus monkey. *Behaviour, 27,* 109–149.

Harlow, H. F. (1953). Mice, monkeys, men, and motives. *Psychological Review, 60,* 23–35.

Harlow, H. F. (1958). The nature of love. *American Psychologist, 13,* 673–685.

Harlow, H. F. (1969). Age-mate or peer affectional system. In D. S. Lehrman, R. A. Hinde, & E. Shaw (Eds.), *Advances in the study of behavior* (Vol. 2, pp. 333–383). New York: Academic Press.

Harlow, H. F., & Harlow, M. K. (1965). The affectional systems. In A. M. Schrier, H. F. Harlow, & F. Stollnitz (Eds.), *Behavior of nonhuman primates* (Vol. 2, pp. 287–334). New York: Academic Press.

Harlow, H. F., Harlow, M. K., & Hansen, E. W. (1963). The maternal affectional system of rhesus monkeys. In H. L. Rheingold (Ed.), *Maternal behavior in mammals* (pp. 254–281). New York: Wiley.

Harlow, H. F., & Lauersdorf, H. E. (1974). Sex differences in passions and play. *Perspectives in Biology and Medicine, 17,* 348–360.

Heils, A., Teufel, A., Petri, S., Stober, G., Riederer, P., Bengel, B., & Lesch, K. P. (1996). Allelic variation of human serotonin transporter gene expression. *Journal of Neurochemistry, 6,* 2621–2624.

Heinz, A., Higley, J. D., Gorey, J. G., Saunders, R. C., Jones, D. W., Hommer, D., Zajicek, K., Suomi, S. J., Weinberger, D. R., & Linnoila, M. (1998). *In vivo* association between alcohol intoxication, aggression, and serotonin transporter availability in nonhuman primates. *American Journal of Psychiatry, 155,* 1023–1028.

Higley, J. D., Hasert, M. L., Suomi, S. J., & Linnoila, M. (1991). A new nonhuman primate model of alcohol abuse: Effects of early experience, personality, and stress on alcohol consumption. *Proceedings of the National Academy of Sciences USA,* 88, 7261–7265.

Higley, J. D., Hommer, D., Lucas, K., Shoaf, S., Suomi, S. J., & Linnoila, M. (in press). CNS serotonin metabolism rate predicts innate tolerance, high alcohol consumption, and aggression during intoxication in rhesus monkeys. *Archives of General Psychiatry.*

Higley, J. D., King, S. T., Hasert, M. F., Champoux, M., Suomi, S. J., & Linnoila, M. (1996). Stability of individual differences in serotonin function and its relationship to severe aggression and competent social behavior in rhesus macaque females. *Neuropsychopharmacology,* 14, 67–76.

Higley, J. D., & Suomi, S. J. (1986). Parental behaviour in primates. In W. Sluckin & M. Herbert (Eds.), *Parental behaviour in mammals* (pp. 152–207). Oxford: Blackwell.

Higley, J. D., & Suomi, S. J. (1989). Temperamental reactivity in nonhuman primates. In G. A. Kohnstamm, J. E. Bates, & M. K. Rothbard (Eds.), *Handbook of temperament in children* (pp. 153–167). New York: Wiley.

Higley, J. D., & Suomi, S. J. (1996). Reactivity and social competence affect individual differences in reaction to severe stress in children: Investigations using nonhuman primates. In C. R. Pfeffer (Ed.), *Intense stress and mental disturbance in children* (pp. 3–58). Washington, DC: American Psychiatric Press.

Higley, J. D., Suomi, S. J., & Linnoila, M. (1996). A nonhuman primate model of Type II alcoholism?: Part 2. Diminished social competence and excessive aggression correlates with low CSF 5-HIAA concentrations. *Alcoholism: Clinical and Experimental Research,* 20, 643–650.

Higley, J. D., Thompson, W. T., Champoux, M., Goldman, D., Hasert, M. F., Kraemer, G. W., Scanlan, J. M., Suomi, S. J., & Linnoila, M. (1993). Paternal and maternal genetic and environmental contributions to CSF monoamine metabolites in rhesus monkeys (*Macaca mulatta*). *Archives of General Psychiatry,* 50, 615–623.

Hinde, R. A. (1976). On describing relationships. *Journal of Child Psychology and Psychiatry,* 17, 1–19.

Hinde, R. A., Rowell, T. E., & Spencer-Booth, Y. (1964). Behavior of socially living monkeys in their first six months. *Proceedings of the Zoological Society of London,* 143, 609–649.

Hinde, R. A., & Spencer-Booth, Y. (1967). The behaviour of socially living rhesus monkeys in their first two and a half years. *Animal Behaviour,* 15, 169–176.

Hinde, R. A., & White, L. E. (1974). Dynamics of a relationship: Rhesus mother–infant ventro–ventro contact. *Journal of Comparative and Physiological Psychology,* 86, 8–23.

Hofer, M. A. (1995). Hidden regulators: Implications for a new understanding of attachment, separation, and loss. In S. Goldberg, R. Muir, & J. Kerr (Eds.), *Attachment theory: Social, developmental, and clinical perspectives* (pp. 203–230). Hillsdale, NJ: Analytic Press.

Immelmann, K., & Suomi, S. J. (1981). Sensitive phases in development. In K. Immelmann, G. W. Barlow, L. Petrinovich, & M. Main (Eds.), *Behavioral development: The Bielefeld Project* (pp. 395–431). New York: Cambridge University Press.

Lesch, K. P., Bengel, D., Heils, A., Sabol, S. Z., Greenberg, B. D., Petri, S., Benjamin, J., Muller, C. R., Hamer, D. H., & Murphy, D. L. (1996). Association of anxiety-related traits with a polymorphism in the serotonin transporter gene regulatory region. *Science,* 274, 1527–1531.

Lesch, L. P., Meyer, J., Glatz, K., Flugge, G., Hinney, A., Hebebrand, J., Klauck, S. M., Poustka, A., Poustka, F., Bengel, D., Mossner, R., Riederer, P., & Heils, A. (1997). The 5-HT transporter gene-linked polymorphic region (5-HTTLPR) in evolutionary perspective: Alternative biallelic variation in rhesus monkeys. *Journal of Neural Transmission,* 104, 1259–1266.

Lorenz, K. (1937). Der Kumpan in der Umwelt des Vogels. *Journal für Ornithologie,* 83, 137–213, 289–413.

Lindburg, D. G. (1971). The rhesus monkey in north India: An ecological and behavioral study. In L. A. Rosenblum (Ed.), *Primate behavior: Developments in field and laboratory research* (Vol. 2, pp. 1–106). New York: Academic Press.

Main, M. (1995). Recent studies in attachment: Overview, with selected implications for clinical work. In S. Goldberg, R. Muir, & J. Kerr (Eds.), *Attachment theory: Social, developmental, and clinical perspectives* (pp. 407–474). Hillsdale, NJ: Analytic Press.

Manson, J. H., & Perry, S. E. (1993). Inbreeding avoidance in rhesus macaques: Whose choice? *American Journal of Physical Anthropology*, 90, 335–344.

Mehlman, P. T., Higley, J. D., Faucher, I., Lilly, A. A., Taub, D. M., Vickers, J., Suomi, S. J., & Linnoila, M. (1994). Low cerebrospinal fluid 5-hydroxyindole-acetic acid concentrations are correlated with severe aggression and reduced impulse control in free-ranging nonhuman primates (*Macaca mulatta*). *American Journal of Psychiatry*, 151, 1485–1491.

Mehlman, P. T., Higley, J. D., Faucher, I., Lilly, A. A., Taub, D. M., Vickers, J. M., Suomi, S. J., & Linnoila, M. (1995). CSF 5-HIAA concentrations are correlated with sociality and the timing of emigration in free-ranging primates. *American Journal of Psychiatry*, 152, 907–913.

Mendoza, S. P., Smotherman, W. P., Miner, M., Kaplan, J., & Levine, S. (1978). Pituitary–adrenal response to separation in mother and infant squirrel monkeys. *Developmental Psychobiology*, 11, 169–175.

Povinelli, D. J., Parks, K. A., & Novak, M. A. (1992). Role reversal by rhesus monkeys, but no evidence of empathy. *Animal Behavior*, 44, 269–281.

Reite, M., Short, R., Seiler, C., & Pauley, J. D. (1981). Attachment, loss, and depression. *Journal of Child Psychology and Psychiatry*, 22, 141–169.

Robertson, J., & Bowlby, J. (1952). Responses of young children to separation from their mothers. *Cours du Centre International de l'Enfance*, 2, 131–142.

Ruppenthal, G. C., Arling, G. L., Harlow, H. F., Sackett, G. P., & Suomi, S. J. (1976). A 10-year perspective on motherless mother monkey mothering behavior. *Journal of Abnormal Psychology*, 88, 341–349.

Ruppenthal, G. C., Harlow, M. K., Eisele, C. D., Harlow, H. F., & Suomi, S. J. (1974). Development of peer interactions of monkeys reared in a nuclear family environment. *Child Development*, 45, 670–682.

Sackett, G. P. (1966). Monkeys reared in isolation with pictures as visual input: Evidence for an innate releasing mechanism. *Science*, 154, 1468–1472.

Schneider, M. L. (1992). Delayed object permanence in prenatally stressed rhesus monkey infants. *Occupational Therapy Journal of Research*, 12, 96–110.

Schneider, M. L., & Suomi, S. J. (1992). Neurobehavioral assessment in rhesus monkey neonates (*Macaca mulatta*): Developmental changes, behavioral

stability, and early experience. *Infant Behavior and Development*, 15, 155–177.

Simpson, M. J. A. (1979). Daytime rest and activity in socially living rhesus monkey infants. *Animal Behaviour*, 27, 602–612.

Simpson, M. J. A., Simpson, A. E., Hooley, J., & Zunz, M. (1981). Infant-related influences on birth intervals in rhesus monkeys. *Nature*, 290, 49–51.

Suomi, S. J. (1979a). Peers, play, and primary prevention in primates. In M. Kent & J. Rolf (Eds.), *Primary prevention in psychopathology: Vol. 3. Social competence in children* (pp. 127–149). Hanover, NH: University Press of New England.

Suomi, S. J. (1979b). Differential development of various social relationships by rhesus monkey infants. In M. Lewis & L. A. Rosenblum (Eds.), *The child and its family: Vol. 2. Genesis of behavior* (pp. 219–244). New York: Plenum Press.

Suomi, S. J. (1981). Genetic, maternal, and environmental influences on social development in rhesus monkeys. In A. B. Chiarelli & R. S. Corruccini (Eds.), *Primate behavior and sociobiology: Selected papers (Part B) of the VIII Congress of the International Primatological Society, 1980* (pp. 81–87). New York: Springer-Verlag.

Suomi, S. J. (1982). Sibling relationships in nonhuman primates. In M. E. Lamb & B. Sutton-Smith (Eds.), *Sibling relationships: Their development and significance* (pp. 284–309). Hillsdale, NJ: Erlbaum.

Suomi, S. J. (1983). Social development in rhesus monkeys: Considerations of individual differences. In A. Oliverio & M. Zappella (Eds.), *The behavior of human infants* (pp. 71–92). New York: Plenum.

Suomi, S. J. (1987). Genetic and maternal contributions to individual differences in rhesus monkey biobehavioral development. In N. A. Krasnagor, E. M. Blass, M. A. Hofer, & W. P. Smotherman (Eds.), *Perinatal development: A psychobiological perspective* (pp. 397–420). New York: Academic Press.

Suomi, S. J. (1991). Up-tight and laid-back monkeys: Individual differences in the response to social challenges. In S. Brauth, W. Hall, & R. Dooling (Eds.), *Plasticity of development* (pp. 27–56). Cambridge, MA: MIT Press.

Suomi, S. J. (1995). Influence of Bowlby's attachment theory on research on nonhuman primate biobehavioral development. In S. Goldberg, R. Muir, & J. Kerr

(Eds.), *Attachment theory: Social, developmental, and clinical perspectives* (pp. 185–201). Hillsdale, NJ: Analytic Press.

Suomi, S. J. (1997). Early determinants of behaviour: Evidence from primate studies. *British Medical Bulletin,* 53, 170–184.

Suomi, S. J. (1998). Conflict and cohesion in rhesus monkey family life. In M. Cox & J. Brooks-Gunn (Eds.), *Conflict and cohesion in families* (pp. 283–296). Mahwah, NJ: Erlbaum.

Suomi, S. J. (in press). Developmental trajectories, early experiences, and community consequences: Lessons from studies with rhesus monkeys. In D. Keating & C. Hertzman (Eds.), *Developmental health: The wealth of nations in the information age.* New York: Guilford Press.

Suomi, S. J., & Harlow, H. F. (1975). The role and reason of peer friendships. In M. Lewis & L. A. Rosenblum (Eds.), *Friendships and peer relations* (pp. 310–334). New York: Basic Books.

Suomi, S. J., & Harlow, H. F. (1976). The facts and functions of fear. In M. Zuckerman & C. D. Spielberger (Eds.), *Emotions and anxiety: New concepts, methods, and applications* (pp. 3–34). Hillsdale, NJ: Erlbaum.

Suomi, S. J., Kraemer, G. W., Baysinger, C. M., & Delizio, R. D. (1981). Inherited and experiential factors associated with individual differences in anxious behavior displayed by rhesus monkeys. In D. G. Klein & J. Rabkin (Eds.), *Anxiety: New research and changing concepts* (pp. 179–200). New York: Raven Press.

Suomi, S. J., & Levine, S. (1998). Psychobiology of intergenerational effects of trauma: Evidence from animal studies. In Y. Danieli (Ed.), *International handbook of multigenerational legacies of trauma* (pp. 623–637). New York: Plenum Press.

Suomi, S. J., Rasmussen, K. L. R., & Higley, J. D. (1992). Primate models of behavioral and physiological change in adolescence. In E. R. McAnarney, R. E. Kriepe, D. P. Orr, & G. D. Comerci (Eds.), *Textbook of adolescent medicine* (pp. 135–139). Philadelphia: Saunders.

Suomi, S. J., & Ripp, C. (1983). A history of motherless mother monkey mothering at the University of Wisconsin Primate Laboratory. In M. Reite & N. Caine (Eds.), *Child abuse: The nonhuman primate data* (pp. 49–77). New York: Alan R. Liss.

Trivers, R. L. (1974). Parent–offspring conflicts. *American Zoologist,* 14, 249–264.

Visalberghi, E. (1990). Tool-use in *Cebus. Folia Primatologica,* 54, 146–154.

Welker, C., Becker, P., Hohman, H., & Schafer-Witt, C. (1987). Social relations in groups of the black-capped capuchin *Cebus apella* in captivity: Interactions of group-born infants during their first 6 months of life. *Folia Primatologica,* 49, 33–47.

Welker, C., Becker, P., & Schafer-Witt, C. (1990). Social relations in groups of the black-capped capuchin (*Cebus apella*) in captivity: Interactions of group-born infants during their second half-year of life. *Folia Primatologica,* 54, 16–33.

Wilson, E. O. (1975). *Sociobiology.* New York: Cambridge University Press.

51 Nongenomic Transmission across Generations of Maternal Behavior and Stress Responses in the Rat

Darlene Francis, Josie Diorio, Dong Liu, and Michael J. Meaney

Individual differences in personality traits appear to be transmitted from parents to offspring. A critical question, however, concerns the mode of inheritance. Concordance studies with mono- and dizygotic twins have provided evidence for a genetic mechanism of transmission even of complex traits (1). In addition, parental behavior influences the development of the offspring (2) and could therefore serve as a mechanism for a nongenomic behavioral mode of inheritance. In the Norway rat (*Rattus norvegicus*), variations in maternal care are associated with the development of individual differences in behavioral and endocrine responses to stress in the offspring (3, 4). In the studies reported here we have examined the possibility that such variations in maternal care might be the mechanism for a behavioral transmission of individual differences across multiple generations.

Mother-pup contact in the rat occurs primarily within the context of a nest bout that begins when the mother approaches the litter, gathers the pups under her, licks/grooms her pups, and nurses her offspring while continuing to occasionally lick/groom the pups, and terminates when the mother leaves the nest (5). Naturally occurring variations in maternal licking/grooming and arched-back nursing (LG-ABN) have been associated with the development of individual differences in hypothalamic-pituitary-adrenal (HPA) and behavioral responses to stress in the offspring (3, 4). As adults, the offspring of high LG-ABN mothers are behaviorally less fearful and show more modest HPA responses to stress than do the offspring of low LG-ABN mothers. The variation in maternal behavior may thus constitute a mechanism for the nongenomic behavioral transmission of fearfulness from parent to offspring. Alternatively, of course, the differences in fearfulness and those in maternal behavior may both be associated with a common genotype so that the observed continu-

ity of individual differences from mother to offspring is mediated by a genomically based pattern of inheritance.

We found that the female offspring of high LG-ABN mothers showed significantly increased licking/grooming of pups in comparison with those of low LG-ABN mothers (12.9 ± 1.0 versus 6.9 ± 1.1; $P < 0.001$) (6), which suggests that individual differences in maternal behavior are transmitted across generations. To determine the mode of transmission we performed a cross-fostering study with the offspring of high and low LG-ABN mothers (7). A primary concern here was that the wholesale fostering of litters between mothers is known to affect maternal behavior (8). To avoid this problem and maintain the original character of the host litter, no more than 2 of 12 pups were fostered into or from any one litter (7). The control groups included (i) the offspring of low LG-ABN mothers fostered to other low LG-ABN mothers as well as offspring of high LG-ABN mothers fostered to other high LG-ABN mothers, (ii) sham-adoption animals, which were simply removed from the nest and fostered back to their biological mothers, and (iii) unmanipulated pups of high or low LG-ABN mothers. The limited cross-fostering design did not affect group differences in maternal behavior. The frequency of pup licking/grooming (Fig. 51.1A) and arched-back nursing across all groups of high LG-ABN mothers was significantly greater than that for any of the low LG-ABN dams, regardless of litter composition.

The biological female offspring of low LG-ABN dams reared by high LG-ABN mothers were significantly less fearful under conditions of novelty (9) than were any of the female offspring reared by low LG-ABN mothers, including the biological offspring of high LG-ABN mothers (Fig. 51.1B). This was also observed for male offspring (10). A separate group of female

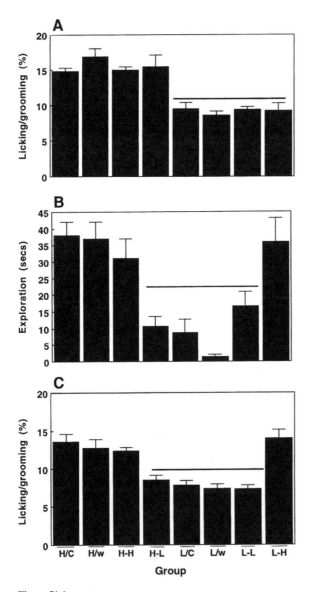

Figure 51.1

(A) Mean ± SEM percentage frequency of licking/grooming in high LG-ABN and low LG-ABN mothers (*n* = 6–8 per group), collapsed over the first 10 days postpartum in the adoption study.[6,7] The biological offspring of high LG-ABN or low LG-ABN mothers were (i) left undisturbed with their mothers, high/control (H/C) and low/control (L/C); (ii) cross-fostered back onto their own mothers, high/w (H/w) and low/w (L/w); (iii) cross-fostered to mothers of the same group, high-high (H-H) and low-low (L-L); and (iv) cross-fostered across groups, high-low offspring was then mated, allowed to give birth, and observed for differences in maternal behavior (6). The effect on maternal behavior followed the same pattern as that for differences in fearfulness. As adults, the female offspring of low LG-ABN dams reared by high LG-ABN mothers did not differ from normal, high LG-ABN offspring in the frequency of pup licking/grooming (Fig. 51.1C) or arched-back nursing (10). The frequency of licking/grooming and arched-back nursing in animals reared by high LG-ABN mothers was significantly higher than in any of the low LG-ABN groups, including female pups originally born to high LG-ABN mothers but reared by low LG-ABN dams.

Postnatal handling of pups is known to increase the frequency of maternal licking/grooming and arched-back nursing (11) and to decrease the response to stress in the offspring (12). Postnatal handling should alter the phenotype of the low LG-ABN offspring, and the behavioral transmission hypothesis would suggest that these effects should then be transmitted to the next generation. To see whether an experimental manipulation that alters maternal behavior would influence the transmission of these individual differences in behavior in subsequent generations, female offspring (F_1) of high or low LG-ABN mothers were mated (6), and the pups (F_2) in one-half of the litters in each group were exposed daily to brief sessions of handling (11). The female offspring of high LG-ABN mothers showed significantly more licking/grooming (Fig. 51.2A) and arched-back nursing than did the offspring of low LG-ABN mothers. Thus, as observed in our earlier study, individual differences in maternal behavior were transmitted across generations. The handling of the pups significantly increased the frequency of maternal licking/grooming and arched-back nursing in the offspring of low LG-ABN mothers but had no effect on the offspring of high LG-ABN mothers (Fig. 51.2A). Thus, the effects of maternal behavior of the low LG-ABN mothers with handled pups was indistinguishable from that of the high LG-ABN mothers. The maternal behavior of the adult female offspring (F_2) showed the same pattern (Fig. 51.2A), and this result is consistent with the transmission of individual differences in maternal behavior across generations. As adults, the handled female offspring of low LG-ABN mothers did not differ from the offspring of high LG-ABN dams in the fre-

(H-L) and low-high (L-H). No more than two pups were cross-fostered from any one litter. The ANOVA revealed a significant group effect ($F = 12.67$; $P < 0.0001$). Post hoc analysis revealed that the frequency of licking/grooming was significantly higher in each of the high LG-ABN groups as compared to any one of the low LG-ABN groups ($P < 0.05$; differences are indicated by a solid horizontal line). (B) Mean $\pm$ SEM time in seconds spent in the inner area of a novel open field (exploration)[9] in the adult female offspring from the cross-fostering study ($n = 6–8$ per group). The ANOVA revealed a significant effect ($F = 3.37$; $P < 0.05$) of the mother, a significant effect of cross-fostering ($F = 11.88$; $P < 0.0001$) and a significant mother $\times$ cross-fostering interaction effect ($F = 7.39$; $P < 0.001$). Post hoc analysis revealed that the time spent in inner area exploration was significantly ($P < 0.01$) higher in the biological offspring of low LG-ABN mothers reared by high LG-ABN mothers (L-H) than in the offspring of high LG-ABN mothers reared by low LG-ABN mothers (H-L). Groups lying below the solid line differ significantly from those above the line. (C) Mean $\pm$ SEM percentage frequency of licking/grooming, collapsed over the first 10 days postpartum in the adult female offspring from the cross-fostering study ($n = 5–7$ per group). The ANOVA revealed a significant effect ($F = 26.28$; $P < 0.0001$) of the mother, a significant effect of cross-fostering ($F = 13.56$; $P < 0.0001$) and a significant mother $\times$ cross-fostering interaction effect ($F = 8.13$; $P < 0.001$). Post hoc analysis revealed that the frequency of maternal licking/grooming was significantly ($P < 0.001$; solid line) higher in the biological offspring of low LG-ABN mothers reared by high LG-ABN mothers (L-H) than in offspring of high LG-ABN mothers reared by low LG-ABN mothers (H-L).

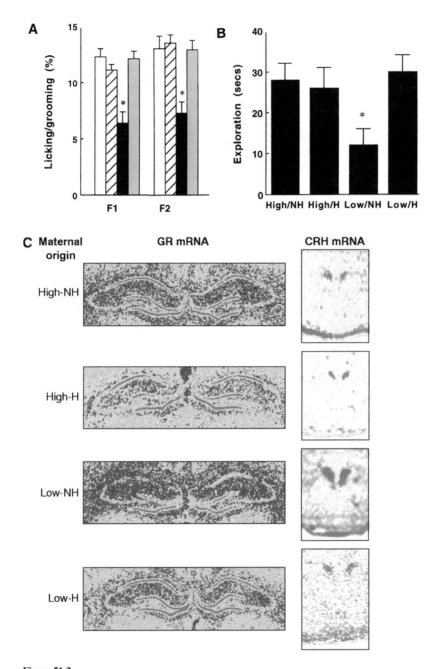

Figure 51.2

(A) Mean ± SEM frequency (as a percentage of total observations) of licking/grooming, collapsed over the first 10 days postpartum in high and low LG-ABN mothers (F_1), with handled (H) or nonhandled (NH) pups ($n = 5-7$ per group). The ANOVA revealed a significant group × pup treatment interaction effect ($F = 7.67$; df = 1, 19; $P < 0.01$). Post hoc analysis showed that the low LG-ABN mothers with nonhandled offspring showed significantly (*, $P < 0.01$) less licking/grooming than any other group, including low LG-ABN mothers with handled offspring. The same group × pup treatment interaction effect ($F = 9.78$; df = 1, 24; $P < 0.001$) in pup licking/grooming was apparent in the lactating female offspring (F_2) of these mothers. Open bar, High-NH; striped bar, High/H; black bar, Low/NH; gray bar, Low/H. (B) Mean ± SEM time in seconds spent in the inner area of a novel open field

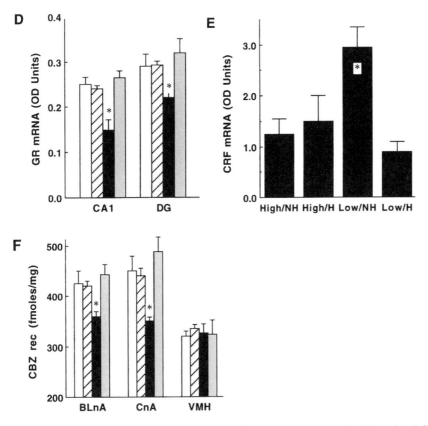

(exploration)[9] in the unmanipulated adult female offspring (F$_3$) of H or NH, high or low LG-ABN (F$_2$) mothers ($n = 8$ to 10 per group). The ANOVA revealed a significant group effect ($F = 3.39$; df = 3, 31; $P < 0.05$). Post hoc analysis revealed that the time spent in inner area exploration was significantly lower in the offspring of the low LG-ABN/NH animals than in any other group (*, $P < 0.05$). (C) A pseudocolor image of representative sections showing relevant brain regions from in situ hybridization studies examining GR mRNA expression in the dorsal hippocampus and CRF mRNA expression in the PVNh in the unmanipulated adult female offspring (F$_3$) of high LG-ABN/NH, high LG-ABN/H, low LG-ABN/NH, and low LG-ABN/H (F$_2$) mothers ($n = 4$ per group). (D) Mean $\pm$ SEM levels of GR mRNA (arbitrary optical density units using [^{35}S]-labeled standards)[14] in Ammon's Horn (CA1) and the dentate gyrus (DG) in the unmanipulated adult female offspring (F$_3$) of high LG-ABN/NH, high LG-ABN/H, low LG-ABN/NH, and low LG-ABN/NH (F$_2$) mothers ($n = 4$ per group). The two-way ANOVA (group × region) revealed a significant group effect ($F = 7.74$; df = 3, 12; $P < 0.01$). Post hoc analysis showed that for both the DG ($P < 0.05$) and the CA1 ($P < 0.002$) regions, GR mRNA levels were significantly lower (*) in the offspring of the low LG-ABN/NH animals than in any other group. Bar shading is the same as in (A). (E) Mean $\pm$ SEM levels of CRF mRNA (arbitrary optical density units using [^{35}S]-labeled standards)[14] in the PVNh in the unmanipulated adult female offspring (F$_3$) of high LG-ABN/NH, high LG-ABN/H, low LG-ABN/NH, and low LG-ABN/NH (F$_2$) mothers ($n = 4$ to 5 per group). The ANOVA revealed a significant group effect ($F = 4.11$; df = 3, 15; $P < 0.05$). Post hoc analysis revealed that in both regions mRNA levels were significantly higher in the offspring of the low LG-ABN/NH animals than in any other group (*, $P < 0.05$). (F) Mean $\pm$ SEM levels of CBZ receptor binding (femtomoles per milligram protein)[15] in the basolateral nucleus (BLnA) and central nucleus (CnA) regions of the amygdala and the ventromedial nucleus of the hypothalamus (VMH) of unmanipulated, adult female offspring (F$_3$) of high LG-ABN/NH, high LG-ABN/H, low LG-ABN/NH, and low LG-ABN/NH (F$_2$) mothers ($n = 4$ per group). The two-way ANOVA (group × region) revealed a marginal group effect ($F = 3.04$; df = 3, 12; $P < 0.10$) and, more important, a significant group × region interactions effect ($F = 3.18$; df = 6, 24; $P < 0.02$). Post hoc analysis showed that for both the basolateral ($P < 0.05$) and the central ($P < 0.002$) regions of the amygdala, CBZ receptor levels were significantly (*, $P < 0.05$) lower in the offspring of the low LG-ABN/NH animals than in other group. Bar shading is the same as in (A).

quency of maternal licking/grooming and arched-back nursing.

The next question concerned the effective transmission of the individual differences in behavioral responses to stress in the unmanipulated offspring (F_3) of these females (F_2). The level of fearfulness under conditions of novelty in the male or female offspring of handled, low LG-ABN mothers, which did not differ from high LG-ABN mothers in measures of maternal behavior, was comparable to that of the offspring of high LG-ABN mothers (Fig. 51.2B). The postnatal handling results suggest that environmental events that affect maternal behavior can alter the pattern of transmission of individual differences in stress reactivity and maternal behavior from one generation to the next.

The effects of variation in maternal care on the development of stress reactivity are mediated by changes in the levels of expression of specific genes in brain regions that regulate behavioral and endocrine responses to stress (3, 4, 13). In comparison to the offspring of low LG-ABN mothers, the adult offspring of high LG-ABN dams showed increased hippocampal glucocorticoid receptor (GR) mRNA expression, increased central benzodiazepine (CBZ) receptor levels in the central and basolateral nuclei of the amygdala, and decreased corticotropin-releasing factor (CRF) mRNA in the paraventricular nucleus of the hypothalamus (PVNh) (3, 4). As adults, the offspring of handled, low LG-ABN mothers showed hippocampal GR mRNA levels that were comparable to those observed in the offspring of either handled (H) or nonhandled (NH) high LG-ABN mothers and were significantly higher than those in the offspring of NH/LG-ABN females (Fig. 51.2, C and D) (14). Moreover, the offspring of the H/low LG-ABN females showed significantly reduced CRF mRNA levels in the paraventricular nucleus of the hypothalamus in comparison to the offspring of the NH/low LG-ABN mothers (Fig. 51.2, C and E) (14). CRF mRNA levels in these animals were comparable to those of the offspring of

H or NH high LG-ABN mothers. In previous studies, we also found that the offspring of high LG-ABN mothers show increased CBZ receptor binding in the amygdala in comparison with the offspring of low LG-ABN mothers (3, 4). As expected, the adult offspring of H/low LG-ABN mothers showed CBZ receptor levels in the central and basolateral nuclei of the amygdala that were comparable to those observed in the offspring of either H or NH high LG-ABN mothers and were significantly higher than those in the offspring of NH/LG-ABN females (Fig. 51.2F) (15).

These findings suggest that individual differences in the expression of genes in brain regions that regulate stress reactivity can be transmitted from one generation to the next through behavior. The studies of Denenberg (16) in rodents suggested that individual differences in behavioral fearfulness to novelty could be transmitted from parent to offspring through a nongenomic mechanism of inheritance. The results of the present study support this idea and suggest that the mechanism for this pattern of inheritance involves differences in maternal care during the first week of life. In humans, social, emotional, and economic contexts influence the quality of the relationship between parent and child (17) and can show continuity across generations (18). Our findings in rats may thus be relevant in understanding the importance of early intervention programs in humans.

References and Notes

1. R. Plomin, J. C. De Fries, G. E. McClearn, M. Rutter, *Behavioral Genetics* (Freeman, New York, ed. 3, 1997).

2. J. Bowlby, *Maternal Care and Mental Health* (World Health Organization, Geneva, 1951); H. F. Harlow, *Am. Psychol.* 13, 673 (1958); S. J. Suomi, *Br. Med. Bull.* 53, 170 (1997); M. Rutter, *Am. Psychol.* 52, 603 (1997); S. Levine and E. B. Thoman, in *Postnatal Development of Phenotype,* S. Kazda and V. H. Denenberg, Eds. (Academia, Prague, 1970).

3. D. Liu et al., *Science* 277, 1659 (1997).

4. C. Caldji et al., *Proc. Natl. Acad. Sci. U.S.A.* 95, 5335 (1998).

5. J. R. Alberts and C. P. Cramer, in *Handbook of Behavioral Neurobiology*, vol. 9, E. M. Blass, Ed. (Plenum, New York, 1989); J. S. Rosenblatt, *Acta Paediatr. Suppl.* 397, 3 (1994); J. M. Stern, *Dev. Psychobiol.* 31, 19 (1997).

6. The animals were derived from Long-Evans hooded rats obtained from Charles River Canada (St. Constant, Québec), mated with males drawn randomly from our colony breeding stock, and maintained under previously described conditions (3, 4). In cases where the offspring of high or low LG-ABN mothers were used in studies, no more than two animals per group were drawn from any single mother. All procedures were performed according to guidelines developed by the Canadian Council on Animal Care and the protocol was approved by the McGill University Animal Care Committee. Mothers and their litters were housed in 46 cm by 18 cm by 30 cm Plexiglas cages and maternal behavior was scored [M. M. Myers, S. A. Brunelli, H. N. Shair, J. M. Squire, M. A. Hofer, *Dev. Psychobiol.* 22, 55 (1989) and (3, 4)] for six 100-min observation periods daily for the first 10 days postpartum by individuals unaware of the origin of the animals. The following behaviors were scored: mother off pups; mother licking/grooming any pup; and mother nursing pups in either an arched-back posture, a "blanket" posture (in which the mother lies over the pups), or a passive posture (in which the mother is lying either on her back or side). The data were analyzed as the percentage of total observations (frequency per total observations × 100) in which animals engaged in the target behavior (3, 4). In order to define populations, we observed the maternal behavior in a cohort of 32 mothers and devised the group mean and standard deviation for each behavior over the first 10 days of life. High LG-ABN mothers were defined as females whose frequency scores for both licking/grooming and arched-back nursing were greater than 1 SD above the mean. Low LG-ABN mothers were defined as females whose frequency scores for both licking/grooming and arched-back nursing were more than 1 SD below the mean. As in our previous reports (3, 4), the frequency of licking/grooming and arched-back nursing were highly correlated ($r > +0.90$). The adult female offspring of high and low LG-ABN dams were then mated and observed for maternal behavior with the use of the same procedures described above over the first 10 days postpartum. As previously reported (3, 4), there were no differences in the percentage of total observations in which the offspring of high or low LG-ABN mothers were observed to be in contact with their pups (53 ± 5 versus $51 \pm 4\%$; NS). Variations in licking/grooming or arched-back nursing were not related to differences in time spent with pups.

7. R. McCarty and J. H. Lee, *Physiol. Behav.* 59, 71 (1996). Female offspring of high or low LG-ABN dams were mated and allowed to give birth. Within 12 hours of birth, dams were removed from the home cage and two animals per litter were cross-fostered. The cross-fostered pups, along with two native pups, were labeled with a permanent marker (Codman pens, Johnson & Johnson) until day 10 of life and were identified by individual differences in the pattern of pelage pigmentation thereafter. All litters were culled to 12 pups. Subsequent studies showed that marking the pups had no effect on maternal licking/grooming; marked pups are licked/groomed no more or less frequently than unmarked pups (10). The dam was returned once the foster pups were introduced into the new litter. The entire procedure took less than 15 min. The data were analyzed using a two-way analysis of variance (ANOVA) (mother × cross-fostering condition).

8. S. Maccari et al., *J. Neurosci.* 15, 110 (1995).

9. Fearfulness under conditions of novelty was studied by means of an open-field test of exploration as previously described (4). Animals were placed one at a time, in a novel, circular open field 1.6 m in diameter for 5 min. The critical measure of exploration was the time (s) spent in the inner area of the novel arena (that is, entire body of the animal being >10 cm away from any wall (>10 cm) enclosing the open field.

10. D. Francis and M. J. Meaney, unpublished data.

11. The handling procedure involved removing the mother and then pups from their cage, placing the pups together in a small container, and returning the animals and their mothers to their cage 15 min later. The manipulation was performed daily for the first 14 days of life, and the animals were tested as fully mature adults. Nonhandled animals were left completely undisturbed until day 12 of life, at which time normal cage maintenance was initiated. Mothers of handled pups consistently showed an increased frequency of maternal licking/grooming [M. H. S. Lee and D. I. Williams,

Anim. Behav. 22, 679 (1974); S. A. Barnett and J. Burn, *Nature* 213, 150 (1967); S. Levine, in *Society, Stress and Disease*, L. Levi, Ed. (Oxford Univ. Press, London, 1975); W. P. Smotherman and R. W. Bell, in *Maternal Influences and Early Behavior*, R. W. Bell and W. P. Smotherman, Eds. (Spectrum, New York, 1980); M. B. Hennessy, J. Vogt, S. Levine, *Physiol. Psychol.* 10, 153 (1982); (3).

12. S. Levine, *Science* 135, 795 (1962); ———, G. C. Haltmeyer, G. G. Karas, V. H. Denenberg, *Physiol. Behav.* 2, 55 (1967); J. L. Hess, V. H. Denenberg, M. X. Zarrow, W. D. Pfeifer, *Physiol. Behav.* 4, 109 (1969); M. X. Zarrow, P. S. Campbell, V. H. Denenberg, *Proc. Soc. Exp. Biol. Med.* 356, 141 (1973); M. J. Meaney, D. H. Aitken, Ch. Van Berkel, S. Bhatnagar, R. M. Sapolsky, *Science* 239, 766 (1988); M. J. Meaney, D. H. Aitken, S. Sharma, V. Viau, A. Sarrieau, *Neuroendocrinology* 5, 597 (1989); M. Vallée et al., *J. Neurosci.* 17, 2626 (1993); S. Bhatnagar, N. Shanks, M. J. Meaney, *J. Neuroendocrinol.* 7, 107 (1995).

13. A. J. Dunn and C. W. Berridge, *Brain Res. Rev.* 15, 71 (1990); M. J. Owens and C. B. Nemeroff, *Pharmacol. Rev.* 43, 425 (1991); P. M. Plotsky, *J. Neuroendocrinol.* 3, 1 (1991); M. F. Dallman et al., *J. Neuroendocrinol.* 4, 517 (1993); G. F. Koob, S. C. Heinrichs, F. Menzaghi, E. M. Pich, K. T. Britton, *Semin. Neurosci.* 6, 221 (1994); S. L. Lightman and M. S. Harbuz, *Ciba Found. Symp.* 172, 173 (1994); J. Schulkin, B. S. McEwen, P. W. Gold, *Neurosci. Biobehav. Rev.* 18, 1 (1994); J. P. Herman and W. E. Cullinan, *Trends. Neurosci.* 20, 78 (1997); J. A. Gray, *The Psychology of Fear and Stress* (Cambridge Univ. Press, Cambridge, 1987); A. L. Malizia et al., Eds., *GABAA Receptors and Anxiety: From Neurobiology to Treatment* (Raven, New York, 1995); P. Roy-Byrne, D. K. Wingerson, A. Radant, D. J. Greenblatt, D. S. Cowley, *Am. J. Psychiatry* 153, 1444 (1996).

14. For all in situ hybridization studies, animals were killed under resting-state conditions directly from the home cage. After rapid decapitation, brains were removed and quickly frozen in isopentane maintained on dry ice. Brains were blocked, and 15-μm cryostat sections were mounted onto poly-D-lysine–coated slides, desiccated under vacuum, and stored at −80°C. CRF mRNA in situ hybridization was performed with a [^{35}S]ATP-labeled 48–base pair (bp) oligonucleotide sequence (CAG TTT CCT GTT GCT GTG AGC TTG CTG AGC TAA CTG CTC TGC CCT GGC) obtained from the Sheldon Biotechnology Center (Montréal, Canada) as previously described (3). Preparation and description of GR riboprobes as well as the in situ hybridization procedure have been described (3). The GR cRNA was transcribed from a 674-bp Pst I–Eco RI fragment of the rat GR cDNA (steroid binding domain, R. Meisfield, University of Arizona), linearized with Ava I, and transcribed with T7 RNA polymerase. The hybridization signal within the parvocellular subregion of the PVNh (CRF mRNA) or the dorsal hippocampus (GR mRNA) was quantified by means of densitometry with an image analysis system (MCID, Imaging Research, Inc., St. Catherines, Ontario). The data are presented as arbitrary optical density (absorbance) units after correction for background. The anatomical level of analysis was verified with the Paxinos and Watson rat brain atlas (19) and Nissl-staining of sections after autoradiography. The hippocampal GR mRNA data were analyzed with a two-way ANOVA (group × region). The CRF mRNA data were analyzed with a one-way ANOVA (group).

15. CBZ receptor binding was measured with in vitro receptor autoradiography as previously described [M. H. Bureau and R. W. Olsen, *J. Neurochem.* 61, 1479 (1993)]. Brain sections were prepared as described above (14) and incubated with [^{3}H]flunitrazepam (84.5 Ci/mmol, New England Nuclear, Boston, MA), with or without 1 μM clonazepam. The sections were left to dry overnight and were then apposed to ^{3}H-sensitive Ultrafilm (Amersham Canada, Montréal, Canada) along with ^{3}H microscales for 14 days. Autoradiograms were analyzed by obtaining optical densities (expressed as mean ± SEM in femtomoles per milligram of protein) that were determined with computer-assisted densitometry using an MCID image analysis system and low activity ^{3}H standards of (19). Autoradiographic data were analyzed with a two-way ANOVA (group × region).

16. V. H. Denenberg and K. M. Rosenberg, *Nature* 216, 549 (1967); V. H. Denenberg, *Psychol. Rev.* 71, 335 (1964).

17. L. Eisenberg, in *Mammalian Parenting: Biochemical, Neurobiological, and Behavioral Determinants,* N. A. Krasnegor and R. S. Bridges, Eds. (Oxford Univ. Press, New York, 1990); T. Field, *Prev. Med.* 27, 200 (1998); A. S. Fleming, *Psychoneuroendocrinology* 13, 189 (1988).

18. M. H. Van Ijzendoorn, *Dev. Rev.* 12, 76 (1992); K. E. Grossman and K. Grossman, in *Attachment Across the Life Cycle,* C. M. Parkes, J. Stevenson-Hinde, P. Marris, Eds. (Routledge, New York, 1993); R. J. Noone, *Fam. Sys.* 2, 116 (1995); L. M. Fairbanks, *Adv. Study Behav.* 25, 579 (1996); L. Miller, R. Kramer, V. Warner, P. Wickramaratne, M. Weissman, *J. Am. Acad. Child Adolesc. Psychiatry* 36, 1134 (1997).

19. G. Paxinos and D. Watson, *The Rat Brain in Stereotaxic Coordinates* (Academic, New York, 1982).

Supported by grants from the Medical Research Council of Canada (MRCC) and the National Institute of Mental Health to M.J.M., as well as an MRCC graduate fellowship (D.L.) and an MRCC Senior Scientist award (M.J.M.). The authors thank B. S. McEwen and M. Hofer for comments on an earlier draft of this paper.

V BIOLOGY OF SOCIAL RELATIONSHIPS AND INTERPERSONAL PROCESSES

B. Social Applications

ii. Personal Ties

52 Neuroendocrine Bases of Monogamy

Larry J. Young, Zuoxin Wang, and Thomas R. Insel

Monogamy as a form of social organization is found in ~3% of mammals, with a higher percentage reported in primates.[1] Monogamy in rodents is characterized by an adult male and female pair sharing a nest and home range, preferential (if not exclusive) copulating with the mate, males participating in parental care, and vigorous defending of the nest against intruders.[2,3] Alternative forms of social organization include polygamy, defined as cohabitation with multiple mates, and promiscuity, characterized by an apparent absence of long-term social relationships. Over the past several years, the neuroendocrine mechanisms underlying the behavioral components of monogamy have been investigated in a group of mouse-like rodents (voles) native to North America. Here we summarize recent research on the neuroendocrine basis of monogamy in rodents and discuss possible genetic mechanisms involved in the evolution of monogamy in voles.

Microtine Rodents: A Comparative Model for Studying Monogamy

North American microtine rodents (voles) present an excellent opportunity for the investigation of the neural substrates underlying monogamy and social attachment. Species within the genus *Microtus* exhibit diverse forms of social organization ranging from minimally parental and promiscuous to biparental and monogamous social structures (Table 52.1). For example, the prairie vole (*Microtus ochrogaster*), which is highly social, forms lasting pair bonds after mating.[4] Pairbonded males prefer the company of the mate and exhibit "selective" aggression toward other members of the species. The breeding pair nests together: both parents provide extensive, prolonged parental care, and the offspring remain in the parental nest for several weeks beyond weaning. By contrast, the montane vole (*Microtus montanus*), which is relatively asocial, nests typically in isolated burrows and breeds promiscuously;[5,6] breeding partners do not form a pair bond after mating, males are not parental, and females abandon the offspring in the second or third postnatal week.

Remarkably, the behavioral differences between these species that have been described in field studies can be demonstrated in the lab. When several individuals are placed in a large cage, prairie voles spend more than 50% of the time in close physical contact with each other, whereas montane voles spend less than 5% of the time in close proximity to other individuals.[7] Experimental paradigms have been developed to study quantitatively various behavioral components of monogamy, such as partner-preference formation, mate guarding and paternal care. In addition, prairie voles and montane voles have been compared using various physiological and anatomical measures to investigate the neural hormones of monogamy. This search has implicated two neuroendocrine hormones, oxytocin (OT) and vasopressin (AVP), that show conspicuous differences in monogamous and nonmonogamous voles.

Oxytocin and Vasopressin: Hormonal Substrates of Monogamy

The central pathways that contain OT and AVP have been implicated in the control of a number of social behaviors in rodents, including sexual behavior, maternal behavior, affiliation, social memory, territorial behavior and aggression (Table 52.2). Specifically, it has been suggested that OT released in the brain at parturition could facilitate the dramatic shift from avoidance of infants to nurturing behavior in female rats and sheep.[21,22] In addition, chronic intracerebroven-

Table 52.1

Comparison of social behavior of the prairie vole and the montane vole

Behavior	Prairie vole	Montane vole
Mating system	Monogamous	Promiscuous
Parental care	Biparental	Maternal
Partner preference	High	Low
"Selective" aggression	High	Low
Social contact	High	Low

Table 52.2

Effects of central administration of oxytocin and vasopressin on social behavior

Behavior	Oxytocin	Vasopressin	Refs
Effects in rodents			
Affiliative behavior	+++	?	[8]
Sexual behavior	+++	?	[9, 10]
Maternal behavior	+++	+	[11, 12]
Social memory	++	+++	[13, 14]
Territorial behavior	?	+++	[15]
Male aggression	?	+++	[16]
Effects in monogamous voles			
Partner preference in females	+++	−	[17, 18]
Partner preference in males	−	+++	[19]
"Selective" aggression	−	+++	[19]
Paternal care	?	+++	[20]

+++, marked effect; ++, moderate effect; +, some effect; −, no effect; ?, effect unknown.

tricular infusion of OT increases social contact in the male rat.[8] Both OT and AVP appear to facilitate the consolidation of memory of socially familiar individuals.[13,14,23] In hamsters, AVP plays a direct role in the expression of territorial aggression in males.[15,16] Because each of these behaviors is a component of monogamy, these neuropeptides are good candidates for influencing pair-bond formation in the monogamous prairie vole.

Prairie voles usually form pair bonds as a consequence of mating. Mating in this species involves 15–30 bouts of copulation during a 24 h period. Because vagino–cervical stimulation in other mammals results in central OT release,[24] it seems likely that the intense mating of the prairie vole could stimulate OT release and facilitate the social attachment of the female vole to her mate. Indeed, in females that do not mate, intracerebroventricular infusion of OT,[18] but not AVP,[17] facilitates the formation of a pair bond, when measured by a partner-preference test (Fig. 52.1). Conversely, intracerebroventricular injection of a specific OT-receptor antagonist, $d(CH_2)_5[Tyr(Me)_2,Thr^4 TyrNH_2^9]$ ornithine vasotocin, before mating prevented the formation of a partner preference.[18] These results suggest that OT, released in response to mating behavior, is sufficient and necessary for the female to form a preference for her mate.

In the male prairie vole, mating also facilitates the formation of a partner preference[19] as well

as paternal behavior.[25] However, in contrast to females, OT appears to have little effect on partner-preference formation in males[19]: mating and the subsequent emergence of these behaviors is associated with a decrease in immunocytochemical staining of AVP fibers in the lateral septum[25] and an increase in AVP mRNA in the cells projecting to the lateral septum.[26] This is consistent with a synaptic release of AVP that is accompanied by increased AVP synthesis (Fig. 52.2). In the male prairie vole, central administration of AVP facilitates the formation of a partner preference, aggression towards strangers[19] and paternal care[20] in the absence of mating (Figs. 52.1,2). Furthermore, a specific vasopressin-receptor antagonist, $d(CH_2)_5[Tyr(Me)]AVP$, blocks the formation of a partner preference and aggression even in males experiencing extended mating bouts. The site of action of the AVP released by the fibers in the lateral

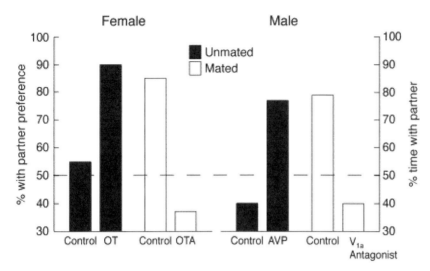

Figure 52.1
Effects of intracerebroventicular oxytocin (OT) and vasopressin (AVP) on partner-preference formation in prairie voles. Oxytocin facilitates the formation of partner preferences in unmated females towards male cagemates when compared with controls, whereas the oxytocin receptor antagonist (OTA) blocks the formation of preferences in mated females.[20] Similar results are found in male prairie voles following administration of AVP or an antagonist of the AVP receptor subtype V_{1a} (ref. 19). These effects are gender-specific: OT has little effect in males and vasopressin does not facilitate partner preference formation in females.

septum is unclear: few AVP receptors are found in this region in the prairie vole,[27] suggesting that diffusion into adjacent areas that are rich in receptors might be required for the facilitation of these behaviors.

The mechanisms underlying this gender dimorphism in the neuroendocrine control of monogamous behaviors are uncertain: there are no sex differences in the distribution or density of either OT or AVP receptors in prairie voles[27,28] and there do not appear to be sex differences in the distribution of OT-immunoreactive cells. However, there are dramatic sex differences in AVP fibers in the lateral septum, with immunoreactive staining in males far exceeding that in females.[29]

Subsequent studies suggest that stress and adrenal corticosterone might also modulate the formation of partner preferences in a sexually dimorphic manner. In female prairie voles, adre-

nalectomy facilitates the formation of a preference for a familiar partner after only 1 h of cohabitation without mating, and corticosterone treatment reverses this effect.[30] By contrast, stress appears to facilitate partner preference in males[31]: males forced to swim before being placed with a female develop a preference for the familiar female in the absence of mating. The interactions of the neurohypophyseal peptides and stress might play an important role in the formation of pair bonds, but the nature of this interaction has yet to be elucidated.

Neuroendocrine Correlates of Monogamy

The pharmacological data demonstrate a role for OT and AVP in monogamous behavior in prairie voles. In non-monogamous species,

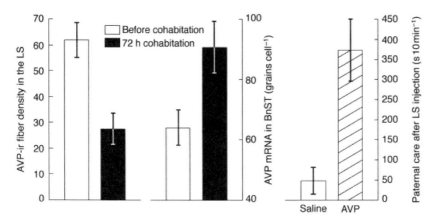

Figure 52.2

Effect of 72 hours of cohabitation (and mating) with a female on AVP-immunoreactive (AVP-ir) fiber density in the lateral septum (LS) of the male prairie vole.[25] The apparent decrease in lateral septum (LS)-fiber AVP content in the male prairie vole is associated with an increase in AVP mRNA synthesis in the cells of the bed nucleus of the stria terminalis (BnST), which project to the LS (left, ref. 27). These observations are consistent with a release of AVP into the LS as a consequence of cohabitation with a female. Direct injections of AVP into the LS (right) potently induced paternal care in sexually naive male prairie voles.[20]

such as montane voles, central administration of OT or AVP is associated with a different behavioral response.[32,33] For example, whereas intracerebroventricular infusion of AVP into a male prairie vole increased aggression toward intruders, the identical treatment in a male montane vole did not affect aggression, but increased autogrooming.[33] Because these species share similar OT and AVP immunoreactive patterns[29] but respond differently to exogenous peptide, the neuroendocrine differences between monogamous and non-monogamous species probably reside post-synaptically rather than pre-synaptically.

The behavioral actions of OT and AVP are mediated by related, seven-transmembrane domain, G-proteincoupled receptors that are located in specific brain regions that are known to modulate social behaviors.[34] The distribution and concentration of OT receptors and AVP receptors of the subtype V_{1a} have been deter-

mined using radioligand–receptor autoradiography. A comparison of the neuroanatomical distribution of the OT and AVP receptors in the prairie vole and montane vole reveals striking species differences (Fig. 52.3).[27,28] Comparison of other vole species supports the suggestion that the pattern of OT and AVP receptor binding is associated with social organization: for example, the monogamous pine vole (*Microtus pinetorum*) shares similar receptor distributions with the prairie vole, whereas the receptor distributions of the promiscuous meadow vole (*Microtus pennsylvanicus*) are similar to those of the montane vole. These differences in OT and AVP receptor distributions appear to be specific because the distribution of other behaviorally relevant receptors, such as the benzodiazapine and μ opiate receptors, is virtually identical between these vole species.[28]

The location of the peptide receptors in the prairie vole brain might provide clues to the

Montane   Prairie

OTR distribution

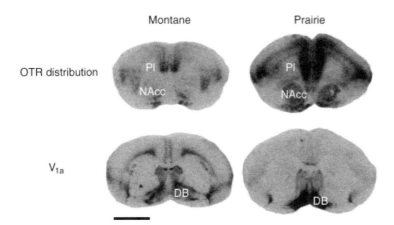

V_{1a}

Figure 52.3
Autoradiographical localization of oxytocin receptor (OTR) and vasopressin-receptor subtype V_{1a} binding in montane and prairie vole brains. Oxytocin (OT) and vasopressin (AVP) receptor autoradiographical studies (top and bottom rows, respectively) were performed on anatomically similar coronal sections from montane and prairie vole brains. The OT receptor autoradiograms are from sections slightly rostral to the V_{1a} receptor sections. Compared with the OTR binding in montane vole brains, binding in prairie vole brains is high in the prelimbic cortex (PI) and the nucleus accumbens (NAcc), whereas V_{1a} receptor binding is intense in the diagonal band (DB). Similar species differences are found throughout the brain. Scale bar, 2.5 mm.

cognitive mechanisms involved in pair bonding. For example, in the prairie vole brain there are high densities of OT receptors in the prelimbic cortex and nucleus accumbens, regions that are involved in the mesolimbic dopamine reward pathway (Fig. 52.3). Montane voles have few receptors in these regions. Therefore, it could be hypothesized that in the female prairie vole OT released upon mating activates this reward pathway, thus conditioning the female to the odor of her mate. Indeed, a dopamine D_2 receptor antagonist prevents the formation of a partner preference whereas a D_2 receptor agonist induces partner preference in female prairie voles (G. Yu, Z. Wang, and T. R. Insel, unpublished). This process, in conjunction with the AVP- or OT-associated consolidation of social memory, might result in the formation of the pair bond with that specific male. In the montane vole, OT would not have these reinforcing properties but pre-

sumably activates other targets (for example, the lateral septum) that are important for nonsocial behaviors.

Molecular Mechanisms Underlying Monogamy

This association between neuropeptide receptor distribution and social behavior suggests a potential mechanism by which social organization might evolve. By altering the neuroanatomical distribution of behaviorally relevant receptors, new brain regions and thus new neural circuits might become responsive to the neuropeptide. This notion is supported by the marked species diversity among mammals in the pattern of OT and V_{1a} receptor distribution and their regulation by gonadal steroids.[35] This phylogenetic plasticity in the regulation of receptor gene-expression might have played a significant role in the evolution of many types of species-specific social behaviors.

How could such differences in receptor distribution develop? Recent research has focused on examining the molecular mechanisms that determine the distribution of OT and AVP binding sites in the brain. Developmental differences in presynaptic innervation are unlikely to contribute to the adult receptor-binding pattern because OT knockout mice have normal OT receptor distribution and concentration.[37] Sequence analysis of the coding regions of the genes that encode OT and V_{1a} receptors reveal similar receptor protein-structures between monogamous and promiscuous vole species.[33,37] Furthermore, analysis of receptor synthesis by in situ hybridization suggests that the species differences in the pattern of receptor binding are due entirely to differences in regional gene expression and not to differential transport from other regions.[33,37] That is, the distribution of receptor mRNA is nearly identical to the distribution of receptor binding sites in both species.

Region-specific gene expression in the brain is determined by the interaction of cis regulatory sequences, usually located in the 5′ flanking region of genes,[38–42] and the action of regulatory proteins or transcription factors. Therefore, analysis of these sequences in the genes encoding OT and V_{1a} receptors might identify potential genetic elements that are important in the control of species-specific, regional gene expression. Comparison of the first 1500 base pairs (bp) of the prairie vole and montane vole OT receptor promoter has revealed variations in potential regulatory elements that might contribute to the species differences in expression of the OT receptor gene.[37] In addition, comparison of the vasopressin receptor gene between these species has revealed more striking differences in the promoter structure: the 5′ flanking region of the prairie vole gene that encodes the vasopressin receptor contains a 450 bp sequence that is absent from this gene in the montane vole, even though the coding sequence for the receptor is 99% homologous between species. An interesting structural feature that is common to the promoters of OT and V_{1a} receptor genes is the presence of long stretches of simple dinucleotide or trinucleotide repeat sequences.[37,43–46] Although present in the 5′ flanking regions of the receptor genes of several species, the length, position and composition of the sequences differ markedly between species. Indeed, it has been suggested that such "microsatellite" sequences are associated with hypermutability of surrounding sequences and might also influence the regulation of gene expression.[47] It is conceivable that diversity in these sequences between species could contribute to the diversity in the regulation of gene expression. Indeed, the unique sequence found in the prairie vole but not in the montane vole, the V_{1a} receptor 5′ promoter contains multiple repetitive sequences. In addition to this diversity in gene sequence, it is possible that species differences in the tissue-specific availability of transcription factors could account for the species-specific expression pattern.

The association between brain OT and V_{1a} receptor binding patterns and monogamy in voles suggests a functional relationship: prairie voles are monogamous because of their regional sensitivity to endogenous OT and AVP. This hypothesis could be tested by altering the pattern of neuropeptide-receptor expression in a species that does not normally express these behaviors. The development of transgenic and viral vector technologies[48] provides exciting opportunities for manipulating receptor gene expression in a targeted manner. Transgenic mice have been created recently using a transgene construct containing the 5′ flanking region of the prairie vole OT-receptor gene spliced upstream of the bacterial reporter gene encoding β-galactosidase.[49] The prairie vole promoter was found to direct the expression of β-galactosidase in several brain regions of the mice that were known to express OT receptor, including the cortex, septum, amygdala and hypothalamus.[50] This study demonstrates that heterologous promoters can be used to drive region-specific gene expression in a targeted manner. Similar experiments are under way with the vasopressin-receptor gene. With the appropriate regulatory sequences identified, it might be possible, using either conventional pronuclear injection techniques or viral vector technology, to create transgenic montane voles that carry a functional OT or V_{1a} receptor transgene with expression driven by prairie vole promoters. This might result in montane voles in which the pattern of neuropeptide-receptor gene expression and potentially, social behavior have been altered. If successful, and provided that the appropriate transcription factors and second-messenger pathways are in place, these experiments should demonstrate the behavioral consequences of altered receptor expression and potentially establish a link between specific genes and monogamy in rodents.

Acknowledgements

The research for the preparation of this manuscript was supported by the grants MH56897 for LY, MH54554 for ZW, and MH56539 and the Whitehall Foundation for TRI.

Selected References

1. Kleiman, D. G. (1977) *Q. Rev. Biol.* 52, 39–69.

2. Dewsbury, D. A. (1981) *The Biologist* 63, 138–162.

3. Dewsbury, D. A. (1987) *Nebraska Symp. Motivation* 35, 1–50.

4. Getz, L. L. et al. (1993) *J. Mammal.* 74, 44–58.

5. Jannett, F. J. (1980) *The Biologist* 62, 3–19.

6. Jannett, F. J. (1982) *J. Mammal.* 63, 495–498.

7. Shapiro, L. E. and Dewsbury, D. A. (1990) *J. Comp. Psychol.* 104, 268–274.

8. Witt, D. M., Winslow, J. T. and Insel, T. R. (1992) *Pharmacol. Biochem. Behav.* 43, 855–861.

9. Witt, D. M. and Insel, T. R. (1991) *Endocrinology* 128, 3269–3276.

10. Arletti, R. et al. (1985) *Horm. Behav.* 19, 14–20.

11. Pedersen, C. A. and Prange, A. J. (1979) *Proc. Natl. Acad. Sci. U.S.A.* 76, 6661–6665.

12. Pedersen, C. A. et al. (1994) *Behav. Neurosci.* 108, 1163–1171.

13. Popik, P., Vetulani, J. and Van Ree, J. M. (1992) *Psycho-pharmacology* 106, 71–74.

14. Dantzer, R. et al. (1988) *Brain Res.* 457, 143–147.

15. Ferris, C. F. et al. (1984) *Science* 224, 521–523.

16. Ferris, C. F. and Potegal, M. (1988) *Physiol. Behav.* 44, 235–239.

17. Insel, T. R. and Hulihan, T. (1995) *Behav. Neurosci.* 109, 782–789.

18. Williams, J. R. et al. (1994) *J. Neuroendocrinol.* 6, 247–250.

19. Winslow, J. T. et al. (1993) *Nature* 365, 545–548.

20. Wang, Z., Ferris, C. F. and DeVries, G. J. (1994) *Proc. Natl. Acad. Sci. U.S.A.* 91, 400–404.

21. Da Costa, A. P. C. et al. (1996) *J. Neuroendocrinol.* 8, 163–177.

22. Pedersen, C. A. et al. (1992) *Ann. New York Acad. Sci.* 652, 58–69.

23. Popik, P., Vos, P. E. and Van Ree, J. M. (1992) *Behav. Pharmacol.* 3, 351–358.

24. Kendrick, K. M. et al. (1988) *Brain Res.* 442, 171–174.

25. Bamshad, M., Novak, M. and DeVries, G. J. (1994) *Physiol. Behav.* 56, 751–758.

26. Wang, Z. et al. (1994) *Brain Res.* 650, 212–218.

27. Insel, T. R., Wang, Z. and Ferris, C. F. (1994) *J. Neurosci.* 14, 5381–5392.

28. Insel, T. R. and Shapiro, L. E. (1992) *Proc. Natl. Acad. Sci. U.S.A.* 89, 5981–5985.

29. Wang, Z. et al. (1996) *J. Comp. Neurol.* 366, 726–737.

30. DeVries, C. A. et al. (1995) *Proc. Natl. Acad. Sci. U.S.A.* 92, 7744–7748.

31. DeVries, C. A. et al. (1996) *Proc. Natl. Acad. Sci. U.S.A.* 93, 11980–11984.

32. Insel, T. R. et al. (1995) *Adv. Exp. Med. Biol.* 395, 227–234.

33. Young, L. J. et al. (1997) *Behav. Neurosci.* 111, 599–605.

34. Barberis, C. and Tribollet, E. (1996) *Crit. Rev. Neurobiol.* 10, 119–154.

35. Insel, T. R. et al. (1993) *J. Neuroendocrinol.* 5, 619–628.

36. Nishimori, K. et al. (1996) *Proc. Natl. Acad. Sci. U.S.A.* 93, 11699–11704.

37. Young, L. J. et al. (1996) *J. Neuroendocrinol.* 8, 777–783.

38. Banerjee, S. A. et al. (1992) *J. Neurosci.* 12, 4460–4467.

39. Hoyle, G. W. et al. (1994) *J. Neurosci.* 14, 2455–2463.

40. Carroll, S. L. et al. (1995) *J. Neurosci.* 15, 3342–3356.

41. Hoesche, C. et al. (1993) *J. Biol. Chem.* 268, 26494–26502.

42. Timmusk, T. et al. (1995) *J. Cell Biol.* 128, 185–199.

43. Bale, T. L. and Dorsa, D. M. (1997) *Endocrinology* 138, 1151–1158.

44. Kubota, Y. et al. (1996) *Mol. Cell. Endocrinol.* 124, 25–32.

45. Murasawa, S. et al. (1995) *J. Biol. Chem.* 270, 20042–20050.

46. Bathgate, R. et al. (1995) *DNA Cell Biol.* 14, 1037–1048.

47. Stallings, R. L. (1995) *Genomics* 25, 107–113.

48. Kaplitt, M. G. and Makimura, H. (1997) *J. Neurosci. Methods* 71, 125–132.

49. Young, L. J. et al. (1996) *Ann. New York Acad. Sci.* 807, 514–517.

50. Young, L. J. et al. (1997) *Horm. Behav.* 31, 221–231.

53 Role of Interleukin-1 Beta in Impairment of Contextual Fear Conditioning Caused by Social Isolation

C. Rachal Pugh, Kien T. Nguyen, Jennifer L. Gonyea, Monika Fleshner, Linda R. Watkins, Steven F. Maier, and Jerry W. Rudy

1 Introduction

Rats exposed to tone-footshock pairings, later display defensive fear responses when re-exposed to either the environmental context where shock occurred (contextual-fear conditioning) or to the tone that preceded shock (auditory-cue fear conditioning). Contextual and auditory-cue fear conditioning are interesting because they are thought to depend on different neural processes. Evidence for this comes from the findings that contextual but not auditory-cue fear conditioning can be disrupted by hippocampal damage [13, 32, 33], adrenalectomy [35], treatment with dehydroepiandrosterone (DHEA) [9] and morphine injection into the nucleus accumbens [44].

Rats that are socially isolated for several hours after conditioning also show impaired contextual but normal auditory-cue fear conditioning [39].

Because of the stressful nature of social isolation, we have previously examined the role of corticosterone in producing this impairment in contextual fear conditioning. This is because the hippocampus (which is critical to contextual fear conditioning) [13, 32, 33] is rich in glucocorticoid receptors [21, 22], and high glucocorticoid levels are thought to impair learning and memory [23]. However, when we attempted to block the isolation induced impairment in contextual fear conditioning with glucocorticoid receptor antagonists, neither Type I, Type II, nor the combination of both Types, was able to attenuate the impairment in contextual fear caused by isolation. Rather, Type I, Type II [34], and Type I and II glucocorticoid receptor antagonists in combination (unpublished data) actually produced impairments in contextual but not auditory-cue fear. In addition, Pugh et al. [35] reported that adrenalectomized rats showed impaired contextual fear conditioning and that this impairment could be eliminated by corticosterone replacement. Finally, post-conditioning corticosterone administration actually enhanced contextual but not auditory-cue fear [40]. Based on these results, it seems unlikely that the isolation induced impairment in contextual fear can be attributed to stress induced corticosterone release.

The present experiments were designed to explore another potential mediator of the impairment in contextual fear caused by isolation, interleukin-1β (IL-1β). IL-1β is a cytokine produced by a number of peripheral cell types and is involved in a variety of immune and inflammatory responses [8, 29, 20].

More recently, IL-1β has also been implicated in neurochemical and behavioral consequences of stressors. For example, immobilization stress increases IL-1β mRNA [24] and bioactivity [41] in the brain, while inescapable tail shock stress increases IL-1β protein levels [26] in brain. IL-1β appears to play a role in these stress responses because central IL-1β administration produces endocrine, neurochemical, and behavioral changes similar to those produced by stressors [42]. Central injection of IL-1 receptor antagonist (IL-1ra) also significantly inhibits both the brain monoamine and pituitary adrenal responses to immobilization stress [43] and the potentiation of fear conditioning and escape learning failure following inescapable tail shock [19].

IL-1β may be a key mediator in the isolation induced impairment in contextual fear because increased levels of IL-1β interfere with long-term potentiation (LTP), an electrophysiological correlate of learning and memory [12, 2]. IL-1β also increases serotonin release in the hippocampus [17, 18], which can depress the expression of LTP [4, 45]. Furthermore, we reported that peripheral lipopolysaccharide (a constituent of cell walls of gram-negative bacteria that increase brain IL-1β gene expression; [14, 15]) administration impairs contextual but not auditory-cue fear, and that this effect is blocked by IL-1ra [36]. For these reasons we explored whether social isolation stress impairs contextual fear by inducing an increase in brain IL-1β.

2 General Methods

2.1 Subjects

Adult (400–450 g) male Sprague–Dawley (Harlan, Indianapolis, IN, USA) rats were housed 4 to a cage at 25°C on a 12 h light/dark cycle (lights on at 06:45 h). Rats were allowed free access to food and water and were given 1 week to acclimate to colony conditions before experimentation began. All experiments were conducted in accordance with protocols approved by the University of Colorado Animal Care and Use Committee.

2.2 Surgery and Microinjections

Rats were anesthetized with Halothane, and using Bregma as a reference, were stereotaxically implanted with chronic stainless steel guide cannulae that terminated in the 3rd ventricle (AP = −0.18, ML = 0, DV = −0.75 from skull). Ventricle placement was verified at the time of surgery as previously described [43]. Cannulae were then secured with dental acrylic, and stainless steel stylets inserted to maintain patency. Rats were allowed 4 weeks to recover.

Microinjections were carried out immediately after conditioning (see below). Rats were gently wrapped in soft towels, and 33-gauge microinjectors attached to calibrated PE-20 tubing were inserted through the indwelling guide cannulae. The distal end of the PE-20 tubing was attached to a 10 µl Hamilton syringe. Five microliters were injected over a 30 s period, and the injector was left in place for 30 s after injection. After each injection, a sterile stylet was inserted into the indwelling guide cannula.

2.3 Drugs

Human recombinant IL-1ra, generously provided by Dr. David Martin of Amgen (Thousand Oaks, CA, USA), was microinjected intracerebroventricularly (ICV) at a dose of 0.25 µg/rat. The 0.25 µg dose was chosen as a central dose because this dose blocks the fever response to peripheral LPS in rats [25]. Vehicle controls received equivolume CSE buffer (Amgen, Thousand Oaks, CA; 10 mM citrate, 140 mM sodium chloride and 0.5 mM EDTA; pH 7).

Human recombinant IL-1β provided by the NIH Biological Response Modifier Program was microinjected at a dose of either 10 or 20 ng/rat. Vehicle controls received equivolume sterile, pyrogen free saline.

2.4 Apparatus

Behavioral conditioning occurred in two identical Igloo ice chests (see [35] for a detailed description). The 2 s, 0.4 mA shock (as measured at the rod floor) unconditioned stimulus (US) was delivered through a removable floor of stainless steel rods 1.5 mm in diameter spaced 1.2 cm center to center. Each rod was wired to a shock generator and scrambler (Lafayette Instruments Model 8240415-SS). Both chambers were cleaned with water before each animal was trained or tested. A 2976-Hz tone presented at 74 dB as measured in the test chamber by a Triplet sound level meter (Model 370 set on the C Scale) served as the auditory conditioned stimulus (CS). Ventilation fans provided background noise (68 dB; measured as above).

2.5 Behavioral Procedures

In all experiments, conditioning occurred between 08:00 and 11:00 h and consisted of two 2 s shocks that were each preceded by a 20 s tone (2976 Hz; 74 dB). The first trial occurred 120 s after the rat was placed into the conditioning chamber. The inter-trial interval was 120 s, and the rats were removed from the conditioning chambers 30 s after the final shock presentation. Thus, a conditioning session lasted approximately 270 s. Isolated rats were placed into individual opaque cages (26 × 16 × 12 cm) with stainless steel wire tops for 5 h following conditioning. Food and water were available to the rats during the isolation period. Conditioned fear was assessed approximately 48 h after conditioning. Contextual fear conditioning was assessed by placing each rat into the original training context for 5 min. Using a time sampling procedure, every 10 s each rat was judged as either freezing or active at the instant the sample was taken. Freezing, the rat's dominant defensive fear response, is an immediate suppression of behavior that is accompanied by immobility, shallow breathing, and a variety of other autonomic changes including an increase in heart rate and pilo-erection. Rats exhibit the freezing response when they are in a potentially harmful situation such as those when the threat of predation is high [7]. Freezing in these experiments was defined as the absence of all visible movement, except for respiration. Scoring began approximately 20 s after the animal was placed into the chamber. Scoring was carried out blind to experimental treatment and inter-rater reliability exceeded 0.98 for all experiments.

The auditory-cue fear conditioning test took place 30 min after all rats had been tested for contextual fear conditioning. To assess auditory-cue fear conditioning, the conditioning chambers were altered by connecting two diagonal corners with a clear Plexiglas panel (34 × 10 × 12 cm) creating a triangular chamber. The rod floors were removed so that the conditioning chambers rested on a clear Plexiglas floor, and a 7 watt 120 V AC clear red light bulb illuminated the chests. During the auditory-cue test, rats were scored for 6 min. To provide a baseline freezing rate in the altered context, the auditory CS was absent for the first 3 min (pre CS period). The tone was then presented during the second 3 min (CS period). Again, rats were judged as either freezing or active every 10 s.

2.6 Tissue Collection

Brains were quickly removed after decapitation, and dissections were performed on metal plates placed on crushed ice. Upon removal, brain structures were immediately frozen in liquid nitrogen. Brain samples, which included the pituitary gland, hypothalamus, hippocampus, and posterior cortex, were stored at $-70°C$ until the time of sonication.

2.7 Tissue Processing

Each tissue was added to 0.25 (pituitary), 0.5 (hypothalamus and hippocampus) or 1.0 (posterior cortex) ml of Iscove's culture media containing 5% fetal calf serum and a cocktail enzyme inhibitor (in mM: 100 amino-n-caproic acid, 10 EDTA, 5 benzamidine-HCl, and 0.2 phenylmethylsulfonyl fluoride). Total protein was mechanically dissociated from tissue using an ultrasonic cell disrupter (Heat Systems, Inc., Farmingdale, NY, USA). Sonication consisted of 10 s of cell disruption at a setting of 10. Sonicated samples were centrifuged at 10 000 rpm at $4°C$ for 10 min. Supernatants were removed and stored at $4°C$ until an enzyme linked immunosorbent assay (ELISA) was performed.

2.8 IL-1β Protein Quantification

Levels of IL-1β protein were determined using a commercially available rat IL-1β ELISA kit (R&D Systems, Minneapolis, MN, USA) as previously described [26]. The validity of this assay has been confirmed using lipopolysaccharide to induce brain IL-1β protein and the results have been previously published [26]. The assay was performed according to manufacturer's instructions. This ELISA kit uses a goat anti-rat IL-1β polyclonal antibody that can recognize both recombinant (r) as well as natural rat IL-1β. No significant cross-reactivity was observed with this antibody to rHuman IL-1 receptor type I, rHuman IL-1 receptor type II, rHuman IL-1 receptor antagonist; rRat IL-1alpha, rRat IL-2, rRat IL-4, rRat interferon-gamma, or rRat tumor necrosis factor alpha; rMouse IL-1 alpha or rMouse IL-1 receptor antagonist, according to manufacturer's data. The detection limit of this assay is typically less than 5 pg/ml, according to manufacturer's data. We, however, have found the limit to be closer to 10 pg/ml, and our assay values are consistently between 20–200 pg/ml. Taking the total amount of protein in each sample into account, the concentration of IL-1β protein in the samples is represented as pg of IL-1β/100 μg of total protein. Furthermore, the intra- and inter-assay coefficients of variance have been found to be <10% according to manufacturer's data. In addition, we have determined the recovery of rRat IL-1β protein from sonicated brain tissue samples and found it to be between 50 and 70%. This was performed by adding a known concentration of rRat IL-1β into brain samples prior to sonication. The tissues were processed as previously described and the ELISA was performed. The recovered values were compared to the values of brain samples without the addition of rRat IL-1β to determine the percentage of recovery.

3 Experiment 1

3.1 Methods and Procedures

Previously, Rudy [39] reported that social isolation after conditioning impaired contextual but not auditory-cue fear conditioning in juvenile rats (35 days old; 100–150 g). The purpose of Experiment 1 was to determine if social isolation would also impair contextual but not auditory-cue fear conditioning in operated adult rats

(400–450 g). Rats were implanted with ICV cannulae and allowed 4 weeks to recover. They were conditioned with 2 tone-shock pairings. Immediately after conditioning, half of the rats were isolated for 5 h ($n = 8$) while the remaining rats were returned to the home cage ($n = 8$). Rats were tested for contextual and auditory-cue fear conditioning 48 h later.

3.2 Results and Discussion

As shown in Fig. 53.1a and b, post-conditioning isolation impaired contextual fear conditioning $F(1, 14) = 32.3$, $P < 0.0001$, but had no effect on auditory-cue fear conditioning, $F < 1$.

In this experiment, the shock paradigm led to substantial freezing in the context where shock occurred. This freezing in the context represents a conditioned response because very little freezing occurred in the altered context before the tone presentation began during the auditory-cue fear conditioning test (Fig. 53.1b). Therefore, any freezing behavior in the original training context must have been controlled by specific associative processes.

These results replicate and add to the generality of Rudy's [39] previous finding that post-conditioning social isolation selectively impairs contextual fear conditioning in juvenile rats. That auditory-cue fear conditioning was not impaired suggests that the impairment in contextual fear conditioning cannot be a result of the isolated rats' inability to express the freezing response. The impairment in contextual fear conditioning also cannot be attributed to motivational or perceptual differences between the groups during conditioning because isolation did not occur until after the conditioning episode was over. Additionally, that isolation occurred after conditioning suggests that it impairs contextual fear conditioning by interfering with some aspect of post-trial memory consolidation processes that are necessary for contextual fear conditioning to occur.

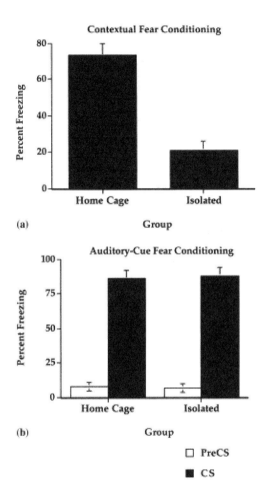

Figure 53.1
(a) Mean percentage freezing during the contextual fear test of rats isolated for 5 h or returned to the home cage after conditioning. Bars represent SE. (b) Mean percentage freezing during the auditory-cue fear conditioning test. Bars: SE.

4 Experiment 2

4.1 Methods and Procedures

If an increase in brain IL-1β activity is involved in producing the impairment in contextual fear conditioning caused by social isolation, then one might expect to observe an increase in brain IL-1β protein levels in isolated rats. To test this hypothesis, rats were conditioned with 2 tone shock pairings. Immediately after conditioning, rats were either isolated ($n = 20$) or returned to the home cage ($n = 16$). At 1 or 3 h after conditioning, both isolated and home cage rats were sacrificed and the hippocampus, hypothalamus, posterior cortex, and pituitary gland were collected to measure IL-1β protein levels. These brain regions were chosen because of their respective involvements in stress responses (pituitary and hypothalamus) and learning and memory processes (hippocampus and posterior cortex).

4.2 Results and Discussion

Social isolation after conditioning induced an increase in IL-1β protein levels in the hippocampus and posterior cortex, but not in the pituitary gland or the hypothalamus (Fig. 53.2). This was confirmed by a series of 2×2 analyses of variance (ANOVAS) for the different brain regions. An Isolation $\times$ Time Point ANOVA for the hippocampal data revealed a main effect of Isolation with isolated rats showing significantly higher IL-1β protein levels than home cage controls, $F(1, 30) = 6.16$, $P < 0.01$. There was no effect of Time Point on IL-1β levels, $F < 1$, and there was no Group $\times$ Time Point interaction, $F < 1$. An Isolation $\times$ Time Point ANOVA for the posterior cortex indicated that isolated rats also showed significantly higher IL-1β protein levels than did home cage controls, $F(1, 30) = 5.22$, $P < 0.05$. Again, there was no

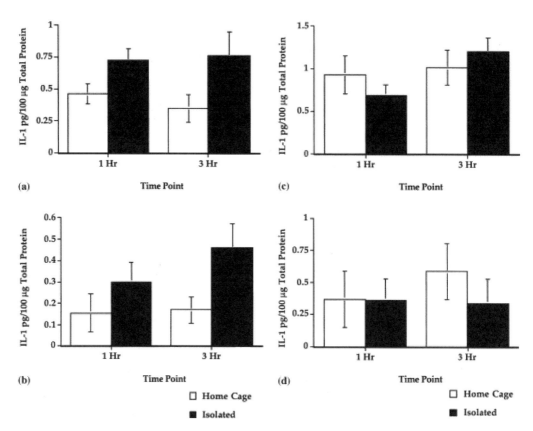

Figure 53.2
(a) IL-1 protein levels in the hippocampus in isolated rates versus home cage controls at 1 and 3 h after conditioning. Bars: SE. (b) IL-1 protein levels in the cortex in isolated rates versus home cage controls at 1 and 3 h after conditioning. Bars: SE. (c) IL-1 protein levels in the hypothalamus in isolated rats versus home cage controls at 1 and 3 h after conditioning. Bars: SE. (d) IL-1 protein levels in the pituitary gland in isolated rats versus home cage controls at 1 and 3 h after conditioning. Bars: SE.

effect of Time Point on IL-1β levels, $F < 1$, and there was no Isolation $\times$ Time Point interaction, $F < 1$. There was no effect of Isolation or Time Point on IL-1β protein levels in the pituitary gland or the hypothalamus, $F < 1$. However, while not statistically significant, there appeared to be a trend towards an increase in IL-1β protein levels in the hypothalamus 3 h after conditioning in home cage controls. This trend however, has not been evident in previous studies and has not been replicated in subsequent measures of IL-1 levels after conditioning (unpublished data).

The finding that social isolation increases central IL-1β protein levels is consistent with the hypothesis that an increase in IL-1β may be involved in producing the impairment in contextual fear conditioning caused by isolation. That the increase in IL-1β protein levels was observed in the hippocampus and posterior cortex is interesting because both of these structures are critically involved in various complex learning and memory paradigms such as contextual fear conditioning [13, 32, 33]. The 1 and 3 h time points were chosen because previous work measuring IL-1β protein levels after 5 h of isolation did not reveal a difference between isolated and home cage controls. However, we reasoned that changes in IL-1β protein levels could happen at anytime during the isolation period and still affect memory consolidation processes. Indeed, in other experiments we have isolated rats for only 1 h and still observed an impairment in contextual fear conditioning [40]. Therefore, 1 and 3 h of isolation were sufficient to produce an impairment in contextual fear conditioning, and these are also the time points where a difference in IL-1β protein levels is most readily detected. The finding that social isolation results in increased central IL-1β protein levels is also consistent with the findings of Shintani et al. [42] and Nguyen et al. [26] that stressors are able to induce IL-1β activity in the uninjured brain.

5 Experiment 3

5.1 Methods and Procedures

If increased IL-1β protein levels in brain induced by isolation are critical to the impairment in contextual fear conditioning caused by isolation, then the central administration of IL-1ra should be able to block the effect of isolation on contextual fear conditioning. To test this hypothesis, rats were implanted with ICV cannulae and allowed 4 weeks to recover. They were conditioned with 2 tone shock pairings. Immediately after conditioning half of the rats were given an ICV injection of IL-1ra ($n = 17$) while the remaining rats were given sterile pyrogen free vehicle ($n = 17$). Half of the rats from each drug condition were isolated for 5 h ($n = 9$) and the other half were returned to the home cage ($n = 8$). Rats were tested for contextual and auditory-cue fear conditioning 48 h later.

5.2 Results and Discussion

Consistent with the hypothesis that isolation impairs contextual fear conditioning by inducing an increase in IL-1β, central IL-1ra (0.25 µg/rat) blocked the effect of social isolation on contextual fear conditioning (Fig. 53.3a). Isolated rats treated with IL-1ra after conditioning showed levels of contextual fear conditioning that were equivalent to home cage controls. Rats that were isolated and given vehicle after conditioning showed substantially less contextual fear conditioning than did all other groups. IL-1ra had no effect on the level of fear conditioning displayed by home cage controls. There were also no differences in auditory-cue fear conditioning between the groups either during the preCS or CS periods (Fig. 53.3b).

An Isolation $\times$ Drug Treatment ANOVA revealed a main effect of group, $F(1, 31) = 7.6$, $P < 0.01$, with isolated rats showing significantly

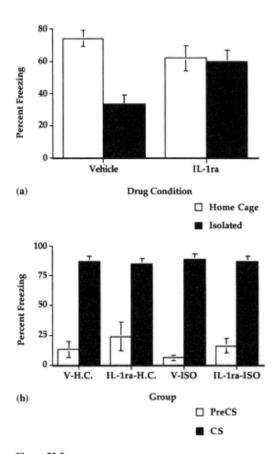

Figure 53.3
(a) Mean percentage of freezing during the contextual fear test of rats given vehicle or IL-1ra (0.25 µg) and isolated or returned to the home cage. Bars: SE. (b) Mean percentage of freezing during the auditory-cue fear conditioning test. Bars: SE.

less contextual fear conditioning than rats returned to the home cage. There was no difference between the 2 drug conditions, $F < 1$. The ANOVA also revealed a significant Group × Drug Treatment interaction, $F(1, 31) = 6.04$, $P < 0.05$. Post hoc comparisons (Newman–Keuls) revealed that isolated rats given vehicle showed significantly less contextual fear conditioning than did isolated rats given IL-1ra ($P < 0.01$). Isolated rats given vehicle also

showed less contextual fear conditioning than did those returned to the home cage and given vehicle, ($P < 0.01$) or IL-1ra ($P < 0.01$). None of the other groups differed from each other in their level of contextual fear conditioning. Isolation × Drug treatment ANOVAS for the preCS and CS period data of the auditory-cue fear conditioning test revealed no differences between the groups during either the preCS or CS test periods ($F < 1$).

The results of the present experiment replicate the previous findings of Rudy [39] and Experiment 1, that social isolation after conditioning impairs contextual fear conditioning but has no effect on auditory-cue fear conditioning. These results also suggest that the increase in IL-1β protein caused by social isolation is necessary to observe the impairment in contextual fear observed in isolated rats. This is because isolated rats given IL-1ra showed levels of contextual fear conditioning equal to those returned to the home cage. This increase in fear conditioning cannot be attributed to a general increase in freezing behavior because rats given IL-1ra and returned to the home cage did not show enhanced levels of fear conditioning. In addition, there were no differences in the amount of fear expressed by the groups during the preCS or CS periods of the auditory-cue fear conditioning test. Importantly, this block of the impairment in fear conditioning caused by isolation cannot be attributed to differences between the groups during conditioning because no manipulations were conducted until after the conditioning episode was over.

6 Experiment 4

6.1 Methods and Procedures

If isolation impairs contextual fear conditioning by inducing an increase in IL-1β protein in brain, then it should be possible to impair contextual fear conditioning by injecting IL-1β centrally. To test the hypothesis that IL-1β is sufficient in itself to produce the impairment in contextual fear conditioning caused by isolation, rats were implanted with ICV cannulae and allowed 4 weeks to recover. Rats were conditioned with two tone-shock pairings, and immediately after conditioning were microinjected with 10 ($n = 6$) or 20 ($n = 8$) ng IL-1β or sterile pyrogen free vehicle ($n = 14$) in a volume of 5 µl. All rats were then returned to the home cage. They were

tested for contextual and auditory-cue fear conditioning 48 h later.

6.2 Results and Discussion

As shown in Fig. 53.4a, central IL-1 administration at a dose of either 10 or 20 ng was sufficient to produce the impairment in contextual fear conditioning observed in isolated rats, $F(2, 25) = 7.1$, $P < 0.01$. Like isolation, neither dose of IL-1β affected auditory-cue fear conditioning (Fig. 53.4b). Post hoc comparisons (Newman–Keuls) indicated that rats given either 10 ng ($P < 0.01$) or 20 ng ($P < 0.05$) of IL-1β showed significantly less contextual fear conditioning than did vehicle-treated controls. There was no effect of central IL-1β administration on auditory-cue fear conditioning during the preCS or CS periods, $F < 1$.

These results indicate that central IL-1β administration by itself is sufficient to produce impairments in contextual fear conditioning similar to that caused by social isolation. As in previous experiments, this effect cannot be attributed to non-specific effects of the drug during conditioning because it was not administered until after the conditioning session was over. This also suggests that IL-1β impairs contextual fear conditioning by interfering with some post-trial memory consolidation processes that are necessary for contextual fear conditioning to occur.

7 General Discussion

The present set of experiments strongly implicates central IL-1β activity in producing the impairment in contextual fear conditioning caused by social isolation. First, 1 and 3 h of isolation after conditioning increased IL-1β protein levels in the hippocampus and posterior cortex but not in the pituitary gland or hypothalamus. Second, central IL-1ra was able to block the impairment in contextual fear conditioning caused by social isolation. Third, like isolation, the administra-

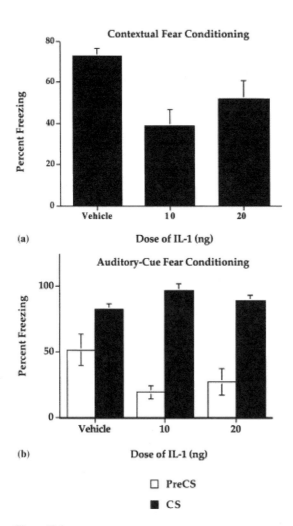

Figure 53.4
(a) Mean percentage of freezing during the contextual fear test of rats given central IL-1 (10 or 20 ng) or vehicle immediately after conditioning. Bars: SE. (b) Mean percentage of freezing during the auditory-cue fear conditioning test. Bars: SE.

tion of central IL-1β was sufficient to impair contextual but not auditory-cue fear conditioning.

The finding that IL-1β administration impairs contextual fear conditioning is consistent with the work of other researchers who have shown that both peripheral immune activation (which leads to increased gene expression of central IL-1β; [15, 14]) and IL-1β administration impair learning and memory processes. For example, we have previously reported that peripheral LPS administration impairs contextual but not auditory-cue fear conditioning, and that this effect could be blocked by IL-1ra [36]. In addition, Aubert et al. [1] have shown that the administration of LPS and IL-1β disrupt the acquisition of an autoshaping task in rats; however, the administration of these agents did not disrupt performance of the task if it had already been acquired. Gibertini et al. [10] reported an impairment in the spatial version of the Morris water escape task caused by the administration of the gram negative *Legionella pneumophila*. This impairment could be blocked by peripherally administered antibodies directed against IL-1 [10]. Finally, Oitzl et al. [28] found a disruptive effect of peripheral IL-1β administration on the spatial version of the Morris water escape task. The present set of experiments are different from these for two reasons. First, given that peripherally administered LPS, IL-1β and anti-IL-1β antibodies are unlikely to cross into the brain, a peripheral site of action is likely in previous studies. In contrast, the present work implicates a central IL-1β site of action. Second, IL-1β (as well as LPS in a previous paper [36]) were not administered until after the learning trials were over. Therefore, all animals in these experiments were equivalent during the actual learning trials. This strongly supports the hypothesis that IL-1β impairs learning and memory processes by disrupting post-trial memory consolidation processes.

The experiments reported here suggest a parallel between peripheral immune activation and stressors. This is because both peripheral immune activation and social isolation increase brain IL-1β, and both also selectively impair contextual fear conditioning. In addition, the impairments caused by both peripheral immune activation and social isolation can be blocked by IL-1ra. Similarities between the neurochemical, endocrine, and behavioral sequelae of immune challenge and stressors have been described frequently [6, 20]. For example, influenza viral infection has been shown to increase plasma corticosterone and brain catecholamine metabolism [5], effects that are also observed in response to stress [43]. Yirmiya [46] has recently reported depressive-like behavior in rats after peripheral immune activation that has also been implicated as a response to stressors [11]. Nguyen et al. [26] showed that inescapable tail shock stress (like endotoxin challenge) increases brain IL-1β protein. It is important to note that the regional distribution of IL-1β changes (like changes in neural activation) are not identical after stress and immune challenge [38]. However, patterns of neural activation differ even between stressors [16], so these differences in patterns of regional IL-1β changes should not be surprising.

Recent evidence suggests that IL-1β can also be present in brain during basal or nonpathological conditions [27, 3, 37]. In fact, Nguyen et al. [26] have demonstrated that IL-1β protein expression exhibits a circadian rhythm. This suggests that IL-1β may play a physiological role in the uninjured brain. Evidence for this comes from the finding that IL-1β may be important in sleep regulation [31, 30]. Also, Besedovsky (personal comunication) has shown that basal levels of IL-1β are neccassary to observe LTP in the hippocampus. While it is presently unclear, these findings leave open the possibility that IL-1β could be involved in learning and memory processes in the absence of stress or immune challenge.

Thus far, we have suggested that isolation is stressful as a result of its social aspects. However, there are other potential explanations of why isolation after conditioning might impair contextual fear conditioning (such as novelty stress). Consistent with the interpretation that it is the social aspect of isolation that is responsible for producing the impairment in contextual fear conditioning, placing two rats from the same home cage into the isolation cage together attenuated the observed impairment (unpublished data).

It is important to note that many of the stressors reported to increase IL-1β activity in the brain have a physical component to them. For example, when increases in IL-1β mRNA [24] and bioactiviy [42] were reported, immobilization stress (which involves forcefully preventing any movement by the rat) was used. Nguyen et al. [26] observed increases in IL-1β protein levels after 100 inescapable tail shocks. Both of these stressors leave open the possibility for injury induced IL-1β activity. In contrast, the stressor used in the present experiments was purely psychological and had no physical components.

It is reasonable to wonder whether there might be any adaptive value to stress-induced IL-1β production producing interference with hippocampal dependent contextual fear conditioning, but not hippocampal independent auditory-cue fear conditioning. We have no definitive answer to this question. However, the hippocampus is a very large structure that is involved in many processes besides learning and memory (such as serving as a site for neuroendocrine integration as well as an integration site for sickness and sickness behaviors [20]). It is possible that the same set of neurons participate in more than one function that the hippocampus serves and that the same neurons that participate in some aspects of learning and memory processes are involved in responding to the stressful situation at hand. To the extent that these neurons are demanded in integrating the stress response, they may be less able to participate in their other cognitive functions.

Acknowledgements

This research was supported by grants NIH MH 5528, NIH MH4505, RSA MH 00314, and NIH F31 MH12148-01, as well as the Undergraduate Research Opportunities Program at the University of Colorado.

References

[1] Aubert A, Vega C, Dantzer R, Goodall G. Pyrogens specifically disrupt the acquisition of a task involving cognitive processing in the rat. Brain Behav Immunol 1995; 9(2):129–48.

[2] Bellinger FP, Madamba S, Siggins GR. Interleukin-1 beta inhibits synaptic strength and long-term potentiation in the rat CA1 hippocampus. Brain Res 1993; 628:227–34.

[3] Coceani F, Lees J, Dinarello CA. Occurrence of interleukin-1 in cerebrospinal fluid of the conscious cat. Brain Res 1988; 446:245–50.

[4] Corradetti R, Ballerini L, Pugliese AM, Pepeu G. Serotonin blocks the long-term potentiation induced by primed burst stimulation in the CA1 region of rat hippocampal slices. Neuroscience 1992; 46:511–8.

[5] Dunn AJ, Powell ML, Meitin C, Small PA. Virus infection as a stressor: influenza virus elevates plasma concentrations of corticosterone, and brain concentrations of MHPG and tryptophan. Physiol Behav 1989; 45:591–4.

[6] Dunn AJ. Interactions between the nervous system and the immune system: Implications for psychopharmacology. In: Psychopharmacology: The Fourth Generation of Progress, New York: Raven Press, 1995. pp. 719–733.

[7] Fanselow MS, Lester LS. A functional behavioristic approach to aversively motivated behavior: predatory imminence as a determinant of the topography of defensive behavior. In: Bolles RC, Beecher MD, editors. Evolution and Learning. Hillsdale, NJ: Erlbaum, 1988:185–211.

[8] Fantuzzi G, Dinarello CA. The inflammatory response in interleukin-1 beta-deficient mice: comparison with other cytokine-related knock-out mice. J Leukocyte Biol 1996; 59(4):489–93.

[9] Fleshner M, Pugh CR, Tremblay D, Rudy JW. DHEA-S selectively impairs contextual-fear conditioning: support for the antiglucocorticoid hypothesis. Behav Neurosci 1997; 111(3):512–7.

[10] Gibertini M, Newton C, Klein TW, Friedman H. Legionella pneumophila-induced visual learning impairment reversed by anti-interleukin-1 beta. Proc Soc Exp Biol Med 1995; 210(1):7–11.

[11] Johnson EO, Kamilaris TC, Chrousos GP, Gold PW. Mechanisms of stress: a dynamic overview of hormonal and behavioral homeostasis. Neurosci Biobehav Rev 1992; 16:115–30.

[12] Katsuki H, Nakai S, Hirai Y, Akaji K, Kiso Y, Satoh M. Interleukin-1 beta inhibits long-term potentiation in the CA3 region of mouse hippocampal slices. Euro J Pharmacol 1990; 181:323–6.

[13] Kim JJ, Fanselow M. Modality-specific retrograde amnesia of fear. Science 1992; 256:675–6.

[14] Laye S, Bluthe RM, Kent S, Combe C, Medina C, Parnet P, et al. Subdiaphragmatic vagotomy blocks induction of IL-1 beta mRNA in mice brain in response to peripheral LPS. Am J Physiol 1995; 268:327–31.

[15] Laye S, Parnet P, Goujon E, Dantzer R. Peripheral administration of lipopolysaccharide induces the expression of cytokine transcripts in the brain and pituitary of mice. Brain Res 1994; 27:157–62.

[16] Li HY, Ericsson A, Sawchenko PE. Distinct mechanisms underlie activation of hypothalamic neurosecretory neurons and their medullary catecholaminergic afferents in categorically different stress paradigms. Proc Natl Acad Sci USA 1996; 93(6):2359–64.

[17] Linthorst AC, Flachskamm C, Holsboer F, Reul JM. Local administration of recombinant human interleukin-1 beta in the rat hippocampus increases serotonergic neurotransmission, hypothalamic-pituitary-adrenocortical axis activity, and body temperature. Endocrinology 1994; 135:520–32.

[18] Linthorst AC, Flachskamm C, Muller-Preuss P, Holsboer F, Reul JM. Effect of bacterial endotoxin and interleukin-1 beta on hippocampal serotonergic neurotransmission, behavioral activity, and free corticosterone levels: an in vivo microdialysis study. J Neurosci 1995; 15:2920–34.

[19] Maier SF, Watkins LR. Intracerebroventricular interleukin-1 receptor antagonist blocks the enhancement of fear conditioning and interference with escape produced by inescapable shock. Brain Res 1995; 695:279–82.

[20] Maier SF, Watkins LR. Cytokines for psychologist: implication of bi-directional immune to brain communication for understanding behavior, mood, and cognition. Psychol Rev 1998; 105(1):83–107.

[21] McEwen BS, Wallach G. Corticosterone binding to hippocampus: nuclear and cytosol binding in vitro. Brain Res 1973; 57(2):373–86.

[22] McEwen BS, Weiss JM, Schwartz LS. Uptake of corticosterone by rat brain and its concentration by certain limbic structures. Brain Res 1969; 16(1):227–41.

[23] McEwen BS, Sapolsky RM. Stress and cognitive function. Curr Opin Neurobiol 1995; 5(2):205–16.

[24] Minami M, Kuraishi Y, Yagaguchi T, Nakai S, Hirai Y, Satoh M. Immobilization stress induces interleukin-1b mRNA in the rat hypothalamus. Neurosci Lett 1991; 123:254–6.

[25] Nava F, Calapai G, DeSarro A, Caputi AP. Interleukin-1 receptor antagonist does not reverse lipopolysaccharide-induced inhibition of water intake in rat. Eur J Pharmacol 1996; 309(3):223–7.

[26] Nguyen KT, Deak T, Owens SF, Kohno T, Fleshner M, Watkins LR, et al. Exposure to acute stress induces brain interleukin-1 protein in the rat. J Neurosci 1998; 18(6):1–7.

[27] Nieto-Sampedro M, Berman MA. Interleukin-1-like activity in rat brain: sources, targets, and effect of injury. J Neurosci Res 1987; 17:214–9.

[28] Oitzl MS, van Oers H, Schobitz B, deKloet ER. Interleukin-1 beta, but not interleukin-6 impairs spatial navigation learning. Brain Res 1993; 613(1):160–3.

[29] O'Neill LA. Molecular mechanisms underlying the actions of the pro-inflammatory cytokine interleukin-1. Royal Irish Academy Medal Lecture. Biochem Soc Trans 1997; 25(1):295–302.

[30] Opp MR, Krueger JM. Anti-interleukin-1b reduces sleep and sleep rebound after sleep deprivation in rats. Amer J Physiol 1994; 266(35):R688–95.

[31] Opp MR, Obal FJ, Kreuger JM. Interleukin-1 alters rat sleep: temporal and dose-related effects. Am J Physiol 1991; 260(29):R52–8.

[32] Phillips RG, LeDoux JE. Differential contribution of amygdala and hippocampus to cued and contextual fear conditioning. Behav Neurosci 1995; 106:274–85.

[33] Phillips RG, LeDoux JE. Lesions of the dorsal hippocampal formation interfere with background but not foreground contextual fear conditioning. Learn Mem 1994; 1:34–45.

[34] Pugh CR, Fleshner M, Rudy JW. Type II glucocorticoid receptor antagonists impair contextual but not auditory-cue fear conditioning in juvenile rats. Neurobiol Learn Mem 1997; 67:75–9.

[35] Pugh CR, Tremblay D, Fleshner M, Rudy JW. A selective role for corticosterone in contextual-fear conditioning. Behav Neurosci 1997; 111(3):503–11.

[36] Pugh CR, Kumagawa K, Fleshner M, Watkins LR, Maier SF, Rudy JW. Selective effects of peripheral lipopolysaccharide administration on contextual and auditory-cue fear conditioning. Brain Behav Immun 1999; 12:212–29.

[37] Quan N, Sundar SK, Weiss JM. Induction of interleukin-1 in various brain regions after peripheral and central injections of lipopolysaccharide. J Neuroimmunol 1994; 49(1–2):125–34.

[38] Rivest S, LaFlamme N, Nappi RE. Immune challenge and immobilization stress induce transcription of the gene encoding the CRF receptor in selective nuclei of the rat hypothalamus. J Neurosci 1995; 15(4):2680–95.

[39] Rudy JW. Post-conditioning isolation disrupts contextual fear conditioning: an experimental analysis. Behav Neurosci 1996; 110:238–46.

[40] Rudy JW, Pugh CR. Time of conditioning selectively influences contextual fear conditioning: further support for a multiple-memory systems view of fear conditioning. J Exp Psychol; Animal Behav Proc 1998; 24(3):316–24.

[41] Shintani F, Nakaki T, Kanba S, Kato R, Asai M. Role of interleukin-1 in stress responses: a putative neurotransmitter. Molec Neurobiol 1995; 10(1):47–71.

[42] Shintani F, Nakaki T, Kanba S, Sato K, Yagi G, Shiozawa M, et al. Involvement of interleukin-1 in immobilization stress-induced increase in plasma adrenocorticotropic hormone and in release of hypothalamic monoamines in the rat. J Neurosci 1995; 15(3):1961–70.

[43] Watkins LR, Wiertelak EP, Maier SF. Delta opiate receptors mediate tail-shock induced antinociception at supraspinal levels. Brain Res 1992; 582:10–20.

[44] Westbrook RF, Good AJ, Kiernan MJ. Microinjection of morphine into the nucleus accumbens impairs contextual learning in rats. Behav Neurosci 1997; 111(5):996–1013.

[45] Villani F, Johnston D. Serotonin inhibits induction of long-term potentiation at commissural synapses in hippocampus. Brain Res 1993; 606:304–8.

[46] Yirmiya R. Endotoxin produces a depressive-like episode in rats. Brain Res 1996; 711:163–74.

Adrenocortical Reactivity and Social Competence in Seven-Year-Olds

Louis A. Schmidt, Nathan A. Fox, Esther M. Sternberg, Philip W. Gold, Craig C. Smith, and Jay Schulkin

1 Introduction

Socially competent children, unlike shy children, display a short latency to approach social novelty, appear to be at "ease" in play groups with unfamiliar peers, and are socially outgoing. Socially competent children also appear to be more successful in regulating the arousal of negative affect during socially evaluative situations compared with shy and socially anxious children. We know, however, comparatively little with regard to how socially competent vs shy children regulate stress during socially evaluative situations.

We (Schmidt et al., 1997) recently found that preschoolers who displayed a high proportion of social wariness while interacting with same-age and same-gender peers exhibited high morning salivary cortisol levels. Also, a number of others have linked high cortisol to fear, distress and related constructs in human infants (Gunnar et al., 1989), shyness and inhibition in children (Kagan et al., 1987; Nachmias et al., 1996), shyness (Bell et al., 1993; Windel, 1994) and agitated depression in adults (Gold et al., 1988a; 1988b), and fearfulness in nonhuman primates (Champoux et al., 1989; Kalin and Shelton, 1989; Levine et al., 1987). The relation between elevated cortisol and fearful and anxious behavioral profiles, however, is not a foregone conclusion. Elevated cortisol has been noted in bold and exuberant children and dominant, rather than submissive, non-human primates (see Gunnar, 1994, for a review).

The purpose of the present study was to extend our previous research on the relation between cortisol and social development in children (e.g. Schmidt et al., 1997) and to clarify some of the apparent inconsistencies on this relation in the extant literature. We examined temporal changes in salivary cortisol in response to a self-presentation task in a group of seven-year-olds, some of whom scored high, average, and low on the Harter (1983) Perceived Social Competence Scale for children. Salivary cortisol was measured pre-task, and 20 and 35 min post-task. We chose to measure cortisol because this stress hormone may provide a window into the origins of emotion regulatory and dysregulatory processes in early school age children during socially evaluative situations. The early school age years are a particularly important period in development as the age point coincides with the child's entry into school and the establishment of peer relationships.

We expected that children who scored high on perceived social competence would display a significantly greater decrease in saliva cortisol following the self-presentation task compared with children who scored relatively lower on the self-report social competence measure. In the present chapter, we report the relation between individual differences in children's self-perceptions of social competence and temporal changes in salivary cortisol in response to the task at age seven.

2 Method

2.1 Subjects

Subjects were 48 children (28 males, 20 females) who were recruited at age four from local area preschools for a larger longitudinal study designed to examine socio-emotional development during the preschool and early school years. The children were unselected for personality differences, primarily Caucasian, from middle class backgrounds, lived in the suburban Washington, DC area, and experienced no pre- or post-natal health problems. Details concerning recruitment and procedures used during the laboratory visit at age four are presented elsewhere (see Fox et al., 1996).

Of the 48 children seen at age four, 39 returned to the laboratory at age seven. The focus of the analyses reported herein is on the salivary cortisol, behavioral, and self-report measures collected at age seven.

2.2 Procedure

Upon arrival at the laboratory, the mother and child were ushered into a testing room and briefed about the procedures. After the child had "settled," a saliva sample was collected from the child. Next, a lycra stretch cap used to collect brain electrical activity (EEG) was attached to the child's head and disposable heart rate electrodes were placed on the child's arms. Baseline behavior, EEG, and heart rate data were collected for 3 min while the child attended to a visual stimulus; the EEG and heart rate data were collected as part of a larger study and are not reported in the present chapter.

We then introduced a self-presentation anxiety task as follows. An experimenter positioned a videocamera in front of the child (approximately 1 m) and told him or her the following:

"In a couple of minutes, we are going to have you give a speech about an embarrassing moment. We will be videotaping you during the speech because we are going to show the tape to a group of 3rd and 4th graders who will be coming in to the lab later."

The experimenter's instructions increased in saliency over time in order to increase anticipatory anxiety. This was accomplished as follows:

After 30 s into the task, the child was reminded by the experimenter that "it is only one more minute until you give the speech!" After 60 s, the child was reminded by the experimenter that "it is only 30 s more until you give the speech; I hope you are ready!" After 70 s, the child was reminded by the experimenter that, "it is only a few more seconds until you give your speech; you must be ready!" On completion of the task, the experimenter told the child, "We are having problems with the camera so you do not have to do the speech unless you want to."

Following the task, the child and mother were moved to an adjacent room for additional testing at which time the child's self-perceptions of social competence were indexed using the Pictorial Scale of Perceived Competence and Social Acceptance for Young Children (Harter, 1983). This scale has a series of pictures which involve various scenarios and which measure different competencies. For example, a child is shown a picture of a little boy with a lot of friends and an experimenter asks the child, "Are you a lot, or a little, like the boy or girl in the picture?" Of particular interest was the scale indexing Perceived Social Competence.

Two saliva samples were collected following the self-presentation task; one saliva sample was collected 20 min post-task; and the other saliva sample was collected 35 min post-task. These time points were selected because activation of the adrenocortical system following a stressor is known to take at least 15 min (see e.g. Stansbury and Gunnar, 1994). All children were tested in the mid-afternoon.

2.3 Salivary Cortisol Collection

The procedures used for collecting saliva in the laboratory were as follows: a dental cotton roll was dipped in sweetened Kool-Aid crystals, the cotton was placed into the child's mouth, and the child was instructed to chew on the cotton. The cotton was removed after approximately 1 min and placed into a needleless syringe. The syringe's plunger was used to compress the cotton, expressing the saliva into a cryogenic tube. The procedures were repeated, if necessary, until at least 500 μl of saliva were collected. All saliva samples were frozen at −80°C until assayed. Similar procedures have been used in our laboratory (Schmidt et al., 1997) as well as elsewhere (see Gunnar et al., 1989).

2.4 Radioimmunoassay (RIA)

The saliva samples were assayed by the Clinical Neuroendocrinology Branch of the National Institute of Mental Health, Bethesda, MD. Samples were thawed, vortexed, and centrifuged for 30 min at $2250 \times g$. Unknown salivary cortisol concentrations were determined with a commercial competitive solid phase RIA (125I) (Coat-A-Count, Diagnostic Products Corporation, Los Angeles, CA, U.S.A), using 200 µl of saliva. Incubation was for 3 h at room temperature. Following aspiration of the liquid, tubes were counted using an ICN Micromedic Systems, Apex Automatic Gamma Counter. Both samples and standards were determined in duplicate, and all samples were performed at the same time in order to eliminate interassay variability. The total binding was 67.7%, and the lower detection limit assay was 0.1 µg dl^{-1}. The intraassay coefficient of variability at the 0.47 µg dl^{-1} level was 2.75%, and at 2.06 µg dl^{-1} was 7.37%.

2.5 Behavioral Coding and Measures

Behaviors were videotaped during the laboratory visit at age seven and subsequently coded by three research assistants who were blind to the hypotheses of the study. Behavior was coded every 10 s for the presence of anxious behaviors (e.g. automanipulatives, nail biting, hair pulling, restlessness, and fidgeting) during the 3 min baseline (i.e. behavior before the task) and the self-presentation task. Reliability among coders was established on a subset of subjects. Kappa's ranged from 0.6 to 0.8 on individual behavioral measures. A separate composite measure of the proportion of anxious behaviors was computed by summing the frequency of anxious behaviors and dividing by the number of codeable epochs within the baseline condition and during the self-presentation task.

Of the 39 children, 36 children had useable behavioral data. Behavioral data from three children were not obtainable during the self-presentation task due to equipment problems.

2.6 Manipulation Check

In order to assess the effectiveness of the self-presentation task to elicit anxiety, a pairwise t-test was performed between the composite measure of anxiety collected during the baseline and self-presentation task. There was a significant within-subjects increase in anxious behavior displayed during baseline (M = 0.39, S.D. = 0.19) to the self-presentation task (M = 1.76, S.D. = 0.68) (pairwise $t(35) = 13.53$, $P = 0.001$), suggesting that the self-presentation task was indeed effective in eliciting behavioral manifestations of anxiety.

2.7 Extreme Groups

We formed three groups of children using the Perceived Social Competence scale: *Group* 1: High Social Competence ($n = 8$) comprised children who scored high on the scale (upper 20%); *Group* 2: Middle ($n = 23$) comprised children who scored around the mean on the scale (middle 60%); and *Group* 3: Low Social Competence ($n = 8$) comprised children who scored low on the scale (bottom 20%).

Of the 39 children seen at age seven, 38 children had useable salivary cortisol data. One child's (who belonged to the high social competence group) salivary cortisol data were not included because his cortisol values exceeded 3 S.D.s above the mean.

3 Results

Table 54.1 presents the means (S.D.s) for the salivary cortisol data collected during pre-task (baseline), and 20 and 35 min post-task for the three groups. A separate ANOVA with Group (high, middle, low) as a between-subjects factor

Table 54.1

Means and (S.D.s) for salivary cortisol measure collected pre-task (baseline) and 20 and 35 min post self-presentation task by the three social competence groups

	Social competence group		
	High (n = 7)	Middle (n = 23)	Low (n = 8)
Salivary cortisol (in μg dl⁻¹)			
Pre-task (baseline)	0.10 (0.08)	0.12 (0.06)	0.12 (0.10)
20 min post-task	0.10 (0.09)	0.07 (0.05)	0.07 (0.04)
35 min post-task	0.04 (0.02)	0.08 (0.06)	0.09 (0.07)

was performed on each time point. The dependent measure was mean salivary cortisol level. There were no significant main effects for Group on salivary cortisol for any of the three time points.

We next examined whether individual differences in children's self-perceptions of social competence were related to temporal changes in salivary cortisol in response to the task. We computed three separate delta salivary cortisol change scores in order to index adrenocortical reactivity in response to the task: (1) 35 min post-task sample–20 min post-task sample; (2) 35 min post-task sample–initial sample; and (3) 20 min post-task sample–initial sample. An ANOVA was performed with Group (high, middle, low) as a between-subjects factor and Change Score (1, 2, 3) as a within-subjects factor, with repeated measures on the second factor. The dependent measure was salivary cortisol reactivity.

The analyses revealed a significant Group × Change Score interaction on salivary cortisol reactivity, $F(4, 70) = 2.85$, $P = 0.03$. In order to decompose this interaction, a separate analysis

of variance (ANOVA) with Group (high, middle, low) as a between-subjects factor was performed on each of the three salivary cortisol change scores. The analyses revealed a significant main effect for Group only on Change Score 1 (i.e. 35 min post-task sample–20 min post-task sample), $F(2, 35) = 4.54$, $P = 0.018$. Figure 54.1 presents the mean differences on this change score for the three groups.

As can be seen in Fig. 54.1, children in the high socially competent group ($M = -0.06$, S.D. $= 0.07$) exhibited a significantly greater decrease in salivary cortisol from 20 to 35 min post-task compared with children in the middle ($M = 0.01$, S.D. $= 0.05$), $t(28) = 2.65$, $P = 0.013$, and the low ($M = 0.02$, S.D. $= 0.05$) groups, $t(13) = 2.50$, $P = 0.027$.

Because of the small number of children who fell into each of the extreme groups, we ascertained the number of children who exhibited an increase vs a decrease in salivary cortisol from 20 to 35 min post-task by social competence group. As shown in Table 54.2, all 7 of the children who fell in the high social competence group exhibited a decrease in salivary cortisol 20 to 35 min post-task [Likelihood Ratio $\chi^2(2) = 6.95$, $P = 0.03$].

It is also important to note that the three groups did not differ on the behavioral measures collected during baseline and during the self-presentation task.

4 Discussion

We found that individual differences in children's self-perceptions of social competence were related to temporal changes in salivary cortisol in response to a task designed to elicit peer self-presentation anxiety. Children who perceived themselves as relatively high in social competence exhibited a significantly greater decrease in salivary cortisol from 20 to 35 min post-task compared with children who perceived themselves as relatively less socially competent. Our

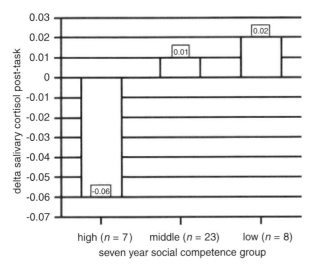

Figure 54.1
Difference between high and low socially competent children and the middle group on delta salivary cortisol (in μg dl^{-1}) from 20–35 min post self-presentation task at age 7. (Note that lower values indicate a decrease in salivary cortisol.)

Table 54.2
Frequency of children displaying an increase vs. decrease in salivary cortisol from 20 to 35 min post self-presentation task by social competence group

	Social competence group		
	High	Middle	Low
Salivary cortisol			
Increase	0	9	4
Decrease	7	14	4

$\chi^2(2) = 6.95$, $P = 0.031$.

findings on salivary cortisol changes in the three social competence groups were specific to the window of time from 20 to 35 min post-task. We did not find significant group differences in baseline salivary cortisol levels, nor in changes in salivary cortisol from baseline to 20 min post-task, or from baseline to 35 min post-task.

What do changes in salivary cortisol between 20 to 35 min following the presentation of a social stressor in socially competent children reflect? We speculate that activation of the adrenocortical system may be linked to the maintenance of fear (see also Schulkin et al., 1994). Activation of the adrenocortical system is known to take at least 15 min following the presentation of a stressor in humans (Stansbury and Gunnar, 1994). Our findings of cortisol changes between 20 to 35 min following the self-presentation task (i.e. stressor) is consistent with this notion. We noted the greatest amount of change in this window of time for the three groups: highly socially competent children showed a significantly greater reduction in salivary cortisol. It is possible that the relative increase in salivary cortisol during this time in children low in social competence may have reflected their inability to regulate negative emotion. Shy children are known to display high salivary cortisol levels (e.g. Kagan et al., 1987; Schmidt et al., 1997). Whereas, the reduction in salivary cortisol in socially competent children following the social stressor may have reflected their ability to regulate negative emotion. Furthermore, the ability to regulate negative emotion and the adrenocortical system may allow socially competent children to approach social situations with less apprehension and to recover faster from social situations which do elicit negative self-evaluation.

There are, in addition, three other points that are worthy of further discussion. First, it is important to point out that, although our task was effective in eliciting an increase in anxiety within-subjects, we did not find significant differences among the three groups on behavioral anxiety during the task. The failure to find behavioral differences among the three groups may have been due to the relatively small number of children in the extreme groups. Future research should considerably increase the number of children in the high and low social competence groups. Second, it is important to note that the present study relied on the child's own self-perceptions of his or her social competence. Traditionally, studies examining the psychophysiology of personality in early school age children have used other informants such as parental report and teacher ratings to index the child's personality, possibly limiting the reliability of the findings. Third, the results of the present study suggest that salivary cortisol responses may be a reliable measure of aspects of socio-emotional development in children. This is a particularly important finding to developmental researchers as they search for relatively non-invasive measures to study complex brain/behavior relations in pediatric populations.

Acknowledgements

This research was supported by a grant from the John D. and Catherine T. MacArthur Foundation's Network on the Transition from Infancy to Childhood and by a grant from the National Institutes of Health (HD 17899) awarded to Nathan A. Fox. We wish to thank the children and mothers for their participation and the following individuals for their assistance with data collection: Lisa Perry-Moss, Anne Schubert, Ariana Shahinfar, Cindy Smith, and Shari Young. Portions of these data were presented at the National Institute of Mental Health Conference for Advancing Research on Developmental Plasticity, Chantilly, Virginia, May 12–15, 1996.

References

Bell, I. R., Martino, G. M., Meredith, K. E., Schwartz, G. E., Siani, M. M., & Morrow, F. D. (1993). Vascular disease risk factors, urinary-free cortisol, and health histories in older adults: Shyness and gender interaction. *Biological Psychology, 35, 37–49.*

Champoux, M., Coe, C. L., Schanber, S. M., Kihn, C. M., & Suomi, S. J. (1989). Hormonal effects of early rearing conditions in the infant rhesus monkey. *American Journal of Primatology, 19, 111–117.*

Fox, N. A., Schmidt, L. A., Calkins, S. D., Rubin, K. H., & Coplan, R. J. (1996). The role of frontal activation in the regulation and dysregulation of social behavior during the preschool years. *Development and Psychopathology, 8, 89–102.*

Gold, P. W., Goodwin, F. K., & Chrousos, G. P. (1988a). Clinical and biochemical manifestations of depression. *New England Journal of Medicine, 319, 348–353.*

Gold, P. W., Goodwin, F. K., & Chrousos, G. P. (1988b). Clinical and biochemical manifestations of depression. *New England Journal of Medicine, 319, 413–420.*

Gunnar, M. R. (1994). Psychoendocrine studies of temperament and stress in early childhood: Expanding current models. In J. E. Bates & T. D. Wachs (Eds.), *Temperament: Individual differences at the interface of biology and behavior* (pp. 175–198). Washington, DC: American Psychological Association.

Gunnar, M. R., Mangelsdorf, S., Larson, M., & Hertsgaard, L. (1989). Attachment, temperament, and adrenocortical activity in infancy: A study of psychoendocrine regulation. *Development Psychology,* 25, 355–363.

Harter, S. (1983). *The Pictorial Scale of Perceived Competence and Social Acceptance for Young Children.* University of Denver.

Kagan, J., Reznick, J. S., & Snidman, N. (1987). The physiology and psychology of behavioral inhibition in children. *Child Development,* 58, 1459–1473.

Kalin, N. H., & Shelton, S. E. (1989). Defensive behaviors in infant rhesus monkeys: Environmental cues and neurochemical regulation. *Science,* 243, 1718–1721.

Levine, S., Wiener, S. G., Coe, C., Bayart, F. S., & Hayashi, K. T. (1987). Primate vocalization: A psychobiological approach. *Child Development,* 58, 1408–1419.

Nachmias, M., Gunnar, M., Mangelsdorf, S., Parritz, R., & Buss, K. (1996). Behavioral inhibition and stress reactivity: The moderating role of attachment security. *Child Development,* 67, 508–522.

Schmidt, L. A., Fox, N. A., Rubin, K. H., Sternberg, E. M., Gold, P. W., Smith, C. C., & Schulkin, J. (1997). Behavioral and neuroendocrine responses in shy children. *Developmental Psychobiology,* 30, 127–140.

Schulkin, J., McEwen, B. S., & Gold, P. W. (1994). Allostasis, amygdala, and anticipatory angst. *Neuroscience and Biobehavioral Reviews,* 18, 385–396.

Stansbury, K., & Gunnar, M. R. (1994). Adrenocortical activity and emotion regulation. In N. A. Fox (Ed.), *The development of emotion regulation: Biological and behavioral considerations* (pp. 108–134). Monographs of the Society for Research in Child Development. Serial No. 240, Vol. 59, Nos. 2–3.

Windel, M. (1994). Temperamental inhibition and activation: hormonal and psychosocial correlates and associated psychiatric disorders. *Personality and Individual Differences,* 17, 61–70.

55 Lonely Traits and Concomitant Physiological Processes: The MacArthur Social Neuroscience Studies

John T. Cacioppo, John M. Ernst, Mary H. Burleson, Martha K. McClintock, William B. Malarkey, Louise C. Hawkley, Ray B. Kowalewski, Alisa Paulsen, J. Allan Hobson, Kenneth Hugdahl, David Spiegel, and Gary G. Berntson

1 Introduction

Humans are social animals, so much so that a basic "need to belong" has been posited (Baumeister and Leary, 1995; Gardner et al., in review; Gardner et al., in press). People form associations and connections with others from the moment they are born. The very survival of newborns depends on their attachment to and nurturance by others over an extended period of time. It should be no surprise that evolution has sculpted the human genome to be sensitive to and succoring of contact and relationships with others. For instance, caregiving and attachment have hormonal (e.g. Uvnäs-Mosberg, 1997) and neurophysiological substrates (cf. Carter et al., 1997). Communication, the bedrock of complex social interaction, is universal and ubiquitous in humans. In the rare instances in which human language is not modeled or taught, language develops nevertheless (e.g. Goldin-Meadow and Mylander, 1983, 1984).

The need to belong does not stop at infancy but rather affiliation and nurturant social relationships appear to be essential for physical and for psychological well-being across the lifespan. Disruptions of social connections, whether through ridicule, separation, divorce, or bereavement, are among the most stressful events people must endure (Gardner et al., in press). Berkman and Syme (1979), for instance, operationalized social connections as marriage, contacts with friends and extended family members, church membership, and other group affiliations. They found that adults with fewer social connections suffered higher rates of mortality over the succeeding 9 years even after accounting for self-reports of physical health, socioeconomic status, smoking, alcohol consumption, obesity, race, life satisfaction, physical activity, and preventive health service usage. House et al. (1982) replicated these findings using physical examinations to assess health status. In their review of five prospective studies, House et al. (1988) concluded that social isolation was a major risk factor for morbidity and mortality from widely varying causes. This relationship was evident even after statistically controlling for known biological risk factors, social status, and baseline measures of health. The negative health consequences of social isolation were particularly strong among some of the fastest growing segments of the population: the elderly, the poor, and minorities such as African-Americans. Astonishingly, the strength of social isolation as a risk factor was comparable to smoking, high blood pressure, obesity, and sedentary lifestyles.

Social isolation and loneliness are associated with poorer mental as well as physical well-being (e.g. Perkins, 1991; Gupta and Korte, 1994; Ernst and Cacioppo, 1999). Conversely, people who report having contact with five or more intimate friends in the prior 6 months are 60% more likely to report that their lives are "very happy," as compared to those who do not report such contact (Burt, 1986). People appear to be cognizant of the importance of social relationships. When asked "what is necessary for happiness?" most rated relationships with friends and family as being the most important factor (Berscheid, 1985).

Although social isolation is multi-dimensional, it generally appears that the intimacy and emotional nourishment provided by at least one other individual are key to buffering the effects of the majority of stressors. In their seminal review, House et al. (1988) concluded that:

... the mere presence of, or sense of relatedness with, another organism may have relatively direct motivational, emotional, or neuroendocrinal effects that promote health either directly or in the face of stress or other health hazards but that operate independently of cognitive appraisal or behavioral coping and adaptation (p. 544).

Our goal here is to provide a preliminary report of an ongoing study of the psychological and physiological differences between individuals differing in social embeddedness. Although there are gripping states of loneliness that everyone experiences transiently in specific circumstances or interactions, some individuals live in the devastating clutches of loneliness even though they are not physically and socially isolated. Our target sample was college undergraduates because (a) this is an active period of dating, mate selection, and sexual activity; (b) habitual patterns of health behaviors and of interacting with others are being established; and (c) social relationships undergo an upheaval when individuals first go to college yet ample opportunities exist for making new acquaintances and friends.

2 Loneliness on College Campus

We tested 2632 male and female undergraduates at The Ohio State University to determine their feelings of loneliness and their living circumstances. Loneliness was unrelated to various features of college life such as the number of roommates with whom they lived, the percent who belonged to organizations, the number of quarters of college completed, the number of hours in college in which they were enrolled, the number of quarters needed to graduate, and the number of hours they exercised weekly. Despite these superficial similarities, lonely individuals clearly felt less connected to the people around them. Loneliness, for instance, was negatively correlated with the extent to which roommates reduced feelings of isolation, and positively re-

lated to feelings of dysphoria and fears of public speaking. Lonely individuals rated their primary roommate less positively than embedded individuals, and lonely individuals who lived in dormitories reported having fewer positive relationships with suitemates, floormates, and hallmates than embedded individuals.

Lonely individuals were slightly though significantly less likely to consume alcohol than socially embedded (i.e. low in loneliness) individuals—a result that is consistent with a study reported recently by Eccles et al. (1997). They conducted a 6-year study of teens' free-time activities, academic performance, and alcohol use in 1259 10th graders from 12 school districts around Detroit. They found that high school athletes had higher grades and stayed in college longer but were also more likely to use alcohol and drugs. The authors noted that athletes tend to form popular cliques who party, and alcohol is part of that entertainment. The same appears true of socially connected students in college.

We recruited approximately 5% from our original sample of 2632 students for more intensive follow-up study. Inclusion criteria included their being enrolled in at least 6 credit hours in the quarter they were tested, none were first quarter freshman or last quarter seniors, none scored higher than mildly dysphoric on the Beck Depression Inventory, none were obese (body mass index < 27), none were speech or needle phobic, none were married or living with a significant other, and all were US citizens. We recruited an equal number of male and female students whose scores on the UCLA loneliness scale (Russell et al., 1980) fell into the top (lonely group), middle (normal group), or bottom quintile (socially embedded group). The middle group was included to allow us to determine whether differences between lonely and socially embedded reflected something special about lonely individuals, something unique about embedded individuals, or something that varied monotonically between these two extreme groups.

3 Differences in Social Capital

We first examined the hypothesis that individuals who were lonely simply had less social capital to offer than others. By social capital, we mean the resources they bring to a social interaction—their physical attractiveness, intelligence, height, weight, age, socioeconomic status, or scholastic achievements. Analyses revealed the groups did not differ on any of these variables.

We next examined the hypothesis that individuals who were lonely reported more traumatic life histories, were dealing with more major life events, or were suffering from more intrusive events. Again, no differences were found among the groups. Instead, the differences among groups were in the way they appraised people and events around them and the way in which they related to others. For instance, lonely individuals reported higher levels of perceived stress, more frequent and more severe hassles, and less severe uplifts than embedded individuals. The lonely and normal participants responded similarly on most of these measures; however, it was the socially embedded group who appeared the least stressed. The same pattern was found on the Profile of Moods States, which revealed embedded individuals reported feeling more vigor and less tension, hostility, confusion, fatigue, and dejection than the normal and lonely groups; of these states, the normal and lonely individuals differed only on feelings of dejection.

The social world also emerged as a less rewarding place for lonely individuals. Lonely relative to embedded individuals, reported comparable social desirability motives but had less secure adult romantic attachment styles. Lonely individuals were also characterized by greater anxiety, anger (including anger-in), and shyness, less sociability, less optimism, and poorer social skills, and they expressed stronger fears of negative evaluation. Lonely individuals were no less assertive than embedded individuals in terms of the likelihood of a behavior, but they reported much higher levels of discomfort and anxiety about being assertive.

This does not mean that lonely individuals do not know how to interact socially; they do so fairly well with their most important contact (though less well with their most frequent contact). Several different measures revealed that lonely, relative to embedded, individuals were more likely to attribute problems in social relationships to others, to view themselves as victims who are already giving as much as they can to their relationships with others. The normal group generally fell between the lonely and embedded groups on these measures.

What happens when you draw upon social capital? Does seeking social support and assistance draw down the balance subsequently available, like a bank account, or does it renew itself through mutually reinforcing interactions? The latter was suggested when we found that lonely individuals drew less upon social capital than normals and embedded individuals. To examine how our participants generally coped with stressors in their lives, we had the participants complete the COPE scale (Carver et al., 1989). The COPE contains 15 subscales of four items each: active coping, planning, seeking instrumental social support, seeking emotional social support, suppression of competing activities, religion, positive reinterpretation and growth, restraint coping, acceptance, focus on venting of emotions, denial, mental disengagement, behavioral disengagement, alcohol/drug use, and humor. The groups were found to differ on four of these subscales: lonely individuals were less likely to actively cope, seek instrumental support from others, or seek emotional support from others and were more likely to behaviorally disengage than were embedded individuals. Apparently, the balance of social capital is not governed like bank accounts, with the total available decreasing with each request for assistance. Instead, they suggest that being a friend in need, especially when the assistance is effective and duly appreciated, may build closer ties between the helper and requester.

4 Differences in Autonomic Activation

If anxiety and anger are especially powerful in lonely individuals, then they might be expected to show greater autonomic activation than embedded individuals. If, however, behavioral or emotional disengagement from the social environment is especially powerful in lonely individuals, then they might be expected to show less autonomic activation than embedded individuals. To examine this issue, participants were tested at the General Clinical Research Center at The Ohio State University Hospitals at approximately the same time in the late afternoon.

Participants completed two social speeches (e.g. asking someone out for a date, describing why you're a likable person), two non-social speeches (e.g. describing the objects in the room, describing the route from your residence to your first class of the week), and a mental arithmetic task (Cacioppo et al., 1995). These five tasks were randomly ordered for each participant. Before each speech task there was a 2-min sitting rest period, and preceding the verbal mental arithmetic task there was a 4-min sitting rest period. The experimental tasks then concluded with the orthostasis task followed by a 4-min sitting rest period and a speech task about one being accused of shoplifting (Saab et al., 1989).

The results, which are displayed in Fig. 55.1, revealed that across tasks the lonely individuals were characterized by lower basal heart rate and lower heart rate reactivity than normal or embedded individuals. Basal blood pressure was comparable across the tasks, although again cardiovascular reactivity tended to be lowest for the lonely individuals. These data are consistent with the notion that lonely individuals are more emotionally withdrawn than normal or embedded individuals when in a new social setting.

5 Differences in Attentional Control

Why might lonely individuals be more emotionally withdrawn in new social settings? Personality differences such as shyness, sociability, negativity, and fear of negative evaluation provide a partial explanation. New social settings can be overwhelming, however, and people must exert voluntary control over their attentional focus to be effective. Do lonely individuals differ in their ability to voluntarily control their attentional focus?

To explore this possibility, participants performed a dichotic listening task (Hugdahl, 1995) while at the Clinical Research Center. The dichotic listening task requires that participants identify the consonant–vowel pair that was presented to their right or left ear. Because the auditory system is predominantly crossed and because language is left-lateralized in most right-handed individuals, right-handed individuals tend to perform better when verbal stimuli are presented to the right than left ear. (All of the participants in our sample were right-handed.) Superimposed on this general right-ear advantage, however, are the effects of attention, as individuals generally perform better whenever verbal stimuli are presented to the ear to which they are focusing their attention, as well.

As expected, there was an overall right-ear advantage across groups and instructional conditions (see Fig. 55.2). In addition, a significant main effect for attentional instruction showed that individuals performed better with left-ear stimuli when they were instructed to focus on stimuli presented to their left ear than in the other conditions. The two-way interaction between attentional instruction and ear was also significant, showing a significant right-ear advantage during the no-instruction and focus on right-ear conditions and a significant left-ear advantage during the focus on left-ear condition.

As can also be seen in Fig. 55.2, lonely individuals tended to show the strongest right-ear

(a)

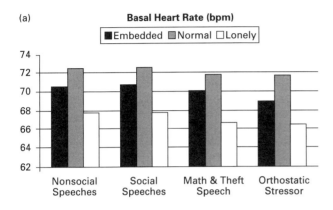

(b)

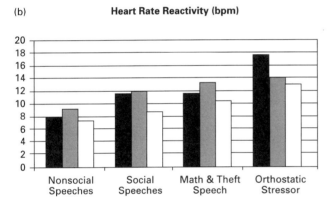

Figure 55.1
Basal heart rate (a) and heart rate reactivity to four classes of stressors (b).

advantage in the no-instruction condition, presumably reflecting the potency of bottom-up (i.e. stimulus-driven) attentional processing. More interestingly, lonely individuals apparently failed to shift to an a priori predicted left-ear advantage in the focus on left-ear condition, despite showing a large right-ear advantage when instructed to shift attention to the right ear. Specific planned contrasts confirmed that all three groups showed a significant right-ear advantage during the focus on right-ear condition, but only the normal and embedded individuals were able to revert to a

significant left-ear advantage in the focus on left-ear condition. Thus, attentional control appeared comparable in lonely and embedded individuals until voluntary attentional control conflicted with automatic attentional processes, at which point lonely individuals showed an attentional deficit. This result raises the possibility that lonely individuals feel overwhelmed and withdraw from the social environment, especially new or complex social environments, because they have less control over the focus of their attention (i.e. they are more distractable).

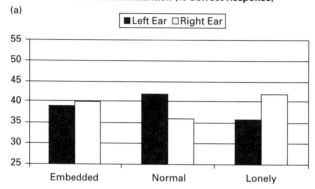

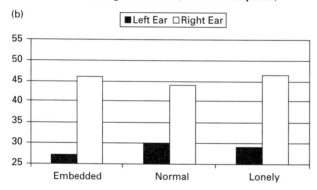

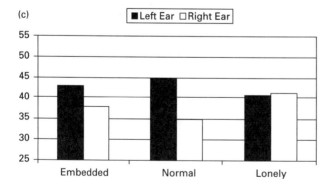

Figure 55.2
Dichotic listening performance under no attentional instruction (a), instructions to attend to the right ear (b), and instructions to attend to the left ear (c).

6 Differences in Neuroendocrine Activation

As noted above, a major objective in this study was to explore potential mechanisms underlying the relationship between social isolation and morbidity and mortality. Our data indicated that lonely, relative to embedded, individuals engaged in comparable or better health behaviors (e.g. cigarette smoking, alcohol consumption, drug abuse, and exercise). Autonomic reactivity to acute psychological stressors also tended to be diminished in lonely, relative to embedded, individuals. Prior research has shown autonomic activation to vary with the quality of a person's social relationship with others, but this prior research has tended to use either more powerful manipulations of social relationships (see review by Gardner et al., in press) or older individuals for whom the cumulative stress of loneliness is higher (see review by Uchino et al., 1996). Thus, both health behaviors and heightened sympathetic tonus remain possible contributors to differences in morbidity and mortality in later life, but these do not play much of a role in young adults.

Given the behavioral and autonomic evidence that lonely individuals disengage from the social environment and the suggestive evidence of their relative inability to override automatic attentional processing, we hypothesized that lonely individuals would show either elevated tonic activation of the hypothalamic–pituitary–adrenocortical system or a muted diurnal pattern. If so, this would provide a potential neurophysiological link between loneliness and later-life morbidity and mortality because the pituitary and adrenal hormones and other neuropeptides play an important role in the modulation of the immune system (Munck et al., 1984).

Cortisol is released in a pulsatile fashion, with major secretory episodes appearing during the early morning with the frequency and amplitude of secretory episodes declining over the course of the day (Van Cauter, 1990). Given the pulsatile nature of cortisol releases, multiple assessments over the course of the day may provide a more reliable assessment of HPA activity. Participants in our study were beeped at nine random intervals during a normal day, at which time they were asked to sit, place a roll of dental cotton in their mouth, and complete a short questionnaire. After each such period, the cotton roll was returned to a test tube, which participants returned to us the following day. Subsequently, assays were performed to quantify salivary cortisol, which is unbound (biologically active) and correlates well with plasma and urinary assessments (Kirschbaum and Hellhammer, 1994).

The salivary cortisol levels across the day, which are depicted in Fig. 55.3, reflected the typical diurnal rhythm, with no differences among groups. Spearman correlations revealed that the mean daily cortisol level was significantly correlated with the participants' perceived stress as well as the number of major life events with which they were dealing. Loneliness was related to mean salivary cortisol levels across the course of a normal day but only when loneliness was chronic. UCLA loneliness scores and state loneliness scores were positively but non-significantly correlated with mean salivary cortisol levels, whereas trait loneliness scores were positively and significantly correlated with mean cortisol levels. The stress of loneliness and associated events may simply take time to alter HPA function.

Our participants attended classes during the morning and afternoon but were left to their own devices in the evenings. Students study during the evening but this is also the most popular time for students to socialize or to think about the absence of satisfactory social interactions. Inspection of Fig. 55.3 reveals that it was during the evening that our participants' trait loneliness was most highly related to salivary cortisol levels despite HPA activity being at its nadir during the evening.

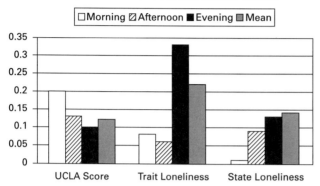

Figure 55.3

Spearman correlations between salivary cortisol and three different measures of loneliness. Salivary cortisol was assayed up to nine random times during a normal day. "Morning" represents the correlation between the mean cortisol during the morning and each loneliness measure. Similarly, "Afternoon" and "Evening" represent the correlation between the mean cortisol during the afternoon and evening, respectively, and each loneliness measure. "Mean" represents the correlation between the mean salivary cortisol across the entire day and each loneliness measure.

7 Differences in the Salubrity of Sleep

The salubrity of nourishing social relationships has been documented previously, but the beneficial effects of nurturant or intimate social relationships are usually attributed to direct assistance or stress buffering (Cohen and McKay, 1984; see Gardner et al., in press). For example, medical students undergoing exams showed stress-induced decrements in immune functioning, but this decline was particularly pronounced for the medical students who reported being lonely (Kiecolt-Glaser et al., 1984; Glaser et al., 1992). The association between trait loneliness and salivary cortisol, particularly in the evening, could be explained in terms of stress buffering or direct effects of social support. Preliminary analyses of diaries completed at random intervals by participants during the course of their day suggested yet another possible means by which social embeddedness contributes to lower levels of salivary cortisol and long-term well being.

We had anticipated that lonely individuals would be socially isolated and would be participating in fewer restorative behaviors (e.g. sleep, exercise, going to the movies, spending time with others, reading, relaxing, praying or meditating). In fact, lonely undergraduates were just as or more likely to engage in these putatively restorative acts than were normal and embedded individuals. Yet they did not show the salubrious effects normals and socially embedded individuals seemed to show. This led us to hypothesize that restorative behaviors were more potent (i.e. salubrious) when individuals felt socially connected than when they felt lonely.

To test the hypothesis that feeling socially embedded enhanced the salubrious effects of restorative behaviors, we measured sleep—a quintessential act of restoration that is performed without immediate social contact, indeed without much explicit awareness at all. Survey data indicated that lonely individuals slept as many hours per day as normal and socially embedded individuals. We used the Pittsburgh Sleep Quality Index (PSQI; Buysse et al., 1989) to assess our participants' reports of sleep disturbances, and we used the Nightcap to measure sleep of a subset of our participants during the night they spent in the Clinical Research Center.

Results from the PSQI, which are depicted in Fig. 55.4, revealed that lonely individuals reported poorer sleep quality, longer sleep latency, longer perceived sleep duration, and greater daytime dysfunction due to sleepiness than embedded individuals. Data from the Nightcap confirmed that lonely individuals slept less efficiently, took slightly longer to fall asleep, evidenced longer REM latency, and awoke more frequently during the night than embedded and normal individuals (see Fig. 55.4). Importantly, the Nightcap recordings revealed that total time asleep did not differ across the groups. Thus, the restorative act of sleep was more efficient and effective in socially embedded than lonely individuals.

To what extent are feelings of loneliness or social embeddedness causal in producing the effects outlined above? Are the elevated anxiety and cortisol levels in individuals high in trait loneliness the result of cumulative stressors or are individuals who are characterized by anxiety or elevated HPA activation likely to feel socially disconnected? Both are possible, and interesting, and either could help account for the higher morbidity and mortality found in socially isolated individuals (House et al., 1988). If only the latter were true, however, there would be little reason to intervene, to try to overcome the feelings of loneliness, to try to reach out and connect with others. Fortunately, there is preliminary evidence for both processes operating.

8 Manipulating Feelings of Loneliness

Uchino et al. (1996) reviewed intervention studies that have been performed to increase social support. A meta-analysis of these studies showed that improving social support and connectedness, especially within families, had beneficial phys-

iological effects (e.g. lowered blood pressure in hypertensives). Such findings are important because they indicate that feelings of loneliness or social embeddedness are not simply markers or epiphenomena, and that loneliness is not an invariant trait but rather is subject to some manipulation.

Although people develop characteristic ways of appraising, attaching, and interacting with others, it is conceivable that how we feel about ourselves in relation to others is the bedrock upon which these appraisals, attachment, and interactive styles are built. If so, then feelings of loneliness may prime memories, associations, and behaviors of alienation and social awkwardness, whereas feelings of connectedness may prime the opposite. That is, how individuals construe and feel about themselves in terms of those around them may be so central to some dimensions of personality (e.g. shyness, sociability, extraversion, agreeableness, fear of negative evaluation) that such construals represent a deep structure that influences the surface manifestations of these personality dimensions. To test this hypothesis, we used hypnosis to *manipulate* feelings of loneliness and embeddedness within-subjects. Twenty high hypnotizable individuals at Stanford University were identified based on high scores on the Harvard Group Scale (scores 9–12) and the Hypnotic Induction Profile (scores 8–10).

Following each hypnotic induction, participants received the suggestion that they felt lonely or socially embedded (the order of which was counterbalanced across participants). In the lonely condition, for instance, participants were told to: "Think of a time in which you felt isolated. You felt lonely. Perhaps you felt like you just didn't belong—that you had no friends. . . ." In the embedded condition, participants were told to: "Think of a time in which you felt a sense of belonging. Perhaps you were a member of a group. Perhaps you had a best friend with whom you felt you could share anything. . . ." After each suggestion, participants completed a set of questionnaires designed to measure

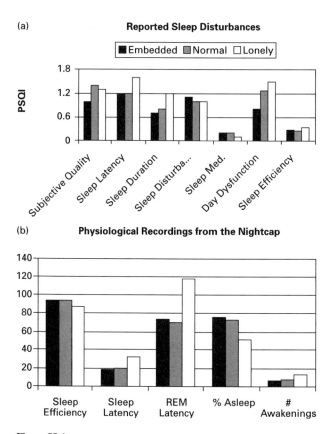

Figure 55.4
Sleep disturbance as indexed by the Pittsburgh Sleep Quality Index, a self-report measure that measures sleep disruptions (a), and Nightcap recordings during the night participants slept in the Clinical Research Center (b).

sociability, optimism, fear of negative evaluation, anger, anxiety, social skills, shyness, self esteem, mood, impact of events, loneliness, and perceived social support.

As would be expected if the manipulations were effective, participants scored higher on loneliness and lower on social support measures in the lonely than embedded condition. More interestingly, the participants' responses to the psychological surveys revealed that they were significantly lower on social skills, sociability, optimism, self esteem, and positivity, and higher

on anger, anxiety, negativity, and fear of negative evaluation in the lonely than embedded condition. Importantly, the participants in the lonely and embedded condition scored comparably on the subscales (intrusion and avoidance) of the impact of events scale—just as had the participants in our cross-sectional study. Thus, the same differences—and lack of differences—we observed between our lonely and embedded groups were replicated within subjects when they were induced to feel very lonely or socially embedded. Together, these results support the hypothesis that how individuals construe and feel about themselves in terms of those around them can affect the surface manifestations of states and traits and, presumably, their physiology.

9 Conclusion

The current research underscores the centrality of social relationships to human existence and experience. For instance, lonely individuals were more anxious, angry, and negative, and less positive, optimistic, comfortable, and secure than embedded individuals, a pattern of findings that was associated with feelings of loneliness whether examined between-subjects or within-subjects. Attentional control appeared comparable in lonely and embedded individuals until voluntary attentional control conflicted with automatic attentional processes, at which point lonely individuals showed an attentional deficit. Interestingly, lonely and embedded individuals were found to have comparable social capital (e.g. attractiveness, SES, intelligence) and social contacts, but lonely individuals, in contrast to embedded individuals, made less use of social capital, expected negative outcomes, were less likely to reach out or to seek help from others, and were more likely to think they were already doing all they could do in their relationships. Loneliness was associated with a range of altered physiological processes, as well, including muted autonomic activation, elevated activation of the HPA axis at least in the subset of individuals who were chronically lonely, and disregulated sleep. These data converge to suggest that the unfulfilled need to belong is associated with complex yearnings for intimacy yet feelings of insecurity and mistrust, anger combined with anger suppression, punishing feelings of isolation coupled with a fear of negative evaluation by others, emotional dysphoria and withdrawal rather than active coping attempts. Given this psychological complex, it is no surprise why daily encounters yield fewer uplifting events and more frequent

hassles for lonely than embedded individuals; across a lifetime, the allostatic load (McEwen and Stellar, 1993) of daily challenges and stressors should be greater, as well.

The social world has tended to be ignored in psychophysiology and in the neurosciences because it falls outside the physical boundaries of the body. Yet our genetic makeup compels us to be social animals, and social contact and relationships are among the most powerful stimuli in the environment. Isolation from the social world is known to be as significant a risk factor as smoking and high blood pressure, but the absence of an obvious physical mechanism has made rigorous scientific analysis difficult. The current research suggests that "social neuroscience" is not an oxymoron, that instead it represents a viable, multi-level integrative approach for understanding the mind and brain. It is also consistent with the notion that the social world in large part defines who we are, how we appraise and relate to events in our lives, and how our biology develops, responds, and ages.

A multi-level integrative approach spanning biological and social levels of organization does not imply dualism (Cacioppo and Berntson, 1992). Multiple levels of analysis do not imply independent (non-reductionistic) determinants. There is a single set of determinants that may be conceptualized at different levels of organization. Hormonal effects, for instance, are mediated by their chemistry but their actions on mating are not optimally organized by chemical/receptor interactions alone. The early American psychologist William James (1890/1950) was among the first to articulate the notion that neurophysiological processes underlie psychological phenomena. James further argued that developmental, environmental, and sociocultural factors influence the neurophysiological processes underlying psychological and social phenomena. Although these influences could be studied as neurophysiological transactions, James recognized that unnecessary diseconomies and conundrums would result if psychological phenomena were described only as neurophysiological events. Social and psychological constructs such as loneliness and social embeddedness, both of which undoubtedly have neurophysiological implementations, are simpler to measure and are more reliably measured using self-report instruments than some physiological processes (e.g. cortisol levels).

There is growing evidence that multi-level analyses spanning neural and social perspectives can foster comprehensive accounts of cognition, emotion, behavior, and health. This is in part because the social environment shapes neural structures and processes and vice versa. Meaney and colleagues (Meaney et al., 1993; Liu et al., 1997), for instance, have found that variations in maternal care influence the development of individual differences in neuroendocrine responses to stress in rats. As adults, the offspring of mothers that exhibited more licking and grooming of pups during the first 10 days of life were also characterized by reduced adrenocorticotropic hormone and corticosterone responses to acute stress. As mothers, these rats also tended to lick and groom their pups. This research raises the possibility that lonely and socially embedded individuals have very different experiences early in life that shape their HPA functioning as well as their social behavior. That is, although the stress of chronic loneliness may affect HPA activation, the reciprocal influence also appears likely.

Our results also raise a number of interesting questions, many of which require experimental and prospective studies to unravel. What does seem clear, however, are that these questions are amenable to social, cognitive, and biological levels of analysis and that the questions are worth asking. As E. O. Wilson (1998) noted,

people must belong to a tribe; they yearn to have a purpose larger than themselves. We are obliged by the deepest drives of the human spirit to make ourselves more than animated dust, and we must have a story to tell about where we came from, and why we are here (p. 6).

Acknowledgements

We wish to thank David Lozano and Dan Litvack of The Ohio State University Social Neuroscience Laboratory for their technical assistance, Robert Stickgold from the Harvard University Neurophysiology Lab and Bita Naouriani from the Stanford University Department of Psychiatry for their assistance in this investigation, the staff of The Ohio State University Residence Halls directed by Steve Kramer for their help, Carolyn Cheney of The Ohio State University Medical Labs for her contributions, and the General Clinical Research Center, including Dana Ciccone, Bob Rice, and the nursing staff headed by Teresa Sampsel, for the assistance and cooperation. This work was supported by training grant MH-19728 from the National Institutes of Mental Health, a National Institute of Health grant to the General Clinical Research Center, MO1-RR00034, and the John D. and Catherine T. MacArthur Foundation.

References

Baumeister, R. F., Leary, M. R., 1995. The need to belong: desire for interpersonal attachment as a fundamental human motivation. Psychol. Bull. 117, 497–529.

Berkman, L. F., Syme, S. L., 1979. Social networks, host resistance, and mortality: a nine-year follow-up study of Alameda County residents. Am. J. Epidemiol. 109, 186–204.

Berscheid, E., 1985. Interpersonal attraction. In: Lindzey, G., Aronson, E. (Eds.), The Handbook of Social Psychology. Random House, New York, NY.

Buysse, D. J., Reynolds, C. F., Monk, T. H., Berman, S. R. et al., 1989. The Pittsburgh Sleep Quality Index: a new instrument for psychiatric practice and research. Psychiatry Res. 28, 193–213.

Burt, R. S., 1986. Strangers, friends, and happiness. GSS Technical Report No. 72. National Opinion Research Center, University of Chicago, Chicago.

Cacioppo, J. T., Berntson, G. G., 1992. Social psychological contributions to the decade of the brain: the doctrine of multilevel analysis. Am. Psychol. 47, 1019–1028.

Cacioppo, J. T., Malarkey, W. B., Kiecolt-Glaser, J. K., Uchino, B. N., Sgoutas-Emch, S. A., Sheridan, J. F., Berntson, G. G., Glaser, R., 1995. Cardiac autonomic substrates as a novel approach to explore heterogeneity in neuroendocrine and immune responses to brief psychological stressors. Psychosom. Med. 57, 154–164.

Carter, C. S., Lederhendler, I. I., Kirkpatrick, B., 1997. The Integrative Neurobiology of Affiliation. New York Academy of Sciences, New York.

Carver, C. S., Scheier, M. F., Weintraub, J. K., 1989. Assessing coping strategies: a theoretically based approach. J. Pers. Social Psychol. 56, 267–283.

Cohen, S., McKay, G., 1984. Social support, stress, and the buffering hypothesis: a theoretical analysis. In: Baum, A., Taylor, S. E., Singer, J. E. (Eds.), Handbook of Psychology and Health. Erlbaum, Hillsdale, NJ, pp. 253–267.

Eccles, J. S., Lord, S. E., Roeser, R. W., Barber, B. L. et al., 1997. The association of school transitions in early adolescence with developmental trajectories through high school. In: Schulenberg, J., Maggs, J. L., Hurrelmann, K. (Eds.), Health Risks and Developmental Transitions During Adolescence. Cambridge University Press, New York, NY, USA, pp. 283–320.

Ernst, J. M., Cacioppo, J. T., 1999. Lonely hearts: Psychological perspectives on loneliness. Appl. Preventive Psychol. 8, 1–22.

Gardner, W. L., Gabriel, S., Diekman, A. B., in press. Interpersonal processes. In: Cacioppo, J. T., Tassinary, L. G., Berntson, G. G. (Eds.), Handbook of Psychophysiology. Cambridge University Press, New York.

Gardner, W. L., Pickett, C., Brewer, M. B., in review. Social exclusion and selective memory: How the need to belong affects memory for social information.

Glaser, R., Kiecolt-Glaser, J. K., Bonneau, R. H., Malarkey, W. et al., 1992. Stress-induced modulation of the immune response to recombinant hepatitis B vaccine. Psychosomatic Medicine 54(1), 22–29.

Goldin-Meadow, S., Mylander, C., 1983. Gestural communication in deaf children: noneffect of parental input on language development. Science 221, 372–374.

Goldin-Meadow, S., Mylander, C., 1984. Gestural communication in deaf children: the effects and non-

effects of parental input on early language development. Monogr. Soc. Res. Child Dev. 49, 1–121.

Gupta, V., Korte, C., 1994. The effects of a confidant and a peer group on the well-being of single elders. Int. J. Aging Hum. Dev. 39, 293–302.

House, J. S., Landis, K. R., Umberson, D., 1988. Social relationships and health. Science 241, 540–545.

House, J. S., Robbins, C., Metzner, H. L., 1982. The association of social relationships and activities with mortality: prospective evidence from the Tecumseh Community Health Study. Am. J. Epidemiol. 116, 123–140.

Hugdahl, K., 1995. Dichotic listening—probing temporal lobe functional integrity. In: Davidson, R. J., Hugdahl, K. (Eds.), Brain Asymmetry. MIT Press, Cambridge, MA, pp. 123–156.

James, W., 1890/1950. Principles of Psychology. Dover, New York.

Kiecolt-Glaser, J. K., Garner, W., Speicher, C. E., Penn, G., Glaser, R., 1984. Psychosocial modifiers of immunocompetence in medical students. Psychosom. Med. 46, 7–14.

Kirschbaum, C., Hellhammer, D. H., 1994. Salivary cortisol in psychoneuroendocrine research: recent developments and applications. Psychoneuroendocrinology 19, 313–333.

Liu, D., Diorio, J., Tannenbaum, B., Caldji, C., Francis, D., Freedman, A., Sharma, S., Pearson, D., Plotsky, P. M., Meaney, M. J., 1997. Maternal care, hippocampal glucocorticoid receptors, and hypothalamic–pituitary–adrenal responses to stress. Science 277, 1659–1662.

Meaney, M. J., Bhatnagar, S., Diorio, J., Larocque, S., Francis, D., O'Donnell, D., Shanks, N., Sharma, S., Smythe, J., Viau, V., 1993. Cellular Molecular Neurobiol. 13, 321–347.

McEwen, B. S., Stellar, E., 1993. Stress and the individual: mechanisms leading to disease. Arch. Internal Med. 153, 2093–2101.

Munck, A., Guyre, P. M., Holbrook, N. J., 1984. Physiological function of glucocorticoids in stress and their relation to pharmacological actions. Endocr. Rev. 5, 25–44.

Perkins, H. W., 1991. Religious commitment, "Yuppie" values, and well-being in post collegiate life. Rev. Religious Res. 32, 244–251.

Russell, D., Peplau, L. A., Cutrona, C. E., 1980. The Revised UCLA Loneliness Scale: concurrent and discriminant validity evidence. J. Pers. Social Psychol. 39, 472–480.

Saab, P. G., Matthews, K. A., Stoney, C. M., McDonald, R. J., 1989. Premenopausal and postmenopausal women differ in their cardiovascular and neuroendocrine responses to behavioral stressors. Psychophysiology 26, 270–280.

Uchino, B. N., Cacioppo, J. T., Kiecolt-Glaser, J. K., 1996. The relationship between social support and physiological process: A review with emphasis on underlying mechanisms and implications for health. Psychol. Bull. 119, 488–531.

Uvnäs-Mosberg, K., 1997. Physiological and endocrine effects of social contact. Ann. N.Y. Acad. Sci. 807, 146–163.

Van Cauter, E., 1990. Diurnal and ultradian rhythms in human endocrine function: a minireview. Hormones Res. 34, 45–53.

Wilson, E. O., 1998. Consilience. Alfred A. Knopf, New York.

56 Neuroendocrine Perspectives on Social Attachment and Love

C. Sue Carter

What Is Love?

Attachment, commitment, intimacy, passion, grief upon separation, and jealousy are but a few of the feelings or emotions sometimes used to describe love (Hatfield and Rapson, 1993; Sternberg and Barnes, 1988). From a scientific perspective, love is a hypothetical construct with many dimensions and interpretations. However, the various emotional states and behaviors associated with love are rarely investigated. In part this is because love has been the domain of poets, novelists, and clinicians, and often is considered beyond the scope of experimental science.

The purpose of this chapter is to review behavioral, neurochemical and anatomical substrates of social attachment, and suggest possible mechanisms through which specific neuroendocrine systems may regulate social attachment. Because scientific study, and especially neurobiological research, demands rigorous experimental control and uses invasive methods, the methods of science are difficult to apply to the personal experiences associated with human love (Porges, 1998). Laboratory rodents, which are preferred subjects in neurobiological research, generally do not show selective social behaviors, and do not lend themselves to studies of love. Various primate species do show social bonds, with features that resemble love, but primates are difficult to study, especially with invasive techniques. Work on maternal bonding has taken advantage of the fact that precocial ungulates, including sheep, are excellent subjects for neurobiological investigation, and do develop selective filial attachments. In addition, monogamous mammals, including prairie voles (*Microtus ochrogaster*) develop adult heterosexual pair bonds which can be studied in the laboratory. Most research on social attachment at present comes from these animal models. In addition, parental behavior and sexual behavior share common features with

attachment and are intimately associated with the concept of love. Therefore, the analysis of parental and sexual behaviors, which can be studied in a variety of species, also offers insight into the neurophysiology of love.

Definitions and Measurements of Love and Attachment

Love and social attachments function to facilitate reproduction, provide a sense of security and reduce feelings of stress or anxiety. The neurobiology of love is interwoven, phylogenetically and ontogenetically, and in adulthood with reproduction and homeostasis (Uvnas-Moberg, 1997).

Attachment is a component of most, if not all, definitions of human love (Bartholomew and Perlman, 1994; Sternberg and Barnes, 1988). Although attachment may exist in the absence of love, it is unlikely that love can exist in the absence of attachment. Attachment as a concept, can be operationalized and studied experimentally, and thus offers a starting point for analyzing the scientific basis of love.

Behavioral theories or models of attachment have focused on either caregiver–infant interactions or adult heterosexual pair bonding. There are similarities between the behaviors associated with parent–infant attachment and adult romantic attachments. In fact, several investigators have suggested that these types of love or attachment share common biological substrates (Fisher, 1992; Hazan and Shaver, 1987; Panksepp et al., 1997).

Attachment is commonly defined as a selective social or emotional bond (Ainsworth, 1989; Bowlby, 1969, 1973, 1980; Hennessy, 1997). Although social bonds cannot be directly measured, the concept of attachment typically has been defined by behavioral or physiological processes. Maintenance of proximity or voluntary contact with an attachment object are the most commonly used behavioral indices of attachment (Carter et al., 1995). Selective or differential behaviors, such allogrooming, directed toward the presumed object of attachment also may be measured. Attachment, especially in primates, sometimes is measured by observing the visual tracking of the attachment object (Kraemer, 1992, 1997). Behavioral tests of attachment usually juxtapose responses toward a familiar individual to those directed toward other forms of social stimuli, such as an unfamiliar conspecific.

Behavioral, endocrine or autonomic responses to separation or reunion also may correlate with or be used to index attachment. In mammals distress vocalizations may increase following separation and decline following reunion. Secretion of hormones of the HPA axis, usually cortisol or corticosterone or adrenocorticotrophic hormone (ACTH), also may follow separation from the attachment figure and HPA activity tends to decline upon reunion (Hennessy, 1997; Levine et al., 1997; Mendoza and Mason, 1997; Reite and Boccia, 1994). Behavioral and endocrine responses to separation, reunion or the presence of a stressor may be discordant or have different time courses (Levine et al., 1989). No single measure of attachment has gained universal acceptance, and existing behavioral and endocrine measures may reflect different, although in some cases related, physiological processes.

Evolutionary and Cross-Species Perspectives on Attachment

Survival and reproduction can depend on the ability to adapt patterns of social and reproductive behavior to environmental and social demands. Social attachments function to facilitate reproduction, provide a sense of security and reduce feelings of stress or anxiety (Fig. 56.1). Mammals generally are social creatures, often living and reproducing in pairs or groups. Pairs and larger groups, such as families or troops, are held together by social bonds or selective social behaviors. The expression of social behavior in general, and social attachment in particular, is species-typical and highly individualized (Carter et al., 1997).

What we now call attachment may have arisen from physiological solutions to simpler problems related to survival or reproduction (Uvnas-Moberg, 1997). Mammalian reproduction requires a particularly intense investment of maternal time and energy, and may involve commitment to a specific infant. A mammalian mother gestates her infant, she may risk her life to give birth, and then, with some human exceptions, provides postnatal care while nourishing the infant with bodily fluids. Lactation is the defining characteristic of Mammalia, and livebirth is a feature of reproduction in eutherian mammals. Hormones, including oxytocin, vasopressin, prolactin, and endogenous opiates, that are involved in sexual behavior, pregnancy, birth, and lactation also have been implicated in the induction of maternal behavior and maternal attachment (Table 56.1). The association between social bonding and reproduction, which is most easily seen in monogamous mammals and in mother–infant interactions, may have contributed, in an evolutionary sense, to the selection of neurochemical systems involved in the occurrence of attachment behaviors. For example, pair bonding in monogamous mammals may be functionally similar to the behavioral patterns that humans associate with social attachments.

Behavioral Models of Social Attachment

Basic Behavioral Systems and Attachment

The tendency to approach or avoid a particular set of social stimuli is fundamental to social behaviors and attachment behaviors. Some stimuli may be inherently positive or may elicit positive responses; other stimuli, particularly

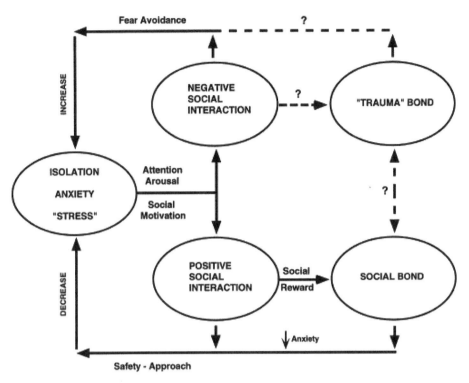

Figure 56.1
Behavioral and emotional correlates of social attachment.

those that are novel, can be innately aversive or fear-inducing. Studies of the physiology of positive social behaviors, including affiliative and reproductive behaviors may be especially relevant to understanding the biology of attachment. Specific physiological states can encourage positive social behaviors, including the formation of attachments and reproduction, while others may promote self-defensive or aggressive behaviors, which are generally, but perhaps not always, incompatible with attachment (Porges, 1998). Peptidergic systems involving oxytocin, and perhaps in some cases vasopressin, may serve to inhibit defensive behaviors associated with stress, anxiety or fear, and allow positive social interactions and the development of social bonds.

Adult Pair Bonds

Heterosexual pair bonds are uncommon in mammals, but are usually found in monogamous species (Kleiman, 1977). Monogamy is presumably favored under conditions when two parents are needed to rear the young, and when it confers reproductive advantages on both parents. Thus, animals that are monogamous provide an opportunity to examine the biology of selective adult social attachments in species where such bonds may facilitate survival and reproduction and, therefore, might have been favored by natural selection.

Monogamous mammals form adult pair bonds with several features that satisfy definitions of

Table 56.1
Experiences or treatments associated with attachment formation

Experience or treatment	Species	Reference
Birth	Sheep	[Keverne et al. (1997)]
Lactation	Sheep	[Keverne et al. (1997)]
	Human	[Uvnas-Moberg (1997)]
Sexual behavior	Prairie vole	[Williams et al. (1992)]
Cohabitation	Prairie vole	[Williams et al. (1992)] [DeVries et al. (1996)]
Stressful experiences	Human	[Simpson and Rholes (1994)]
	Prairie vole	[DeVries et al. (1996)]
Corticosterone treatment	Prairie vole	[DeVries et al. (1996)]
Vasopressin treatment	Prairie vole	[Winslow et al. (1993)]
Oxytocin treatment	Sheep	[Keverne and Kendrick (1992)]
	Prairie vole	[Williams et al. (1994)]

attachment and which on the surface resemble love. Monogamy in mammals does not follow taxonomic boundaries, and has been reported in various species of primates, canids and a few rodent species (Carter et al., 1995; Dewsbury, 1988; Gubernick et al., 1994; Kleiman, 1977). Experiments on the physiology of pair bonding are rare in larger mammals, and at present most of what is known regarding the neuroendocrinology of pair bonding comes from rodents.

Caregiver–Infant Attachments

Attachment, especially in primates, often is studied in terms of the behavioral, emotional or hormonal changes that accompany separation

from an attachment figure or reunion with or attempts to reunite with the object of an attachment. In humans and other primates, it is assumed that the attachment object, often the mother or another caretaker, serves as a secure base which is reliably available, can shield the infant from threats and may provide the infant with resources, such as food. These assumptions are the core of the theories of Bowlby (1969, 1973, 1980) and Ainsworth (1989). However, most of this literature looks at attachment from the perspective of the infant.

When Are Attachments Formed?

Evidence for attachment formation comes from behavioral changes associated with mammalian birth, lactation and sexual interactions (Table 56.1). In addition, novel or stressful experiences may encourage increased social behaviors and attachment. Comparatively high levels of HPA axis activity or other indications of sympathetic arousal, and the subsequent release of oxytocin have been measured under conditions that commonly precede or are associated with the formation of social bonds.

Birth

Mammalian birth is a uniquely stressful experience. In the mother the physiological events preceding and during parturition involve exceptionally high levels of adrenal activity and catecholamines and the subsequent release of peptides, including endogenous opioids, oxytocin and vasopressin (Keverne and Kendrick, 1992; Landgraf et al., 1991). Infants also experience parturitional stress or birth trauma and probably experience increased exposure to maternal oxytocin during labor. Hormonal experiences associated with birth may affect the tendency of young animals to form social bonds, although such effects remain to be demonstrated.

The Postpartum Period and Lactation

The postpartum period in mammals is characterized by lactation. Lactation is further associated with both maternal and infant attachment. Lactation is a dynamic process, which involves the pulsatile release of oxytocin. In addition, production of vasopressin, prolactin, and the endogenous opioids may be elevated, with concurrent reduced reactivity in the HPA axis (Altemus et al., 1995; Carter and Altemus, 1997; Lightman 1992). Lactation may provide additional opportunity for maternal bonding, perhaps allowing oxytocin to reinforce attachments initially formed during parturition.

The postpartum period and lactation also provide infants with opportunities to develop a social attachment with their mother. In addition, milk contains comparatively high levels of hormones including oxytocin (Leake et al., 1981) and prolactin (Grosvenor et al., 1990). In infants the digestive system is more permeable than in adults. There is evidence in rats that milk-borne prolactin has long-term effects on neuroendocrine development. The behavioral effects of milk-borne oxytocin have not been studied, but hormones in milk could provide another level of regulation for the developing nervous system, possibly influencing the offspring's subsequent management of stressful experiences (Carter, 1988).

Oxytocin injections, given peripherally to the mother, can facilitate nipple attachment by young rat pups, suggesting that oxytocin may change the olfactory characteristics of the parent and thus the response of a young animal to its mother (Singh and Hofer, 1978). Rat pups also show preferences for specific odors that are associated with exposure to their mothers. Preferences for the mother do not develop in animals that are pretreated with oxytocin antagonists (Nelson and Panksepp, 1996). Thus, oxytocin may act on both the mother and infant to influence the response of young animals to their mother.

Sexual Behavior and Attachment

In species that form heterosexual pair bonds, including prairie voles, sexual interactions are associated with the formation of social attachments (Carter et al., 1995). Sexual behavior also can be physiologically stressful for both sexes. Adrenal steroids, vasopressin, oxytocin and endogenous opioids are released during sexual behavior (Carter, 1992; Meisel and Sachs, 1994; Pfaff et al., 1994).

Stressful Experiences and Attachment

Threatening situations may encourage return to a secure base or otherwise strengthen social bonds (Bowlby, 1969; Panksepp et al., 1985). The literature on human and animal behavior consistently implicates stress, threatening situations, and hormones of the HPA axis in the formation of attachments.

Stress or corticosterone facilitates pair bond formation in male prairie voles (DeVries et al., 1996). Although female prairie voles did not form pair bonds with familiar males following stressful treatments, stress did encourage the development of preferences for other females, consistent with the communal breeding pattern of this species (DeVries and Carter, unpublished data). Steroid hormones, including glucocorticoids can influence the synthesis of, release of, and/or receptors for neuropeptides. In addition, steroid and peptide hormones may regulate or interact with each other to influence behavior (Table 56.2).

Neophobia and Attachment

Hormones can reduce fear or behavioral inhibition and permit the expression of social behaviors, such as those necessary for pair bonding, maternal behavior (Fleming et al., 1989; McCarthy et al., 1992; Numan, 1994), or sexual behavior (Carter, 1992). The neurochemical processes that are capable of overcoming neophobia

Table 56.2
Mechanisms through which steroids and/or peptides may influence attachment

---

Developmental regulation of:

species-typical traits

sexual dimorphism in nervous system

alterations in peptide sensitivity or reactivity by altering:

    hormones or neurotransmitters

    and/or their receptors

In adulthood:

peptide synthesis and/or release

peptide receptors and/or binding

altering behaviors that release peptides

peptide–peptide interactions

steroid–steroid interactions

steroid–peptide–neurotransmitter interactions

hormonal effects on the autonomic nervous system

---

also may be needed to permit the formation of new social attachments. Prosocial behavior or social contact is facilitated and aggression is diminished following central oxytocin treatments in estrogen-treated female prairie voles (Witt et al., 1990). Increases in social contact also follow oxytocin treatment in both male and female rats (Witt et al., 1992). In addition, in sexually-naive male rats a brief (15 min) heterosexual interaction is followed by an approximate doubling of serum oxytocin levels; this change was not seen in sexually-experienced males for which this situation may have been less novel (Hillegaart et al., 1997). Oxytocin treatments may reduce anxiety as measured by exploration of a novel environment in rats (McCarthy et al., 1992; Uvnas-Moberg, 1997). In humans (Chiodera et al., 1991) and prairie voles (DeVries et al., 1997), oxytocin inhibited the secretion of glucocorticoids (Fig. 56.3). Social contact also can inhibit HPA axis activity in prairie voles (DeVries et al., 1995, 1996). In reproductively naive prairie voles, either oxytocin (ICV) or social contact

produced a 50% decline in corticosterone, which occurred within 30–60 min. In male prairie voles either mating (Insel et al., 1995) or vasopressin treatment (Dharmadhikari et al., 1997) is associated with increased exploration in the open arm of a plus maze, a measure often considered indicative of reduced anxiety.

These findings suggest that stressful conditions and anxiety are associated with the formation of new social bonds. In addition, under a variety of conditions oxytocin and/or vasopressin may function to reduce neophobia or anxiety, while concurrently promoting positive social behaviors including social attachment.

Endocrine Theories of Social Attachment: Overview

Data from a variety of species and different paradigms implicate oxytocin and vasopressin in social attachment and in related prosocial and reproductive behaviors, including parental and sexual behaviors. Some, but not all, of the behavioral effects of oxytocin are similar to those seen after vasopressin treatment. In addition, vasopressin, but not oxytocin, has been associated with agonistic and territorial behaviors, including mate guarding (Winslow et al., 1993). The endogenous opioids also have been implicated in attachment and in the response to separation, but the nature of this effect is currently uncertain and beyond the scope of this review (Panksepp et al., 1997; Shapiro et al., 1989).

Reproduction and social attachment are intimately connected. Steroid hormones fluctuate throughout the reproductive life of mammals and could coordinate social behaviors, including attachment formation, with specific reproductive events. Thus, hormones of the hypothalamic–pituitary–gonadal (HPG) axis are candidates for roles in the physiology of attachment. However, at present there is no evidence of a direct role for HPG axis hormones in the initiation of social attachments (Carter et al., 1995, 1997). In contrast, hormones of the HPA axis are associated with the formation of social attachments. Evidence regarding this hypothesis will be described below.

Oxytocin and Vasopressin: Background

Oxytocin and Vasopressin: Structure and Synthesis

Oxytocin and vasopressin are small peptides, consisting of nine amino acids, configured as a six amino acid ring with a three amino acid tail. Oxytocin and vasopressin differ from each other in two amino acids and may have evolved from a common ancestral peptide (Acher, 1996). The gene for these two peptides occupies the same chromosome. There is abundant evidence for functional interactions among these peptides (Barberis and Tribollet, 1996; Carter et al., 1995; De Wied et al., 1993; Engelmann et al., 1996; Pedersen et al., 1992). Both oxytocin and vasopressin have been described as mammalian hormones, although structurally similar peptides, such as vasotocin, mesotocin and isotocin, are found in other vertebrates (Acher and Chauvet, 1988; Moore, 1992) and invertebrates (Van Kesteren et al., 1992).

Large, magnocellular neurons in the supraoptic nucleus (SON) and paraventricular nucleus (PVN) are the major source of circulating oxytocin and vasopressin. Oxytocin and vasopressin, in conjunction with their carrier proteins, are transported from magnocellular neurons in the SON and PVN to the posterior pituitary (hypophysis), where they are stored and secreted into the blood stream. In addition oxytocin and vasopressin are released within the central nervous system (CNS) from smaller, parvocellular neurons, located in the PVN and other brain areas. The release of peptides within the CNS and posterior pituitary can occur independently, although central and peripheral release patterns also may be coordinated (Kendrick et al., 1986).

In addition to the oxytocin that is produced in the SON and PVN, cell bodies producing oxytocinergic fibers also have been identified in the bed nucleus of the stria terminalis (BNST), the anterior commissural nucleus and the spinal cord (Sofroniew, 1983). The latter fibers terminate within the CNS or release oxytocin into the cerebrospinal fluid. Oxytocin is also produced in nonneural tissue. Oxytocin gene expression increases in the PVN and SON during lactation and around birth or under hormonal conditions that mimic birth (Crowley et al., 1995; Lightman and Young, 1987, 1989; van Tol et al., 1988).

As with oxytocin the most abundant sources of vasopressin are found in the PVN and SON. Vasopressin is synthesized and released within the nervous system by parvocellular neurons in the PVN. Vasopressinergic cell bodies also have been identified in the suprachiasmatic nucleus (SCN), medial amygdala (MAMY), BNST and other areas of the caudal brain stem. Androgens facilitate the synthesis of vasopressin, particularly in the MAMY and lateral septum (LS) (DeVries and Villalba, 1997; Van Leeuwen et al., 1985), accounting for clear sex differences in the abundance of vasopressin in the CNS.

Receptors for Oxytocin and Vasopressin

The behavioral functions of peptides, like most other hormones, depend on their capacity to bind to specific receptors. One receptor has been identified for oxytocin, while at least three receptor subtypes are responsible for the functions of vasopressin (Barberis and Tribollet, 1996; Ostrowski, 1998). V1a receptors are found throughout the CNS and cardiovascular system. V1b receptors are most abundant in the pituitary gland, and tend to occur in low densities in the CNS, often in conjunction with oxytocin receptors. V2 receptors are most abundant in the kidney.

Within the CNS oxytocin and vasopressin receptors are found in the olfactory system, limbic–hypothalamic system, brain stem and spinal cord areas that regulate reproductive and autonomic functions. The distributions of oxytocin and vaso-pressin receptors within the CNS vary across development and among mammalian species (Barberis and Tribollet, 1996; Patchev and Almeida, 1995; Patchev et al., 1993; Insel et al., 1994, 1997; Wang et al., 1996, 1997; Witt et al., 1991). The densities and patterns of distribution of oxytocin binding in specific brain areas also can be influenced by steroid hormones, including estrogen, progesterone, androgens and gluco-corticoids (Insel et al., 1993; Johnson, 1992; Liberzon et al., 1994; Liberzon and Young, 1997; Schumacher et al., 1990; Tribollet et al., 1990; Witt et al., 1991). Patterns of vasopressin recep-tor binding in the CNS are similar in males and females. There is at present no evidence that adult gonadal hormones can influence patterns of vasopressin receptor distribution. However, developmental hormonal experiences can alter adult gene expression for both oxytocin and vasopressin receptors (Ostrowski, 1998). The ca-pacity of peptides to respond to developmental processes provides a mechanism through which individual experiences could influence adult so-cial behavior. Oxytocin and vasopressin also are capable of binding to each other's receptors (Barberis and Tribollet, 1996), further compli-cating the analysis of mechanisms through which oxytocin and vasopressin affect behavior.

Classic Functions of Oxytocin

Oxytocin is released peripherally from the pos-terior pituitary in pulses that trigger muscular contractions necessary for birth. During lacta-tion oxytocin contracts myoepithelial tissue in the breast to produce milk let-down. In general the functions of oxytocin receptors in specific areas of the nervous system remain to be deter-mined. However, many brain regions containing oxytocin receptors have been implicated in sen-sory processing, memory, behavior, reproduc-tion and/or homeostasis. Oxytocin is particularly associated with the functions of the parasympa-

thetic component of the autonomic nervous sys-tem (ANS) (Dreifuss et al., 1992; Sawchenko and Swanson, 1982; Swanson and Sawchenko, 1980; Uvnas-Moberg, 1994). Oxytocin also plays a role in the regulation of the HPA axis (Uvnas-Moberg, 1998) although like many of its be-havioral effects, the HPA modulatory effects of oxytocin are species specific.

Classic Functions of Vasopressin

The classic functions of vasopressin also are those attributed to its peripheral actions. Vaso-pressin is named for its capacity to increase blood pressure and has various effects on cardiovascu-lar function (Berecek, 1991). However, neuro-hypophyseal vasopressin also acts within the kidney to conserve water and thus vasopressin sometimes is called the anti-diuretic hormone (ADH). Vasopressin has many functions reflect-ing its capacity to be released within and acts within the CNS. Vasopressin has been implicated in attention and various forms of learning and memory (De Wied et al., 1991, 1993; Engelmann et al., 1996). In rats centrally-active vasopressin, in conjunction with CRH, determines the release of ACTH by the anterior pituitary (Whitnall, 1993). ACTH, in turn, regulates the release of glucocorticoids from the adrenal cortex. Vaso-pressin is a central component of the sympathetic nervous system, but also may regulate para-sympathetic nervous system function (Dreifuss et al., 1992; Engelmann et al., 1996; Porges, 1998).

Hormonal Effects on Pair Bonding

Prairie voles, small arvicoline rodents from the midwestern United States, have proven particu-larly amenable to the experimental analysis of pair bond formation. Prairie voles live in pairs and show well-defined behavioral preferences for their familiar partner (Getz et al., 1981). Pair bonding in this species is assessed by allowing an experimental animal to chose between a stimulus animal made familiar by association or cohabitation, or a comparable stranger (Carter et al., 1995). Both monogamous and nonmonogamous species of voles are found within the genus *Microtus,* allowing valuable intrageneric comparisons (Dewsbury, 1988; Insel, 1997).

Oxytocin

Reliable partner preferences can develop following a period of nonsexual cohabitation, but preferences occur more quickly when a male and female are allowed to mate (Williams et al., 1992). Mating or vaginal cervical stimulation is known to release oxytocin (Carter, 1992). In addition, we have observed increased social contact in female prairie voles treated with oxytocin (ICV) (Cho et al., in press; Witt et al., 1990) (Fig. 56.3). We hypothesized that the release of oxytocin might facilitate pair bonding, and this hypothesis was confirmed. In female prairie voles central oxytocin treatments hastened pair bonding; conversely oxytocin antagonists interfered with partner preference formation following either oxytocin-treatments or prolonged cohabitation (Cho et al., in press; Insel and Hulihan, 1995; Williams et al., 1994).

In female prairie voles facilitative effects of centrally-administered oxytocin on pair bonding have been seen following either chronic infusions, using a miniature osmotic pump implanted 24 h prior to exposure to a partner (Williams et al., 1994), or following acute ICV injections, given immediately prior to brief (1 h) exposure to the partner (Cho et al., in press). In addition, peripheral pulses, but not single injections of oxytocin, facilitate pair bonding in female prairie voles (Cushing and Carter, 1998). In male prairie voles acute oxytocin treatments given ICV also can facilitate partner preference formation (Cho et al., in press). These results indicate that in prairie voles exogenously administered oxytocin is capable of inducing pair bonding in both sexes. These data also support the hypothesis that for females endogenous oxytocin, released during either mating or cohabitation, plays a role in pair bond formation. The role of endogenous oxytocin in males remains less certain, possibly because males are more dependent than females on vasopressin (Insel and Hulihan, 1995).

Vasopressin

Vasopressin can also facilitate the onset of partner preferences. In male prairie voles chronic (Winslow et al., 1993) or acute (Cho et al., in press) vasopressin treatments facilitate the selection of a particular female partner. Acute vasopressin injections also can facilitate partner preference formation in female prairie voles. Testosterone treatments can increase vasopressin synthesis and mating influences vasopressin levels in males (DeVries and Villalba, 1997), offering further support for the hypothesis that endogenous vasopressin plays a role in pair bonding in male prairie voles.

Vasopressin, at least when administered as a chronic infusion, has the added ability to induce mate guarding and territoriality in males; mate guarding in this species is important to maintaining the integrity of pair bonds, since females in estrus (even when apparently pair bonded) sometimes will mate with strangers (Carter et al., 1995). Both male and female prairie voles become aggressive following sexual experience (Getz et al., 1981; Winslow et al., 1993); however, the onset of postcopulatory aggression is less predictable and slower in females. In male prairie voles aggression usually appears within 24 h of the onset of mating, while in females mating is not necessary and defensive aggression to strangers is most reliably induced by a period of a week or more of cohabitation with a male (Bowler and Carter, unpublished data). These and other findings suggest gender differences in the role of peptides in pair bonding in this species (Carter et al., 1995).

Stress and Corticosterone

Stressful experiences facilitate the onset of partner preferences in male prairie voles (DeVries et al., 1996). Male prairie voles formed new pair bonds quickly following either exposure to a stressor (3 min of swimming) or corticosterone injections. Under comparable conditions stressed females did not form new pair bonds with males (DeVries et al., 1995), but did develop preferences for females that were present immediately following exposure to the stressor (DeVries and Carter, unpublished data). Prairie voles are both monogamous and communal. Males have no opportunity to mate within their natal family, and must leave the family to reproduce. For female prairie voles, conditions of environmental stress could produce physiological signals encouraging a return to the security of the family nest; unlike males, females may produce litters within the natal nest (McGuire et al., 1993). Thus stress may encourage the rapid formation of social preferences in both sexes, even when the object of the attachment is not necessarily a member of the opposite sex.

Catecholamines and Pair Bonding

Based on the known functions of the catecholamines, and especially dopamine, it is likely that catecholamines are involved in pair bond formation. Dopamine agonists release oxytocin, and interactions between oxytocin and dopamine are reported in rats (Kovacs et al., 1998; Sarnyai and Kovacs, 1994). In addition, high levels of oxytocin receptor binding have been reported in the nucleus accumbens in prairie voles, but not in montane voles (Insel and Shapiro, 1992). Preliminary studies suggest that inhibitions of dopaminergic activity (acting on the D2 receptor) can interfere with pair bonding in prairie voles (Wang Z, personal communication). Dopamine, acting in the nucleus accumbens, is considered important for a reward system in other species. Interactions between oxytocin and catechol-amines may provide a mechanism for rewarding or reinforcing pair bonding. Catecholamines, including dopamine and norepinephrine, may be necessary to activate or reward various behavioral processes, including arousal and selective attention, and also may regulate the effects of oxytocin and vasopressin in the CNS (Pedersen, 1997).

Separation Distress and Social Buffering

Separation from an attachment figure is associated with various behavioral and physiological changes (Hennessy, 1997; Reite and Field, 1985; Reite and Boccia, 1994). In young animals vocalizations, in either the audible or ultrasonic range, often increase following separation. Measurements of these vocalizations have been used as indices of distress and may be indicative of attachment (Panksepp et al., 1997).

Physiological changes, including increased secretion of glucocorticoids and/or ACTH, cardiovascular measures or immune system parameters, also have been described following social separation in primates (Reite and Boccia, 1994). Cortisol responses have been used to assess the intensity of separation distress and/or to examine the hypothesis that the presence of a partner may provide a form of social buffering (Hennessy, 1997).

Squirrel monkeys are small New World primates that usually live in unisex groups. Behavioral changes in squirrel monkeys do occur following the removal of companions, although these responses may reflect general arousal or physiological adjustments to being alone, rather than the loss of a particular companion. A number of studies have attempted to document physiological consequences following social separation in squirrel monkeys (Hennessy, 1997; Mendoza and Mason, 1997; Mason and Mendoza, 1998). Although basal cortisol levels are very high in squirrel monkeys, procedures associated with capturing one member of a pair can further elevate cortisol levels; however, this response is not affected by the presence or absence of social companions. Thus, although squirrel monkeys appear highly social, physiological measures do not suggest selective pair bonding or stress buffering by companions.

Social separation in both male and female prairie voles is followed by an increase in glucocorticoid (corticosterone) levels (Williams and Carter, unpublished data). When reunited with a partner, corticosterone levels dropped to below baseline in previously paired males and females. However, if previously paired animals and separated animals were placed with an unfamiliar animal of the opposite sex corticosterone levels remained elevated (DeVries et al., 1995). Separation from the mother also induces increased corticosterone levels in infant prairie voles, but not montane voles. Such findings suggest that adult separation responses may be related to those seen in infants.

Experiments on separation distress have tested the capacity of peptides to prevent behavioral changes during separation. The intense calling behavior of isolated domestic chicks declines following various treatments, including injections of oxytocin/vasotocin, opioids that stimulate mu receptors, and prolactin (Panksepp et al., 1997). Opiate injections also diminish distress vocalizations in guinea pigs (Herman and Panksepp, 1987). The separation cries of infant rats did not show the predicted decline following opiate treatments (Winslow and Insel, 1991a). However, in rat pups separation cries were inhibited by central treatments with oxytocin or vasopressin (Insel and Winslow, 1991; Winslow and Insel, 1993). In squirrel monkeys there also is evidence that both vasopressin and oxytocin are capable of reducing isolation calling, although the effects were dependent on social status and high doses of the peptides (1 or 5 µg, ICV) were necessary to obtain behavioral effects (Winslow and Insel, 1991b).

As reviewed throughout this chapter, oxytocin has been implicated in the formation of at-

tachments. In addition, oxytocin is capable of regulating the HPA axis (DeVries et al., 1997; Uvnas-Moberg, 1998). The data described above suggest the hypothesis that reductions or fluctuations in oxytocin activity also might account for some of the symptoms of social separation. Oxytocin is well positioned to influence both the behavioral and autonomic symptoms that follow the loss of an attachment object.

Parental Behavior

Overview

The most accepted form of enduring social bond is maternal attachment. The concept of mother love (Harlow, 1986) implies a selective behavioral response by the parent to its offspring. Because of the intimate relationship between parental responses and attachments, and the conservative nature of hormone and behavior relationships, understanding parental behavior, even in cases when the behaviors are not selectively directed to a particular infant, may provide insights into the physiology of social attachment.

Hormones that regulate birth and lactation are particularly important in caregiver–child attachments (Keverne, 1995; Keverne et al., 1997; Keverne and Kendrick, 1992). Oxytocin and to a lesser extent vasopressin have been implicated in both maternal behavior and maternal attachment. Catecholamines are involved in response to novelty, arousal, selective attention, certain kinds of learning, and may play a role in the development of attachments and/or may reinforce or reward the expression of these attachments. In addition, catecholamines, endogenous opioids and prolactin affect parental behavior, possibly by modulating the rewarding aspects of this behavior (Panksepp, 1981; Panksepp et al., 1994, 1997), or by pacing of mother–infant interactions (Bridges, 1990), or through their documented abilities to influence the release or actions of other peptides, including oxytocin (Keverne et al., 1997; Parker et al., 1991).

Parental Attachment

Selective maternal attachment has been described in sheep and other precocial ungulates, which must follow their mother at birth (Keverne and Kendrick, 1992). In sheep maternal behavior is usually directed only toward the ewe's own lamb and unfamiliar lambs are physically rejected. Vaginal–cervical stimulation and suckling, which release both oxytocin and endogenous opioids, have been implicated in maternal bonding (Keverne et al., 1997). Oxytocin injections can cause ewes to become attached to an unfamiliar lamb presented at the time oxytocin is released or injected. Oxytocin antagonists block filial bonding in sheep. These experiments offer clear evidence that sheep can develop selective social attachments and implicates oxytocin in this form of social bonding.

Maternal Behavior

Maternal behavior shares many behavioral features with attachment. In addition, there is striking concordance between physiological and anatomical substrates of parental behavior and those thus far implicated in filial attachment (Keverne, 1995; Keverne et al., 1997).

Mammalian parental behavior is usually measured by approach and positive caregiving behaviors directed by adult animals to young conspecifics. It has been proposed that maternal behavior is facilitated when the tendency to approach infants is stronger than the tendency to avoid infants. It is further suggested that reproductively naive rats of both sexes have an inherent tendency to avoid potentially aversive novel stimuli, such as those presumably presented by rat pups (Fleming et al., 1980, 1989; Numan, 1994). Hormones associated with birth, or other factors involved in repeated pup exposures, such as habituation to pup odors, are believed to in-

hibit this fear-based system, thus permitting the expression of maternal responses.

Hormones of Pregnancy and Parturition
Both maternal responses and lactation are facilitated by the hormonal events of pregnancy and birth, which include prolonged exposure to comparatively high levels of progesterone and estrogen, a subsequent dramatic prepartum decline in progesterone, and increases in oxytocin and prolactin (Bridges, 1990; Pedersen, 1997; Pedersen and Prange, 1979). However, hypotheses regarding hormonal causes of parental behavior are complicated by the fact that apparently normal parental behavior is observed in virgin females, even after removal of the ovary and uterus, as well as in males of many species (Brown, 1993; Gubernick and Nelson, 1989). Thus, the experiences of pregnancy and birth may facilitate, but are not essential for, parental behavior.

Adrenal Steroids
The role of hormones of the adrenal axis in maternal behavior has received comparatively little attention. However, glucocorticoid levels rise in late pregnancy, and hormones of the HPA axis have been implicated in parturition. In human females, high levels of cortisol on days 2 or 3 postpartum were correlated with positive maternal behaviors and attitudes (Corter and Fleming, 1995; Fleming et al., 1987). Cortisol levels also were correlated with positive responses to odors from infants, suggesting a role for cortisol in sensory processes. Research in rats also provides circumstantial evidence for a role for adrenal steroids in maternal behavior (McCarthy et al., 1992).

Oxytocin
Because oxytocin is a predominantly mammalian hormone with a critical role in both birth and lactation, it was an obvious candidate for involvement in maternal attachment. In fact, over 20 years ago oxytocin was suggested as the hormone of mother love (Klopfer, 1971, 1996; Newton, 1973).

ICV treatment with oxytocin has the capacity to facilitate the onset of maternal responsiveness in virgin females, acting within 30 min or less (Pedersen, 1997; Pedersen and Prange, 1979). In this species, treatment with oxytocin antagonists (OTA) (Pedersen, 1997), antibodies to oxytocin (Fahrbach et al., 1985) or lesions of oxytocin producing neurons (Insel and Harbaugh, 1989) inhibit the induction of maternal behavior. There also is evidence that oxytocin is released in or acts upon brain areas associated with maternal behavior under conditions, such as parturition, when maternal behavior also increases (Keverne and Kendrick, 1992; Kendrick et al., 1988).

Oxytocinergic pathways that originate within the hypothalamus and project to the ventral tegmental area (VTA) are necessary for maternal behavior (Numan and Sheehan, 1997; Pedersen, 1997). Mesolimbic dopaminergic projections originating in the VTA also facilitate maternal behavior. Pedersen (1997) speculates that interactions between oxytocin and dopamine contribute to the positive effects of oxytocin on maternal behavior and serve to reinforce this behavior. Oxytocin also may modulate the release of norepinephrine, which in turn could potentiate or reinforce maternal behavior.

In rats, oxytocin also has been shown to have anxiolytic and anti-nociceptive effects (Uvnas-Moberg, 1997); these properties of oxytocin may indirectly facilitate maternal behavior by increasing tolerance for pups. These and other studies (Numan, 1994; Pedersen, 1997; Uvnas-Moberg, 1997) suggest a critical role for endogenously produced oxytocin in maternal behavior in rats.

Research on maternal behavior in rats indirectly implicates corticosterone in the behavioral effects of oxytocin. For example, in one study oxytocin injections were only effective in females that were tested ≈ 2 h after being placed in a novel environment. Oxytocin treatments given immediately upon introduction to a novel setting and those given after a 24 h habituation period did not significantly facilitate maternal behavior (Fahrbach et al., 1985). In addition, the original

studies of the behavioral effects of ICV oxytocin in rats were done in animals that were later shown to have a respiratory infection; oxytocin was less effective in healthy animals (Pedersen and Prange, 1979; Pedersen et al., 1992), possibly in part because the healthier animals did not experience elevated corticosterone. Alternatively, it was suggested that the animals with respiratory infections may have been anosmic, and thus less fearful of pups. Studies by Wamboldt and Insel (1987) showed that either removal of the olfactory bulbs or anosmia induced by peripheral treatments with zinc sulfate made animals more responsive to oxytocin treatments. This study was interpreted as evidence for a role for olfactory-based neophobia in maternal behavior. However, treatments that created anosmia, including surgery or zinc sulfate infusions of the olfactory mucosa, were presumably stressful and also may have been associated with elevated glucocorticoid production. In rats, glucocorticoid receptors are present on a subset of oxytocin neurons (Jirikowski et al., 1993). Thus, it is possible that elevated adrenal hormones potentiate the behavioral effects of oxytocin in rats, possibly by increasing oxytocin receptor binding (Liberzon and Young, 1997; Liberzon et al., 1994). The effects of oxytocin also might act in conjunction with anosmia to facilitate maternal behavior. Increased oxytocinergic activity or anosmia, in turn, might reduce neophobia or anxiety (Uvnas-Moberg, 1997), thus permitting the expression of maternal behavior.

In what was apparently the first experiment aimed at studying the effects of oxytocin on primate maternal behavior, two nulliparous female rhesus monkeys received ICV injections of oxytocin or saline. Oxytocin treatment was followed by an increase in the frequency of touching, watching or lip-smacking that was directed toward infants, and a decrease in agonistic yawns and facial threats directed toward the observers (Holman and Goy, 1995). These findings, although preliminary, are consistent with research from other mammals, and offer support for the hypothesis that oxytocin is capable of facilitating primate social behaviors.

Indirect evidence implicates oxytocin in human maternal behavior. Oxytocin production during breast-feeding is correlated with personality traits and behaviors generally associated with parental behavior. For example, basal levels of oxytocin are positively related to calmness, while pulsatile patterns of oxytocin production are associated with a desire to please, give and interact socially (Uvnas-Moberg et al., 1990). In one study of Swedish women, those who had acute caesarean sections had fewer oxytocin pulses during the postpartum period and also were less likely than vaginally-delivered women to describe themselves as exhibiting a calm personality and high levels of sociality (Nissen et al., 1996). This correlational study does not distinguish cause and effect, since it is possible that calm women were less likely to require caesarean sections and/or that oxytocin pulses induced calmness or increased sociality; either case could implicate oxytocin since insufficient endogenous production of oxytocin may be associated with a need for caesarean sections. In a more experimental study, women were encouraged to place their infants to the breast immediately following birth; women whose infants made early contact with the breast, subsequently spent more time with their babies and talked more to their infants than women who did not experience this form of contact (Widstrom et al., 1990). These, and other correlational studies in humans by Uvnas-Moberg (1997, 1998), support the hypothesis that oxytocin released during labor and lactation may influence human maternal responsivity and perhaps attachment. Direct or experimental tests of this hypothesis in humans are not available.

Vasopressin

ICV vasopressin also can facilitate maternal behavior, but acts more slowly than oxytocin requiring more than 1 h to significantly affect behavior (Pedersen and Prange, 1979). Because direct effects of peptides on behavior are often rapid, the comparatively slow actions of vasopressin in the induction of maternal behavior could suggest that the observed effects are mediated by intermediary processes. Injections of a selective vasopressin receptor (V1a) antagonist can inhibit maternal behavior (Pedersen, 1997). Vasopressin-deficient Brattleboro rats show lower levels of parental care (Wideman and Murphy, 1990). In addition, vasopressinergic activity increases in the hypothalamus in late pregnancy (Caldwell et al., 1987; Landgraf et al., 1991). In monogamous prairie voles central vasopressin content in males, but not females, is elevated following mating and under conditions when male parental behavior is particularly likely (Bamshad et al., 1993, 1994; DeVries and Villalba, 1997).

Sexual Behavior

Sexual behavior and attachment are related, but not synonymous concepts. Sexual activity can occur in the absence of social attachment and many forms of attachment do not involve sexual behavior. In humans the most desired sexual partner often is the object of strong feelings of attachment, but exceptions may exist to this pattern.

In monogamous mammals, pair bonds provide a social matrix for sexual behavior. Mating also promotes social preferences (Williams et al., 1992), possibly because oxytocin and/or vasopressin are released during sexual interactions (Carter, 1992). Males and females tend to show intrasexual aggression which may serve as mate guarding (Insel et al., 1995; Winslow et al., 1993). In addition, established pairs often show mating preferences for familiar partners. But even in socially monogamous or pair bonding mammals, such as prairie voles, absolute sexual exclusivity is rare and both sexes may engage in extra-pair copulations (Carter et al., 1995).

Although the expression of sexual behavior and attachment are not identical, these behaviors do share several features, possibly because they share common neuroendocrine substrates. Sex steroids have been implicated in sexual behavior in a variety of mammalian species, permitting mating and fertilization to be coordinated with gonadal functions (Meisel and Sachs, 1994; Pfaff et al., 1994). Thus, although research on the endocrinology of sexual behavior has been focused on the effects of gonadal steroids, it is becoming evident that the strength of the relationship between gonadal steroids and reproductive behaviors varies within and among species. Interactions between the HPA and HPG axes may allow reproduction to be adapted to environmental demands. Steroid hormones alone are not adequate to explain many aspects of sexual behavior. Peptide hormones, including oxytocin and vasopressin, which are regulated in part by steroid hormones, may provide mechanisms for coordinating the appearance of sexual behavior with the demands of the social and physical environment (Carter, 1992).

Mechanisms through which Peptides and Steroids May Influence Attachment

Ontogenetic Influences on Attachment

Steroid exposures during development have the capacity to produce both structural and behavioral changes (Gorski, 1990), including changes that may alter the propensity for social behavior. For example, in prairie voles prenatal steroid treatments (either testosterone or corticosterone) are associated with an increased preference for familiar versus unfamiliar partners, while postnatal treatments with these same hormones were associated with a preference for strangers (Roberts et al., 1996). Prenatal stressors or treatments with stress hormones also can affect adult patterns of social and sexual behaviors in rats (Ward and Ward, 1986) and guinea pigs (Sachser and Kaiser, 1996). Thus social preferences, upon which attachments are formed, can be develop-

mentally altered by stress and/or steroid hormones (Table 56.2).

Dramatic changes in both peptides and peptide receptor binding can be detected in the immediate postnatal period (Al-Shamma and DeVries, 1996; Tribollet et al., 1991; Wang et al., 1997). Both steroid and peptide hormones are capable of altering gene expression for peptide receptors. Thus, peptidergic systems, including oxytocin and vasopressin, can be affected by the developmental history of an organism. Peptide treatments either in development (Boer, 1993; Boer et al., 1994; Meyerson et al., 1988; Swabb and Boer, 1994) or in adulthood (Poulain and Pittman, 1993) may alter the sensitivity of the nervous system to subsequent hormonal experiences. For example, in rat treatment with vasopressin during the first week of life is capable of reducing gene expression for the oxytocin receptor in the PVN during adulthood (Ostrowski, 1998; Vaccari et al., 1996). Since vasopressin is part of the HPA axis and is sensitive to androgens, this finding suggests that developmental changes associated with perinatal stress or gender-dependent androgenization could alter the subsequent sensitivity of the oxytocinergic system.

We have begun to examine more directly the hypothesis that peptides have a developmental role in social attachment (Stribley and Carter, 1998). Males, and to a much lesser extent females, that were exposed to vasopressin injections during the 1st week of life were as adults more aggressive toward intruders than were untreated animals. However, animals that were treated with either vasopressin or a vasopressin antagonist continued to show the capacity in adulthood to develop a preference for a familiar partner. Thus, the mate guarding component of monogamy, but apparently not the tendency to form social attachments, was sensitive to vasopressin during development.

In adult rats, exposure to either vasopressin or oxytocin sensitizes animals to respond behaviorally to subsequent treatments with previously ineffective doses of vasopressin (Poulain and Pittman, 1993). Steroid-peptide or peptide-peptide interactions may have long term consequences for the development of neural systems that predispose a given species (Insel, 1997) or individual within a species to form social attachments.

Sex Differences in Attachment

Although changes in gonadal hormones during adulthood have not yet been strongly implicated in adult attachment formation, the substrates for social interactions generally seem to have sexually dimorphic components.

Vasopressin content is strongly determined by androgens, although the vasopressin receptors may not be sexually dimorphic. Thus, it is likely that at least some sexually dimorphic behaviors, including aggression, are determined by the availability of vasopressin (DeVries and Villalba, 1997; Wang, 1995).

In contrast, at least in rats, the effects of oxytocin on reproductive behaviors may be influenced by sex steroids, including ovarian hormones (Caldwell, 1992; Schumacher et al., 1990). Thus, for female rats the behavioral effects of oxytocin may vary according to the estrous condition of the female. Male rats also are capable of high levels of oxytocin binding and like females respond to estrogen with increased levels of oxytocin binding in the hypothalamus; testosterone also increases oxytocin binding in male rats and is more effective than estrogen in this regard (Johnson, 1992). These somewhat unexpected findings, although done in a species that does not show pair bonds, do not suggest that sexual dimorphism in oxytocin binding is likely to explain gender differences in social behavior or social attachment.

Male and female prairie voles differ in the stimuli to which they direct social preferences (DeVries et al., 1997). Pair bonds also form more quickly and last slightly longer following separation in female versus male prairie voles. In addition, in prairie voles stressful experiences have

different effects on heterosexual pair bond formation in males and females (DeVries et al., 1995, 1996). In this species, oxytocin and vasopressin treatments have regionally specific effects on neuronal activation, as indexed by cFOS expression (Gingrich et al., 1997). Treatment with oxytocin increased cFOS expression in the BNST, while vasopressin treatment was associated with increased activity in the nucleus accumbens. In prairie voles sex differences in the response to peptides also were seen in the gender-specific activational effects of vasopressin on postcopulatory aggression (Winslow et al., 1993) and exploratory behavior (Dharmadhikari et al., 1997). In male, but not female, prairie voles vasopressin injections were associated with increased cFOS in the central amygdala (CAMY) (Gingrich et al., 1997). In turn, the vasopressinergic effects on the CAMY can regulate autonomic functions at least in rats (Roozendaal et al., 1993) providing a potentially sexually dimorphic substrate for social engagement.

Species Variations in Peptide Receptors

The expression of attachment behaviors varies widely among species, and the mechanisms responsible for these behaviors also must have species-specific components. Peptide hormones, including oxytocin and vasopressin, with species-typical patterns of peptide production, receptor distributions and functions (Insel and Shapiro, 1992; Insel et al., 1997; Wang, 1995; Wang et al., 1996, 1997; Witt et al., 1991; Young et al., 1996), are particularly well positioned to influence behaviors, such as pair bonding, that vary among different species (Carter et al., 1995, 1997).

Both general patterns of oxytocin receptor expression and binding and receptor responses to steroids differ among species (Insel and Shapiro, 1992; Insel et al., 1994; Insel et al., 1997; Tribollet et al., 1992; Witt, 1997; Young et al., 1996). For example, estrogen increases oxytocin binding within the VMH in rats, but not in prairie voles (Witt et al., 1991).

Species differences in peptide receptor activity are presumably an important source of interspecific variation in the behavioral effects of oxytocin and vasopressin. Species-typical variations in peptide receptors are apparent in early development. For example, vasopressin receptor binding increased rapidly in the 2nd week of life in the LS of nonmonogamous montane voles, but not prairie voles (Wang et al., 1997). Insel et al. (1997) and Young et al. (1996) have compared the genes for oxytocin receptors in prairie voles and montane voles, and found that these receptors are virtually identical in genetic structure. However, promoter elements can regulate the expression of these receptor genes in particular tissues; subtle, but potentially important species differences in base sequences may be responsible for the interspecific variations in peptide receptor distributions. Based on rodent work, especially in voles, Wang et al. (1996) suggest that neuroendocrine systems may evolve by changes in receptor distribution rather than by restructuring the presynaptic pathway. Comparisons among related vole species with very different patterns of social behavior offer insights into the role of peptides and their receptors in species-typical social behaviors (Insel, 1997).

Ontogenetic experiences, including levels of perinatal stress and varying amounts of parent-young interaction could contribute to the development of species-typical patterns of social behavior. An example of the consequences of perinatal exposure to stress hormones again comes from work with prairie voles; in this species corticosterone treatments during the perinatal period altered both social and reproductive behaviors. In female prairie voles postnatal treatments with corticosterone were associated with an increased preference for unfamiliar partners versus siblings, lower levels of alloparenting, and increased masculinization of sexual behavior (indexed by mounting behavior in females). Stressful experiences, including the absence of the father, also inhibit alloparenting in female prairie voles from a population captured in Illi-

nois (Roberts et al., 1997, 1998). However, even within prairie voles, intraspecific population differences exist in social behaviors, including juvenile alloparental behavior and other indices of communal breeding. Prairie voles reared from populations captured in Illinois are both monogamous and communal, while those from populations captured in Kansas show some features of monogamy, but are not communal (Roberts et al., 1998). When prairie voles were reared with both parents present, alloparental behavior was much more common in Illinois versus Kansas animals; this behavioral difference in alloparenting disappeared when animals were reared only by their mothers. Animals from both populations formed pair bonds, although voles from the Illinois population were slightly more tolerant of unfamiliar animals than were Kansas voles.

Intraspecific variation provides a model for the analysis of factors that can contribute to sociality, and more specifically to social attachment. In both cases, differences based on developmental experiences would be expressed within genetic constraints. Behavioral flexibility, such as that seen in prairie voles, and possibly mediated by peptide–steroid interactions during development, allows animals to individually adapt their social systems to accommodate early experiences and environmental demands.

Species Variation in Adrenal Corticoids

Species differences in the tendency to form social bonds also may be related to variations in HPA axis activity. For example, prairie voles have serum levels of adrenal corticoids that are 5–10× those found in nonmonogamous montane voles (Carter et al., 1995; Taymans et al., 1997). Marmosets and tamarins, which form pair bonds, also have exceptionally high levels of adrenal corticoids (Chrousos et al., 1982). Squirrel monkeys also have elevated basal corticosteroids (Hennessy, 1997; Mendoza and Mason, 1997); although squirrel monkeys do not form heterosexual pair bonds, they do form cohesive same-sex social groups. Guinea pigs can secrete very high levels of adrenal corticoids under stress, and, although not considered monogamous, also are capable of developing social attachments. In fact in male guinea pigs, death, possibly mediated by changes in the ANS, has been observed when social stress is followed by subsequent isolation from a specific social partner (Sachser and Lick, 1989, 1991; Sachser et al., 1998).

Not all pair bonding species have exceptional levels of adrenal corticoids. For example, monogamous titi monkeys do not seem to fit this pattern (Mendoza and Mason, 1997; Mason and Mendoza, 1998). However, in many cases exceptionally high levels of activity in the HPA axis, measured as increased glucocorticoid secretion, are associated with or precede well-defined patterns of social attachment. Correlations between HPA axis activity and attachment offer support for a role for hormones of the HPA axis, and specifically the glucocorticoids in the events which eventually lead to pair bonding (Fig. 56.2).

Steroid–Peptide Interactions

Steroid Effects on Peptide Production

Oxytocin synthesis and release are sensitive to gonadal steroids, including estrogens and androgens (Caldwell, 1992; Rhodes et al., 1981). For example, an estrogen-sensitive promotor has been identified on the oxytocin gene (Zingg et al., 1995). Treatment with a regimen of ovarian steroids that approximates the hormonal profile during late pregnancy and near the time of parturition (chronic estrogen and progesterone followed by progesterone withdrawal) increases oxytocin gene expression in rats (Crowley et al., 1995). Glucocorticoid levels also are high in late pregnancy and may decline at delivery. Progesterone and the glucocorticoids have similar chemical structures and share many physiological and behavioral properties, and in some cases have similar affects on peptide binding (Patchev et al., 1993); these steroids could act separately or in concert to influence behavior.

Vasopressin synthesis, especially within the MAMY and BNST, is increased by androgens, producing a sexually dimorphic distribution of vasopressin, especially in neural processes that project to the LS (DeVries and Villalba, 1997; Wang, 1995; Wang and DeVries, 1994; Wang et al., 1994). Vasopressin content, detected by immunocytochemistry, declines slowly after castration, with a time course that resembles the postcastrational loss of sexual interest in male rats. In many cases the effects of androgen require aromatization to estrogen, and it is often difficult to determine the relative contributions of estrogens and androgens.

Steroid Effects on Peptide Receptors

Steroid hormones can influence oxytocin receptor binding in the CNS, particularly in the olfactory–limbic–hypothalamic axis, which has been implicated in social and sexual behaviors (Johnson, 1992). For example, there is recent evidence that progesterone is capable of binding to the rat oxytocin receptor on membranes and thus inhibiting the functions of the oxytocin receptor (Grazzini et al., 1998). This effect was highly specific and not observed following treatment with estrogen or the synthetic glucocorticoid, dexamethasone. In addition, this effect was species specific, since human oxytocin receptors, expressed in a cell line, were inhibited by a progesterone metabolite (5 beta-dihydroprogesterone), but not by progesterone itself.

The concurrent presence of multiple steroid and peptide receptors in a given neural system, or even within the same cell, offers mechanisms through which steroid hormones may regulate peptidergic functions (Axelson and Van Leeuwen, 1990; DeVries and Villalba, 1997; Jirikowski et al., 1993). In rats, gonadal and/or adrenal steroids also can cause an increase in hippocampus (Liberzon et al., 1994; Liberzon and Young, 1997), and in some, but not all areas of the hypothalamus (Patchev et al., 1993). For example, pretreatment with a synthetic glucocorticoid (dexamethasone) increased oxytocin

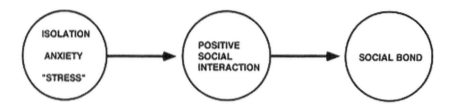

BEHAVIORAL OR EMOTIONAL RESPONSE

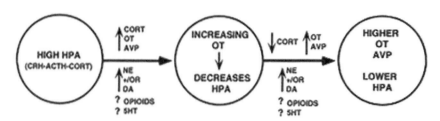

NEUROENDOCRINE MODULATION

Figure 56.2
Behavioral, emotional and neuroendocrine correlates of social attachment. HPA, hypothalamic–pituitary–adrenal axis; CRH, corticotropin-releasing hormone; ACTH, adrenocorticotropic hormone; CORT, glucocorticoids including corticosterone and cortisol; OT, oxytocin; AVP, arginine vasopressin; opioids, endogenous opioids; 5HT, serotonin.

receptor ligand binding in the BNST, LS and AMY, but decreased binding in the ventromedial hypothalamus. Site-specific modulation of peptide binding by specific steroid hormones or combinations of steroid hormones could account for at least some of the regulatory effects of steroids or stress on maternal and sexual behavior.

Steroid Effects on the Production of Co-localized Peptides

Oxytocin and vasopressin are commonly co-localized with other peptides. For example, in rats corticotropin releasing hormone (CRH), cholecystokinin (CCK) and dynorphin have been observed in magnocellular oxytocinergic neu-

rons, while angiotensin II, galanin and dynorphin are found in vasopressinergic neurons (Levin and Sawchenko, 1993; Meister et al., 1990). The production of these additional peptides is steroid-dependent and provides a mechanism through which steroids may modulate the functions of oxytocin and vasopressin.

Behavior as an Intermediary in Steroid–Peptide Interactions

Steroid hormones also may act on behavioral systems which in turn regulate the release of neuropeptides. For example, estrogen increases female sexual behavior (Pfaff et al., 1994), while androgens, in some cases converted to estrogen, increase male sexual behavior (Meisel and Sachs, 1994). Sexual behavior, in turn, can release oxytocin and vasopressin (Carter, 1992; Kendrick and Keverne, 1989). Nonsexual social contact and other forms of somatosensory stimulation also are capable of releasing oxytocin and other peptides (Uvnas-Moberg, 1994, 1997, 1998), providing a possible mechanism for the formation of social attachments, such as those that accompany nonsexual cohabitation (Williams et al., 1994).

Peptide–Peptide Interaction

Oxytocin and Vasopressin

Behavioral studies indicate that some behavioral effects of oxytocin and vasopressin are similar, while in other cases these peptides are functionally antagonistic (Bohus et al., 1978; De Wied et al., 1991, 1993; Engelmann et al., 1996; Pedersen et al., 1992). For example in rats, passive avoidance (De Wied et al., 1991), and locomotor and autonomic functions (Roozendaal et al., 1993) have indicated that oxytocin and vasopressin can have either similar or apparently opposite effects.

Research on vasopressin has concentrated on the assumption that behavioral effects of this peptide are due to actions at receptors of the V1a type, while work with oxytocin has assumed that the functions of this peptide were due to effects at the oxytocin receptor. However, because oxytocin and vasopressin are similar in structure, with the exception of two amino acids, these peptides have the potential for agonistic or antagonistic interactions with each other's receptors (Carter and Altemus, 1997; Carter et al., 1995). In addition, gene expression for the V1b receptor recently has been measured in CNS areas that contain V1a and oxytocin receptors, opening the possibility for dynamic interactions with the V1b receptor (Barberis and Tribollet, 1996; Ostrowski, 1998)

De Wied et al. (1991, 1993) have suggested that an additional receptor system, beyond the well-characterized V1a and oxytocin receptors, exists and that this receptor is capable of recognizing both peptides. For example, the role of the V1b receptor in behavior remains poorly defined. Alternatively, oxytocin and vasopressin may serve as ligands for each other's receptors. Evidence from tissue culture supports this hypothesis, and also indicates that vasopressin has a strong affinity for oxytocin receptors (Barberis and Tribollet, 1996). In some cases the receptors for oxytocin and vasopressin are in different tissues, providing mechanisms through which specific functions could be regulated by either different peptides or different concentrations of a particular peptide. In addition, site-specific effects of steroids on peptide binding could specify the differential functions of vasopressin and oxytocin. Different cells of origin and patterns of endogenous release, such as more dramatic pulses in oxytocin versus vasopressin, could affect these systems. In addition, although the full peptide molecule is usually considered necessary for the physiological functions of vasopressin and oxytocin, smaller portions or fragments of these peptides can have behavioral functions, allowing further mechanisms for cellular specification of functions (De Wied et al., 1993).

Recent research from our laboratory suggests that while either oxytocin or vasopressin is sufficient to increase social contact, both oxytocin and vasopressin are necessary to facilitate partner preference formation in prairie voles (Cho et al., in press). In this study males or females were allowed to cohabit for one h with a stimulus animal of the opposite sex and then tested for preferences for the familiar (cohabitating) partner or an otherwise comparable stranger. Using this paradigm, large doses of 100 ng (ICV) of oxytocin and vasopressin produced high levels of social contact and strong partner preferences in both male and female prairie voles. Earlier studies, using chronic treatments (osmotic minipumps) and longer periods of cohabitation had suggested that partner preference development in female prairie voles was more sensitive to oxytocin (Insel and Hulihan, 1995; Williams et al., 1994), while males responded more readily to vasopressin (Winslow et al., 1993). The methodologies in the two studies have not been compared directly. Whether the effects of oxytocin and vasopressin on pair bonding in prairie voles are due to effects on different or common receptors remains to be determined (see below).

Peptides and the Autonomic Nervous System

Hormones act on the ANS to integrate attention, emotional states and social communication, with other physiological and environmental demands. The ANS is essential for social attachment and love and also contains receptors for oxytocin and vasopressin. The various subcomponents of the ANS suggest sites at which peptides such as oxytocin and vasopressin could act to regulate these behaviors.

The polyvagal theory of Porges (1995, 1997) differentiates between a phylogenetically more modern smart vagal system, which is unique to mammals, and a more primitive vegetative vagal system, found throughout the vertebrates. According to this theory, the smart and vegetative vagal systems and, in addition, the sympathetic nervous system must interact to regulate social engagement and reproductive behaviors. The smart vagus plays a role in social engagement and the appetitive components of behavior. The source nuclei of the smart vagus, the nucleus ambiguus, contain receptors for both oxytocin and vasopressin. In contrast, the phylogenetically older vegetative vagus may regulate consummatory behaviors, such as lordosis. The source nuclei for the vegetative vagus, the dorsal motor nucleus of the vagus, contains primarily oxytocin receptors. The polyvagal theory predicts that although oxytocin and vasopressin might be acting on different target tissues, both could influence emotional systems involved in autonomic functions and social attachment.

Sensory feedback to the CNS from the visceral organs travels through vagal afferents to the nucleus tractus solitarius, providing a mechanism through which oxytocin may influence visceral experiences and bodily states. Vasopressin from the PVN also communicates with the sensory part of the dorsal vagal complex. The influence of oxytocin and/or vasopressin on visceral states could influence feedback from peripheral tissues to the brain via vagal afferents. A perceived change in visceral state would result which could affect the probability that social interactions or attachments would occur.

Thus, the ANS is an important site for peptidergic effects on emotional behavior. Because functions of the brain stem and the ANS are fundamental to virtually all other behavioral states, understanding the effects of peptides on this system may be especially critical to our understanding of physiological influences on attachment. Many components of human behavior, such as motor patterns involved in sexual behavior or parenting are regulated, at least in part, by cognitive processes. However, the decision to engage in a given behavior and various mood states are strongly determined by visceral processes or autonomic states, which may in turn motivate the occurrence of specific behaviors. Peptides, including oxytocin and vasopressin, regulate these visceral state or emotional feelings.

Vasopressin also is a component of the sympathoadrenal axis, capable in rats of increasing the secretion of ACTH and thus glucocorticoids (Whitnall, 1993). Central vasopressin allows increased activity in the sympathetic nervous system and also is associated with the functions of the smart vagus, including behavioral mobilization and social communication and engagement. Centrally-active vasopressin also can raise the set-point of vagal reflexes facilitating sympathetic activity (Porges, 1997). These vasopressinergic-vagal functions might facilitate social engagement and attachment particularly under conditions of stress or states of visceral arousal.

Oxytocin has been associated with stress-reduction. In humans (Carter and Altemus, 1997; Chiodera et al., 1991; Uvnas-Moberg, 1997, 1998) and in prairie voles (DeVries et al., 1997) oxytocin, but not vasopressin, treatments inhibit sympathoadrenal activity, including the release of adrenal corticoids. The effects of oxytocin on pair bonding or other forms of social attachment may be related to the autonomic role of oxytocin in stress reduction.

A Working Model for the Role of Steroids and Neuropeptides in Social Attachment

Behavioral-emotional Models of Attachment

Stressful experiences (such as pregnancy and parturition), anxiety, neophobia and isolation often precede the formation of social attachments (Figs. 56.1 and 56.2). These circumstances may increase social drive or motivation and subsequent social interactions. Positive social interactions in turn could be rewarding and in species or individuals that possess the capacity to form attachment, positive social bonds would follow. Both positive social interactions and social bonds could function to provide a sense of safety and reduce anxiety or stress.

In contrast, if social interactions were negative, fear or anxiety might increase. Depending on the gender, species, history of the individual, intensity of the experience, and so forth, negative or traumatic social interactions could feed back to heighten fear or anxiety and prevent the formation of social attachments. However, under certain conditions traumatic events may result in strong social attachments. In some cases, trauma bonds might be formed even in the absence of a concurrent reduction in anxiety or fear.

Neuroendocrine Correlates of Attachment

Traits

The propensity to form attachments is a species-typical trait. Based on somewhat limited mam-malian data, it appears that social bonding is particularly common in species, including monogamous or highly social mammals, that are glucocorticoid-insensitive and thus capable of producing exceptionally high serum levels of glucocorticoids. At present the best known animal models of glucocorticoid-insensitivity are New World primates or rodents, many of which, such as prairie voles or marmosets, also are capable of developing social attachments.

States

Attachment formation and other forms of social behavior also are state-dependent. For example, maternal–infant attachment usually follows the extreme physiological challenges associated with pregnancy and parturition. Metabolically demanding behaviors, such as sexual activity or exercise, may precede attachment formation. In addition, both glucocorticoids and oxytocin can be anxiolytic in rats (Uvnas-Moberg, 1998). High levels of steroids, opioids, oxytocin and/or vasopressin may induce a physiological process or social motivation that increases the probability of social interactions. Our research with prairie voles indicates that either oxytocin or vasopressin can increase social contact, while it appears that both peptides may be needed to allow social bonding (Cho et al., in press). In addition, serotonin or catecholamines, possibly through effects on arousal or attention, could facilitate social interactions (Fig. 56.2).

It has recently been shown in rats that oxytocin is capable of facilitating conditioned place preferences (Liberzon et al., 1997). In addition, oxytocin is capable of reinforcing the tendency of young rats to develop a preference for maternal odors (Nelson and Panksepp, 1996). The mechanisms underlying these effects may be shared with those responsible for the development of selective social behaviors in monogamous rodents.

Positive social interactions are associated with an increase in oxytocin and a state-dependent decline in HPA axis activity. Oxytocin is capable of facilitating both social contact and social attachment, at least in prairie voles. In addition, positive social behaviors, perhaps mediated in part through oxytocin or vasopressin, may feed back to inhibit HPA axis activity and reduce sensations of anxiety or fear.

Social interactions, if negative, might cause an increase in HPA axis activity or prevent the subsequent decline in glucocorticoids that can follow positive social interactions. Intensely negative interactions or threatening experiences might reduce the probability of subsequent attachment formation or result in an avoidance of individuals associated with the negative situation. Alternatively, attachments may form in the presence of traumatic experiences. Whether such trauma bonds are due to neuroendocrine changes that are similar to those described for positive social attachments or rely on different processes, for example related to the release of exceptionally high levels of CRH, vasopressin or catecholamines, remains to be determined.

Gender and Social Attachment
Males and females often show different patterns of social behavior and especially social bonding. Females may develop social bonds more quickly than males, while pair bonding in males is more likely to include an aggressive component. In most mammals females are more likely than males to have higher basal levels of HPA axis activity and glucocorticoids. In one species, the golden hamster, in which males have higher levels of cortisol, females are notably more asocial than males. Female golden hamsters become very aggressive after mating (Carter and Schein, 1971), sometimes leading to the death of the male partner, rather than the formation of social bonds.

Research with prairie voles suggests that the neuroendocrinology of social attachments is sexually dimorphic, with males more likely than females to form heterosexual pair bonds in the presence of a stressful experience or high levels of HPA activity. In male prairie voles the in-

duction of aggression toward strangers, which accompanies mating and pair bonding, seems to be particularly sensitive to vasopressin. The fact that vasopressin synthesis, especially in the limbic system, is androgen-dependent makes vasopressin a particularly likely candidate for social processes that are sexually dimorphic. Thus, species-typical, gender differences may be expected in parameters of this model.

Hypotheses
Steroid–peptide interactions, involving hormones of the HPA axis, and vasopressin and oxytocin, provide neuroendocrine substrates for species-typical social behaviors and emotions. Other peptides or neurotransmitters, including for example, endogenous opioids and monoamines, may regulate social attachment by modulating the central release or effects of oxytocin and vasopressin, as well as the functions of the HPA axis. In addition, opioids and monoamines could modulate social interactions and attachment by influencing arousal, attention, motivation and reward. Several components of this system can be modified by gonadal hormones and may be sexually dimorphic.

Unexplored Research Questions

The Nature of Social Attachment

Awareness that social attachment could have physiological substrates is recent, and there are far more questions than answers. For example, is attachment one process or many? Do attachments that form slowly, during long-term associations, including lactation or nonsexual cohabitation, have the same physiology as those that form quickly, for example during an acute experience, such as birth or sexual interactions? Are the mechanisms involved in the formation of a social attachment also responsible for the maintenance of the attachment? How are the physiological changes associated with social separation or social distress related to social attachment? Do social attachments formed at different ages or in different species depend on comparable or different mechanisms? Is attachment based on the same neuroendocrine substrates that regulate maternal behavior? Are the appetitive or motivational components of attachment similar to the consummatory components? Do the factors that regulate the formation of maternal attachment or pair bonds also regulate the response to the absence of a parent or partner?

Learning and Attachment

Does social attachment represent a novel class of learning, perhaps related to imprinting or other forms of prepared learning? Do processes underlying conditioned emotional responses, such as those associated with fear or avoidance, share neural substrates with social attachment?

Species Differences in the Propensity to Attachment

What are the mechanisms that allow some species to form selective social attachments, while other related species do not? Do observed species differences in steroid hormones, peptide concentrations and/or receptors account for these differences?

Peptides

With regard to attachment formation, do oxytocin and vasopressin have a similar mechanism of action? Do these peptides work on common tissues or do they have different sites of action? Do different peptide experiences convey different behavioral messages? For example, would acute exposure to oxytocin promote a search for social contact, while chronic exposure might signal social satiety or safety and reduce social motivation? Similarly, do peripherally-active versus centrally-active peptides have comparable effects? How do various peptides, including the endoge-

nous opiates, oxytocin and vasopressin, interact with each other to influence attachment behaviors? What is the role of other hormones, peptides or neurotransmitters, for example CRH, dopamine, norepinephrine, serotonin, CCK, dynorphin, and so forth, in the regulation of these behaviors?

Steroids

What is the role of steroid hormones in the regulation of peptidergic effects on social attachment? How do various steroids including estrogen, testosterone, progesterone and corticosterone affect this system and how do they interact with each other? Are steroid hormones from the adrenal cortex particularly important in specifying the occurrence of social bonds? Are the behavioral consequences for social attachment of acute and chronic stress different?

Methodological Issues and the Study of Hormonal Correlates of Human Attachment

Although animal research supports the hypothesis that oxytocin and vasopressin may influence social attachment, very little human research directly addresses this issue. Because neurohypophyseal hormones do not readily pass the blood–brain barrier, it is generally assumed that oxytocin and vasopressin released from the posterior pituitary gland cannot easily return to the brain. Animal research, however, suggests that oxytocin and vasopressin can affect behavior through actions both within the CNS and in the periphery. To study the CNS effects of oxytocin and vasopressin the hormones must be given in relatively high doses, with potential peripheral side effects, or the peptides must be administered directly into the CNS; even in animal research this presents technical problems for behavioral studies. Intranasal preparations of oxytocin and vasopressin agonists are available and have been used in some behavioral studies, but the effectiveness of these treatments in reaching CNS peptide receptors is uncertain. At present effective, selective agonists or antagonists, that easily pass the blood–brain barrier, have not been used in behavioral studies. Blood levels of peptide hormones do not necessarily reflect central activity, and although peptides can be measured in cerebral-spinal fluid, the relevance of such studies to dynamic behaviors is limited. In addition, peptide hormone assays are technically difficult. Thus, direct knowledge of the behavioral effects of oxytocin and vasopressin has been difficult to obtain.

Clinical Implications of a Peptidergic Theory of Social Attachment

The presence or absence of attachments has broad consequences across the life span. Like other mammals, humans rely on positive social interactions for both safety and reproduction. It has been argued that the tendency to form pair bonds or social attachments is a universal human characteristic (Fisher, 1992; Hazan and Shaver, 1987). Social support has documented health benefits, and the absence of positive social interactions or social bonds typically is associated with both physical and mental illness (Amini et al., 1996; House et al., 1988; Klaus et al., 1995; Knox and Uvnas-Moberg, 1998; Reite and Boccia, 1994; Ryff and Singer, 1998; Sperling and Berman, 1994).

Forced social separations or the absence of social attachments can trigger stress, anxiety, fear and even depression. The behaviors and physiological changes associated with bereavement or grief are similar to those used to define depression (Reite and Boccia, 1994). Understanding the nature of physiological processes that regulate social attachment also could be of value in the treatment or prevention of disorders, such as depression or schizophrenia, which can involve dysfunctional social attachment (Kirkpatrick, 1997).

In primate (including human) infants the absence of adequate maternal care has been associated with growth retardation, social withdrawal, inadequate interpersonal relatedness and inhibited verbal communication (Harlow, 1986). This complex of symptoms has even been recognized in human development as a medical syndrome, termed Reactive Attachment Disorder of Infancy (Shaffer and Campbell, 1994). Although the concept of attachment disorder has begun to generate treatment strategies, the relationship between this disorder and normal human attachment remains to be described.

It has been proposed that autism, which can be characterized by atypical social behavior and a failure to form social attachments, may involve abnormal activity in endogenous peptidergic systems. For example, a variety of clinical studies have implicated opioids in autism (Bouvard et al., 1995). Treatment with naltrexone produces some clinical benefits and alters biochemical profiles in a subset of autistic children. More recent studies also have begun to explore the role of oxytocin in autism (Insel, 1997). Studies in autistic adults suggest that deficits in oxytocin may be correlated with some symptoms of autism (Modahl et al., 1998) and there is a report that increased gregariousness may follow oxytocin treatments. However, the possible role for either oxytocin or opioids in selective human social attachments remains unexplored.

Other neurochemicals, such as endogenous opioids, catecholamines and serotonin, also can influence the release and actions of oxytocin and vasopressin. For example, psychoactive drugs, such as Prozac, which affect serotoninergic systems, can influence peptidergic systems (Li et al., 1993). The clinical effects of these chemicals in the context of attachment are largely unknown.

Visceral or Autonomic Sensations and Attachment

The information carried by the ANS is perceived as rather nonspecific or "vague." Emotional feelings have long been associated with visceral sensations, and popular culture abounds with concepts like love sickness, heartaches, and the way to a man's heart is through his stomach. Humans often express confusion regarding the source or meaning of emotional experiences, and the neurobiology of visceral experiences may be related to this perceived uncertainty. Vagal pathways in modern mammals evolved from ancient structures responsible for both oxygenating the brain and for regulating "vegetative" functions of the digestive organs (Porges, 1995, 1997; Uvnas-Moberg, 1994, 1997, 1998). Since it is possible to measure many aspects of autonomic functions in humans, understanding the role of peptides in the ANS offers a promising window to the brain and a better understanding of emotion.

Stress and Attachment

It is well known that social attachments can form during or immediately following the experience of common threat, such as those reported by soldiers in war (Milgram, 1986). Attachments also can develop toward abusive or inadequate social partners or caretakers (Bowlby, 1969; Hatfield et al., 1989; Kraemer, 1992, 1997). A recent review of the role of stress in human attachment concludes that stressors trigger the need for proximity and attachment behaviors, and surmises that some degree of strong, yet manageable stress may be necessary for very strong bonds to form (Simpson and Rholes, 1994).

Forced isolation, anxiety, fear, and other forms of stressful conditions are associated with increased levels of HPA activity (Fig. 56.2). Such conditions or experiences normally tend to encourage social interactions. Both the human (Simpson and Rholes, 1994) and animal literature (reviewed here) suggests an association between HPA activation and stressful experiences and the development of social attachments. The role of hormones of the HPA axis in attachment is probably not linear, since both animals and

humans under extreme conditions may become either self-protective or immobilized (Porges, 1998). Excessively stressful conditions, such as those that could compromise survival or in the face of intense grief may lead to a breakdown of social relationships (Reite and Boccia, 1994). Thus, the association between chronic or extreme stress could inhibit subsequent attachment. However, our work with rodents suggests that within a homeostatic range, stress-related physiological processes, including hormones of the HPA axis, can promote the development of social bonds (DeVries et al., 1996). In addition, positive social interactions, including social bonds, may help to create physiological states that are anxiolytic or stress reducing.

Oxytocin, perhaps released by positive social interactions, has the capacity to produce both acute and chronic reductions in the activity of the HPA axis (Carter and Altemus, 1997; Uvnas-Moberg, 1997, 1998) (Fig. 56.3). Studies of lactating women support this hypothesis in humans (Altemus et al., 1995). Thus, oxytocin, with both central and peripheral processes, is part of an endogenous homeostatic or in some cases anti-stress system. This system has the concurrent capacity to increase social attachment and other positive social behaviors (Fig. 56.3), providing the additional indirect benefits of sociality.

The role of vasopressin in human social behavior is more difficult to characterize. Vasopressin is believed to be similar to the ancestral peptide from which oxytocin and vasopressin were derived. Vasopressin binds to several types of receptors, including the oxytocin receptor. Vasopressin has been implicated in territoriality, agonistic behaviors and HPA arousal, and may be part of a more primitive adaptive system for mobilization and self-defense (Carter et al., 1995; Moore, 1992). In some cases the functions of vasopressin are apparently similar to those of oxytocin. However, as described above, under other conditions oxytocin and vasopressin may have antagonistic actions. Dynamic and complex interactions between oxytocin and vasopressin,

a. COHABITATION INHIBITS CORTICOSTERONE LEVELS

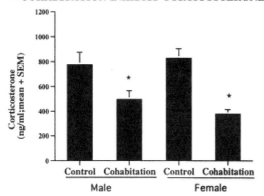

b. OXYTOCIN INHIBITS CORTICOSTERONE

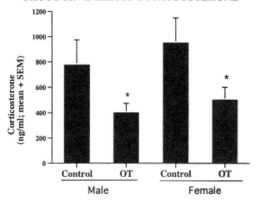

c. OXYTOCIN FACILITATES PAIR BONDING

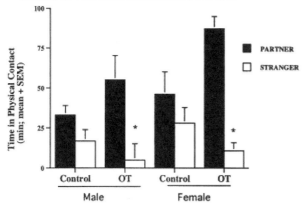

Figure 56.3
(a) Cohabitation inhibits corticosterone levels. (b) Oxytocin inhibits corticosterone. (c) Oxytocin faciltates pair bonding.

working in the presence of a more slowly changing steroid background, could help to regulate underlying human visceral states and emotions.

Awareness of the importance of peptides, including oxytocin and vasopressin, in human behavior is comparatively recent, but of considerable importance. Many aspects of daily life can affect the release of the peptides. For example, social or sexual contact, food intake (Uvnas-Moberg, 1994), the use of steroid hormones, or drugs of abuse or alcohol (Kovacs et al., 1998; Sarnyai and Kovacs, 1994), are only a few examples of experiences that have been shown to influence the endogenous production, release or actions of these peptides. In addition, developmental research suggests various mechanisms through which peptides and steroids could retune neural systems that are implicated in attachment. Thus, peptidergic systems capable of affecting attachment are subject to change in the face of environmental challenges.

Oxytocin and vasopressin are directly and indirectly manipulated by various medical practices. For example, large doses of "Pitocin" a synthetic version of oxytocin, are routinely used to hasten childbirth, with unexplored effects on the social behavior or propensity to attachment of both the mother and child (Boer, 1993). Long labors, caesarean sections and the decision to breast or bottle feed are indirectly peptidergic manipulations. Remarkably little attention has been given to the behavioral or hormonal consequences of these peptide-related events which can have profound effects on behavioral, homeostatic and emotional systems for both the parent and the child (Carter, 1988; DiPietro et al., 1987; Worobey, 1993).

Conclusions

The expression of attachments must incorporate genetic potentials and limitations associated with species variations, sex differences and individual experiences. Such changes require both short-term and long-lasting modifications of the nervous system. Steroids, neuropeptides and their interactions provide potential substrates for behavioral processes including those that are necessary for social attachment. Steroid hormones can regulate synthesis, release and receptor binding for oxytocin and vasopressin. These effects vary according to the species, gender and age of the subject, as well as by brain region.

In mammals, rodents provide the most accessible laboratory models for physiological research. Our recent awareness of the novel physiology of monogamous rodents provides an opportunity to explore the neurobiology of attachment, and thus one aspect of love. Such studies in turn have identified important candidate systems and molecules which may be central to understanding the biology of attachment and love.

Gonadal steroids, including androgens and estrogens, have species-typical developmental effects on neural systems that have been implicated in social attachment and may mediate both genetic and environmental influences on the propensity to form attachments. Gonadal hormones can regulate both oxytocinergic and vasopressinergic functions, and the expression of other peptides and neurotransmitters, which in turn also can modulate oxytocin and vasopressin. However, social attachments apparently can occur in the absence of gonadal steroids. At present direct evidence for an activational role for gonadal hormones in social attachment is inconclusive.

Sex differences in social behavior and the propensity to develop social attachments may reflect the organizational effects of steroids during development. High levels of vasopressinergic activity in males, regulated both developmentally and in adulthood by sex differences in androgens, could account for some gender differences in social behaviors. In addition, early exposure to vasopressin is capable of modifying subsequent aggression. Social and reproductive behaviors in males typically involve high levels of physical activity and vigilance. Vasopressin, which plays a role in pair bonding and defensive aggression, also can continue to function during mobilized behavioral states, possibly providing an explanation for male–female differences in social attachment.

There is a recurrent association between increased activity in the hypothalamic–pituitary–adrenal (HPA) axis and the subsequent expression of social behaviors and attachments. The HPA axis and adrenal steroids are particularly responsive to social and environmental demands. As described above, under certain conditions, stressful experiences and HPA axis activity are followed by increased sexual, parental and social behaviors and the formation of social bonds. Adrenal steroid–neuropeptide interactions involving oxytocin or oxytocin receptors may regulate the development of social attachments, while concurrently modulating the HPA axis. Positive social behaviors, perhaps mediated through a central oxytocinergic system, may modulate the activity of the HPA axis and the ANS, accounting for health benefits that are attributed to attachment.

Acknowledgements

I wish to acknowledge the generous advice of Stephen Porges who helped in the development of many of the organizing principles used to structure this review. I am thankful to Courtney DeVries for her help in understanding the role of the HPA axis in pair bonding, and to Bruce Cushing, Diane Witt, Leah Gavish, Luci Roberts, Mary Cho, Katie Bowler, John Stribley, Susan Taymans, Jessie Williams, Zuoxin Wang, and Tom Insel for their collaborations and for allowing me in some cases to discuss their unpublished data. I am particularly grateful to Bruce Cushing and Nancy Cushing for help with the references and in finding time to complete this review and to Tom Insel for his excellent editorial comments on this manuscript. Manuscript preparation and the animal research described here from my laboratory were sponsored by the National Institutes of Health, National Institute of Mental Health, National Science Foundation and the Department of Defense.

References

Acher, R. (1996) Molecular evolution of fish neurohypophysial hormones: neutral and selective evolutionary mechanisms. *General and Comparative Endocrinology* 102, 17–172.

Acher, R. and Chauvet, J. (1988) Structure, processing and evolution of the neurohypophysial hormone-neurophysin precursors. *Biochimie* 70, 1197–1207.

Ainsworth, M. D. S. (1989) Attachments beyond infancy. *American Psychologist* 44, 709–716.

Altemus, M., Deuster, P. A., Gallivan, E., Carter, C. S. and Gold, P. W. (1995) Suppression of hypothalamic-pituitary–adrenal responses to exercise stress in lactating women. *Journal of Clinical Endocrinology and Metabolism* 80, 2954–2959.

Al-Shamma, H. A. and DeVries, G. J. (1996) Neurogenesis of the sexually dimorphic vasopressin cells of the bed nucleus of the stria terminalis and amygdala of rats. *Journal of Neurobiology* 29, 91–98.

Amini, F., Lewis, T., Lannon, R., Louie, A., Baumbacher, G., McGuinness, T. and Schiff, E. Z. (1996) Affect, attachment, memory: contributions toward psychobiologic integration. *Psychiatry* 59, 213–239.

Axelson, J. F. and Van Leeuwen, F. W. (1990) Differential localization of estrogen receptors in various vasopressin synthesizing nuclei of the rat brain. *Journal of Neuroendocrinology* 2, 209–216.

Bamshad, M., Novak, M. A. and DeVries, G. J. (1993) Species and sex differences in vasopressin innervation of sexually naive and parental prairie voles, *Microtus ochrogaster* and meadow voles, *Microtus pennsylvanicus. Journal of Neuroendocrinology* 5, 247–255.

Bamshad, M., Novak, M. A. and DeVries, G. J. (1994) Cohabitation alters vasopressin innervation and paternal behavior in prairie voles, *Microtus ochrogaster. Physiology and Behavior* 56, 751–758.

Barberis, C. and Tribollet, E. (1996) Vasopressin and oxytocin receptors in the central nervous system. *Critical Reviews in Neurobiology* 10, 119–154.

Bartholomew, K. and Perlman, D. (1994) *Attachment Processes in Adulthood. Advances in Personal Relationships*, Vol. 5. Jessica Kingsley Publishers, London.

Berecek, K. H. (1991) Role of vasopressin in central cardiovascular regulation. In: Kunos, G. and Ciriello, J. (Eds.). *Central Neural Mechanisms in Cardiovascular Regulation*, Vol. 2. Birkhauser, Boston, pp. 1–34.

Boer, G. J. (1993) Chronic oxytocin treatment during late gestation and lactation impairs development of rat offspring. *Neurotoxicology and Teratology* 15, 383–389.

Boer, G. J., Quak, J., DeVries, M. C. and Heinsbroek, R. P. W. (1994) Mild sustained effects of neonatal vasopressin and oxytocin treatment on brain growth and behavior of the rat. *Peptides* 15, 229–236.

Bohus, B., Kovacs, G. L., Greven, H. M. and De Wied, D. (1978) Oxytocin, vasopressin and memory: opposite effects on consolidation and memory processes. *Brain Research* 157, 414–417.

Bouvard, M. P., Leboyer, M., Launay, J.-M., Recasens, C., Plumet, M.-H., Waller-Perotte, D., Tabuteau, F., Bondoux, D., Dugas, M., Lensing, P. and Panksepp, J. (1995) Low-dose naltrexone effects on plasma chemistries and clinical symptoms in autism: a double-blind, placebo-controlled study. *Psychiatric Research* 58, 191–201.

Bowlby, J., 1969. Attachment and Loss: vol. 1 *Attachment*. Hogarth Press, London.

Bowlby, J., 1973. Attachment and Loss: vol. 2 *Separation*. Hogarth Press, London.

Bowlby, J., 1980. Attachment and Loss: vol. 3 *Loss*. Hogarth Press, London.

Bridges, R. S. (1990) Endocrine regulation of parental behavior in rodents. In: Krasnegor, N. A. and Bridges, R. S. (Eds.). *Mammalian Parenting*. Oxford University Press, New York, pp. 93–117.

Brown, R. E. (1993) Hormonal and experiential factors influencing parental behaviour in male rodents: an integrative approach. *Behavioral Processes* 30, 1–28.

Caldwell, J. D. (1992) Central oxytocin and female sexual behavior. *Annals of the New York Academy of Science* 652, 166–179.

Caldwell, J. D., Greer, E. R., Johnson, M. F., Prange, A. J. Jr and Pedersen, C. A. (1987) Oxytocin and vasopressin immunoreactivity in hypothalamic and extrahypothalamic sites in late pregnant and postpartum rats. *Neuroendocrinology* 46, 39–47.

Carter, C. S. (1988) Patterns of infant feeding, the mother–infant interaction and stress management. In: Field, T. M., McCabe, P. M. and Schneiderman, N. (Eds.). *Stress and Coping Across Development*. Erlbaum, Hillsdale, NJ, pp. 27–46.

Carter, C. S. (1992) Oxytocin and sexual behavior. *Neuroscience and Biobehavioral Reviews* 16, 131–144.

Carter, C. S. and Altemus, M. (1997) Integrative functions of lactational hormones in social behavior and stress management. *Annals of the New York Academy of Science* 807, 164–174.

Carter, C. S. and Schein, M. W. (1971) Sexual receptivity and exhaustion in the female golden hamster. *Hormones and Behavior* 2, 191–200.

Carter, C. S., DeVries, A. C. and Getz, L. L. (1995) Physiological substrates of mammalian monogamy: the prairie vole model. *Neuroscience and Biobehavioral Reviews* 19, 303–314.

Carter, C. S., Lederhendler, I. I. and Kirkpatrick, B., 1997. The Integrative Neurobiology of Affiliation. *Annals of the New York Academy of Science* 807.

Chiodera, P., Salvarani, C., Bacchi-Modena, A., Spallanzani, R., Cigarini, C., Alboni, A., Gardini, E. and Coiro, V. (1991) Relationship between plasma profiles of oxytocin and adrenocorticotropic hormone during suckling or breast stimulation in women. *Hormones and Research* 35, 119–123.

Cho, M. M., DeVries, C. A. and Carter, C. S. The effects of oxytocin and vasopressin on partner preferences in male and female prairie voles (*Microtus ochrogaster*) (in press).

Chrousos, G. P., Renquist, D., Brandon, D., Eil, C., Pugeat, M., Vigersky, R., Cutler, G. B. Jr, Loriaux, D. L. and Lipsett, M. B. (1982) Glucocorticoid hormone resistance during primate evolution: receptor-mediated mechanisms. *Proceedings of the National Academy of Science USA* 79, 2036–2040.

Corter, C. M. and Fleming, A. S. (1995) Psychobiology of maternal behavior in human beings. In: Bornstein, M. H. (Ed.). *Handbook of Parenting: Biology and Ecology of Parenting*. Lawrence Erlbaum, Mahwah, NJ, pp. 87–116.

Crowley, R. S., Insel, T. R., O'Keefe, J. A., Kim, N. B. and Amico, J. A. (1995) Increased accumulation of oxytocin messenger ribonucleic acid in the hypothalamus of the female rat: induction by long term estradiol and progesterone administration and subsequent progesterone withdrawal. *Endocrinology* 136, 224–231.

Cushing, B. S. and Carter, C. S. (1998) Peripheral pulses of oxytocin facilitate partner preference and increase probability of mating in female prairie voles. *Society for Behavioral Neuroendocrinology Abstracts* 30, 148.

DeVries, A. C., DeVries, M. B., Taymans, S. E. and Carter, C. S. (1995) The modulation of pair bonding by corticosterone in female prairie voles (*Microtus ochrogaster*). *Proceedings of the National Academy of Science USA* 92, 7744–7748.

DeVries, A. C., DeVries, M. B., Taymans, S. E. and Carter, C. S. (1996) The effects of stress on social preferences are sexually dimorphic in prairie voles. *Proceedings of the National Academy of Science USA* 93, 11980–11984.

DeVries, A. C., Cho, M. M., Cardillo, S. and Carter, C. S. (1997) Oxytocin can suppress the HPA axis in prairie voles. *Society for Neuroscience Abstracts* 22, 1851.

DeVries, G. F. and Villalba, C. (1997) Brain sexual dimorphism and sex differences in parental and other social behaviors. *Annals of the New York Academy of Science* 807, 273–286.

De Wied, D., Elands, J. and Kovacs, G. (1991) Interactive effects of neurohypophyseal neuropeptides with receptor antagonists on passive avoidance behavior: mediation by a cerebral neurohypophyseal hormone receptor? *Proceedings of the National Academy of Science USA* 88, 1494–1498.

De Wied, D., Diamant, M. and Fodor, M. (1993) Central nervous system effects of neurohypophyseal hormones and related peptides. *Frontiers in Neuroendocrinology* 14, 251–302.

Dewsbury, D. A. (1988) The comparative psychology of monogamy. *Nebraska Symposium in Motivation* 35, 1–50.

Dharmadhikari, A., Lee, Y. S., Roberts, R. L. and Carter, C. S. (1997) Exploratory behavior correlates with social organization and is responsive to peptide injections in prairie voles. *Annals of the New York Academy of Science* 807, 610–612.

DiPietro, J. A., Larson, S. K. and Porges, S. W. (1987) Behavioral and heart rate difference between breast-fed and bottle-fed neonates. *Developmental Psychology* 23, 467–474.

Dreifuss, J. J., Dubois-Dauphin, M., Widmer, H. and Ragggenbass, M. (1992) Electrophysiology of oxytocin actions on central neurons. *Annals of the New York Academy of Science* 652, 46–57.

Engelmann, M., Wotjak, C. T., Neumann, I., Ludwig, M. and Landgraf, R. (1996) Behavioral consequences of intracerebral vasopressin and oxytocin: focus on learning and memory. *Neuroscience and Biobehavioral Reviews* 20, 341–358.

Fahrbach, S. E., Morrell, J. I. and Pfaff, D. W. (1985) Possible role for endogenous oxytocin in estrogen-facilitated maternal behavior in rats. *Neuroendocrinology* 40, 526–532.

Fisher, H. E. (1992) *Anatomy of Love.* Fawcett Columbine, New York.

Fleming, A. S., Vaccarino, F. and Luebke, C. (1980) Amygdaloid inhibition of maternal behavior in the nulliparous female rat. *Physiology and Behavior* 25, 731–743.

Fleming, A. S., Steiner, M. and Anderson, V. (1987) Hormonal and attitudinal correlates of maternal behavior during the early postpartum period. *Journal of Reproductive and Infant Psychology* 5, 193–205.

Fleming, A. S., Cheung, U., Myhal, N. and Kessler, Z. (1989) Effects of maternal hormones on timidity and attraction to pup-related odors in female rats. *Physiology and Behavior* 46, 449–453.

Getz, L. L., Carter, C. S. and Gavish, L. (1981) The mating system of the prairie vole *Microtus ochrogaster:* field and laboratory evidence for pair-bonding. *Behavioral Ecology and Sociobiology* 8, 189–194.

Gingrich, B. S., Huot, R. L., Wang, Z. and Insel, T. R. (1997) Differential fos expression following microinjection of oxytocin or vasopressin in the prairie vole brain. *Annals of the New York Academy of Science* 807, 504–505.

Gorski, R. A. (1990) Structural and sexual dimorphisms in the brain. In: Krasnegor, N. A. and Bridges, R. S. (Eds.). *Mammalian Parenting: Biochemical, Neurobiological and Behavioral Determinants.* Oxford University Press, New York, pp. 61–90.

Grazzini, E., Guillon, G., Mouillac, B. and Zingg, H. H. (1998) Inhibition of oxytocin receptor function by direct binding of progesterone. *Nature* 392, 609–612.

Grosvenor, C. E., Shah, G. V. and Crowley, W. R. (1990) Role of neurogenic stimuli and milk prolactin in the regulation of prolactin secretion during lactation.

In: Krasnegor, N. A. and Bridges, R. S. (Eds.). *Mammalian Parenting: Biochemical, Neurobiological and Behavioral Determinants*. Oxford University Press, New York, pp. 324–342.

Gubernick, D. J. and Nelson, R. J. (1989) Prolactin and paternal behavior in the biparental California mouse, *Peromyscus californicus*. *Hormones and Behavior* 23, 203–210.

Gubernick, D. J., Schneider, K. A. and Jeannotte, L. A. (1994) Individual differences in the mechanisms underlying the onset and maintenance of paternal behavior and the inhibition of infanticide in the monogamous biparental California mouse, *Peromyscus californicus*. *Behavioral Ecology and Sociobiology* 34, 225–231.

Harlow, C. M. (1986) *Learning to Love: The Selected Papers of HF Harlow*. Praeger, New York.

Hatfield, E. and Rapson, R. L. (1993) *Love, Sex and Intimacy*. Harper Collins, New York.

Hatfield, E., Brinton, C. and Cornelius, J. (1989) Passionate love and anxiety in young adolescents. *Motivation and Emotions* 13, 271–289.

Hazan, C. and Shaver, P. R. (1987) Romantic love conceptualized as an attachment. *Journal of Personal and Social Psychology* 52, 511–524.

Hennessy, M. B. (1997) Hypothalamic–pituitary–adrenal responses to brief social separation. *Neuroscience and Biobehavioral Reviews* 21, 11–29.

Herman, B. H. and Panksepp, J. (1987) Effects of morphine and naloxone on separation distress and approach attachment: Evidence for opiate mediation of social affect. *Pharmacology and Biochemical Behavior* 9, 213–220.

Hillegaart, V., Alster, P., Uvnas-Moberg, K. and Ahlenius, S. (1997) Heterosexual interactions promote oxytocin secretion in sexually naive, but not experienced, male Wistar rats. *Annals of the New York Academy of Science* 807, 530–533.

Holman, S. D. and Goy, R. W. (1995) Experiential and hormonal correlates of care-giving in rhesus macaques. In: Pryce, C. R., Martin, R. D. and Skuse, D. (Eds.). *Motherhood in Human and Nonhuman Primates*. Karger, Basel, pp. 87–93.

House, J. S., Landis, K. R. and Umberson, D. (1988) Social relationships and health. *Science* 241, 540–545.

Insel, T. R. (1997) A neurobiological basis of social attachment. *American Journal of Psychiatry* 154, 726–735.

Insel, T. R. and Harbaugh, C. R. (1989) Lesions of the hypothalamic paraventricular nucleus disrupt the initiation of maternal behavior. *Physiology and Behavior* 45, 1033–1041.

Insel, T. R. and Hulihan, T. J. (1995) A gender-specific mechanism for pair bonding: oxytocin and partner preference formation in monogamous voles. *Behavioral Neuroscience* 109, 782–789.

Insel, T. R. and Shapiro, L. E. (1992) Oxytocin receptor distribution reflects social organization in monogamous and polygamous voles. *Proceedings of the National Academy of Science USA* 89, 5981–5985.

Insel, T. R. and Winslow, J. T. (1991) Central administration of oxytocin modulates the infant rat's response to social isolation. *European Journal of Pharmacology* 203, 149–152.

Insel, T. R., Preston, S. and Winslow, J. T. (1995) Mating in the monogamous male: behavioral consequences. *Physiology and Behavior* 57, 615–627.

Insel, T. R., Wang, Z. and Ferris, C. F. (1994) Patterns of brain vasopressin receptor distribution associated with social organization in microtine rodents. *Journal of Neuroscience* 14, 5381–5392.

Insel, T. R., Young, L. and Wang, Z. (1997) Molecular aspects of monogamy. *Annals of the New York Academy of Science* 807, 302–316.

Insel, T. R., Young, L. J., Witt, D. and Crews, D. (1993) Gonadal steroids have paradoxical effects on brain oxytocin receptors. *Journal of Neuroendocrinology* 5, 619–628.

Jirikowski, G. F., McGimsey, W. C., Caldwell, J. D. and Sar, M. (1993) Distribution of oxytocinergic glucocorticoid target neurons in the rat hypothalamus. *Hormones and Metabolic Research* 25, 543–544.

Johnson, A. E. (1992) The regulation of oxytocin receptor binding in the ventromedial hypothalamic nucleus of gonadal steroids. *Annals of the New York Academy of Science* 652, 357–373.

Kendrick, K. M. and Keverne, E. B. (1989) Effects of intracerebroventricular infusions of naltrexone and phentolamine on central and peripheral oxytocin release and on maternal behaviour induced by vaginocervical stimulation in the ewe. *Brain Research* 505, 329–332.

Kendrick, K. M., Keverne, E. B., Chapman, C. and Baldwin, B. A. (1988) Microdialysis measurement of oxytocin, aspartate gamma-aminobutyric acid and glutamate release from the olfactory bulb of the sheep during vaginocervical stimulation. *Brain Research* 411, 171–174.

Kendrick, K. M., Keverne, E. B., Hinton, M. R. and Goode, J. A. (1986) Cerebrospinal fluid levels of acetylcholinesterase, monoamines and oxytocin during labour, parturition, vaginocervical stimulation, lamb separation and suckling in sheep. *Neuroendocrinology* 44, 149–156.

Keverne, E. B. (1995) Neurochemical changes accompanying the reproductive process: their significance for maternal care in primates and other mammals. In: Pryce, C. R., Martin, R. D. and Skuse, D. (Eds.). *Motherhood in Human and Nonhuman Primates.* Karger, Basel, pp. 69–77.

Keverne, E. B. and Kendrick, K. M. (1992) Oxytocin facilitation of maternal behavior in sheep. *Annals of the New York Academy of Science* 652, 83–101.

Keverne, E. B., Nevison, C. M. and Martel, F. L. (1997) Early learning and the social bond. *Annals of the New York Academy of Science* 807, 329–339.

Kirkpatrick, B. (1997) Affiliation and neuropsychiatric disorders: the deficit syndrome of schizophrenia. *Annals of the New York Academy of Science* 807, 455–468.

Klaus, M. H., Kennell, J. H. and Klaus, P. H. (1995) *Bonding.* Addison-Wesley, Reading, MA.

Kleiman, D. (1977) Monogamy in Mammals. *Quarterly Reviews in Biology* 52, 39–69.

Klopfer, P. H. (1971) Mother love: What turns it on? *American Scientist* 59, 404–407.

Klopfer, P. H. (1996) Mother love revisited: On the use of animal models. *American Scientist* 84, 319–321.

Knox, S. S. and Uvnas-Moberg, K. (1998) Social isolation and cardiovascular disease: an atherosclerotic pathway? *Psychoneuroendocrinology* 23, 877–890.

Kovács, G. L., Sarnyai, Z. and Szabó, G. (1998) Oxytocin and addiction: a review. *Psychoneuroendocrinology* 23, 945–962.

Kraemer, G. W. (1992) A psychobiological theory of attachment. *Behavioral Brain Science* 15, 493–511.

Kraemer, G. W. (1997) Psychobiology of early social attachment in rhesus monkeys. *Annals of the New York Academy of Science* 807, 401–418.

Landgraf, R., Neumann, I. and Pittman, Q. J. (1991) Septal and hippocampal release of vasopressin and oxytocin during late pregnancy and parturition in the rat. *Neuroendocrinology* 54, 378–383.

Leake, R. D., Wietzman, R. E. and Fisher, D. A. (1981) Oxytocin concentrations during the neonatal period. *Biology of the Neonate* 39, 127–131.

Levin, M. C. and Sawchenko, P. E. (1993) Neuropeptide co-expression in the magnocellular neurosecretory system of the female rat: evidence for differential modulation by estrogen. *Neuroscience* 54, 1001–1018.

Levine, S., Coe, C. and Wiener, S. G. (1989) Psychoneuroendocrinology of stress: a psychobiological perspective. In: Brush, F. R. and Levine, S. (Eds.). *Psychoneuroendocrinology.* Academic Press, New York, pp. 341–380.

Levine, S., Lyons, D. M. and Schatzberg, A. F. (1997) Psychobiological consequences of social relationships. *Annals of the New York Academy of Science* 807, 210–218.

Li, Q., Levy, A. D., Cabrera, T. M., Brownfield, M. S., Battaglia, G. and Van de Kar, L. D. (1993) Long-term fluoxetine, but not desipramine, inhibits the ACTH and oxytocin responses to the 5-HT1a agonist, 8-OH-DPAT, in male rats. *Brain Research* 630, 148–156.

Liberzon, I. and Young, E. A. (1997) Effects of stress and glucocorticoids on CNS oxytocin receptor binding. *Psychoneuroendocrinology* 22, 411–422.

Liberzon, I., Trujillo, K. A., Akil, H. and Young, E. A. (1997) Motivational properties of oxytocin in the conditioned place preference paradigm. *Neuropychopharmacology* 17, 353–359.

Liberzon, I., Chalmers, D. T., Mansour, A., Lopez, J. F., Watson, S. J. and Young, E. A. (1994) Glucocorticoid regulation of hippocampal oxytocin receptor binding. *Brain Research* 650, 317–322.

Lightman, S. L. (1992) Alterations in hypothalamic-pituitary responsiveness during lactation. *Annals of the New York Academy of Science* 652, 340–346.

Lightman, S. L. and Young, W. S. (1987) Vasopressin, oxytocin, dynorphin, enkephalin, and corticotrophin releasing factor mRNA stimulation in the rat. *Journal of Physiology* 394, 23–29.

Lightman, S. L. and Young, W. S. (1989) Lactation inhibits stress–mediated secretion of corticosterone and oxytocin and hypothalamic accumulation of corticotropin–releasing factor and enkephalin messenger ribonucleic acids. *Endocrinology* 124, 2358–2364.

Mason, W. A. and Mendoza, S. P. (1998) Generic aspects of primate attachments: parents, offspring and mates. *Psychoneuroendocrinology* 23, 765–778.

McCarthy, M. M., Kow, L. M. and Pfaff, D. W. (1992) Speculations concerning the physiological significance of central oxytocin in maternal behavior. *Annals of the New York Academy of Science* 652, 70–82.

McGuire, B., Getz, L. L., Hofmann, J. E., Pizzuto, T. and Frase, B. (1993) Natal dispersal and philopatry in prairie voles (*Microtus ochrogaster*) in relation to population density, season, and natal social environment. *Behavioral Ecology and Sociobiology* 32, 293–302.

Meisel, R. L. and Sachs, B. D. (1994) The physiology of male sexual behavior. In: Knobil, E. and Neill, D. (Eds.). *The Physiology of Reproduction*, 2. Raven Press, New York, pp. 3–105.

Meister, B., Villar, M. J., Ceccatelli, S. and Hokfelt, T. (1990) Localization of chemical messengers in magnocellular neurons of the hypothalamic supraoptic and paraventricular nuclei: an immunohistochemical study using experimental manipulations. *Neuroscience* 37, 603–633.

Mendoza, S. P. and Mason, W. A. (1997) Attachment relationships in New World primates. *Annals of the New York Academy of Science* 807, 203–209.

Meyerson, B. J., Hoglund, U., Johansson, C., Blomqvist, X. and Ericson, H. (1988) Neonatal vasopressin antagonist treatment facilitates adult copulatory behavior in female rats and increases hypothalamic vasopressin content. *Brain Research* 473, 344–351.

Milgram, N. A. (1986) *Stress and Coping in Time of War: Generalizations from the Israeli Experience.* Brunner-Mazel, New York.

Modahl, C., Green, L.-A., Fein, D., Morris, M., Waterhouse, L., Feinstein, C. and Levin, H. (1998) Plasma oxytocin levels in autistic children. *Biological Psychiatry* 43, 270–277.

Moore, F. L. (1992) Evolutionary precedents for behavioral actions of oxytocin and vasopressin. *Annals of the New York Academy of Science* 652, 156–165.

Nelson, E. and Panksepp, J. (1996) Oxytocin mediates acquisition of maternallly associated odor preferences in preweanling rat pups. *Behavioral Neuroscience* 110, 583–592.

Newton, N. (1973) Interrelationships between sexual responsiveness, birth, and breast feeding. In: Zubin, J. and Money, J. (Eds.). *Contemporary Sexual Behavior: Critical Issues in the 1970s.* Johns Hopkins University Press, Baltimore, pp. 77–98.

Nissen, E., Uvnas-Moberg, K., Svensson, K., Stock, S., Widstrom, A. M. and Winberg, J. (1996) Different patterns of oxytocin, prolactin but not cortisol release during breastfeeding in women delivered by caesarean section or by the vaginal route. *Early Human Development* 45, 103–118.

Numan, M. (1994) Maternal behavior. In: Knobil, E. and Neill, D. (Eds.). *The Physiology of Reproduction*, 2. Raven Press, New York, pp. 221–302.

Numan, M. and Sheehan, T. P. (1997) Neuroanatomical circuitry for mammalian maternal behavior. *Annals of the New York Academy of Science* 807, 101–125.

Ostrowski, N. L. (1998) Oxytocin receptor mRNA expression in rat brain: implications for behavioral integration and reproductive success. *Psychoendocrinology* 23, 989–1004.

Panksepp, J. (1981) Brain opioids—A neurochemical substrate for narcotic and social dependence. In: Cooper, S. J. (Ed.). *Theory of Psychopharmacology.* Academic Press, New York, pp. 49–175.

Panksepp, J., Nelson, E. and Siviy, S. (1994) Brain opioids and mother–infant social motivation. *Acta Paediatrica Supplement* 397, 40–46.

Panksepp, J., Nelson, E. and Bekkedal, M. (1997) Brain systems for the mediation of social separation-distress and social-reward. *Annals of the New York Academy of Sciences* 807, 78–100.

Panksepp, J., Siviy, S. and Normansell, L. (1985) Brain opioids and social emotions. In: Reite, M. and Fields, T. (Eds.). *The Psychobiology of Attachment and Separation.* Academic Press, San Diego, pp. 3–49.

Parker, S. L., Armstrong, W. E., Sladek, C. D., Grosvenor, C. E. and Crowley, W. R. (1991) Prolactin stimulates the release of oxytocin in lactating rats: evidence for a physiological role via an action at the neural lobe. *Neuroendocrinology* 53, 503–510.

Patchev, V. K. and Almeida, O. F. X. (1995) Corticosteroid regulation of gene expression and binding characteristics of vasopressin receptors in the rat brain. *European Journal of Neuroscience* 7, 1579–1583.

Patchev, V. K., Schlosser, S. F., Hassan, A. H. S. and Almeida, O. F. X. (1993) Oxytocin binding sites in rat limbic hypothalamic structures: site specific modulation by adrenal and gonadal steroids. *Neuroscience* 57, 537–543.

Pedersen, C. A. (1997) Oxytocin control of maternal behavior. Regulation by sex steroids and offspring stimuli. *Annals of the New York Academy of Science* 807, 126–145.

Pedersen, C. A., Caldwell, J. D., Peterson, G., Walker, C. H. and Mason, G. A. (1992) Oxytocin activation of maternal behavior in the rat. *Annals of the New York Academy of Science* 652, 58–69.

Pedersen, C. A. and Prange, A. J. Jr. (1979) Induction of maternal behavior in virgin rats after intracerebroventricular administration of oxytocin. *Proceedings of the National Academy of Science USA* 76, 6661–6665.

Pfaff, D. W., Schwartz-Giblin, S., McCarthy, M. M. and Kow, L. M. (1994) Cellular and molecular mechanisms of female reproductive behaviors. In: Knobil, E. and Neill, D. (Eds.). *The Physiology of Reproduction*, 2. Raven Press, New York, pp. 107–220.

Porges, S. W. (1995) Orienting in a defensive world: mammalian modifications of our evolutionary heritage. A polyvagal theory. *Psychophysiology* 32, 301–318.

Porges, S. W. (1997) Emotion: an evolutionary by-product of the neural regulation of the autonomic nervous system. *Annals of the New York Academy of Science* 807, 62–77.

Porges, S. W. (1998) Love: an emergent property of the mammalian autonomic nervous system. *Psychoneuroendocrinology* 23, 837–861.

Poulain, P. and Pittman, Q. (1993) Oxytocin pre-treatment enhances arginine vasopressin-induced motor disturbances and arginine vasopressin-induced phosphoinositol hydrolysis in rat septum: a cross-sensitization phenomenon. *Journal of Neuroendocrinology* 5, 33–39.

Reite, M. and Field, T. (1985) *The Psychobiology of Attachment and Separation*. Academic Press, New York.

Reite, M. and Boccia, M. L. (1994) Physiological aspects of adult attachment. In: Sperling, M. B. and Berman, W. H. (Eds.). *Attachment in Adults*. Guilford Press, New York.

Rhodes, C. H., Morrell, J. I. and Pfaff, D. W. (1981) Changes in oxytocin content in magnocellular neurons of the rat hypothalamus following water deprivation and estrogen treatment. *Cellular and Tissue Research* 126, 47–55.

Roberts, R. L., Zullo, A. S. and Carter, C. S. (1997) Sexual differentiation in prairie voles: the effects of corticosterone and testosterone. *Physiology and Behavior* 62, 1379–1383.

Roberts, R. L., Zullo, A., Gustafson, E. A. and Carter, C. S. (1996) Perinatal steroid treatments alter alloparental and affiliative behavior in prairie voles. *Hormones and Behavior* 30, 576–582.

Roberts, R. L., Williams, J. R., Wang, A. K. and Carter, C. S. (1998) Cooperative breeding and monogamy in prairie voles: influence of the sire and geographic variation. *Animal Behavior* 55, 1131–1140.

Roozendaal, B., Schoorlemmer, G. H. M., Koolhaas, J. M. and Bohus, B. (1993) Cardiac, neuroendocrine, and behavioral effects of central amygdaloid vasopressinergic and oxytocinergic mechanisms under stress-free conditions in rats. *Brain Research Bulletin* 32, 573–579.

Ryff, C. D. and Singer, B. (1998) The concept of positive human health. *Psychological Inquiries* 9, 1–19.

Sachser, N., Dürschlag, M. and Hirzel, D. (1998) Social relationships and the management of stress. *Psychoneuroendocrinology* 23, 891–904.

Sachser, N. and Kaiser, S. (1996) Prenatal social stress masculinizes the females' behaviour in guinea pigs. *Physiology and Behavior* 60, 589–594.

Sachser, N. and Lick, C. (1989) Social stress in guinea pigs. *Physiology and Behavior* 46, 137–144.

Sachser, N. and Lick, C. (1991) Social experience, behavior and stress in guinea pigs. *Physiology and Behavior* 50, 83–90.

Sarnyai, Z. and Kovacs, G. L. (1994) Role of oxytocin in the neuroadaptation to drugs of abuse. *Psychoneuroendocrinology* 19, 85–117.

Sawchenko, P. E. and Swanson, L. W. (1982) Immunohistochemical identification of neurons in the paraventricular nucleus of the hypothalamus that project to the medulla or to the spinal cord in the rat. *Journal of Comparative Neurology* 205, 260–272.

Schumacher, M., Coirini, H., Pfaff, D. W. and McEwen, B. S. (1990) Behavioral effects of progesterone associated with rapid modulation of oxytocin receptors. *Science* 250, 691–694.

Shaffer, D. and Campbell, M. (1994) Reactive attachment disorder of infancy or early childhood. In: Frances, A. and Pincus, H. A. (Eds.). *Diagnostic and Statistical Manual of Mental Disorders: DSM-IV,* 4. American Psychiatric Association, Washington, DC, pp. 16–118.

Shapiro, L. E., Meyer, M. E. and Dewsbury, D. A. (1989) Affiliative behavior in voles: effects of morphine, naloxone, and cross-fostering. *Physiology and Behavior* 46, 719–723.

Simpson, J. A. and Rholes, W. S. (1994) Stress and secure base relationships in adulthood. *Advances in Personal Relatioships* 5, 181–204.

Singh, P. J. and Hofer, M. A. (1978) Oxytocin reinstates maternal olfactory cues for nipple orientation and attachment in rat pups. *Physiology and Behavior* 20, 385–389.

Sofroniew, M. W. (1983) Vasopressin and oxytocin in the mammalian brain and spinal cord. *Trends in Neuroscience* 6, 467–472.

Sperling, M. B. and Berman, W. H. (1994) *Attachment in Adults.* Guilford Press, New York, NY.

Sternberg, R. J. and Barnes, M. I. (1988) *The Psychology of Love.* Yale University Press, New Haven, CT.

Stribley, J. and Carter, C. S. (1998) Postnatal vasopressin exposure increases aggression in adult prairie voles. *Society for Behavioral Neuroendocrinology Abstracts* 30, 114.

Swabb, D. F. and Boer, G. J. (1994) Neuropeptides and brain development: current perils and future potential. *Journal of Developmental Physiology* 5, 67–75.

Swanson, L. W. and Sawchenko, P. E. (1980) Paraventricular nucleus: a site for the integration of neuroendocrine and autonomic mechanisms. *Neuroendocrinology* 31, 410–417.

Taymans, S. E., DeVries, A. C., DeVries, M. B., Nelson, R. J., Friedman, T. C., Castro, M., Detera-Wadleigh, S., Carter, C. S. and Chrousos, G. P. (1997) The hypothalamic–pituitary–adrenal axis of prairie voles (*Microtus ochrogaster*): evidence for target tissue glucocorticoid resistance. *General and Comparative Endocrinology* 106, 48–61.

Tribollet, E., Audigier, S., Dubois-Dauphin, M. and Dreifuss, J. J. (1990) Gonadal steroids regulate oxytocin receptors but not vasopressin receptors in the brain of male and female rats. An autoradiographical study. *Brain Research* 511, 129–140.

Tribollet, E., Goumaz, M., Raggenbass, M., Dubois-Dauphin, M. and Dreifuss, J. J. (1991) Early appearance and transient expression of vasopressin receptors in the brain of rat fetus and infant: an autoradiographical and electrophysiological study. *Developmental Brain Research* 58, 13–24.

Tribollet, E., Dubois-Dauphin, M., Dreifuss, J. J., Barberis, C. and Jard, S. (1992) Oxytocin receptors in the central nervous system: distribution, development, and species differences. *Annals of the New York Academy of Science* 652, 29–38.

Uvnas-Moberg, K. (1994) Role of efferent and afferent vagal nerve activity during reproduction: integrating function of oxytocin on metabolism and behavior. *Psychoneuroendocrinology* 19, 687–695.

Uvnas-Moberg, K. (1997) Physiological and endocrine effects of social contact. *Annals of the New York Academy of Science* 807, 146–163.

Uvnas-Moberg, K., Windstrom, A. M., Nissen, E. and Bjorvell, H. (1990) Personality traits in women 4 days post partum and their correlation with plasma levels of oxytocin and prolactin. *Journal of Psychosomatic Obstetrics and Gynaecology* 11, 261–272.

Uvnas-Moberg, K. (1998) Oxytocin may mediate the benefits of positive social interaction and emotions. *Psychoneuroendocrinology* 23, 819–835.

Vaccari, C. S., Carter, C. S. and Ostrowski, N. L. (1996) Neonatal exposure to arginine vasopressin alters adult vasopressin V1a and oxytocin receptor mRNA expression in rat brain. *Society for Neuroscience Abstracts* 26, 81.

Van Kesteren, R. E., Smit, A. B., Dirkds, R. W., Dewith, N. D., Deraerts, W. P. M. and Joosse, J. (1992) Evolution of the vasopressin/oxytocin superfamily: characterization of a cDNA encoding a vasopressin-related precursor, preproconopressin, from the mollusc *Lymnaea stagnalis. Proceedings of the National Academy of Science USA* 89, 4593–4597.

Van Leeuwen, F. W., Caffe, A. R. and DeVries, G. J. (1985) Vasopressin cells in the bed nucleus of the stria terminalis of the rat: sex differences and the influence of androgens. *Brain Research* 325, 391–394.

Van Tol, H. H. M., Bolwerk, E. L. M., Liu, B. and Burbach, J. P. H. (1988) Oxytocin and vasopressin gene expression in the hypothalamo-neurohypophyseal system of the rat during the estrous cycle, pregnancy, and lactation. *Endocrinology* 123, 945–951.

Wamboldt, M. and Insel, T. R. (1987) The ability of oxytocin to induce short latency maternal behavior is dependent on peripheral anosmia. *Behavioral Neuroscience* 101, 439–441.

Wang, Z. (1995) Species differences in the vasopressin-immunoreactive pathways in the bed nucleus of the stria terminalis and medial amygdaloid nucleus in prairie voles (*Microtus ochrogaster*) and meadow voles (*Microtus pennsylvanicus*). *Behavioral Neuroscience* 109, 305–311.

Wang, Z. and DeVries, G. J. (1994) Testosterone effects on paternal behavior and vasopressin immunoreactive projections in prairie voles (*Microtus ochrogaster*). *Brain Research* 631, 156–160.

Wang, Z., Smith, W., Major, D. E. and DeVries, G. J. (1994) Sex and species differences in the effects of cohabitation on vasopressin messenger RNA expression in the bed nucleus of the stria terminalis in prairie voles (*Microtus ochrogaster*) and meadow voles (*Microtus pennsylvanicus*). *Brain Research* 650, 212–218.

Wang, Z., Young, L. J., Liu, Y. and Insel, T. R. (1997) Species differences in vasopressin receptor binding are evident early in development: comparative anatomic studies in prairie and montane voles. *Journal of Comparative Neurology* 378, 535–546.

Wang, Z., Zhou, L., Hulihan, T. and Insel, T. R. (1996) Immunoreactivity of central vasopressin and oxytocin pathways in microtine rodents: a quantitative comparative study. *Journal of Comparative Neurology* 366, 726–737.

Ward, I. L. and Ward, O. B. (1986) Sexual behavior differentiation: effects of prenatal manipulations in rats. In: Adler, N., Pfaff, D. and Goy, R. W. (Eds.). *Handbook of Behavioral Neurobiology: Reproduction*. Plenum Press, New York, pp. 77–98.

Whitnall, M. H. (1993) Regulation of the hypothalamic corticotropin-releasing hormone neurosecretory system. *Progress in Neurobiology* 40, 573–629.

Wideman, C. H. and Murphy, H. M. (1990) Vasopressin, maternal behavior and pup well-being. *Current Psychology Research Reviews* 9, 285–295.

Widstrom, A. M., Wahlberg, V., Matthiesen, A. S., Eneroth, P., Uvnas-Moberg, K., Werner, S. and Winberg, J. (1990) Short-term effects of early suckling on

maternal behaviour and breast-feeding performance. *Early Human Development* 21, 153–163.

Williams, J. R., Catania, K. C. and Carter, C. S. (1992) Development of partner preferences in female prairie voles (*Microtus ochrogaster*): the role of social and sexual experience. *Hormones and Behavior* 26, 339–349.

Williams, J. R., Insel, T. R., Harbaugh, C. R. and Carter, C. S. (1994) Oxytocin centrally administered facilitates formation of a partner preference in female prairie voles (*Microtus ochrogaster*). *Journal of Neuroendocrinology* 6, 247–250.

Winslow, J. T. and Insel, T. R. (1991a) Endogenous opioids: do they modulate the rat pup's response to social isolation? *Behavioral Neuroscience* 105, 253–263.

Winslow, J. T. and Insel, T. R. (1991b) Vasopressin modulates male squirrel monkeys' behavior during social separation. *Euopean Journal of Pharmacology* 200, 95–101.

Winslow, J. T., Hastings, N., Carter, C. S., Harbaugh, C. R. and Insel, T. R. (1993) Selective aggression and affiliation increase following mating in a monogamous mammal: a role for central vasopressin in pair bonding. *Nature* 365, 545–548.

Winslow, J. T. and Insel, T. R. (1993) Effects of central vasopressin administration to infant rats. *European Journal of Pharmacology* 233, 101–107.

Witt, D. M. (1997) Regulatory mechanisms of oxytocin-mediated sociosexual behavior. *Annals of the New York Academy of Science* 807, 22–41.

Witt, D. M., Carter, C. S. and Insel, T. R. (1991) Oxytocin receptor binding in female prairie voles: endogenous and exogenous oestradiol stimulation. *Journal of Neuroendocrinology* 3, 155–161.

Witt, D. M., Carter, C. S. and Walton, D. (1990) Central and peripheral effects of oxytocin administration in prairie voles (*Microtus ochrogaster*). *Pharmacology and Biochemical Behavior* 37, 63–69.

Witt, D. M., Winslow, J. T. and Insel, T. R. (1992) Enhanced social interactions in rats following chronic, centrally infused oxytocin. *Pharmacology and Biochemical Behavior* 43, 855–861.

Worobey, J. (1993) Effects of feeding method on infant temperament. *Advances in Child Development* 24, 37–61.

Young, L. J., Juot, B., Nilsen, R., Wang, Z. and Insel, T. R. (1996) Species differences in central oxytocin receptor gene expression: comparative analysis of promoter sequences. *Journal of Neuroendocrinology* 8, 777–783.

Zingg, H. H., Rozen, F., Chu, K., Larcher, A., Arslan, A., Richard, S. and Lefebure, D. (1995) Oxytocin and oxytocin receptor gene expression in the uterus. *Recent Progress in Hormone Research* 50, 255–273.

V BIOLOGY OF SOCIAL RELATIONSHIPS AND INTERPERSONAL PROCESSES

B. Social Applications

iii. Affiliation and Sexuality

57 A Role for Central Vasopressin in Pair Bonding in Monogamous Prairie Voles

James T. Winslow, Nick Hastings, C. Sue Carter, Carroll R. Harbaugh, and Thomas R. Insel

Monogamous social organization is characterized by selective affiliation with a partner, high levels of paternal behaviour and, in many species, intense aggression towards strangers for defence of territory, nest and mate.[1,2] Although much has been written about the evolutionary causes of monogamy, little is known about the proximate mechanisms for pair bonding in monogamous mammals.[2,3] The prairie vole, *Microtus ochrogaster,* is a monogamous, biparental rodent which exhibits long-term pair bonds characterized by selective affiliation (partner preference) and aggression.[4,5] Here we describe the rapid development of both selective aggression and partner preferences following mating in the male of this species. We hypothesized that either arginine-vasopressin (AVP) or oxytocin (OT), two nine-amino-acid neuropeptides with diverse forebrain projections, could mediate the development of selective aggression and affiliation. This hypothesis was based on the following observations: (1) monogamous and polygamous voles differ specifically in the distribution of forebrain AVP and OT receptors;[6,7] (2) AVP innervation in the prairie vole brain is sexually dimorphic and important for paternal behaviour;[8] (3) central AVP pathways have been previously implicated in territorial displays and social memory;[9,10] and (4) central OT pathways have been previously implicated in affiliative behaviours.[11] We now demonstrate that central AVP is both necessary and sufficient for selective aggression and partner preference formation, two critical features of pair bonding in the monogamous prairie vole.

To characterize the development of selective aggression in prairie voles, sexually naive adult males were tested in a resident–intruder paradigm similar to that used with mice.[12] Naive males, that is, males without female exposure, explored a novel male intruder but showed little attack behaviour. Within 24 h of mating, males showed a qualitative change in their behaviour towards an intruder, with vigorous attacks and threats and decreased defensive behaviour (Fig. 57.1). This increase in aggression seemed to be sustained and selective. Either with or without further exposure to a female, males continued to show attack behaviour 1 week later (Fig. 57.1). Attacks against the mate were not observed either during or after the initial 24-h mating experience, although females other than the partner were attacked as intruders (Fig. 57.1). Sexually naive males rarely show offensive aggression towards a conspecific female.

Mating seemed to be critical to the rapid induction of aggression, as males within 24 h of social but not sexual experience rarely show attack behaviour (Fig. 57.1). Mating has previously been shown in the female to help the development of a partner preference, critical for pair bonding in this species.[13] The development of aggression, essential for mate guarding and nest defence, may also be associated with pair bonding. In support of this hypothesis, no similar transition to aggression was seen in males of the closely related montane vole (*Microtus montanus*) which does not pair bond.[14] Montane males exhibited few attacks and threats when tested serially ($n = 7$) before mating (9.7 ± 2.9), 24 h after mating (4.7 ± 1.6) or while living with a female as part of a breeding pair (5.8 ± 1.9).

To investigate a role for either AVP or OT in the induction of aggression, male prairie voles were injected intracerebroventricularly (i.c.v) with either cerebrospinal fluid (CSF), the vasopressin-1a receptor (V_{1a}) antagonist [1-(β-mercapto-β,β-cyclopentamethylene propionic acid), 2-(O-methyl)tyrosine]-arginine-vasopressin (d(CH$_2$)$_5$[Tyr(Me)] AVP) or the OT receptor antagonist d(CH$_2$)$_5$-[Tyr(Me)$_2$, Thr^4, Tyr-NH$_2$^{9}]-ornithine vasotocin (OTA) just before 24 h of exposure to a sexually receptive female. After either CSF or OTA injection, males showed

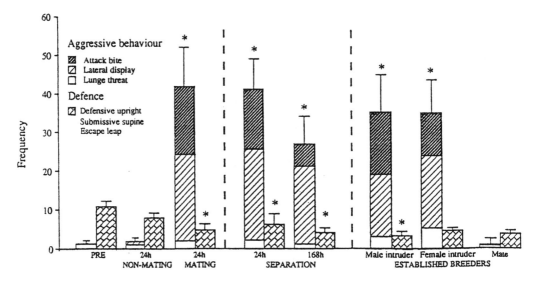

Figure 57.1

Mean ($\pm$ SEM) frequency of aggressive and defensive behaviour in 6-min resident–intruder tests. Before exposure to a female (Pre), sexually naive prairie vole males ($n = 17$) exhibit minimal aggressive and moderate defensive behaviour towards a novel male intruder. Tested 24 h later, a subset of these same males ($n = 8$) show a similar response to an intruder if housed in the interim with a female without mating (Non-mating). Another subset ($n = 9$) that mated with females (Mating) exhibit a significant increase in aggression ($F(6, 48) = 7.44$, $P < 0.05$) when tested after 24 h with the female (Dunnett's t-test, $t_D = 3.97$, $P < 0.05$) or after subsequent separation from their mates for 24 h ($t_D = 4.10$, $P < 0.05$) or 168 h ($t_D = 2.61$, $P < 0.05$). These same males respond to an intruder with comparable levels of aggression after being reunited with their mates for at least 1 week. (Established breeder) ($t_D = 3.28$, $P < 0.05$). Aggression seems to be selective in that it is directed at both males and novel females, but rarely at the mate. A concurrent decrease in defensive behaviour is observed post-mating ($F(6, 48) = 3.89$, $P < 0.05$). An asterisk signifies difference ($P < 0.05$) from baseline frequency (Pre) in composite score of aggressive or defensive behaviour by within-subjects post hoc Dunnett's t-test. *Methods.* For aggression testing, socially reared males (60–75 days old) were isolated for at least 3 days to avoid potential effects of social status in communal cages. For the resident–intruder model, an intruder male was placed in the home cage of the experimental animal for 6 min. Each male was tested at baseline and then tested with a different intruder for subsequent tests. For groups with female exposure, the female was removed before adding the intruder male. Behaviour was recorded on videotape and scored using a computer-assisted data acquisition system by a rater blind to group assignment. Behaviour was operationally defined as previously described[22] with reported means indicating frequency over the 6-min test.

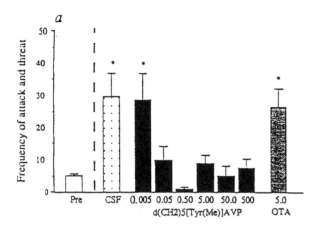

Antagonist treatment (ng, i.c.v.)

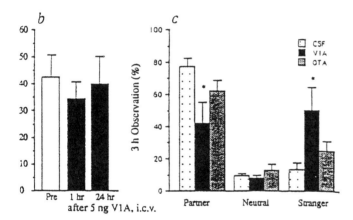

Established breeder   Partner preference

Figure 57.2

A V_{1a} antagonist given i.c.v. before mating blocked the induction of aggression in the male prairie vole. (a) Before female exposure, males showed low levels of aggression (attacks and threats) in the resident–intruder paradigm as described for Figure 57.1. Aggression increased after 24 h with a sexually receptive female if the male received i.c.v. injection of CSF, the OT antagonist OTA, or the lowest dose (5 pg) of V_{1a} antagonist $d(CH_2)_5[Tyr(Me)]AVP$ ($F(7, 54) = 4.68$, $P = 0.0004$; CSF: Newman-Keuls post hoc comparison, $q_r = 8.97$, $P < 0.05$; 5 pg OTA: $q_r = 8.25$, $P < 0.05$; 5 pg V_{1a}: $q_r = 8.33$, $P < 0.05$). Males receiving all other doses of antagonist failed to increase aggressive behaviour above baseline frequency. Antagonist injection did not alter the number of males mounting females in the first 6 h (χ^2(d.f. = 7) = 2.186, $P = 0.945$; range = 62.5–83.3%) or frequency of mounts ($F(3, 19) = 0.82$, $P = 0.50$). (b) When given to breeder males with established aggression at baseline, $d(CH_2)_5[Tyr(Me)]AVP$ (5.0 ng, i.c.v.) had no effect on the number of attacks or threats ($F(2, 20) = 0.227$, $P = 0.80$). (c) After 24 h of

(continued on p. 896)

mating-induced aggression (Fig. 57.1). Males injected with a wide range of V_{1a} antagonist doses failed to exhibit aggression after 24 h with a sexually receptive female (minimum effective dose 50.0 pg i.c.v.) (Fig. 57.2a). This failure could not be attributed to blockade of mating, as reproductive behaviour was unaffected by any dose of the antagonist (see Fig. 57.2 legend). Furthermore, the V_{1a} antagonist did not seem to be anti-aggressive *per se*. Breeder males with established selective aggression showed no decrease in attack or threat behaviour either 1 or 24 h after i.c.v. injection of the antagonist (5.0 ng) (Fig. 57.2b). Thus, AVP antagonism seemed to block the transition to aggression, not its expression.

To determine if the V_{1a} antagonist blocked the development of selective affiliation as well as aggression, males were tested for a partner prefer-

ence after 24 h of mating. Injections and mating were as above, but after 24 h of mating each male was moved to the neutral cage of a three-chamber partner preference apparatus[13] with access to two adjoining cages, one with the mate (partner), the other with a novel female. Each female was loosely tethered to restrict movement out of her own cage. Males injected with CSF or OTA (5 ng, i.c.v.) before mating showed a significant preference for the mate 24 h later (Fig. 57.2c). After V_{1a} antagonist injection (5 ng, i.c.v.), males spent as much time with the stranger as the mate.

These results imply that physiological actions of endogenous AVP are essential for the induction of selective aggression and partner preference. But in initial studies in which we administered AVP (5–500 ng) as a single i.c.v. injection to sexually naive males, we observed no

mating, a partner preference was observed in males injected with either CSF ($t = 6.71, P = 0.0005$) or OTA ($t = 3.061, P = 0.03$), but not in d(CH$_2$)$_5$[Tyr(Me)]AVP ($t = 0.29$, NS) injected males. Treatment groups differed in time with the partner ($F(2, 16) = 4.09, P = 0.04$) and time with the stranger ($F(2, 16) = 4.21, P = 0.03$) due, in each case, to significant differences between the d(CH$_2$)$_5$[Tyr(Me)]AVP- and CSF-injected voles ($t_D = 2.86, P < 0.05$ in each case). Groups did not differ in activity as measured by number of entries into each of the chambers ($F(2, 16) = 0.54$, NS). *Methods.* Before exposure to sexually receptive females, sexually naive males were given a baseline intruder aggression test as described for Figure 57.1. Each male then received a single i.c.v. injection of either artificial CSF (BioFluids, Inc., Rockville, MD; $n = 13$); the OT antagonist OTA (Peninsula; $n = 8$)[23]; or the V_{1a} antagonist d(CH$_2$)$_5$[Tyr(Me)]AVP (Peninsula; $n = 6$–8 per dose).[24] *Ex vivo* studies after central injection of d(CH$_2$)$_5$[Tyr(Me)]AVP (50 ng, i.c.v.) demonstrated persistent blockade of AVP-receptor binding for 18 h in the vole brain (data available on request), a time course which agrees with previous behavioural data in hamsters,[25] our own behavioural data in voles (see figure 57.3b), as well as the time course of OTA activity.[26] Injections (2 µl) were given to halothane-anesthetized voles using a 30-G needle attached via polyethylene-20 tubing to a 10 µl Hamilton syringe. Because the vole skull is lightly calcified, injections could be reliably given percutaneously by using a cranial band for placement over the lateral ventricle.[27] To verify placement, each injection included 10% india ink (v/v) and staining of the entire ventricular system was required at necropsy for inclusion of behavioural data (< 10% rejected). After the injection, males were given sexually receptive females (ovariectomized and injected subcutaneously with 1.0 µg oestradiol benzoate for 2–4 days). Behaviour was recorded for the next 24 h with time-lapse videotaping. Females were then removed and males received a repeat intruder test. Aggression was scored as for figure 57.1. Reproductive behaviour scored from the time-lapse videotapes included latency to first mount and number of mounts. In an independent study, males ($n = 19$) were similarly injected with CSF, OTA or d(CH$_2$)$_5$[Tyr(Me)]AVP just before mating, and about 24 h later they were assessed for partner preference as previously described[13] by measuring time in partner's (that is, mate's), stranger's (novel sexually receptive female) or neutral (uninhabited) cage over 3 h using time-lapse videotaping with 12:1 reduction. Partner preference was assessed by a paired *t*-test comparing time in partner's versus time in stranger's cage for each treatment, followed by a between-subject's factorial ANOVA to compare treatment groups on each measure.

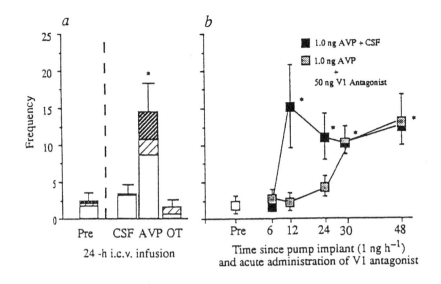

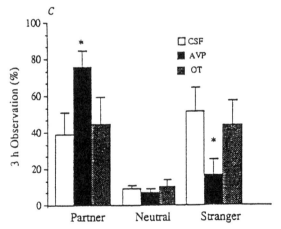

Figure 57.3
Central infusion of AVP increases aggression and induces partner preference. (a) After 24 h i.c.v. infusion of AVP (0.5 ng h^{-1}) but not CSF or OT (0.5 ng h^{-1}), aggression towards an intruder increases in male prairie voles. Groups did not differ before infusion (Pre), but in post-infusion resident–intruder tests, frequency of aggression was higher in AVP- than in either CSF- or OT-treated males ($F(2, 22) = 4.98$, $P = 0.02$). (Figure 57.1 legend; asterisk signifies $P < 0.05$ comparison with CSF). (b) In a separate study, aggression (attacks + threats) increased above baseline within 12 h of beginning AVP infusion (1.0 ng h^{-1}). Asterisk signifies significant ($P < 0.05$) difference from baseline (Pre) aggression. Administration of a V$_{1a}$ antagonist (50 ng, i.c.v.) at the start of infusion delayed the AVP-induced aggression by 18 h, yielding a temporal pattern significantly different from controls that received CSF i.c.v. instead of V$_{1a}$ antagonist i.c.v. at the start of AVP infusion ($F(5, 60) = 3.06$, $P < 0.05$). (c) In a third group, during central infusion of CSF, OT or AVP (0.5 ng h^{-1}), each male was housed with a non-receptive female "partner" for 24 h. In

(continued on p. 898)
(continued on p. 898)

increase in aggression (data not shown). As the effects of sociosexual experience seemed to be mediated over several hours and the clearance of centrally injected AVP has been reported to be within minutes,[15] a single injection of agonist may be insufficient to mimic physiological changes in AVP. To achieve prolonged elevated brain concentrations of peptide, we administered AVP (and OT) i.c.v. by osmotic mini-pump for 48 h to voles receiving neither sexual nor social experience. Males became aggressive after AVP (0.5 ng h^{-1}) but not after OT (0.5 ng h^{-1}) or CSF infusion (Fig. 57.3a). This dose of AVP increased AVP concentrations in the septum threefold (0.94 ± 0.29 pg per mg tissue versus 0.31 ± 0.10 pg per mg tissue comparing AVP and CSF group; $n = 9$) using a standard radioimmunoassay (kit from Peninsula) with microdissected tissue after a 24-h infusion. Aggression appeared with 12 h of starting AVP administration and seemed to be mediated via a V_{1a} receptor, as prior injection with the V_{1a} antagonist delayed the initiation of aggression by 18 h (Fig. 57.3b). The aggressive behaviour after AVP seemed to be qualitatively similar to that seen post-mating, although the intensity of attacks was slightly less with exogenous peptide, possibly due to the encumbrance of the mini-pump. Nevertheless, the data demonstrate that activation of the V_{1a} receptor is both necessary and sufficient for the development of selective aggression in the male prairie vole.

To determine if exogenous AVP also induced a partner preference, a separate group of males received i.c.v. infusion of AVP, OT or CSF by mini-pump while being housed with an ovariectomized (that is, non-receptive) female for 24 h. In a 3-h choice test, CSF- and OT-injected males showed no preference (spent roughly equal times in partner's cage and that of the novel female). Males injected with AVP (0.5 ng h^{-1}) spent 75.4% of the available time with the partner and 16.7% with the stranger (Fig. 57.3c). The groups did not differ on number of entries into the two cages ($F(2, 22) = 0.40$, not significant (NS)), suggesting that activity level was not affected by AVP.

Our results, implicating AVP in the development of selective aggression and partner preference, are consistent with recent data suggesting an important role for AVP in mediating parental behaviour in prairie voles.[8] Thus, it seems that AVP may be integral to several of the behaviours characterizing monogamous social organization in general and the process of pair bonding in particular. Studies in non-monogamous mam-

a subsequent preference test, CSF- and OT-treated males spent equal time with a novel female (stranger) and the partner ($t = 0.51$, NS and 0.17, NS for CSF and OT, respectively). AVP-infused males spent more time with the partner than the stranger ($t = 3.26$, $P = 0.01$), with a significant overall treatment difference in time with the partner ($F(2, 22) = 3.3$, $P = 0.05$) attributed to a difference between AVP- and CSF-treated males ($t_D = 2.38$, $P = 0.05$). *Methods.* AVP, OT or CSF was given to sexually naive males using a chronic i.c.v. infusion technique. Following a baseline resident–intruder test, voles were anaesthetized with chloropent (chloral hydrate (40 mg ml^{-1}) plus pentobarbital (10 mg ml^{-1})) (0.3 ml 100 g^{-1}) and stereotaxically fitted with a 25-G L-shaped cannula into the left lateral ventricle. The extra-cranial end of the cannula was fixed to the skull with dental cement and connected to PE20 tubing attached to an osmotic mini-pump (Alzet). The pump with attached tubing had been filled with CSF, OT or AVP (peptides from Peninsula) 18 h previously and primed by incubation in sterile saline at 37°C. After recovery from anaesthesia, males were returned to their home cages and tested for aggression towards an intruder at various times thereafter. In an initial study (a), AVP ($n = 9$), OT ($n = 8$) or CSF ($n = 8$) was administered via mini-pump and aggression was assessed 24 h later. In a second study (b), either CSF ($n = 6$) or d(CH$_2$)$_5$[Tyr(Me)]AVP (50 ng, $n = 6$) was administered through the cannula at the time of implantation to determine the time course and specificity of AVP effects. In a third study (c), males ($n = 25$) were implanted with pumps, housed with females for 24 h and then assessed for partner preference as described for figure 57.2.

mals have implicated AVP in social memory in rats,[10] territorial marking in hamsters[9] and aggression in mice.[16,17] There are also extensive data demonstrating AVP effects on memory and learning, thermoregulation, and grooming—effects with only an indirect relationship to affiliative behaviours, particularly in commonly used research animals such as rats and mice which do not pair bond (see, for instance, ref. 18). In a species that forms long-term selective bonds, however, memory of a mate, huddling for thermal comfort and grooming are important aspects of affiliation.

Our results are consistent with the hypothesis that the activation of central AVP pathways by mating is an essential neural correlate of pair bonding in the male prairie vole. Oxytocin and not AVP increases in CSF after ejaculation in the rat, a polygynous rodent,[19] whereas in male prairie voles AVP is apparently released after mating.[20] AVP secretion has previously been described with sexual arousal in human males,[21] but the extent to which any single peptide subserves any aspect of social bonding in humans remains entirely speculative.

References

1. Kleiman, D. G. *Q. Rev. Biol.* 52, 39–69 (1977).

2. Clutton-Brock, T. H. *Proc. R. Soc. Lond.* 236, 339–372 (1989).

3. Dewsbury, D. A. in *American Zoology Nebraska Symposium on Motivation* (ed. Leger, D. W.) 1–50 (Univ. Nebraska Press, Lincoln, 1988).

4. Getz, L. L., Carter, C. S. & Gavish, L. *Behav. Ecol. Sociobiol.* 8, 189–194 (1981).

5. Carter, C. S., Getz, L. L. & Cohen-Parsons, M. in *Advances in the Study of Behavior* (eds. Rosenblatt, J. S., Beer, C., Busnel, M. C. & Slater, P. J. B.) 109–145 (Academic, New York, 1986).

6. Insel, T. & Shapiro, L. *Proc. Natl. Acad. Sci. U.S.A.* 89, 5981–5985 (1992).

7. Insel, T. R. et al. *Regul. Peptides* 45, 127–131 (1993).

8. Bamshad, M., Novak, M. & De Vries, G. *J. Neuroendocr.* 5, 247–256 (1993).

9. Ferris, C. F., Albers, H. E., Wesolowski, S. M. & Goldman, B. D. *Science* 224, 521–523 (1984).

10. Dantzer, R., Bluthe, R.-M., Koob, G. F. & Le Moal, M. *Psychopharmacology* 91, 363–368 (1987).

11. Insel, T. R. *Psychoneuroendocrinology* 17, 3–33 (1992).

12. Miczek, K. A. & Winslow, J. T. in *Experimental Psychopharmacology* (eds. Greenshaw, A. J. & Dourish, C. T.) 27–113 (Humana, Clifton, New Jersey, 1987).

13. Williams, J. R., Catania, K. C. & Carter, C. S. *Horm. Behav.* 26, 339 (1992).

14. Jannett, F. J. *Biologist* 62, 3–19 (1980).

15. Jones, P. M. & Robinson, I. C. A. F. *Neuroendocrinology* 34, 297–302 (1982).

16. Roche, K. E. & Leshner, A. I. *Science* 204, 1343–1344 (1979).

17. Compaan, J. C., Buijs, R. M., Pool, C. W., de Ruiter, A. J. H. & Koolhaas, J. M. *Br. Res. Bull.* 30, 1–6 (1993).

18. De Wied, D., Elands, J. & Kovaks, G. *Proc. Natl. Acad. Sci. U.S.A.* 88, 1494–1498 (1991).

19. Hughes, A. M., Everitt, B. J., Lightman, S. L. & Todd, K. *Br. Res.* 414, 133–137 (1987).

20. Bamshad, M., Novak, M. & De Vries, G. *Soc. Neurosci. Abstr.* 18, 152.10 (Soc. for Neuroscience, Anaheim, California, 1992).

21. Murphy, M. R., Seckl, J. R., Burton, S., Checkley, S. A. & Lightman, S. L. *J. Clin. Endocr. Metab.* 65, 738–741 (1987).

22. Pierce, J. D. J., Pellis, V. C., Dewsbury, D. A. & Pellis, S. M. *Aggressive Behav.* 17, 337–349 (1991).

23. Elands, J. et al. *Eur. J. Pharmac.* 147, 197–207 (1987).

24. Kruszynski, M. et al. *J. Med. Chem.* 23, 364 (1980).

25. Ferris, C. F., Singer, E. A., Meenan, D. M. & Albers, H. E. *Eur. J. Pharmac.* 154, 153–159 (1988).

26. Witt, D. M. & Insel, T. R. *Endocrinology* 128, 3269–3276 (1991).

27. Popick, F. R. *Life Sci.* 18, 197–204 (1975).

58 Prior Exposure to Oxytocin Mimics the Effects of Social Contact and Facilitates Sexual Behaviour in Females

B. S. Cushing and C. S. Carter

Sexual reproduction in vertebrates involves species-specific social interactions. These interactions range from brief encounters between males and females lasting long enough for mating to occur, typical of many polygynous species, to the formation of life-long pair-bonds that characterize monogamy. Although the mechanisms responsible for the establishment of positive social behaviour remain largely unknown, there is growing evidence that the neuropeptide oxytocin plays a role in the initiation and maintenance of various mammalian social behaviours. Oxytocin can facilitate maternal behaviour (1, 2), social attachments (3), pair-bond formation (4), and sexual behaviour in both males (5–7) and females (8). Neuroendocrine processes underlie species-typical patterns of social and reproductive behaviours, and there appears to be a recurrent association between oxytocin and positive social interactions.

Much of the research on the neuroendocrinology of reproductive behaviour has been conducted in domestic laboratory animals, such as rats, that are polygynous. Research in rats has suggested that oxytocin facilitates sexual behaviour and that the actions of oxytocin depend on prior exposure to oestrogen (7–9). In rats oestradiol enhances the effects of oxytocin through the up-regulation of oxytocin receptors (OTR) (10). While this pattern is well established in rats the social consequences of exposure to oxytocin and the patterns of brain receptors for the peptide vary among species and social systems (11, 12).

Like most laboratory animals, rats have been artificially selected for their ability to mate in the absence of a complex social system. Research in animals with more complex social systems, for example monogamous rodents, such as prairie voles (*Microtus ochrogaster*), offer new perspectives regarding the behavioural effects of neuropeptides. The formation of long-term pair-bonds is a defining feature of monogamy and oxytocin plays a central role in pair-bond development in prairie voles (13). Unlike rats, in prairie voles central injections of oxytocin did not facilitate sexual receptivity in oestradiol-pretreated females (11), although oxytocin-treated females were more social and less aggressive. In addition, treatment with an oxytocin antagonist did not inhibit sexual activity (14). Finally, in contrast to most polygynous mammals, prairie voles do not experience a spontaneous oestrus cycle. In sexually naive female prairie voles social interaction with an unfamiliar male normally triggers an endocrine cascade that leads to social bonding and sexual behaviour. Social contact with, and urinary cues from, an unfamiliar male stimulates the release of gonadotropin-releasing hormone (GnRH) which leads to the release of luteinizing hormone (LH), which in turn leads to ovarian activation and the production of oestrogen, and the eventual induction of sexual receptivity (15–17). In prairie voles sexual receptivity usually occurs within 48 h of the initiation of extended contact with a novel male.

Although oestrogen is required to stimulate lordosis, the onset of behavioural oestrus and the threshold for responding to oestrogen can be modulated by the social history of the female; e.g. sexually experienced female prairie voles require a much lower threshold of exogenous oestradiol to stimulate sexual receptivity than do sexually naive females (18). Additionally, while male siblings do not induce sexual receptivity, extended contact with male siblings enhances subsequent female sensitivity to oestrogen, causing females to respond as if they were sexually experienced. Since social experience appears to have a direct effect on sexual activity and oxytocin is involved in regulating social interactions, we hypothesized that oxytocin might substitute for and/or mediate the effects of social experiences. Based upon the hypothesis that contact with a sibling male, like other forms of social behaviour, may be mediated by oxytocin, we further hypothesized that prior exposure to exogenous oxytocin would enhance sexual receptivity in females. To test this hypothesis we substituted injections of oxytocin for social contact with males. Since several days of cohabitation with male siblings were necessary to enhance the response of a female to oestrogen, females were given five daily injections of oxytocin prior to testing. Two experiments were conducted to test this hypothesis.

Materials and Methods

Animals

Animals in the study were third or fourth generation prairie voles derived from wild-caught animals originally captured near Urbana, Illinois. Animals were weaned at 21 days of age and housed in same-sex pairs in single-sex animal rooms. Animals were provided with Purina high fibre rabbit chow and water *ad lib.* and maintained on a 14 h:10 h light:dark cycle. All experimental females were sexually naive, no exposure to males since weaning, and were tested between 60 and 90 days of age. Sexually experienced males were used as stimulus animals. Females were randomly assigned to experiments and treatment groups.

Procedures

Experiment 1

Experiment 1 was designed to determine whether pretreatment with oxytocin would increase the probability of females mating or decrease the latency to mate in females that were placed with males and allowed to come into natural oestrus. Beginning 6 days prior to testing females were either handled once a day (n = 15) or received either s.c. injection of isotonic saline (50 μl)

(n = 14) or 20 μg of oxytocin (in 50 μl of isotonic saline) (n = 17) for 5 days. On the sixth day females were placed in a transparent cage (29 × 19 × 12.7 cm) with a sexually experienced male. Behaviour was then monitored for at least 48 h by time lapse video recording using a 12:1 reduction. Forty-eight h was chosen because it represents a length of time greater than the previously reported latency to mate in prairie voles (19). Video tapes were later scored by experimentally-blind observers, who had demonstrated at least a 95% inter-observer reliability. The number of pairs mating and the latency to mate were recorded. Nine pairs that did not mate (three oxytocin + three of each type of control) were monitored for an additional 24 h. The two control groups did not differ (six of 14 saline *versus* six of 15 handled controls mated); therefore these data were combined for analysis (control, Fig. 58.1). The likelihood of mating was compared using a 2 × 2 Contingency χ^2, while latency to mate was analysed using an unpaired *t*-test.

Experiment 2

Experiment 2 was designed to determine whether prior treatment with oxytocin enhances subsequent sensitivity of females to exogenous oestradiol. Females were assigned to one of six treatments; n = 8 per group. As described in experiment 1, four of the groups received a daily s.c. injection of either 20 μg of oxytocin (in 50 μl of isotonic saline) or isotonic saline (50 μl) for 5 days. Beginning 1 day after the fifth injection of oxytocin or saline females received a s.c. injection, once a day for 2 days, of either 0.5 μg oestradiol benzoate (OB) (in 50 μl of sesame oil) or sesame oil only. The groups were intact females receiving oxytocin followed by 2 days of oil (oxytocin/OIL), saline followed by OB (SAL/OB), or oxytocin followed by OB (oxytocin/OB), or ovariectomized (OVX) females receiving oxytocin followed by OB (OVX/oxytocin/OB). An additional two groups received only the OB in-

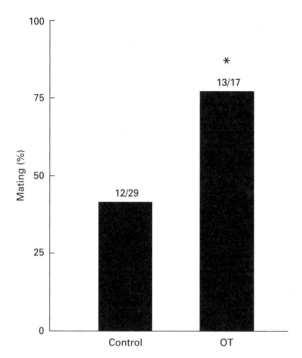

Figure 58.1
Shows the percentage of control versus oxytocin-pretreated females that mated during a 48 h cohabitation period with a male. Oxytocin-pretreated females were significantly more likely to mate than females that did not receive oxytocin. * Significantly different from the control group ($P < 0.05$).

jections; one was OB and the other was OVX (OVX/OB). Ovariectomies were performed under anaesthesia and aseptic conditions at least 14 days prior to testing. The dose of OB was selected based upon previous studies showing that this low dose stimulates sexual receptivity in sexually experienced females, but not sexually naive females (20, 21). One day after the second OB or oil injection each female was placed with a sexually experienced male for 15 min. If a female did not mate during this period she was placed with a second male for another 15 min. This methodology has been previously shown to effectively index sexual receptivity in oestrogen-primed females (20, 22). More than 80% of the

females that mated did so with the first male. The percentages of females that showed lordosis during either test are reported here. Data were analysed using a Contingency χ^2 test.

Results

Experiment 1

Experiment 1 tested the capacity of oxytocin to influence subsequent responses to endogenous reproductive hormones. Sexually naive females were pretreated with oxytocin (n = 17), isotonic saline (n = 14), or handled only (n = 15) and then placed with an unfamiliar male and allowed to come into natural oestrus. There was no difference between control groups (six of 14 saline versus six of 15 handled) so these data were combined for analysis. Females that had received prior treatment with oxytocin were significantly more likely to come into behavioural oestrus and mate than were control females ($\chi^2 = 5.32$, df = 1, P < 0.05) (Fig. 58.1). However, of the females that did mate, there was no difference in the latency to mate between the two groups (oxytocin mean = 38.7 ± 4.37 h; control mean = 35.02 ± 6.9 h, t = 1.60, df = 23, ns). None of the nine pairs that did not mate within 48 h, and were videotaped for an additional 24 h, mated during this additional time. This suggests that if mating does not occur within the 48 h it is unlikely to occur within the next day.

Experiment 2

Experiment 2 tested the capacity of oxytocin to influence the subsequent response of sexually naive females to exogenous oestradiol benzoate (OB). As previously reported (20), treatment with OB (0.5 µg) did not enhance sexual receptivity in sexually naive females. There were no significant differences in the occurrence of sexual behaviour between females that received oxytocin followed by oil (oxytocin/OIL) or saline followed by OB (SAL/OB), or females that received only OB ($\chi^2 = 0.0$, df = 1, ns; $\chi^2 = 2.59$, df = 1, ns, respectively). Pretreatment with oxytocin increased the sensitivity of females to subsequent effects of OB; females treated with oxytocin followed by OB were significantly more likely to display lordosis than females that received OB only or saline pretreatments ($\chi^2 = 15.0$, df = 1, P < 0.01; $\chi^2 = 4.27$, df = 1, P < 0.05). This effect was seen in both OVX and gonadally intact females (Fig. 58.2). These results support the hypothesis that in female prairie voles prior exposure to oxytocin, even in the absence of social contact, can facilitate sexual receptivity, probably by increasing sensitivity to oestrogen. These data also support the more

general hypothesis that oxytocin can mimic the behavioural effects of social experience.

Discussion

The present results suggest that in prairie voles the willingness of a female to mate, which is modulated by the social history of the female, can also be mediated by prior exposure to oxytocin. This study differs from those in rats in which oxytocin was given following exposure to oestrogen and immediately prior to behavioural testing. In rats oxytocin can cause the release of follicle stimulating hormone (FSH) and LH (23), which in turn may increase the production of ovarian steroids, or can act centrally to replace or enhance the effects of progesterone (24). However, progesterone is not necessary for sexual receptivity in prairie voles (25). The absence of a difference between intact and OVX females indicates that in prairie voles the release of endogenous gonadal hormones is not essential for the actions of oxytocin to occur. It is unlikely that the behavioural effects of oxytocin are a direct effect of the peptide at the time of testing, because oxytocin has a half-life of minutes (26), and here the oxytocin treatments were stopped several days prior to testing.

The effects of oxytocin described in this study were seen following peripheral (s.c.) administration of oxytocin, and fall within the range of doses used in other studies (23, 27). These findings suggest that s.c. administration of oxytocin can trigger many of the same responses that occur following the release of or administration of oxytocin within the central nervous system (CNS) (27–30). While this study did not directly address the mechanism of the action of oxytocin, this peptide could be acting directly on the CNS or through effects on peripheral tissues. Although it is generally assumed that systemic oxytocin does not readily cross the blood–brain-barrier, a small fraction of peripherally injected oxytocin does reach the brain (26, 31–33); thus, the

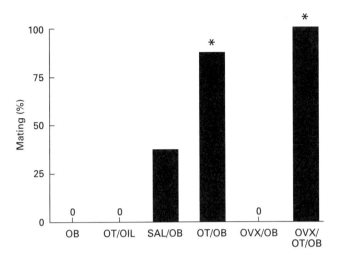

Figure 58.2
Pretreatment with oxytocin (OT) increased the probability that females would mate, as indexed by lordosis, when treated with low doses of oestradiol benzoate (OB). Data are shown as the percentage of females in each group that mated when placed with a sexually experienced male. The test groups reported here include intact females that received only OB; oxytocin followed by oil (oxytocin/OIL); saline followed by OB (SAL/OB); oxytocin followed by OB (oxytocin/OB); or ovariectomized females that received only OB (OVX/OB); or oxytocin followed by OB (OVX/oxytocin/OB). More than 80% of the females that mated did so with the first male, oxytocin alone did not facilitate lordosis and only females pretreated with oxytocin followed by OB showed a significant increase ($P < 0.05$) in lordosis compared to females treated with OB only. * Significantly different from OB treatment.

observed behavioural changes might reflect the effects of oxytocin on the CNS. In addition, peripherally-injected oxytocin may influence behaviour through actions on peripheral tissues. For example, oxytocin could be stimulating uterine/cervical contractions, which in turn could feed back to the nervous system to facilitate sexual responses. This idea is supported by research in rats in which the effects of oxytocin on female sexual receptivity were blocked by removal of the uterus or by severing its afferent neurons (34). Prairie voles have unusually high levels of corticosterone (35) and oxytocin has been shown to acutely reduce corticosterone levels in prairie voles (36). High levels of stress hormones may inhibit various aspects of reproduction, and either socially-induced and/or oxytocin-induced

reductions in circulating glucocorticoids might indirectly increase the sensitivity of females to oestradiol. However, measurements of corticosterone levels in females receiving oxytocin treatments comparable to those used here did not indicate that glucocorticoids were lowered by prior exposure to peripheral oxytocin, at least at the time of behavioural testing.

In prairie voles sexual maturity is only achieved after exposure to a novel male, and oestrus occurs at concentrations of oestradiol that are much lower than those reported in other species (20). A significant component of sexual maturity is the ability to respond to naturally occurring levels of sex steroids. Therefore, completion of puberty in prairie voles is tied to exposure to males and may be oxytocin-dependent.

It is possible that oxytocin plays a similar role in the onset of puberty in species that experience a spontaneous oestrous cycle. For example, in cultured bovine ovarian tissue oxytocin facilitated the production of oestrogens and progesterone in granulosa cells (37). However, once puberty has been completed oxytocin may no longer be necessary.

In conclusion, the present results support the hypothesis that oxytocin not only has an important role in social behaviour, but that it also plays a role in the integration of species-typical social and sexual responses. Additionally, the behavioural effects of oxytocin described in this study were apparent several days following oxytocin treatment, and appear to have been mediated by changes in sensitivity to oestrogen.

Acknowledgements

We wish to thank Nancy Cushing for her help with this project and comments on the manuscript. All work was conducted within OPRR and USDA guidelines and under protocols approved by the University of Maryland Animal Care and Use Committee. This research was supported by grants from the National Institutes of Health (HD 32675 and MH 01050) to CSC.

References

1. Keverne EB, Kendrick KM. Oxytocin facilitation of maternal behavior in sheep. *Ann NY Acad Sci* 1992; 652:83–101.

2. Pedersen CA, Ascher JA, Monroe YL, Prange AJ Jr. Oxytocin induces maternal behavior in virgin female rats. *Science* 1982; 216:648–649.

3. Carter CS. Neuroendocrine perspectives on social attachment and love. *Psychoneuroendocrinology* 1998; 23:779–818.

4. Carter CS, DeVries AC, Getz LL. Physiological substrates of mammalian monogamy: the prairie vole model. *Neurosci Biobehav Rev* 1995; 19:303–314.

5. Arletti R, Benelli A, Bertolini A. Oxytocin involvement in male and female sexual behavior. *Ann NY Acad Sci* 1992; 652:180–193.

6. Carter CS. Oxytocin and sexual behavior. *Neurosci Biobehav Rev* 1992; 16:131–144.

7. Witt DM. Regulatory mechanisms of oxytocin-mediated sociosexual behavior. *Ann NY Acad Sci* 1997; 807:287–301.

8. Caldwell JD, Prange AJ, Pedersen CA. Oxytocin facilitates the sexual receptivity of estrogen-treated female rats. *Neuropeptides* 1986; 7:175–189.

9. McCarthy MM, Kleopoulos SP, Mobbs CV, Pfaff DW. Infusion of antisense oligodeoxynucleotides to the oxytocin receptor in the ventromedial hypothalamus reduces estrogen-induced sexual receptivity and oxytocin receptor-binding in the female rat. *Neuroendocrinology* 1994; 59:432–440.

10. Johnson AE, Coirini H, Ball GF, McEwen BS. Anatomical localization of the effects of 17β-estradiol on oxytocin receptor binding in the ventromedial hypothalamus nucleus. *Endocrinology* 1989; 124:207–211.

11. Witt DM, Carter CS, Walton DM. Central and peripheral effects of oxytocin administration in prairie voles (*Microtus ochrogaster*). *Pharmacol Biochem Behav* 1990; 37:63–69.

12. Insel TR, Young L, Wang Z. Molecular aspects of monogamy. *Ann NY Acad Sci* 1997; 807:302–316.

13. Williams JR, Insel TR, Harbaugh CR, Carter CS. Oxytocin centrally administered facilitates formation of a partner preference in female prairie voles (*Microtus ochrogaster*). *J Neuroendocrinol* 1994; 6:247–250.

14. Witt DM, Carter CS, Insel TRJ. Oxytocin receptor binding in female prairie voles: endogenous and exogenous oestradiol stimulation. *J Neuroendocrinol* 1991; 3:155–161.

15. Dluzen DE, Ramirez VD, Carter CS, Getz LL. Male vole urine changes luteinizing hormone-releasing hormone and norepinephrine in female olfactory bulb. *Science* 1981; 212:573–575.

16. Carter SC, Witt DM, Schneider J, Harris ZL, Volkening D. Male stimuli are necessary for female sexual behavior and uterine growth in prairie voles (*Microtus ochrogaster*). *Horm Behav* 1987; 21:74–82.

17. Carter SC, Witt DM, Manock SR, Adams KA, Bahr JM, Carlstead K. Hormonal correlates of sexual behavior. *Physiol Behav* 1989; 46:941–948.

18. Morgan L, Hite RF, Cushing BS. Exposure to male siblings facilitates the response to estradiol in sexually naive female prairie voles. *Physiol Behav* 1997; 61:955–956.

19. Roberts RL, Cushing BS, Carter CS. Intraspecific variation in the induction of female sexual receptivity in prairie voles. *Physiol Behav* 1998; 64:209–212.

20. Cushing BS, Hite R. Effects of estradiol on sexual receptivity, wheel-running behavior, and vaginal estrus in virgin prairie voles. *Physiol Behav* 1996; 60:829–832.

21. Cushing BS, Marhenke S, McClure PA. Estradiol concentration and the regulation of locomotor activity. *Physiol Behav* 1995; 58:953–956.

22. Carter CS, Witt DM, Auski T, Casten L. Estrogen and the induction of lordosis in the female and male prairie voles (*Microtus ochrogaster*). *Horm Behav* 1987; 21:65–73.

23. Evans JJ, Robinson G, Catt KJ. Gonadotrophin-releasing activity of neurohypophysial hormones: I. Potential for modulation of pituitary hormone secretion in rats. *J Endocrinol* 1989; 122:99–106.

24. Gorzalka BB, Lester GL. Oxytocin-induced facilitation of lordosis behaviour in rats is progesterone-dependent. *Neuropeptides* 1987; 10:55–65.

25. Dluzen DE, Carter CS. Ovarian hormones regulating sexual and social behaviors in female prairie voles (*Microtus ochrogaster*). *Physiol Behav* 1979; 23:597–600.

26. Engelmann M, Wotjak CT, Neumann I, Ludwig M, Landgraf R. Behavioral consequences of intracerebral vasopressin and oxytocin: focus on learning and memory. *Neurosci Biobehav Rev* 1996; 20:341–358.

27. Liberzon I, Trujillo KA, Akil H, Young EA. Motivational properties of oxytocin in the conditioned place preference paradigm. *Neuropsychopharmacology* 1997; 17:353–359.

28. Argiolas A, Gessa GL. Central functions of oxytocin. *Neurosci Biobehav Rev* 1991; 15:217–231.

29. McCarthy MM, Kow LM, Pfaff DW. Speculations concerning the physiological significance of central oxytocin in maternal behavior. *Ann NY Acad Sci* 1992; 652:70–82.

30. Petersson M, Alster P, Lundeberg T, Uvnäs-Moberg K. Oxytocin causes a long-term decrease of blood pressure in female and male rats. *Physiol Behav* 1996; 60:1311–1315.

31. Mens WBJ, Witter A, van Wimersma Greidanus TB. Penetration of neurohypophyseal hormones from plasma into cerebrospinal fluid (CSF): half-times of disappearance of these neuropeptides from CSF. *Brain Res* 1983; 262:143–149.

32. Ermish A, Rühle HJ, Landgraf R. Hess J. Blood-brain-barrier and peptides. *J Cerebral Blood Flow Metabol* 1985; 5:350–357.

33. Kendrick KM, Keverne EB, Baldwin BA, Sharman DF. Cerebrospinal fluid levels of acetylcholinesterase, monoamines and oxytocin during labour, parturition, vaginocervical stimulation, lamb separation and suckling in sheep. *Neuroendocrinology* 1986; 44:149–156.

34. Moody KM, Steinman JL, Komisaruk BR, Adler NT. Pelvic neurectomy blocks oxytocin-facilitated sexual receptivity in rats. *Physiol Behav* 1994; 56:1057–1060.

35. DeVries AC, DeVries MB, Taymans SE, Carter CS. The modulation of pair bonding by corticosterone in female prairie voles (*Microtus ochrogaster*). *Proc Natl Acad Sci USA* 1995; 92:7744–7748.

36. DeVries AC, Cho MM, Cardillo LL, Carter CS. Oxytocin can suppress the HPA axis in prairie voles. *Soc Neurosci* 1997; 22:1851.

37. Sirotkin AV, Nitray JJ. The interrelationships between nonapeptide and steroid-hormone secretion by bovine granulosa-cells *in vitro*. *Steroid Biochem Mol Biol* 1992; 43:529–534.

Psychological State and Mood Effects of Steroidal Chemosignals in Women and Men

Suma Jacob and Martha K. McClintock

Although behavioral pheromones are well established in many invertebrate and vertebrate species (for recent review, see McClintock, 2000), we have evidence in humans for only priming pheromones which regulate endocrine function (Stern and McClintock, 1998). According to the classic definition, pheromones are airborne chemical signals produced by an individual of a species that trigger a neuroendocrine response or control behavior, endocrine state, or development in another member of the same species (Karlson and Luscher, 1959). Despite the lack of isolated chemicals that fulfill these criteria, there is a popular notion that human behavioral pheromones exist, and many companies market fragrances purported to contain pheromones.

To date, human behavioral pheromone research has been conceptually limited to identifying releasing pheromones, chemosignals that trigger specific emotional and/or behavioral responses. The focus has been on sociosexual behaviors comparable to sex attraction in silkworm moths, hamsters, and rhesus monkeys (Michael, Keverne, and Bonsall, 1971; Schneider, 1974; Singer, 1991; Singer, Macrides, Clancy, and Agosta, 1986; Wood, 1998) and mating reflexes in pigs and rats (Sachs, 1999; Signoret, Baldwin, Fraser, and Hafez, 1975). With primates, Michael and colleagues promoted the concept that some chemosignals are releaser pheromones and used the term "copulin" for vaginal aliphatic acids which putatively triggered sexual behavior of male rhesus monkeys (Michael et al., 1971). Later, it was argued that these compounds were neither sufficient nor necessary for copulation in this species, particularly when the rhesus monkeys were not confined to a small enclosure (Goldfoot, Kravetz, Goy, and Freeman, 1976). Likewise, aliphatic acids did not increase intercourse rates when human married couples were studied in their homes (Morris and Udry, 1978)

nor did they change aspects of social behavior (Cowley, Johnson, and Brooksbank, 1991).

In another study, it was reported that women were more likely to have intercourse if they wore extract of women's axillary secretions, pooled from across all phases of the menstrual cycle (Cutler, 1987; Cutler and Stine, 1988). Similarly, an unidentified compound is reported to increase sociosexual activity of male subjects (Cutler et al., 1998; critiqued by Preti and Wysocki, 1999). In neither case did researchers examine whether these were chemosignals simply operating by learned associations with consciously perceived odors, nor did they determine whether it was the subjects themselves or their partners who were affected, making it difficult to investigate their sex specificity and mechanism of action.

Another line of research has investigated the effects of animal pheromones on human behavior. Androstenone, a 16-androstene steroid, is a behavioral releaser pheromone in swine; it is present in boar saliva and triggers an immobile mating stance in the gilt. It and its related compound, androstenol, are present in human sweat and urine. This led many researchers to speculate about the roles of these steroids in human social interactions (reviewed by Gower and Ruparelia, 1993). A variety of human behaviors in the presence of androstenol have been reported, yet they do not create a coherent picture. Androstenol increased the number of conversations that women reported having with men (Cowley et al., 1991) and companies market fragrances with it claiming that "the pheromone" increases women's interest in sex. In marked contrast, others report that it decreases women's sense of their own attractiveness and depresses their mood (Filsinger, Fabes, and Hughston, 1987), as does living near a pig farm, a natural source of these steroids (Schiffman, Miller, Suggs, and Graham, 1995a).

At the high concentrations in these studies, the odor of androstenol or androstenone was consciously detectable, confounding any interpretation that these steroids act simply as pheromones and not as odors (Doty, 1981; Grammer, 1993; Schaal and Porter, 1991). The idea that olfaction and conscious odor associations may mediate these reported effects is supported by the fact that groups of subjects who found the odor of androstenol unpleasant versus those who found it pleasant often reported diverging behavior (Filsinger, Braun, and Monte, 1985; Filsinger, Braun, and Monte, 1990; Gilbert and Wysocki, 1987; Kirk-Smith, Booth, Carroll, and Davies, 1978). Furthermore, recent work in domestic pigs shows that the vomeronasal organ (VNO), a pheromone detection organ, is not necessary for the detection of androstenone or the production of sexual behavior associated with androstenone in estrous females (Dorries, Adkins Regan, and Halpern, 1997). Since olfactory sensitivity to androstenone is sexually dimorphic in the pig, these releaser pheromone effects may be mediated via the olfactory system. This illustrates the controversy surrounding the role of the vomeronasal versus the olfactory system in the processing of pheromonal chemicals in animals as well as humans. Therefore, based on our current understanding, it is neither necessary nor sufficient to define a pheromone according to its actions via the vomeronasal system.

Nonetheless, putative human pheromones have been identified based on scientific claims about their effects on the human vomeronasal organ (Berliner, 1994; Monti-Bloch and Grosser, 1991; Monti-Bloch, Jennings-White, Dolberg, and Berliner, 1994). In particular, two steroids have been isolated from human skin (Berliner, 1994; Preti and Wysocki, 1999) and identified because of their sex-specific and sex-exclusive effects on the surface potential of the human vomeronasal epithelium and not on the olfactory epithelium when delivered by intranasal cannula (Monti-Bloch and Grosser, 1991). Compound ER-670 (later revealed to be Δ4,16-androstadien-3-one in U.S. Patent No. 5,278,141) only affected women by increasing their VNO surface potential almost sixfold compared to the effects of control substances (propylene glycol or clove oil), whereas compound ER-830 (1,3,5,(10),16-estratetraen-3-ol in the same patent) affected just men by producing a similar ninefold increase. These and other patented steroids were also reported to change skin conductance and temperature as well as increase the percentage of alpha wave cortical activity (Monti-Bloch et al., 1994). Although little else is known about estratetraenol, Δ4,16-androstadien-3-one belongs to the odorous 16-androstene steroid family and is part of the steroid metabolic pathway in the adrenals or gonads. It also can be measured in peripheral plasma of men and women at 98 and 36 ng/100 ml, respectively (Brooksbank, Brammall, Cunningham, Shaw, and Camps, 1972).

Surface potential changes in the putative VNO have been cited as an indicator of the mechanism by which these steroids affect psychosocial behavior (Kodis, Moran, and Houy, 1998). However, we fully recognize that whether humans have a functional vomeronasal system remains highly controversial and inconclusive (Dulac and Axel, 1995, 1998; Preti and Wysocki, 1999). An epithelial surface potential is not necessarily a receptor potential, nor is the goal of our study to provide evidence that humans have a functional vomeronasal system in addition to the olfactory system. Our work does, however, provide a specific starting point for determining whether these two steroids have sex-exclusive effects on psychological state and whether these effects are related to conscious chemosensory processing. Even if these steroids ultimately fail to fulfill an eventual set of criteria required of human pheromones, this research contributes to a better understanding of the effects of steroids and chemical signals affecting mood and psychological state.

Our experiments sought to test whether two specific steroids could modulate aspects of mood, psychopharmacological "drug-like" states, or physical state. We believe it unlikely that human chemosignals or pheromones would be an aphrodisiac chemical signal bearing an irresistible or urgent message, although most previous research has been limited to such a narrow view. Few aspects of human behavior are triggered or "released" in such a stereotyped way by any sensory signal. Instead, human behavior is complex and highly dependent on learning and the context of the social and physical environment, as are the pheromone systems of other mammals (McClintock, 1998, 2000). Moreover, even when a sensory signal is simple, human behavioral responses are rarely stereotyped. We cannot expect humans to behave like moths flying up the concentration gradient toward the desirable source.

Therefore, our working hypothesis was that if behavior-influencing, communicative chemosignals existed, they would activate basic human drive states or produce a generalized subcortical effect which changes the underlying tone or valence for perceiving external stimuli or interactions. In either case, the effects of these signals may be overridden by cortical inputs also controlling the behavioral response. Under this hypothesis, behavior is expected to be more weakly associated with chemosignals than psychological state. Direct effects on psychological state could be accomplished in several ways such as affecting particular neurotransmitter systems in the brain (similar to the psychoactive effects of specific drug classes), acting to activate or inhibit certain brain circuits involved in emotion or motivation, or by influencing arousal, attention, or memory biasing systems.

The hypothesis that emotional effects are mediated by specific neural circuits related to chemosensation is supported by the mammalian literature. Both vomeronasal and olfactory inputs project to regions of the amygdala and hypothalamus in several species (Risold and Swanson, 1995; Wysocki and Meredith, 1987). Both brain areas are closely related to changes in emotional tone (Aggleton, 1993). They also play a primary role in the regulation of physical states such as

body temperature, autonomic nervous system tone, appetite, and reproductive function. Thus, investigating changes in emotional state as well as a variety of somatic states is fundamental for characterizing the full range of potential effects that these steroids might produce.

Since there are no peer-reviewed studies on the behavioral effects of these steroids, we used the psychopharmacological battery which is the best-known model for studying the psychological effects of specific compounds on behavior. Researchers have already used psychopharmacological or neuropsychological test batteries to examine the effects of steroid treatments (Fingerhood, Sullivan, Testa, and Jasinski, 1997; Hines and Sandberg, 1996; Schmidt, Nieman, Danaceau, Adams, and Rubinow, 1998). Research on pharmacological agents has already established reliable and valid methods to determine whether the psychological effects of a chemical substance are similar to those of specific classes of psychoactive drugs. Therefore, we used these existing methodologies to determine whether the steroids of interest have effects similar to those of pharmacological agents operating via specific neurotransmitter systems. This is a novel approach for examining psychological effects of potential signals for natural human chemical communication. In sum, our goal was to determine whether these steroids have detectable drug-like or emotional effects, and if they released simple, sex-specific emotional or somatic behavior within a laboratory or everyday context.

We examined whether androstadienone or estratetraenol affected the psychological state or mood of men and women. These steroids are reported to have sex-exclusive effects on the brain: the male-typic steroid (androstadienone) affects only women and the female-typic steroid (estratetraenol) affects only men (Berliner, 1994; Monti-Bloch and Grosser, 1991; Monti-Bloch et al., 1994). This sex specificity is typical of signals used by animals as part of sociosexual interactions between males and females (Agosta, 1992). Thus, we tested the hypothesis that these steroids have sex-specific effects on psychological state potentially involved in sociosexual interactions between men and women. If so, can these changes in psychological state be detected immediately, within minutes, or over a longer time course, within hours? We assessed the potential effects of androstadienone or estratetraenol on behavior using well-validated and standardized measures of: (1) specific emotions as well as mood states, (2) pharmacologically induced (drug-like) states, and (3) physical states.

Experiment 1

Methods

Participants

Twenty volunteers (10 women and 10 men) participated in a study which we described as investigating odorants, including compounds commercially marketed in perfumes. Participants were blind to our specific hypotheses and the identity of all compounds, although they were aware that they could receive control odors or chemicals used in perfumes. All were university students or staff 27.0 ± 1.5 years of age (range 20–48 years) and in good health, with no history of any respiratory or reproductive disease. Participants had no sinus problems while in the study and were not currently smokers. Their ethnic backgrounds were 65% White/Caucasian, 30% East or South Asian, and 5% Black/African American.

Carrier and Steroid Stimuli

We presented the same steroid compounds used to elicit surface potentials of the vomeronasal epithelium and that justified patent claims (U.S. Patent No. 5,278,141): Δ4,16-androstadien-3-one (A; 0.00025 M concentration in propylene glycol or PG) and 1,3,5,(10),16-estratetraen-3-ol (E; 0.00025 M concentration in PG), or carrier odorant alone (PG). We obtained these steroids from Steraloids, Inc., a company not affiliated with

patenting these steroids for perfume use. Standard purity of the steroids was determined by a single spot with thin-layer chromatography (approximately 98% pure, personal communication with Steraloids, Inc., NH). We chose propylene glycol as the carrier odorant and control stimulus because it was used in previous experiments with these steroids (Monti-Bloch and Grosser, 1991).

After finding that nasal sprays of propylene glycol caused discomfort, we decided to apply the odorants directly to the skin above the upper lip (as have other putative human pheromone studies: Preti, Cutler, Garcia, Huggins, et al., 1986; Russell, Switz, and Thompson, 1980; Stern and McClintock, 1998) as well as on the neck above the carotid area, where it was less likely to be wiped off and where perfumes are typically worn. This was done to cover several possible routes of detection which were ecologically valid and did not focus on the potential function of the vomeronasal organ. Participants were required to leave the stimulus on until they completed their last questionnaire.

To achieve compound concentration in the nasal cavity comparable to the studies on which patent claims were based, our fluid concentration was greater than those administered directly to the putative VNO by intranasal cannula (Monti-Bloch and Grosser, 1991). Our concentration also mitigated falsely accepting the null hypothesis because our concentrations were higher than those used in the Berliner (1994) and Monti-Bloch studies (1994). We applied approximately 9 nm of the steroid above the lip and under the nose of each participant. The application Q-tip was dipped into an Eppendorf tube containing 130 µl of either the control or the steroid solutions. The amount remaining above the lip of the participant was determined in a separate experiment using 28 solution applications performed by four different testers. By centrifuging the Q-tip after application, the total amount of solution left on the Q-tip and in the tube could be subtracted from the amount in the tube prior to

Descriptors	Total Number of Responses Made:					
	Androstadienone + PG		Estratetraene + PG		PG alone	
	Male	Female[a]	Male	Female	Male	Female[b]
☐ No Smell	7	6	8	8	6	8
▨ Chemical[c]	3	0	1	1	1	2
▧ Muskey Smell[d]	0	3	0	0	0	0
▧ Sweet/Sour/ Bitter	0	0	1	0	3	0
■ Floral	0	0	0	1	0	1

[a]one female did not respond
[b]one female reported both a chemical and a floral smell
[c]reported as "rubbing alcohol," "lighter fluid," "ammonia," and "dishwasher soap"
[d]reported as "musky," "clothes," or "like my male roommates"

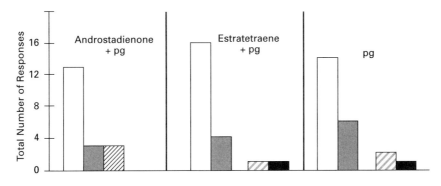

Figure 59.1
Smell association responses of 20 participants for androstadienone with propylene glycol (PG), estratetraene with PG, and PG alone.

application. The amount remaining on the participant was 35.8 ± 3.3 µl of a 0.00025 M steroid solution, approximately 9 nm of steroid.

Most participants reported that they could not smell the solutions, i.e., the carrier odorant propylene glycol with or without the nanomolar amounts of the steroids. In the carrier control session, "no smell" was reported by 60% of the males and 80% of the females (see Fig. 59.1). The six participants who reported that control carrier had an odor, described it as having faint or fleeting smells of rubbing alcohol, ammonia, medicine, vinegar, floral, or sweetness.

For the androstadienone solution, most participants again reported it had no smell (70% of the males and 66.7% of the females; see Fig. 59.1). Three male participants reported that the androstadienone in propylene glycol smelled faintly like rubbing alcohol, chemistry lab, or dish soap, whereas three females described the mixture as smelling slightly musky, "like a male roommate" or "clothes."

Most participants (80% of the males and 80% of the females) reported that they could not smell estratetraenol (Fig. 59.1). Two males said that the mixture of propylene glycol with estratetraenol reminded them of lighter fluid or sweets whereas two females described it to smell like rubbing alcohol or a faint floral scent. In this experiment, the sample size is not large enough to determine whether those detecting a smell had different psychological responses.

Design
We used a within-subjects design, with a randomized, double-blind treatment order. Participants were asked to come to our human subject room (75.1 $\pm$ 3°F with 15 room air changes per hour) for three sessions. All sessions were identical in procedure except for the testing solution that was used. At least 1 day intervened between each session for each subject.

Psychological Measures and Testing Procedures
We utilized the most well-established and validated scales available for assessing subjective effects of exogenous or drug-like substances on mood and psychological state (for reviews, see de Wit and Griffiths, 1991; Fischman and Foltin, 1991) in order to measure the impact of these steroids on psychological state. The following scales have considerable internal consistency, reliability, and have been utilized in a wide range of experimental designs.

POMS The Profile of Mood States (POMS, McNair, Lorr, and Droppleman, 1971) was originally developed as a fairly rapid assessment of transient and fluctuating affective states. POMS was selected because it is an established measure that is sensitive to mood changes related to olfactory cues (Schiffman, Sattely-Miller, Suggs, and Graham, 1995b), to drug-induced changes in mood (de Wit and Griffiths, 1991; Fischman and Foltin, 1991), to hormonal state influences (Kraemer, Dzewaltowski, Blair, Rinehardt, and Castracane, 1990), and to normal transient mood shifts in a wide range of circumstances (Cockerill, Nevill, and Lyons, 1991; Der and Lewington, 1990; Horswill, Hickner, Scott, Costill, and Gould, 1990; Lieberman, Corkin, Spring, Grow-

don, and Wurtman, 1982/83; Williams, Krahenbuhl, and Morgan, 1991).

The POMS scale we used in this study had 72 items in an adjective checklist format. Participants rate their current feelings at the moment on a scale from 0 ("not at all") to 4 ("extremely"). From this extensive checklist, previous research has empirically derived eight factors: Anxiety, Depression, Anger, Vigor, Fatigue, Confusion, Friendliness, and Elation.

ARCI The Addiction Research Center Inventory is a standardized questionnaire that contains 49 true/false statements (ARCI, Haertzen, 1974a, b). The questionnaire was originally developed to provide scales that distinguish the sensations and perceptions uniquely associated with specific drugs or classes of drugs (Bigelow, 1991; Fischman and Foltin, 1991). The ARCI has five empirically derived scales: the Morphine-Benzedrine Group (MBG) scale which reflects drug euphoria, the Lysergic Acid Diethylamide (LSD) scale which reflects drug dysphoria and mental confusion, the Pentobarbital-Chlorpromazine-Alcohol Group (PCAG) scale which measures level of sedation, the Amphetamine Group (A) which measures amphetamine-like stimulant effects, and the Benzedrine Group (BG) scale which measures stimulant-like effects or intellectual efficacy.

VAS Visual Analog Scales (VAS) are often used to assess momentary changes in affect (Folstein and Luria, 1973). We utilized an established scale used in psychopharmacological research (Brauer and de Wit, 1997; de Wit, Clark, and Brauer, 1997; Kirk, Doty, and de Wit, 1998; Zacny, Bodker, and de Wit, 1992) that measures participants' responses to six adjectives ("stimulated," "high," "anxious," "sedated," "down," and "hungry"). Participants made vertical marks on a horizontal line (100 mm) under each adjective to indicate how they felt at that moment, from "not at all" to "extremely."

Procedure

In order to measure immediate mood responses, participants filled out this battery of psychometric scales approximately 6 min after the odorant was initially applied while seated at a desk in the laboratory subject room. They were also asked how they felt, an open-ended question designed to elicit descriptors of their experience that were not included in the psychometric scales.

After they returned to their everyday lives, participants were to fill out the same battery at 2, 4, and 9 h after initial exposure to the solutions. Each participant was given three specific times of day to fill out the battery, corresponding to these intervals, and asked to do so as soon as possible after the specified time if inflexible activities intervened (e.g., driving). Compliance was excellent; participants completed their batteries at 2.4 ± 0.1, 4.5 ± 0.1, and 9.5 ± 0.3 h after initial exposure to the solutions.

Normalizing Data

One goal of our analyses was to test the time course of the responses. Response distributions from many subscales were significantly skewed to the right when assessed relative to time; scores from the early intervals were higher than later scores. To normalize the data, we did log transformations of the raw scores.

Because the various questionnaires used different response scales, we expressed all data as z-scores so that the subscale responses could be accurately compared with each other. In addition, this allowed us to standardize individual differences in scale use and typical mood level. Each participant's z-score for his or her response to a given steroid at a particular interval was calculated with reference to his or her four responses under the control condition. By graphing the distributions and calculating descriptive statistics, we confirmed that these transformed values formed a normal distribution, and that both log transformation and z-scoring were necessary steps in normalizing the data prior to doing any parametric statistics.

Data Reduction

Psychopharmacological studies using the POMS, ARCI, and VAS scales typically test each subscale for statistical significance and then make inferences based on robust patterns across all subscales. They report significant changes on several different subscales each measuring the same mood or state (e.g., Brauer and de Wit, 1997). Indeed, descriptive statistics and preliminary analyses of our data revealed robust patterns of mood changes for several subscales.

Nonetheless, other disciplines prefer limiting the number of statistical tests, which is accomplished by data reduction prior to targeted statistical analysis. We used factor analysis with varimax rotation, an empirical data-reduction method used widely in the social sciences. Factor analyses extract a small number of components by isolating clusters of highly intercorrelated variables as factors. Varimax rotation is a method of orthogonal rotation of the axes in a factor analysis which simplifies the factor structure.

First we identified the significant factors (components) in the entire set of all subscale scores from males and females obtained at all four intervals after application of the solutions. Because our focus was on potential differences caused by the presence of a steroid, we used a difference score, calculated by subtracting the steroid response from the carrier response, matching scores within each individual and at testing interval ($T = 21$ test variables; $S = 160$ testing sessions in which all these variables were used in the same test battery). We confirmed that the factors were virtually identical when we used the unnormalized, raw scores for each person at each interval ($T = 21$ test variables; $S = 240$ testing sessions in which all these variables were used in the same test battery), demonstrating that the same factors were manifest both in the difference in response and in the absolute responses to the steroids.

Three significant factors were identified based on eigenvalues greater than 1.00 as well as the

Table 59.1
Factor loadings (varimax rotation) of androstadienone and estratetranol with respect to control for women and men in Experiment 1

	Alertness (Factor 1)	Negative-Confused mood (Factor 2)	Positive-Stimulated mood (Factor 3)	
Eigenvalue	6.10501	2.07676	1.96475	
Rotated variable		Factor loadings[a]		Uniqueness
Vigor (POMS)	−0.60153	—	0.53482	0.18225
Sedative (PCAG-ARCI)	0.81354	—	—	0.15043
Sedated (VAS)	0.79618	—	—	0.23822
Intellectual efficacy (BG-ARCI)	−0.70299	—	—	0.15248
Fatigue (POMS)	0.52539	0.60098	—	0.16959
Confusion (POMS)	—	0.60896	—	0.3262
Dysphoric (LSD-ARCI)	—	0.62941	—	0.37598
Anger (POMS)	—	0.72781	—	0.32087
Depression (POMS)	—	0.78214	—	0.16417
Anxiety (POMS)	—	0.79909	—	0.25281
Euphoric (MBG-ARCI)	—	—	0.81916	0.11096
Elation (POMS)	—	—	0.78381	0.18829
Stimulant (A-ARCI)	—	—	0.69284	0.21098
Friendliness (POMS)	—	—	0.67724	0.28338

scree plot. The critical values for identifying significant rotated loading on a factor were set at < -0.500 and $> +0.500$ to ensure that Factors had only those subscales with the highest level of intercorrelation (Table 59.1). Factor 1 had an eigenvalue of 6.11 and was a composite measure of Alertness. Factor 2, with an eigenvalue of 2.08, was a measure of Negative-Confused mood and Factor 3, with an eigenvalue of 1.96, measured Positive-Stimulated mood.

Statistical Analyses
For each of the three factors, an unpaired t test was used to assess sex differences in participants' immediate response to a steroid when they were in the controlled setting of the laboratory. Sex differences in the long-term effects of exposure to steroids, while participants were in their natural everyday environments, were explored with a repeated-measures analysis of variance for responses at 2, 4, and 9 h after initial exposure. Analyses were done on each of the three factors with sex of participant as a between-subjects variable and treatment and time as within-subjects variables.

Results

Immediate Responses
When exposed to androstadienone, men and women had a significantly different response in Positive-Stimulated mood (Factor 3; $t = 2.22$, $P \leq 0.04$). Women experienced higher Positive-Stimulated mood in comparison to propylene glycol alone, while men reported lower levels (see Fig. 59.2). There were no significant sex differences in Negative-Confused mood responses nor in Alertness.

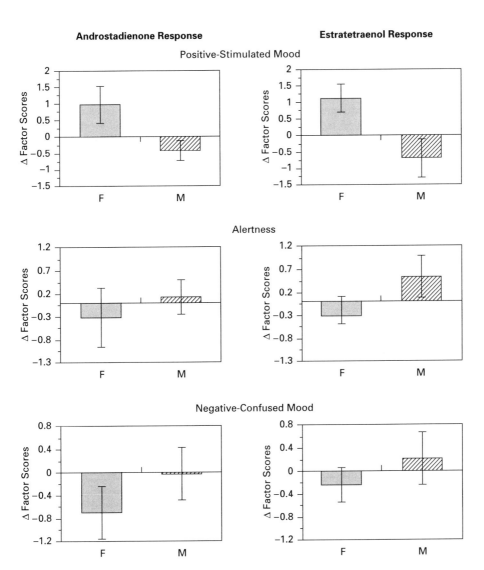

Figure 59.2
Factor scores ($\pm$ SEM) of the responses to steroids approximately 6 min after stimulus application within the lab for women versus men. Values on the ordinate represent the differential effect of treatment for each factor derived by factor analysis and varimax rotation (e.g., factor score under androstadienone condition—control factor score). A factor score is the mean of its component subscales, each expressed as a z-score (where 0 is each subject's average subscale response during the control condition).

When exposed to estratetraenol, men and women again had significantly different responses in Positive-Stimulated mood ($t = 2.55$, $P \leq 0.02$). Women again experienced higher Positive-Stimulated mood relative to their responses to propylene glycol, a finding not concordant with reports that women do not respond physiologically to estratetraenol on the surface potential of vomeronasal epithelium (Berliner, 1994; Monti-Bloch and Grosser, 1991; Monti-Bloch et al., 1994). Men experienced lower Positive-Stimulated mood (see Fig. 59.2) rather than the increase predicted by previous research. As with androstadienone, there was neither a significant difference in Negative-Confused responses nor a difference in Alertness. This pattern of sex differences in mood does not support a simple sex-specific or sex-exclusive model (Berliner, 1994; Monti-Bloch and Grosser, 1991; Monti-Bloch et al., 1994).

Long-Term Effects

When men and women were in a nonlaboratory setting, there were no significant differences in any of the three factors. For all three factors, there were: (a) no main effects of steroid, (b) no interactions with sex of participant, and (c) no interactions with time interval. Although no significant long-term effects were detected with these factors, a visual inspection of coherent sets of the subscales (Elation-POMS, Euphoric-MBG-ARCI, Stimulant-A-ARCI, and High-VAS) revealed that effects may extend beyond immediate exposure. For example, examining the stimulant or drug-high response revealed that women experienced a greater response with the steroids that did not decline until 4.5 h (see Fig. 59.3, Stimulant-A-ARCI and High-VAS), although men did not display any longterm effects (see Fig. 59.4). Future studies need to further examine these as well as other potential longer term effects, but the most robust effects appear to occur within minutes of steroid exposure measured in the laboratory.

Open-Ended Descriptors of Responses

When asked to describe how they felt after the compounds had been applied, 80% of women exposed to androstadienone stated they felt one or more of the following ways: warm, heavy, spacy, sharp, nauseous, or light-headed. When exposed to estratetraenol, 80% said they felt heavy, warm, chesty, irritable, or drowsy. Approximately 50% of the men felt warm or irritable after androstadienone exposure and 60% of men felt warm or stimulated with estratetraenol. When exposed to propylene glycol alone participants used these adjectives more rarely (only 5% used irritable and 40% used warm). Future research is needed to quantify these self reports of physical perceptions.

Discussion

Our results from Experiment 1 show that these steroids had an effect on aspects of Positive-Stimulated mood, and not on Negative-Confused mood or alertness. Emotional responses did not parallel the reported sex-specific physiological effects of the steroids on the vomeronasal epithelium of men and women (Berliner, 1994; Monti-Bloch and Grosser, 1991). Although our dependent measures have no direct link with the VNO, we purposely tested the identical compounds that were reported to have sex-specific effects: androstadienone, which activated only women's vomeronasal surface epithelium but not that of men, and estratetraenol which had the converse sex-specific effects. If the VNO were the only sensory pathway for chemosignals, one might hypothesize that androstadienone stimulus information only reaches the female brain and would produce psychological effects only in women, whereas estratetraenol would signal only to the male brain and produce exclusively male psychological changes. In contrast to this sex-specific hypothesis our results showed that women had Positive-Stimulated mood response to both androstadienone and estratetraenol

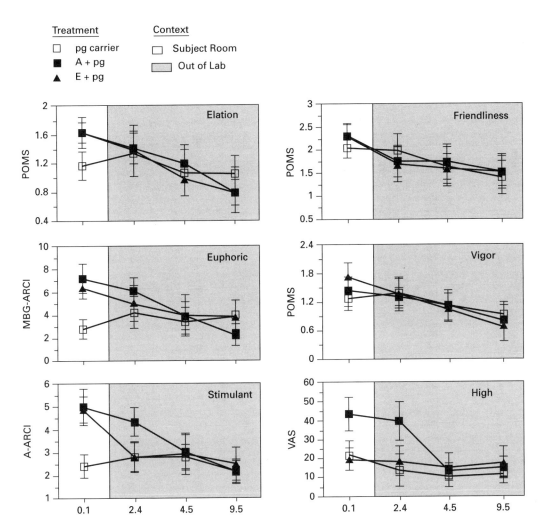

Figure 59.3
Time course of individual subscales included in Positive-Stimulated mood factor plus the High-VAS subscale for women ($M \pm$ SEM).

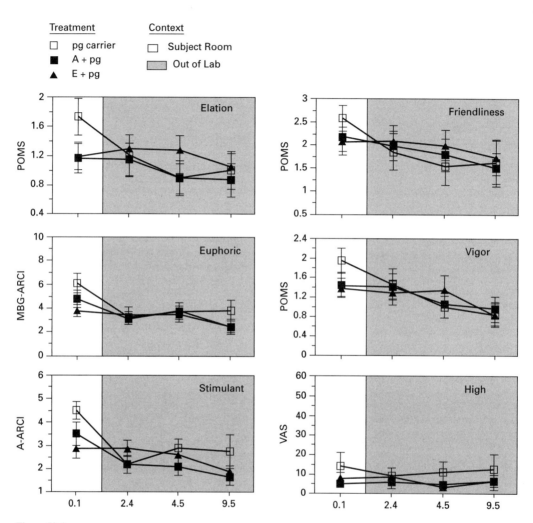

Figure 59.4
Time course of individual subscales included in Positive-Stimulated mood factor plus the High-VAS subscale for men ($M \pm$ SEM).

within 6 min of initial exposure. Similarly, the vomeronasal epithelium of men responded only to estratetraenol (Berliner, 1994; Monti-Bloch and Grosser, 1991). However, men also responded to androstadienone, with a decrease in Positive-Stimulated mood, a response different from that of women.

There are several possible explanations for the lack of parallel results. Differences in methodologies and procedures of our study could have precluded sex-specific effects. For example, we may have presented these steroids in a mode or concentration that affects additional and alternative sensory processing systems. Alternatively, our psychological measures could be more sensitive than measuring surface potential and thus the effects of estratetraenol on female vomeronasal epithelium and androstadienone on male epithelium may have gone undetected by previous methodologies. Finally, it is highly likely that both steroids could produce their psychological effects via systems that do not involve the vomeronasal organ, as with androstenone, the pig pheromone (Dorries et al., 1997).

At the low concentrations we used, most people could not verbalize differences in odors of the stimuli when they were presented on sequential days. Thus, our data suggest that chemical signals may not need to be detected consciously and identified as odors in order to exert their effects. The carrier-odor mask was weak and a few women subjects did verbally describe an odor when given androstadienone. This interpretation is consistent with the fact that women have superior olfactory acuity and ability to verbalize odors (Doty, Snyder, Huggins, and Lowry, 1981). Nonetheless, estratetraenol did alter Positive-Stimulated mood in a similar way without being detected as an odor. In order to control for odor effects while keeping the chemical concentration the same, the next experiment used a stronger odor as a mask to ensure that stimuli were verbally indistinguishable. Doing so was the only way to ensure that any psychological effects could not be attributed to conscious emotional associations with its odor.

Long-term mood effects were not significantly different for men and women but future studies should more closely examine long-term effects within each sex because our within-sex sample size is small. In addition, it may be that these compounds do modulate a specific circuit or aspect of brain function, but in the richer, more variable context of everyday life, other variables may have a more prepotent effect on determining experienced mood, despite unconscious responses to the stimuli.

Experiment 2

We now focused on the immediate response of women to androstadienone in order to replicate the findings from Experiment 1. In Experiment 2, we used more stringent controls and refined the experimental design. Our primary goal was to determine whether immediate mood changes in women were still evident when androstadienone was not subjectively detectable or distinguishable as an odor. Even though the nanomolar amounts of androstadienone used in our initial study were only detectable by 30% of the women, we wanted to prevent conscious detectability by masking androstadienone with the strong odor of clove oil in propylene glycol. If our androstadienone effects disappeared, this would indicate that the effects are more likely olfactory associations than specific pheromonelike influences and that future research should focus on learned emotional associations with the detectable odor of androstadienone. If effects were sustained even when the steroid was not olfactorily detectable, androstadienone may have effects on humans even when they are not aware of its presence. This would be comparable to other known examples of pheromonal phenomena in humans (Stern and McClintock, 1998) or to effects of unconscious olfactory processing (Kirk-Smith,

Van Toller, and Dodd, 1983). Despite the long-term interest in 16-androstenes as putative human pheromones, Experiment 2 is the first to investigate their effects using standardized psychological tests while their odor was masked and not verbally distinguished.

Noting individual differences in mood when subjects began our laboratory protocol, we added a measure of their baseline mood so we could measure the effects of androstadienone in terms of a change from each woman's mood when she began her testing session. In addition, we utilized stricter screening criteria, standardized sessions to same time of day within subjects to minimize effects of circadian rhythm, added additional visual analogue measures to test social emotions and open-ended responses from Experiment 1, and tested a larger sample of women to avoid incorrectly accepting the null hypothesis.

Methods

Participants
Thirty-one women participated and were blind to our hypotheses. They were told that we were studying changes in olfactory perception and psychological response within the menstrual cycle. The women were university students or staff with a mean age of 23 ± 1.2 years (range 18–48 years) and in good health, with no history of respiratory or reproductive disease, psychiatric illness, or current sinus problems. These women identified themselves exclusively as heterosexual on a sexual orientation checklist that included "heterosexual," "homosexual," "bisexual," or "other (please describe)" as choices. They were not smokers, 29 of them were nulliparous, and women were not excluded from the study if they had previously used hormonal birth control.

Masking Odor, Carrier, and Steroid Stimuli
We selected clove oil as the olfactory masking component because (1) it has been reported to have no effect on the surface potential of the vomeronasal organ (unlike androstadienone; Monti-Bloch and Grosser, 1991), (2) it is considered to be a botanical or natural odor rather than a synthetic or chemical odor, (3) it produces overall pleasant odor ratings, (4) it is not closely associated with perfume or cologne fragrances, and (5) it is a standard odor used to demonstrate normal olfaction (Dorries, Schmidt, Beauchamp, and Wysocki, 1989; Doty, McKeown, Lee, and Shaman, 1995). Therefore, we presented a 0.00025 M concentration of $\Delta4,16$-androstadien-3-one within a carrier odorant of 1% clove oil propylene glycol solution, or the 1% carrier odorant alone to the 31 women. We used the same method of presentation as in Experiment 1.

To validate our masking methods, we studied a larger sample of women, each in the periovulatory phase of her menstrual cycle when olfactory sensitivity is highest (Doty et al., 1981) in order to cover the full range of individual differences in ability to recognize verbally the odor of androstadienone. This sample of women was asked to describe the odor of two solutions when presented with approximately 36 μl above their upper lip at least 24 h apart: (1) clove oil + propylene glycol as the carrier (1:99 solution) and (2) this same odor carrier with androstadienone (250 μM concentration). The women were told that the solutions had complex odors and were encouraged to use as many descriptors as they needed to describe the odor.

The distribution of descriptors for the two solutions was essentially identical (see Fig. 59.5). Both were described almost exclusively in terms of food or plant smells, and occasionally as a chemical smell such as alcohol. Only 5% of descriptors referred to humans in any way (e.g., my grandmother's kitchen), and human sweat was mentioned in less than 4% of descriptors and then only as a qualifier. This was true whether or not the solutions contained androstadienone. Thus, we conclude that a 1% clove oil in propylene glycol solution successfully masked the verbally conscious attributes of androstadienone's odor when 9 nm was applied.

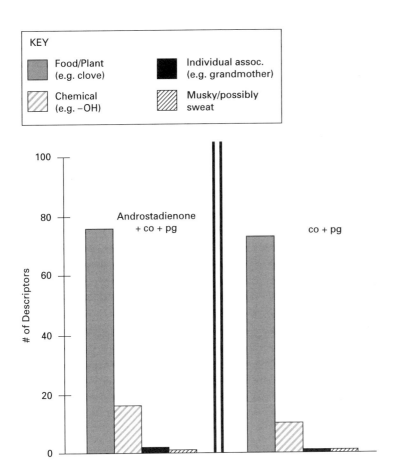

Figure 59.5
Odor profile summarizing the descriptors of masked olfactory stimuli with the larger sample of women in Experiment 2 under Methods ($N = 45$ women). Food/plant descriptions include spices, fruits, flowers, woods, or baked goods. Chemical descriptors include rubbing alcohol, lighter fluid, ammonia, and dishwasher soap.

Design

We used a within-subjects, double-blind design that was randomized for order of treatment administration. Participants were asked to come to our small human subject room (10×10 feet, $74.3 \pm 2°F$ with 15 air changes per hour) for sessions with at least 1 day between sessions. Sessions were identical in procedure, environment, and experimenter interaction except for the odorant solution used. Each participant was tested by the same tester. Three testers followed an identical protocol, adhered closely to a script, and demonstrated high interrater reliability.

Shortly after the participant arrived, she was seated at her own desk in the human subject room, approximately 4 feet from the tester. The tester administered the battery of psychological tests following a timed protocol, applied the odorant, and then administered the battery again at approximately 0.1 and 1 h after exposure to the odorant mixture. To decrease the effects of circadian rhythms and to control for related confounds, each participant had all sessions at the same time of day (± 1 h variation within subject, testing times occurred between 8 AM and 10 PM).

Once seated at her desk, the participant was allowed to read catalogues and nature magazines or play low-key computer games during the intervals when she was not doing activities required by the protocol. All participants were required to remain in the testing room throughout the 1-h testing interval. Nineteen participants (62%) also remained in the human subject room until after a battery of questionnaires 2 h postapplication. The other 12 participants, because of scheduling conflicts, were allowed to fill out their 2-h battery outside the laboratory after returning to their everyday lives (demarcated by gray shading in Figs. 59.7–59.9). This procedural difference had no significant statistical effects or interactions in our reported results.

Psychological Measures and Testing Procedures

To test our alternative hypotheses about the psychological effects of androstadienone, we utilized the same standardized psychometric tests from Experiment 1: (1) Profile of Mood States (POMS, McNair et al., 1971), (2) psychopharmacological mood state (Addiction Research Center Inventory, ARCI, Haertzen, 1974a, b), and (3) the original Visual Analog Scales (Brauer and de Wit, 1997; de Wit et al., 1997; Zacny et al., 1992).

We added a number of VAS items in order to test some of the open-ended descriptions from the first experiment and published anecdotal reports. Based on descriptors reported spontaneously by women in our initial experiment, we asked participants to respond to the following items: sociosexual perceptions ("social," "relaxed," and "sensual"), confidence and affiliative perceptions ("self-assured" and "open"), and physical or arousal states ("warm," "heavy," "nauseous," "light-headed," "irritated," "spacy," "sharp," "focused," and "energetic").

Menstrual Cycle Status

Menstrual cycle information was gathered for all 31 women based on dates of menses onset. Twelve of the women were also collecting detailed daily data on their basal body temperature, vaginal secretions, menses, and urinary LH measures. The other 19 women retrospectively reported the dates of menses onset. During their sessions, most women (74%) were in the periovulatory phase, 11% were in the preovulatory phase, and 15% were in the postovulatory phase. The effects of phase on psychological response were not investigated because of the asymmetric distribution of cycle phases. Since nothing is known about changes in mood responses to this particular steroid within different phases of the menstrual cycle, subjects in all cycle phases were included in the analyses, with the knowledge that effects of menstrual cycle variability, if any, had been minimized.

Normalizing Data

Given the shorter time course of this experiment, changes in response were not strongly positively

Table 59.2
Factor loadings (varimax rotation) of masked androstadienone with respect to clove oil for women in Experiment 2

	General mood state (Factor 1)	Stimulant/euphoric drug state (Factor 2)	
Eigenvalue	6.27652	3.38635	
Rotated variable		Factor loadings	Uniqueness
Anxiety (POMS)	0.64924	—	0.26193
Anger (POMS)	0.61256	—	0.23443
Irritated (VAS)	0.51544	—	0.20246
Friendliness (POMS)	−0.73062	—	0.3051
Elation (POMS)	−0.74577	—	0.18686
Stimulant (A-ARCI)	—	0.80045	0.24281
Euphoric (MBG-ARCI)	—	0.7916	0.2409
Intellectual efficacy (BG-ARCI)	—	0.75991	0.22251

skewed; they approximated a normal distribution and no log transformation was required. z-score normalization was still required to combine measures from different subscales so that subscale responses could later be added together to obtain factor scores. We calculated each participant's z-score for their response to androstadienone on a given subscale with reference to all measures of that subscale during the control condition. After z-transformations, all scales and factors were graphed and descriptive statistics calculated to confirm a normal distribution.

Data Reduction
As in Experiment 1, we used Factor Analysis with varimax rotation for data reduction prior to targeted statistical analysis. The 14 new VAS items were included in the Factor Analyses with the original VAS, POMS, and ARCI items in order to present a more complete psychological profile of any effects and possibly link the open-ended reports with our preexisting standardized measures.

We identified the significant factors (components) from the entire set of subscale scores from women over all tested time intervals. Because our focus was on mood changes caused by the presence of a single steroid, we used mood changes from baseline at each time interval. Similar to the previous experiment, differences caused by the presence of a steroid were calculated by subtracting the steroid response from the carrier response, matching scores within each individual and at testing interval ($T = 33$ test variables; $S = 93$ testing sessions in which all these variables were used within the same test battery).

In this laboratory experiment of affects of androstadienone on women alone, two significant factors were identified based on the scree plot with eigenvalues greater than 1.0. As with Experiment 1, the critical values for identifying significant loading on a factor were set at < -0.500 and $> +0.500$ to ensure that the factors analyzed for this study had only those subscales with the highest level of intercorrelation (Table 59.2). Factor 1 with an eigenvalue of 6.28 was a bipolar measure of positive/negative mood. Factor 2 with an eigenvalue of 3.39 measured a stimulated and euphoric drug-like state. Note that these factors are similar to those of the previous experiment, but they are not identical. This may be because we added new visual analog items and were exclusively testing women with androsta-dienone in a strong odor carrier rather than both steroids and both sexes in a weak odor carrier during a longer time course.

Statistical Analyses

To test our hypothesis that women have a psy-chological state change in response to androsta-dienone, even when it is not olfactorially identifiable, we used repeated-measures analysis of variance to assess the 0.1-, 1-, and 2-h re-sponses to strong odor masked androstadienone versus the strong odor control. Analyses were done on both factors with no between-subjects variables, and treatment and time as within-subjects variables. Those measures that did not contribute to the factors and had high unique-ness values (greater than 0.40) or were related to published anecdotal reports (Kodis et al., 1998) were graphically examined.

Results

Mood and Alertness Factors

Even though subjects did not identify or describe smelling androstadienone, the steroid had a sig-nificant effect on general mood (main effect of treatment: $F(1, 30) = 4.34$, $P \leq 0.05$) indepen-dent of the passage of time (see Fig. 59.6). By examining the graphs of the subscales included in the general mood factor, it is evident that being in the experiment itself was influential, causing an increase in negative mood and a drop in positive mood. Androstadienone prevented these mood effects and sustained the general mood which the women had at the beginning of their testing session (see Figs. 59.7–59.9). Over time in the testing session, subjects also tended to expe-rience a decrease in a drug-like state ($F(2, 60) = 2.9$, $P \leq 0.06$) but androstadienone did not have a main effect, nor an interaction with time in this factor.

Although factor analyses are useful for isolat-ing highly intercorrelated variables and limiting the number of analyses, it is also important to

look at the subscales within the factors inde-pendently in order to visualize the time course of the main effects (see Figs. 59.7 and 59.8). Under the control condition, there was a gradual in-crease in anxiety, anger, and irritation that did not occur or was prevented under the androsta-dienone condition. Similarly, there was a decrease under the control condition with elation or posi-tive mood (POMS) that was prevented in the same subjects under the androstadienone condi-tion. Euphoric (MBG-ARCI) subscale may show time course effects but stimulant (A-ARCI) and intellectual efficacy subscales do not appear to be affected differentially over time. As a preliminary analysis, we also graphed the time course of the VAS scales that did not correlate strongly with main factors or were related to published anec-dotal reports. Androstadienone did increase two physical response measures (heavy and sensual) but did not affect any of the self-confidence or affiliative measures (Fig. 59.9). Future experi-ments should examine whether androstadienone affects such physical perceptions.

Discussion

Although masked by the odor of clove oil and not consciously detectable, 9 nm of androsta-dienone modulated the general mood state of women within a laboratory setting. We use the term modulated because it did not have a direct effect itself, but rather appears to have modu-lated the subjects' response to the testing session. During the tedious 2-h study protocol when they were exposed to clove oil, women's mood dete-riorated. Androstadienone, however, both main-tained their initial levels of positive mood and prevented the increase in negative mood which occurred when they were exposed only to clove oil and propylene glycol.

Androstadienone's effects were detected almost immediately. After 6 min of exposure, women maintained their baseline levels of positive mood, all of which had begun to drop when they were in the testing room exposed to only the clove-

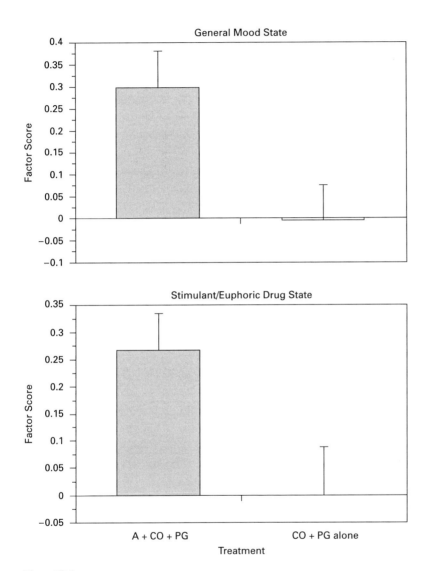

Figure 59.6
Female responses ($N = 31$) on General Mood State and Stimulant Drug State factors over all time intervals ($M \pm$ SEM). A factor score is the mean of its component subscales, each expressed as a z-score.

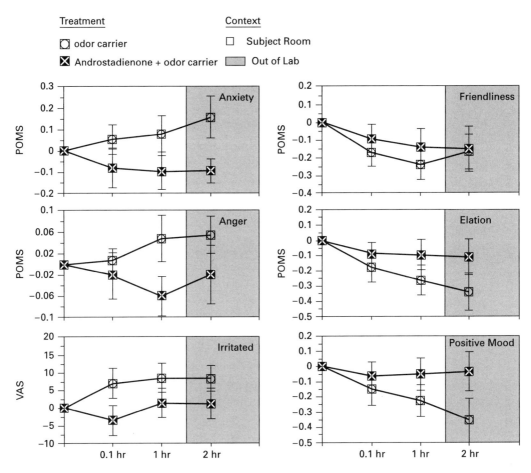

Figure 59.7
Time course of subscales related to General Mood State factor for women plus a composite POMS-Positive Mood Score (not included in Factor Analysis because it is a composite score of elation minus depression; $M \pm$ SEM).

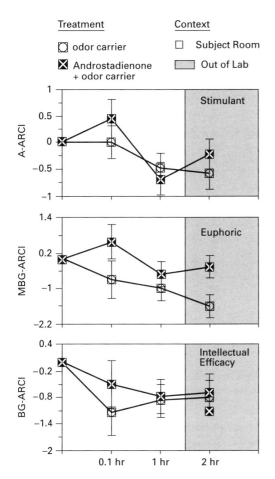

Figure 59.8
Time course of subscales related to Euphoric-Stimulated State factor ($M \pm$ SEM).

scented carrier. At this time, the women also felt less negative than they did under the carrier condition. That these protective effects were sustained for 2 h is indicated by a lack of an interaction between treatment and time of assessment: Women maintained both their positive mood and their relative absence of a negative mood, a conclusion based on the concordance of results from diverse psychological scales (VAS,

POMS, and ARCI) as well as the combined factor score.

These general mood responses paralleled those detected in Experiment 1. Androstadienone modulated women's mood in a positive direction across two experiments (Experiment 1, separate positive and negative mood scales; Experiment 2, one bipolar scale of positive and negative mood). Androstadienone prevented an increase in negative mood and maintained or increased positive mood when presented in two different olfactory contexts. The drug-like effects were not as strong or striking as in Experiment 1, but the direction of change was similar; the drop in stimulant/euphoric pharmacologically induced drug-like effect was only a trend in this study, as were the ameliorative effects of androstadienone. Differences could be attributed to variation in experimental and olfactory context of the two studies. The odor of the carrier was strong in this experiment (1% clove oil solution) and weak in the previous one (only propylene glycol). In Experiment 2, psychological response to clove oil could influence the response to the unperceived androstadienone. This is similar to Experiment 1, when a few subjects did consciously perceive androstadienone in propylene glycol, and when detectable, the odor may have influenced their psychological responses. Moreover, the stricter experimental protocol that rigorously controlled social interactions within the testing room also may have contributed to the differences.

In this experiment, women did not verbally discriminate between the odors of the steroid-containing solutions and clove oil/propylene glycol carrier solutions; they gave the same odor descriptors for each. Therefore, we can conclude that androstadienone had its unique effects on the psychological state of women without identification or conscious detection as an odor. Our current results, however, do not enable us to determine whether mood or physical state changes are evidence of more general, unconscious olfactory processing or are unique to specialized processing of pheromonal information relevant to

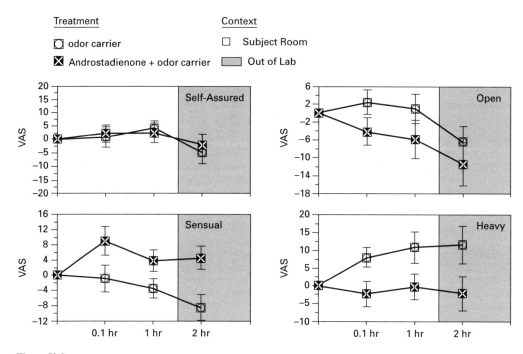

Figure 59.9
Time course of specific Visual Analog responses that were added to the second experiment ($M \pm$ SEM). The VAS items Heavy and Sensual had high uniqueness proportions in the factor analysis (e.g., greater than 0.4112).

social behavior. This hypothesis would best be tested by a neuroimaging study of specific brain mechanisms of sensory processing and psychological response. Moreover, because learning and conditioning can take place in both conscious and unconscious states (Kirk-Smith et al., 1983), we will also need to conduct controlled studies to determine if these psychological responses are a result of previous learning or experience.

Conclusions

The results from both experiments do not support the hypothesis that androstadienone simply mimics a single, characterized, drug-like state. Rather, the steroids had effects on a general pattern of mood state that were detectable from a suite of psychological scales. This is consistent with the model that this chemical information is processed along with other sensory inputs and related to more complex changes in psychological state and consequently behavior. Throughout our psychological measures and observations, these steroids did not appear to act as simple, sex-specific or stereotyped behavior releasers, neither immediately within a laboratory setting nor in a normal, everyday context.

The pattern of results in these experiments supports our hypothesis that androstadienone and possibly other steroid chemosignals modulate human psychological state in a complex manner. Human behaviors and psychological states are multifaceted and are determined by the interplay of a wide variety of stimuli. Therefore, it is unlikely that androstadienone, or any other potential communicative chemical signal, is sufficient for triggering stereotyped behavior when a person is also responding to a rich social and physical environment (McClintock, 1971, 1998, 2000). These compounds would be unique among human sensory stimuli if they could trigger complex behavior in a fixed-action pattern.

Although many people are interested in how these steroids affect sexual behavior, we did not want to limit this experiment to a single social context because animal pheromones have been shown to influence a wide repertoire of behaviors (e.g., territorial behavior and maternal/child recognition). We started with an isolated compound rather than a known behavioral effect. Since our results do show a psychological state response during routine activities, it would be interesting to explore how these steroids affect psychological state or behavior in specific social or even sexual contexts. It is interesting that steroidal effects were more evident in primary moods that do not necessarily relate to social interactions (e.g., elation which was included in the significant factors in both studies) versus subscales specifically related to social moods (e.g., friendliness which was included in the significant factors in both studies, see Figs. 59.3 and 59.7). Further work is required to determine which specific aspects of physical condition made women feel more sensual and heavy (Fig. 59.9). It could be related to underlying mood states, physical state changes that are associated with the autonomic nervous system or sexuality, or unconscious associations with this kind of stimulus. Although sexual effects are generally implied by marketing claims with perfumes containing these steroids, our reported general effects on mood suggest that simple, stereotyped releaser effects on sexual behavior would be unlikely. While we did not find any evidence for effects on self-confidence or affiliative states, the possibility exists that steroidal effects in psychological states may influence more complex social interactions.

We believe that it is premature to call these steroids human pheromones. Because the existence of behavioral pheromones in humans can be established only with converging lines of independent evidence, future work is now warranted to establish the specific contexts in which these steroids affect behavior, their receptor mechanisms within the perinasal region, the pathways by which they produce their psychological effects, and at what concentrations they are naturally produced and released. Chemical communication could exist in humans without a functional vomeronasal system. Future work needs to be done considering any potential role of the main olfactory system, nervus terminalis, trigeminal system, and portal neuroendocrine systems. A systemic effect from steroid uptake through mucous membranes could produce psychological state changes, although the dose we used is probably not sufficient to produce effects in this manner during such a short time. Furthermore, we need to confirm whether these chemicals are released from human skin under normal conditions. It has not yet been shown that their release is sexually dimorphic or in sufficient quantity to produce a behavioral effect. If released in a natural context, it may be critical that pheromones are not isolated but associated with carrier proteins or a cocktail of other chemicals and scents. Future behavioral research must address these complexities.

If these steroids ever meet a given set of criteria for being pheromones, we feel that they should be considered modulator chemical signals (McClintock, 1971, 1998, 2000), rather than stereotyped behavior releasers as defined in the animal literature. We use the term, "modulator," to describe this heretofore unexplored type of behavioral chemosignal. This type of behavioral chemosignal has functional effects that differ from those of primer and signaling pheromones. Modulator chemosignals change how individuals behave or react to their current situation by influencing psychological state, for example, the conditions of our controlled laboratory experiment. These steroids do not simply signal information about another person's presence, condition, or status that the receiver may or may not act upon. Modulators modulate the psychological state or behavior of the recipient, rather than release a new behavioral pattern or simply change long-term neuroendocrine state. Modulators would be the type of chemosignals or pheromones most likely to guide human behavior in an appropriate context, if indeed pheromones have a nonvestigial role in human psychology.

Finally, if these kinds of chemosignals are to be considered a part of an evolved human social behavior, and not just an epiphenomenon or drug-like effect, we must address the question of their adaptive advantage or function. It is premature, however, to generate hypotheses about the evolutionary advantage or specific effects of fitness with such a human chemical communication system. We first need to clearly understand and define the phenotype on which selection could have acted. If androstadienone proves to have an effect that attenuates negative emotions in a context when people are close to each other, it could promote social interactions that have beneficial effects on health and reproductive fitness. If it has purely a psychopharmacological effect of an exogenous steroid, then it is not likely to be a single trait that has evolved because of specific consequences.

We propose that modulating chemosignals could affect (1) the state or mood of the individual and (2) regulation of multisensory inputs during exposure. Together, these contribute to the final common paths that will determine the actual action or the perception of other sensory information. In many situations, the changes induced by modulating chemosignals may indeed be unconscious changes. Future research needs to focus on how psychological state and mood are affected by various unconscious olfactory stimuli as well as putative pheromonal stimuli. Our results indicate that if androstadienone is a behavioral chemosignal affecting women, it is clearly not a releaser pheromone within our ex-

perimental setting. Even if these or related steroids are eventually proven not to be human pheromones, their behavioral effects must still be conceptualized as modulating multidetermined behavior, not as a sole triggers or simple releasers.

Acknowledgments

This work was supported by the Mind-Body Network of the John D. and Catherine T. MacArthur Foundation, the NIH MERIT Award R37 MH41788 to Martha K. McClintock, and the Olfactory Research Fund's Tova Fellowship to Suma Jacob. We thank Davinder Hayreh, Sheila Garcia, and Natasha Spencer for their commitment and long-term help with data collection and processing. We appreciate Harriet de Wit's assistance with creating the psychological test battery. Special thanks to Bethanne Zelano for her superb graphing abilities and support during the completion of this work.

References

Aggleton, J. (1993). The contribution of the amygdala to normal and abnormal emotional states. *Trends Neurosci.* 16, 328–333.

Agosta, W. C. (1992). *Chemical Communication: The Language of Pheromones.* Sci. Am. Library, New York.

Berliner, D. L. (1994). Fragrance compositions containing human pheromones, U.S. Patent 5,278,141.

Bigelow, G. E. (1991). Human drug abuse liability assessment: Opioids and analgesics. *Br. J. Addiction* 86, 1615–1628.

Brauer, L. H., and de Wit, H. (1997). High dose pimozide does not block amphetamine-induced euphoria in normal volunteers. *Pharmacol. Biochem. Behav.* 56, 265–272.

Brooksbank, B. W., Brammall, M. A., Cunningham, A. E., Shaw, D. M., and Camps, F. E. (1972). Estimation of corticosteroids in human cerebral cortex after death by suicide, accident, or disease. *Psycholog. Med.* 2, 56–65.

Cockerill, I. M., Nevill, A. M., and Lyons, N. (1991). Modelling mood states in athletic performance. *J. Sports Sci.* 9, 205–212.

Cowley, J. J., Johnson, A. L., and Brooksbank, B. W. L. (1991). Human exposure to putative pheromones and changes in aspects of social behavior. *J. Steroid Biochem. Mol. Biol.* 39, 647–659.

Cutler, W. B. (1987). Female essence (pheromones) increases sexual behavior of young women. XVIII meeting of the International Society of Psychoneuroendocrinology.

Cutler, W. B., and Stine, R. (1988). Female essence increases heterosexual activity of women. The annual meeting of the American Fertility Society.

de Wit, H., Clark, M., and Brauer, L. H. (1997). Effects of d-amphetamine in grouped versus isolated humans. *Pharmacol. Biochem. Behav.* 57, 333–340.

de Wit, H., and Griffiths, R. R. (1991). Testing the abuse liability of anxiolytic and hypnotic drugs in humans. *Drug Alcohol Depend.* 28, 83–111.

Der, D. F., and Lewington, P. (1990). Rational self-directed hypnotherapy: A treatment for panic attacks. *Am. J. Clin. Hypnosis* 32, 160–167.

Dorries, K. M., Adkins Regan, E., and Halpern, B. P. (1997). Sensitivity and behavioral responses to the pheromone androstenone are not mediated by the vomeronasal organ in domestic pigs. *Brain Behav. Evol.* 49(1), 53–62.

Dorries, K. M., Schmidt, H. J., Beauchamp, G. K., and Wysocki, C. J. (1989). Changes in sensitivity to the odor androstenone. *Dev. Psychobiol.* 22, 423–436.

Doty, R. L. (1981). Olfactory communication in humans. *Chem. Senses* 6, 351–376.

Doty, R. L., McKeown, D. A., Lee, W. W., and Shaman, P. (1995). A study of the test-retest reliability of ten olfactory tests. *Chem. Senses* 20, 645–656.

Doty, R. L., Snyder, P. J., Huggins, G. R., and Lowry, L. D. (1981). Endocrine, cardiovascular, and psychological correlates of olfactory sensitivity changes during the human menstrual cycle. *J. Comp. Physiol. Psychol.* 95, 45–60.

Dulac, C., and Axel, R. (1995). A novel family of genes encoding putative pheromone receptors in mammals. *Cell* 83, 195–206.

Dulac, C., and Axel, R. (1998). Expression of candidate pheromone receptor genes in vomeronasal neurons. *Chem. Senses* 23, 467–475.

Filsinger, E. E., Braun, J. J., and Monte, W. C. (1985). An examination of the effects of putative pheromones on human judgments. *Ethol. Sociobiol.* 6, 227–236.

Filsinger, E. E., Braun, J. J., and Monte, W. C. (1990). Sex differences in response to the odor of alpha androstenone. *Percept. Motor Skills* 70, 216–218.

Filsinger, E. E., Fabes, R. A., and Hughston, G. (1987). Introversion-extraversion and dimensions of olfactory perception. *Percept. Motor Skills* 64, 695–699.

Fingerhood, M., Sullivan, J., Testa, M., and Jasinski, D. (1997). Abuse liability of testosterone. *J. Psychopharmacol.* 11, 59–63.

Fischman, M. W., and Foltin, R. W. (1991). Utility of subjective-effects measurements in assessing abuse liability of drugs in humans. *Br. J. Addiction* 86, 1563–1570.

Folstein, M. F., and Luria, R. (1973). Reliability, validity, and clinical application of the visual analogue mood scale. *Psychol. Med.* 3, 479–486.

Gilbert, A. N., and Wysocki, C. J. (1987). The National Geographic smell survey results. *Nat. Geographic Mag.* 172, 514–524.

Goldfoot, D., Kravetz, M., Goy, R., and Freeman, S. (1976). Lack of effect of vaginal lavages and aliphatic acids on ejaculatory responses in rhesus monkeys: Behavioral and chemical analyses. *Horm. Behav.* 7, 1–27.

Gower, D. B., and Ruparelia, B. A. (1993). Olfaction in humans with special reference to odorous 16-androstenes: Their occurrence, perception, and possible social, psychological, and sexual impact. *J. Endocrinol.* 137, 167–187.

Grammer, K. (1993). 5-α-androst-16en-3α-on: A male pheromone? A brief report. *Ethol. Sociobiol.* 14, 201–207.

Haertzen, C. (1974a). Addiction research inventory. National Institute of Mental Health, Washington, DC.

Haertzen, C. (1974b). *An overview of the Addiction Research Center Inventory (ARCI): An Appendix and Manual of Scales.* Natl. Inst. on Drug Abuse, Rockville, MD.

Hines, M., and Sandberg, E. (1996). Sexual differentiation of cognitive abilities in women exposed to diethylstilbestrol (DES) prenatally. *Horm. Behav.* 30, 354–363.

Horswill, C. A., Hickner, R. C., Scott, J. R., Costill, D. L., and Gould, D. (1990). Weight loss, dietary carbohydrate modifications, and high intensity, physical performance. *Med. Sci. Sports Exec.* 22, 470–476.

Karlson, P., and Luscher, M. (1959). "Pheromones": A new term for a class of biologically active substances. *Nature* 183, 55–56.

Kirk, J. M., Doty, P., and de Wit, H. (1998). Effects of expectancies on subjective responses to oral delta-9-tetrahydrocannabinol. *Pharmacol. Biochem. Behav.* 59, 287–293.

Kirk-Smith, M., Booth, D. A., Carroll, D., and Davies, P. (1978). Human social attitudes affected by androstenol. *Res. Commun. Psychol. Psychiatry Behav.* 3, 379–384.

Kirk-Smith, M. D., Van Toller, C., and Dodd, G. H. (1983). Unconscious odour conditioning in human subjects. *Biol. Psychol.* 17, 221–231.

Kodis, M., Moran, D., and Houy, D. (1998). *Love Scents.* Dutton, New York.

Kraemer, R. R., Dzewaltowski, D. A., Blair, M. S., Rinehardt, K. F., and Castracane, V. D. (1990). Mood alteration from treadmill running and its relationship to beta-endorphin, corticotropin, and growth hormone. *J. Sports Med. Phys. Fitness* 30, 241–246.

Lieberman, H. R., Corkin, S., Spring, B. J., Growdon, J. H., and Wurtman, R. J. (1982/83). Mood, performance and pain sensitivity: Changes induced by food constituents. *J. Psychiatric Res.* 17, 135–145.

McClintock, M. K. (1971). Menstrual synchrony and suppression. *Nature* 229, 244–245.

McClintock, M. K. (1998). On the nature of mammalian and human pheromones. *Ann. N. Y. Acad. Sci.* 855, 390–392.

McClintock, M. K. (2000). Human pheromones: Primers, releasers, signallers or modulators? In K. Wallen and J. E. Schneider (Eds.), *Reproduction in Context.* pp. 335–420. MIT Press, Cambridge, MA.

McNair, D. M., Lorr, M., and Droppleman, L. F. (1971). Profile of Mood States (Manual). Educational and Industrial Testing Service, San Francisco.

Michael, R. P., Keverne, E. B., and Bonsall, R. W. I.-B. R. H., Inst. of Psychiatry, Beckenham, England (1971). Pheromones: Isolation of male sex attractants from a female primate. *Science* 172, 964–966.

Monti-Bloch, L., and Grosser, B. I. (1991). Effect of putative pheromones on the electrical activity of the human vomeronasal organ and the olfactory epithelium. *J. Steroid Biochem. Mol. Biol.* 39, 573–582.

Monti-Bloch, L., Jennings-White, C., Dolberg, D., and Berliner, D. (1994). The human vomeronasal system. *Psychoneuroendocrinology* 19, 673–686.

Morris, N. M., and Udry, J. R. (1978). Pheromonal influences on human sexual behaviour: An experimental search. *J. Biosocial Sci.* 10, 147–157.

Preti, G., Cutler, W. B., Garcia, C. R., Huggins, G. R., et al. (1986). Human axillary secretions influence women's menstrual cycles: The role of donor extract of females. *Horm. Behav.* 20(4), 474–482.

Preti, G., and Wysocki, C. J. (1999). Human pheromones: Releasers or primers: Fact or myth. In *Advances in Chemical Signals in Vertebrates 8.* pp. 315–331. Plenum Press, New York.

Risold, P. Y., and Swanson, L. W. (1995). Evidence for a hypothalamothalamocortical circuit mediating pheromonal influences on eye and head movements. *Proc. Natl. Acad. Sci. USA* 92, 3898–3902.

Russell, M. J., Switz, G. M., and Thompson, K. (1980). Olfactory influences on the human menstrual cycle. *Pharmacol. Biochem. Behav.* 13, 737–738.

Sachs, B. D. (1999). Airborne aphrodisiac odor from estrous rats: Implication for pheromonal classification. In R. Johnston, D. Müller-Schwarz, and P. Sorensen (Eds.), *Chemical Signals in Vertebrates 8.* pp. 333–342. Plenum Press, New York.

Schaal, B., and Porter, R. H. (1991). "Microsmatic humans" revisited: The generation and perception of chemical signals. In J. S. R. Peter, J. B. Slater, Colin Beer, Manfred Milinski (Eds.), *Advances in the Study of Behavior,* Vol. 20, pp. 135–199. Academic Press, San Diego.

Schiffman, S. S., Miller, E. A. S., Suggs, M. S., and Graham, B. G. (1995a). The effect of environmental odors emanating from commercial swine operations on the mood of nearby residents. *Brain Res. Bull.* 37, 369–375.

Schiffman, S. S., Sattely-Miller, E. A., Suggs, M. S., and Graham, B. G. (1995b). The effect of pleasant odors and hormone status on mood of women at midlife. *Brain Res. Bull.* 36, 19–29.

Schmidt, P., Nieman, L., Danaceau, M., Adams, L., and Rubinow, D. (1998). Differential behavioral effects of gonadal steroids in women with and in those without premenstrual syndrome. *N. Engl. J. Med.* 338, 209–216.

Schneider, D. (1974). The sex-attractant receptor of moths. *Sci. Am.* 231, 28–35.

Signoret, J. P., Baldwin, B. A., Fraser, D., and Hafez, E. S. E. (1975). The behavior of the swine. In E. S. E. Hafez (Ed.), *The Behavior of Domestic Animals*. Williams & Wilkins, Baltimore.

Singer, A. G. (1991). A chemistry of mammalian pheromones. *J. Steroid Biochem. Mol. Biol.* 39, 627–632.

Singer, A. G., Macrides, F., Clancy, A. N., and Agosta, W. C. (1986). Purification and analysis of a proteinaceous aphrodisiac pheromone from hamster vaginal discharge. *J. Biol. Chem.* 261, 13323–13326.

Stern, K., and McClintock, M. K. (1998). Regulation of ovulation by human pheromones. *Nature* 392, 177–179.

Williams, T. J., Krahenbuhl, G. S., and Morgan, D. W. (1991). Mood state and running economy in moderately trained male runners. *Med. Sci. Sports Exerc.* 23, 727–731.

Wood, R. I. (1998). Integration of chemosensory and hormonal input in the male Syrian hamster brain. *Ann. N. Y. Acad. Sci.* 855, 362–372.

Wysocki, C. J., and Meredith, M. (1987). *The Vomeronasal System.* In T. Finger and W. Silver (Eds.), *Neurobiology of Taste and Smell.* pp. 125–150. Wiley, New York.

Zacny, J. P., Bodker, B. K., and de Wit, H. (1992). Effects of setting on the subjective and behavioral effects of d-amphetamines in humans. *Addictive Behav.* 17, 27–33.

D. I. Perrett, K. J. Lee, I. Penton-Voak, D. Rowland, S. Yoshikawa, D. M. Burt, S. P. Henzi, D. L. Castles, and S. Akamatsu

Testosterone-dependent secondary sexual characteristics in males may signal immunological competence[1] and are sexually selected for in several species.[2,3] In humans, oestrogen-dependent characteristics of the female body correlate with health and reproductive fitness and are found attractive.[4–6] Enhancing the sexual dimorphism of human faces should raise attractiveness by enhancing sex-hormone-related cues to youth and fertility in females,[5,7–11] and to dominance and immunocompetence in males.[5,12,13] Here we report the results of asking subjects to choose the most attractive faces from continua that enhanced or diminished differences between the average shape of female and male faces. As predicted, subjects preferred feminized to average shapes of a female face. This preference applied across UK and Japanese populations but was stronger for within-population judgements, which indicates that attractiveness cues are learned. Subjects preferred feminized to average or masculinized shapes of a male face. Enhancing masculine facial characteristics increased both perceived dominance and negative attributions (for example, coldness or dishonesty) relevant to relationships and paternal investment. These results indicate a selection pressure that limits sexual dimorphism and encourages neoteny in humans.

Computer-graphic techniques can be used to construct "average" male and female faces by digitally blending photographs of individuals of the same sex[14] (Fig. 60.1). Sexual dimorphism in face shape can then be enhanced or diminished[14,15] (Fig. 60.2). We presented such manipulations of both Japanese and Caucasian face stimuli to Japanese subjects in Japan and Caucasian subjects in Scotland.

The amount of transformation (that is, masculinization or feminization) that was applied by subjects to obtain the most attractive face shape

was compared with a mean of 0% predicted by the null hypothesis (that altering sex-related characteristics would not affect attractiveness) and predicted by the hypothesis that attractiveness is averageness.[16] The face shape selected by Caucasian subjects as most attractive (from the shape range available) was significantly feminized for both the Caucasian female face (mean level of feminization was 24.2%; $t_{49} = 7.6$, $P < 0.001$) and the Japanese female face continua (mean 10.2%; $t_{49} = 2.3$, $P = 0.027$). Japanese subjects also selected significantly feminized versions of the female stimuli for both the Japanese (mean 22.9%; $t_{41} = 7.6$, $P = 0.001$) and the Caucasian (mean 15.3%; $t_{41} = 4.5$, $P = 0.001$) female face continua.

Three-way analysis of variance (ANOVA) of the level of transform applied by subjects to define attractive face shapes revealed no main effect of subject sex ($F_{1,88} = 1.58$, $P = 0.21$), population of subjects ($F_{1,88} = 0.32$, $P = 0.57$) or type of stimulus face (Japanese/Caucasian; $F_{1,88} = 1.42$, $P = 0.24$). The only significant interaction between main effects was that between subject population and type of stimulus face ($F_{1,88} = 17.06$, $P < 0.001$), which was attributable to the greater degree of feminization preferred for stimulus faces of the subject's own population (Fig. 60.3a).

Previous studies show cross-population consistency in judgements of attractiveness.[9,11,14,17] Our study shows cross-cultural (between-population) agreement in the preference for feminized to average face shapes, which refutes the averageness hypothesis.[14,16] The study also indicates effects of experience on judgements of female attractiveness as a greater degree of feminization was preferred for faces from the subject's own population than for faces from a different population. Both generalization and cultural specificity of judgements of attractiveness may result

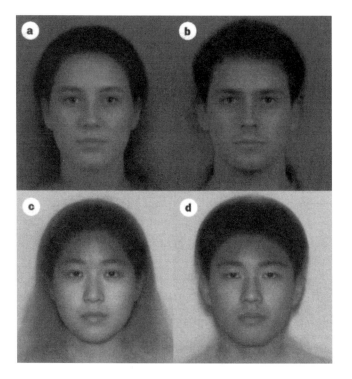

Figure 60.1
Composite "average" facial images. (a) "Caucasian" female face; (b) "Caucasian" male face; (c) "Japanese" female face; (d) "Japanese" male face.

from learning. We find cues to female attractiveness relate to the way that female faces differ from males. Sensitivity to the consistent sex differences in faces (and hence female attractiveness) could be learned through exposure to male and female exemplars. Most differences learned this way will generalize between populations as they reflect the common action of sex hormones during growth. Subjects, however, may become more sensitive to the sexual dimorphism of faces within the subject's own population because of increased exposure to population-specific male–female variations.

For the male face stimuli, the shape selected by Caucasian subjects as most attractive (from

the shape range available) was significantly feminized for both the Caucasian male face (mean level of feminization was 15%; $t_{49} = 4.22$, $P < 0.001$) and the Japanese male face continua (mean 9%; $t_{49} = 2.2$, $P = 0.03$). Japanese subjects also selected significantly feminized versions of the male stimuli for both the Japanese (mean 20%; $t_{41} = 6.5$, $P < 0.001$) and the Caucasian (mean 17%; $t_{41} = 4.8$, $P < 0.001$) male face continua. For the male stimuli, three-way ANOVA revealed there was no main effect of subject sex ($F_{1,88} = 0.18$, $P = 0.67$), subject population ($F_{1,88} = 2.94$, $P = 0.09$) or type of stimulus face ($F_{1,88} = 0.02$, $P < 0.89$) and no significant interactions between effects.

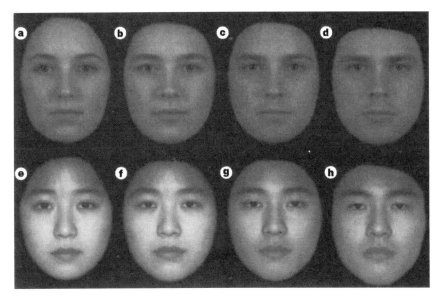

Figure 60.2
Facial images of Caucasian and Japanese females and males that were "feminized" and "masculinized" 50% in shape. (a) Caucasian female, feminized; (b) Caucasian female, masculinized. (c) Caucasian male, feminized; (d) Caucasian male, masculinized. (e) Japanese female, feminized; (f) Japanese female, masculinized. (g) Japanese male, feminized; (h) Japanese male, masculinized.

Asymmetries in the facial outline (from the hairline), which remain after cropping, could contribute to judgements. With a different set of Caucasian faces (19 male, 17 female, 30–35 years old), symmetrical composites were made by averaging component faces and their mirror reflections. Caucasian subjects ($n = 67$, age range 15–40, 23 female) made forced-choice judgements of attractiveness of symmetrical average stimuli that were 50% masculinized or feminized. Masculinization of face shape decreased attractiveness of male (87% of subjects; Binomial test $P = 0.001$) and female faces (78%; $P < 0.001$), whereas feminization increased attractiveness of male (64%; $P < 0.05$) and female faces (53%; $P < 0.05$).

Males have larger faces than females. However, standardizing the distance between pupils removes this size difference. We prepared composite images from a new set of Caucasian faces (26 male, 17 female, 18–21 years old) without standardizing the inter-pupil separation. Manipulation of these composites maintained sexual dimorphism in face shape and size. Caucasian subjects ($n = 135$, age range 15–71, 65 female) ranked average images that were masculinized and feminized by 50% for attractiveness. Masculinization of the average shape decreased attractiveness of male (74% of subjects; $P < 0.000005$) and female (76%; $P < 0.000005$) faces, whereas feminization increased attractiveness rankings for male (58%; $P = 0.029$) and female (60%; $P < 0.013$) faces.

Thus, preference for feminized face shapes over average male and female face shapes was found with interactive and forced-choice methods using

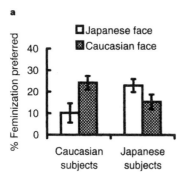

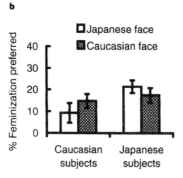

Figure 60.3
The effect of feminization of face shape on judgements
of female and male attractiveness. (a) Female stimuli;
(b) male stimuli. Overall, subjects preferred a feminine
face shape to an average shape both within and between populations. The degree of feminization preferred was greater within than between populations for
female faces.

different face sets, even when the potential
contributions by symmetry and size dimorphism
were controlled.

To interpret preferences, 50% masculinized,
50% feminized and cropped average images (Fig.
60.2) were rated for perceived characteristics by
a new set of subjects. Twenty Caucasian subjects
(age range 18–50, 10 female) were presented with
four sets of three images that represented the end
points of each continuum and the average. Subjects were asked to rank stimuli from one set
on seven characteristics (masculinity, dominance,

warmth, emotionality, honesty, intelligence and
age). The order of testing of characteristics and
image sets was randomized. An additional 20
subjects (age range 19–61, 10 female) ranked the
stimuli on three further characteristics (cooperativeness, assertiveness and "good parent").

For Caucasian and Japanese male faces, increasing the masculinity of face shape across the
three set members increased ranking of perceived
dominance, masculinity and age but decreased
ranking of perceived warmth, emotionality, honesty, cooperativeness and quality as a parent
(Friedman's $\chi^2 \geq 15.6$, degrees of freedom
(d.f.) $= 2$, $P < 0.0005$, for each rated dimension). Increasing masculinity affected the Japanese and Caucasian female face sets in the same
way for all characteristics ($\chi^2 \geq 8.1$, d.f. $= 2$,
$P < 0.017$, each dimension), except for "good
parent" with the Caucasian female faces, where
the rank order was average, feminized and
masculinized ($\chi^2 \geq 6.7$, d.f. $= 2$, $P < 0.035$). Increasing masculinity did not consistently decrease
apparent intelligence (Caucasian male and female
faces, $P > 0.5$; Japanese female face, $P = 0.07$;
Japanese male face, $P = 0.02$) or increase attributions of assertiveness (Japanese and Caucasian
female faces, $P > 0.5$; Japanese male face, $P =
0.058$; Caucasian male face, $P = 0.157$).

The preference for male face shapes that
are slightly feminized may reflect the effects of
masculinity on perceived age. Whereas status
and height are valued in males,[9,18] youth benefits judgements of attractiveness for both female[9,11,19] and male[19] faces. For both males
and females, enhancing sexual dimorphism in
face shape develops cues to characteristics which,
from a biological perspective, appear beneficial
(that is, youth and fertility in females[7–11] and
dominance in males[12,13,18]). For males, however, enhancing masculinity in face shape also
predisposes some negative personality attributions. Such attributions, although stereotypic,
may predict behaviour; ratings of perceived dishonesty from facial appearance correlate with
the face owner's willingness to participate in

deceptive behaviour.[20] Indeed, increasing testosterone level in males is associated with more troubled relationships (including increased infidelity, violence and divorce).[21] Feminization of male face shape may increase attractiveness because it "softens" particular features[10,22] that are perceived to be associated with negative personality traits.

Together, the results indicate that judgements of male attractiveness reflect multiple motives.[22] Females may adopt different strategies, giving preference to characteristics that are associated with dominance and an effective immune system,[12,13] or to characteristics that are related to paternal investment.

Sexual dimorphism in any species reflects compromises among diverse selection pressures. In humans, the greater upper body musculature and more rugged skeletal anatomy of males relative to females may reflect advantages in male–male competition and hunting. Because male attractiveness is an important determinant of relationships and sexual partnerships,[23] the reduction in attractiveness of male face shape with masculinization represents a further selection pressure. This would act against "run away" fisherian sexual selection for extreme male characteristics,[1] and is consistent with the relative lack of sexual dimorphism in humans.[24]

The preferences found here indicate a selection pressure on the evolution of face shape that acts against pronounced differences between males and females and, as more-feminine face shapes are perceived as younger, the preferences would encourage a youthful, neotonous appearance in the species generally.

Methods

Preparation of Composite Facial Images

Japanese faces (students at Otemon-Gakuin University; 28 male, age 20–23 years, mean 21.6 years; 28 female, age 20–22 years, mean 21.4 years) were photographed under standard lighting conditions with neutral facial expression. Similar photographs were prepared for Caucasian faces (students at St. Andrews University, 25 male, age 19–23 years, mean 21.0 years; 30 female, age 19–22 years, mean 20.6 years). Photographs were converted to digital format (Kodak Photo-CD) and 174 feature points on salient facial landmarks (for example, nose-tip) were defined manually for each face.[14,15] The average face shapes of the male and female Japanese and Caucasian face subsets were calculated from the feature points. The position of eye centres was standardized for corresponding average male and female face shapes. Each original face image was then warped to the shape of the corresponding average face and the resultant reshaped face images were blended together by averaging colour and intensity values of pixels at corresponding image locations[14,15] (Fig. 60.1). The vector difference between corresponding feature points on the male and female averages was increased or decreased by 50% to create feminized and masculinized shapes. The image of the composite face was then warped into these new face shapes to create image pairs with identical texture but enhanced or diminished sexually dimorphic differences in face shape. The size of all male and female face images was matched by standardization of inter-pupil distance. The resulting composite images were cropped around the face and faded into a black background (Fig. 60.2). Cropping removed the hair, ears and neck, which were not consistent in shape or visibility in component images because of differing hairstyles and clothing.

Procedure

A Silicon Graphics Indigo[2] Maximum Impact (4 MB TRAM) was used to create smooth continua between 50% masculinized and 50% feminized face pairs (Fig. 60.2) as the end points, and the cropped average as the midpoint. The point along a shape continuum was controlled interactively by the position of the computer mouse. The appropriate image was calculated in real-time using texture mapping hardware. Stimuli were presented in 24-bit colour at the centre of an 800×800 pixel window. Fifty Caucasian subjects (research staff and students from St. Andrews University; age 19–31 years, 25 female) and 42 Japanese subjects (research staff and students from ATR and Doshisha University; age 18–44 years, 19 female) were instructed to select the most attractive face from the continuum. Each continuum was presented twice to allow left/right counterbalancing of the end points, making a total of eight trials in randomized order.

Acknowledgements

This work was supported by Unilever Research and the ESRC. We thank A. Whiten, R. Byrne, R. Barton, J. Lycett, S. Reicher, D. Carey, M. Ridley, J. Graves, and D. Symons for comments.

References

1. Kirkpatrick, M. & Ryan, M. J. The evolution of mating preferences and the paradox of the lek. *Nature* 350, 33–88 (1991).

2. Andersson, M. Female choice for extreme tail length in a widowbird. *Nature* 299, 818–820 (1992).

3. Møller, A. P. Female swallow preference for symmetrical male sexual ornaments. *Nature* 357, 238–240 (1992).

4. Singh, D. Body shape and women's attractiveness—the critical role of waist-to-hip ratio. *Hum. Nature* 4, 297–321 (1993).

5. Barber, N. The evolutionary psychology of physical attractiveness: sexual selection and human morphology. *Ethol. Sociobiol.* 16, 395–424 (1995).

6. Manning, J. T., Scutt, D., Whitehouse, G. H. & Leinster, S. J. Breast asymmetry and phenotypic quality in women. *Evol. Hum. Behav.* 18, 223–236 (1997).

7. Symons, D. *The Evolution of Human Sexuality* (Oxford Univ. Press, 1979).

8. Cunningham, M. R. Measuring the physical in physical attractiveness: quasi-experiments on the sociobiology of female facial beauty. *J. Pers. Soc. Psychol.* 50, 925–935 (1986).

9. Buss, D. M. Sex differences in human mate preferences: evolutionary hypotheses tested in 37 cultures. *Behav. Brain Sci.* 122, 1–49 (1989).

10. Johnston, V. S. & Franklin, M. Is beauty in the eye of the beholder? *Ethol. Sociobiol.* 14, 183–199 (1993).

11. Jones, D. Sexual selection, physical attractiveness, and facial neoteny. *Curr. Anthropol.* 36, 723–748 (1995).

12. Grammer, K. & Thornhill, R. Human (*Homo sapiens*) facial attractiveness and sexual selection: the role of symmetry and averageness. *J. Comp. Psychol.* 108, 233–242 (1994).

13. Thornhill, R. & Gangestad, S. The evolution of human sexuality. *Trends Ecol. Evol.* 11, 98–102 (1996).

14. Perrett, D. I., May, K. A. & Yoshikawa, S. Facial shape and judgements of female attractiveness. *Nature* 368, 239–242 (1994).

15. Rowland, D. A. & Perrett, D. I. Manipulating facial appearance through shape and color. *IEEE Comput. Graph. Appl.* 15, 70–76 (1995).

16. Langlois, J. H. & Roggman, L. A. Attractive faces are only average. *Psychol. Sci.* 1, 115–121 (1990).

17. Cunningham, M. R., Roberts, A. R., Barbee, A. P. & Druen, P. B. "Their ideas of beauty are, on the whole, the same as ours": consistency and variability in the cross-cultural perception of female attractiveness. *J. Pers. Soc. Psychol.* 68, 261–279 (1995).

18. Jackson, L. A. *Physical Appearance and Gender: Sociobiology and Sociocultural Perspectives* (State Univ. New York Press, Albany, 1992).

19. Deutsch, F. M., Zalenski, C. M. & Clark, M. E. Is there a double standard of ageing? *J. Appl. Soc. Psychol.* 16, 771–785 (1986).

20. Berry, D. S. & Wero, J. L. F. Accuracy of face perception: a view from ecological psychology. *J. Pers.* 61, 497–519 (1993).

21. Booth, A. & Dabbs, J. Testosterone and men's marriages. *Social Forces* 72, 463–477 (1993).

22. Cunningham, M. R., Barbee, A. P. & Pike, C. L. What do women want? Facialmetric assessment of multiple motives in the perception of male facial attractiveness. *J. Pers. Soc. Psychol.* 59, 61–72 (1990).

23. Gangestad, S. W. & Thornhill, R. The evolutionary psychology of extrapair sex: the role of fluctuating symmetry. *Ethol. Hum. Behav.* 18, 69–88 (1997).

24. Martin, R. D. & May, R. M. Outward signs of breeding. *Nature* 293, 7–9 (1990).

61 Nature Needs Nurture: The Interaction of Hormonal and Social Influences on the Development of Behavioral Sex Differences in Rhesus Monkeys

Kim Wallen

The relative influence of biological and social factors on the development of human behavioral and cognitive sex differences remains unresolved. One view stresses the social construction of human behavioral sex differences and disputes whether biological sex differences, beyond those directly related to reproduction, contribute to the formation of behavioral sex differences (Bleier, 1984; Fausto-Sterling, 1992). Although no credible researcher argues the contrary, that biological factors solely and completely determine human behavioral sex differences, it is certainly the case that others have emphasized biological processes and focused less often on socialization processes (Barash, 1979; Reinisch, 1974). The more common biologically based view is that biological processes induce predispositions to engage in specific behaviors which can be shaped and modified by specific social experience (Collaer and Hines, 1995). However, this view still leaves unresolved the extent to which either biological processes or socialization influences specific behavioral patterns. One facet of this ongoing debate has been to attempt to relate the results of studies of behavioral sex differences in animals to the development of human sex differences. While animal studies offer a large body of evidence supporting biological influences on the development of sexually dimorphic behavior (Baum, 1979; Adkins-Regan, 1989; Goy and McEwen, 1980; Collaer and Hines, 1995), they have presented less evidence for the effect of social context on the development of behavioral sex differences. One reason for the paucity of evidence of socialization influences is undoubtedly because biological forces more strongly canalize some aspects of behavioral development in nonhumans than is the case for humans. However, there is evidence in animals that even such a clearly biological trait as the number of neurons in the corpus callosum as well as other areas of the male and female nervous system are exquisitely sensitive to the social context of rearing (Juraska and Kopcik, 1988; Juraska, 1991; Moore, Dou, and Juraska, 1992). Such findings suggest that the lack of evidence for socialization influences on the development of sex differences in animals reflects more the researcher's research emphasis than a fundamental difference between humans and animals. Similarly, the less complete evidence of biological influences on human behavioral sex differences results partly from ethical considerations which preclude the sort of precise physiological manipulations possible with animals. Thus most human evidence results from experiments of nature which alter some aspect of the typical developmental sequence. However, such "accidents of nature" lack the precision and control possible in animal experimentation. Looking at close nonhuman primate relatives offers the opportunity to investigate these issues in species likely to produce information more relevant to the human condition. In this regard the rhesus monkey provides an ideal opportunity to systematically investigate the interaction between biological predispositions and social influences on the development of behavioral sex differences.

Rhesus monkeys in nature live in complex social groups integrated around a complex matrilineal social structure (Lindburg, 1971). Adult patterns of behavior are strongly sexually differentiated in regard to mating behavior, infant care, and patterns of social interaction. In addition, rhesus monkey infant and juvenile development has been studied in a wide range of social contexts ranging from total social isolation to complex age-graded groups of more than 100 animals. This rich data set on the relation between the developmental environment and behavioral sex differences is complemented by 25 years of studies in which the pre- and postnatal hormonal environment has been manipulated in different dosages, through different hormones, and at different developmental times. Integration of these two bodies of developmental data provides insight into the relative contributions of hormonal influences and early social experience on the development of behavioral sex differences. These studies provide a model system for understanding how sex differences develop and demonstrate that neither nature nor nurture determines the developmental trajectory, but, instead, it is the interaction between biological predispositions and the characteristics of the rearing environment which determines the form of behavior displayed during development. In contrast to this view, the first fully developed description of juvenile rhesus monkey behavioral sex differences argued for constitutional differences between male and female infant rhesus monkeys which led directly to juvenile behavioral sex differences and ultimately shaped adult sexual roles (Harlow, 1965). Harlow's study provides the starting point for this review as it not only attempted to develop a complete description of the development of juvenile behavioral sex differences, but also described their relationship to adult behavior.

Harlow described developmental patterns of male assertiveness and aggressivity as a developmental training ground for adult male rhesus monkey sexual assertiveness. In a complementary manner females were shown to display passivity and accommodation, which would ultimately prepare females for their assumed accommodating role in adult rhesus monkey sexuality. This integrated view of the development and function of behavioral sex differences relied upon several assumptions about rhesus monkey juvenile and adult behavior which have subsequently been shown to be inaccurate. Thus the view of male assertiveness and female accommodation and passivity presented by Harlow, which has substantially influenced thinking on behavioral sex differences in both nonhuman primates and humans, needs reevaluation. This reevaluation requires first reviewing the schema presented by Harlow more than 30 years ago and investigating the assumptions inherent in that view of adult sexual behavior and developmental sex differences.

Our current understanding of adult rhesus monkey sexual behavior has changed substantially from the view 30 years ago and this affects the possible relationship between juvenile behavioral sex differences and adult sexuality. Additionally, as described below, it is apparent that the type and magnitude of behavioral sex differences are functions of the specific conditions of rearing. Finally, the interaction between the developmental social context and the prenatal and early postnatal hormonal environment is considered.

Adult Sexual Behavior in Rhesus Monkeys

Harlow proposed that juvenile sex differences in a variety of social and protosexual behaviors subserved the development of the adult heterosexual affectional system and adult sexual roles (Harlow, 1965). Evaluating this proposition first requires an understanding of adult rhesus monkey sexual behavior as described by Harlow and in comparison to our current understanding.

While Harlow's description of adult rhesus monkey sexual behavior is quite brief, consisting of two paragraphs (Harlow, 1965), he acknowledged that "Sexual behavior is generally initiated by the female" (p. 235), through approaching, grooming, or sexually presenting to the male. However, he also wrote that after a female lies down near a male she "... passively awaits until he approaches or establishes contact before assuming the female sexual posture" (p. 235), suggesting a more active role of the male in sexual initiation. The female's passive acceptance of the male was clearly integral to Harlow's notion of the role juvenile behavioral sex differences played in the development of adult heterosexuality as he later emphasized juvenile female behaviors of passivity and rigidity as critical to the development of male heterosexual behavior, stating, "... the female infant's tendency to respond to approach by passivity, withdrawal, and rigidity with buttocks presentation and head aversion increases the likelihood that the approaching male will establish dorsoventral contact" (p. 243). Thus the developmental passivity of the female allows the male to "discover" the appropriate adult sexual posture. However, this view of adult rhesus monkey sexuality reflects a limited set of circumstances under which the male controls the sexual interaction.

The earliest detailed description of rhesus monkey sexual behavior under semi-free ranging conditions emphasized the role of the female in initiating and actively maintaining sexual interactions with males (Carpenter, 1942). Carpenter's description, later reinforced by Altmann (1962), describes several active behavioral patterns, in addition to sexual presentations used by females to encourage male sexual activity. However, during the 1960s and 1970s studies of rhesus monkey sexual behavior almost exclusively used pairs of males and females (pair-tests) tested in time-limited tests in enclosures marginally larger than the pair of animals (Wallen, 1990). It was from studies under such conditions that Harlow obtained his description of adult rhesus monkey sexual behavior. This testing environment divorces heterosexual behavior from the typical rhesus monkey social context in which females outnumber males and much of the social structure is built around matrilineal relations. Pair-tests have generally emphasized the role that the male appears to play in initiating sexual activity and find that male behavior rather than female behavior varies more consistently with female hormonal state (Michael, Zumpe, and Bonsall, 1982). In contrast, at least one investigator using pair-tests reported reliable changes in female initiation of proximity in relation to the female's ovarian cycle in pair-tests (Goy and Resko, 1972). However, the predominant view resulting from laboratory studies is one of male initiation of sexual behavior with female behavior primarily relegated to attracting the male and responding to his sexual overtures (Keverne, 1976; Michael and Bonsall, 1979; Michael, Zumpe, and Bonsall, 1982; Keverne, 1982).

Precise studies on captive groups of rhesus monkeys which preserve male:female sex ratios comparable to those found in free-ranging groups (Wallen, 1990; Lindburg, 1971) have provided a quite different picture of rhesus monkey heterosexual behavior (Cochran, 1979; Gordon, 1981; Wilson, Gordon, and Collins, 1982; Wallen, Winston, Gaventa, and Davis-DaSilva, 1984; Wallen, 1990, 1995). In captive-group studies the active solicitation by females of males is readily apparent (Cochran, 1979; Wallen et al., 1984), with more than 90% of all sexual interactions initiated by the female (Wallen et al., 1984). In addition, the pattern of behavior shown by the female is certainly not passive, but involves active pursuit of the male (Wallen, 1990). Even when a male and female are sitting closely together the female will actively solicit mounting and copulation through the rapid staccato hand and head movements described for semi-free ranging rhesus monkeys on Cayo Santiago more than 50 years ago (Carpenter, 1942). Thus outside of the very limited social environment of the laboratory pair-test, the evidence overwhelmingly supports active female initiation of sexual behavior with male accommodation and responsiveness to female sexual overtures. If we are to understand the developmental pathway leading to adult rhesus monkey heterosexual activity, it is the male responsivity to female initiation which requires an ontogenetic precursor, not female accommodation of male initiation. However, it may be the case that female rhesus monkeys interact with males with much more passivity and hesitancy as juveniles, but become sexual initiators after puberty. Similarly, juvenile males may actively initiate social interactions with females, but stop initiating as adults and become sensitive and responsive to female initiation. Alternatively, the character of juvenile sex differences may be as sensitive to the social environment as is the character of adult heterosexual interaction. This is, in fact, the case as juvenile sex differences vary with rearing context.

Rearing Context and Juvenile Behavioral Sex Differences

In keeping with the emphasis on experimental control which dominated the experimental psychology of the 1950s and 1960s, laboratory environments for rearing monkeys rarely attempted to duplicate the social complexity of free-ranging populations, but instead simplified the young monkey's social environment to isolate specific variables of interest. As part of Harlow's emphasis on the development of affectional systems in monkeys, young rhesus monkeys were typically separated from their mothers soon after birth and surrogate reared with differing degrees of exposure to comparably treated peers. Social behavior of these monkeys was assessed by observing their behavior in a playroom with a consistent group of peers for 20 min to 2 hr 5 days per week. This "normal" laboratory rearing environment produced the first demonstration of reliable sex differences in juvenile behavior: sex differences which seemed to fit with the predominant view of adult sex role behavior in rhesus monkeys (Harlow, 1965). Although presented as a "normal" developmental pathway, it is now evident that this is not the case. However, it is still unclear how consistently specific behavioral sex differences are expressed under different rearing conditions, whether all are equally sensitive to social context, and how the prenatal hormonal environment interacts with the social context of rearing to influence their expression. This discussion will be limited primarily to the signature behavioral patterns Harlow viewed as critical to the development of adult heterosexuality. As described in Table 61.1, these patterns represent the primary behavioral sex differences seen in juvenile rhesus monkeys and most have been studied in social-developmental contexts ranging from the peer-playpen situation of Harlow

and colleagues to large age-graded heterosexual groups of rhesus monkey (Lovejoy and Wallen, 1988; Wallen, Maestripieri, and Mann, 1995). The following section presents evidence of the occurrence of behavioral sex differences in each of these behavioral patterns in relation to the social context of rearing.

Passivity, Rigidity, and Withdrawal

In the peer-playroom rearing condition (Peer-Group reared) Harlow (1965) reported that females displayed significantly more passivity, rigidity, and withdrawal than did infant and juvenile males. These sex differences were evident within the first 2 months of life and remained evident throughout the 1st year of life. Harlow (1965) argued that this constellation of behaviors expressed more frequently by females facilitated the development of appropriate male sexual posturing leading to the differentiation of adult male and female sexual roles. Specifically, Harlow viewed infants as primarily showing immature mounts and the stereotypical adult footclasp mount was something that males gradually learned during development. The propensity of females to display passivity and rigidity allowed males to discover the appropriate mounting posture through a process of trial and error. There are several difficulties with this conceptualization, even within the context of the Peer-Group rearing condition employed by Harlow. First, although passivity and rigidity might contribute to male exploration of female peers, it is difficult to see how increased female withdrawal would facilitate such development. Second, there is no mechanism proposed for how this female passivity lead to male discovery of the appropriate mounting posture. These males never achieve vaginal intromissions as juveniles, and rarely, if at all, as adults (Wallen, Beilert and Slimp, 1977; Goy and Wallen, 1979). Thus vagino-penile stimulation cannot be what guides the male's development. If the reinforcing property of the mount was penile stimulation, then even immature

Table 61.1
Behavioral patterns reported by Harlow to differ between infant males and females

Behavior name[a]	Description[b]
Passivity	"... the monkey sits quietly and is relatively unresponsive when approached by another animal."
Withdrawal	"... monkey actively avoids the approach of another, and if the approach continues, the withdrawing animal commonly assumes a prone position with the head oriented away from the approaching monkey."
Rigidity	"This also occurs in response to the approach of another monkey and is characterized by a fixed, hardened rigidity, with the head averted."
Threat	"... Stiffening posture, staring at the other monkey, flattening of hair on top of head, retracting the lips, and baring the teeth."
Female sex posturing (present)	"... elevation of the buttocks and the tail, lowering of the head and shoulders, backward orientation of the face ..."[c]
Rough and tumble play	"... monkey infants wrestle and roll and engage in sham biting although none is ever hurt."
Immature sexual behavior (abortive mounting)	"Rubbing and thrusting responses directed towards a second infant."
Dorsoventral mounting (foot-clasp mounting)	"... dorso-ventral positioning of the female, mounting with hands clasping the female's buttocks and feet clasping the female's ankles or legs ..."[c]

a. Names in parentheses represent names for these same behaviors used by other researchers.
b. From Harlow, 1965.
c. From Harlow's description of adult sexual behavior. In the paper's context this was apparently applied to the infant's behavior. Though data for these behaviors are shown, there is no specific description of the behaviors for infants.

mounts which involve penile rubbing on another animal would provide such stimulation. Thus female passivity is not sufficient to develop male sexual posturing and the alternative mechanism, that males are predisposed to engage in foot-clasp mounting, is not proposed. The last problem with the developmental schema proposed by Harlow did not become evident until some years later when it was found that males reared in groups where females displayed high levels of these behaviors were very poor adult copulators at best (Wallen, Beilert and Slimp, 1977; Goy and Wallen, 1979). Moreover, when these signature patterns of female passivity, rigidity, and withdrawal are studied under social conditions other than Peer-Group rearing they are not consistently displayed or there is no sex difference in their occurrence.

Two of these patterns of behavior, rigidity, and withdrawal have been studied in small mother–infant groups with continuous access and large outdoor-housed age-graded rhesus monkey groups with multiple adult males and females. The findings are quite consistent: sex differences in these behaviors are found only in the Peer-Group rearing environment with limited daily social contact. Table 61.2[1] compares the occurrence of these behaviors by infants reared in large outdoor-housed age-graded monkey groups with multiple adult males and females (Social-Group reared) to their occurrence in Harlow's environment and other environments constructed in the laboratory. When rhesus monkeys are reared in large age-graded groups, rigidity is not observed in the behavioral repertoire of either male or female yearlings (Lovejoy and Wallen,

Table 61.2
Comparison of the occurrence of behavioral sex differences during the first or second year of life under different experimental rearing conditions in comparison to their occurrence in large age-graded social groups

	Social group[a] 24 hr/day access	Rearing condition										
		Peer-group rearing						Mother-peer rearing			
		Heterosexual < 2 hr/day[b]		Isosexual 30 min/day[c]		Heterosexual 30 min/day[d]		Heterosexual 24 hr/day[e]		Isosexual 24 hr[f]	
	Sex diff	Sex diff	Effect[g]	Sex diff	Effect	Sex diff	Effect	Sex diff	Effect	Sex diff	Effect
Rigidity	NO[h]	F > M	↑ Sex D	—[i]	—	—	—	—	—	—	—
Passivity	—	F > M	↑ Sex D	—	—	—	—	—	—	—	—
Withdrawal	F ≈ M	F > M	↑ Sex D	—	—	—	—	—	—	—	—
Threat	F ≈ M	M > F	↑ Sex D	M > F	↑ Sex D	M > F	↑ Sex D	F ≈ M	None	—	—
Presenting	F ≈ M	F > M	↑ Sex D	M > F	↑ Male	F ≈ M	None	F ≈ M	None	M > F?	↑ Sex D?
R&T play[j]	M > F	M > F	↑ Male	M > F	↓ Male	—	—	M > F	None	M > F	None
Mount											
Immature	—	M > F	↑ Sex D	—	—	—	—	M > F	None	—	—
Foot-clasp	M > F	M > F	↓ Male	—	—	—	—	M > F	None	M > F	↓ Sex D

a. Age-graded, heterosexual outdoor-housed groups (e.g., Lovejoy and Wallen, 1988; Wallen, Maestripieri, and Mann, 1995).
b. Harlow, 1965.
c. Goldfoot and Wallen, 1978.
d. Wallen, Goy, and Goldfoot, 1981.
e. Goy, Wallen, and Goldfoot, 1974; Wallen, Goy, and Goldfoot, 1981.
f. Goldfoot et al., 1984.
g. Effect, The effect the rearing condition has on the magnitude of sex differences. ↑ Sex D, Difference between males and females is greater than that seen in the social group condition. ↓ Male or ↑ Male, the frequency of male expression of the behavior was increased or decreased under that rearing condition. None, no apparent affect of rearing condition in comparison to social-group rearing.
h. NO, Included in behavioral scoring lexicon, but never observed to occur.
i. (—) Data for this behavioral measure not collected under this rearing condition or collected, but not analyzed for possible sex differences.
j. R&T, rough and tumble.

1988). Withdrawal is displayed, but at comparable frequencies by male and female infants (Lovejoy and Wallen, 1988; Wallen, Maestripieri, and Mann, 1995). Similarly male and female rhesus monkey infants withdraw from each other at comparable frequencies when reared for the 1st year of life with continuous access to their mothers and three to five other infants (Mother-Peer reared; Wallen, Goldfoot, and Goy, 1981). Thus rigidity and withdrawal do not appear to be prototypical behaviors foreshadowing adult female sex roles, as both Social-Group reared and Mother-Peer reared females either do not display these behaviors or display them at frequencies comparable to males, yet they develop into fully sexually competent adults. Similarly, males growing up in environments where females do not display the heightened levels of submissiveness described by Harlow develop complete adult heterosexual behavior. In contrast, Peer-Group males who grow up in groups where females display high levels of these behaviors are generally not sexually competent as adults (Goy and Wallen, 1979). Thus it seems unlikely that these behaviors are related at all to the development of heterosexuality. As discussed in the next section, it seems more likely that the sex differences reported by Harlow reflect heightened agonistic behavior between infants resulting from the limited daily social contact of the Peer-Group rearing environment and the absence of comforting adults to which infants can retreat when peer interactions become too intense.

Evidence in support of the notion that sex differences in rigidity and withdrawal reflect differences in the agonism inherent in different environments comes from a study which observed small groups of rhesus monkey mothers and infants under conditions where infant peer contact was continuous or limited to 30 min per day (Wallen, Goldfoot, and Goy, 1981). Two findings from this study are relevant here. During the 1st year of life, when all infants had continuous access to their mothers, infants receiving 30 min of daily peer contact withdrew from peers significantly more frequently than did infants having continuous access to peers. After weaning at 1 year of age infants were observed for 30 min daily with their natal peers. In these observations only the infants receiving 30 min of daily peer access in their 1st year of life withdrew from peers. In addition, females withdrew almost twice as frequently as males, a significant difference in withdrawal frequency (Wallen, Goldfoot, and Goy, 1981). Thus the occurrence of withdrawal and its sexual differentiation appears to be limited to conditions where peers have very limited opportunity for social contact. Under rearing conditions providing continuous daily peer contact, withdrawal, like rigidity, rarely is observed or is not differentially displayed by males and females. These results suggest that infant rhesus monkeys require long periods of daily interaction in order to develop stable and nonantagonistic social relations. Even the presence of a mother is not sufficient to prevent the development of heightened agonism between peers if the infants have insufficient opportunity to establish consistent social relations. Unanswered by these data is why females appear to be more profoundly affected by limited opportunity for social interaction. Both males and females were limited to 30 min for social interaction, yet it is the females who displayed increased submissiveness. Threat behavior, another behavioral pattern which Harlow viewed as critically sexually differentiated, offers a possible solution to this problem.

Threat

In the Peer-Group rearing condition males threaten peers significantly more frequently than do females during the 1st year of life (Harlow, 1965). However, as shown in Table 61.2, when infants are reared in groups with their mothers, threatening between peers is infrequent and males and females threaten with comparable frequencies (Goy, Wallen, and Goldfoot, 1974; Wallen, Goldfoot, and Goy, 1981; Lovejoy and

Wallen, 1988; Wallen, Maestripieri, and Mann, 1995). This failure to find a sex difference in threatening is not even affected by the amount of daily peer access as long as the mother is present. During the 1st year of life infants living with their mothers, but receiving 30 min of daily peer access, did not threaten each other more frequently than did Mother-Peer reared infants with continuous access to peers (Wallen, Goldfoot, and Goy, 1981). However, when the infants were weaned, the infants who had received 30 min of daily peer access during their 1st year of life now threatened peers significantly more frequently than did those who had continuous peer access during their 1st year. In addition, the display of threats by these limited peer-access yearlings was sexually differentiated, with males displaying 30 times as many threats as females with almost 75% of these threats directed toward female peers (Wallen, Goldfoot, and Goy, 1981). In contrast, those infants receiving continuous access to peers during their 1st year continued to display low frequencies of threat when removed from their mothers and limited to 30 min of daily social contact with peers. Thus the presence of the mother appeared to moderate threatening between males and their female peers, but this influence disappeared as soon as the infants were removed from the mother and left to their own devices to regulate their social behavior. These results also suggest that the frequency of threatening by males is influenced by the presence of female peers.

Further support for this notion is provided from studies in which infant males and females were reared in isosexual groups allowing independent assessment of the behavior of males and females without the presence of the other sex (Table 61.2). Threatening by males reared during the 1st year of life in isosexual peer groups was one-third the frequency seen in heterosexually Peer-Group reared male infants (Goldfoot and Wallen, 1978). In contrast, isosexual rearing of females had no measurable effect on their threatening behavior with almost identical mean frequencies displayed by heterosexually and isosexually reared females (Goldfoot and Wallen, 1978). Although the isosexually reared male threat frequency was almost 75% greater than that of isosexual females, it was not indicated in this research report whether this was a significant difference. Thus it is not certain whether the absence of female peers in the Peer-Group rearing condition eliminates the sex difference in threat reported by Harlow. It is clear, however, that the magnitude of the sex difference is markedly reduced (from 318% more frequent threatening by heterosexually reared males to 73% greater frequency for isosexually reared males) when female peers are not present during the 1st year of life. However, both of the sex differences are substantially greater than that seen in Social-Group reared infants where males and females display threats at comparable frequencies (Table 61.2).

These results demonstrate that high frequencies of threat behavior, instead of being a hallmark of infant male development, sensitively reflect the social conditions of rearing. The degree of sex difference in this behavior ranges from markedly and significantly higher frequencies of male threat under heterosexual Peer-Group rearing to marginal sex difference in isosexual Peer-Group rearing, to no detectable evidence of any sex difference in threat behavior in Mother-Peer rearing with continuous social access or Social-Group rearing (Harlow, 1965; Goldfoot and Wallen, 1978; Wallen, Goldfoot, and Goy, 1981; Lovejoy and Wallen, 1988; Wallen, Maestripieri, and Mann, 1995). In his original discussion of infant rhesus monkey threatening, Harlow argued for a constitutional difference between males and females to account for the higher male frequency by stating: "It is extremely difficult for us to believe that these differences are cultural, for we cannot imagine how our inanimate surrogate mothers could transmit culture to their infants" (Harlow, 1965, p. 240). Clearly he was correct on the inability of surrogate mothers to transmit culture. However, the data now strongly support the view that threatening behavior during development is strongly culturally influenced, with the socializing influence coming from the infants themselves. This analysis, however, leaves unresolved why males threaten female peers more frequently when the social environment is devoid of adult moderating influences or the infants have very short periods for social interaction. This raises the possibility that a predisposition to harass and dominate one's peers is sexually dimorphic and expressed more regularly in males than females. A complete understanding of the predisposition to threaten others awaits studies directed specifically at this issue.

Present

The present, or female sexual posture as Harlow referred to it, was reported to be displayed more frequently by females than males during early development in Peer-Group reared rhesus monkeys (Harlow, 1965). This sex difference was regarded as indicating heterosexual development and thus a sign of "normal" development. However, when observed under a variety of social rearing conditions this behavior is found to be highly variable in its expression (Table 61.2). In Social-Group reared infants presents are displayed at comparable frequencies by both males and females (Lovejoy and Wallen, 1988; Wallen, Maestripieri, and Mann, 1995). This is also the case in Mother-Peer reared infants regardless of whether they receive 30 min or 24 hr of daily access to peers (Wallen, Goldfoot, and Goy, 1981).

Rearing infants in single-sex groups (isosexual rearing), however, has the effect of dramatically increasing the frequency that males display presents whether or not they are Peer-Group or Mother-Peer reared (Table 61.2). In contrast isosexual rearing had no measurable effect on the display of presents by infant females, resulting in a reversal of the sex difference reported by Harlow. Thus for this behavior social context appears to influence whether presents are displayed more frequently by females, by males, or at similar frequencies by both sexes.

Although infant presents are morphologically similar to the adult sexual posture, it seems unlikely that the display of presents during infancy is related to adult sexuality in any clear way. Isosexually reared males, who display presents at much higher frequencies than heterosexually reared males (Goldfoot, Wallen, Neff, McBrair, and Goy, 1984), differ in only minor ways in their adult sexual behavior from heterosexually reared males (Berkovitch, Roy, Sladky, and Goy, 1988). In fact, it seems likely that infantile presents reflect a submissive response to agonistic interactions rather than protosexual behavior. The increased presenting by isosexually reared males probably reflects the fact that males occupy all dominance positions in isosexual groups, whereas male average rank is higher than female average rank in heterosexual peer groups (Goldfoot et al., 1984). Thus isosexual males present more on average than their heterosexually reared brethren because there are more low-ranking isosexual males. This is borne out by the finding that low-ranking heterosexually reared males display significantly more presents than do high-ranking heterosexually reared males (Goldfoot et al., 1984). Like withdrawal and rigidity, it seems likely that the high levels of presents displayed by heterosexual Peer-Group reared females reflects both high levels of agonism in such groups and a lower average social status requiring more submissive behavior. It is unlikely that these behaviors are related to the development of adult female sexuality. The reason that females have a lower average social rank in groups without adults and limited opportunity for social interaction remains unanswered.

Rough and Tumble Play

The rough wrestling play reported by Harlow to be displayed more frequently by males than females has been found to be one of the most robust sex differences in infant and juvenile behavior (Table 61.2). In every rearing environment where play was studied, males displayed rough and tumble play more frequently than did females. The only effects of rearing condition were an increased frequency of rough and tumble play displayed by Peer-Group reared males in comparison to Social-Group reared males and somewhat lower play frequencies in isosexually reared males. This latter finding suggests either that the presence of females stimulates males to play or, as in the case of presenting, lower-ranking monkeys engage in less play than do higher-ranking monkeys. In this view the reduction in play by isosexually reared males reflects the fact that they occupy all dominance ranks within their groups, resulting in more low-ranking males than would be found among heterosexually reared males. This can only be a partial explanation since isosexually reared females did not show any evidence of increased rough and tumble play, even though they occupied the highest social ranks in their groups. Thus the specific form of this sex difference appears to be only weakly modulated by the specific social context of rearing.

It has been argued that rough and tumble play is a principal indicator of appropriate social development in rhesus monkey males (Harlow and Lauersdorf, 1974). However, the relationship between play and appropriate social development is not linear. Peer-Group reared males engage in rough and tumble play at very high frequencies, yet develop poor adult sexual behavior (Wallen, Bielert, and Slimp, 1977; Goy and Wallen, 1979). In contrast, rearing environments which produce the most sexually competent males are characterized by moderate levels of rough and tumble play in comparison to that displayed by Peer-Group reared males (Wallen, Bielert, and Slimp, 1977; Goy and Wallen, 1979). Thus it appears that too much, as well as too little, rough and tumble play probably reflects an inadequate social environment. As has been previously suggested (Goy and Wallen, 1979), very high levels of rough and tumble play may reflect juvenile

antagonism rather than play per se. Whatever the relationship between rough and tumble play and social development, it remains a consistent difference in juvenile behavior between males and females, which appear the least sensitive to the social context of rearing.

Mounting

Infant male rhesus monkeys separated from their mothers at birth or 30 days later and Peer-Group reared display immature sexual responses, also called abortive mounts, at much higher frequencies than females during the 1st year of life (Harlow, 1965). Under these rearing conditions this is the primary protosexual behavior displayed by infant males. The foot-clasp mount typical of adult male sexual behavior is rarely seen under these rearing conditions with Harlow writing that (at this age) "There is no semblance of normal sex posturing in either the male or female infant monkey" (Harlow, 1965, p. 243). Later he would write that the "... double foot clasp of the female's legs ... is not an infant male posture" (Harlow and Lauersdorf, 1974). However, it is now apparent that the specific form of mounting displayed by infant male rhesus monkeys, and, to some extent, infant female monkeys is strongly affected by the early rearing environment (Goy, Wallen, and Goldfoot, 1974; Wallen, Bielert, and Slimp, 1977; Goy and Wallen, 1979; Wallen, Goy, and Goldfoot, 1981; Goldfoot et al., 1984). In contrast to Peer-Group reared males, Mother-Peer reared males display primarily foot-clasp mounts after the first 3 months of life (Goy, Wallen, and Goldfoot, 1974). Yearling Social-Group reared males display foot-clasp mounts almost exclusively (Lovejoy and Wallen, 1988; Wallen, Maestripieri, and Mann, 1995), whereas less than 2% of the mounts displayed by yearling Peer-Group reared males are foot-clasp mounts (Goy, Wallen, and Goldfoot, 1974).

This difference in the expression of foot-clasp mounting in males reared with their mothers during the 1st year of life may result in part from the mother's presence, but primarily is a consequence of continuous access to peers. Only one of six infant male rhesus monkeys reared with their mothers during the 1st year of life, but with peer access limited to 30 min per day, displayed foot-clasp mounts to peers. In contrast, all six males reared under identical conditions except with 24 hr access to peers displayed foot-clasp mounts to peers at high frequencies (Wallen, Goldfoot, and Goy, 1981). Males under both rearing conditions did not differ in their overall level of mounting (abortive and foot-clasp mounts combined), solely in the expression of foot-clasp mounting. Similarly, infant males reared without mothers, but with continuous access to peers during the 1st year of life routinely display foot-clasp mounts (Wallen, Thornton, and Goy, unpublished). Thus the expression of foot-clasp mounting reflects the character of peer relations, rather than being a pattern with a fixed developmental schedule. Under conditions of high peer agonism, such as Peer-Group rearing, this mount pattern is rarely displayed. Under conditions of low agonism, primarily resulting from continuous opportunity for peer interaction, foot-clasp mounting is displayed readily and more frequently by males than females (Table 61.2).

The sexual composition of the rearing group also influences the expression of foot-clasp mounting and the magnitude of the sex difference (Table 61.2). When infant rhesus monkeys are Peer-Group reared in isosexual groups, as with Peer-Group reared rhesus monkeys, neither males nor females regularly displayed foot-clasp mounts (Goldfoot and Wallen, 1979). However, females reared in isosexual Mother-Peer groups displayed significantly more foot-clasp mounts than females reared in heterosexual Mother-Peer groups (Goldfoot et al., 1984). In contrast, though the sex difference in foot-clasp mounting seen in Mother-Peer reared infants remains, the degree of difference is reduced as isosexually reared Mother-Peer males displayed lower foot-

clasp mount frequencies than heterosexually reared males (Goldfoot et al., 1984). Thus rearing infants in same-sexed groups altered the expression of foot-clasp mounting by males and females, but did not alter the direction of the sex difference in mounting seen in Social-Group reared infants. In addition, the reduced level of foot-clasp mounting by isosexually reared males had no apparent effect on these males' adult sexual behavior (Berkovitch, Roy, Sladky, and Goy, 1988). The reduction in mounting in isosexually reared males, again, may simply reflect that males occupy all dominance positions and low-ranking males mount less than high-ranking males (Goldfoot et al., 1984). Similarly, the increase in mounting by isosexually reared females may reflect that females occupy all social ranks in isosexual groups and higher-ranking females display more foot-clasp mounts, even when reared in heterosexual groups (Goldfoot et al., 1984).

Hormonal Environment and Juvenile Sex Differences

In male rhesus monkeys testicular androgen secretion starts around Day 40 of gestation and continues, with varying levels, through 3 months after birth (Resko, 1985; Mann, Davis-DaSilva, Wallen, Coan, Evans, and Collins, 1984). Genital differentiation occurs soon after the onset of prenatal testicular function and males are born with fully differentiated genitalia, unlike the case in some short gestation mammals like the rat, where a substantial portion of genital differentiation occurs in the early neonatal period. A small number of studies have investigated the effects of eliminating neonatal androgen secretion in male rhesus monkeys, but not the effects of suppressing prenatal testicular function (Mann et al., 1984; Mann, Gould, and Wallen, 1992). The complementary studies, administering malelike levels of androgen prenatally to genetic females, have been pursued for more than 25 years and offer substantial evidence of the capacity of androgens to alter juvenile behavioral sex differences. Though these studies have used both Peer-Group and Mother-Peer rearing, the most extensive body of literature is in Mother-Peer reared monkeys, which is the primary focus of the following section. Research on the effects of the early hormonal environment on the development of behavior have not reported all of the measures originally described by Harlow as sexually dimorphic. Instead this research primarily focused on rough and tumble play and patterns of mounting, with some investigation of threatening and presenting. Thus this review will focus on these behavioral patterns in relation to the timing and duration of pre- and postnatal hormonal manipulations.

Neonatal Manipulation of Testicular Function in Male Rhesus Monkeys

Early attempts to eliminate neonatal testicular function used castration either on the day of birth or 90 days later (Goy, 1978). These studies reported no effect of the elimination of early testicular function on the development of mounting or rough and tumble play (Table 61.3; Goy, 1978). More recently, testicular function has been suppressed, starting within 3 days of birth, using a gonadotropin releasing-hormone antagonist, which suppresses gonadotropin release (Leal, Williams, Danforth, Gordon, and Hodgen, 1988). The 10 males treated this way have been Social-Group reared in two large outdoor-housed age-graded social groups. Elimination of neonatally secreted testicular androgen had no detectable effect on threatening, presenting, mounting, or rough and tumble play (Table 61.3; Wallen, Maestripieri, and Mann, 1995). Testicular-suppressed males displayed mounting and play behaviors significantly more frequently than control females and at levels comparable to control males. The only clear effect of neonatal testicular suppression was on aspects of the mother–infant relationship between the testicular-suppressed males and their mothers. Mothers of testicular-suppressed males groomed their infants significantly longer than either control males or females (Wallen, Maestripieri, and Mann, 1995). This study also included males whose neonatal testicular function had been suppressed and androgen exogenously replaced. By accident, the replacement therapy resulted in the administration of supraphysiological levels of androgen. These males provided further evidence that neonatal androgen influences the mother–infant relationship, as these males followed their mothers significantly less frequently and spent significantly less time in proximity to their mothers than did testicular-suppressed males (Wallen, Maestripieri, and Mann, 1995). Thus the effects of neonatal testicular secretions are subtle and do not affect the occurrence of mounting and rough and tumble play, but instead seem limited to effects on aspects of the mother–infant relationship (Wallen, Maestripieri, and Mann, 1995).

Prenatal Hormonal Manipulations in Rhesus Monkeys

Prenatal administration of androgens to genetic males, as summarized in Table 61.3, had no discernible effect on their juvenile behavior (Goy, 1981) presumably due to the males' own testicular secretions. In contrast to the lack of effects of prenatal androgens in males and the minimal effects of early neonatal androgen manipulations, exposing genetic female rhesus monkeys to prenatal androgen profoundly alters their juvenile behavior to be more like that of genetic males whether they are Peer-Group or Mother-Peer reared (Table 61.3; Goy, 1970, 1978, 1981; Goy, Bercovitch, and McBrair, 1988). Prenatal administration of androgens for more than 35 days to Peer-Group reared females increased frequencies of both rough and tumble play and foot-clasp mounting, but had no clear effect on threatening behavior, which is sexually dimorphic in this rearing environment (Goy, 1970). Studies

Table 61.3
Effects of different prenatal and neonatal hormonal treatments in genetic male and female rhesus monkeys on various patterns of juvenile social behavior

	Threat	Present	Rough play	Foot-clasp mounting
Social-Group reared				
Genetic males				
Neonatal testicular suppression (GnRH[a] antagonist)[b]	No effect	No effect	No effect	No effect
Peer-Group reared				
Genetic females				
Long androgen treatment (≥ 35 days of treatment)[c]	No effect	NR[d]	Increase	Increase
Mother-Peer reared				
Genetic males				
Prenatal androgen treatment (15–80 days of treatment)[e]	NR[e]	No effect	No effect	No effect
Neonatal castration[b]	NR	No effect	No effect	No effect
Genetic females				
Long androgen treatment (≥ 35 days of treatment)[e]	NR	No effect	Increase	Increase
Short-early androgen treatment (Days 40–64 gestation)[f]	NR	NR	No effect	Increase
Short-late androgen treatment (Days 115–139 gestation)[f]	NR	NR	Increase	Increase
Brief androgen treatment (15 days of treatment starting at 40, 50, or 60 days of gestation)[e]	NR	No effect	No effect	No effect

a. GnRH, gonadotropin-releasing hormone.
b. Wallen, Maestripieri, and Mann, 1995.
c. Goy, 1970.
d. NR, Data not reported for this measure.
e. Goy, 1978, 1981.
f. Goy, Bercovitch, and McBrair, 1988.

of Mother-Peer reared monkeys have varied both the duration and the timing of prenatal androgen treatments and have demonstrated that timing and duration influence the development of sex differences in behavior (Table 61.3). Prenatal androgen treatments 35–80 days in duration extensively masculinized the expression of both rough and tumble play and foot-clasp mounting, but had no effect on the occurrence of presents to peers (Goy, 1981). In addition these long prenatal androgen treatments also extensively masculinized and defeminized the external genitals of the females, producing a penis and scrotum almost indistinguishable from those of

normal genetic males and the complete elimination of a vaginal opening (Goy, Uno, and Sholl, 1989). Similarly extensive modification of the external genitalia can be produced with 15 or 25 days of prenatal androgen exposure if the treatment is started by 40 days of gestation (Goy, Bercovitch, and McBrair, 1988; Goy, Uno, and Sholl, 1989). A comparable 25-day treatment starting after Day 100 of gestation had no discernible effect on genital anatomy (Goy, Bercovitch, and McBrair, 1988). Thus the modification of the external genitalia is exquisitely sensitive to the timing of androgen exposure. The behavioral consequences of prenatal androgen exposure were similarly affected by treatment timing, as well as treatment duration.

Fifteen-day prenatal androgen treatments started on Gestation Day 40, while they extensively masculinized and defeminized female genitalia, had no discernible effect on any measure of juvenile behavior (Goy, 1981). Starting these 15-day treatments later in gestation reduced their effect on genital differentiation, but they still had no apparent behavioral effect. Increasing treatment duration from 15 to 25 days markedly altered the effect of the hormones on behavioral development. A 25-day prenatal androgen treatment started on Day 40 of gestation extensively masculinized and defeminized the fetal female's genitalia and also significantly increased the expression of juvenile foot-clasp mounting (Table 61.3; Goy, Bercovitch, and McBrair, 1988). However, this 25-day treatment had no apparent effect on the occurrence of rough play, with these genitally masculinized females displaying rough play at frequencies no different than their control female peers. Presenting, a behavior not found to be sexually dimorphic in Mother-Peer reared males and females, not surprisingly was unaffected by this prenatal androgen treatment. Administering the same 25-day prenatal androgen treatment, but starting later in gestation (Gestation Day 115), produced strikingly different effects than the earlier 25-day treatment. Females exposed to 25 days of androgen late in gestation were not noticeably genitally modified by the treatment, but their juvenile behavior was extensively masculinized (Table 61.3; Goy, Bercovitch, and McBrair, 1988). These females displayed significantly higher levels of both foot-clasp mounting and rough and tumble play than control females and higher levels of rough and tumble play than females exposed to the same androgen levels earlier in gestation. Again, not surprisingly this treatment had no effect on presenting to peers.

Considered together, these studies, varying the duration and timing of prenatal androgen exposure to genetic females, demonstrate that the specific anatomical and behavioral effects are the consequence of the specific pattern of exposure. By altering the timing of exposure during gestation it has been possible to separate androgenic effects on the differentiation of the genitalia from their effects on behavioral differentiation. Whether similar effects can be obtained by varying the time when prenatal testicular function is suppressed in genetic males remains to be seen in studies currently in progress.

Nature Needs Nurture: The Interaction between Predispositions and Social History

This chapter set out to delineate the relative role that social context plays in determining the expression of behavioral sex differences in rhesus monkeys and their relation to adult sexual behavior. Harlow's pioneering work, which provided the first comprehensive description of juvenile behavioral sex differences, demonstrates that it is not possible to understand either the extent or the function of behavioral sex differences by focusing on what was essentially a single rearing environment. Only when a range of rearing environments encompassing many important aspects of the species-typical social organization of rhesus monkeys were investigated was it possible to identify those behavioral sex differences which primarily occur in a specific social context and those which occur across a wide range of social contexts. Table 61.4 summarizes the social factors that have been varied between rearing environments and their effect on the behaviors under discussion. Rigidity is an example of a submissive behavior where its expression as a behavioral sex difference is limited to a very specific social context. While this behavior is displayed very frequently by Peer-Group reared females, it is almost never observed in other rearing environments. Its expression, like other submissive behaviors, is strongly affected by the amount of time peers have to interact. The expression of presenting as a sexually differentiated response is

Table 61.4
Summary of effects of various social and hormonal variables on the occurrence of various juvenile social behaviors reported to be sexually dimorphic in at least one social rearing environment

	Submission	Threat/ aggression	Presenting	Rough play	Foot-clasp mounting
Social context variables					
Limited access time to peers	↑ Female	↑ Male	↑ Female	↑ Male	↓ Male
Unlimited access time to peers	↓ Female	↓ Male	↓ Female	↓ Male	↑ Male
Limiting group to same-sex peers	↓ Female	↓ Male	↑ Male	↓ Male	↓ Male ↑ Female
Adding presence of mothers during first year	↓ Female	↓ Male	↓ Female	↓ Male	↑ Male
Hormonal exposure variables					
Suppressing male neonatal testicular function	No effect	No effect	No effect	No effect	No effect
Exposing genetic males to prenatal androgen	No effect	No effect	No effect	No effect	No effect
Exposing genetic females to long prenatal androgen	↓ Female	No effect	No effect	↑ Female	↑ Female
Exposing genetic females to short early prenatal androgens	Unknown	Unknown	Unknown	No effect	↑ Female
Exposing genetic females to short late prenatal androgens	Unknown	Unknown	Unknown	↑ Female	↑ Female

also almost exclusively influenced by social context, and it also is influenced by both peer-access time and the sexual composition of the group (Table 61.4). No developmental hormonal treatment has been found to affect its expression, yet in some social contexts it is displayed more frequently by females, in other social contexts, more frequently by males, and in still other contexts there is no difference between males and females in its display. Thus whether presenting is found to be sexually dimorphic and the direction of the dimorphism depend upon the social context and not the duration or amount of exposure to a specific prenatal hormonal environment.

Other behaviors exhibit a clear interaction between the prenatal hormonal environment and the social context of development. Mounting is readily modified by specific prenatal hormonal treatments, yet the degree of the difference between males and females depends upon the social environment (Table 61.4). In all cases, males display this behavior more frequently than females, but the magnitude of the difference is strongly affected by the sexual composition of the rearing environment, with a greater sexual dimorphism in this behavior in heterosexual groups than in isosexual groups. The smaller difference between the sexes in isosexual groups is the result of both increased mounting by females and decreased mounting by males. Thus the prenatal hormonal environment shapes the predisposition to engage in mounting of peers, but this predisposition must be nurtured by a specific social context for full expression. Limit social contact between peers early in life and the foot-clasp mount rarely develops, no matter what hormonal environment a genetic male or female is exposed to. The expression of this behavior is strictly the result of an interaction between propensities influenced by hormones and the extent to which the social environment promotes the expression of these propensities.

In contrast to mounting, rough and tumble play appears to be a behavior which is less dependent upon a specific social context for its expression than upon a specific pattern of prenatal hormonal exposure. Rough and tumble play occurs in all social environments reported here with males expressing it more frequently than females. As inferred from present data, the propensity to exhibit rough and tumble play is seemingly sensitive to very specific and brief hormonal exposure. Furthermore, prenatal hormonal environments which increase mounting by females can have no measurable effect on rough and tumble play, whereas any prenatal treatment which increases rough and tumble play also increases mounting. However, even this behavior, which is strongly affected by the prenatal hormonal environment, is still modulated to some degree by social context (Table 61.4). The sexual composition of the rearing environment affects the expression of rough and tumble play by males, but not females. Isosexual rearing decreases the occurrence of rough and tumble play by males, but, unlike mounting, isosexual rearing has no effect on the expression of play by females. Thus the predisposition to engage in rough and tumble play appears to be largely determined by the prenatal hormonal environment. However, the actual expression of this predisposition is a consequence of the social context of rearing, though the capacity of the social environment to markedly alter the expression of play behavior appears much more limited than behaviors such as threat, presenting, and even mounting.

Harlow presented the first integrated view of the relationship between developmental behavioral sex differences and their function in preparing for adult behavioral sex roles. We now know that the view Harlow offered, while appropriate given the information available in 1965, neither reflected a sufficient range of developmental variability nor accurately reflected adult rhesus monkey sex roles. Unfortunately, though we now know that the conception of passive females and assertive males leading each to discover its appropriate role in sexual behavior is incorrect, we still do not know the functional relationship between juvenile behavioral sex differences and adult sexual behavior, except that males who do not develop foot-clasp mounting are poor copulators in adulthood. Maybe there is no relationship between juvenile and adult behavior beyond this simple relationship, which actually encapsulates a great deal of social complexity during development. Alternatively, these behavioral sex differences may serve specific social needs of the infant monkeys themselves and are only incidentally related to adult social behavior. This view of infant behavior, as serving the infants' needs, suggests why some of these behaviors vary so greatly across different rearing environments. Each social rearing context provides a different set of social challenges to the infant requiring a different set of behavioral responses. An infant spending 23.5 hr per day in a single cage and 30 min with five other rambunctious infants, and no adults, faces a markedly different set of social problems than does an infant living all day with its protective mother, one or more siblings, and an assorted collection of aunts, great aunts, and a few adult males. We should not be surprised that the behavior of infants in these two contexts is markedly different in many ways. Maybe more surprising is that some behaviors, play and mounting, are remarkably consistent across such differing social contexts. The finding that these behaviors, play and mounting, are also strongly affected by the prenatal hormonal environment indicates the importance of these behaviors to normal development.

If it is true that nature needs nurture, that a hormonally induced behavioral predisposition can only be expressed in a supportive social environment, then the complement is also true; nurture requires nature. Some may view this chapter as suggesting that some behavioral sex differences, such as threatening, are strictly the result of a specific social context and thus are socially constructed sex differences. In one sense this is true because without that specific social context the behavioral sexual dimorphism would not occur. However, in another sense, the fact that a behavioral sexual dimorphism occurs only within a specific social context does not eliminate the need to consider an underlying sex difference in predisposition to engage in specific behaviors. The finding that rigidity and withdrawal are only expressed at higher frequencies by females in a Peer-Group rearing condition is not a demonstration that this sex difference is solely the result of a specific social context. Such a view, of complete social construction, ignores the finding that it is females, but not males, who consistently display these patterns more frequently. The existence of the sex difference in a single social context does not provide a mechanism to produce the consistency in the behavioral response to that environment. It is this consistency between the sexes within a constant social environment which argues for an underlying, albeit possibly small, constitutional difference between males and females. This could be something as simple as males physically maturing more rapidly than females, allowing them to use their greater size to intimidate smaller females. It could be something more complicated, such as a different style of social interaction which only is canalized into increased submission when there is limited opportunity for social interaction in the absence of adult authority figures. These examples are, of course, pure speculation, but illustrate that the social lability of a behavioral sex difference still requires rigorous investigation of possible predispositions which interact with social context to shape behavioral expression. It is only in the human case, where a sex difference in behavior is verbally mandated, "boys don't cry" for example, that consideration of underlying predispositions may be irrelevant. In all other cases, social context and biological predispositions are indispensable components in the development of behavioral sex differences.

Acknowledgments

This chapter is dedicated to Robert W. Goy, without whose insight and ground-breaking work this attempt at synthesis would not have been possible. Not only has he provided the critical evidence necessary for the thesis presented here, but also personally shaped my own thinking on these issues when I first worked in his laboratory 30 years ago. His continued input and guidance over the ensuing years are greatly appreciated. This chapter attempts to continue the line of thinking so well argued in his many papers on the development of behavioral sex differences and many of the ideas presented here owe a great intellectual debt to Bob. Any errors or omissions are solely mine. Preparation of this chapter was supported in part by NIMH RSDA Award K02-MH01062 and NIMH Research Award R01-MH50268.

Note

1. In the text and Table 61.2, differences between males and females have been taken from the original author's analyses in each rearing condition. When an author stated that there was a sex difference in behavior this was regarded as accurate whether or not the author reported the statistical support for the conclusion. Cases where an explicit comparison was not made between males and females and the reported means were clearly comparable were regarded as the lack of a sex difference. In one case, presenting in Mother-Peer reared subjects reared in isosexual groups (Goldfoot et al., 1984), the explicit comparison between males and females is not reported, but isosexual male presenting frequencies were severalfold higher than isosexual female frequencies during the 1st year of life. This is shown as a sex difference with a question mark to indicate that this sex difference is not verified.

References

Adkins-Regan, E. (1989). Sex hormones and sexual orientation in animals. *Psychobiology* 16, 335–347.

Altmann, S. A. (1962). A field study of the sociobiology of rhesus monkeys, *Macaca mulatta. Ann. N. Y. Acad. Sci.* 102, 338–435.

Barash, D. (1979). *The Whisperings Within.* Harper and Row, New York.

Baum, M. J. (1979). Differentiation of coital behavior in mammals: A comparative analysis. *Neurosci. Biobehav. Rev.* 3, 265–284.

Bercovitch, F. B., Roy, M. M., Sladky, K. K., and Goy, R. W. (1988). The effects of isosexual rearing on adult sexual behavior in captive male rhesus macaques. *Arch. Sex. Behav.* 17, 381–388.

Bleier, R. (1984). *Science and Gender.* Pergamon, New York.

Carpenter, C. R. (1942). Sexual behavior of free-ranging rhesus monkeys (*Macaca mulatta*). II. Periodicity of estrus, homosexual, autoerotocism and nonconformist behavior. *J. Comp. Psychol.* 33, 143–162.

Cochran, C. G. (1979). Proceptive patterns of behavior throughout the menstrual cycle in female rhesus monkeys. *Behav. Neurol. Biol.* 27, 342–353.

Collaer, M. L., and Hines, M. (1995). Human behavioral sex differences—A role for gonadal hormones during early development. *Psych. Bull.* 118, 55–107.

Fausto-Sterling, A. (1992). *Myths of Gender,* Revised ed. Basic Books, New York.

Goldfoot, D. A., and Wallen, K. (1978). Development of gender role behaviors in heterosexual and isosexual groups of infant rhesus monkeys. *In* D. J. Chivers and J. Herbert (Eds.), *Recent Advances in Primatology. I. Behaviour,* pp. 155–159. Academic Press, London.

Goldfoot, D. A., Wallen, K., Neff, D. A., McBrair, M. C., and Goy, R. W. (1984). Social influences on the display of sexually dimorphic behavior in rhesus monkeys: Isosexual rearing. *Arch. Sex. Behav.* 13, 395–412.

Gordon, T. P. (1981). Reproductive behavior in the rhesus monkey: Social and endocrine variables. *Am. Zool.* 21, 185–195.

Goy, R. W. (1970). Early hormonal influences on the development of sexual and sex-related behavior. *In*

F. O. Schmitt (Ed.), *The Neurosciences: Second Study Program,* pp. 196–207. Rockefeller Univ. Press, New York.

Goy, R. W. (1978). Development of play and mounting behaviour in female rhesus virilized prenatally with esters of testosterone and dihydrotestosterone. *In* D. J. Chivers and J. Herbert (Eds.), *Recent Advances in Primatology. I. Behaviour,* pp. 449–462. Academic Press, London.

Goy, R. W. (1981). Differentiation of male social traits in female rhesus macaques by prenatal treatment with androgens: Variation in the type of androgen, duration, and timing of treatment. *In* M. J. Novy and J. A. Resko (Eds.), *Fetal Endocrinology,* pp. 319–339. Academic Press, New York.

Goy, R. W., and McEwen, B. S. (1980). *Sexual Differentiation of the Brain.* The MIT Press, Cambridge, MA.

Goy, R. W., and Resko, J. A. (1972). Gonadal hormones and behavior of normal and pseudohermaphroditic nonhuman female primates. *Rec. Prog. Hormone Res.* 28, 707–733.

Goy, R. W., and Wallen, K. (1979). Experimental variables influencing play, foot-clasp mounting, and adult sexual competence in male rhesus monkeys. *Psychoneuroendocrinology* 4, 1–12.

Goy, R. W., Bercovitch, F. B., and McBrair, M. C. (1988). Behavioral masculinization is independent of genital masculinization in prenatally androgenized female rhesus macaques. *Horm. Behav.* 22, 552–571.

Goy, R. W., Uno, H., and Sholl, S. A. (1989). Psychological and anatomical consequences of prenatal exposure to androgens in female rhesus. *In* H. Nagasawa (Ed.), *Toxicity of Hormones in Perinatal Life,* pp. 1127–1142, CRC Press, Boca Raton.

Goy, R. W., Wallen, K., and Goldfoot, D. A. (1974). Social factors affecting the development of mounting behavior in male rhesus monkeys. *In* W. A. Sadler (Ed.), *Reproductive Behavior,* pp. 223–247. Plenum, New York.

Harlow, H. F. (1965). Sexual behavior in the rhesus monkey. *In* F. A. Beach (Ed.), *Sex and Behavior,* pp. 234–265. Krieger, New York.

Harlow, H. F., and Lauersdorf, H. E. (1974). Sex differences in passion and play. *Perspec. Biol. Med.* 17, 348–60.

Juraska, J. M. (1991). Sex differences in "cognitive" regions of the rat brain. *Psychoneuroendocrinology* 16, 105–109.

Juraska, J. M., and Kopcik, J. R. (1988). Sex and environmental influences on the size and ultrastructure of the rat *corpus callosum. Brain Res.* 450, 1–8.

Keverne, E. B. (1976). Sexual receptivity and attractiveness in the female rhesus monkey. *In* D. S. Lehrman, R. A. Hinde, and E. Shaw (Eds.), *Advances in the Study of Behavior,* Vol. 7, pp. 155–200. Academic Press, New York.

Keverne, E. B. (1982). Olfaction and the reproductive behavior of nonhuman primates. *In* C. T. Snowdon, C. H. Brown, and M. R. Petersen (Eds.), *Primate Communication,* pp. 396–412, Cambridge Univ. Press, Cambridge, MA.

Leal, J. A., Williams, R. F., Danforth, D. R., Gordon, K., and Hodgen, G. D. (1988). Prolonged duration of gonadotropin inhibition by a third generation GnRH antagonist. *J. Clin. Endocrinol. Metab.* 67, 1325–1327.

Lindburg, D. G. (1971). The rhesus monkey in North India: An ecological and behavioral study. *In* L. A. Rosenblum (Ed.), *Primate Behavior: Developments in Field and Laboratory,* pp. 1–137. Academic Press, New York.

Lovejoy, J., and Wallen, K. (1988). Sexually dimorphic behavior in group-housed rhesus monkeys (*Macaca mulatta*) at 1 year of age. *Psychobiology* 16, 348–356.

Mann, D. R., Davis-DaSilva, M. A., Wallen, K., Coan, P., Evans, D. E., and Collins, D. C. (1984). Blockade of neonatal activation of the pituitary-testicular axis with continuous administration of a GnRH agonist in male rhesus monkeys. *J. Clin. Endocrinol. Metab.* 59, 207–211.

Mann, D. R., Gould, K. G., and Wallen, K. (1992). Use of gonadotropin releasing hormone (GnRH) analogues to influence sexual and behavioral development. *Symposium on Modes of Action of GnRH and GnRH Analogues.* Serona Symposium Series, USA.

Michael, R. P., and Bonsall, R. W. (1979). Hormones and the sexual behavior of rhesus monkeys. *In* C. Beyer (Ed.), *Endocrine Control of Sexual Behavior,* pp. 279–302. Raven Press, New York.

Michael, R. P., Zumpe, D., and Bonsall, R. W. (1982). Behavior of rhesus during artificial menstrual cycles. *J. Comp. Physiol. Psychol.* 96, 875–885.

Moore, C. L., Dou, H., and Juraska, J. M. (1992). Maternal stimulation affects the number of motor neurons in a sexually dimorphic nucleus of the lumbar spinal cord. *Brain Res.* 572, 52–56.

Reinisch, J. R. (1974). Fetal hormones, the brain and human sex differences: A heuristic integrative review of the recent literature. *Arch. Sex. Behav.* 3, 51–69.

Resko, J. A. (1985). Gonadal hormones during sexual differentiation in vertebrates. *In* R. W. Goy (Ed.), *Handbook of Behavioral Neurobiology. VII. Reproduction,* pp. 21–42. Plenum, New York.

Wallen, K. (1990). Desire and ability: Hormones and the regulation of female sexual behavior. *Neurosci. Biobehav. Rev.* 14, 233–241.

Wallen, K. (1995). The evolution of female sexual desire. *In* P. R. Abramson and S. D. Pinkerton (Eds.), *Sexual Nature Sexual Culture,* pp. 57–79. Univ. of Chicago Press, Chicago.

Wallen, K., Bielert, C. F., and Slimp, J. (1977). Foot-clasp mounting in prepubertal rhesus monkeys: Social and hormonal influences. *In* S. Chevalier-Skolnikoff and F. Poirier (Eds.), *Primate Bio-social Development,* pp. 439–461. Garland, New York.

Wallen, K., Goldfoot, D. A., and Goy, R. W. (1981). Peer and maternal influences on the expression of foot-clasp mounting by juvenile male rhesus monkeys. *Dev. Psychobiol.* 14, 299–309.

Wallen, K., Maestripieri, D., and Mann, D. R. (1995). Effects of neonatal testicular suppression with a GnRH antagonist on social behavior in group-living juvenile rhesus monkeys. *Horm. Behav.* 29, 322–337.

Wallen, K., Winston, L., Gaventa, S., Davis-DaSilva, M. A., and Collins, D. C. (1984). Periovulatory changes in female sexual behavior and patterns of steroid secretion in group-living rhesus monkeys. *Horm. Behav.* 18, 431–450.

Wilson, M. E., Gordon, T. P., and Collins, D. C. (1982). Variation in ovarian steroids associated with the annual mating period in female rhesus (*Macaca mulatta*). *Biol. Reprod.* 27, 530–539.

V BIOLOGY OF SOCIAL RELATIONSHIPS AND INTERPERSONAL PROCESSES

B. Social Applications

iv. Aggression and Social Order

62 The Search for the Age of "Onset" of Physical Aggression: Rousseau and Bandura Revisited

Richard E. Tremblay, Christa Japel, Daniel Perusse, Pierre McDuff, Michel Boivin, Mark Zoccolillo, and Jacques Montplaisir

Introduction

There is no original sin in the human heart, the how and why of the entrance of every vice can be traced.
—Rousseau, 1762/1911:56

People are not born with preformed repertoires of aggressive behaviours; they must learn them in one way or another.
—Bandura, 1973:61

Based on the results of a relatively large number of longitudinal studies over the past two decades, it has often been concluded that childhood aggression is one of the best predictors of adolescent and adult aggression (e.g. Reiss and Roth, 1993; Huesmann et al., 1996; Coie and Dodge, 1998). This conclusion has launched a quest for the age of onset of aggression and the pathways which lead to aggression. If aggressive behaviour is learned (Lefkowitz et al., 1977; Bandura, 1973; Eron, 1990; Huesmann, 1997), if it is a stable behaviour (Olweus, 1979; Parke and Slaby, 1983; Coie and Dodge, 1998), if its age of onset can be identified, and if its antecedents can be recognized, then one can hope that preventive interventions will nip its development in the bud.

Defining Aggression

A major problem with this quest is the operational definition of aggression (de Wit and Hartup, 1974; Farrington, 1997). Studies on aggression attract much interest from the public and policy makers because fear of becoming the victim of violent aggression is a major issue in our modern societies. However, most of the longitudinal studies of aggression during childhood have not been assessing the type of aggression which people fear most, namely physical aggression. The peer, parent and self-rating scales of "aggression" in these studies typically include only a few physical aggression items among a majority of items which refer to disruptive behaviours such as disobedience, attention seeking, impulsivity, opposition, competition, hyperactivity, rejection, association with bad friends, vandalism, lying and stealing (e.g. Pekarik et al., 1976; Lefkowitz et al., 1977; Achenbach and Edelbrock, 1986; Tremblay, 1991; Tremblay et al., 1991). Thus, many developmental studies continue to confound physical aggression with verbal aggression, indirect aggression, opposition, hyperactivity, competition, and other disruptive or troublesome behaviours. Many studies lump together all these behaviours and label them externalizing, delinquent or antisocial (Coie and Dodge, 1998).

There are at least six important advantages in differentiating physical aggression from other aggressive, disruptive and antisocial behaviours. First, the concreteness of physical aggression makes it somewhat easier to measure than most other social or antisocial behaviours. Second, there is a relatively large consensus that physical aggression, i.e. aggression that causes bodily harm, is a socially undesirable behaviour. The consensus is less clear for aggressive behaviour that is not physical in nature. For example, most parents would be proud to hear their son described as an aggressive tennis player or an aggressive debater. Fewer would take pride in a physically aggressive debater or tennis player. A consensus concerning aggression that is not physical, and thus inflicts mental harm, would not be as easy to reach and would be more difficult to measure. Third, one would expect that most individuals who tend to inflict bodily harm to others also tend to inflict mental harm, but individuals who tend to inflict mental harm to others do not necessarily inflict bodily harm. Fourth, from a developmental perspective, one would expect that the capacity to inflict bodily harm to others would precede the capacity to inflict mental harm. Fifth, although there is a large consensus that physical aggression should be inhibited, it is still omnipresent in our modern societies. Finally, interventions may need to be tailored to the type of aggressive behaviour one wants to prevent.

Physical Aggression from School Entry to Adulthood

Data on the prevalence of serious violent crimes from the National Youth Survey (Elliott, 1994) indicate that both black and white males and females in the United States become more and more at risk of committing serious physical aggressions from 12 to 17 years of age. This phenomenon has been observed in other data sets (Farrington, 1987) and appears to support the conclusion that the likelihood of physical aggression increases as children grow older. Loeber and Hay's (1997) retrospective and prospective data from a sample of Pittsburgh males, first assessed when they were in seventh grade, showed that as children grow older, more and more start to display minor aggression, fighting and violence.

These data also lend credence to recent models of pathways for the development of antisocial behaviour. For example, the data seem to support a model where fighting in males is preceded by temper tantrums, which were themselves preceded by disobedience (Patterson et al., 1992). Loeber and colleagues (1994; Loeber and Stouthamer-Loeber, 1998) presented a more complex model, but still one that shows minor aggression and physical fighting being preceded by disobedience and stubborn behaviour.

This image of children being more inclined to initiate physical aggression as they grow older fits an image of children born good and becoming bad under the influence of their environment, which dates back to at least Jean-Jacques Rous-

seau's (Rousseau, 1911 [1762]) model of child development, and the more recent social learning hypothesis of aggression (Bandura, 1973). However, it does not fit well with average levels of physical aggression obtained from the few studies that have focused specifically on the development of physical aggression during the elementary school years. For example, in their prospective longitudinal study of North Carolina children, using both teacher and self-reports, Cairns, Cairns, and colleagues (Cairns and Cairns, 1994; Cairns et al., 1989) found that the mean frequency of physical aggressions decreased with relative steadiness from 10 to 18 years of age. We obtained a similar developmental trend with a sample of 1037 males from low socioeconomic areas of Montréal whose physical aggression was rated by teachers from 6 to 15 years of age (Figure 62.1). Similar results have also been obtained in the Pittsburgh Youth Study (Loeber and Hay, 1997) and from cross-sectional studies (Choquet, 1996; Tremblay et al., 1996).

It could be argued that although most children are less and less physically aggressive with time, a minority of children commence or increase the frequency of their physical aggression as they grow older. Nagin and Tremblay (in press) have addressed this issue by attempting to identify the developmental trajectories of teacher-rated physical aggression in a sample of low socioeconomic area boys followed from six to 15 years of age. They found that 14% of the boys appeared to never have been physically aggressive, 4% showed a high frequency of physical aggression from six to 15 years of age, 28% started with a high level of physical aggression at age six and became less and less physically aggressive with time, while the majority (53%) had a low level of physical aggression at age six and also became less and less aggressive with time. In contrast with hypotheses concerning late onset of antisocial behaviour (Patterson et al., 1989; Moffitt, 1993), Nagin and Tremblay did not find any group that could be labelled "late onset" for physical aggression, i.e. boys with an "onset" and maintenance of a

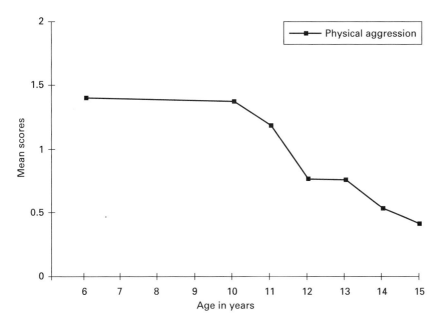

Figure 62.1
Boys' teacher-rated physical aggression from age 6–15 years.

moderate or high level of physical aggression for a significant number of years after age six.

These results certainly challenge the idea that physical aggression is a behaviour with a frequency that increases with age. They also challenge the notion that there is a significant group of children who show chronic physical aggression during late childhood or adolescence after having had low levels of aggression throughout childhood.

Physical Aggression during the Preschool Years

Because the mean frequency of physical aggression, for any type of developmental trajectory of physical aggression, appears to be at its highest in kindergarten (Nagin and Tremblay, in press), the search for the "onset" of physical aggression must logically focus on the preschool years. Al-

though de Wit and Hartup (1974) made a convincing plea for studying the early development of aggression more than 20 years ago, there are surprisingly very few longitudinal studies which have tried to chart the development of physical aggression during the preschool years.

Two longitudinal studies of small samples of children found relatively high levels of continuity in physical aggression, i.e. children tend to maintain the same relative level of physical aggression from around the end of the second year after birth onward. Keenan and Shaw (1994) observed a sample of 89 boys and girls of low socioeconomic status mothers. Direct observations of behaviour during laboratory assessments when the children were 18 and 24 months of age yielded significant inter-age Pearson correlations of 0.23, 0.30 and 0.45 respectively for physical aggression towards mothers, objects and examiners. Cummings et al. (1989) assessed the physical aggression of 22 boys and 21 girls by direct observations in a play situation with a friend at 2 and 5 years of age. They found high correlations for boys ($r = 0.59$) and somewhat lower correlations for girls ($r = 0.36$). These two studies indicate levels of continuity of physical aggression similar to those observed in older children. Other studies of preschool children's aggression have used less specific definitions of aggression. For example, Kingston and Prior (1995: 349) describe their focus on aggression in the following way: "we focus on the development and correlates of what we call, for brevity, 'aggressive behaviour' but which incorporates both verbally and physically aggressive behaviour.... More specifically, our definition of aggression includes behaviours such as temper outbursts; damage or destruction to property; verbal and physical threats; bullying; fights; hurting others by hitting, biting or scratching; and frequent disobedience." Competitive behaviour was also included in their aggression scale for two- to four-year-olds. Because such studies do not distinguish physical aggression from verbal aggression, disobedience, competition and temper tantrums, they cannot inform us on the age of onset and stability of physical aggression.

The fact that longitudinal studies show relatively high correlations of physical aggression scores between two and five years of age (continuity) does not tell us if the frequency of physical aggression is increasing or decreasing (stability) during the preschool years. The first descriptions of these developmental trends can be found in a number of cross-sectional studies undertaken by the child development pioneers of the 1920s and 1930s (e.g. Bridges, 1931; Dawe, 1934; Murphy, 1937) who targeted conflicts and tantrums in small samples of children. These studies suggested that with age, physical aggression decreased, while verbal aggression and conflicts increased. A recent cross-sectional study of a large representative sample of Canadian children also indicated that, according to maternal reports, the frequency of physical aggression declined from

two to 11 years of age (see Figure 62.2), while the frequency of indirect aggression increased (Tremblay et al., 1996).

Again, if the frequency of physical aggression is at its highest at the end of the second year after birth, when is the age of "onset" of physical aggression?

Published studies of physical aggression during the first two years after birth are extremely rare. In a British longitudinal study of 49 second-born children, Dunn and Munn (1985) observed physical aggression of the subjects towards their eldest sibling at ages 14, 18 and 24 months. The observed trend indicated an increase in physical aggression. In a cross-sectional study of social interactions in French day-care centres, Restoin (1985; Restoin et al., 1985) reported an increase in the proportion of physical aggressions, compared with other forms of social interactions, from the end of the first to the end of the second year after birth. That study also showed a decrease in physical aggression from the end of the second year after birth to the end of the third year.

In an attempt to trace the development of physical aggression in the first 17 months after birth, we studied the frequency of different forms of physical aggression reported by mothers for their 17-month-old child, and tried to identify the age of onset of these behaviours.

Method

Subjects

A total of 511 mothers were interviewed when one of their children (260 girls, 251 boys) was 17 months old ($M = 16.86$, $\text{SD} = 0.60$). These mothers were part of a population sample of 572 mothers living in the main urban areas of the province of Québec and recruited in the fall of 1996. Demographic characteristics of the 511 mothers differed slightly from a subsequent population sample representing mothers of all newborns in the Province of Québec in the spring of

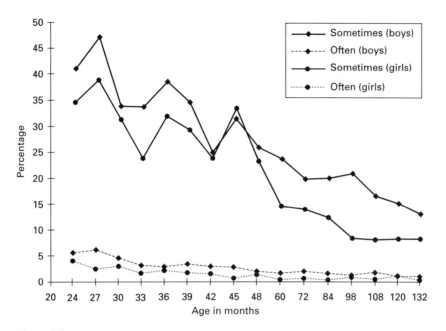

Figure 62.2
Hitting, biting, and kicking (boys and girls aged 2–11 years).

1998 (Table 62.1). The mothers and fathers of the 1996 sample were more educated and had a higher family income than those recruited in 1998. However, the samples did not differ on variables such as the parents' age and the number of children in the family.

Instruments

The "person most knowledgeable" about the child (PMK), which in 98% of the cases was the mother, was asked to indicate whether the child never, sometimes, or often manifests a variety of behaviours. The behaviour questionnaire presented to parents was developed by the senior author for the Canadian Longitudinal Survey of Children and Youth from a variety of sources (Statistics Canada and HRDC, 1995). It consists of items measuring dimensions such as hyperactivity, physical aggression, inattention, anxiety

and prosocial behaviour. Since the original questionnaire contained only three items pertaining to physical aggression, these items were replaced by 11 items yielding a more detailed picture of physical aggression at 17 months. These items are: takes away things from others; pushes to get what he/she wants; threatens to hit; hits; bites; kicks; physically attacks; fights; starts fights; bullies; and is cruel. Furthermore, for each of these 11 items, mothers were asked to indicate at what age the child had manifested the behaviour for the first time.

Results and Discussion

Frequency of Physical Aggressions at 17 Months

Table 62.2 shows the percentage of 17-month-old boys and girls whose mother reported that

Table 62.1
Sociodemographic characteristics of the samples

Characteristics	1996 sample (n = 511) (%)	1998 sample (n = 787) (%)	(χ^2)
Family income			7.33*
<$30 000	23.2	30.2	
$30 000–$60 000	44.1	39.7	
>$60 000	32.7	30.1	
Educational level of the mother			12.78*
No high school diploma	9.6	16.1	
High school diploma	32.7	33.0	
Vocational/trade school diploma	11.8	10.6	
College diploma	17.1	13.6	
University degree	28.9	26.7	
Educational level of the father			22.66**
No high school diploma	12.8	20.3	
High school diploma	31.1	35.6	
Vocational/trade school diploma	13.0	8.0	
College diploma	15.3	13.3	
University degree	27.9	22.8	
Number of brothers and sisters			0.55
None	42.1	40.0	
1 brother or sister	37.6	39.1	
2 or more	20.4	20.8	
	M	*M*	*t*
Age of mother	29.77	29.38	−1.36
Age of father	32.25	32.02	−0.71

Notes: * $p < 0.5$, ** $p < 0.001$.

they had sometimes or often manifested each of the behaviours. It can be seen that taking away things from others is a highly prevalent behaviour at 17 months of age. Half of the children are reported by their mothers to sometimes take away things from others, and 17.7% are reported to often show this behaviour. The inclusion of this behaviour in a scale of physical aggression could be questioned since it involves a minimum level of physical aggression. However, direct ob-

servations of these behaviours (see e.g. Restoin, 1985) show that children often resist, and sometimes strongly resist, by holding on to the object while the other is trying to pull it away. The same event involving adolescents or adults could lead to a robbery charge.

The second most frequently reported physical aggression at 17 months is pushing others to get what the child wants (40.1% sometimes, 5.9% often). This behaviour probably happens most

Table 62.2

Prevalence of physically aggressive behaviour by 17 months of age

Behaviours	Some-times	Often	Total
(1) Takes away things from others	52.7	17.7	70.4
(2) Pushes to get what he/she wants	40.1	5.9	46.0
(3) Bites	24.3	2.9	27.2
(4) Kicks	20.4	3.9	24.3
(5) Fights	19.8	3.3	23.1
(6) Threatens to hit	19.8	2.7	22.5
(7) Physically attacks	19.4	1.2	20.6
(8) Hits	14.7	0.6	15.3
(9) Starts fights	11.0	1.4	12.4
(10) Bullies	7.6	0.6	8.2
(11) Cruel	3.3	0.6	3.9

often in the same context as the previous behaviour (taking away things from others) but appears to indicate a higher level of physical aggression. Instead of only pulling on an object the other is holding, the child actually physically pushes the other. Taking away things and pushing to get these things are clearly the most frequent behaviours of the physical aggression items presented to the mothers. These results replicate direct observation studies of children which conclude that object struggles are the most frequent agonistic behaviours among young children (e.g. Hay and Ross, 1982; Restoin et al., 1985).

Biting, kicking, fighting, threatening to hit and physically attacking others are reported for one in four to one in five of the children. Although few mothers endorsed the most serious descriptors, there were still 8.2% who reported their 17-month-old child to bully and 3.9% who described their child as cruel.

Table 62.3 presents a breakdown of the total percentage from Table 62.2 into males and females, and whether or not a sibling is present.

The clearest result from Table 62.3 is the effect of having a sibling. Since the subjects were 17 months old, it can be assumed that the siblings were almost always older. Observational studies of sibling interactions have shown that younger siblings between 14 and 24 months tend to initiate physically aggressive interactions (Dunn and Munn, 1985). For both males and females, having a sibling clearly increased the likelihood of mothers reporting physically aggressive behaviour, except for boys' biting, and boys and girls being cruel.

No significant differences in the use of physical aggression were observed between boys and girls who had siblings, except for the kicking item which was more frequent for boys. However, a number of significant differences were observed between males and females who did not have siblings. Behaviours such as taking away things from others and biting were more prevalent among boys without siblings than girls without siblings. The interaction effect between sex and presence of sibling was seen most clearly (lines 12 and 13 of Table 62.3) when we calculated the percentage of boys and girls who had received a positive rating on at least one of the 11 items, or one of the 10 items left after having excluded the most frequent, and possibly less physically aggressive item (taking away things from others). To our knowledge, this is the first time that such an interaction has been observed. It suggests that sex differences in physical aggression at that age are highly dependent on context. It is also noteworthy that the presence of the interaction depends on the type of physical aggression that is being assessed.

Cumulative Onset of Physical Aggression

When mothers reported that their 17-month-old child had sometimes or often manifested one of the physically aggressive behaviours, we followed up by asking at what age they had manifested the behaviour for the first time. This gave an estimate of the age of onset for each of these

Table 62.3
Prevalence (%) of physically aggressive behaviour by 17 months of age

	Boys		Girls	
	Sibs	No sibs	Sibs	No sibs
(1) Takes away things from others	79.0	68.2[b]	74.5	54.7[b]
(2) Pushes to get what he/she wants	59.1	38.0	50.4	30.2
(3) Threatens to hit	25.2	21.3	24.2	17.8
(4) Hits	21.0	15.7	15.0	7.4
(5) Bites	29.4	29.7[b]	30.1	17.7[b]
(6) Kicks	37.8[a]	15.8	25.1[a]	31.1
(7) Physically attacks	23.1	15.7	26.8	13.1
(8) Fights	32.9	9.1	30.7	12.1
(9) Starts fights	16.1	8.3	16.3	5.6
(10) Bullies	9.8	5.6	9.9	6.5
(11) Cruel	2.8	3.7	3.3	6.6
(12) Any one of 1 to 11	93.7	89.9[c]	90.8	68.2[c]
(13) Any one of 1 to 11	80.4	69.5[c]	80.4	49.5[c]

Notes: a. Boys with siblings differ from girls with siblings ($p < 0.05$); b. Boys without siblings differ from girls without siblings ($p < 0.05$); c. Boys without siblings differ from girls without siblings ($p < 0.01$).

behaviours. These are of course retrospective data which resemble the earlier reported data from the Pittsburgh Youth Study (Loeber and Stouthamer-Loeber, 1998), where parents and early adolescents were asked to recall the age of onset of minor aggressions, fighting and serious violent behaviours. However, there is an important difference, in that the period of recall for the infants is 10 to 12 months compared with 10 to 12 years when parents of adolescents or adolescents are questioned.

Figure 62.3 shows the cumulative age of onset of pushing, hitting and kicking. Some children are reported to start these behaviours before their first birthday. But the action really starts in the first few months after that first birthday. The cumulative onset rate of pushing is faster than that of kicking and hitting. Pushing appears to precede kicking, and the latter appears to precede hitting. If we change the label on the X axis

from months to years, the developmental trend could easily be mistaken for the one described by Loeber and Stouthamer-Loeber (1998) for the cumulative onset of minor aggression, fighting and serious violence from three to 16 years of age.

Figure 62.4 illustrates a breakdown of the "kicking" onset curve for males and females with and without siblings. A survival analysis revealed significant differences between the four groups with respect to their "kicking" onset curve (log rank $(3, 511) = 23.98$, $p < 0.000$). While the cumulative onset curve of the four groups was similar up to the age of 12 months, group differences became evident between 13 and 17 months of age. Boys with siblings had the steepest cumulative onset curve followed by girls with siblings. The cumulative onset curve of the boys without siblings was much less steep and was similar to the curve for girls without siblings.

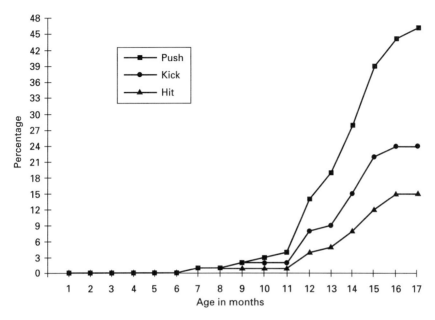

Figure 62.3
Cumulative onset of physically aggressive behaviour.

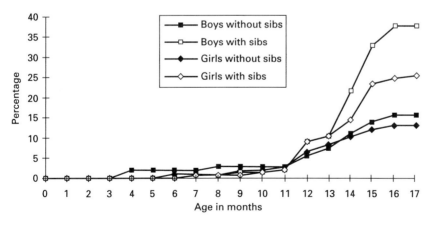

Figure 62.4
Cumulative onset of kicking others for boys and girls with and without siblings.

Conclusion

Mothers' reports on the frequency of physical aggression of their 17-month-old child and the age of onset of these behaviours provide evidence that physical aggression by humans can appear before the end of the first year after birth, and that the rate of cumulative onset increases substantially from 12 to 17 months. By that age, onset of physical aggression is reported for close to 80% of the children. From other studies, it appears that the peak in terms of total frequency of physical aggressions is reached by the end of the second year after birth. After this peak of the "terrible twos," the frequency of physical aggression appears to show a continuous decline up to adulthood (see Figure 62.2).

This view of the mean developmental trend of physical aggression makes it difficult to understand how we could support the idea of "onset" of physical aggression during the elementary school years, during adolescence, or during adulthood. The large majority of children will have had a period of relatively frequent physical aggression during the first two to three or four years of life. By school entry, most children seem to fit the "desistors" category. If there are children who increase the frequency of their physical aggressions after the preschool age, the term "relapse" may be more adequate than the term "onset" to describe these children. There are probably some children who never used physical aggression during the preschool years. It is most likely that most of them do not use physical aggression as they grow older. Some might, however, and it would be extremely interesting to understand what triggers a meaningful onset of chronic physical aggression or an isolated incident of serious physical aggression, after an early childhood without physical aggression. However, to study this category of individuals, we clearly would need good data from early childhood onward for an extremely large sample.

The search for the onset of aggression has focused on middle childhood and adolescence. Developmental models of antisocial behaviour usually describe physical aggression as the outgrowth of prior problems, such as opposition, disobedience and hyperactivity. Yet studies of infants indicate that onset of physical aggression is probably as early as the forms of opposition and disobedience, which have been included in these models. By the end of the second year after birth, physical aggression appears to be a normative behaviour. While most children have learned to inhibit physical aggression by their entry into kindergarten, a minority have not, and some of these children may become lifelong chronic cases. These chronic cases are extremely resistant to therapeutic interventions, and they may well be those who showed higher levels of physical aggression during the first 24 months after birth. Thus, there may be two main developmental trajectories of physical aggression, the childhood limited and the life-course persistent. The childhood-limited trajectory would include those who desist before school entry, and those who desist during elementary school or early adolescence (see Nagin and Tremblay, in press). Understanding the causes and consequences of earlier and later desistance should be an important research focus.

The fact that most children appear to learn to inhibit physical aggression between birth and three or four years of age, added to the fact that those who appear not to have learned to inhibit physical aggression during that period will have great difficulty learning to do so later on, may be an indication that there is a sensitive period for learning to inhibit physically aggressive behaviour. If this were the case, then the first three or four years of life should provide the best window of opportunity to prevent the development of chronic physical aggression. To our knowledge, most preventive interventions in the preschool years have not made learning to inhibit physical aggression a main component of their curriculum. In fact, the focus of research over the past few decades, largely inspired by the social learning hypothesis (Bandura, 1973), has been on how children learn to aggress, rather than on how children learn not to physically aggress. The answer to the latter question may be extremely useful to answer the former question and develop preventive interventions.

The study of aggression is slowly taking a life-course perspective. The focus over the years has shifted from adults to adolescents and to children. The next step should be early childhood. To make this shift, we need to better define not only what we mean by aggression, but also what we mean by physical aggression and by chronic physical aggression.

Notes for Future Research

(1) Some of the questions that need to capture our attention: Why do most toddlers use physical aggression? Why do most children learn to inhibit physical aggression? Why do some children fail to learn to inhibit physical aggression? Why do some relapse? (during childhood, during adolescence, during adulthood). Why do some individuals never use physical aggression, even under the most appropriate conditions? Do some start using physical aggression only after early childhood? If so, why?

(2) It will be difficult to prove that there are really late-onset cases of physical aggression. It is most likely they are those cases for which we simply have not recorded their earlier physical aggression. If there are late-onset cases, there are probably very few. This will make them still harder to detect. We must not confuse them with occasionals, that is those who at any one point in time can show a short period of extreme (e.g. killing someone) or less extreme (e.g. child beating or wife abuse) physical aggression, but are not and have not been chronic cases.

(3) Are there real desistors? Most humans appear to be desistors after early childhood, but most can at any one point in time act in a physically aggressive way. Most humans have physically aggressed at one point in time and are capable of doing it again. When we talk of early or late onset, we need to clearly define onset of exactly what kind of behaviour, over which period of time, and in which context.

(4) If there were a significant number of individuals who were never physically aggressive during early childhood but started displaying serious physical aggression later on in life (late onset: during late childhood, adolescence, or adulthood), one could hypothesize that experimentation with physical aggression during infancy and toddlerhood is a means of learning to effectively inhibit physical aggression.

(5) To create adequate models of the life-span development of physical aggression and physical violence, we will need to chart the course of physical aggression during early childhood and study the mechanisms which underlie the different trajectories.

(6) To completely characterize these developmental trajectories we will naturally also have to follow the course of physical aggression from early childhood to adulthood.

Acknowledgement

Funds for the infancy study reported in this paper were provided by Québec's Ministry of Health and Social Services, and Canada's Social Sciences and Humanities Research Council. Data were collected by Santé Québec (Mireille Jetté, coordinator). R. E. Tremblay is supported by the Molson Foundation and the Canadian Institute of Advanced Research. The Research Unit on Children's Psychosocial Maladjustment is funded by the University of Montréal, Laval University, McGill University, and Québec's Fond FCAR.

References

Achenbach TM, Edelbrock C (1986) *Manual for the Teacher's Report Form and Teacher Version of the Child Behaviour Profile.* Burlington, VT: University of Vermont, Department of Psychiatry.

Bandura A (1973) *Aggression: A Social Learning Analysis.* New York: Holt.

Bridges KMB (1931) *The Social and Emotional Development of the Pre-school Child.* London: Kegan Paul.

Cairns RB, Cairns BD (1994) *Life Lines and Risks: Pathways of Youth in Our Time.* New York: Cambridge University Press.

Cairns RB, Cairns BD, Neckerman HJ, Ferguson LL, Gariépy JL (1989) Growth and aggression, 1: Childhood to early adolescence. *Developmental Psychology* 25(2):320–330.

Choquet M (1996) La violence des jeunes: Données épidémiologiques. In Rey C, ed. *Les adolescents face à la violence.* Paris: Syros, pp 51–63.

Coie JD, Dodge KA (1998) Aggression and antisocial behaviour. In Damon W, Eisenberg N, eds. *Handbook of Child Psychology: Social, Emotional, and Personality Development,* Vol. 3. Toronto: Wiley, pp 779–862.

Cummings EM, Iannotti RJ, Zahn-Waxler C (1989) Aggression between peers in early childhood: Individual continuity and developmental change. *Child Development* 60(4):887–895.

Dawe HC (1934) An analysis of 200 quarrels of preschool children. *Child Development* 5:139–157.

de Wit J, Hartup WW (1974) *Determinants and Origins of Aggressive Behaviour.* The Hague, Netherlands: Mouton.

Dunn J, Munn P (1985) Becoming a family member: Family conflict and the development of social understanding in the second year. *Child Development* 56: 480–492.

Elliott DS (1994) Serious violent offenders: Onset, developmental course and termination: the American Society of Criminology 1993 Presidential Address. *Criminology* 32(1):1–21.

Eron LD (1990) Understanding aggression. *Bulletin of the International Society for Research on Aggression* 12:5–9.

Farrington DP (1987) Epidemiology. In Quay HC, ed. *Handbook of Juvenile Delinquency.* New York: Wiley, pp 31–61.

Farrington DP (1997) Key issues in studying the biosocial bases of violence. In Raine A, Farrington D, Brennan P, Mednick SA, eds. *Biosocial Bases of Violence.* New York: Plenum Press, pp 293–300.

Hay DF, Ross HS (1982) The social nature of early conflict. *Child Development* 53:105–113.

Huesmann LR (1997) Observational learning of violent behaviour: social and biosocial processes. In Raine A, Farrington D, Brennan PA, Mednick SA, eds. *Biosocial Bases of Violence.* New York: Plenum Press, pp 69–88.

Huesmann LR, Becker JV, Dutton MA, Coie J, Gladue B, Hawkins D, Susman E (1996) *Reducing Violence: A Research Agenda,* Report of the Human Capital Initiative. American Psychological Association.

Keenan K, Shaw DS (1994) The development of aggression in toddlers: a study of low-income families. *Journal of Abnormal Child Psychology* 22(1):53–77.

Kingston L, Prior M (1995) The development of patterns of stable, transient, and school-age onset aggressive behaviour in young children. *Journal of the American Academy of Child and Adolescent Psychiatry* 34:348–358.

Lefkowitz MM, Eron LD, Walder LO, Huesmann LR (1997) *Growing Up to be Violent. A Longitudinal Study of the Development of Aggression.* New York: Pergamon Press.

Loeber R, Hay DF (1997) Key issues in the development of aggression and violence from childhood to early adulthood. *Annual Review of Psychology* 48:371–410.

Loeber R, Hay DF (1994) Developmental approaches to aggression and conduct problems. In Rutter M, Hay DF, eds. *Development through Life: A Handbook for Clinicians.* Oxford: Blackwell Scientific Publications, pp 488–516.

Loeber R, Stouthamer-Loeber M (1998) Development of juvenile aggression and violence. Some common misconceptions and controversies. *American Psychologist* 53(2):242–259.

Moffitt TE (1993) Adolescence-limited and life-course persistent antisocial behaviour: a developmental taxonomy. *Psychological Review* 100(4):674–701.

Murphy LB (1937) *Social Behaviour and Child Personality.* New York: Columbia University Press.

Nagin D, Tremblay RE (In press) Trajectories of boys' physical aggression, opposition, and hyperactivity on the path to physically violent and non violent juvenile delinquency. *Child Development.*

Olweus D (1979) Stability of aggressive reaction patterns in males: a review. *Psychological Bulletin* 85:852–875.

Parke RD, Slaby RG (1983) The development of aggression. In Mussen PH, ed. *Handbook of Child Psychology,* Vol. 4: *Socialization, Personality and Social Development.* New York: Wiley, pp 547–641.

Patterson GR, DeBaryshe BD, Ramsey E (1989) A developmental perspective on antisocial behaviour. *American Psychologist* 44:329–335.

Patterson GR, Reid JB, Dishion TJ (1992) *Antisocial Boys.* Eugene, OR: Castalia.

Pekarik EG, Prinz RJ, Liebert DE, Weintraub S, Neale JN (1976) The Pupil Evaluation Inventory: A sociometric technique for assessing children's social behaviour. *Journal of Abnormal Child Psychology* 4:83–97.

Reiss AJ, Roth JA (eds) (1993) *Understanding and Preventing Violence.* Washington, DC: National Academy Press.

Restoin A (1985) Aspects fonctionnels et ontogénétiques des comportements de communication chez le jeune enfant. Concomitants chronobiologiques. Unpublished Grade de docteurs et sciences naturelles, Université de Franche-Comté, Besançon, France.

Restoin A, Montagner H, Rodriguez D, Girardot JJ, Laurent D, Kontar F, Ullmann V, Casagrande C, Talpain B (1985) Chronologie des comportements de communication et profils de comportement chez le jeune enfant. In Tremblay RE, Provost MA, Strayer FF, eds. *Ethologie et développement de l'enfant* Paris: Editions Stock/Laurence Pernoud, pp 93–130.

Rousseau JJ (1911) *Emile.* London: J. M. Dent and Sons (Original work published 1762).

Statistics Canada, and HRDC (1995) *National Longitudinal Survey of Children: Overview of Survey Instruments for 1994–95 Data Collection—Cycle 1.* Ottawa: Statistics Canada and Human Resources Development Canada.

Tremblay RE (1991) Aggression, prosocial behaviour and gender: three magic words but no magic wand. In Pepler D, Rubin K, eds. *The Development and Treatment of Aggression.* Hillsdale, NJ: Lawrence Erlbaum, pp 71–78.

Tremblay RE, Boulerice B, Harden PW, McDuff P, Pérusse D, Pihl RO, Zoccolillo M (1996) Do children in Canada become more aggressive as they approach adolescence? In Human Resources Development Canada and Statistics Canada, eds. *Growing up in Canada: National Longitudinal Survey of Children and Youth.* Ottawa: Statistics Canada, pp 127–137.

Tremblay RE, Loeber R, Gagnon C, Charlebois P, Larivée S, LeBlanc M (1991) Disruptive boys with stable and unstable high fighting behaviour patterns during junior elementary school. *Journal of Abnormal Child Psychology* 19:285–300.

CSF 5-HIAA and Aggression in Female Macaque Monkeys: Species and Interindividual Differences

G. C. Westergaard, S. J. Suomi, J. D. Higley, and P. T. Mehlman

Introduction

Many studies have shown that men with psychopathological syndromes associated with impaired impulse control, severe aggression, and social incompetence exhibit low central nervous system (CNS) serotonin (5-HT) activity, as reflected in low cerebrospinal fluid (CSF) concentrations of the major 5-HT metabolite 5-hydroxyindoleacetic acid (5-HIAA) (Brown et al. 1979, 1982; Linnoila et al. 1983; Kruesi et al. 1990b; Virkkunen et al. 1994a, 1994b). Included among these pathological patterns are high rates of criminality, alcohol dependence and abuse, and premature mortality from murder and suicide (Ballenger et al. 1979; Banki et al. 1981; Borg et al. 1985; Moss 1987; Roy et al. 1989; Virkkunen et al. 1989). Although the relationship among CSF 5-HIAA, impaired impulse control, severe aggression, and social competence is less well-documented in women than in men, the limited literature base suggests consistent findings for both sexes (e.g., see review in Linnoila and Virkkunen 1992).

Prospective studies of male macaques with low CSF 5-HIAA concentrations show that they develop psychopathological patterns that parallel deleterious impulse control deficits seen in human males with low CSF 5-HIAA concentrations. Included are severe aggression, impulsive risk-taking, and violence leading to trauma and early mortality (Higley et al. 1992a, 1994, 1996b, 1996c; Mehlman et al. 1994, 1995, 1997; Higley and Linnoila 1997). It is important to note that male macaques with low CSF 5-HIAA concentrations do not necessarily show higher rates of overall aggression than do macaques with high CSF 5-HIAA concentrations, but instead these monkeys show higher rates of only the most violent and severe forms of aggression involving chases and physical assaults (Higley et al. 1992a, 1994, 1996b, 1996c; Mehlman et al. 1994, 1995,

1997; Higley and Linnoila 1997). Non-human primate males with low CSF 5-HIAA concentrations also show deficits in social functioning as evidenced by infrequent social interactions, and social isolation as measured by time in interactions and distances from conspecifics (Higley et al. 1992a, 1996b, 1996c; Mehlman et al. 1994, 1995, 1997). As is the case in humans, the behavioral implications of low CSF 5-HIAA in non-human primates are less well-documented in females than in males, although there is limited evidence from laboratory studies that the negative correlation between 5HT turnover and aggression, and the positive correlation between 5HT turnover and sociality, may generalize to both sexes (Higley et al. 1996a, 1996d; also see Raleigh and McGuire 1994; Shively et al. 1995). A primary purpose of the present study was to assess the degree to which the above findings in males are also present in females.

A second purpose of this study was to investigate the generalizability of the relationship between low CSF 5-HIAA concentrations and aggression. The correlation between low CSF 5-HIAA concentration and aggression in human and non-human primate males is a well-replicated phenomenon, suggesting a powerful and evolutionarily ancient biological characteristic. Comparative studies indicate that the correlation between severe aggression and low CNS serotonin, whether naturally occurring or pharmacologically induced, may represent a generalized trend across species. For example, when Popova and colleagues (Popova et al. 1991a) selectively bred wild rats over 24–27 generations for "domestication," they found a parallel increase in both tameness and midbrain and hypothalamic 5-HIAA across generations, with the mean level in the midbrain and the cortices higher in the "domesticated" rats than in the aggressive rats. Similarly, silver foxes selected for over 30 years for domestication have higher serotonin concentrations in the midbrain and hypothalamus, and higher 5-HIAA concentrations in the midbrain, hypothalamus and hippocampus when they are compared to nonselected wild silver foxes bred in captivity over the same time span (Popova et al. 1991b). The present study was designed to assess the generalizability of the relationship between low CSF 5-HIAA concentrations, aggression, and sociality using two closely related non-human primate species with known differences in temperament and sociality. We included both rhesus and pigtailed macaques because these primates share a wide range of morphological and genetic characteristics, have well-characterized social dominance hierarchies, and because preliminary observations indicated lower rates of wounding in the pigtail species relative to the rhesus species.

A third goal of the present study was to investigate the relationship between social dominance and 5HT functioning. Human studies show that social competence and social dominance are positively correlated with serotonin functioning (Kruesi et al. 1990a; Madsen 1994). While it was once held that for non-human primates high social dominance was based on high levels of aggression, recent studies have shown that social dominance is actually independent of fighting skills, body size, or overall rates of violent behavior (Raleigh and McGuire 1991; Higley et al. 1996a, 1996d). Indeed, in males, subordinate subjects are actually more likely to exhibit severe aggression, direct it towards inappropriate targets, and show fewer affiliative actions than are high-ranking subjects (Raleigh and McGuire 1991). These findings indicate that acquiring and maintaining social dominance is largely a function of an individual's ability to establish and maintain relationships with kin and other conspecifics to use as support during social challenges (Chapais 1986, 1988; Raleigh and McGuire 1986; Raleigh et al. 1991; Higley and Suomi 1996). Several studies have shown that non-human primates with low CSF 5-HIAA concentrations are less likely to acquire and maintain social domi-

nance ranking than are those with high CSF 5-HIAA concentrations (Higley et al. 1994, 1996a, 1996d; Raleigh et al. 1983; however, see Yodyingyuad et al. 1985), a finding that is consistent with the prediction of an overall pattern of impaired social competence in subjects with reduced serotonin functioning.

In the present study, we examined the correlation between CSF 5-HIAA and aggression using female rhesus (*Macaca mulatta*) and pig-tailed (*Macaca nemestrina*) macaques. We chose to study female primates in order to assess whether the findings of our previous studies with males generalized to females. Given our previous findings, we speculated that the relationship between interindividual differences in CNS serotonin turnover and aggression found within species might also explain between-species differences in agonistic behavior. With this in mind we tested the following three hypotheses. First, that female rhesus macaques would have lower CSF 5-HIAA concentrations and be more aggressive than would female pigtailed macaques. Second, that like males, females of both species would exhibit an inverse relationship between interindividual differences in CSF 5-HIAA concentrations and rates of severe aggression. Third, that subjects with high CSF 5-HIAA concentrations would more likely be higher in social dominance within their respective groups than would subjects with low CSF 5-HIAA concentrations.

Materials and Methods

Subjects and Design

The subjects were 31 female rhesus macaques and 30 age-matched female pigtailed macaques. Monthly censuses using field observations were utilized to obtain the ages for the rhesus macaque subjects. The exact ages for the pig-tailed macaques were not available and thus were estimated by weight regressions and dental eruptions, a procedure used in other studies (Sirianni

1985). At the onset of this study, the mean ages for the rhesus and pigtailed macaques were 23 and 29 months, respectively. Prior to this study all subjects were reared in species-typical social groups. In the present research, we tested subjects in two housing conditions. In the first housing condition, subjects were individually housed in standard laboratory cages for 1 year. Physiological sampling was limited to the period when the subjects were single-caged and occurred twice during this period. Behavior sampling occurred during the second housing condition when the subjects were maintained in unisex groups of four to six animals each with balanced group sizes across the two species. Each social group cage measured $3.3 \times 3.3 \times 2.6$ m and featured a mesh outdoor wall, allowing ambient light and temperature. Behavioral sampling began after a 3-month habituation period to social-housing conditions.

Physiological Data

Prior to group formations, while the monkeys were in single cages, two cisternal CSF samples (3 ml) were drawn at approximately 6-month intervals from anesthetized subjects (ketamine, 10 mg/kg, IM) between 1400 and 1500 hours. Samples were quick frozen at $-70°$C, and later assayed for 5-HIAA and homovanillic acid (HVA) using high performance liquid chromatography with electrochemical detection (Scheinin et al. 1983). All inter-assay and intra-assay coefficients of variation for CSF assays were <10%. We also recorded potential confounds such as temperature and time between capture, anesthesia, and CSF sampling. Because the animals were single-caged, they were captured readily, with no between-species difference in time to capture. We recorded animal weights using a commercial scale accurate to $+0.25$ kg.

Behavioral Data

We obtained frequency data using 15-min focal-animal sampling (Altmann 1974), randomized by order, representational by season and time of day, and totaling 210 observation hours (3 h per subject). The ethogram described grooming and agonistic behaviors, the latter recorded as either low-intensity aggression or high-intensity aggression. Grooming was used as a measure of social affiliation and was scored when a subject gave or received movement of fingers and mouth through another's pelage (Mehlman et al. 1995). Categories for agonism followed those established for rhesus macaques and related species (Altmann 1962; van Hooff 1967) and were identical to those used in our other studies (e.g., Higley et al. 1996c). Displacements and stationary threats were scored as low-intensity aggression. Displacements occurred when a subject moved toward another subject and the latter subject retreated. Stationary threats included all threats, such as stares, open-mouth threats, head bobs, ground slaps, etc., that were displayed while the subject remained stationary (Mehlman et al. 1994). High-intensity aggression consisted of chases and physical assaults, the former occurring when a subject chased another and it fled (often screaming and exhibiting submission), and the latter occurring for all contact aggression (i.e., when the subject pushed, hit, slapped, wrestled with, or bit another monkey). To control for the possibility that high-intensity aggression was simply a function of high overall rates of aggression or generalized activity, we derived a variable designated "escalated aggression" by calculating the proportion of all aggressive acts that were characterized by high-intensity aggression. Prior to analysis, we converted the absolute frequency of each agonistic and affiliative act into a rate of occurrence for each hour of observation per subject.

Wounding Data

Rates of wounding were sampled during routine daily status checks by trained observers blind to the biochemical data. The observer recorded the number and location of all wounds thought to have occurred through agonistic actions.

Social Dominance Data

Social dominance rankings were obtained by assessing the directionality of outcomes for each subject when in naturalistic agonistic encounters with another subject, an established method to assess social dominance in non-human primates (McGuire et al. 1986; Higley and Suomi 1996; Higley et al. 1996d). A subject was considered more dominant than another monkey when it won more encounters than it lost with the other monkey.

Observer Reliability

To establish inter-observer reliability, simultaneous observation sessions were conducted periodically throughout the study. During these sessions two observers concurrently scored the same subject for a 15-min period. The resultant scores were combined in an overall reliability test. The reliability of all behaviors was shown by Cohen's kappa values to be greater than 0.70. Observers were blind to all biochemical data and to the specific hypotheses being tested.

Analysis of Physiological Data

To prepare CSF 5-HIAA data for between-species analyses we first examined and ruled out all confounds except time-to-sample. When the females from the two species were compared, there were no weight differences [$t(35) = 0.41$, $P > 0.68$]. We did find that time-to-sample was significantly correlated with CSF 5-HIAA in one sample and nearly reached significance in the other. To partial out this effect, time-to-sample was residualized out of the data in the two sample sets. Because there were mean differences in each metabolite between the two species, multiple regression was used to correlate the biochemical values with behavior, with species simultaneously entered as one of two independent variables in each behavior-biochemical analysis. Partial correlations are reported, and the associated degrees of freedom have been adjusted accordingly.

Results

Between-species Comparisons of CSF 5-HIAA and HVA

Monoamine metabolite levels for the two samples (time 1 and time 2) were highly correlated [for 5-HIAA: $r(50) = 0.77$, $P < 0.001$; for HVA: $r(53) = 0.54$, $P < 0.001$]. Therefore, we formulated a mean for both 5-HIAA and HVA in order to assess species differences in correlations between biochemical values with behavior. We found significantly lower mean CSF 5-HIAA concentrations, and significantly higher CSF HVA concentrations, for rhesus macaques than for pigtailed macaques [mean 5-HIAA concentration per subject = 202.4 pmol/ml for rhesus macaques versus 302.3 pmol/ml for pigtailed macaques, $t(59) = 8.99$, $P < 0.0001$; mean HVA concentration per subject = 1224.4 pmol/ml for rhesus macaques versus 926.1 pmol/ml for pigtailed macaques, $t(59) = 5.58$, $P < 0.0001$; see Fig. 63.1]. Because on average the pigtailed subjects were older than the rhesus subjects, we performed a second analysis using only animals of the same age. This analysis indicated that between-species differences in CSF 5-HIAA values remained significant when we used only same-aged animals [$t(35) = 6.70$, $P < 0.0001$]. Between-species differences in CSF HVA values approached statistical significance when we controlled for between-species differences in subject age [$t(35) = 1.78$, $P < 0.08$]. As has been reported in other studies (Agren et al. 1986), when species differences were statistically controlled, there was a significant positive correlation between CSF 5-HIAA and CSF HVA ($r = 0.41$, $P > 0.0001$, $df = 2/60$).

Between-species Comparisons in Behavior

Between-species comparisons indicated significantly higher rates of high-intensity and escalated aggression for rhesus macaques than for pigtailed macaques [for high-intensity aggres-

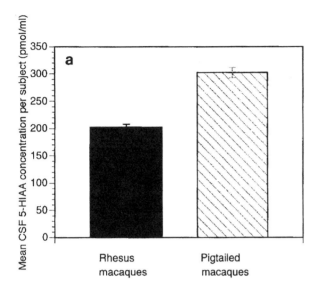

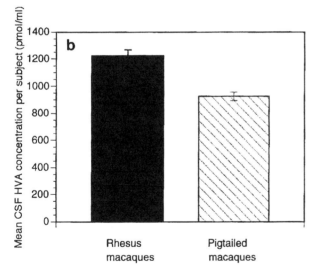

Figure 63.1
Mean CSF 5-HIAA (a) and CSF HVA (b) concentrations per subject for female rhesus and pig-tailed macaques. Standard error bars are also shown for each measure. For rhesus macaques, $n = 31$. For pigtailed macaques, $n = 30$. Values represent the mean of two samples taken when the animals were individually housed. Samples were drawn at approximately 6-month intervals from anesthetized subjects (ketamine 10 mg/kg, IM) between 1400 and 1500 h.

Table 63.1
Summary of behavioral and wounding data for female rhesus and pig-tailed macaques

Category	Rhesus macaques (mean per subject)	Pigtailed macaques (mean per subject)
Low-intensity aggression	9.42	6.48
High-intensity aggression	13.01*	1.69
Escalated aggression	0.57*	0.21
Grooming	2.47	2.28
Wounding	2.68*	0.73

Hourly rate per subject shown for low-intensity aggression, high-intensity aggression and grooming. Escalated aggression represents the proportion of all aggressive acts characterized to high-intensity aggression. Wounding represents the total number of wounds attributed to agonistic actions during gang-caged housing. For rhesus macaques, $n = 31$. For pig-tailed macaques, $n = 30$.
*Statistically significant difference between species, unpaired t-test, $P < 0.0004$, two-tailed.

sion: mean frequency per hour $= 13.01$ for rhesus macaques versus 1.69 for pigtailed macaques; $t(59) = 6.24$, $P < 0.0001$; for escalated aggression: mean incidence of high-intensity aggression per aggressive act $= 0.57$ for rhesus macaques versus 0.21 for pigtailed macaques; $t(59) = 10.19$, $P < 0.0001$; see Table 63.1]. Consistent with these findings, examination of wounding rates indicated a significantly higher incidence of wounding for rhesus macaques than for pigtailed macaques [mean number of wounds per subject $= 2.68$ for rhesus macaques versus 0.73 for pigtailed macaques, $t(59) = 3.74$, $P < 0.0004$]. Further examination indicated no between-species differences in rates of grooming and low-intensity aggression ($P > 0.10$).

Within-species Comparisons of CSF 5-HIAA and HVA with Behavior

Within-species correlations of CSF 5-HIAA and other measures indicated that with species held

statistically constant, there was a significant negative correlation between 5-HIAA and escalated aggression ($r = -0.35$, $P < 0.004$, $df = 2/60$; see Fig. 63.2) and a significant positive correlation between CSF 5-HIAA and social dominance ranking ($r = 0.41$, $P < 0.04$, $df = 2/60$). CSF 5-HIAA was not significantly correlated with rates of low-intensity aggression, high-intensity aggression, grooming, or wounding. CSF HVA was not significantly correlated with any of the aggression measures, grooming, wounding, or social dominance ranking ($P > 0.20$).

Social Dominance Ranking and Behavior

We next examined the relationship between social dominance ranking and social behavior. This analysis indicated that with species held statistically constant, there were significant negative relationships between social dominance ranking and low-intensity aggression ($r = -0.36$, $P < 0.007$, $df = 2/60$), high-intensity aggression ($r = -0.52$, $P < 0.002$, $df = 2/60$), and escalated aggression ($r = -0.53$, $P < 0.02$, $df = 2/60$). Social dominance ranking was not significantly correlated with grooming or wounding ($P > 0.40$).

Discussion

Each of the three hypotheses was supported. Concerning our first hypothesis, we found that female rhesus macaques exhibited lower CSF 5-HIAA concentrations and higher rates of high-intensity aggression, escalated aggression, and wounding than did female pigtailed macaques. Our second hypothesis was also supported. Replicating what has been found in studies of male primates (Higley et al. 1992a, 1994, 1996b, 1996c; Mehlman et al. 1994, 1995, 1997; Higley and Linnoila 1997), there was a within-species interindividual negative correlation between escalated aggression and CSF 5-HIAA concentrations. Low-intensity, restrained aggression was not correlated with CNS serotonin turnover. We also found support for our third hypothesis, as in

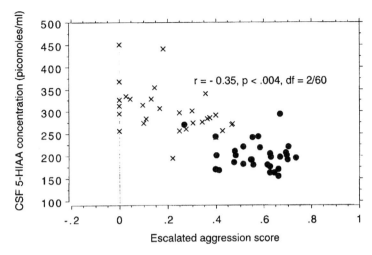

Figure 63.2
Scatterplot showing the correlation between CSF 5-HIAA concentrations and escalated aggression scores for female rhesus and pigtailed macaques. Escalated aggression scores (range = 0.00–0.74) were derived by calculating the proportion of all aggressive acts that were characterized by high-intensity aggression. ● Rhesus monkeys, × pigtailed macaques.

both species females with high CSF 5-HIAA concentrations exhibited high social dominance ranks relative to females with low CSF 5-HIAA concentrations.

In related research, Higley and colleagues (Higley et al. 1996a) found that female rhesus macaques with low CSF 5-HIAA concentrations are wounded more often than are subjects with high CSF 5-HIAA concentrations. While this study used rates of wounding as the dependent measure for aggression, others have directly investigated aggressive behavior and CNS serotonin functioning in females. For example, Raleigh and McGuire (1994) found that when dominance ranking is controlled CSF 5-HIAA is inversely related to rates of inappropriate aggression in female and male vervet monkeys. Similarly, Shively and colleagues found that the rate of aggression was negatively correlated with prolactin response to a fenfluramine challenge in cynomolgus macaques (Shively et al. 1995). Our

findings and those above indicate that high concordance rates for violent and unrestrained aggression, aggressive trauma, and impaired CNS serotonin functioning are not limited to males but instead are present in both sexes.

It is noteworthy that the rate of low-level, restrained aggression (aggression typically used to defend status) did not correlate with CSF 5-HIAA; rather, low concentrations of CSF 5-HIAA correlated with escalated aggression. This finding replicates an often-reported finding with male subjects, and illustrates the importance of CNS serotonin functioning in impulse control (Mehlman et al. 1994; Higley et al. 1996c).

In the present study, we found a parallel species difference, with rhesus macaques, who are reportedly one of the more aggressive macaque species (Bernstein and Gordon 1974), exhibiting lower CSF 5-HIAA concentrations, higher rates of serious and escalated aggression, and a higher incidence of wounding, when compared to the more placid and friendly pigtailed macaques. Within-species analyses showed that for both species, low CSF 5-HIAA concentrations were negatively correlated with high intensity aggression and wounding indicating that this relationship is present in multiple species, as well as humans (see also Raleigh and McGuire 1994; Shively et al. 1995). The present findings underscore the phylogenetic importance of serotonin in controlling violent aggression. Given the apparent deleterious effects of possessing low CNS serotonin functioning, it is an interesting research question as to why this phenotype has endured across evolutionary history. While somewhat speculative, differences in aggressive behavior and CSF 5-HIAA concentration between rhesus and pigtailed macaques may be linked to species differences in adaptation to different environments and associated evolutionary pressures. Rhesus macaques live in larger social groups and inhabit a wider variety of marginal limited resource habitats than do pigtailed macaques. The resulting increased competition for resources may have led to higher rates of aggression in rhesus over evolutionary history and suggests a possible adaptive purpose for the high rates of aggression in this species. This interpretation also underscores the possibility that under some conditions and environments, low CNS serotonin functioning may have adaptive functions.

Although the mean age was 6 months lower for the rhesus females, these differences are not likely to account for the observed species differences as younger animals typically have higher CSF 5-HIAA concentrations and are less likely to receive serious wounds than are older animals (Higley et al. 1992b, 1996e). Hence, we would expect any age differences to have biased our results so that rhesus would have higher CSF 5-HIAA concentrations. Moreover, when the same comparison was made using only same-aged rhesus and pigtailed macaques, the difference remained significant.

The within-species positive correlation between social dominance and CSF 5-HIAA concentra-

tions replicates several studies showing a positive relationship between social dominance ranking and CSF 5-HIAA (Raleigh et al. 1986, 1992; Higley and Suomi 1996; Higley et al. 1996a, 1996d). Social dominance ranking is widely held to be a measure of competent social behavior in non-human primates and, unlike in rodents, social dominance does not appear to be directly related to fighting skills or overall aggression levels (Raleigh and McGuire 1994; Higley et al. 1996a, 1996c, 1996d; however, see Yodyingyuad et al. 1985; Shively et al. 1995). The present findings replicate an earlier study in rhesus macaques, where high CSF 5-HIAA concentrations taken from subjects isolated in single cages predicted the subsequent acquisition of high social dominance rank (Higley et al. 1996a). It is possible that the correlation between serotonin functioning and social dominance rank may be, at least in part, a cause-and-effect relationship, as pharmacological manipulations that increase serotonin functioning also increase the frequency of affiliative social behaviors and social dominance rank. Further, pharmacological manipulations that decrease serotonin functioning also decrease the frequency of affiliative social behaviors and social dominance rank (Raleigh et al. 1980, 1986, Raleigh 1987; Raleigh and McGuire 1991).

The positive interindividual correlation between the two repeated CSF 5-HIAA samples is one of our most replicated findings. Our studies and others that have repeatedly sampled CSF in the same individuals have shown that interindividual differences in CSF 5-HIAA concentrations are stable over time and across situations (Higley and Linnoila 1997). Such findings suggest that as a potential risk factor, trait-like impaired CNS serotonin functioning, as reflected in chronically low CSF 5-HIAA concentrations, may underlie the risk for aggression and other impulse control deficits.

In summary, we found that CSF 5-HIAA concentrations correspond negatively with rates of escalated aggression, and positively with social dominance in female macaques. These relationships were robust both between and within the two species studied. These results support the view that CNS 5HT functioning is related to violent aggression and social dominance in female primates, and they complement previous studies that have focused on the relationship among serotonergic functioning, violent aggression, and social competence in men and free-ranging rhesus macaque males. We conclude that the negative correlation between 5HT turnover and aggression generalizes to both sexes and represents a phylogenetically ancient evolutionary trend.

Acknowledgements

We gratefully acknowledge the contributions of Alan Dodson, Keri Holmes, Anne Hurley, Stephen Lindell, Alecia Lilly, Courtney Shannon, Kathy Weld, and Kristen Zajicek during the design and data collection phases of this study. This research was conducted with support from NIH grants 5U42RR05083 and R24 RR09983. The LABS of Virginia, Inc. Institutional Animal Care and Use Committee approved a research protocol for this study in accordance with and as required by the Animal Welfare Act.

References

Agren H, Mefford IN, Rudorfer MV, Linnoila M, Potter WZ (1986) Interacting neurotransmitter systems: a non-experimental approach to the 5-HIAA-HVA correlation in human CSF. Psychiatry Res 20:175–193.

Altmann J (1974) Observational study of behavior: sampling methods. Behaviour 49:227–267.

Altmann SA (1962) A field study of the sociobiology of rhesus monkeys, *Macaca mulatta*. Ann NY Acad Sci 102:338–435.

Ballenger JC, Goodwin FK, Major LF, Brown GL (1979) Alcohol and central serotonin metabolism in man. Arch Gen Psychiatry 36:224–227.

Banki CM, Molnar G, Fekete I (1981) Correlation of individual symptoms and other clinical variables with cerebrospinal fluid amine metabolites and tryptophan in depression. Arch Psychiatr Nervenkrank 229:345–353.

Bernstein IS, Gordon TP (1974) The function of aggression in primate societies. Am Sci 62:304–311.

Borg S, Kvande H, Liljeberg P, Mossberg D, Valverius P (1985) 5-Hydroxyindoleacetic acid in cerebrospinal fluid in alcoholic patients under different clinical conditions. Alcohol 2:415–418.

Brown GL, Goodwin FK, Ballenger JC, Goyer PF, Major LF (1979) Aggression in humans correlates with cerebrospinal fluid amine metabolites. Psychiatry Res 1:131–139.

Brown GL, Ebert MH, Goyer PF, Jimerson DC, Klein WJ, Bunney WEJ, Goodwin FK (1982) Aggression, suicide, and serotonin: relationships to CSF amine metabolites. Am J Psychiatry 139:741–746.

Chapais B (1986) Why do male and female rhesus monkeys affiliate during the birth season? In: Rawlins RG, Kessler M (eds) The Cayo Santiago macaques. SUNY Press, Chicago, pp 173–200.

Chapais B (1988) Rank maintenance in female Japanese macaques: experimental evidence for social dependency. Behaviour 102:41–59.

Higley JD, Linnoila M (1997) Low central nervous system serotonergic activity is traitlike and correlates with impulsive behavior: a nonhuman primate model investigating genetic and environmental influences on neurotransmission. Ann NY Acad Sci 836:39–56.

Higley JD, Suomi SJ (1996) Effect of reactivity and social competence on individual responses to severe stress in children: investigations using nonhuman primates. In: Pfeffer CR (ed) Intense stress and mental disturbance in children. American Psychiatric Press, Washington, D.C., pp 1–69.

Higley JD, Mehlman P, Taub D, Higley SB, Vickers JH, Suomi SJ, Linnoila M (1992a) Cerebrospinal fluid monoamine and adrenal correlates of aggression in free-ranging rhesus monkeys. Arch Gen Psychiatry 49:436–441.

Higley JD, Suomi SJ, Linnoila M (1992b) A longitudinal assessment of CSF monoamine metabolite and plasma cortisol concentrations in young rhesus monkeys. Biol Psychiatry 32:127–145.

Higley JD, Linnoila M, Suomi SJ (1994) Ethological contributions: experiential and genetic contributions to the expression and inhibition of aggression in primates. In: Hersen M, Ammerman RT, Sisson L (eds) Handbook of aggressive and destructive behavior in psychiatric patients. Plenum Press, New York, pp 17–32.

Higley JD, King ST, Hasert MF, Champoux M, Suomi SJ, Linnoila M (1996a) Stability of interindividual differences in serotonin function and its relationship to aggressive wounding and competent social behavior in rhesus macaque females. Neuropsychopharmacology 14:67–76.

Higley JD, Mehlman PT, Higley SB, Fernald B, Vickers J, Lindell SG, Taub DM, Suomi SJ, Linnoila M (1996b) Excessive mortality in young free-ranging male nonhuman primates with low cerebrospinal fluid 5-hydroxyindoleacetic acid. Arch Gen Psychiatry 53:537–543.

Higley JD, Mehlman PT, Poland RE, Taub DT, Vickers J, Suomi SJ, Linnoila M (1996c) CSF testosterone and 5-HIAA correlate with different types of aggressive behaviors. Biol Psychiatry 40:1067–1082.

Higley JD, Suomi SJ, Linnoila M (1996d) A nonhuman primate model of type II alcoholism? Part 2. Diminished social competence and excessive aggression correlates with low cerebrospinal fluid 5-hydroxyindoleacetic acid concentrations. Alcoholism Clin Exp Res 20:643–650.

Higley JD, Suomi SJ, Linnoila M (1996e) A nonhuman primate model of type II excessive alcohol consumption? Part 1. Low cerebrospinal fluid 5-hydroxyindoleacetic acid concentrations and diminished social competence correlate with excessive alcohol consumption. Alcohol Clin Exp Res 20:629–642.

Kruesi MJ, Rapoport JL, Hamburger S, Hibbs E, Potter WZ, Lenane M, Brown GL (1990a) Cerebrospinal fluid monoamine metabolites, aggression, and impulsivity in disruptive behavior disorders of children and adolescents. Arch Gen Psychiatry 47:419–426.

Kruesi MJ, Swedo S, Leonard H, Rubinow DR, Rapoport JL (1990b) CSF somatostatin in childhood psychiatric disorders: a preliminary investigation. Psychiatry Res 33:277–284.

Linnoila VM, Virkkunen M (1992) Aggression, suicidality, and serotonin. J Clin Psychiatry 53:46–51.

Linnoila M, Virkkunen M, Scheinin M, Nuutila A, Rimon R, Goodwin FK (1983) Low cerebrospinal fluid 5-hydroxyindoleacetic acid concentration differentiates impulsive from nonimpulsive violent behavior. Life Sci 33:2609–2614.

Madsen D (1994) Serotonin and social rank among human males. In: Masters RD, McGuire MT (eds) The neurotransmitter revolution. Southern Illinois University Press, Carbondale, pp 146–158.

McGuire MT, Brammer GL, Raleigh MJ (1986) Resting cortisol levels and the emergence of dominant status among male vervet monkeys. Horm Behav 20:106–117.

Mehlman PT, Higley JD, Faucher I, Lilly AA, Taub DM, Suomi S, Linnoila M (1994) Low CSF 5-HIAA concentrations and severe aggression and impaired impulse control in nonhuman primates. Am J Psychiatry 151:1485–1491.

Mehlman P, Higley JD, Faucher I, Lilly AA, Taub DM, Vickers JH, Suomi S, Linnoila M (1995) Correlation of CSF 5-HIAA concentration with sociality and the timing of emigration in free-ranging primates. Am J Psychiatry 152:907–913.

Mehlman PT, Higley JD, Fernald BJ, Sallee FR, Suomi SJ, Linnoila M (1997) CSF 5-HIAA, testosterone, and sociosexual behaviors in free-ranging male rhesus macaques in the mating season. Psychiatry Res 72:89–102.

Moss HB (1987) Serotonergic activity and disinhibitory psychopathy in alcoholism. Med Hypoth 23:353–361.

Popova NK, Kulikov AV, Nikulina EM, Kozlachkova EY, Maslova GB (1991a) Serotonin metabolism and serotonergic receptors in Norway rats selected for low aggressiveness towards man. Aggress Behav 17:207–213.

Popova NK, Voitenko NN, Kulikov AV, Avgustinovich DF (1991b) Evidence for the involvement of central serotonin in mechanism of domestication of silver foxes. Pharmacol Biochem Behav 40:751–756.

Raleigh MJ (1987) Differential behavioral effects of tryptophan and 5-hydroxytryptophan in vervet monkeys: influence of catecholaminergic systems. Psychopharmacology 93:44–50.

Raleigh MJ, McGuire MT (1986) Animal analogues of ostracism: biological mechanisms and social consequences. Ethol Sociobiol 7:53–66.

Raleigh MJ, McGuire MT (1991) Bidirectional relationships between tryptophan and social behavior in vervet monkeys. Adv Exp Med Biol 294:289–298.

Raleigh MJ, McGuire MT (1994) Serotonin, aggression, and violence in vervet monkeys. In: Masters RD, McGuire MT (eds) The neurotransmitter revolution. Southern Illinois University Press, Carbondale, pp 129–145.

Raleigh MJ, Brammer GL, Yuwiler A, Flannery JW, McGuire MT (1980) Serotonergic influences on the social behavior of vervet monkeys (Cercopithecus aethiops sabaeus). Exp Neurol 68:322–334.

Raleigh MJ, Brammer GL, McGuire MT (1983) Male dominance, serotonergic systems, and the behavioral and physiological effects of drugs in vervet monkeys (Cercopithecus aethiops sabaeus). In: Miczek KA (ed) Ethopharmacology: primate models of neuropsychiatric disorders. Liss, New York, pp 185–197.

Raleigh MJ, Brammer GL, Ritvo ER, Geller E, McGuire MT, Yuwiler A (1986) Effects of chronic fenfluramine on blood serotonin, cerebrospinal fluid metabolites, and behavior in monkeys. Psychopharmacology 90:503–508.

Raleigh MJ, McGuire MT, Brammer GL, Pollack DB, Yuwiler A (1991) Serotonergic mechanisms promote dominance acquisition in adult male vervet monkeys. Brain Res 559:181–190.

Raleigh MJ, Brammer GL, McGuire MT, Pollack DB, Yuwiler A (1992) Individual differences in basal cisternal cerebrospinal fluid 5-HIAA and HVA in monkeys. The effects of gender, age, physical characteristics, and matrilineal influences. Neuropsychopharmacology 7:295–304.

Roy A, De JJ, Linnoila M (1989) Cerebrospinal fluid monoamine metabolites and suicidal behavior in depressed patients. A 5-year follow-up study. Arch Gen Psychiatry 46:609–612.

Scheinin M, Chang WH, Jimerson DC, Linnoila M (1983) Measurement of 3-methoxy-4-hydroxyphenylglycol in human plasma with high-performance liquid chromatography using electrochemical detection. Anal Biochem 132:165–170.

Shively CA, Fontenot MB, Kaplan JR (1995) Social status, behavior, and central serotonergic responsivity in female cynomolgus monkeys. Am J Primatol 37:333–340.

Sirianni JS (1985) Growth and development of the pigtailed macaque. CRC Press, Boca Raton.

van Hooff JARAM (1967) The facial displays of the catarrhine monkeys and apes. In: Morris D (ed) Primate ethology. Aldine Publishing Company, Chicago, pp 7–68.

Virkkunen M, De Jong J, Bartko J, Linnoila M (1989) Psychobiological concomitants of history of suicide attempts among violent offenders and impulsive fire setters. Arch Gen Psychiatry 46:604–606.

Virkkunen M, Kallio E, Rawlings R, Tokola R, Poland RE, Guidotti A, Nemeroff C, Bissette G, Kalogeras K, Karonen SL, Linnoila M (1994a) Personality profiles and state aggressiveness in Finnish alcoholic, violent offenders, fire setters, and healthy volunteers. Arch Gen Psychiatry 51:28–33.

Virkkunen M, Rawlings R, Tokola R, Poland RE, Guidotti A, Nemeroff C, Bissette G, Kalogeras K, Karonen SL, Linnoila M (1994b) CSF biochemistries, glucose metabolism, and diurnal activity rhythms in alcoholic, violent offenders, fire setters, and healthy volunteers. Arch Gen Psychiatry 51:20–27.

Yodyingyuad U, de la Riva C, Abbott DH, Herbert J, Keverne EB (1985) Relationship between dominance hierarchy, cerebrospinal fluid levels of amine transmitter metabolites (5-hydroxyindoleacetic acid and homovanillic acid) and plasma cortisol in monkeys. Neuroscience 16:851–858.

64 Developmental Exposure to Vasopressin Increases Aggression in Adult Prairie Voles

John M. Stribley and C. Sue Carter

Arginine vasopressin (AVP) is a nonapeptide hormone primarily synthesized in the paraventricular nucleus and the supraoptic nucleus of the hypothalamus. In the brain, AVP predominantly binds to a G protein-coupled, V_{1a} receptor subtype having seven transmembrane domains. V_1 receptors depend on phosphatidyl inositol hydrolysis and intracellular calcium mobilization as part of the second messenger system for transcriptional activation and gene expression. In addition, there are numerous areas within the brain that receive AVP fiber projections from the paraventricular nucleus, including the amygdala, hippocampus, and posterior pituitary. Additional sites of AVP synthesis include the locus ceruleus and the bed nucleus of the stria terminalis, which sends neural projections to the lateral septum and the lateral habenular nucleus, among others (see refs. 1–4).

AVP and related peptides have well documented effects on a variety of systems associated with the physiological and behavioral defense of homeostasis. For example, AVP is necessary for water retention and affects blood pressure and other aspects of cardiovascular function (5). In rats, AVP influences the regulation of the hypothalamic-pituitary-adrenal axis, and it is likely that the central release of AVP is sensitive to stressful experiences (6, 7). In addition, AVP can enhance avoidance learning and some forms of memory (8). AVP also can influence the expression of territorial aggression in hamsters (9) and mate guarding in male prairie voles (*Microtus ochrogaster*) (10).

Although experiments conducted to determine the effects of AVP in adult animals are common, less is known regarding the role of this peptide during development (11, 12). Prairie voles offer an attractive model system both for the study of aggression and for the analysis of the developmental effects of AVP. In adult prairie voles, AVP affects several of the behavioral characteristics that define monogamy (13, 14), including high levels of social contact (15), male parental care (16, 17), the development of partner preferences (9, 10), and mating-induced aggressive behavior (10, 18). In addition, intracerebroventricular injection of AVP in adult male prairie voles has been shown to increase exploratory activity in an elevated plus maze (19).

AVP cell bodies and receptors are present well before birth (20), suggesting that this system is functional during the postnatal period (21). In this paper, we hypothesized that the behavioral systems, which are regulated by AVP in adulthood, might also be responsive to developmental changes in AVP. This hypothesis was tested in prairie voles by manipulating the functional levels of AVP during the early postnatal period and by assessing subsequent behavioral changes in adult animals.

Methods

Hormone Treatment

Prairie voles used in this study were fourth generation descendants of a stock originally captured near Urbana, IL. The animals were housed under a 14:10 light/dark cycle, in polycarbonate mouse cages. Purina rabbit chow and water were provided ad libitum. On the first postnatal day, prairie vole pups were sexed, weighed, and toe-clipped for identification. Males and females were randomly assigned to one of six different groups ($n = 8$–10 per group). Experimental animals were generated from 10 independent breeding pairs over six generations. Only one male and one female pup per litter received hormone treatments, and like-sex siblings received either saline (controls) or no treatment (stimulus animals) in each generation. Over the first seven postnatal days, each animal either received (*a*) 120 ng of AVP; (*b*) 12 ng of AVP; (*c*) 1.2 ng of AVP; (*d*) 0.5 ng of [d(CH$_2$)$_5$Tyr(Me)]AVP [an AVP antagonist (AVPA)], each in 50 µl of saline; or (e) 50 µl of saline; or (f) was left untreated and unhandled. To limit the number of groups in this experiment, only one type and dose of AVP antagonist was chosen. The AVP antagonist used here is known to be selective for the V$_{1a}$ receptor subtype found in the brain and has been used at this dose level to successfully block the behavioral effects of both mating and AVP in adult prairie voles (10, 15). Although the AVP antagonist used in the aforementioned studies was administered directly into the intracerebral ventricles of adult animals, it was assumed in our study that peripheral injections of 0.05 ng of AVP antagonist would be suitable given the size of the neonates (1/10 of adult size) and their altricial state. It is known that the blood–brain barrier in altricial species is not fully formed at birth (22) and there is mounting physiological and behavioral evidence (23–30) to suggest that AVP can pass and perhaps play a facilitatory role in the blood–brain barrier of neonatal and adult rats, respectively (31–34). In our study, all of the pharmacological agents were injected intraperitoneally once per day by using a 30-gauge, 0.5-inch hypodermic needle affixed to a 100-µl Hamilton syringe. Treated animals were returned to their litters after each injection. All animals were weaned and paired with a same-sex sibling on postnatal day 31.

Behavior Tests and Analysis

At 90 days of age, each subject was tested for activity and general exploration in an elevated plus maze (5-min test as described in refs. 18 and 19). Plus-maze activity levels were calculated as a percentage of the entries into the open arms divided by the sum of the open- and closed-arm entries. Twenty-four hours later, each subject was placed for 5 min in a clean polycarbonate mouse cage (12 × 18 × 28 cm) with an unfamiliar, same-sex conspecific of approximately the same body weight. All agonistic behaviors (lunges, bites,

and lateral displays as defined in ref. 10) were recorded, and the total frequency of these behaviors is presented here as an index of aggression. Treatment effects were analyzed by using Kruskal–Wallis tests, and pairwise comparisons were made by using Mann–Whitney U tests with a level of significance of $P < 0.05$. The percentage data for animals displaying at least one act of aggression toward an unfamiliar, same-sex conspecific were analyzed by using the Yate's Corrected χ^2 test with a level of significance assigned at $P < 0.05$.

Results

Males

Aggression frequencies in adult, sexually naïve, male prairie voles were significantly affected by neonatal treatment with AVP ($\chi^2 = 19.2$; df = 5; $P = 0.002$). Males that were injected neonatally (Fig. 64.1A) with 120 ng of AVP were significantly more aggressive than were males receiving no treatment, saline, 12 ng of AVP, or the AVP antagonist, AVPA (pairwise comparisons; Mann–Whitney U test; $P < 0.05$). Further, the percentage of animals within the 120-ng AVP dose group that displayed any form of aggression toward an unfamiliar male conspecific was significantly higher (Yate's corrected χ^2; $P < 0.05$) when compared with the control groups. Males that received 1.2 ng of AVP also were more aggressive than males that were not treated or those receiving AVPA, but the behavior of the 1.2-ng AVP group did not differ significantly from the other AVP-treated males.

Subsequent behavioral tests of these animals supported the assumption that the capacity of neonatal AVP to increase aggression was not restricted to male–male aggression, because aggression also was seen in encounters with females. Additionally, in males, aggression induced by 120 ng of AVP continued to be shown throughout the lives of the animals, and was not further

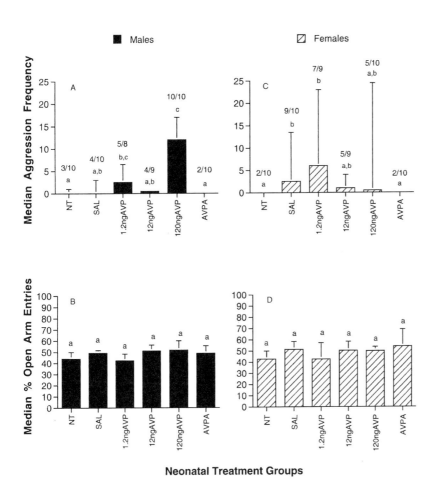

Figure 64.1

Median aggression frequency (+75% quartile range) exhibited by sexually naïve, adult male (A) and female (C) prairie voles in a 5-min test with a comparable like-sex stimulus animal. Experimental animals received either no treatment (NT); one daily intraperitoneal injection of 50 μl of physiological saline (SAL); or 1.2 ng of AVP, 12 ng of AVP, 120 ng of AVP, or 0.5 ng of AVPA, each suspended in 50 μl of saline over the first 7 postnatal days of life. Columns sharing letters in common are not significantly different (Mann–Whitney U; $P > 0.05$). The ratio of animals showing aggression within each group is noted above each bar. Median percentage entries into the open arm of an elevated plus maze by sexually naïve, adult male (B) and female (D) experimental prairie voles during a 5-min test. There were no group differences on this measure (Mann–Whitney U; $P > 0.05$).

increased by sexual experience. Tendencies to display exceptionally low levels of aggression also were consistent throughout the lives of AVPA animals. In contrast, exploratory behavior (Fig. 64.1B) was not significantly affected by treatments with either AVP or AVPA (Kruskal–Wallis; $\chi^2 = 3.8$; df $= 5$; $P = 0.58$).

Females

In a concurrent study of female prairie voles, only the lowest dose of postnatal AVP tended to increase the expression of aggression in sexually naïve, adult females (Fig. 64.1C; Kruskal–Wallis; $\chi^2 = 13.1$; df $= 5$; $P = 0.022$). As in males, neonatal treatments did not alter exploratory behavior (Fig. 64.1D). Further pairwise comparisons revealed that females in the 1.2-ng AVP dose group were significantly more aggressive relative to the untreated and AVPA-treated control groups (Fig. 64.1C). Saline-treated females also showed an increase in aggression in comparison to untreated or AVPA-treated females, but did not differ from AVP-treated females. Although a few individual females exhibited intense levels of aggression within several of the AVP-treated groups, females in general were less aggressive than their male counterparts.

Discussion

It has been proposed that hormones, which are essential for normal physiological functions in the adult, may play an important role during development by fine tuning their respective receptors or neuroendocrine pathways (35–37). The results from our study suggest that in male prairie voles the neural substrates underlying the expression of aggression are sensitive to exposure to AVP during the early postnatal period and that AVP may be a component of the developmental mechanisms regulating aggression later in life. Furthermore, the heightened level of aggression observed in AVP-treated animals was

secondary neither to increased activity patterns nor to any other observed behavioral impairments. Aggression is rare in sexually naïve, adult male prairie voles; however, after mating, prairie voles exhibit a long-lasting, permanent increase in aggression (38, 39). AVP is implicated in the induction of aggression both during development and in adulthood, although whether the same cellular mechanisms are responsible for increasing aggression in both cases remains to be determined. For example, it is possible that both mating (40) and developmental exposure to AVP sensitizes AVP receptors to become more responsive to subsequent exposure to this peptide.

The vasopressinergic system in prairie voles appears to be sexually dimorphic (41), with a higher concentration of immunoreactive AVP localized in the lateral septum and lateral habenular nucleus of males. Our study confirms that male and female prairie voles responded differently to AVP challenges during early postnatal development. For example, in female prairie voles, we observed that postnatal treatment with either the lowest dose of AVP or the injections with the saline vehicle was associated with increased aggression in adulthood. On the contrary, males responded with increased aggression only at the highest dose of AVP given. One possible explanation is that females are more sensitive to handling stress, perhaps as mediated through corticosterone during early postnatal development, whereas males are more sensitive to AVP. Interestingly, both males and females exhibited virtually no aggression when treated with AVPA, suggesting that some level of endogenous AVP production as a result of handling may be directly or indirectly associated with the development of aggression in males and females, respectively. Alternatively, among those groups of females that were aggressive, only a few individual females were exceptionally aggressive, accounting for the high level of variability we observed within the respective groups and, thus, may require a larger sample size to be used in future studies.

It is generally assumed that perinatal androgens play a role in mammalian sexual differentiation. However, a sex difference with respect to the behavioral effects of AVP suggests that some aspects of the sexual differentiation of the system responsible for aggression may be present at birth. The developmental effects of androgens on aggression remain to be studied in prairie voles. However, in adult prairie voles, castration does not inhibit aggression, and aggression appears to be independent of gonadal steroids (N. Hastings and C.S.C., unpublished observations).

Recent experiments with prairie voles have implicated adrenal steroids, not gonadal hormones, in the process of behavioral masculinization in this species (42, 43). For example, postnatal treatments with corticosterone, rather than testosterone, were associated with increased mounting in female prairie voles, and neonatal castration did not reduce the tendency of males of this species to mount in response to adult androgens.

Our study suggests the more general hypothesis that peptides may mediate the effects of environmental cues on subsequent adult patterns of aggression. Mechanisms such as these could confer selective advantages by allowing individual experiences capable of releasing AVP to produce long-lasting adjustments in physiological and behavioral systems. For example, postnatal fluid restriction (drought) could increase the endogenous production of AVP and, thus, increase subsequent aggressive behavior. Under harsh environmental conditions, a more aggressive behavioral response to other animals, especially potential competitors, might be advantageous. Alternatively, under more benign conditions, endogenous AVP might remain low, permitting lower levels of aggression, especially in reproductively naïve animals.

The clinical implications of developmental exposure to AVP or related peptides are largely unknown. Analogues of AVP such as desmopressin or lysine vasopressin have been used to treat nocturnal enuresis (bed wetting) in normal children (44) or to enhance learning and memory in mentally disabled children (45, 46), respectively. Particularly disturbing is the fact that nicotine, a potent releaser of AVP (47–50), can freely pass both the placental and blood–brain barriers of fetuses and their mothers alike (51, 52). Given the recent rise in cigarette use among young girls and pregnant teenagers in the United States (53), it is important to understand the links among nicotine, vasopressin, and various conduct disorders observed in children of smoking mothers (54–59).

Given the structural similarity between oxytocin and AVP, these peptides can affect each other's receptors. Oxytocin (Pitocin) is widely used to facilitate parturition and in some cases is used as a lactational aid. Developmental exposure to oxytocin might act as either an agonist or an antagonist on the vasopressinergic system. The long-term effects of such manipulations have not been fully examined (30).

Acknowledgments

We thank Bruce Cushing, Nancy Cushing, Edward Lee, Kinnari Patel, and Sophia Fuentes for their help with this project. All work was conducted within the guidelines established by the Animal Care and Use Committee of the University of Maryland. This research was supported by grants from the National Institutes of Health to C.S.C.

References

1. Barberis, C. & Tribollet, E. (1996) *Crit. Rev. Neurobiol.* 10, 119–154.

2. Boer, G. J., Buijs, R. M., Swaab, D. F. & De Vries, G. J. (1980) *Peptides* 1, Suppl. 1, 203–209.

3. Ervin, M. G., Kullama, L. K., Ross, M. G., Leake, R. D. & Fisher, D. A. (1993) *Reg. Pept.* 45, 203–208.

4. Ostrowski, N. L., Lolait, S. J., Bradley, D. J., O'Carroll, A. M., Brownstein, M. J. & Young, W. S. (1992) *Endocrinology* 131, 533–535.

5. Berecek, K. H. (1991) in *Central Neural Mechanisms in Cardiovascular Regulation,* eds. Kunos, G. & Ciriello, J. (Birkhauser, Boston), pp. 1–34.

6. Aguilera, G., Lightman, S. L. & Kiss, A. (1993) *Endocrinology* 132, 241–248.

7. Yates, F. E., Russell, S. M., Dallman, M. F., Hedge, G. A., McCann, S. M. & Dhariwal, A. P. S. (1971) *Endocrinology* 88, 3–15.

8. Engelmann, M., Wotjak, C. T., Neumann, I., Ludwig, M. & Landgraf, R. (1996) *Neurosci. Biobehav. Rev.* 20, 341–358.

9. Ferris, C. F., Albers, H. E., Wesolowski, S. M., Goldman, B. D. & Luman, S. E. (1984) *Science* 224, 521–523.

10. Winslow, J. T., Hastings, N., Carter, C. S., Harbaugh, C. R. & Insel, T. R. (1993) *Nature (London)* 365, 545–548.

11. Van Tol, H. H. M., Snijdewint, F. G. M., Boer, G. J. & Burbach, J. P. H. (1986) *Neurosci. Lett.* 65, 1–6.

12. Varlinskaya, E. I., Petrov, E. S., Robinson, S. R. & Smotherman, W. P. (1994) *Behav. Neurosci.* 108, 395–409.

13. Carter, C. S., DeVries, A. C. & Getz, L. L. (1995) *Neurosci. Biobehav. Rev.* 19, 303–314.

14. Kleiman, D. (1977) *Quart. Rev. Biol.* 52, 39–69.

15. Cho, M. M., DeVries, A. C., Williams, J. R. & Carter, C. S. *Behav. Neurosci.,* in press.

16. Wang, Z. X., Zhou, L., Hulihan, T. & Insel, T. R. (1996) *J. Comp. Neurol.* 366, 726–737.

17. Wang, Z. X., Ferris, C. F. & DeVries, G. J. (1994) *Proc. Natl. Acad. Sci. USA* 91, 400–404.

18. Insel, T. R., Preston, S. & Winslow, J. T. (1995) *Physiol. Behav.* 57, 615–627.

19. Dharmadhikari, A., Lee, Y. S., Roberts, R. L. & Carter, C. S. (1997) *Ann. N.Y. Acad. Sci.* 807, 260–272.

20. DeVries, G. F. & Villalba, C. (1997) *Ann. N.Y. Acad. Sci.* 807, 273–286.

21. Wang, Z., Young, L. J., Kiu, Y. & Insel, T. R. (1997) *J. Comp. Neurol.* 378, 535–546.

22. Johanson, C. E. (1980) *Brain Res.* 190, 3–16.

23. Bluthe, R. M., Schoenen, J. & Dantzer, R. (1990) *Brain Res.* 519, 150–157.

24. Chen, X. F., Chen, Z. F., Liu, R. Y. & Du, Y. C. (1988) *Peptides* 9, 717–721.

25. Dantzer, R., Bluthe, R. M., Koob, G. F. & Le Moal, M. (1987) *Psychopharmacology* 91, 363–368.

26. De Vries, G. J., Buijs, R. M. & Swaab, D. F. (1981) *Brain Res.* 218, 67–78.

27. De Wied, D., Elands, J. & Kovacs, G. (1991) *Proc. Natl. Acad. Sci. USA* 88, 1494–1498.

28. Popik, P. & Van Ree, J. M. (1993) *Behav. Neural Biol.* 59, 63–68.

29. Strupp, B. J., Bunsey, M., Bertsche, B., Levitsky, D. A. & Kesler, M. (1990) *Behav. Neurosci.* 104, 268–276.

30. Swabb, D. F. & Boer, G. J. (1983) *J. Dev. Physiol.* 5, 67–75.

31. Banks, W. A. & Kastin, A. J. (1985) *Psychoneuroendocrinology* 10, 385–399.

32. Brust, P. (1986) *J. Neurochem.* 46, 534–541.

33. Brust, P., Shaya, E. K., Jeffries, K. J., Dannals, R. F., Ravert, H. T., Wilson, A. A., Conti, P. S., Wagner, H. N., Gjedde, A., Ermisch, A. & Wong, D. F. (1992) *J. Neurochem.* 59, 1421–1429.

34. Ermisch, A., Ruhle, H. J., Landgraf, R. & Hess, J. (1985) *J. Cereb. Blood Flow Metab.* 5, 350–357.

35. Csaba, G. (1986) *Experientia* 42, 750–759.

36. Boer, G. J., Snijdewint, G. M. & Swaab, D. F. (1988) *Prog. Brain Res.* 73, 245–264.

37. Handelmann, G. E. (1988) *Prog. Brain Res.* 73, 523–533.

38. Getz, L. L., Carter, C. S. & Gavish, L. (1981) *Behav. Ecol. Sociobiol.* 8, 189–194.

39. Gavish, L., Carter, C. S. & Getz, L. L. (1983) *Anim. Behav.* 31, 511–517.

40. Insel, T. R., Wang, Z. X. & Ferris, C. F. (1994) *J. Neurosci.* 14, 5381–5392.

41. Bamshad, M., Novak, M. A. & DeVries, G. J. (1993) *J. Neuroendocrinology* 5, 247–255.

42. Roberts, R. L., Zullo, A. S., Gustafson, E. A. & Carter, C. S. (1996) *Horm. Behav.* 30, 576–582.

43. Roberts, R. L., Zullo, A. S. & Carter, C. S. (1997) *Physiol. Behav.* 62, 1379–1383.

44. Moffatt, M. E. (1997) *Dev. Behav. Ped.* 18, 49–56.

45. Andersen, L. T., David, R., Bonnet, K. & Dancis, J. (1979) *Life Sci.* 24, 905–910.

46. Eisenberg, J., Chazan-Gologorsky, S., Hattab, J. & Belmaker, R. H. (1984) *Biol. Psychiatry* 19, 1137–1141.

47. Andersson, K., Siegel, R., Fuxe, K. & Eneroth, P. (1983) *Acta Physiol. Scand.* 118, 35–40.

48. Husain, M. K., Frantz, A. G., Ciarachi, F. & Robinson, A. G. (1975) *J. Clin. Endocrinol. Metab.* 41, 1113–1117.

49. Matta, S. G., Foster, C. A. & Sharp, B. M. (1993) *Endocrinology* 132, 2149–2156.

50. Seyler, L. E., Pomerleau, O. F., Fertig, J. B., Hunt, D. & Parker, K. (1986) *Pharmacol. Biochem. Behav.* 24, 159–162.

51. Riah, O., Courriere, P., Dousset, J. C., Todeschi, N. & Labat, C. (1998) *Cell. Mol. Neurobiol.* 18, 311–318.

52. Spector, R. & Goldberg, M. J. (1982) *J. Neurochem.* 38, 594–596.

53. Matthews, T. J. (1998) *Natl. Vit. Stat. Rep.* 47, 1–9.

54. Milberger, S., Biederman, J., Faraone, S. V., Chen, L. & Jones, J. (1996) *Am. J. Psychiatry* 153, 1138–1142.

55. Pomerleau, O. F. (1992) *Am. J. Med.* 93(1A), 2S–7S.

56. Pomerleau, O. F., Downey, K. K., Stelson, F. W. & Pomerleau, C. S. (1995) *J. Subst. Abuse* 7, 373–378.

57. Rantakallio, P., Laara, E., Isohanni, M. & Moilanen, I. (1992) *Int. J. Epidem.* 21, 1106–1113.

58. Wakschlag, L. S., Lahey, B., Loeber, R., Green, S., Gordon, R. & Leventhal, B. L. (1997) *Arch. Gen. Psychiatry* 54, 670–676.

59. Weitzman, M., Gortmaker, S. & Sobol, A. (1992) *Pediatrics* 90, 342–349.

65 CSF Testosterone and 5-HIAA Correlate with Different Types of Aggressive Behaviors

J. Dee Higley, Patrick T. Mehlman, Russell E. Poland, David M. Taub, James Vickers, Stephen J. Suomi, and Markku Linnoila

Introduction

Recent psychobiological studies on aggressive behaviors have focused on central nervous system (CNS) serotonin and testosterone functioning as major biological variables of interest (Archer 1991; Brown and Linnoila 1990; Dabbs et al. 1987; Kruesi et al. 1990, 1992; Virkkunen et al. 1994a, 1994b). Few studies, however, have attempted to assess simultaneously possible differential contributions of serotonin and testosterone metabolism to expressing and inhibiting aggressive behaviors (Virkkunen et al. 1994a, 1994b). Understanding the possible differential roles of serotonin and testosterone in the control of aggressive and violent behaviors could be of importance for designing strategies to prevent violence, while not affecting other types of adaptive behaviors such as assertiveness. Eichelman's review on the current state of psychiatry in understanding and treating violent behaviors emphasized the need to differentiate between categories of aggressive behaviors and their underlying neural substrates (Eichelman 1992). Determining which behaviors correlate with serotonin turnover rate and which correlate with testosterone concentrations could serve to demarcate functional differences in types of aggression and could also suggest novel approaches to classify, treat, and prevent inappropriate behaviors.

Studies Linking Serotonin Turnover Rate to Aggression and Impulsivity

Studies on humans show a consistent pattern: men who engage in impulsive, unplanned acts of interpersonal violence or arson exhibit a lower mean cerebrospinal fluid (CSF) concentration of 5-hydroxyindoleacetic acid (5-HIAA), the major metabolite of serotonin, than the population average (Brown et al. 1979, 1982; Lidberg et al. 1985; Limson et al. 1991; Linnoila et al. 1983, 1989; Roy et al. 1988; Virkkunen et al. 1994a, 1994b). Similarly, recent studies have shown a negative correlation between CSF 5-HIAA concentrations and excessive and inappropriate aggression in nonhuman primates (Higley et al. 1992, 1994, in press; Mehlman et al. 1994, 1995; Raleigh and McGuire 1994).

In both humans and nonhuman primates, interindividual differences in CSF 5-HIAA show traitlike stability beginning early in life, and they continue to correlate across time and settings (Bertilsson et al. 1982; Cohen et al. 1974; Kraemer and McKinney 1979; Riddle et al. 1986; Träskman-Bendz et al. 1984). Similarly, a number of studies have shown that plasma testosterone concentrations are relatively stable over time (Dabbs 1990; Ehrenkranz et al. 1974; Mattsson et al. 1980; Olweus 1986; Olweus et al. 1980). Such findings led us to postulate that CSF 5-HIAA and testosterone, along with the aggressive behaviors associated with each of the respective biochemicals, would show long-term interindividual stability.

Serotonin—Aggression or Impulsivity

Several recent reviews have concluded that reduced CNS serotonin functioning is one of the biological variables underlying impaired impulse control (Cloninger 1986; Soubrié 1986; Coccaro 1992; Csernansky and Sheline 1993; López-Ibor 1991; Stein et al. 1993). One reason to focus on the relationship between reduced serotonin functioning and violence is findings from animal studies that show a relationship between diminished central serotonin functioning and impaired inhibition of responses that require individuals to wait or withhold a response or risk punishment or injury (Soubrié 1986; Higley et al. 1992; Mehlman et al. 1994), and studies in humans that show that ratings of impulsivity are positively correlated with lifetime risk for violence, hostility, irritability, and suicide (Apter et al. 1990; Banki and Arato 1983a, 1983b). For individuals with low CSF 5-HIAA concentrations, the impact of impaired impulse control is not limited to aggressive behaviors; instead, impulsivity appears to be a traitlike personality characteristic. Indeed, on various, well-validated personality inventories, individuals with reduced serotonin functioning, as measured by low CSF 5-HIAA or plasma prolactin concentrations following a fenfluramine challenge, often score high on items measuring impulsivity (Banki and Arato 1983a, 1983b; Coccaro 1989, 1992; Roy et al. 1988; but see also Fishbein et al. 1989; Kruesi et al. 1990; Limson et al. 1991; Moss et al. 1990). As might be expected, individuals with lower than average CSF 5-HIAA frequently exhibit other behavioral problems that may be indicative of impaired impulse control, such as excessive alcohol consumption, polysubstance abuse, suicide attempts, and among violent criminals, high rates of recidivism (Banki and Arato 1983a, 1983b; Brown et al. 1979, 1982; Limson et al. 1991; Virkkunen et al. 1989). In Brown and colleagues' studies on violent marines (Brown et al. 1979, 1982), the men with the lowest CSF 5-HIAA concentrations also exhibited impulse control problems, such as repeated rule infractions and high scores on the Minnesota Multiphasic Personality Inventory (MMPI) scale for psychopathic deviance (Brown et al. 1979, 1982). Thus, one might postulate that impulsivity should correlate with excessive or inappropriate aggression and violence.

Studies Linking Testosterone to Aggression and Social Dominance

High testosterone, unlike low serotonin turnover rate, is seldom linked with impulsivity (see, for example, Mattsson et al. 1980; Olweus et al. 1980; however see Daitzman and Zuckerman 1980); rather, in terms of aggression, it shows a more general relationship to competitiveness, a drive for social dominance, or an overall aggressive motivation (Archer 1991; Buchanan et al. 1992; Christiansen and Knussmann 1987; Olweus 1984, 1986). The significant positive correlations between testosterone and aggression occur most often when both are measured during competitive events or during social status challenge (Mazur 1983; Rose et al. 1971; Scaramella and Brown 1978) or in response to provocation or threat (Olweus et al. 1980, 1988; Olweus 1986). Most individuals with high testosterone are not violent but are restrained in their use of aggression, expressing their aggression in settings or using methods that are socially acceptable, which may be a function of what the aggression is used for, i.e., maintenance of social status and defense of competitive challenge. Moreover, correlations between testosterone and behavior are not limited to aggression. Testosterone also shows correlations with seemingly positive traits such as toughness (Dabbs et al. 1987), social dominance (Booth et al. 1989; Christiansen and Knussmann 1987; Ehrenkranz et al. 1974; Lindman et al. 1987; Rose et al. 1971), social assertiveness (Lindman et al. 1987), and competitiveness and physical vigor (Booth et al. 1989; Mattsson et al. 1980). These findings and others (e.g., Archer 1991; Olweus et al. 1980, 1988; Soubrié 1986) suggest that testosterone may be correlated with aggressive motives and competitiveness, rather than violence per se. CNS serotonin functioning, as indicated by CSF 5-HIAA, on the other hand, may function to limit aggression to proper time, setting, and intensity.

A Working Model

One possible interpretation of these data is that testosterone and serotonin may contribute differentially to the expression of aggressive behaviors, with testosterone contributing to aggressive drive and motivation and serotonin regulating the threshold, intensity, and resulting frequency of the behavioral expression. Thus, individuals with above average testosterone but normal serotonin may express aggression in a variety of settings, but generally, would not express violence or unrestrained aggression. They would also be expected to exhibit more assertive behaviors that characterize socially dominant males, such as mounting of other male monkeys (Richards 1974). Individuals with lower than average serotonin functioning would be expected to exhibit impaired impulse control, resulting in a low threshold to display aggression and ultimately in more frequent violence. High testosterone, however, because it increases aggressive motivation, would further augment the propensity to engage in aggression in subjects with low CSF 5-HIAA. Furthermore, once an aggressive act had begun, subjects with low CSF 5-HIAA would exhibit deficits in stopping the aggression before it escalated into violence that has a high probability to produce injury.

Methodological Issues

Most studies of testosterone and aggression have measured either plasma total testosterone or salivary testosterone concentrations. Measuring plasma total testosterone as an estimate of central androgen functioning is problematic, however, since in plasma the free fraction accessible to the central nervous system is only about 2% (Pardridge 1986; Sannikka et al. 1983). Although a few studies have quantified free testosterone as a measure of central androgen functioning, Eichelman indicates that, "Central probe studies of testosterone sensitivity may be more productive than the measurement of peripheral levels" (Eichelman 1992, p. 490). It is likely that a relatively accurate reflection of CNS androgen activity is obtained by quantifying CSF free testosterone; however, to date no studies have investigated the relationship between plasma and CNS testosterone in nonhuman primates. A major purpose of this study was to investigate the correlation between plasma testosterone and CSF free testosterone in rhesus monkeys.

Purposes and Hypotheses for the Study

Over the past 3 years we have conducted a longitudinal research project investigating the genetic and environmental antecedents of various kinds of aggressive behaviors and their underlying biological substrates using a nonhuman primate model. Our research subjects are free-ranging, young adolescent male rhesus monkeys (*Macaca mulatta*). In three published studies (Higley et al. 1992; Mehlman et al. 1994, 1995), we found a relationship between low CSF 5-HIAA and aggression in young prepubescent male nonhuman primates. In these studies, we found that both the number and severity of scars and wounds, as well as the relative incidence of aggressive behaviors that place individuals at risk for injury, i.e., aggression that escalates to dangerous levels of severity, were strongly negatively correlated with CSF 5-HIAA. Overall rates of aggression, however, particularly restrained aggression used to defend social status, were *not* correlated with CSF 5-HIAA (Mehlman et al. 1994). Plasma testosterone, on the other hand, was not correlated with aggression that placed individuals at risk for injury (Higley et al. 1992; Mehlman et al. 1994). An indirect corroboration of these findings comes from studies on nonhuman primates showing that administering exogenous testosterone increases the rate of aggressive encounters but not the rate of physical injury (Rejeski et al. 1990). In our earlier study (Mehlman et al. 1994), there was evidence that the negative correlation between CSF 5-HIAA and escalated aggression may have been related to higher levels of traitlike impulsivity and perseveration in the subjects with lower than average CSF 5-HIAA. In this study, we used a measure of impulsivity—spontaneous, unprovoked, long leaps at great heights between treetops—and correlated it with CSF 5-HIAA. This measure is obtained outside of aggressive contexts and is also independent of overall motor activity and playfulness. Whereas monkeys with higher than average CSF 5-HIAA moved carefully from tree to tree, seldom making dangerous leaps, the monkeys with lower than average CSF 5-HIAA were more likely to use dangerous, long, unprovoked leaps when moving between trees (Mehlman et al. 1994). One purpose of the present study was to attempt to replicate the negative correlation between long, spontaneous leaps and CSF 5-HIAA. To date, both studies that have assessed aggression and CSF 5-HIAA have investigated prepubescent male monkeys. Another purpose was to assess the relationship between aggression and low CSF 5-HIAA in older subjects, i.e., young adolescent males.

Based on our working model and previous findings (Higley et al. 1992; Mehlman et al. 1994, 1995) we hypothesized the following: 1) CSF free testosterone would correlate positively with overall rates of aggression and nonsexual male mounting, a measure of high social dominance (Richards 1974), but not with behaviors indicative of impulsivity (impulsive leaps—unprovoked, spontaneous, long, dangerous leaps between trees) nor with impulsive, uncontrolled aggression that escalates into bites, assaults, wounds, and prolonged chase sequences (escalated aggression). 2) CSF 5-HIAA concentrations would correlate negatively with impulsive leaps and escalated aggression, but not with overall rates of aggression. 3) Impulsive leaps would correlate positively with escalated aggression, but not with overall rates of aggression. 4) Interindividual differences in CSF 5-HIAA, homovanillic acid (HVA), free testosterone, and measures of violence would remain relatively stable between years. 5) Although plasma and CSF free testosterone concentrations should correlate positively with each other, CSF testosterone concentrations would be more strongly correlated with aggressive behavior than peripheral measures such as plasma testosterone concentrations.

What follows is a 2-year longitudinal study of adolescent male rhesus monkeys. In the spring of 1991 and again in the spring of 1992, a CSF and blood sample was obtained from each subject.

Following the CSF sampling, systematic behavioral data were collected from each of the subjects during the summer of both years and interindividual differences on all measures were correlated between years.

Methods

Subjects

The 1992 subjects were 24 adolescent male rhesus macaques with a mean age of 45.3 months (mid to late adolescence), captured in the spring of 1992, chosen from a large population of 4500 rhesus monkeys maintained as a free-ranging, food-provisioned breeding colony on a semitropical, 475-acre island. As in other natural macaque populations, the colony was organized into multimale and multifemale social groups (number of groups = 35, median group size = 50; adult sex ratio = 2.5 females to 1 male) distributed in separate but overlapping home ranges. Physiological and behavioral samples had been obtained from 17 of the same 24 subjects 1 year earlier in May, 1991 and from June through August, 1991, respectively, and form the basis of our longitudinal comparisons. The 1991 data are described in detail in a previous publication (Mehlman et al. 1994).

Conditions of Capture

To perform physical examinations and routine medical procedures, the monkeys living on the island are captured three to four times each year in 10 large corrals (diameter = 10–25 m, wall height = 4 m) that normally serve as free-access food stations. On the day previous to the start of the 5-day capture–sampling period, all corrals are baited with food and entrance to each is closed. The monkeys voluntarily jump into the corrals, but are precluded from exiting by the high walls. While in the corrals, monkeys have ad libitum access to food and water. Typically, only a portion of each social group jumps into a corral, and the monkeys remain in the corral until the technical crew is ready to capture them (the length of time monkeys spend in a corral is a function of the number of monkeys that jump into the corrals and the number that can be processed each day during a 5-day capture period). During the captures, the technical staff nets each monkey individually, anesthetizes it with ketamine hydrochloride, and removes it from the corral. In May, 1992, 17 of the 24 subjects were randomly selected and captured during the first 3 days of the 5-day capture period. To increase our sample size, 5 additional subjects that had been previously sampled were selected at random, and captured using a CO_2-propelled rifle with ketamine darts. All 17 of the 1991 subjects that were used in the longitudinal comparison were captured in corrals during the first 3 days of the 5-day capture period (Mehlman et al. 1994).

Selection of Subjects

The 24 1992 study subjects were trapped from a larger study population of adolescent males who have been CSF-sampled since the autumn of 1989. The 17 subjects that were randomly captured by voluntarily jumping into corrals did not differ in mean CSF 5-HIAA and CSF free or plasma testosterone concentrations from the overall population of subjects that we captured previously (Higley et al. 1992; Mehlman et al. 1994). The 5 subjects who were randomly captured by darting had similar CSF free and plasma testosterone and CSF 5-HIAA concentrations when compared with the remaining 17 subjects.

Physiological Measures

All samples were obtained between 0800 and 1600 hours. To obtain the samples, each subject was anesthetized using ketamine hydrochloride (10 mg/kg, IM), and weighed on a commercial scale (± 0.25 kg); the CSF samples were drawn immediately thereafter. Two milliliters of CSF were obtained from the cisterna magna of each subject using a 22-gauge needle and a 5-cc syringe, gently vortexed to assure complete mixing, and aliquoted into two 1-mL samples. The samples were immediately placed on dry ice. Blood samples were simultaneously obtained, immediately centrifuged, and the plasma was placed on dry ice and stored for subsequent assay. Both the CSF and plasma samples were stored at $-80°C$. One of each subject's CSF samples was assayed for HVA and 5-HIAA, using high-performance liquid chromatography with electrochemical detection according to the method of Scheinin et al. (Scheinin et al. 1983). The second 1-mL aliquot of CSF and the plasma were assayed for testosterone using a radioimmunoassay procedure (Rahe et al. 1990). All intra- and interassay coefficients of variation were less than 10%. The monoamine metabolite concentrations are reported in picomoles per milliliter, and the plasma and CSF free testosterone concentrations are reported in micrograms and nanograms per deciliter, respectively. To control for possible confounds on CSF and plasma concentrations, records were kept of: 1) the elapsed minutes from when the technician initially entered the corral until the CSF was obtained; 2) time of day when sample was obtained; and 3) day of the week when each sample was obtained.

Behavioral Observations

After capture and sampling, each subject was fitted with a radio transmitter collar emitting a unique frequency. Subjects were then released with other members of their group within their home range area. Thereafter, subjects were located in the field by a radio telemetry receiver and observed visually, either aided or unaided by binoculars depending on the distance from the observer. Behavioral observations were conducted from 1 June to the end of August, 1992 by one observer who was trained by the second author (PTM). The data collected in 1991 were collected during the same seasonal period by PTM and an observer that was not present in 1992. The second observer in 1991 was also trained by PTM. As in 1991, assessment of the 1992 interrater reliability for overall aggression using Cohen's kappa indicated a consistency .95 or better agreement. Aggression occurred too infrequently to separately assess reliability for the different aggression categories. The behavioral observers were blind to the biochemical data.

Behavioral data were collected on each subject during seven 60-min sessions, randomized for subject order and time of day. The sessions were distributed across the day to represent a daily profile (one session from 0700 to 1000 hours, two sessions from 1000 to 1200 hours, one session from 1200 to 1400 hours, one session from 1400 to 1600 hours, and two sessions from 1600 to 1900 hours). Behavioral categories for agonism (aggression and submission) followed those established for rhesus monkeys and related macaques (Altmann 1962; Mehlman et al. 1994).

Observations of aggression were recorded as frequency data, falling into one of four categories of increasing intensity: 1) displacements, 2) stationary threats, 3) chases, and 4) physical assaults. Displacements were recorded when the subject physically moved toward another monkey and the latter moved from its position (usually occurring in the context of feeding or drinking). Stationary threats included all threat gestures, such as stares, open-mouth threats, head bobs, ground slaps, etc., that were displayed while the subject remained in a stationary position. Chases were recorded when the subject chased another monkey and the other monkey fled (often screaming and exhibiting submissive gestures). Physical assaults were recorded for all contact aggression, i.e., when the subject bit, hit, or slapped another individual. When a sequence of aggressive behaviors was observed (e.g., stationary threat, chase, and then bite) only the most intense aggressive act was recorded (e.g., physi-

cal assault). To control for rate of activity and frequency of social encounters, a derived variable, "escalated aggression," was calculated by dividing the total number of chases and physical assaults by the total number of aggressive acts (1–4 above). For any subject, the escalated aggression score therefore represented the proportion of aggressive acts that escalated into the two most intense forms of aggression. Receiving aggressive acts were also recorded (received aggression), using the same scale. Observations of submissive behavior were recorded as frequency data, categorized as: 1) displaced and/or avoid, 2) flee and/or receive contact aggression, 3) bared teeth "fear" grimace, or 4) freeze-crouch. Social dominance was measured by measuring the direction of male–male mounting. Mounting of other males was recorded as either nonsexual (no thrusting or anal penetration) or sexual (thrusting, penetration, or ejaculation).

Unprovoked leaping behavior was scored as frequency data, falling into one of three categories of increasing danger: 1) short leaps, 2) medium leaps, and 3) long leaps. Only those leaps occurring at a height of 7 meters or greater were scored (judged to be high enough to be potentially harmful if a fall occurred). Leaps were only scored if they were unprovoked, and not part of a social or aggressive sequence. Leaps estimated to traverse less than 1 m of open space were scored as short. Leaps between 1 and less than 3 m were scored as medium and leaps of greater than 3 m were scored as long. Because the overall rate of activity could influence the rate of leaping and thus the raw frequency of long leaps, a derived variable, "% long leaps—long leap ratio," was calculated by dividing the total number of long leaps by the total number of all leaps; it therefore represents the proportion of overall leaping that could be considered the most dangerous to the subject. Thus, the two dependent variables used to measure leaping were long leap ratio and other leap ratio (short + medium leaps divided by total leaps).

Data Analyses

In 1992, we were unable to obtain valid monoamine metabolite concentrations from 3 of the 24 subjects due to technical problems; CSF free testosterone was obtained from all 24 subjects. Testosterone and each of the monoamine metabolites were correlated with the potential confounding variables: time of day, day of week, time from entering corral to obtain sample, months of age, and weight, using Pearson's product-moment correlations. None of the biological variables were correlated with the time of day when the sample was obtained, day of the week when sample was obtained, or elapsed time between start of capture process and when sample was obtained. Only age and weight (estimates of developmental status) demonstrated any correlation with some of the biochemical analyses and behaviors. Because age and weight were highly correlated ($r = .81$, $p < .0001$, df = 1/23), and both were correlated with the same dependent variables, age was used as an independent variable to represent developmental status. Multiple regression was used when developmental status was correlated with the biochemical analyses and behaviors. The confounding variable (age) was entered into the multiple regression first and we report the partial correlation with its associated adjusted degrees of freedom. When analyzing the correlation between the biochemical and behavioral variables, if there were no significant relationships with age, weight, or the other confounds, univariate Pearson's product-moment correlations were used.

To code the data to perform dimensional analyses of the behaviors, the subjects were assigned to one of four categories: 1. low CSF 5-HIAA/low CSF testosterone; 2. low CSF 5-HIAA/high CSF testosterone; 3. high CSF 5-HIAA/low CSF testosterone; and 4. high CSF 5-HIAA/high CSF testosterone, with the a priori criterion for statistical comparisons that each category must have at least 4 subjects. These categories were made by first performing a median split of the CSF 5-

HIAA and then CSF testosterone and coding each half of the split as high or low. The high–low codings from each subject for 5-HIAA and testosterone were then combined to produce categories of high/high, high/low, low/high, and low/low. Because CSF testosterone was correlated with age, before performing the median splits age was first factored out of CSF testosterone using multiple regression, and the residuals were then used to perform the codings. The initial splits produced only 3 subjects with low CSF 5-HIAA and low CSF testosterone. To assure at least 4 subjects in each cell, the split was modified to include the next lowest CSF 5-HIAA subject whose testosterone value was also low. This produced a sample subset of $n = 4$ subjects with low CSF 5-HIAA/low CSF testosterone; $n = 7$ subjects with low CSF 5-HIAA/high CSF testosterone; $n = 5$ subjects with high CSF 5-HIAA/low CSF testosterone; and $n = 5$ subjects with high CSF 5-HIAA/high CSF testosterone. Table 65.1 gives the means/SDS and mean ranks for CSF 5-HIAA and CSF testosterone for each category. These four dimensional categories were then used as independent variables to code the data, and between-group univariate analyses of variance (ANOVAs) were used to perform the analyses. Where the data structure violated the ANOVA requirement of homogenous variances, Kruskal–Wallis nonparametric tests were used. To assess developmental changes in means between 1991 and 1992, a repeated measures ANOVA was employed.

Results

Relationships between Age/Weight and CSF Free and Plasma Testosterone and Monoamine Metabolites

The descriptive statistics for each variable can be found in Table 65.2. CSF free and plasma testosterone and HVA were both correlated with age (CSF testosterone: $r = .59$, $p < .003$, df =

Table 65.1

Means and SD for the dimensional codings of CSF 5-HIAA and testosterone

	CSF 5-HIAA			CSF testosterone		
Dimensional category	Dimensional mean $\pm$ SD	Mean dimensional rank for testosterone	Dimensional mean $\pm$ SD	Mean dimensional rank for testosterone	Mean $\pm$ SD (age-residualized)
Low CSF 5-HIAA/ low CSF testosterone	170.4 ± 37.2	5.8	72.9 ± 51.9	7.3	-24.5 ± 25.7
Low CSF 5-HIAA/ high CSF testosterone	182.7 ± 25.4	6.9	131.6 ± 96.9	15.4	44.1 ± 83.2
High CSF 5-HIAA/ low CSF testosterone	233.7 ± 18.8	17.0	63.6 ± 23.8	4.4	-42.2 ± 15.9
High CSF 5-HIAA/ high CSF testosterone	227.8 ± 26.0	15.0	78.0 ± 32.9	14.4	11.2 ± 20.6

Because the variances were nonhomogeneous, the mean for each dimensional rank is also given for both 5-hydroxyindoleacetic acid (5-HIAA) and testosterone. To calculate mean dimensional ranks, subjects were ranked from the highest to the lowest concentration for each biochemical and the mean biochemical rank was then calculated for each of the four dimensional categories. Because cerebrospinal fluid (CSF) testosterone was correlated with age, and the dimensional categories used the age-residualized CSF testosterone values, a third column showing the mean age-residualized CSF testosterone values and SDs is included. Four categories, each based on the combined median splits of CSF 5-HIAA and age-controlled testosterone, are shown (see data analyses for explanation).

$1/23$; plasma testosterone: $r = .52$, $p < .01$, df $= 1/23$; HVA: $r = -.55$, $p < .008$, df $= 1/20$). CSF 5-HIAA was not correlated with any of the confounding variables. There were no other significant correlations between the biochemicals and day of week, time of day, time to obtain sample, or any of the other confounding variables.

Relationships between CSF Free and Plasma Testosterone and Monoamine Metabolite Concentrations

CSF free and plasma testosterone were positively correlated ($r = .63$, $p < .002$, df $= 1/23$). When age was statistically controlled, CSF free and plasma testosterone were not correlated with either of the monoamine metabolites (HVA: $r = -.07$, $p > .75$, df $= 2/20$; 5-HIAA: $r = -.21$, $p > .33$, df $= 2/20$). With age statistically

controlled, there was a significant correlation between HVA and 5-HIAA ($r = .64$, $p = .004$, df $= 2/20$).

Relationships between Behaviors and CSF Free Testosterone Concentration

With age statistically controlled, CSF free testosterone was positively correlated with overall aggression ($r = .61$, $p = 0.01$, df $= 2/23$), and total received aggression ($r = .44$, $p = 0.04$, df $= 2/23$), and total leaping ($r = .51$, $p < .02$, df $= 2/23$) (Table 65.3). Total submissive behaviors were positively correlated with CSF free testosterone ($r = .55$, $p < .05$, df $= 2/23$). The total submissive behaviors–CSF free testosterone correlation did not remain significant, however, when 2 outliers whose values were more than 2 SD from the rest of the subjects were removed. With age controlled, CSF testosterone was

Table 65.2
Descriptive statistics for each variable

	Biological variables					
	Age	Weight	CSF testosterone	CSF HVA	CSF 5-HIAA	Plasma testosterone
Mean	46.4	7.0	79.3	1467.4	212.7	84.9
SD	9.1	1.7	52.0	318.2	47.2	116.6
n	24	24	24	21	21	24

	Leaping				
	Short leaps	Medium leaps	Long leaps	Total leaps	Long leap ratio
Mean	13.9	22.3	13.9	46.9	.23
SD	7.0	12.9	14.4	22.1	.17
n	24	24	24	24	24

	Agonism				
	Overall aggression	Escalated aggression	Nonescalated aggression	Received aggression	Submissiveness
Mean	25.4	9.9	73.9	3.5	2.6
SD	14.8	8.6	16.4	4.2	3.2
n	24	24	24	24	24

	Male mounting		
	Nonsexual	Sexual	Number of thrusts
Mean	.21	2.4	4.7
SD	.42	1.9	2.0
n	24	24	24

Age is reported in months; weight is in kilograms; cerebrospinal fluid (CSF) monoamine metabolites are reported in picomoles per milliliter, plasma testosterone in micrograms/100 mL, and CSF free testosterone in ng/100 mL. Abbreviations are as follows: 5-HIAA, 5-hydroxyindoleacetic acid; HVA, homovanillic acid; *n*, number of subjects sampled. Long leap ratio is calculated by dividing long leaps by total leaps.

Table 65.3
Correlations of CSF free and plasma testosterone and monoamine metabolites, weight, and age with behaviors recorded in the field

	Age	Weight	CSF testosterone (age-controlled)	CSF HVA (age-controlled)	CSF 5-HIAA	Plasma testosterone
Total aggression (r)	−.07	.14	.63[a]	−.15	−.37	−.09
Probability	.73	.52	.02[a]	.61	.11	.73
df	1/23	1/23	2/23	2/20	1/20	2/23
Escalated aggression (r)	−.16	−.10	−.21	.11	−.66[a]	−.01
Probability	.46	.63	.43	.72	.009	.97
df	1/23	1/23	2/23	2/20	1/20	2/23
Total received aggression (r)	−.46[a]	−.40[a]	.60[a]	.09	−.07	.28
Probability	.03[a]	.05[a]	.008[a]	.84	.97	.22
df	1/23[a]	1/23[a]	2/23[a]	2/20	1/20	2/23
Total submission (r)	−.61[a]	−.48[a]	.39	.07	−.14	.31
Probability	.002[a]	.02[a]	.06	.91	.56	.11
df	1/23	1/23	2/23	2/20	1/20	1/23
Other leaps (r)	−.13	−.12	.41	−.36	−.35	−.09
Probability	.53	.58	.15	.18	.22	.74
df	1/23	1/23	2/23	2/20	1/20	2/23
Long leap ratio (r)	.12	.20	−.22	−.07	−.44[a]	.09
Probability	.57	.35	.40	.91	.05[a]	.73
df	1/23	1/23	2/23	2/20	1/20	2/23
Nonsexual mounts (r)	.04	.06	.67[a]	−.17	.11[a]	−.10
Probability	.84	.78	.003[a]	.57	.64[a]	.70
df	1/23	1/23	2/23[a]	2/20	1/20[a]	2/23
Sexual mounts (r)	.21	.07	.04	−.43	−.48[a]	−.44
Probability	.33	.76	.87	.11	.03[a]	.08
df	1/23	1/23	2/23	2/20	1/20[a]	2/23
Mean number of thrusts per sexual mount (r)	.20	.29	.25	.21	−.38	.20
Probability	.34	.17	.31	.43	.09	.40
df	1/23	1/23	2/23	2/20	1/20	2/23

The reported correlations are Pearson's product–moment correlation coefficients or partial correlations with age as the first factor in a multiple regression. All plasma hormones and monoamines that showed significant correlations with weight and age (Table 65.2) had the effects statistically partialled out entering age as an independent variable along with the variable to be correlated (e.g., age was partialled out of "total submission" before the latter was tested with the hormones and monoamine metabolites). Abbreviations: CSF, cerebrospinal fluid; HVA, homovanillic acid; 5-HIAA, 5-hydroxyindoleacetic acid.
a. Significant correlations ($p \leq .05$). Nonsignificant trends are noted by probability levels ($p \leq .10$).

correlated with nonsexual mounting ($r = .64$, $p < .03$, df $= 2/23$). Escalated aggression and long leap ratio were not correlated with CSF free testosterone ($p > .40$, df $= 2/23$). Although there were positive trends, when age was statistically controlled, plasma testosterone was not significantly correlated with any of the aggressive behaviors ($p > .20$).

Relationships between Behaviors and Monoamine Metabolite Concentrations

CSF 5-HIAA was negatively correlated with escalated aggression ($r = -.66$, $p = 0.007$, df $= 1/20$; see Figure 65.1), and long leap ratio ($r = -.44$, $p = 0.04$, df $1/20$; see Figure 65.2). With age controlled, CSF 5-HIAA was negatively correlated with sexual mounts of other males ($r = -.48$, $p < .03$), and it was weakly correlated with the number of thrusts while mounting ($r = -.38$, $p < .09$). It was not correlated with nonsexual mounts ($p > .60$). CSF 5-HIAA and CSF HVA were not correlated with any of the other behaviors.

Analyses of Behaviors by CSF Testosterone and Monoamine Metabolite Quartiles

Exhibit Aggression
There were significant effects for the parametric and Kruskal–Wallis' ANOVAs for the individual aggression categories threats ($F = 4.03$, df $= 3$, 20; $p < .03$), chases ($F = 14.34$, df $= 3$, 20; $p < .0001$), and assaults ($F = 10.71$, df $= 3$, 20; $p < .02$) (Table 65.4). The ANOVAs were also significant for the derived categories escalated aggression ($F = 13.78$, df $= 3$, 20; $p < .0001$; see Figure 65.3) and total aggression ($F = 4.78$, df $= 3$, 20; $p < .02$). Further analysis of the significant ANOVAs for threats, chases, and assaults showed that subjects having the combinations of low CSF 5-HIAA and high CSF testosterone generally engaged in more of each type of aggression than subjects with high CSF 5-HIAA and high CSF testosterone ($p < .05$). Subjects

with low CSF 5-HIAA and high CSF testosterone engaged in more chases and assaults than subjects with low CSF 5-HIAA and low CSF testosterone, and rates of each of the above forms of aggression in low CSF 5-HIAA subjects were unaffected by testosterone. Similarly, although rates of bites were too infrequent to perform formal statistics, no subject with high CSF 5-HIAA bit another animal. Also, rates of biting were twice as high in subjects with the combination of low CSF 5-HIAA and high CSF testosterone than in subjects with low CSF 5-HIAA and low CSF testosterone. Further analysis of total aggression showed a pattern similar to threats. Subjects having the combination of low CSF 5-HIAA and high CSF testosterone exhibited higher rates of total aggression than subjects with high CSF 5-HIAA from either the low- or high-testosterone categories (see Figure 65.3). Further analysis of escalated aggression showed that subjects with low CSF 5-HIAA engaged in higher rates of escalated aggression than subjects with high CSF 5-HIAA ($p < .05$). CSF testosterone, on the other hand, was unrelated to rates of escalated aggression.

Receive Aggression
When age was controlled, there was a statistically significant ANOVA for receive threats ($F = 4.73$, df $= 3$, 20; $p < .02$), and a significant Kruskal–Wallis for receive aggressive chases ($F = 3.11$, df $= 3$, 20; $p = .05$). Further analysis showed that subjects with low CSF 5-HIAA received more threats than subjects with high CSF 5-HIAA ($p < .05$), and high testosterone reduced the rate of threats that were received by subjects having low CSF 5-HIAA, although this observation was only of trend level significance ($p < .10$). Similarly, high testosterone reduced the number of chases subjects received, with subjects having low CSF testosterone and low CSF 5-HIAA receiving more chases than subjects with low CSF 5-HIAA and high CSF testosterone ($p < .05$), and only subjects with low CSF testosterone and low CSF 5-HIAA received assaults.

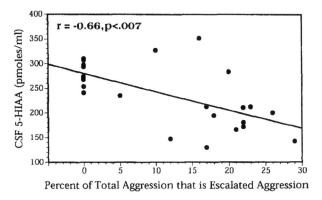

Figure 65.1
Correlation of cerebrospinal fluid (CSF) 5-hydroxyindoleacetic acid (5-HIAA) with escalated aggression (a measure of severe, unprovoked aggression—see text for full definition). CSF 5-HIAA concentrations are reported in picomoles per milliliter. Escalated aggression is reported as a percentage of overall total aggression. The reported correlation is a Pearson's product–moment correlation coefficient.

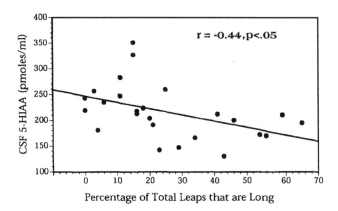

Figure 65.2
Correlation of cerebrospinal fluid (CSF) 5-hydroxyindoleacetic acid (5-HIAA) with long leaps (a measure of impulsivity—see text for full definition). CSF 5-HIAA concentrations are reported in picomoles per milliliter. Long leaps are reported as a percent of total leaps. The reported correlation is a Pearson's product-moment correlation coefficient.

Table 65.4
Means and SD for each of the aggressive, submissive, and leaping behaviors grouped by the CSF 5-HIAA and testosterone dimensional codings

	Low CSF testosterone		High CSF testosterone	
	Low 5-HIAA	High 5-HIAA	Low 5-HIAA	High 5-HIAA
Aggression/social dominance				
Displacements	1.750/2.363	2.20/2.387	2.571/2.76	1.60/1.517
Threats	16.25/6.85	12.20/5.718	24.714/11.8	9.20/3.962
Chases	3.25/2.986	0.0/0.0	6.714/2.628	0.40/0.548
Assaults	0.0/0.0	0.0/0.0	1.143/1.215	0.20/0.447
Bites	0.25/0.5	0.0/0.0	0.571/0.787	0.0/0.0
Total aggression	21.5/12.699	14.40/8.105	35.713/19.19	11.40/6.474
Escalated aggression	0.137/0.108	0.0/0.0	0.213/0.018	0.430/0.072
Nonsexual male–male mounts	0.0/0.0	0.140/0.140	0.130/0.13	0.60/0.60
Receive aggression				
Displaced	0.75/0.957	1.20/1.643	0.571/1.134	2.4/4.827
Receive threats	3.50/2.89	1.20/1.63	2.490/0.78	1.20/2.67
Receive chases	0.75/0.5	0.40/0.894	0.14/0.378	0.40/0.894
Receive assaults	0.25/0.5	0.0/0.0	0.0/0.0	0.0/0.0
Receive total aggression	5.25/9.347	2.80/4.617	3.204/2.292	4.0/8.391
Submission				
Avoiding	2.25/3.30	1.20/1.64	2.14/3.34	2.80/5.17
Lipsmacks	0.0/0.0	0.0/0.0	0.50/0.54	0.20/0.44
Grimaces	0.50/0.51	0.0/0.0	0.30/0.35	1.40/1.51
Crouch	0.25/0.50	0.40/0.89	0.14/0.38	0.18/3.49
Flight	0.50/0.58	0.20/0.45	0.14/0.37	0.20/0.44
Leaping				
Short	14.75/8.098	14.80/7.155	13.714/9.482	18.0/5.612
Medium	30.5/19.018	22.40/9.555	22.714/12.737	26.60/19.424
Long	26.0/23.58	7.00/4.899	25.857/16.181	6.80/8.044
Total leaps	71.25/48.238	44.20/20.548	62.286/30.788	51/40/31.397
Long leap ratio	0.348/0.124	0.139/0.093	0.40/0.217	0.09/0.09

Abbreviations: CSF, cerebrospinal fluid; 5-HIAA, 5-hydroxyindoleacetic acid.

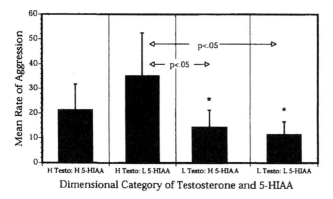

Dimensional Category of Testosterone and 5-HIAA

Figure 65.3
Means and standard deviations for rates of overall aggression categorized by each of the four dimensional codings of high or low cerebrospinal fluid (CSF) testosterone and 5-hydroxyindoleacetic acid (5-HIAA). To code the data for dimensional analyses of the behaviors, the subjects were assigned to one of four categories: 1. low CSF 5-HIAA/ low CSF testosterone; 2. low CSF 5-HIAA/high CSF testosterone; 3. high CSF 5-HIAA/low CSF testosterone; and 4. high CSF 5-HIAA/high CSF testosterone (see text for further explanation). * Significantly different $(P < .05)$ from the group with low CSF 5-HIAA/high CSF testosterone. Low CSF 5-HIAA appeared to augment the effect of high testosterone on overall aggressiveness, with subjects having both high testosterone and low 5-HIAA concentrations exhibiting more overall aggression than subjects from the two categories with low testosterone. Testo, testosterone; L, low; H, high.

Submissive Behaviors

In response to aggression, no subject with low CSF 5-HIAA/high testosterone exhibited submissive or appeasement signals such as lipsmacks $(F = 3.11, df = 3, 20; p = .05)$, and fear grimaces $(F = 3.86, df = 3, 20; p < .03)$.

Other Social Dominance Behaviors

The ANOVA for nonsexual mounting of males was also statistically significant $(F = 8.01, df = 3, 20; p < .05)$. Subjects with high CSF 5-HIAA and high CSF testosterone mounted other males more often than subjects from any other condition. Indeed, subjects with low CSF 5-HIAA and low testosterone never mounted other males (see Table 65.4).

Leaping between Trees

There were significant ANOVAs for age-controlled long leaps $(F = 5.50, df = 3, 20; p < .009)$ and long leap ratio $(F = 5.50, df = 3, 20; $

$p < .009)$. Subjects with low CSF 5-HIAA made more long leaps than subjects with high CSF 5-HIAA $(p < .05)$. For long leap ratio, in all comparisons, subjects with low CSF 5-HIAA had a higher percentage of long leaps $(p < .05)$ than subjects with high CSF 5-HIAA $(p < .05)$. Testosterone was unrelated to long leaps and long leap ratio. ANOVAs for short and medium leaps were not statistically significant.

Relationships between Behaviors

Long leap ratio was significantly correlated with escalated aggression $(r = .48, p = 0.02, df = 1/23)$ (Table 65.5). As might be expected, within behavioral categories there were also significant correlations: overall aggression was correlated with escalated aggression $(r = .45, p = 0.03, df = 1/23)$. With age statistically controlled, total received aggression was positively correlated with total submissive behaviors $(r = .86, p < $

Table 65.5
Correlations between behaviors collected in the field

	Escalated aggression	Total receive aggression	Total submission (weight-controlled)	Other leaps	Long leap ratio	Nonsexual mounts	Sexual mounts
Total aggression (r)	.46[a]	.33	−.02	.03	.65[a]	.35[a]	.64[a]
Probability	.03[a]	.12	.94	.91	.006[a]	.10[a]	.0007[a]
df	1/23	1/23	1/23	1/23	1/23	1/23	1/23[a]
Escalated aggression (r)		.11	.03	.04	.53[a]	.33[a]	.18[a]
Probability		.62	.90	.90	.008[a]	.13[a]	.40[a]
df		1/23	1/23	1/23	1/23	1/23	1/23
Total receive aggression (r)			.81[a]	−.03	.03	.32	.37
Probability			.0001[a]	.91	.88	.13	.08
df			1/23	1/23	1/23	1/23	1/23
Total submission (r)				−.10	−.21	.27	.01
Probability				.65	.33	.21	.98
df				1/23	1/23	1/23	1/23
Other leaps (r)					.02	.31	.27
Probability					.93	.14	.21
df					1/23	1/23	1/23
Nonsexual mounting (r)							.12
Probability							.58
df							1/23

The reported correlations are Pearson's product–moment correlation coefficients.
a. Significant correlations ($p \leq .05$). Nonsignificant trends are noted by probability levels ($p \leq .10$).

.0001, df = 2/23). Overall aggression was also correlated with long leap ratio ($r = .65$, $p < .006$, df = 1/23).

Biochemical Changes between Years

The ANOVAs for plasma and CSF free testosterone were both statistically significant with 1992 plasma concentrations over three times higher and 1992 CSF concentrations four times higher than concentrations in 1991 (plasma: $F = 11.6$, df = 1, 41; $p < .003$; means/SD: 1991, 23.7/10.1 μg/100 mL; 1992, 66.3/86.4 μg/100 mL; CSF: $F = 5.15$, df = 1, 41; $p < .003$; means/SD: 1991, 19.8/16/2 ng/100 mL; 1992, 85.8/66.8 ng/100

mL). The between-year ANOVA for CSF HVA was also statistically significant, with concentrations lower in 1992 than in 1991 ($F = 12.5$, df = 1, 29; $p < .003$; Means/SD: 1991, 1613.0/97.0 pmol/mL; 1992, 1443.2/58/6 pmol/mL). The between-year ANOVA for CSF 5-HIAA was not statistically significant ($p > .9$).

Changes in Behaviors between Years

Of the behaviors, total submissive behaviors and long leap ratio were both statistically different between years. Submissive behaviors decreased with increasing age ($F = 12.5$, df = 1, 29; $p < .003$; total mean frequency/SD: 1991, 17.3/3.2;

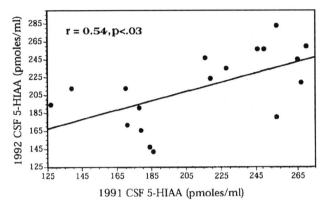

Figure 65.4
Correlation of interindividual differences in cerebrospinal fluid (CSF) 5-hydroxyindoleacetic acid (5-HIAA) between the first and second year of the study. CSF 5-HIAA concentrations are reported in picomoles per milliliter. The reported correlation is a Pearson's product–moment correlation coefficient.

1992, 3.9/1.8, and the percent of leaps that were long and dangerous increased between years ($F = 7.1$, df = 1, 29; $p < .02$; mean percentage/ SD: 1991, 12/03; 1992, 26/05). Total aggression, total leaps, escalated aggression, total receive aggression, and long leap ratios were not significantly different between years ($p > .4$).

Stability of Interindividual Differences between Years

Interindividual differences in CSF 5-HIAA concentrations were stable between 1991 and 1992 samples ($r = .54$, $p < .03$, df = 1/16; see Figure 65.4). With age statistically controlled, HVA was also correlated between years ($r = .62$, $p < .02$, df = 2/16). Between-year correlations for CSF testosterone, plasma testosterone, and each of the behaviors failed to reach a level of statistical significance ($p > .4$).

Discussion

The results of our study provide support for four of the five hypotheses, and partial support for

the hypothesis of stability of interindividual differences across time. These results also replicate our earlier findings (Higley et al. 1992; Mehlman et al. 1994), which showed that monkeys with low CSF 5-HIAA concentrations exhibit increased wounding, high levels of escalated aggression, and increased impulsivity, as measured by dangerous, unprovoked long leaps.

Testosterone and Behavior

In support of our first hypothesis, when testosterone was considered in the absence of CSF 5-HIAA, total rates of aggression and nonsexual male mounting were positively correlated with CSF free testosterone, but they were not correlated with CSF 5-HIAA concentrations. Total aggression included socially assertive behaviors such as displacements, stares, and threats, behaviors which are typically exhibited by animals maintaining or establishing social dominance, and low-intensity aggressive behaviors that have little probability of injury. Social dominance is often seen as a measure of social competence in rhesus monkeys (Higley and Suomi in press). Escalated aggression was not, however, correlated with CSF testosterone. These findings indicate that while subjects with higher than average central testosterone exhibit more aggression, the aggressive encounters are terminated before they escalate into dangerous forms of aggression. These findings are also consistent with Rose and colleagues' (Rose et al. 1971) study of social dominance and aggression in nonhuman primates, where they found that assertive, less violent forms of aggression used to support social dominance were correlated with circulating testosterone, whereas more violent forms of aggression were not. Similarly Rejeski and colleagues (Rejeski et al. 1988, 1990) found that injecting monkeys with testosterone-related anabolic steroids increased aggression more in high than in low dominant monkeys. In addition, although the lower-ranking monkeys increased their aggression, they also showed a concomitant increase in levels of social submission following the injections. Our findings are also consistent with the findings from studies of human aggression and testosterone, where correlations are most frequently found between testosterone and aggression when social status is challenged such as during competitive events (Scaramella and Brown 1978), or in response to provocation or threat (Olweus et al. 1980, 1988). The aggression expressed in these socially acceptable settings is generally restrained and not conducive to physical injuries. Indeed, in his review of testosterone and aggression, Mazur (1983) concludes, "It seems as plausible to link testosterone to dominance behavior (which is often unaggressive in humans) as to aggression per se" (p. 574). In certain population samples, however, CSF testosterone concentrations may be positively correlated or secondarily associated with violence (Virkkunen et al. 1994b). On the other hand, in the same population sample, CSF 5-HIAA was negatively correlated with impulsivity and unprovoked violence (Virkkunen et al. 1994b).

Plasma testosterone was not correlated with any of the aggressive behaviors, whereas CSF free testosterone was correlated with a number of the aggressive behaviors. This finding is consistent with our last hypothesis, that CSF free testosterone would better correlate with aggressive behaviors than plasma testosterone, and suggests that CSF free testosterone is the preferred variable to be used in exploring relationships between testosterone and behavior.

Serotonin and Behavior

In support of our second hypothesis, when CSF 5-HIAA was considered in the absence of CSF free testosterone, impulsivity and persevering in aggression, as measured by long leap ratio and escalated aggression, respectively, were both negatively correlated with CSF 5-HIAA, but not with testosterone, consistent with other studies. For example, Olweus found that aggression in response to threat or provocation was correlated with testosterone; unprovoked aggression was not related to testosterone (Olweus 1986). Our findings are also supportive of our third hypothesis: escalated aggression is related to impaired impulse control. Unprovoked, escalated aggression was strongly correlated with measures associated with impulsivity. When our derived measure of impulsivity, long leap ratio, was correlated with escalated aggression, a strong positive correlation was found. On the other hand, escalated aggression was not correlated with overall leaping, indicating that individuals with increased escalated aggression were not simply more active and thus more likely to engage in a number of behaviors including aggression. There was, however, a positive correlation between overall aggression and the long leap ratio. This is not altogether unexpected, since the overall aggression category includes bites, chases, and other high-risk aggressive acts that comprise the escalated aggression variable, and overall aggression was positively correlated with escalated aggression. Indeed, when behaviors characterizing escalated aggression (i.e., bites, chases, and assaults) were subtracted from overall aggression, there was no longer a significant correlation between aggression and the long leap ratio ($r = .15$, $p > .50$, $n = 20$). These findings suggest that excessive violence may characterize aggressive encounters in monkeys that possess a low threshold to initiate aggression. Once aggression starts, it escalates into severe forms of aggression due to the subjects' perseverance, which is associated with impaired impulse control. They are also consistent with other research showing that impulsive violence, but not overall aggressivity, is correlated with diminished central serotonin functioning (Coccaro et al. 1989; Linnoila et al. 1983). This finding of a correlation between low CSF 5-HIAA and high rates of spontaneous, unprovoked long leaps is also consistent with a growing body of research showing a correlation between impulsivity and diminished central serotonin functioning in adult humans (see for example recent reviews, Coccaro 1992; Csernansky and Sheline 1993; López-Ibor 1991; Stein et al. 1993). Not all studies have found this relationship. For example, in a study of prepubertal human males (Kruesi et al. 1990), impulsivity was not correlated with CSF 5-HIAA. Kruesi, discussing this apparent incongruence with studies in adults, suggested that the range of impulsivity in his subjects was truncated, which may have prevented detecting the relationship between impulsivity and CSF 5-HIAA.

In the present study, CSF 5-HIAA was also positively correlated with sexual mounting of other males, and there was a nearly significant correlation between CSF 5-HIAA and the number of thrusts that males made during a sexual mount. While not part of our hypotheses, this suggests a possible role for serotonin in some forms of sexual behavior, a topic that we are currently investigating.

Dimensional Analyses

Dimensional analyses suggested that the frequency of most aggressive behaviors is highest in subjects characterized by both high CSF testosterone and low 5-HIAA concentrations. This finding might indicate that in general, the effect of low CSF 5-HIAA on most forms of aggression was augmented by high concentrations of CSF testosterone. CSF 5-HIAA concentration was generally inversely correlated to modest or high rates of most forms of aggression, such as rates of threats, chases, assaults, bites, and total aggression. Nevertheless, rates of these behaviors were highest when low CSF 5-HIAA and high CSF testosterone coexisted. Indeed, in the absence of low CSF 5-HIAA and high CSF testosterone, chases, assaults, and bites never occurred. On the other hand, escalated aggression, aggression with a high probability of trauma and injury, was higher in both groups with low CSF 5-HIAA than in groups with high CSF 5-HIAA. CSF testosterone did not affect rates of escalated aggression. Signals of submission typically used to terminate low-level aggression were used more often by males with high CSF 5-HIAA. For example, only males with high CSF 5-HIAA exhibited lipsmacking, and males with high CSF 5-HIAA exhibited more fear grimaces than subjects with low CSF 5-HIAA, although testosterone appeared to augment this later effect. Perhaps this is why subjects with low CSF 5-HIAA and low CSF testosterone were threatened, assaulted, and chased most frequently, i.e., they do not make appropriate social signals to prevent aggression. Testosterone again appeared, however, to mediate some of the effects of low CSF 5-HIAA, with rates of threats and chases less frequent when high concentrations of testosterone were present. It is also noteworthy that there was no correlation between CSF testosterone and CSF 5-HIAA. These findings suggest that serotonin and testosterone have relatively independent influences on aggression and its control.

The presence of both high CSF testosterone and high CSF 5-HIAA appeared to be necessary for high rates of nonsexual male mounting to occur, suggesting that high CSF 5-HIAA and high CSF testosterone increase the probability of high social dominance. Indeed, in the absence of both, male mounting did not occur. These findings are consistent with other studies showing that high central serotonin turnover rate (Higley et al. 1994, in press; Raleigh et al. 1983, 1991; Raleigh and McGuire 1994), and high testosterone (Rose et al. 1971) are correlated with high social dominance ranking. Nevertheless, this is the first study to suggest that the combination of both high CNS serotonin and testosterone is important for at least one measure of social dominance ranking, male mounting. On the other hand, subjects with low CSF 5-HIAA were more likely to make impulsive dangerous leaps, suggesting that the function of serotonin is not limited to the inhibition of aggressive impulses only. In a similar fashion, CSF testosterone did not contribute to impulsive leaps, suggesting that the investigated behaviors, the effect of testosterone is limited to aggressive and competitive motivation.

Continuity of Interindividual Differences

As predicted, interindividual differences in CSF 5-HIAA and HVA were both positively correlated between years. This is to our knowledge the first demonstration that in natural settings, free of the highly controlled laboratory constraints, CSF 5-HIAA and HVA concentrations in nonhuman primates show long-term stability. Although a number of studies have investigated stability of individual differences in infant and prepubescent primates, this is also to our knowledge the first demonstration of temporal stability in CSF 5-HIAA over a long period of time in nonhuman adolescent primates. These findings suggest that for CNS serotonin and dopamine, individuals possess a predictable inherent response bias that may result in differential responses between individuals even when exposed to the same stimuli.

On the other hand, we did not find a correlation between years for testosterone or any of the behaviors. This may have been because some of the subjects migrated to new social groups. Also, unlike our within-year analyses, the sample size of repeatedly sampled subjects was small (only 17 subjects), and both may have impeded our capacity to detect a correlation between years. A second potential reason for our failure to find between-year correlations in testosterone and the behaviors is that with the onset of puberty some of the subjects underwent developmental shifts between the 2 years. Indeed, both plasma and CSF testosterone showed an average three- or fourfold increase, respectively, and on the average, the subjects gained more than one third of their 1991 body weight between two samplings. As Kagan points out in his critique of developmental data analyses (Kagan 1979), to detect individual differences in a developmental phenomenon that matures in a nonlinear fashion, during a hypothetical point in development (such as at puberty), all subjects must be at the same maturational point. During nonlinear developmental changes, detecting continuity between samples may prove problematic because some individuals may be in the early and others may be in the late stages of puberty. In such cases, even with age held statistically constant, intraindividual continuities may be obscured by the maturational changes. It may be that with continued samplings when all subjects reach similar developmental points both CSF free testosterone and aggression may show long-term interindividual stability. Alternatively, Olweus (Olweus et al. 1980, 1988) showed that when studying plasma testosterone, the majority of studies that have demonstrated stable interindividual differences across time obtained multiple samples and used average testosterone concentrations in their correlations. It may be that as with plasma testosterone, for CSF free testosterone multiple sampling is required to adequately elucidate any underlying correlations between behaviors. We are currently obtaining repeated samples from the same individuals to assess this issue.

Conclusion

The present findings suggest that testosterone-mediated aggression may serve functional and possibly positive purposes among healthy non-human primates with normal central serotonin function and that impulsive, dysregulated aggression that escalates to physically damaging proportions is strongly associated with low CSF 5-HIAA. They also suggest that multivariate predictors for identifying a predisposition to violent behaviors should include impulsivity and CSF 5-HIAA, as well as aggressiveness and testosterone. An optimal balance between the two systems is probably needed for a rhesus monkey male to successfully maintain a dominant status in its social group. Our findings also suggest that CSF testosterone, rather than plasma free testosterone, may be the preferred variable in exploring testosterone–aggression relationships. Finally, interindividual differences in the turnover rates of central serotonin and dopamine both show long-term, traitlike interindividual stability.

Acknowledgments

The authors wish to thank Alan Dodson, Beth Fernald, Sue Higley, Ted King, Stephen Lindell, and Scott Cheslak for their help and assistance in data collection and manuscript preparation. The subjects included in this research are part of a breeding colony supported by the Food and Drug Administration; the authors wish to acknowledge FDA contract 223-89-1101 made to Laboratory Animal Breeders and Services, Inc., which supports the colony, and to thank the FDA for its authorization to conduct the research. A research protocol was approved by LABS' Institutional Animal Care and Use Committee, in accordance with and as required by the Animal Welfare Act.

References

Altmann SA (1962): A field study of the sociobiology of rhesus monkeys, *Macaca mulatta. Ann N Y Acad Sci* 102:338–435.

Apter A, van Praag HM, Plutchik R, Sevy S, Kern M, Brown SL (1990): Interrelationships among anxiety, aggression, impulsivity, and mood: A serotonergically linked cluster? *Psychiatry Res* 32:191–199.

Archer J (1991): The influence of testosterone on human aggression. *Br J Psychol* 82:1–28.

Banki CM, Arato M (1983a): Amine metabolites, neuroendocrine findings, and personality dimensions as correlates of suicidal behavior. *Psychiatry Res* 10:253–261.

Banki CM, Arato M (1983b): Relationship between cerebrospinal fluid amine metabolites, neuroendocrine findings and personality dimensions (Marke–Nyman scale factors) in psychiatric patients. *Acta Psychiatr Scand* 67:272–280.

Bertilsson L, Tybring G, Braithwaite R, Träskman-Bendz L, Åsberg M (1982): Urinary excretion of 5-hydroxyindoleacetic acid—No relationship to the level in cerebrospinal fluid. *Acta Psychiatr Scand* 66:190–198.

Booth A, Shelley G, Mazur A, Tharp G, Kittok R (1989): Testosterone, and winning and losing in human competition. *Horm Behav* 23:556–571.

Brown GL, Linnoila MI (1990): CSF serotonin metabolite (5-HIAA) studies in depression, impulsivity, and violence. *J Clin Psychiatry* 51(suppl):31–43.

Brown GL, Goodwin FK, Ballenger JC, Goyer PF, Major LF (1979): Aggression in humans correlates with cerebrospinal fluid amine metabolites. *Psychiatry Res* 1:131–139.

Brown GL, Ebert MH, Goyer PF, et al. (1982): Aggression, suicide, and serotonin: Relationships to CSF amine metabolites. *Am J Psychiatry* 139:741–746.

Buchanan CM, Eccles JS, Becker JB (1992): Are adolescents the victims of raging hormones? Evidence for activational effects of hormones on moods and behavior at adolescence. *Psychol Bull* 111:62–107.

Christiansen K, Knussmann R (1987): Androgen levels and components of aggressive behavior in men. *Horm Behav* 21:170–180.

Cloninger CR (1986): A unified biosocial theory of personality and its role in the development of anxiety states. *Psychiatric Dev* 3:167–226.

Coccaro EF (1989): Central serotonin and impulsive aggression. *Br J Psychiatry Suppl*: 52–62.

Coccaro EF (1992): Impulsive aggression and central serotonergic system function in humans: An example of a dimensional brain-behavior relationship. *Int Clin Psychopharmacol* 7:3–12.

Coccaro EF, Siever LJ, Klar HM, et al. (1989): Serotonergic studies in patients with affective and personality disorders: Correlates with suicidal and impulsive aggressive behavior. *Arch Gen Psychiatry* 46:587–599.

Cohen DJ, Shaywitz BA, Johnson WT, Bowers MD (1974): Biogenic amines in autistic and atypical children. *Arch Gen Psychiatry* 31:845–853.

Csernansky JG, Sheline YI (1993): Abnormalities of serotonin metabolism and nonpsychotic psychiatric disorders. *Ann Clin Psychiatry* 5:275–281.

Dabbs JM (1990): Salivary testosterone measurements: Reliability across hours, days, and weeks. *Physiol Behav* 1:83–86.

Dabbs JM, Frady RL, Carr TS, Besch NF (1987): Saliva testosterone and criminal violence in young adult prison inmates. *Psychosom Med* 49:174–182.

Daitzman RJ, Zuckerman M (1980): Disinhibitory sensation seeking, personality, and gonadal hormones. *Person Individ Diff* 1:103–110.

Ehrenkranz J, Bliss E, Sheard MH (1974): Plasma testosterone: Correlation with aggressive behavior and social dominance in man. *Psychosom Med* 36:469–475.

Eichelman B (1992): Aggressive behavior: From laboratory to clinic *quo vadit? Arch Gen Psychiatry* 49:488–492.

Fishbein DH, Lozovsky D, Jaffe JH (1989): Impulsivity, aggression, and neuroendocrine responses to serotonergic stimulation in substance abusers. *Biol Psychiatry* 25:1049–1066.

Higley JD, Suomi SJ (1996): Effect of reactivity and social competence on individual responses to severe stress in children: Investigations using nonhuman primates. In Pfeffer CR (ed), *Severe Stress and Mental Disturbance in Children*. Washington, DC: American Psychiatric Press, pp. 3–58.

Higley JD, Mehlman P, Taub D, et al. (1992): Cerebrospinal fluid monoamine and adrenal correlates of aggression in free-ranging rhesus monkeys. *Arch Gen Psychiatry* 49:436–441.

Higley JD, Linnoila M, Suomi SJ (1994): Ethological contributions: Experiential and genetic contributions to the expression and inhibition of aggression in primates. In Hersen M, Ammerman RT, Sisson L (eds), *Handbook of Aggressive and Destructive Behavior in Psychiatric Patients*. New York: Plenum Press, pp 17–32.

Higley JD, King ST, Hasert MF, Champoux M, Suomi SJ, Linnoila M (1996): Stability of interindividual differences in serotonin function and its relationship to aggressive wounding and competent social behavior in rhesus macaque females. *Neuropsychopharmacology* 14:67–76.

Kagan J (1979): The form of early development. Continuity and discontinuity in emergent competences. *Arch Gen Psychiatry* 36:1047–1054.

Kraemer GW, McKinney WT (1979): Interactions of pharmacological agents which alter biogenic amine metabolism and depression—An analysis of contributing factors within a primate model of depression. *J Affect Disord* 1:33–54.

Kruesi MJ, Rapoport JL, Hamburger S, et al. (1990): Cerebrospinal fluid monoamine metabolites, aggression, and impulsivity in disruptive behavior disorders of children and adolescents. *Arch Gen Psychiatry* 47:419–426.

Kruesi MJ, Hibbs ED, Zahn TP, et al. (1992): A 2-year prospective follow-up study of children and adolescents with disruptive behavior disorders. Prediction by cerebrospinal fluid 5-hydroxyindoleacetic acid, homovanillic acid, and autonomic measures. *Arch Gen Psychiatry* 49:429–435.

Lidberg L, Tuck JR, Åsberg M, Scalia-Tomba GP, Bertilsson L (1985): Homicide, suicide and CSF 5-HIAA. *Acta Psychiatr Scand* 71:230–236.

Limson R, Goldman D, Roy A, et al. (1991): Personality and cerebrospinal fluid monoamine metabolites in alcoholics and controls. *Arch Gen Psychiatry* 48:437–441.

Lindman R, Järvinen P, Vidjeskog J (1987): Verbal interactions of aggressively and nonaggressively predisposed males in a drinking situation. *Aggress Behav* 13:187–196.

Linnoila M, Virkkunen M, Scheinin M, Nuutila A, Rimon R, Goodwin FK (1983): Low cerebrospinal fluid 5-hydroxyindoleacetic acid concentration differentiates impulsive from nonimpulsive violent behavior. *Life Sci* 33:2609–2614.

Linnoila M, DeJong J, Virkkunen M (1989): Monoamines, glucose metabolism, and impulse control. *Psychopharmacol Bull* 25:404–406.

López-Ibor JJ (1991): The functional approach of biological research in psychiatry. *Acta Neurochir Suppl (Wien)* 52:149–153.

Mattsson A, Schalling D, Olweus D, Löw H, Svensson J (1980): Plasma testosterone, aggressive behavior, and personality dimensions in young male delinquents. *J Am Acad Child Psychiatry* 19:476–490.

Mazur A (1983): Hormones, aggression, and dominance in humans. In Svare BB (ed), *Hormones and Aggressive Behavior*. New York: Plenum Press, pp 563–576.

Mehlman PT, Higley JD, Faucher I, et al. (1994): Low CSF 5-HIAA concentrations and severe aggression and impaired impulse control in nonhuman primates, *Am J Psychiatry* 151:1485–1491.

Mehlman P, Higley JD, Faucher I, et al. (1995): Correlation of CSF 5-HIAA concentrations with sociality and the timing of emigration in free-ranging primates. *Am J Psychiatry* 152:907–913.

Moss HB, Yao JK, Panzak GL (1990): Serotonergic responsivity and behavioral dimensions in antisocial personality disorder with substance abuse. *Biol Psychiatry* 28:325–338.

Olweus D (1984): Development of stable aggressive reaction patterns in males. *Adv Study Aggress* 1:103–137.

Olweus D (1986): Aggression and hormones: Behavioral relationship with testosterone and adrenaline. In Olweus D, Block J, Radke-Yarrow M (eds), *Development of Antisocial and Prosocial Behavior*. New York: Academic Press, pp 51–72.

Olweus D, Mattsson A, Schalling D, Löw H (1980): Testosterone, aggression, physical, and personality dimensions in normal adolescent males. *Psychosom Med* 42:253–269.

Olweus D, Mattsson A, Schalling D, Löw H (1988): Circulating testosterone levels and aggression in adolescent males: A causal analysis. *Psychosom Med* 50:261–272.

Pardridge WM (1986): Serum bioavailability of sex steroid hormones. *Clin Endocrinol Metab* 15:259–278.

Rahe RH, Karson S, Howard NS, Rubin RT, Poland RE (1990): Psychological and physiological assessments on American hostages freed from captivity in Iran. *Psychosom Med* 52:1–16.

Raleigh MJ, McGuire MT (1994): Serotonin, aggression, and violence in vervet monkeys. In Masters RD, McGuire MT (eds), *The Neurotransmitter Revolution*. Carbondale, IL: Southern Illinois University Press, pp 129–145.

Raleigh MJ, Brammer GL, McGuire MT (1983): Male dominance, serotonergic systems, and the behavioral and physiological effects of drugs in vervet monkeys (*Cercopithecus aethiops sabaeus*). In Miczek KA (ed), *Ethopharmacology: Primate Models of Neuropsychiatric Disorders*. New York: Liss, pp 185–197.

Raleigh MJ, McGuire MT, Brammer GL, Pollack DB, Yuwiler A (1991): Serotonergic mechanisms promote dominance acquisition in adult male vervet monkeys. *Brain Res* 559:181–190.

Rejeski WJ, Brubaker PH, Herb RA, Kaplan JR, Koritnik D (1988): Anabolic steroids and aggressive behavior in cynomolgus monkeys. *J Behav Med* 11:95–105.

Rejeski WJ, Gregg E, Kaplan JR, Manuck SB (1990): Anabolic-androgenic steroids: Effects on social behavior and baseline heart rate. *Health Psychol* 9:774–791.

Richards SM (1974): The concept of dominance and methods of assessment. *Anim Behav* 22:914–930.

Riddle MA, Anderson GM, McIntosh S, Harcherik DF, Shaywitz BA, Cohen DJ (1986): Cerebrospinal fluid monoamine precursor and metabolic levels in children treated for leukemia: Age and sex effects and individual variability. *Biol Psychiatry* 21:69–83.

Rose RM, Holaday JW, Bernstein IS (1971): Plasma testosterone, dominance rank and aggressive behaviour in male rhesus monkeys. *Nature* 231:366–368.

Roy A, Adinoff B, Linnoila M (1988): Acting out hostility in normal volunteers: Negative correlation with levels of 5HIAA in cerebrospinal fluid. *Psychiatry Res* 24:187–194.

Sannikka E, Terho P, Suominen J, Santti R (1983): Testosterone concentrations in human seminal plasma and saliva and its correlation with non-protein-bound and total testosterone levels in serum. *Int J Androl* 6:319–330.

Scaramella TJ, Brown WA (1978): Serum testosterone and aggressiveness in hockey players. *Psychosom Med* 40:262–265.

Scheinin M, Chang WH, Kirk KL, Linnoila M (1983): Simultaneous determination of 3-methoxy-4-hydroxyphenylglycol, 5-hydroxyindoleacetic acid, and homovanillic acid in cerebrospinal fluid with high-performance liquid chromatography using electrochemical detection. *Anal Biochem* 131:246–253.

Soubrié P (1986): Reconciling the role of central serotonin neurons in human and animal behavior. *Behav Brain Sci* 9:319–364.

Stein DJ, Hollander E, Liebowitz MR (1993): Neurobiology of impulsivity and the impulse control disorders. *J Neuropsychiatry Clin Neurosci* 5:9–17.

Träskman-Bendz L, Åsberg M, Bertilsson L, Thoren P (1984): CSF monoamine metabolites of depressed patients during illness and other recovery. *Acta Psychiatr Scand* 69(Suppl):333–342.

Virkkunen M, De Jong J, Bartko J, et al. (1989): Relationship of psychobiological variables to recidivism in violent offenders and impulsive fire setters. A follow-up study. *Arch Gen Psychiatry* 46:600–603.

Virkkunen M, Kallio E, Rawlings R, et al. (1994a): Personality profiles and state aggressiveness in Finnish alcoholic, violent offenders, fire setters, and healthy volunteers. *Arch Gen Psychiatry* 51:28–33.

Virkkunen M, Rawlings R, Tokola R, et al. (1994b): CSF biochemistries, glucose metabolism, and diurnal activity rhythms in alcoholic, violent offenders, fire setters, and healthy volunteers. *Arch Gen Psychiatry* 51:20–27.

66 Reduced Prefrontal Gray Matter Volume and Reduced Autonomic Activity in Antisocial Personality Disorder

Adrian Raine, Todd Lencz, Susan Bihrle, Lori LaCasse, and Patrick Colletti

Brain imaging research on antisocial, violent offenders is beginning to reveal potentially important functional abnormalities in these subjects. Ranging from small pilot studies of 4 cases[1] to group studies of more than 40 cases,[2] there is increasing evidence that poor prefrontal functioning is a characteristic of violent, antisocial persons as indicated by both positron emission tomography[3–5] and single-photon emission computed tomography.[6,7] Nevertheless, few if any of these studies control for comorbidity of substance abuse, schizophrenia-spectrum disorders, and other psychiatric comorbidity, and all have been conducted on selected samples derived from psychiatric hospitals, prisons, or forensic settings. Unlike these functional imaging findings, there have been no prior magnetic resonance imaging (MRI) studies of structural brain deficits in antisocial groups, and nothing is known about brain abnormalities in noninstitutionalized violent offenders.

In contrast, studies of patients with neurological disorders have provided provocative insights into which structural brain mechanisms, when damaged, may predispose some persons to irresponsible, antisocial, and psychopathic behavior. Ranging from single case studies[8] to series of neurological patients,[9,10] those who have suffered demonstrable damage to both gray and white matter within the prefrontal region of the brain acquire an antisocial, psychopathic-like personality. These patients also show autonomic arousal and attention deficits to socially meaningful events,[9,11] a finding consistent with the role played by the prefrontal cortex in modulating emotion, arousal, and attention[10,12,13] and with the somatic marker hypothesis that appropriate autonomic functioning is critical to experiencing emotional states that guide prosocial behavior and good decision making.[11] On the other hand, not all persons with prefrontal lesions show antisocial, psychopathic behavior.

While these "acquired sociopaths"[11] provide intriguing links between ostensible brain damage and the onset of antisocial personality disorder (APD), it could be argued that these findings have little relevance to "life-course persistent"[14] offenders in the community who have consistent antisocial behavior throughout their lives, yet have not suffered gross brain damage. It has been speculated that these developmental sociopaths possess much more subtle prefrontal dysfunction than the blunt macroscopic damage in the acquired sociopath,[11] but there have been no tests of this hypothesis. Specifically, it is not known whether (1) antisocial persons in the community have subtle structural deficits to the prefrontal cortex in the absence of discernable lesions; (2) these prefrontal deficits are restricted to gray matter as opposed to white matter; (3) prefrontal structural and autonomic functional deficits are specific to APD as opposed to other forms of psychopathology; (4) autonomic deficits are independent of, or conversely linked to, prefrontal deficits; and (5) prefrontal and autonomic deficits account for variance in antisocial personality over and above that explained by psychosocial risk factors.

This chapter attempts to address these 5 questions by conducting structural MRI on volunteers from the community with APD and by making volumetric assessments of prefrontal gray and white matter. Skin conductance and heart rate activity during a social stressor were also measured to assess whether persons with APD show reduced autonomic activity in a socially meaningful context, and also to assess whether antisocial persons with prefrontal structural deficits are especially characterized by reduced electrodermal activity.[11] In addition, psychosocial and demographic risk factors for violence were measured to assess whether brain and autonomic deficits predict group membership after controlling for these factors.

Box 66.1
Subjects and methods

Subjects

All subjects were drawn from 5 temporary employment agencies in Los Angeles, Calif. This recruitment strategy was used because pilot data had shown that this community group had relatively high rates of violence perpetration.[15] Subject groups were as follows: 21 men with a diagnosis of APD (APD group), 34 men who had neither APD nor alcohol or other drug dependence (control group), and 27 men with substance dependence (substance-dependent group), who had a lifetime diagnosis of drug or alcohol dependence but not APD. Full demographic, cognitive, physical, and criminal measures for the 3 groups are presented in Table 66.1. All subjects who read a description of the study and who wished to participate were included. Subjects were otherwise unselected, with the exception of the following exclusion criteria: age younger than 21 years or older than 45 years, nonfluency in English, history of epilepsy or claustrophobia, use of a pacemaker, and metal implants. In addition, one subject was excluded a priori because brain scanning revealed major atrophy of the right superior temporal gyrus. Full informed, written consent was obtained from all subjects in accordance with institutional review board procedures at the University of Southern California, Los Angeles. Subjects were paid $5.50/h for participation and were informed that the study concerned the biological basis to personality and behavior problems, including criminal behavior.

Because the APD group had comorbid clinical conditions other than alcohol and substance abuse, a psychiatric control group was formed ($n = 21$) by matching the 21 subjects in the APD group with 21 subjects from the control and substance-dependent groups to assess whether brain and psychophysiological differences were an artifact of psychiatric comorbidity. Twenty-one subjects in the psychiatric control group were matched with the 21 subjects in the APD group on schizophrenia-spectrum disorders, affective disorders, anxiety disorders, and other personality disorders that do not fall under the category of APD; results of this matching

are presented in Table 66.2. There were no significant differences between groups using the χ^2 test ($P > .35$ in all cases), with the psychiatric control group having slightly higher rates than the APD group for all diagnoses.

Diagnostic, Cognitive, Physical, and Psychosocial Assessment

All diagnoses were made using *DSM-IV* criteria[16] and ascertained using the Structured Clinical Interview for Axis I *DSM-IV* Disorders[17] and the Structured Clinical Interview for *DSM-IV* Axis II Personality Disorders.[18] Diagnoses were made by research assistants who had participated in a standardized training and quality assurance program for diagnostic assessment.[19] Subjects also completed an alcohol use questionnaire.

Estimated intelligence was based on 5 subtests (vocabulary, arithmetic, digit span, digit symbol, and block design) of the Wechsler Adult Intelligence Scale (Table 66.1).[20] Degree of right vs left hand preference was assessed using the abbreviated Oldfield Inventory (Table 66.1),[21] with high scores indicating a stronger preference for right-handedness. History of head injury was defined as head trauma resulting in hospitalization (Table 66.1). The 10 demographic and psychosocial measures were derived from a structured psychosocial interview with the participant,[15] with social class measured using the Hollingshead classification system.[22] A physical examination was conducted after psychophysiological testing to derive measures of height, weight, and head circumference (Table 66.1). Body mass index (a measure of obesity) was calculated as weight in kilograms divided by the square of height in meters (Table 66.1).

Violence and Assessment of Psychopathy

Perpetration of serious violence was measured using an adult extension of the self-report delinquency measure used in the National Youth Survey (Table 66.1),[15,23] and was defined as acts

Box 66.1

(continued)

that caused bodily injury or trauma or were life-threatening. Eight items fit this definition: history of an attack on a spouse or girlfriend causing bruises or bleeding, attack on relative or friend causing bruises or bleeding, attack on a stranger causing bruises or bleeding, rape, using a weapon in a fight, using force or a weapon to rob, firing a gun at someone, and attempted murder or murder.

To help minimize false negatives (denial of violence by truly violent offenders), a certificate of confidentiality was obtained from the Secretary of Health, Education, and Welfare, Washington, DC, that protected the research investigators under section 303(a) of Public Health Act 42 from being subpoenaed by any federal, state, or local court in the United States to release the self-reported crime data. Consequently, subjects were protected from the possible legal action that could be taken against them for crimes they committed and admitted in the interview, but which were not detected and punished by the criminal justice system.

Psychopathic personality was assessed using the Hare Psychopathy Checklist[24] with collateral interview information from the Interpersonal Measure of Psychopathy[25] and from criminal history transcripts obtained from the Department of Justice. The scale ranges from 0 (low psychopathy) to 40 (high psychopathy).

Psychophysiological Assessment

Heart rate and skin conductance was recorded during a social stressor using a Grass model 7 polygraph with a constant 0.5 V potential across electrodes. Skin conductance was recorded from the distal phalanges of the first and second fingers of the left hand using silver/silver chloride electrodes (1 cm in diameter) (Sensor Medics Corp, Yorba Linda, Calif) and physiological saline (0.9% sodium chloride) in Unibase (Warner Chilcott Laboratories, Morris Plains, NJ) as the electrolyte, with the skin contact area delineated using double-sided adhesive masking tape with a hole 1 cm in diameter. Heart rate was monitored using silver/silver chloride electrodes and a standard lead-I configuration, with conductivity gel (Medi-Trace; Graphic

Control Corp, Buffalo, NY) serving as the electrolyte. During the social stressor, subjects were told to spend 2 minutes preparing a speech about their faults,[26] followed by a 2-minute period in which they gave their speech to the experimenter while being videotaped. Heart rate and skin conductance levels were sampled each minute and averaged across the 4-minute stress paradigm (see below) to create indices of electrodermal and cardiovascular activity.

Magnetic Resonanace Imaging

Structural MRIs were conducted on a scanner (S15/ACS; Phillips, Selton, Conn) with a magnet of 1.5-T field strength. After an initial alignment sequence of 1 midsagittal and 4 parasagittal scans (spin echo T1-weighted image acquisition, $TR = 600$ milliseconds, $TE = 20$ milliseconds) to identify the anterior commissure–posterior commissure plane, 128 three-dimensional T1-weighted gradient-echo coronal images ($TR = 34$ milliseconds; $TE = 12.4$ milliseconds; flip angle, 35°; overcontiguous slices, 1.7 mm; matrix, 256×256; field of view, $= 23$ cm) were obtained in the plane directly orthogonal to the anterior commissure–posterior commissure line.

Three-dimensional brain images were reconstructed using a SPARC workstation and semiautomated software (CAMRA S200 ALLEGRO) used for segmentation of gray matter, white matter, and cerebrospinal fluid. Segmentation of gray and white matter was performed using a thresholding algorithm, with the operator blind to group membership applying a cutoff value to the signal intensity histogram to optimally differentiate white matter from gray matter, areas of which were defined using an automated seeding algorithm on each slice. The left hemisphere (right side) in Figure 66.1 shows the seed volume of interest circumscribing the entire cortex (in yellow), illustrating segmentation of gray matter and cerebrospinal fluid. The right hemisphere (left side) shows the seed volume of interest for the white matter (red border), illustrating segmentation of gray and white matter.

Box 66.1

(continued)

The prefrontal region was defined as all of the cortex anterior to the genu of the corpus callosum, and was divided into left and right hemispheres along the longitudinal fissure (Figure 66.1). Interrater reliability (intraclass correlation coefficient) based on 23 scans (raters blind to each other's ratings and group membership) were as follows: left prefrontal gray matter (0.99), right prefrontal gray matter (0.99), left prefrontal white matter (0.93), right prefrontal white matter (0.94), and total brain volume (0.99).

Statistical Analyses

One-way analysis of variance, χ^2, repeated-measures multivariate analysis of variance, and follow-up t tests were used to assess group differences on antisocial, demographic, MRI, and psychophysiological variables. All tests of significance are 2-tailed with an α level of .05. The procedure used by Rom[27] a sequentially rejective method, was used to correct for type 1 errors in t test comparisons. The repeated-measures analyses of variance used the multivariate approach and were conducted on left and right hemisphere volume measures in a 3 (groups) $\times$ 2 (left and right hemisphere) design for gray and white matter separately. The ability of measures to predict group membership was assessed using logistic regression and the Wald χ^2 statistic by using a classification cutoff of 0.5, and with the Nagelkerke statistic used for variance estimation. Brain and autonomic variables were entered using a stepwise forward procedure (Wald χ^2) with an entry probability of .05 and a removal probability of .10, while all psychosocial risk factors were entered simultaneously in one block, and brain and autonomic variables were entered in a stepwise forward procedure. Effect sizes were calculated using Cohen's d.[28]

Results

Antisocial, Demographic, and Substance Abuse Measures

The APD group reported having committed a greater number of serious violent crimes than both the control group ($\chi^2_1 = 9.3$, $P = .002$) and the substance-dependent group ($\chi^2_1 = 6.4$, $P = .01$) (Table 66.2). Specifically, 52.4% of the persons with APD reported having attacked a stranger and having caused bruises or bleeding, with rates of 42.9% for rape, 38.1% for firing a gun at someone, and 28.6% for attempted or completed homicide. Persons in the APD group were more likely than both those in the control group ($\chi^2 = 18.1$, $P = .0001$) and those in the substance-dependent group ($\chi^2 = 4.5$, $P = .03$) to have been arrested by the police (see Table 66.1). Persons in the APD group also scored 1.4 SDs above the mean of persons in the substance-dependent group on psychopathy ($t_{52} = 8.9$, $P = .0001$), who in turn scored 1.0 SDs higher than the control group ($t_{44} = 4.7$, $P = .0001$) (Table 66.1).

Groups were closely comparable in age, social class, ethnicity, intelligence, handedness, history of head injury, weight, and head circumference ($P > .56$ in all cases; see Table 66.2). As predicted by recent findings on aggressive children,[29] persons in the APD group were significantly taller than those in the control group ($t_{53} = 2.4$, $P = .02$).

Antisocial personality disorder and substance-dependent groups were compared in terms of alcohol and other substance use disorders (sedatives, hypnotics, anxiolytics, cannabis, stimulants, opioids, cocaine, hallucinogens, phencyclidine, polysubstances, and other substances) both in severity (abuse vs dependence) and current usage (Table 66.3). Of 18 χ^2 anal-

Table 66.1
Characteristics of the study groups*

Characteristic	Group			Statistic
	Control ($n = 34$)	Substance-dependent ($n = 26$)	APD ($n = 21$)	
Demographic				
Age, y	30.4 (6.7)	30.2 (6.2)	31.9 (6.8)	$F_{2,78} = 0.5, P = .63$
Social class	35.6 (9.9)	34.2 (11.7)	34.7 (8.9)	$F_{2,78} = 0.1, P = .87$
White race, %	47.1	53.8	38.1	$\chi_2^2 = 1.2, P = .57$
Cognitive and physical				
Full-scale intelligence	100.9 (15.2)	100.0 (19.1)	98.4 (12.8)	$F_{2,78} = 0.2, P = .86$
Handedness†	34.1 (10.0)	32.6 (11.4)	35.4 (9.4)	$F_{2,78} = 0.4, P = .66$
Height, cm	176.4 (7.3)	180.3 (7.8)	181.2 (7.0)	$F_{2,78} = 4.0, P = .02$
Weight, kg	80.1 (13.7)	82.2 (15.5)	83.9 (8.5)	$F_{2,78} = 0.46, P = .64$
Body mass index, kg/m^2	25.7 (4.0)	25.2 (4.0)	25.6 (2.6)	$F_{2,78} = 0.15, P = .86$
Head circumference, cm	146.0 (4.4)	145.9 (4.3)	146.8 (4.1)	$F_{2,78} = 0.2, P = .82$
History of head injury, %	23.5	34.6	23.8	$\chi_2^2 = 4.8, P = .58$
Criminal				
Psychopathy	14.2 (5.5)	20.1 (6.0)	28.5 (5.7)	$F_{2,78} = 38.4, P = .0001$
Serious violent crimes	1.2 (2.2)	1.1 (1.3)	3.9 (3.8)	$\chi_2^2 = 10.8, P = .004‡$
Arrests, %	14.7	40.7	71.4	$\chi_2^2 = 17.9, P = .0001$

* All data are given as mean (SD) unless otherwise indicated. APD indicates antisocial personality disorder.
† High scores indicate greater degree of right-handedness.
‡ Kruskal–Wallis χ^2.

yses, one was marginally significant, with persons in the APD group having rates of cocaine dependence higher than those in the substance-dependent group ($\chi_4^2 = 6.1$, $P = .05$). Groups did not differ in age of onset of drug use (APD group, mean [SD], 16.4 [4.8]; substance-dependent group, 16.6 [3.6]; $t_{45} = 0.2$, $P = .87$).

Antisocial personality disorder and substance-dependent groups were also compared on frequency of alcohol usage, the results of which are given in Table 66.4. Groups did not differ significantly on number of times alcohol was used in the past week and past month, number of drinks taken when drinking, and largest number of drinks taken on one occasion.

MRI Prefrontal Volumes

Persons with APD showed a significant reduction in the volume of prefrontal gray matter, but not white matter (Figure 66.2). A repeated-measures multivariate analysis of variance on gray matter showed a main effect for group ($F_{2,78} = 3.7$, $P = .02$). The APD group had lower prefrontal gray volumes than both the control group ($t_{53} = 2.2$, $P = .03$) and the substance-dependent group ($t_{45} = 2.5$, $P = .009$). In contrast, groups did not differ on white matter prefrontal volume ($F_{2,78} = 1.4$, $P = .25$). There was a main effect of hemisphere on prefrontal gray matter volume ($F_{1,78} = 119.5$, $P = .0001$),

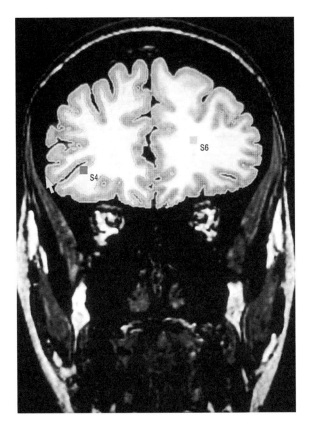

Figure 66.1
Coronal slice of the prefrontal cortex illustrating the seeding program for calculation of gray and white volumes.

indicating increased right relative to left prefrontal gray matter volume, but no group × hemisphere interaction for gray ($F_{2,78} = 1.9$, $P = .16$) or white matter volumes ($F_{2,78} = 1.4$, $P = .26$). The APD group had an 11.0% reduction (9.01 cc) in prefrontal gray matter volume compared with the control group, and a 13.9% reduction (11.9 cc) compared with the substance-dependent group.

When prefrontal gray matter was expressed as a function of whole-brain volume, groups were again found to differ significantly ($F_{2,28} = 4.5$, $P = .01$). Persons with APD had lower mean (SD) prefrontal gray matter to whole-brain ratios (0.075 [.015]) compared with both the control group (0.086 [.012]; $t = 2.6$, $P = .01$) and the substance-dependent group (0.086 [.014]; $t = 2.6$, $P = .01$). Conversely, groups did not differ on prefrontal white matter whole-brain volume ($F_{2,78} = 1.3$, $P = .28$).

Autonomic Activity

Persons with APD also showed reduced autonomic activity during the social stressor (Figure 66.3). An analysis of variance on skin conduc-

Table 66.2
Rates of psychiatric disorder in the APD group and the psychiatric control group, together with χ^2 analyses*

Disorder	Group		χ^2, P
	Psychiatric control ($n = 21$)	APD ($n = 21$)	
Schizophrenia spectrum†	38.1	33.3	$\chi^2_1 = 0.10, P = .74$
Affective‡	52.4	38.1	$\chi^2_1 = 0.87, P = .35$
Anxiety§	23.8	19.0	$\chi^2_1 = 0.14, P = .71$
Other personality disorders‖	33.3	23.8	$\chi^2_1 = 0.46, P = .73$

* APD indicates antisocial personality disorder.
† Includes schizotypal personality, paranoia, schizoid personality, psychosis, and schizophrenia.
‡ Includes major depression, bipolar depression, and other depressive disorders.
§ Includes phobia, panic, and generalized anxiety.
‖ Includes borderline, histrionic, narcissistic, avoidant, dependent, and obsessive-compulsive disorders.

tance showed a main effect for group ($F_{2,78} = 4.6$, $P = .01$), with persons with APD showing lower mean (SD) skin conductance (5.4 [2.5]) compared with both the control group (7.9 [3.4]; $t_{53} = 2.8$, $P = .007$) and the substance-dependent group (7.4 [0.5]; $t_{45} = 2.6$, $P = .01$). Similarly, there was a main effect of group on heart rate levels ($F_{2,78} = 6.8$, $P = .002$). Persons with APD had lower heart rates (69.0 [8.0] beats/min) compared with both the control group (77.6 [8.1] beats/min; $t_{53} = 3.8$, $P = .001$) and with the substance-dependent group (76.8 [9.8] beats/ min; $t_{45} = 3.6$, $P = .004$).

Are autonomic deficits in persons with APD related to their prefrontal gray deficits? Those with APD were divided at the median on prefrontal gray volume to create high (n = 10) or low (n = 11) prefrontal gray matter groups. Means (SD) for low and high prefrontal gray matter groups, respectively, were as follows: skin conductance, 4.2 (2.5) vs 6.6 (2.1) microsiemens; and heart rate, 71.6 (8.2) vs 66.5 (7.4) beats per minute. Compared with persons with APD with high prefrontal gray matter volume, those with APD with low prefrontal gray matter volume had reduced skin conductance activity ($t_{18} = 2.3$, $P = .03$), but not reduced heart rates ($t_{18} = 1.5$,

$P > .16$), indicating that prefrontal gray deficits were linked to electrodermal, but not cardiovascular, deficits within the APD group.

Possible Diagnostic Confounds

Although differences between the APD group and the substance-dependent group indicated that prefrontal and autonomic deficits are not an artifact of comorbidity for alcohol and substance dependence in persons with APD, it is possible that these deficits could be attributed to comorbid affective and schizophrenia-spectrum disorders also present in persons with APD who have been shown to have prefrontal structural deficits.[30-35] This possibility was tested by comparing subjects from the APD group with subjects from the psychiatric control group who were matched for these disorders. Subjects from the APD group had lower mean (SD) prefrontal gray volumes compared with the psychiatric control group (73.51 [17.9] vs 86.19 [12.3] cc, respectively; $F_{1,40} = 7.2$, $P = .01$), lower prefrontal gray matter to whole-brain ratios (0.075 [.015] vs 0.089 [0.011] cc, respectively; $t_{40} = 3.4$, $P = .002$), lower heart rates (69.0 [8.0] vs 77.2 [9.9] beats per minute, respectively; $t = 2.9$, $P = .007$),

Table 66.3
Lifetime rates of substance abuse and other psychiatric disorders in the substance-dependent and APD groups*

| | Group | | |
| | Substance-dependent ($n = 26$) | APD ($n = 21$) | χ^2,† P |
Disorder			
Alcohol use			0.2_4, .90
Abuse	23.1	28.6 ⌐	
Dependence	65.4	61.9	0.05_2, .82
Yes in past month	11.5	9.5 ⌐	
Use of sedatives, hypnotics, and anxiolytics			1.7_4, .42
Abuse	7.7	4.8 ⌐	
Dependence	3.8	14.3	1.3_2, .26
Yes in past month	0.0	4.8 ⌐	
Cannabis use			1.8_4, .41
Abuse	23.1	38.1 ⌐	
Dependence	50.0	47.6	0.11_2, .74
Yes in past month	23.1	19.0 ⌐	
Stimulant use			2.1_4, .35
Abuse	11.5	23.8 ⌐	
Dependence	7.7	14.3	NA
Yes in past month	0.0	0.0 ⌐	
Opioids			1.7_4, .43
Abuse	3.8	4.8 ⌐	
Dependence	3.8	14.3	2.6_2, .11
Yes in past month	0.0	9.5 ⌐	
Cocaine			6.1_4, .05
Abuse	7.7	4.8 ⌐	
Dependence	30.8	66.7	0.02_2, .89
Yes in past month	3.8	4.8 ⌐	
Hallucinogens/PCP			2.71_4, .26
Abuse	23.1	33.3 ⌐	
Dependence	3.8	14.3	1.3_2, .26
Yes in past month	0.0	4.8 ⌐	
Polysubstance use			2.6_4, .27
Abuse	0.0	4.8 ⌐	
Dependence	0.0	4.8	NA
Yes in past month	0.0	0.0 ⌐	

Table 66.3
(continued)

	Group		
Disorder	Substance-dependent ($n = 26$)	APD ($n = 21$)	χ^2,† P
Other			2.0_4, .38
Abuse	3.8	9.5 ⎤	
Dependence	0.0	4.8 ⎟	NA
Yes in past month	0.0	0.0 ⎦	

* APD indicates antisocial personality disorder group; NA, not applicable.
† χ^2 Analyses are conducted on psychiatric disorder categorization and substance use in the past month. Subscript numbers indicate degrees of freedom.

Table 66.4
Comparisons of alcohol use in substance-dependent and APD groups*

	Group		
Alcohol use	Substance-dependent ($n = 26$)	APD ($n = 21$)	t,† P
Times used in past week	1.73 (1.61)	1.76 (2.02)	0.1_{45}, .95
Times used in past month	6.62 (5.55)	7.75 (8.53)	0.5_{45}, .59
No. of drinks when drinking	4.08 (4.11)	3.00 (2.85)	1.0_{45}, .31
Largest no. of drinks on 1 occasion	10.96 (9.94)	6.85 (7.52)	1.5_{45}, .13

* All data are given as mean (SD) unless otherwise indicated. APD indicates antisocial personality disorder.
† Subscript numbers indicates degrees of freedom.

and lower skin conductance (5.44 [2.5] vs 7.46 [2.7] microsiemens, respectively; $t = 2.5$, $P = .022$). Groups did not differ on prefrontal white matter ($F_{1,40} = 0.9$, $P = .34$). The APD group showed a 14.7% reduction (12.7 cc) in prefrontal gray matter volume compared with the psychiatric control group.

Prediction of Group Membership

In a logistic regression in which subjects from the APD group were compared with those from the control group, the 3 prefrontal and autonomic variables (prefrontal gray matter/whole-brain volume, heart rate, and skin conductance) predicted 50.8% of the variance in group membership ($\chi^2_{10} = 25.3$, $P = .005$) and predicted group membership with an accuracy of 76.9%. Similarly, in predicting whether a person would belong to the APD or substance-dependent group, these measures accounted for 50.2% of the variance ($\chi^2 = 21.6$, $P < .001$) and correctly classified 76.1% of group members.

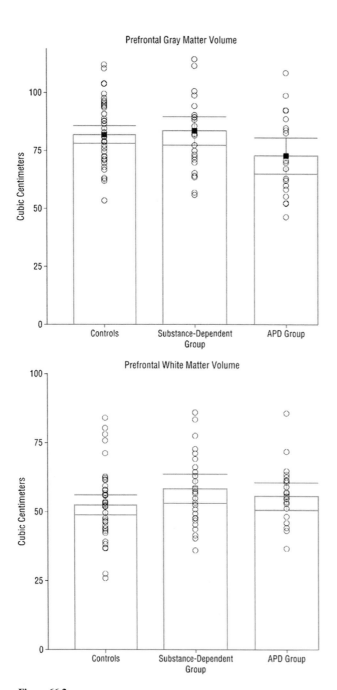

Figure 66.2
Scatterplots, means, and SE bars for volumes of prefrontal gray (top) and white (bottom) matter for subjects in the control group ($n = 34$), substance-dependent group ($n = 26$), and the antisocial personality disorder (APD) group ($n = 21$).

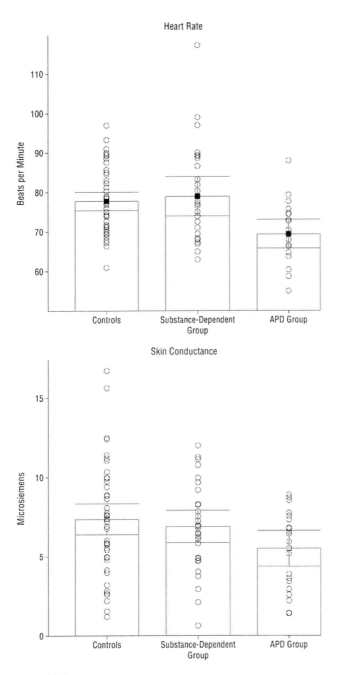

Figure 66.3
Scatterplots, means, and SE bars for heart rate levels and skin conductance during the social stressor for the control group ($n = 34$), the substance-dependent group ($n = 26$), and the antisocial personality disorder (APD) group ($n = 21$).

Independence of Deficits from Height and Psychosocial Factors

The reduction in prefrontal gray in the APD group was not attributable to the significant group difference between the APD and control groups in height, or a combination of minor group differences in physical and cognitive factors including head circumference, history of head injury, and intelligence. After entry of these variables in a single block in a logistic regression comparing the APD group (n = 21) with the control group (n = 34), effects remained significant for prefrontal gray matter/whole-brain volume ($\chi_1^2 = 4.8$, $P = .03$, d = 0.64), heart rate ($\chi_1^2 = 11.1$, $P < .001$, d = 1.04), and skin conductance ($\chi_1^2 = 7.4$, $P = .007$, d = 0.81). Similarly, after controlling for these variables, APD (n = 21) vs substance-dependent (n = 26) group differences remained significant for prefrontal gray matter/whole-brain volume ($\chi^2 = 7.2$, $P = .008$, d = 0.86), heart rate ($\chi^2 = 7.3$, $P = .007$, d = 0.86), and skin conductance ($\chi^2 = 9.1$, $P = .003$, d = 0.99).

Prefrontal and autonomic deficits were independent of psychosocial risk factors in the APD group. This was demonstrated by first entering all 10 demographic and psychosocial risk factors for APD (parental social class, early parental divorce, parental verbal arguments, parental criminality, parental physical fights, family size, physical abuse, sexual abuse, being raised in an institution, and being raised by foster parents) into a logistic regression in a single block, after which APD vs control group differences remained significant for prefrontal gray matter volume ($\chi_1^2 = 5.7$, $P = .02$, d = 0.70), heart rate ($\chi_1^2 = 8.5$, $P = .004$, d = 0.88), and skin conductance ($\chi_1^2 = 4.6$, $P = .04$, d = 0.62). In a similar analysis comparing the APD with the substance-dependent group, effects remained significant for prefrontal gray matter volume ($\chi_1^2 = 6.3$, $P = .02$, d = 0.79), heart rate ($\chi_1^2 = 7.6$, $P = .006$, d = 0.88), and skin conductance ($\chi_1^2 = 4.1$, $P = .05$, d = 0.62) after controlling for psychosocial measures. These analyses indicate that prefrontal and autonomic deficits in persons with APD cannot be attributed to psychosocial risk factors.

The prefrontal and autonomic deficits added substantially to the prediction of APD vs control group membership over and above psychosocial measures. The 10 psychosocial variables in this logistic regression accounted for 41.3% of the variance. After the additional entry of the 3 prefrontal gray matter, heart rate, and skin conductance measures into the regression equation, the amount of group variance explained increased significantly ($\chi_3^2 = 24.4$, $P < .001$) to 76.7%. Prediction of group membership increased from 73.0% correctly classified to 88.5% after including prefrontal and autonomic measures. Similarly, in a comparison of APD vs substance-dependent groups, the psychosocial variables explained 23.8% of the variance, which increased significantly ($\chi_3^2 = 18.3$, $P < .004$) to 60.0% after entry of the 3 prefrontal and autonomic variables, while accuracy of group prediction increased from 71.4% to 82.6%.

References

1. Volkow ND, Tancredi L. Neural substrates of violent behavior: a preliminary study with positron emission tomography. *Br J Psychiatry.* 1987; 151:668–673.

2. Raine A, Buchsbaum MS, La Casse L. Brain abnormalities in murderers indicated by positron emission tomography. *Biol Psychiatry.* 1997; 42:495–508.

3. Goyer PF, Andreason PJ, Semple WE, Clayton AH, King AC, Compton-Totm BA, Schulz SC, Cohen RM. Positron-emission tomography and personality disorders. *Neuropsychopharmacology.* 1994; 10:21–28.

4. Volkow ND, Tancredi LR, Grant C, Gillespie H, Valentine A, Mullani N, Wang GJ, Hollister L. Brain glucose metabolism in violent psychiatric patients: a preliminary study. *Psychiatry Res.* 1995; 61:243–253.

5. Raine A, Meloy JR, Bihrle S, Stoddard J, Lacasse L, Buchsbaum MS. Reduced prefrontal and increased subcortical brain functioning assessed using positron emission tomography in predatory and affective murderers. *Behav Sci Law.* 1998; 16:319–332.

6. Amen DG, Stubblefield M, Carmicheal B, Thisted R. Brain SPECT findings and aggressiveness. *Ann Clin Psychiatry.* 1996; 8:129–137.

7. Kuruoglu AC, Arikan Z, Vural G, Karatas M, Arac M, Isik E. Single photon emission computerised tomography in chronic alcoholism: antisocial personality disorder may be associated with decreased frontal perfusion. *Br J Psychiatry.* 1996; 169:348–354.

8. Damasio H, Grabowski T, Frank R, Galaburda AM, Damasio AR. The return of Phineas Gage: clues about the brain from a skull of a famous patient. *Science.* 1994; 264:1102–1105.

9. Damasio AR, Tranel D, Damasio H. Individuals with psychopathic behavior caused by frontal damage fail to respond autonomically to social stimuli. *Behav Brain Res.* 1990; 41:81–94.

10. Stuss DT, Benson DF. The frontal lobes. New York, NY: Raven Press; 1986.

11. Damasio AR. *Descartes' Error: Emotion, Reason, and the Human Brain.* New York, NY: GP Putnam's Sons; 1994.

12. Davidson RJ. Parsing affective space: perspectives from neuropsychology and psychophysiology. *Neuropsychology.* 1993; 7:464–475.

13. Raine A, Reynolds G, Sheard C. Neuroanatomical mediators of electrodermal activity in normal human subjects: a magnetic resonance imaging study. *Psychophysiology.* 1991; 28:548–555.

14. Moffitt TE. Adolescence-limited and life-course persistent antisocial behavior: a developmental taxonomy. *Psychol Rev.* 1993; 100:674–701.

15. Raine A. Structural and functional brain imaging correlates of violence. Paper presented at: Annual Meeting of the American College of Neuropsychopharmacology; December 8–12, 1997; Walkoloa, Hawaii.

16. American Psychiatric Association. *Diagnostic and Statistical Manual of Mental Disorders, Fourth Edition.* Washington, DC: American Psychiatric Association; 1994.

17. First MB, Spitzer RL, Gibbon M, Williams JBW. *Structured Clinical Interview for Axis I DSM-IV Disorders.* Version 2.0. New York, NY: New York State Psychiatric Institute; 1994.

18. First MB, Spitzer RL, Gibbon M, Williams JBW, Benjamin L. *Structured Clinical Interview for DSM-IV Axis II Personality Disorders.* Version 2.0. New York, NY: New York State Psychiatric Institute; 1994.

19. Ventura J, Liberman RP, Green MF, Shaner A, Mintz J. Training and quality assurance with Structured Clinical Interviews for DSM-IV (SCID-I/P). *Psychiatry Res.* 1998; 79:163–173.

20. Wechsler D. *Wechsler Adult Intelligence Scale: Revised.* San Antonio, Tex: Psychological Corporation; 1981.

21. Bryden MP. Measuring handedness with questionnaires. *Neuropsychologia.* 1977; 15:617–624.

22. Hollingshead AB. *Four Factor Index of Social Status.* New Haven, Conn: Yale University; 1975.

23. Elliott DS, Ageton S, Huizinga D, Knowles B, Canter R. *The Prevalence and Incidence of Delinquent Behavior: 1976–1980 National Youth Survey, Report No. 26.* Boulder, Colo: Behavior Research Institute; 1983.

24. Hare RD. *The Hare Psychopathy Checklist: Revised.* New York, NY: Multi-Health Systems; 1991.

25. Kosson DS, Steuerwald BL, Forth A, Kirkhart KJ. A new method for assessing the interpersonal behavior of psychopathic individuals: preliminary validation studies. *Psychol Assess.* 1997; 9:89–101.

26. Rozanski A, Bairey CN, Krantz DS, Friedman J, Resser KJ, Morell M, Hilton-Chalfen S, Hestrin L, Bietendorf J, Berman DS. Mental stress and the induction of silent myocardial ischemia in patients with coronary artery disease. *N Engl J Med.* 1988; 318:1005–1012.

27. Rom DD. A sequentially rejective test procedure based on a modified Bonferroni inequality. *Biometrika.* 77:663–666.

28. Cohen J. *Statistical Power Analysis for the Behavioral Sciences.* 2nd ed. Hillsdale, NJ: Lawrence Erlbaum; 1988.

29. Raine A, Reynolds C, Venables PH, Mednick SA, Farrington DP. Fearlessness, stimulation-seeking, and large body size at age 3 years as early predispositions to childhood aggression at age 11 years. *Arch Gen Psychiatry.* 1998; 55:745–751.

30. Buchsbaum MS, Bairey CN, Krantz DS, Friedman J, Resser KJ, Morell M, Hilton CS, Hestrin L, Bietendorf J, Berman DS. Ventricular volume and asymmetry in schizotypal personality disorder and schizophrenia assessed with magnetic resonance imaging. *Schizophrenia Res.* 1997; 27:45–53.

31. Raine A, Sheard S, Reynolds GP, Lencz T. Prefrontal structural and functional deficits associated

with individual differences in schizotypal personality. *Schizophrenia Res.* 1992; 7:237–247.

32. Cannon TD. Abnormalities of brain structure and function in schizophrenia: implications for aetiology in pathophysiology. *Ann Med.* 1996; 28:533–539.

33. Gur RE, Cowell P, Turetsky BI, Gallacher F, Cannon T, Bilker W, Gur RC. A follow-up magnetic resonance imaging study of schizophrenia: relationship of neuroanatomical changes to clinical and neurobehavioral measures. *Arch Gen Psychiatry.* 1998; 55:145–152.

34. Siever LJ. Brain structure/function and the dopamine system in schizotypal personality disorder. In: Raine A, Lencz T, Mednick SA, eds. *Schizotypal Personality.* New York, NY: Cambridge University Press; 1995:272–286.

35. Drevets WC, Price JL, Simpson JR, Todd RD. Subgenual prefrontal cortex abnormalities in mood disorders. *Nature.* 1997; 386:824–827.

V BIOLOGY OF SOCIAL RELATIONSHIPS AND INTERPERSONAL PROCESSES

B. Social Applications

v. Individual Differences in Social Behavior

67 Asymmetric Frontal Brain Activity, Cortisol, and Behavior Associated with Fearful Temperament in Rhesus Monkeys

Ned H. Kalin, Christine Larson, Steven E. Shelton, and Richard J. Davidson

Considerable evidence demonstrates that individual differences in temperament are associated with differences in brain and peripheral physiological functioning (e.g., Davidson & Tomarken, 1989; Kagan, Reznick, & Snidman, 1988). Thus, temperament can no longer be viewed simply as a stable trait-like behavioral and emotional style but should be considered as a constellation of stable behavioral, emotional, and physiological characteristics. How these different characteristics interact and the mechanisms underlying the formation of individual differences in temperament are important questions that remain to be answered. To begin to unravel these issues, we have used rhesus monkeys to more completely characterize the physiological concomitants of behavioral responses associated with fearful temperaments. Eventually, this information will guide studies aimed at elucidating the mechanisms underlying the development of individual differences in fear-related temperaments.

Findings from human studies suggest that asymmetric electrical activity of frontal brain regions is associated with different emotional and temperamental styles (see Davidson, 1995, for review). For example, individuals with accentuated activation in right prefrontal regions report more dispositional negative affect (Tomarken, Davidson, Wheeler, & Kinney, 1992) and a larger increase in negative affect in response to negative laboratory eliciters (Wheeler, Davidson, & Tomarken, 1993) compared with individuals displaying left prefrontal activation. Studies in young children demonstrate that the trait of behavioral inhibition, which in its extreme form is thought to be an early marker of fearful temperament, is associated with relative right prefrontal asymmetric brain activation (Davidson, 1992). Other studies have demonstrated that increased sympathoadrenal activity occurs in adults and children with fearful traits. In some, but not all studies, extremely inhibited children have been shown to have increased sympathetic activ-

ity as well as increased levels of the stress-related hormone cortisol (Kagan et al., 1988).

Studies from our laboratory have demonstrated that rhesus monkeys display stable fear-related behaviors that are similar to those observed in humans with fearful temperaments. Using a paradigm that reliably elicits these responses, we have shown an association between individual differences in nonstressed levels of cortisol and extreme behavioral inhibition (Kalin, Shelton, Rickman, & Davidson, 1998). Our studies of asymmetric frontal electrical activity in rhesus monkeys also have demonstrated similarities in this measure between rhesus monkeys and humans. As in humans, rhesus monkeys display asymmetric anterior brain electrical activity. Both monkeys (Davidson, Kalin, & Shelton, 1993) and humans (Tomarken, Davidson, Wheeler, & Doss, 1992) exhibit marked individual differences in the degree of relative right and left frontal electrical activity, which in both species have been demonstrated to be a stable characteristic of an individual. These behavioral and electrophysiological similarities between rhesus monkeys and humans support the feasibility of using rhesus monkeys to understand the behavioral correlates and neurobiological substrates of individual differences in asymmetric frontal activation (Kalin, 1993). We previously demonstrated in monkeys that the anxiolytic benzodiazepine, diazepam, increases relative left frontal electrical activity while decreasing the occurrence of fear-related behaviors (Davidson, Kalin, & Shelton, 1992; Kalin & Shelton, 1989). In addition, diazepam had its greatest effect on shifting frontal activity to the left in monkeys that were dispositionally more fearful (Davidson et al., 1993). This finding suggests the possibility that individual differences in fearful temperament and asymmetric frontal brain electrical activity may be related to asymmetric functioning of endogenous benzodiazepine systems.

In both humans and monkeys, asymmetric brain electrical activity is recorded noninvasively from the scalp surface. The methods used to process the brain electrical activity data are identical in both species. In adult humans, power in the alpha band (8–13 Hz) has been used as the primary dependent measure because it has been shown to vary inversely with cortical activation (e.g., Davidson, Chapman, Chapman, & Henriques, 1990). In our studies with human infants and children (e.g., Davidson & Fox, 1989), we have used power in a theta frequency band (4–8 Hz) in view of the well-known developmental changes in the frequency distribution of the electroencephalogram (e.g., Niedermeyer, 1993). In humans, the frequency of the dominant background rhythm gradually increases until it attains its maximum value (approximately 10 Hz) at about 10 years of age. Similar developmental changes are likely to occur in the brain electrical activity of rhesus monkeys. In previous work, we determined that the peak of the power spectrum in monkeys 1 year of age was between 4 and 8 Hz (Davidson et al., 1992). Accordingly, we used the same frequency band in the present study, given that the age of the monkeys studied was similar to those tested previously (Davidson et al., 1992).

Because both asymmetric frontal electrical activity and cortisol have been independently demonstrated to be associated with a fearful temperamental style, the current study was designed to examine the relation between individual differences in asymmetric frontal electrical activity and circulating levels of cortisol in a large sample of rhesus monkeys. We also studied the extent to which individual differences in these parameters are associated with stable, fear-related behavioral traits. We hypothesized that rhesus monkeys with extreme relative right frontal activity would have higher nonstressed cortisol levels and would be more fearful when compared with monkeys with extreme left frontal activity. The relation between brain electrical measures and cortisol was examined both con-temporaneously as well as predictively. For the latter, we hypothesized that measures of asymmetric prefrontal activation would predict basal cortisol levels when assessed 2 years after the collection of the initial brain electrical data.

Method

Experimental Design

Subjects were 50 rhesus monkeys (*Macaca mulatta;* 29 male, 21 female). All monkeys were maintained on a 12-hr light–dark cycle (lights on 0600 to 1800 hr) at the Wisconsin Regional Primate Center and the Harlow Primate Laboratory (Madison, WI). Animal housing and experimental procedures were in accordance with institutional guidelines.

At 8 months of age, 15 monkeys were manually restrained and the electroencephalogram (EEG) was recorded. Restraint was achieved by holding monkeys on a table in a darkened room. At 1 year of age, EEG measurements were collected from 50 monkeys, which included the 15 monkeys that were assessed at 8 months. In addition, blood was sampled for cortisol and behavior was assessed using the human intruder paradigm (Kalin & Shelton, 1989). Animals received four human intruder tests at weekly intervals, which assessed defensive responses in three different contexts, each lasting 9 min. First, monkeys were separated from their mothers and placed in a cage alone (A), during which animals respond with distress-related coo calls. Next, freezing duration was assessed as elicited by a human entering the room and presenting his or her profile to the monkey, ensuring never to engage the monkey in eye contact (NEC). Finally, defensive aggressive responses, such as barking and hostility, were elicited by having the human stare directly at the animal (ST; Kalin & Shelton, 1989; Kalin, Shelton, & Takahashi, 1991). Behavior and vocalizations were scored from videotapes using a scoring system developed in our laboratory (Kalin & Shelton, 1989). Vocalization data were collected as the frequency of occurrence, and other behavior was scored as duration of occurrence during 9-min periods of either A, NEC, or ST. Based on the EEG data collected from the 50 monkeys at this age, extreme left and right frontal groups and a middle group were selected. Monkeys with EEG asymmetry scores more than .7 standard deviations greater than the mean were classified as extreme left frontals ($n = 12$; 5 males, 7 females), and those with asymmetry scores more than .7 standard deviations less than the mean were classified as right frontal ($n = 11$; 3 males, 8 females). The middle group was formed using $-.35$ standard deviation and .35 standard deviation as the cutoffs ($n = 16$; 8 males, 8 females). These cutpoints are similar to those used in related human research (Tomarken, Davidson, Wheeler, & Kinney, 1992). After selection, the extreme left and right frontal animals were maintained for follow-up at 3 years of age when blood was resampled for cortisol determinations.

EEG Recording and Quantification

Left and right frontal and parietal and mastoid gold-cup electrodes were placed according to the standard 10/20 system. The five active leads (left and right frontal, and parietal and right mastoid) were referenced to the left mastoid, and the linked mastoids were mathematically derived. All electrode impedances were below 5K ohms. We used a mathematically derived averaged mastoid reference rather than a physically linked mastoid reference because of the possible contribution of slight impedance differences between the mastoids affecting the effective spatial location of the reference when they are physically linked. When an averaged mastoid reference is mathematically derived, the data are recorded referenced to a single mastoid. The other mastoid is then recorded as an active channel. In this way, the high input impedance of the amplifiers prevents any slight difference in electrode impedances

from affecting the recorded signal at the scalp surface. This is the preferred method for quantitative EEG analysis when asymmetric effects are the subject of analysis (Pivik et al., 1993). EEG was amplified using Grass Model 12 EEG amplifiers (Grass Instrument Company, Quincy, MA), with a gain of 20,000 and a band-pass filter of 0.1 to 200 Hz. A minimum of 20 artifact-free s of EEG was required per condition, per monkey. There was a mean of 70.95 artifact-free s of EEG per condition.

EEG signals were passed through active anti-aliasing, low-pass filters set at 210 Hz with a 36 dB/octave roll-off. The output of the filters was digitized on-line at 500 Hz with an 80486 PC-clone (Diversified Systems, Madison, WI), equipped with a 12-bit, 32-channel A/D board and signal-acquisition software and stored on magnetic tape cartridges.

All data were edited for artifact on a high-resolution graphics monitor. EEGs from each of the scalp leads during all artifact-free periods were analyzed. Epochs of EEG 2 s in duration were extracted through a Hamming window. A Fast Fourier Transform (FFT) was applied to each chunk of EEG, with epochs overlapping by 50%. The FFT output was in μV^2. Data were aggregated into band power for the 4–8-Hz band and expressed as $\mu V^2/Hz$ based on our previous research with rhesus monkeys (Davidson et al., 1992, 1993). EEG data were log-transformed to normalize the distribution of power values. For each monkey, asymmetry scores were calculated by subtracting the left from the right frontal power. Because power is inversely related to activation, lower asymmetry scores indicated greater relative right frontal activation.

Blood Sampling and Cortisol Radioimmunoassay

Blood was sampled at 1 and 3 years of age. At 1 year, one sample was obtained, whereas at 3 years, two samples were obtained on different days. To control for diurnal variation as well as potential environmental disturbance, all samples were collected during the circadian peak between 0830 and 1030 hr and under nonstressed conditions. Blood was collected (2 ml) by femoral venipuncture into glass tubes containing 4.5 mg ethylenediaminetetraacetate (EDTA) within 5 min ($M = 2.22$ min) after the monkey was removed from its cage. Previous studies from our laboratory demonstrated that sampling within this time frame resulted in levels that were significantly lower than those induced by stress (Kalin, Shelton, & Turner, 1992). Blood was immediately placed on ice until plasma was separated by centrifugation at 4°C for 10 min at 4,000 rpm and stored at −70°C until assayed. Plasma cortisol concentration was determined using a cortisol RIA kit (Pantex Corp., Santa Ana, CA). The intra-assay variability was 10.4% with an interassay variability of 11.3% and a detection limit (ED90) of 1.0 ug/dl.

Data Analysis

First, we hypothesized that individual differences in asymmetric frontal activity would be stable within monkeys. To test this, we performed intraclass correlations on the frontal asymmetry scores (log-right minus log-left power) collected from the 15 monkeys sampled both at 8 months and 1 year of age.

We hypothesized that increased right frontal asymmetry scores would be correlated with higher levels of cortisol and defensive behaviors and that cortisol levels also would be directly related to defensive behaviors. Because the experiment contained male and female monkeys, we established that gender did not affect cortisol levels. Spearman rank-order correlations were performed on data collected from the 50 animals at 1 year of age among (a) frontal asymmetry scores and plasma cortisol levels, (b) frontal asymmetry scores and defensive behaviors (average NEC-induced freezing duration, A-induced cooing, ST-induced barking, and ST-induced hostility), and (c) cortisol and the defensive behaviors.

Next, an extreme-groups analysis was used to further understand the differences between left and right frontally activated animals. Between the extreme left and right frontal groups, t tests were performed on measures of cortisol and individual defensive behaviors. The middle group was also used in a one-way analysis of variance (ANOVA) to determine the extent to which the two extreme groups differed from the middle asymmetry group. The inclusion of this group allowed for the specification of whether either or both extreme groups differed from the middle group control. One-way ANOVAs were computed on both the cortisol levels and defensive behaviors. Post hoc contrasts were performed when appropriate.

At the Year 3 resampling time, the sample size of the left and right frontal groups had decreased to 10 and 9 monkeys, respectively. Based on the Year 1 data, we expected that right frontal monkeys would continue to have cortisol levels greater than those in the left frontal group. First, we tested the stability of cortisol values within monkeys between 1 and 3 years of age by correlating the Year 1 value with the mean of the Year 3 cortisol values (an intraclass correlation was not computed because the Year 3 cortisols were significantly higher than those at 3 years of age). Next, one-tailed t tests were performed between the laterality groups for the two separately collected cortisol values as well as on their mean values.

Results

Stability of Individual Differences in Frontal Asymmetry and Relations among EEG, Behavior, and Cortisol

As can be seen in Figure 67.1, frontal asymmetry scores (log right minus log left, 4–8 Hz power) derived from the 15 monkeys at 8 months and 1 year of age showed stability over time as reflected in a significant intraclass correlation (ICC = .58, $p < .05$).

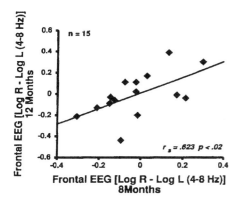

Figure 67.1
The stability of individual differences in asymmetric brain activity in 15 monkeys assessed by intraclass correlation (ICC = .58, $P < .05$) repeatedly at 8 and 12 months of age. Spearman rank = order correlation is shown.

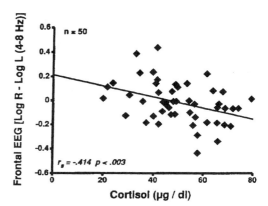

Figure 67.2
The relation between asymmetric frontal activity (lower scores indicate greater relative right-sided activity) and plasma cortisol concentration in 50 monkeys at 1 year of age. EEG, electroencephalogram.

The data collected from the entire group of 50 monkeys at 1 year of age revealed a significant inverse relation between frontal asymmetry scores and plasma cortisol levels ($r = -.41$, $p < .003$; Figure 67.2). Animals with greater relative right-sided prefrontal activation (i.e., lower asymmetry scores) had higher levels of plasma cortisol.

Correlations between the frontal asymmetry score and measures of freezing duration, defensive aggression (barking and hostility), and cooing were not significant. However, cortisol concentrations were correlated with ST-induced barking ($r = .46$, $p < .01$; Figure 67.3A) and ST-induced hostility ($r = .37$, $p < .01$; Figure 67.3B). Neither A-induced coos nor NEC-induced freezing were significantly correlated to cortisol.

Extreme EEG Asymmetry, Cortisol, and Behavior Assessed at 1 Year

The analyses comparing the extreme left and right frontal groups revealed that, compared to left frontal monkeys, the right frontal monkeys

had significantly higher cortisol concentrations: $58.02 \pm SE$ 3.17 ug/dl vs. $40.60 \pm SE$ 3.36 ug/dl; $t(21) = -3.76$, $p < .0006$; see Figure 67.4. In addition, right frontal monkeys were more hostile during ST: right = $81.23 \pm SE$ 13.54 s, left = $43.28 \pm SE$ 9.81 s; $t(21) = -2.30$, $p < .04$; see Figure 67.5, and froze for longer durations during A and NEC conditions. The only statistically significant difference in freezing occurred during the A period: right = $24.1 \pm SE$ 7.28 s, left = $7.1 \pm SE$ 4.05 s; $t(21) = -2.08$, $p < .05$; see Figure 67.5.

The data also were analyzed using the middle group to compare with the two extreme groups. The one-way ANOVA for cortisol comparing the left, middle, and right frontal asymmetry groups revealed a significant main effect for group, $F(2, 36) = 5.70$, $p < .007$; Figure 67.4. Post hoc comparisons revealed that the middle and right frontal groups did not significantly differ from each other. However, the extreme left frontal monkeys had cortisol concentrations that were significantly lower than both the middle ($p < .02$) and the right frontal groups ($p < .01$).

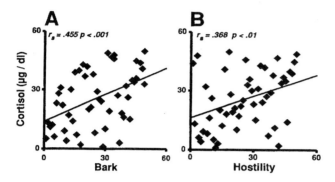

Figure 67.3
The relation between plasma cortisol concentrations and ST-induced barking (A), and cortisol and ST-induced hostility (B) in 50 monkeys at 1 year of age.

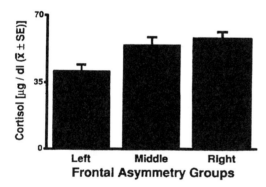

Figure 67.4
Plasma cortisol concentrations in right $(n = 11)$ and left $(n = 12)$ extreme activation groups as well as the middle group $(P < .0006)$.

Among the three frontal asymmetry groups, significant differences were not found for freezing duration, cooing, barking, and hostility.

Cortisol Concentrations in Left and Right Extreme Laterality Groups Assessed 2 Years Later

Cortisol values measured at 1 year of age were significantly correlated with the mean of the two values measured at 3 years $(r = .51, \ p < .05)$. At 3 years of age, cortisol levels continued to be significantly different between the left and right frontal groups on Day 1 of sampling, $22.76 \pm SE = 1.78$ ug/dl and $32.80 \pm SE = 1.78$ ug/dl, respectively; $t(17) = -2.26, \ p < .02$. On Day 2 of sampling, cortisol differences between the groups were in the same direction (left frontal $= 25.59$ ug/dl vs. right frontal $= 31.86$ ug/dl) but were not statistically different, $t(17) = -1.16, \ p = .13$. When comparing the means of the two samples, significant differences were found between the left and right frontal groups: left $= 24.17 \pm SE \ 2.73$ ug/dl vs. right $= 32.33 \pm SE \ 3.44$ ug/dl; $t(17) = -1.87, \ p < .04$; see Figure 67.6.

Discussion

The findings from this study demonstrate important relations among extreme asymmetric frontal brain electrical activity, nonstressed levels of cortisol, and trait-like, fear-related behaviors in young rhesus monkeys. The data underscore the similarities between humans and monkeys in these dimensions and further strengthen the rationale for using rhesus monkeys to explore

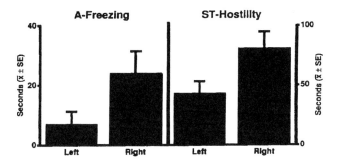

Figure 67.5
Differences in A-induced freezing and ST-induced hostility in animals in the left compared to the right frontal asymmetry groups. A, monkeys in a cage alone; ST, monkeys stared at by the humans.

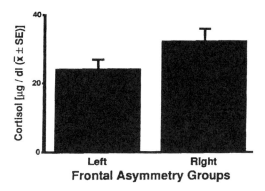

Figure 67.6
The mean cortisol concentrations of two samples collected on different days at 3 years of age for animals in the extreme left ($n = 10$) and extreme right ($n = 9$) frontal asymmetry groups ($P < .04$).

mechanisms underlying the development of individual differences in fearful temperamental styles in humans.

In earlier studies, we demonstrated that fear-related behavioral responses, such as freezing and defensive aggression, are relatively stable characteristics of individual animals (Kalin & Shelton, 1989). In another study using a small group of animals, we found that individual differences in patterns of frontal asymmetric activity were

stable over time (Davidson et al., 1992). The data from this study replicate the earlier finding and confirm the stability of intraindividual differences in asymmetric frontal brain electrical activity. A similar pattern of stability in frontal brain electrical asymmetry has also been demonstrated in humans (Tomarken, Davidson, Wheeler, & Doss, 1992).

Correlational analyses performed at 1 year of age revealed that this stable characteristic of brain activity was associated with nonstressed plasma cortisol concentrations. Monkeys with greater left frontal activation had lower cortisol levels, whereas higher cortisol levels tended to occur in monkeys with greater right frontal activation. When the monkeys were divided into extreme left and right frontal asymmetric groups, the same finding was apparent, with left frontal monkeys having cortisol levels that were significantly lower than right frontal monkeys. Additional analyses of the data comparing the middle asymmetry group with the two extreme groups demonstrated that the difference in cortisol between the two extreme groups was due to reduced levels in the left frontal group. This finding underscores the importance of including a middle group and suggests a different interpretation than the traditional view that increased fearfulness is necessarily associated with increased cortisol levels. Perhaps humans who are less fearful and have greater left frontal asymmetry also have lower levels of cortisol.

When the extreme left and right frontal groups were resampled approximately 2 years later, similar group differences in cortisol concentrations were found. Taken together, these findings support a linkage between indexes of brain activity that have been linked to temperament and circulating levels of the stress-related hormone cortisol. The data from the follow-up measures of cortisol, obtained 2 years after the measures of brain electrical activity were acquired, indicated that the relation between asymmetric frontal electrical activity and nonstressed cortisol levels is long lasting.

Though robust differences in nonstressed cortisol were obtained between monkeys with extreme left versus right frontal activation, a comparison of plasma cortisol levels in a small sample of left- and right-frontally activated humans in an earlier study did not reveal a reliable group difference (Kang et al., 1991). The lack of consistent findings between this and the current study could be due to a number of factors. In the human study, only women were studied and they were considerably older than the relative age of the monkeys studied in the present study. In addition, many of the women, especially those in the extreme left frontal group, were taking oral contraceptives, which are known to affect cortisol concentrations (Coenen, Thomas, Borm, & Rolland, 1995; Kirschbaum, Pirke, & Hallhammer, 1995; Reinberg et al., 1996). In the present study, monkeys were manually restrained for the recording of brain electrical activity. This is likely a more stressful situation than that used in the recording of brain activity in humans and also could have contributed to differences between the two studies. Future studies in monkeys that use chaired animals habituated to the chairing procedure for EEG recording would help to determine if the stress of manual restraint is a key component in uncovering relations between frontal brain electrical asymmetries and cortisol.

Based on human studies, we hypothesized that defensive behavioral traits indicative of fear and anxiety would be associated with extreme right frontal brain activity. Correlational analyses between EEG asymmetry and these behaviors, at 1 year of age, were not significant. We also failed to find this relation in an earlier study that used a smaller group of monkeys (Davidson et al., 1993). However, the extreme-groups analytic approach demonstrated that, compared with humans with left frontal activity, those monkeys with extreme right frontal activity engaged in greater amounts of freezing and defensive aggression. When these data were analyzed with the additional middle asymmetry group, the differences were no longer significant. This was due to the large range of variability in the behavioral responses of the middle group and should not diminish the importance of the findings from the two-way extreme group comparison. In general, the finding that extreme right frontal monkeys display more intense defensive responses is consistent with findings in human children and adults, demonstrating that right frontal asymmetry is associated with increased behavioral and emotional distress (see Davidson, 1995, for review).

From the data collected at 1 year of age, we also examined the relations between cortisol concentrations and the various defensive behaviors. Based on earlier work in behaviorally inhibited children (Kagan et al., 1988) and monkeys with a propensity to freeze (Kalin et al., 1998), we expected that individual differences in freezing behavior would be positively correlated with cortisol levels. In the present study, nonstressed cortisol concentrations were positively correlated with the amount of hostility, or defensive aggression, displayed toward the staring human intruder. However, cortisol was not correlated with freezing duration. A possible explanation for the differences found between these studies could be that a single cortisol measurement can only grossly reflect a system that has a dynamic pattern of change. Alternatively, the relation between nonstressed levels of cortisol and defensive behaviors may be a general one that is not specifically linked to one type of defensive behavior. Despite these variations in the specific type of defensive behavior associated with cortisol, together the human and monkey studies suggest that non-stressed cortisol concentrations are generally related to individual differences in a constellation of behavioral responses all associated with fearful temperaments.

The findings from the current study are the first to link individual differences in asymmetric frontal electrical activity with circulating levels of cortisol. This is of importance because both parameters have been independently associated with fear-related temperamental styles. However, the extent to which the relation between extreme right frontal asymmetry and nonstressed cortisol levels is associational or causally linked remains to be determined. The finding that the differences in cortisol were attributable to extreme left frontal activity is interesting and should be pursued. Although the brain neural circuitry that ultimately regulates the release of cortisol has been established, little is known regarding the mechanisms underlying frontal asymmetric electrical activity. Consistent with the findings from the current study, a study in humans suggests a preferential role for the right hemisphere in emotion-induced release of cortisol (Wittling & Pfluger, 1990; see review in Wittling, 1995). Future studies in monkeys will be aimed at elucidating the mechanisms underlying this relation as well as those regulating emotion-related asymmetric frontal electrical activity.

References

Coenen, C. M., Thomas, C. M., Borm, G. F., & Rolland, R. (1995). Comparative evaluation of the androgenicity of four low-dose, fixed-combination oral contraceptives. *International Journal of Fertility & Menopausal Studies, 40* (Suppl. 2), 92–97.

Davidson, R. J. (1992). Anterior cerebral asymmetry and the nature of emotion. *Brain and Cognition, 20,* 125–151.

Davidson, R. J. (1995). Cerebral asymmetry, emotion and affective style. In R. J. Davidson & K. Hugdahl (Eds.), *Brain asymmetry* (pp. 361–387). Cambridge, MA: MIT Press.

Davidson, R. J., Chapman, J. P., Chapman, L. P., & Henriques, J. B. (1990). Asymmetrical brain electrical activity discriminates between psychometrically-matched verbal and spatial cognitive tasks. *Psychophysiology, 27,* 528–543.

Davidson, R. J., & Fox, N. A. (1989). Frontal brain asymmetry predicts infants' response to maternal separation. *Journal of Abnormal Psychology, 98,* 127–131.

Davidson, R. J., Kalin, N. H., & Shelton, S. E. (1992). Lateralized effects of diazepam on frontal brain electrical asymmetries in rhesus monkeys. *Biological Psychiatry, 32,* 438–451.

Davidson, R. J., Kalin, N. H., & Shelton, S. E. (1993). Lateralized response to diazepam predicts temperamental style in rhesus monkeys. *Behavioral Neuroscience, 107,* 1106–1110.

Davidson, R. J., & Tomarken, A. J. (1989). Laterality and emotion: An electrophysiological approach. In F. Boller & J. Grafman (Eds.), *Handbook of neuropsychology.* (pp. 419–441) Amsterdam: Elsevier.

Kagan, J., Reznick, J. S., & Snidman, N. (1988, April 8). Biological bases of childhood shyness. *Science, 240,* 167–171.

Kalin, N. H. (1993). The neurobiology of fear. *Scientific American, 268,* 94–101.

Kalin, N. H., & Shelton, S. E. (1989). Defensive behaviors in infant rhesus monkeys: Environmental cues and neurochemical regulation. *Science, 243,* 1718–1721.

Kalin, N. H., Shelton, S. E., Rickman, M., & Davidson, R. J. (1998). Individual differences in freezing and cortisol in infant and mother rhesus monkeys. *Behavioral Neuroscience, 112,* 251–254.

Kalin, N. H., Shelton, S. E., & Takahashi, L. K. (1991). Defensive behaviors in infant rhesus monkeys: Ontogeny and context-dependent selective expression. *Child Development, 62,* 1175–1183.

Kalin, N. H., Shelton, S. E., & Turner, J. G. (1992). Effects of b-carboline on fear-related behavioral and neurohormonal responses in infant rhesus monkeys. *Biological Psychiatry, 31,* 1008–1019.

Kang, D. H., Davidson, R. J., Coe, C. L., Wheeler, R. W., Tomarken, A. J., & Ershler, W. B. (1991). Frontal brain asymmetry and immune function. *Behavioral Neuroscience,* 105, 860–869.

Kirschbaum, C., Pirke, K. M., & Hellhammer, D. H. (1995). Preliminary evidence for reduced cortisol responsivity to psychological stress in women using oral contraceptive medication. *Psychoneuroendocrinology,* 20, 509–514.

Niedermeyer, E. (1993). Maturation and the EEG: Development of waking and sleep patterns. In E. Niedermeyer & F. Lopes da Silva (Eds.), *Electroencephalography: Basic principles, clinical applications and related fields* (pp. 167–191). Baltimore: Williams and Wilkins.

Pivik, T., Broughton, R., Coppola, R., Davidson, R. J., Fox, N. A., & Nuwer, R. (1993). Guidelines for quantitative electroencephalography in research contexts. *Psychophysiology,* 30, 547–558.

Reinberg, A. E., Touitou, Y., Soudant, E., Bernard, D., Bazin, R., & Mechkouri, M. (1996). Oral contraceptives alter circadian rhythm parameters of cortisol, melatonin, blood pressure, heart rate, skin blood flow, transepidermal water loss, and skin amino acids of healthy young women. *Chronobiology International,* 13, 199–211.

Tomarken, A. J., Davidson, R. J., Wheeler, R. E., & Doss, R. C. (1992). Individual differences in anterior brain asymmetry and fundamental dimensions of emotion. *Journal of Personality and Social Psychology,* 62, 676–687.

Tomarken, A. J., Davidson, R. J., Wheeler, R. E., & Kinney, L. (1992). Psychometric properties of resting anterior EEG asymmetry: Temporal stability and internal consistency. *Psychophysiology,* 29, 576–592.

Wheeler, R. W., Davidson, R. J., & Tomarken, A. J. (1993). Frontal brain asymmetry and emotional reactivity: A biological substrate of affective style. *Psychophysiology,* 30, 82–89.

Wittling, W. (1995). Brain asymmetry in the control of autonomic-physiologic activity. In R. J. Davidson & K. Hugdahl (Eds.), *Brain asymmetry* (pp. 305–357). Cambridge, MA: MIT Press.

Wittling, W., & Pfluger, M. (1990). Neuroendocrine hemisphere asymmetries: Salivary cortisol secretion during lateralized viewing of emotion-related and neutral films. *Brain and Cognition,* 14, 243–265.

Frontal Brain Electrical Activity in Shyness and Sociability

Louis A. Schmidt

Some people in social situations appear quite reserved and quiet. Are these people reserved because they prefer to be alone rather than with others (i.e., they are introverts) or because they feel anxious and tense during social interactions and these feelings inhibit their ability to act in such situations (i.e., they are shy)? Are shyness and sociability so highly interrelated that being high on one trait means being low on the other? Cheek and Buss (1981) asked these very questions and noted that the answer to the latter question is yes, by definition, if shyness is defined as nothing more than a tendency to avoid people, as this is the reverse of sociability. If shyness and sociability are defined independently, however, then the extent to which they are related becomes an empirical question.

Cheek and Buss (1981) examined this issue. They developed short self-report measures of shyness and sociability and noted that undergraduates' responses to the two measures were only modestly related. Cheek and Buss then asked, if a person is shy, does it make any difference in behavior whether the person is high or low in sociability? They selected subjects who self-reported high and low shyness and sociability and observed them while interacting with unfamiliar peers. Cheek and Buss found that high-shy/high-social undergraduates exhibited more overt behavioral anxiety during the social interaction compared with undergraduates in the other three groups.

Using a design identical to that reported by Cheek and Buss (1981), Fox and I (Schmidt & Fox, 1994) recently examined the extent to which shyness and sociability were distinguishable on the basis of autonomic measures. We found that different combinations of shyness and sociability were distinguishable on two separate autonomic measures (mean heart rate and heart rate variability) just prior to an anticipated novel social encounter. Undergraduates classified as high-shy/high-social exhibited a significantly faster and more stable heart rate in anticipation of a novel social interaction than undergraduates in the other three groups.

It is also important to note that the Cheek and Buss (1981) measurement model concerning the relative independence of shyness and sociability has been independently replicated both with children (Asendorpf & Meier, 1993) and cross-culturally, most recently in German (Czeschlik & Nurk, 1995) and Portuguese (Neto, 1996) translations. Together, these sets of data suggest that shyness and sociability are distinct traits not only at the construct level, but at the empirical level as well, and are distinguishable across different measures, ages, and cultures. The purpose of the present study was to extend previous research by examining whether shyness and sociability are distinguishable on the basis of measures of frontal brain electrical activity.

Frontal Activation–Emotion Models

Davidson and Fox (Davidson, 1993; Fox, 1991, 1994) have articulated a theoretical model of emotion in which emotions are (a) organized around approach-avoidance tendencies and (b) differentially lateralized in the frontal region of the brain. The left frontal area is involved in the experience of positive emotions such as joy, interest, and happiness; the experience of positive affect facilitates and maintains approach behaviors (e.g., sociability). The right frontal region is involved in the experience of negative emotions such as fear and disgust; the experience of negative emotion facilitates and maintains avoidance behaviors (e.g., shyness). Utilizing frontal electroencephalogram (EEG) measures to index ongoing brain activity during the processing of different affects, Davidson and Fox have found empirical support for the model (for reviews, see

Davidson, 1993; Fox, 1991, 1994). Left frontal EEG asymmetries are routinely associated with the processing of positive affects, and right frontal EEG asymmetries are consistently linked with the processing of negative affects. Davidson and his colleagues have also used this model in an attempt to understand individual differences in adult personality.

In a series of studies with adults, Davidson and his colleagues have noted a relation between the pattern of resting frontal EEG activity and individual differences in affective-personality style. For example, adults who exhibit greater relative resting right frontal EEG activity are known to rate negative affective films more intensely negative compared with adults who exhibit greater relative resting left frontal EEG activity (Tomarken, Davidson, & Henriques, 1990). Also, individuals who exhibited a stable pattern of greater relative resting right frontal EEG activity over 3 weeks reported more intense negative affect in response to negative emotional film clips, whereas individuals who displayed a stable pattern of greater relative resting left frontal EEG activity reported more intense positive affect in response to positive emotional film clips (Wheeler, Davidson, & Tomarken, 1993). More recently, Davidson's group found that the pattern of resting frontal EEG activity was related to subjects' subjective report of motivational-affective style (Sutton & Davidson, 1997). Individuals with greater relative resting left frontal EEG activity were likely to score high on a psychometric measure indexing behavioral approach tendencies. Davidson and his colleagues (Davidson & Rickman, 1999) have speculated that these sets of findings suggest that the pattern of resting EEG activity from the anterior portion of the scalp may reflect a predisposition to experience positive and negative emotion and may distinguish individual differences in personality.

It is important to note that, traditionally, frontal EEG asymmetry scores have been computed by right frontal EEG power minus left frontal EEG power, with negative scores reflect-

ing greater relative right activation.[1] Using this metric, there are at least two ways right frontal asymmetry can be exhibited and at least two ways left frontal asymmetry can be exhibited. Right frontal EEG asymmetry could result from (a) a reduction in EEG power in the right lead, with EEG power in the left lead remaining constant (an example of right EEG hyperactivation), or (b) constant EEG power in the right lead accompanied by an increase in EEG power in the left lead (an example of left EEG hypoactivation). Left frontal EEG asymmetry could result from (a) a reduction in EEG power in the left lead, with EEG power in the right lead remaining constant (an example of left EEG hyperactivation), or (b) constant EEG power in the left lead accompanied by an increase in EEG power in the right lead (an example of right EEG hypoactivation). The difference between these varying patterns of frontal EEG asymmetry is not trivial, as different patterns appear to have different psychological meanings.

For example, Henriques and Davidson (1991) found a pattern of greater relative resting right frontal EEG asymmetry in depressed adults; right frontal asymmetry was a function of left hypoactivation. Henriques and Davidson speculated that left frontal EEG hypoactivation in depression reflects lack of approach and an absence of positive affect rather than the presence of heightened negative affect. Fox and I (Schmidt & Fox, 1996) recently found a pattern of greater relative resting left frontal EEG asymmetry in a sample of aggressive toddlers; left frontal EEG asymmetry was a function of right hypoactivation. We hypothesized that right frontal hypoactivation reflects heightened approach and an inability to experience the consequences of negative emotion, traits characteristic of some forms of aggression (e.g., proactive).

Together, these findings suggest that not only the pattern of resting frontal EEG asymmetry, but also the pattern in resting absolute EEG power in each frontal hemisphere may distinguish individual differences in personality: Resting frontal EEG asymmetry may reflect the type (i.e., valence) of emotion experienced, and resting frontal absolute EEG power may reflect the intensity of the affective experience (see, e.g., Dawson, 1994; Schmidt & Fox, 1998, 1999). Utilizing these models relating frontal activation to emotion, the present study examined whether shyness and sociability and different combinations of shyness and sociability are distinguishable on the basis of the pattern of resting frontal EEG asymmetry and power.

The Present Study

Resting EEG was recorded for 6 min from undergraduates who self-reported high and low shyness and sociability. The following predictions were tested. Because shyness is presumably characterized and maintained by the experience of heightened negative emotion, the first prediction was that high-shy subjects would exhibit significantly greater relative right frontal EEG activity compared with low-shy subjects. Second, because sociability is presumably characterized and maintained by the experience of heightened positive emotion, high-social subjects were predicted to display significantly greater relative left frontal EEG activity compared with low-social subjects. Third, the high-shy/low-social and low-shy/high-social subtypes were predicted to exhibit the greatest magnitude in asymmetries in resting frontal EEG activity. The high-shy/low-social subtype would exhibit significantly greater relative right frontal EEG activity compared with the other subtypes because of the relative balance between positive and negative emotion that characterizes and maintains this subtype: the presence of heightened negative emotion and the absence of positive emotion. The low-shy/high-social subtype would exhibit significantly greater relative left frontal EEG activity because of the relative balance between positive and negative emotion that characterizes and maintains this subtype: the presence of heightened positive

emotion and the absence of negative emotion. The fourth prediction was that the high-shy/high-social and high-shy/low-social subtypes would both exhibit greater relative right frontal EEG activity because shyness is presumably characterized and maintained by the presence of more negative than positive affect; however, the two shy subtypes would be distinguishable on resting power in the left, but not right, frontal lead because the high-shy/high-social subtype is presumably characterized and maintained by the experience of more positive affect compared with the high-shy/low-social subtype.

Method

Subjects

Subjects were 271 right-handed (Oldfield, 1971) undergraduate women who were recruited from psychology courses at McMaster University ($M = 20.97$ years, $SD = 3.19$ years). The sample was restricted to women because of the disproportionate number of women who had completed and returned a screening survey that included self-report measures of shyness and sociability (Cheek, 1983; Cheek & Buss, 1981). The relation between shyness and sociability in the total sample was $r = -.32$; it is important to note that this correlation is similar to or lower than the correlations reported in many previous studies (e.g., Bruch, Gorsky, Collins, & Berger, 1989; Cheek & Buss, 1981; Schmidt & Fox, 1994). In addition, left-handed individuals were excluded because evidence indicates that they may differ from right-handers in hemispheric specialization of emotion (Heller & Levy, 1981).

Self-report Measures

Shyness was assessed using the revised 13-item Cheek and Buss Shyness Scale (Cheek, 1983; Cheek & Buss, 1981). Items from this scale include "I find it hard to talk to strangers" and "I feel inhibited in social situations." Sociability was assessed using the 5-item Cheek and Buss Sociability Scale (Cheek & Buss, 1981). Items from this scale include "I like to be with other people" and "I prefer working with others rather than alone." Items on both scales are scored on a scale from 0 (*extremely uncharacteristic*) to 4 (*extremely characteristic*). Reliability and validity data for these two scales are reported in Cheek and Buss (1981) and Bruch et al. (1989).

Procedure

Subject Selection From the larger sample of 271, 40 women were selected for high (approximately the upper 30%) and low (approximately the lower 30%) self-ratings of shyness and sociability. The 40 women included 10 in each of the subtypes: high-shy/high-social, high-shy/low-social, low-shy/high-social, and low-shy/low-social. The selected subjects were called and asked to participate in a follow-up study. All were tested within 1 month of completing the screening survey and received $10 remuneration for their participation.

As a test of whether subjects' self-report ratings of shyness and sociability remained stable from the initial screening to laboratory testing, all subjects completed the shyness and sociability scales at the time of their laboratory visit. Each subject's shyness and sociability scores fell within the initial cutoff values used to define her particular group.

EEG Recording Upon arrival at the laboratory, the subject was briefed about the procedures and consent was obtained. Baseline EEG was recorded for 6 min (3 min with eyes open, 3 min with eyes closed) while the subject was seated. The subject was instructed to simply "relax" during the EEG testing. EEG was recorded using a Lycra stretchcap (Electro-Cap, Inc.). The cap electrodes were positioned according to the International 10/20 Electrode Placement System (Jasper, 1958). The experimenter used the blunt end of a Q-tip in combination with an abrasive gel (Omni-prep) and gently abraded each electrode surface. Each electrode

site was then filled with a small amount of electrolyte gel, which served as a conductor. Electrode impedances below 10 K ohms per site were considered acceptable, as were impedance differences of up to 500 ohms between homologous sites.

EEG was recorded from six scalp locations: left and right mid-frontal (F3, F4), parietal (P3, P4), and occipital (O1, O2) regions. These sites represent the left and right hemispheres and anterior and posterior regions of the brain. EEG activity in posterior sites served as a comparison in order to ensure that group differences in resting EEG power were specific to the frontal region. All electrodes were referenced to the central vertex (Cz). Electro-oculographic (EOG) activity was also recorded, using two Beckman miniature electrodes, which were placed on the external canthus and the supraorbital area of the right eye. The EOG signal was input into a separate channel and was used to facilitate subsequent EEG artifact editing.

The seven channels were amplified by individual SA Instrumentation Bioamplifiers. The filter settings for the seven channels were set at 1 Hz (high pass) and 100 Hz (low pass). The data from all seven channels were digitized on-line at a sampling rate of 512 Hz.

EEG Data Reduction and Analysis The EEG data were rereferenced to an average reference configuration and visually scored for artifact due to eyeblinks, eye movements, and other motor movements, using software (EEG Analysis Program) developed by James Long Company (Caroga Lake, New York). This program removes data from all channels if artifact is present on any one channel. The amount of artifact-edited EEG data was examined among subjects in order to ensure that it did not systematically vary within and between subjects.

All artifact-free EEG data were analyzed using a discrete Fourier transform (DFT), with a Hanning window of 1-s width and 50% overlap. Power (microvolts squared) was derived from the

DFT output in the alpha band (8 to 13 Hz). An aggregate measure of EEG was computed by weighting the amount of EEG power data from the eyes-open and eyes-closed conditions by the number of chunks (DFT windows analyzed) used in the analysis. This weighting procedure produces a more reliable estimate of EEG activity than analyzing eyes-open and eyes-closed conditions separately (Tomarken, Davidson, Wheeler, & Kinney, 1992).

Data Analysis An analysis of variance (ANOVA) was performed to examine whether shyness and sociability were distinguishable on the basis of regional EEG power. In this analysis, shyness (high vs. low) and sociability (high vs. low) were between-subjects factors, and region (frontal vs. parietal vs. occipital) and hemisphere (left vs. right) were within-subjects factors. The dependent measure was resting EEG alpha power (8 to 13 Hz).

Results

The results of the analyses revealed a significant Shyness × Sociability × Region × Hemisphere interaction, $F(2, 72) = 4.49$, $p < .05$. This interaction was decomposed by performing a separate ANOVA for each region, with shyness (high vs. low) and sociability (high vs. low) as between-subjects factors and hemisphere (left vs. right) as a within-subjects factor. The analyses revealed significant effects on EEG power only for the frontal region. There were no significant main effects or interactions found for EEG power in the parietal and occipital regions, so data from these sites are not described further. Figure 68.1 presents the mean differences in left and right resting frontal EEG alpha power for the four groups.

The analyses revealed separate significant Shyness × Hemisphere and Sociability × Hemisphere interactions ($ps < .01$). These interactions were decomposed by computing a traditional frontal EEG asymmetry score[2] and examining

frontal asymmetry differences between high- and low-shy subjects and high- and low-social subjects. As predicted, high-shy subjects ($M = -0.059$, $SD = 0.096$) exhibited significantly greater relative resting right frontal EEG activity compared with low-shy subjects ($M = +0.173$, $SD = 0.205$), $t(38) = 4.58$, $p < .01$; high-social subjects ($M = +0.160$, $SD = 0.217$) exhibited significantly greater relative resting left frontal EEG activity compared with low-social subjects ($M = -0.047$, $SD = 0.100$), $t(38) = 3.88$, $p < .01$.

The analysis also revealed a significant Shyness × Sociability × Hemisphere interaction for resting frontal EEG alpha power ($p < .01$). Again, this interaction was decomposed by computing a traditional frontal EEG asymmetry score and comparing the different subtypes. Between-subjects t tests revealed that, as predicted, the high-shy/low-social subtype ($M = -0.098$, $SD = 0.121$) exhibited significantly greater relative right frontal EEG activity compared with the low-shy/low-social subtype ($M = +0.004$, $SD = 0.031$), $t(18) = 2.59$, $p < .02$, and the low-shy/high-social subtype ($M = +0.341$, $SD = 0.158$), $t(18) = 7.00$, $p < .01$. The frontal EEG asymmetry difference between the high-shy/low-social subtype and high-shy/high-social subtype ($M = -0.021$, $SD = 0.038$) only approached significance, $t(18) = 1.93$, $p = .07$. In addition, the low-shy/high-social subtype, as predicted, exhibited significantly greater relative left frontal EEG activity compared with the low-shy/low-social and high-shy/high-social subtypes, $t(18) = 6.63$, $p < .01$, and $t(18) = 7.06$, $p < .01$, respectively.

The next analysis examined whether the two shy subtypes, although not distinguishable on the traditional frontal EEG asymmetry measure, were distinguishable on absolute frontal EEG power. As can be seen in Figure 68.1, although the high-shy/high-social and high-shy/low-social subtypes both exhibited greater relative right frontal EEG activity, the two shy subtypes differed significantly on the pattern of EEG power

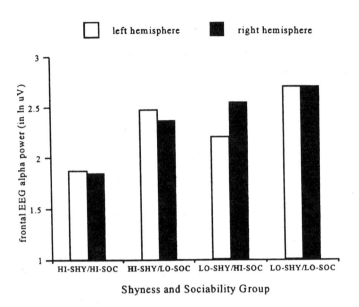

Figure 68.1
Differences in left and right resting frontal electroencephalogram (EEG) alpha (8–13 Hz) power in undergraduates reporting high and low shyness and sociability. HI-SHY, high in shyness; LO-SHY, low in shyness; HI-SOC, high in sociability; LO-SOC, low in sociability. Note that EEG power is inversely related to activity. Thus, lower power reflects higher activation.

only in the left frontal lead. Planned comparisons of EEG power in the left frontal site revealed that, as predicted, the high-shy/high-social subtype ($M = 1.87$, $SD = 0.42$) displayed significantly less EEG power (i.e., more activity) in the left frontal site compared with the high-shy/low-social subtype ($M = 2.47$, $SD = 0.74$), $t(18) = 2.22$, $p < .05$. These two subtypes did not differ on EEG power in the right frontal lead.

Discussion

Are Shyness and Sociability Distinguishable on the Basis of Resting Frontal Brain Activity?

Shyness was associated with resting right frontal EEG asymmetry. Individuals who scored high on

subjective measures of shyness exhibited greater relative resting right frontal EEG activity compared with their low-shy counterparts. Also, sociability was associated with resting left frontal EEG asymmetry. Individuals who scored high on subjective measures of sociability displayed greater relative resting left frontal EEG activity compared with their low-social counterparts. These data are consistent with the notion that shyness and sociability are separable not only at the construct level, but at the empirical level as well. The present findings also extend previous work in this area, which has found that shyness and sociability are distinguishable on behavioral (Cheek & Buss, 1981) and autonomic (Schmidt & Fox, 1994) measures. This extension to electrocortical measures perhaps suggests that shyness and sociability may be subserved by different neurophysiological substrates.

If a Person Is Shy, Does Sociability Make Any Difference for the Pattern of Resting Frontal Brain Activity?

Different combinations of shyness and sociability were distinguishable on measures of resting frontal EEG asymmetry and absolute power. High-shy/low-social subjects were distinguishable from low-shy/high-social and low-shy/low-social subjects on resting frontal EEG asymmetry. High-shy/low-social subjects exhibited significantly greater relative resting right frontal EEG activity compared with their low-shy/high-social and low-shy/low-social counterparts. This finding is consistent with predictions derived from the model combining frontal EEG and emotion. According to this model, the high-shy/low-social subtype would exhibit the greatest asymmetry in resting right frontal EEG activity; this subtype is presumably characterized and maintained by a greater degree of negative affect relative to positive affect compared with the other three subtypes.

It is also important to note that although the high-shy/high-social and high-shy/low-social subtypes both exhibited greater relative right resting frontal EEG activity, they did not differ significantly on the frontal EEG asymmetry measure. The two shy subtypes were, however, distinguishable on the measure of absolute EEG power in the frontal hemispheres. They differed significantly on EEG power only in the left, but not the right, frontal lead. These findings provide further empirical support for the theoretical notion that there may be different types of shyness, each of which has distinct behavioral (Cheek & Buss, 1981) and psychophysiological (Schmidt & Fox, 1994) correlates. Taken together, the results of the present study extend these previous findings on differences among shy subtypes to electrocortical measures and suggest that not only the pattern of frontal EEG asymmetry, but also the pattern of absolute EEG power in each frontal hemisphere, is important in distinguishing subtypes of shyness.

A final note concerning the low-shy/high-social subtype is also warranted. The results revealed that this subtype was distinguishable from the other three subtypes on the basis of resting frontal EEG asymmetry. Low-shy/high-social subjects exhibited significantly greater relative resting left frontal EEG activity compared with subjects in the other three subtypes. This finding is also consistent with the frontal activation–emotion model: The low-shy/high-social subtype is presumably characterized and maintained by a greater degree of positive affect relative to negative affect compared with the other three subtypes.

What Do Differences in Frontal EEG Asymmetry and Power Reflect?

It has been argued (Dawson, 1994; Schmidt & Fox, 1998, 1999) that the pattern of frontal EEG asymmetry may reflect the type (i.e., valence) of emotional experience, whereas the pattern of frontal EEG power may reflect the intensity with which the emotion is experienced. Some researchers (Cheek & Buss, 1981; Schmidt & Fox, 1999) have suggested that high-shy/high-social individuals are characterized by an approach-avoidance conflict. It is possible that the pattern of greater relative resting right frontal EEG activity that is characteristic of both shy subtypes reflects a predisposition (perhaps a diathesis) to experience intense negative emotion. This diathesis is expressed differently in the two shy subtypes, however, in how they experience positive affect. Meeting real or imagined social stressors may lead to an approach-avoidance conflict in people who are high in both shyness and sociability because of the experience of competing positive and negative emotions: a desire to affiliate with others, but a fear of doing so. In contrast, people who are high in shyness and low in sociability may experience relatively less conflict in such situations because they do not have the same desire to affiliate with others.

A final methodological point is worthy of discussion. Some previous studies (e.g., Sutton & Davidson, 1997) have used only a frontal EEG difference score (asymmetry) and related it to individual differences in personality. If the present study had been limited to the use of a frontal EEG difference measure, it would have shown little about how absolute EEG power in each frontal lead contributes to the difference score. Considering absolute power in each hemisphere made it possible to distinguish the high-shy/high-social and high-shy/low-social subtypes on the basis of the pattern of absolute EEG power in the left frontal lead. Because the pattern of absolute EEG power in each frontal hemisphere may have unique psychological meaning, the results of the present study highlight the importance of considering the contribution of absolute EEG power in each frontal hemisphere in distinguishing individual differences in personality. Future studies should examine the pattern of resting frontal EEG asymmetry and absolute power in distinguishing personality subtypes in general, and shyness and sociability in particular, in both men and women, as well as in children. Also, behavioral measures of shyness and sociability and issues of stability should be incorporated into this work.

Acknowledgments

This research was supported by a grant from the McMaster University Faculty of Science. I wish to thank John Kihlstrom, Todd Riniolo, Ariana Shahinfar, and two anonymous reviewers for their helpful comments on earlier versions, and Nicole Conrad and Lori Francis for their help with data collection, reduction, and analyses.

Notes

1. EEG power is thought to be inversely related to activation, with lower power reflecting greater cortical activation (Lindsley & Wicke, 1974).

2. This score was calculated as right frontal power minus left frontal power, with negative scores reflecting greater relative right frontal EEG activity.

References

Asendorpf, J. B., & Meier, G. H. (1993). Personality effects on children's speech in everyday life: Sociability-mediated exposure and shyness-mediated reactivity to social situations. *Journal of Personality and Social Psychology, 64,* 1072–1083.

Bruch, M. A., Gorsky, J. M., Collins, T. M., & Berger, P. A. (1989). Shyness and sociability reexamined: A multi-component analysis. *Journal of Personality and Social Psychology, 57,* 904–915.

Cheek, J. M. (1983). *The Revised Cheek and Buss Shyness Scale.* Unpublished manuscript, Wellesley College, Wellesley, MA.

Cheek, J. M., & Buss, A. H. (1981). Shyness and sociability. *Journal of Personality and Social Psychology, 41,* 330–339.

Czeschlik, T., & Nurk, H. C. (1995). Shyness and sociability: Factor structure in a German sample. *European Journal of Psychological Assessment, 11,* 122–127.

Davidson, R. J. (1993). The neuropsychology of emotion and affective style. In M. Lewis & J. M. Haviland (Eds.), *Handbook of emotion* (pp. 143–154). New York: Guilford Press.

Davidson, R. J., & Rickman, M. (1999). Behavioral inhibition and the emotional circuitry of the brain: Stability and plasticity during the early childhood years. In L. A. Schmidt & J. Schulkin (Eds.), *Extreme fear, shyness and social phobia: Origins, biological mechanisms, and clinical outcomes* (pp. 67–87). New York: Oxford University Press.

Dawson, G. (1994). Frontal electroencephalographic correlates of individual differences in emotional expression in infants. In N. A. Fox (Ed.), The development of emotion regulation: Behavioral and biological considerations. *Monographs of the Society for Research in Child Development, 59*(2–3, Serial No. 240), 135–151.

Fox, N. A. (1991). If it's not left, it's right: Electroencephalograph asymmetry and the development of emotion. *American Psychologist, 46,* 863–872.

Fox, N. A. (1994). Dynamic cerebral processes underlying emotion regulation. In N. A. Fox (Ed.), The development of emotion regulation: Behavioral and biological considerations. *Monographs of the Society for Research in Child Development, 59*(2–3, Serial No. 240), 152–166.

Heller, W., & Levy, J. (1981). Perception and expression of emotion in right-handers and left-handers. *Neuropsychologia, 19,* 263–272.

Henriques, J. B., & Davidson, R. J. (1991). Left frontal hypoactivation in depression. *Journal of Abnormal Psychology, 100,* 535–545.

Jasper, H. H. (1958). The ten-twenty electrode system of the International Federation. *Electroencephalography and Clinical Neurophysiology, 10,* 371–375.

Lindsley, D. B., & Wicke, J. D. (1974). The EEG: Autonomous electrical activity in man and animals. In R. Thompson & M. N. Patterson (Eds.), *Bioelectrical recording techniques* (pp. 3–83). New York: Academic Press.

Neto, F. (1996). Correlates of Portuguese college students' shyness and sociability. *Psychological Reports, 78,* 79–82.

Oldfield, R. C. (1971). The assessment and analysis of handedness: The Edinburgh Inventory. *Neuropsychologia, 9,* 97–113.

Schmidt, L. A., & Fox, N. A. (1994). Patterns of cortical electrophysiology and autonomic activity in adults' shyness and sociability. *Biological Psychology, 38,* 183–198.

Schmidt, L. A., & Fox, N. A. (1996). Frontal EEG correlates of dysregulated social behavior in children [Abstract]. *Psychophysiology, 33,* S8.

Schmidt, L. A., & Fox, N. A. (1998). The development and outcomes of childhood shyness: A multiple psychophysiological measure approach. In R. Vasta (Ed.), *Annals of child development* (Vol. 13, pp. 1–20). London: Kingsley.

Schmidt, L. A., & Fox, N. A. (1999). Conceptual, biological, and behavioral distinctions among different types of shy children. In L. A. Schmidt & J. Schulkin (Eds.), *Extreme fear, shyness and social phobia: Origins, biological mechanisms, and clinical outcomes* (pp. 47–66). New York: Oxford University Press.

Sutton, S. K., & Davidson, R. J. (1997). Prefrontal brain asymmetry: A biological substrate of the behavioral approach and inhibition systems. *Psychological Science, 8,* 204–210.

Tomarken, A. J., Davidson, R. J., & Henriques, J. B. (1990). Resting frontal brain asymmetry predicts affective responses to films. *Journal of Personality and Social Psychology, 59,* 791–801.

Tomarken, A. J., Davidson, R. J., Wheeler, R. E., & Kinney, L. (1992). Psychometric properties of resting anterior EEG asymmetry: Temporal stability and internal consistency. *Psychophysiology, 29,* 576–592.

Wheeler, R. E., Davidson, R. J., & Tomarken, A. J. (1993). Frontal brain asymmetry and emotional reactivity: A biological substrate of affective style. *Psychophysiology, 30,* 82–89.

69 Selective Alteration of Personality and Social Behavior by Serotonergic Intervention

Brian Knutson, Owen M. Wolkowitz, Steve W. Cole, Theresa Chan, Elizabeth A. Moore, Ronald C. Johnson, Jan Terpstra, Rebecca A. Turner, and Victor I. Reus

Research indicates that individual differences in human personality can be summarized by three to five independent dimensions (1). Status on each of these dimensions is stable over the adult lifespan (2) and typically shows heritabilities on the order of 50% (3). However, the physiological substrates underlying these personality dimensions have not yet been elucidated. Spurred by advances in psychopharmacology, several theorists have proposed that brain biogenic amine mechanisms may contribute to the phenotypic expression of some of these dimensions, particularly those which involve affective and motivational processes (4–6).

Consistent with these speculations, clinical studies of psychiatric patients suggest that low brain serotonin activity may be related to psychiatric disorders involving hostile affect and aggressive behavior. For instance, people with a history of impulsively violent behavior (e.g., arsonists, violent criminals, people who die by violent methods of suicide) have low CSF serotonin metabolite levels (7). In addition, patients with violent histories (e.g., with antisocial personality disorder) show signs of compromised brain serotonin function, as assessed by neuroendocrine probes (8). Finally, pharmacological interventions that augment serotonergic efficacy can reduce hostile sentiment and violent outbursts in aggressive psychiatric patients (9).

In contrast, the impact of serotonergic interventions on hostile personality characteristics in normal individuals has received less investigation. Impairment of brain serotonin function by means of precursor depletion can induce depressive affect (10, 11) and may potentiate hostile behavior (12, 13) in normal control subjects. At the time this study was conducted, no one had investigated whether augmentation of brain serotonin would affect hostility variables in normal volunteers. If enhancement of brain serotonergic function reduces hostility, might such effects remain focal only to hostility variables, or might they be attributable to broader changes in affective personality variables? For example, might administration of a selective serotonin reuptake inhibitor (SSRI) reduce negative affect (including sadness, anxiety, and other negative emotions in addition to hostility) or increase positive affect? To address these questions, we used a pharmacologically selective intervention to alter brain serotonin function in normal subjects and observed subsequent changes in standard affective personality variables over 4 weeks.

A second but related body of research suggests that brain serotonin function also plays a role in the social behavior of nonhuman primates. For instance, rhesus monkeys with low CSF serotonin metabolite levels show more spontaneous aggression toward conspecifics, receive more wounds, and die at a younger age (14, 15), while those with high CSF serotonin metabolite levels show greater proximity to and grooming of peers and have a greater number of neighbors living nearby (16). Serotonergic interventions change primate social behavior in ways that are consistent with these naturally occurring correlations. For example, chronic administration of agents that eventually deplete serotonin (i.e., fenfluramine) increases aggression and locomotor activity in male vervet monkeys (17), while serotonergic augmentation through either dietary increases in serotonin precursors (i.e., tryptophan) or a pharmacological blockade of serotonin reuptake (i.e., fluoxetine) reduces aggression, vigilance, and locomotion (18) and increases proximity to and grooming of peers (19). To address the hypothesis that augmentation of central serotonergic function would increase affiliative behavior in humans, we observed the effects of our serotonergic intervention on the social behavior of normal humans in the context of a cooperative dyadic puzzle task.

Method

Subjects and Treatment

We examined the effects of a serotonergic reuptake blockade on personality and social behavior in a double-blind protocol by randomly assigning 51 medically and psychiatrically healthy volunteers to treatment with either an SSRI, paroxetine, 20 mg/day p.o. (N = 25), or placebo (N = 26). Paroxetine was selected because of its relatively potent and specific inhibition of the serotonin reuptake mechanism in comparison with other SSRIs (20), although any SSRI may have secondary effects on other monoamine systems (21). Volunteers were recruited by advertisements in a local weekly newspaper. They gave written informed consent and were screened to exclude subjects with a history of or with first-degree relatives with a history of axis I disorders or dysthymia, as determined by the Structured Clinical Interview for DSM-III-R—Non-Patient Edition (22). Volunteers were also screened to exclude subjects with a history of psychotropic medication or substance abuse and subjects taking concurrent medications (including birth control pills in the case of women). Volunteers were informed of the possibility of physical side effects but not of the hypotheses. After complete description of the study, written informed consent was obtained from volunteers. One man and one woman in the paroxetine group did not complete the experiment because of side effects, while a second woman in the control group did not complete the experiment because of scheduling conflicts, leaving a total of 23 volunteers in the SSRI group (nine women and 14 men) and 25 in the placebo group (11 women and 14 men). The mean ages of SSRI-treated (mean = 26.7 years, SD = 2.9) and placebo-treated (mean = 27.9, SD = 4.2) volunteers did not differ.

Psychometric Measures

Standard psychometric and behavioral measures were administered at three times: at baseline, after 1 week of treatment, and after 4 weeks of treatment (i.e., at the end of the study). At each assessment, hostility was assessed with the assaultiveness and irritability subscales of the Buss-Durkee Hostility Inventory (23), as suggested by Siever and Trestman (24). To determine whether changes in hostility could be accounted for by more general changes in affective dimensions of personality, we also administered the Positive and Negative Affect Scales. Prior research has shown that different negative affects (e.g., hostility, fear) tend to be correlated in incidence, as do different positive affects (e.g., happiness, excitement). However, negative and positive affects tend to be uncorrelated with each other rather than inversely correlated, and so they are conceptualized as independent trait dimensions (25). To enhance the sensitivity of all psychometric measures to change over time, participants were asked to respond to the questionnaires in terms of their experience during the previous week.

Behavioral Measures

Objective behaviors were elicited at each assessment in the context of a standardized dyadic puzzle task. The task was designed to elicit face-valid social behaviors that could be reliably coded within the context of a cooperative interaction and subsequently compared across repeated measurement occasions. During the task, each subject collaborated with a partner in planning and implementing solutions for different spatial puzzles (also known as tangrams). Subject pairs were given 10 minutes to combine a set of seven puzzle pieces into configurations that matched as many target shapes as possible, with the stipulation that only one partner could touch the puzzle pieces at a time. Pairs always consisted of one SSRI- and one placebo-treated subject, and novel partners were assigned at each assessment. Neither the subjects nor the experimenter knew the experimental condition of pair members. One of the subjects in the SSRI group did not participate in the baseline puzzle task because of scheduling conflicts.

Puzzle-solving sessions were videotaped without volunteers' knowledge by a hidden camera placed behind a one-way mirror, so as to preserve the authenticity of the volunteers' nonverbal behavior. At the end of the experiment, an interviewer explained the rationale for the hidden camera and offered volunteers an opportunity to have their behavioral records removed from the analyses and deleted. None chose this option; all released their behavioral records for analysis. Coders who were blind to the volunteers' condition subsequently scored the videotapes for various objective social behaviors indicative of cooperation. Specifically, making suggestions while a partner handled the puzzle pieces was considered cooperative, but issuing commands while the partner handled the puzzle pieces was not. In addition, grasping the pieces with the intent of arriving at a unilateral solution was not considered cooperative. Coders attained significant agreement (intraclass $r = 0.73$, $p < 0.001$) on an aggregate measure composed of these behaviors (i.e., behavioral aggregate = (number of suggestions–number of commands)–number of unilateral grasps), which served as the index of affiliative behavior in subsequent analyses.

Plasma Measures

To determine whether individual differences in SSRI bioavailability might exist and potentially influence results, we assayed paroxetine levels in peripheral blood after 4 weeks of treatment. Assays were performed on samples of venous blood drawn at baseline and week 4. The baseline sample was drawn following an overnight fast, and the week 4 sample was also drawn following an overnight fast, 10 hours after the final dose of paroxetine. Plasma paroxetine was quantitated from these samples by using liquid

chromatography with fluorescence detection following precolumn derivatization with dansyl chloride (26). Intra- and interassay coefficients of variation were all less than 10%.

Physical Symptoms

Participants rated the severity of 16 physical side effects (e.g., nausea, insomnia, trembling) on 7-point Likert scales in a semistructured interview format. Differences between groups in physical symptoms were analyzed by separate variance t tests with a Bonferroni correction (p for 32 comparisons = 0.0016).

Statistical Analysis

Exploratory data analysis revealed that plasma paroxetine levels varied dramatically among treated individuals (range = 0–44 ng/ml, with an approximate fivefold variation across the interquartile range: 5–24 ng/ml) and that changes in both psychometric and behavioral indices were strongly correlated with changes in plasma paroxetine level. Thus, psychometric and behavioral data were analyzed in two ways: 1) with a traditional group-based approach (i.e., a 2-by-3 [treatment-by-time within] repeated measures analysis of variance), and 2) with a similar statistical model that substituted continuous changes in plasma paroxetine levels for the dichotomous grouping variable as a predictor of psychometric and behavioral changes (27). Five individuals in the SSRI-treated group showed plasma paroxetine levels below 5 ng/ml, suggesting either failure to comply with the treatment regimen or negligible bioavailability. Thus, these individuals were excluded a priori from the group-based (but not plasma-based) analyses. All individuals were included in the plasma analysis, and the plasma change value assigned to control subjects was 0, since they did not take the medication.

Differential rates of change in the SSRI-treated and placebo-treated groups were assessed by a series of pairwise contrasts on change scores from

Table 69.1

Changes in psychometric and behavioral scores from baseline to weeks 1 and 4 for normal volunteers receiving placebo or an SSRI

	Score							
	Change from baseline to week 1				Change from baseline to week 4			
	Placebo		SSRI		Placebo		SSRI	
Variable	Mean[a]	SD	Mean[a]	SD	Mean[a]	SD	Mean[a]	SD
Hostility[b]								
Assaultiveness	0.11	0.80	−0.47[c]	0.76	0.39	0.95	−0.39[c]	0.93
Irritability	0.29	0.70	−0.04	0.97	0.42	0.85	−0.23[c]	1.10
Affect[d]								
Negative	0.24	0.95	−0.51[c]	1.02	0.32	1.35	−0.50[c]	1.02
Positive	0.05	0.85	−0.50	1.14	0.08	1.05	−0.11	1.06
Affiliative behavior	−0.34	1.15	0.47[c]	1.02	−0.53	1.40	0.03	1.10

a. Standardized.
b. Buss-Durkee Hostility Inventory.
c. Significant difference from placebo group ($p < 0.05$).
d. Positive and Negative Affect Scales.

one time point to another. Specifically, effects related to early physiological changes were assessed by a planned contrast comparing changes from baseline to week 1 across groups. Effects related to later physiological changes were assessed by a second planned contrast comparing changes from baseline to week 4 across groups. Finally, differential effects of early and later physiological changes were assessed by a third planned contrast comparing changes from week 1 to week 4. All data were standardized by using the pooled mean and standard deviation of scores at baseline. All a priori hypothesis tests were two-tailed and used p < 0.05 as the significance criterion.

Results

Preliminary analyses of psychometric variables, behavioral variables, and physical symptoms with sex and treatment as dual factors yielded no significant interactions of sex with treatment

(although women did have significantly lower assaultiveness scores on the Buss-Durkee Hostility Inventory than did men at all assessment points). Thus, sex was not included as a factor in the analyses that follow in order to preserve adequate statistical power to test the hypotheses. Results for group analyses are listed in table 69.1, while results for plasma analyses are listed in table 69.2.

Psychometric Measures

Group analyses indicated that assaultiveness scores on the Buss-Durkee Hostility Inventory declined significantly for the SSRI-treated group relative to placebo control subjects at both week 1 and week 4 (treatment-by-time interaction: F = 5.04, df = 2, 82, p < 0.01) (table 69.1). While omnibus tests did not indicate a statistically significant decrement in irritability scores on the Buss-Durkee Hostility Inventory for the SSRI-treated group overall (treatment-by-time

Table 69.2

Relationship of plasma paroxetine levels to changes in psychometric and behavioral scores from baseline to weeks 1 and 4 for normal volunteers receiving placebo or an SSRI

Variable	Analysis[a]								
	Omnibus test			Change from baseline to week 1			Change from baseline to week 4		
	F	df	p	F	df	p	F	df	p
Hostility[b]									
Assaultiveness	3.12	2, 92	0.05	2.07	1, 46	0.16	4.71	1, 46	0.03
Irritability	3.81	2, 92	0.03	2.85	1, 46	0.10	7.56	1, 46	0.01
Affect[c]									
Negative	5.12	2, 92	0.01	6.06	1, 46	0.02	9.12	1, 46	<0.01
Positive	1.56	2, 92	0.22	2.44	1, 46	0.13	<1.00	1, 46	0.79
Affiliative behavior	5.88	2, 90	<0.01	10.69	1, 45	<0.01	5.49	5, 45	0.02

a. F ratio tests for time-by-plasma paroxetine level interaction.
b. Buss-Durkee Hostility Inventory.
c. Positive and Negative Affect Scales.

interaction: $F = 2.45$, df $= 2, 82$, $p < 0.10$), pairwise contrasts suggested a significant reduction at week 4. There were no significant group differences in changes in either assaultiveness or irritability scores on the Buss-Durkee Hostility Inventory from week 1 to week 4. Plasma-based analyses indicated that decreases in assaultiveness and irritability scores on the Buss-Durkee Hostility Inventory at week 4 were both significantly related to increased plasma paroxetine at the end of the experiment (table 69.2).

Group analyses also indicated that negative affect scores on the Positive and Negative Affect Scales decreased for the SSRI-treated group relative to placebo subjects at both week 1 and week 4 (treatment-by-time interaction: $F = 3.30$, df $= 2, 82$, $p < 0.05$). There were no significant group differences in changes in negative affect scores from week 1 to week 4. Plasma-based analyses also revealed that reductions in negative affect scores at week 1 and week 4 were significantly related to plasma paroxetine at the end of the experiment (table 69.2 and figure 69.1). Un-

like negative affect scores, positive affect scores did not change significantly as a function of SSRI treatment (treatment-by-time interaction: $F = 1.38$, df $= 2, 82$, $p = 0.26$), and changes in positive affect scores were not related to plasma paroxetine levels at the end of the experiment.

Analyses of covariance were conducted to determine whether global decreases in negative affect scores on the Positive and Negative Affect Scales could account for more focal changes in assaultiveness and irritability scores on the Buss-Durkee Hostility Inventory from baseline to the treatment period (the average of weeks 1 and 4) (28). Statistically controlling for changes in negative affect scores rendered relationships between plasma paroxetine levels and changes in assaultiveness and irritability scores on the Buss-Durkee Hostility Inventory nonsignificant. However, the relationship between plasma paroxetine and changes in negative affect scores remained statistically significant despite control for changes in assaultiveness scores ($F = 7.17$, df $= 1, 45$, $p < 0.01$) and irritability scores ($F = 4.63$, df $=$

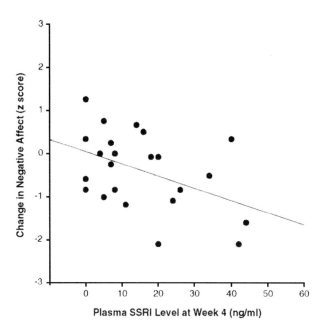

[a]r=–0.44, N=23, p<0.05. Change scores were calculated as the mean
of week 1 and week 4 scores minus baseline.

Figure 69.1
Correlation of changes in negative affect with plasma paroxetine levels at the end of the experiment for normal volunteers receiving an SSRI.[a]

1, 45, p < 0.05). Similar results obtained when items directly related to hostility were removed from the negative affect scale. Thus, in this group, SSRI-induced reductions in negative affect scores on the Positive and Negative Affect Scales (including feelings not directly related to hostility such as anxiety and depression) could statistically account for more specific reductions in assaultiveness and irritability scores on the Buss-Durkee Hostility Inventory.

Behavioral Measure

Group analyses indicated that the SSRI-treated group showed more affiliative behavior in the puzzle task than the placebo-treated group at week 1, but not at week 4 (treatment-by-time interaction: F = 3.17, df = 2, 80, p < 0.05). However, the SSRI- and placebo-treated groups did not show differential change in their affiliative behavior from week 1 to week 4. Plasma-based analyses indicated that affiliative behavior at both week 1 and week 4 was significantly related to plasma paroxetine levels at the end of the experiment (table 69.2 and figure 69.2).

Physical Symptoms

Of all physical symptoms assessed, the SSRI-treated group reported significantly more sleepi-

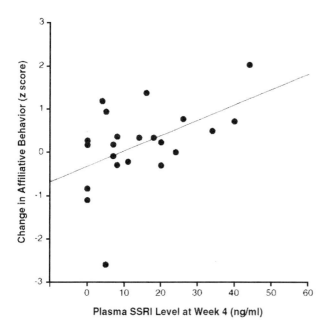

[a]r=0.65, N=22, p<0.01. Change scores were calculated as the mean of week 1 and week 4 scores minus baseline.
[b]One subject's behavioral data were not available because of scheduling conflicts.

Figure 69.2
Correlation of changes in affiliative behavior with plasma paroxetine levels at the end of the experiment for normal volunteers receiving an SSRI.[a,b]

ness at week 1 and significantly delayed orgasms at week 4 (men and women combined). Increased sleepiness at week 1 was not significantly correlated with changes in the psychometric or behavioral variables at week 1, and delayed orgasm at week 4 was not significantly correlated with changes in psychometric or behavioral variables at week 4. Thus, these physical symptoms were not included as covariates in any of the preceding analyses. However, increased sleepiness at week 1 (but not delayed orgasm at week 4) was significantly correlated with plasma paroxetine levels at the end of the experiment ($r = 0.51$, $N = 23$, $p < 0.05$).

Discussion

These data indicate that SSRI administration can modulate some aspects of personality in normal human volunteers. Furthermore, these changes show some functional selectivity. First, SSRI administration reduced psychometric assaultiveness relative to placebo; this finding extends the generalizability of clinical observations that SSRIs can reduce hostile sentiment and violent outbursts in aggressive psychiatric patients (29). Second, SSRI administration reduced negative affect relative to placebo, and this shift could statistically account for reductions in assaultiveness, which suggests that SSRIs may modulate a broader range of affective variables than those strictly related to hostility. Third, SSRI administration did not significantly alter positive affect, which indicates that global effects on arousal (as in the case of sedation) could not account for the observed reductions in negative affect. While changes in positive affect did show a nonsignificant trend toward diminution at week 1, the change was not significant and was unrelated to plasma paroxetine levels at the study's conclusion. Overall, these findings support theories which posit that separable neurochemical substrates modulate the expression of negative and positive affect (30, 31).

Besides modulating psychometric indices of negative affect, SSRI administration also enhanced behavioral indices of social affiliation in a cooperative task. While collaboratively solving a puzzle, SSRI-treated partners scored higher on an affiliative behavioral composite consisting of increased suggestions, decreased commands, and decreased unilateral solution attempts at week 1 of testing. It is unclear why this group difference did not persist until week 4, but affiliative behavior at week 4 nevertheless remained correlated with plasma paroxetine levels. Drops in affiliative behavior for both groups across time may have diminished potential group differences at week 4. These findings in human volunteers complement primate studies in which chronic SSRI treatment of male vervet monkeys enhanced a constellation of affiliative behaviors, which in turn led to increased status (19). However, affiliative behavior may raise one's status only in certain social contexts (e.g., in the absence of a preexisting dominance hierarchy, in the presence of peers who reciprocate affiliative behavior [32, 33]). Thus, while this work suggests that chronic SSRI administration can enhance affiliative behavior of normal volunteers in a cooperative task with novel partners, more research is needed on interpersonal effects of SSRI treatment in other types of social scenarios (e.g., competitive).

Analyses across time points suggested that both psychometric and behavioral effects at week 1 did not change appreciably by week 4. This may indicate that early SSRI-induced physiological changes (i.e., increased synaptic availability of serotonin) are at least sufficient to initiate psychometric and behavioral effects in normal subjects. However, it is not clear whether the persistence of these effects until week 4 is also due to early physiological changes or to later ones more commonly associated with antidepressant response (e.g., autoreceptor desensitization). Further, our data do not address whether the observed effects would persist or dwindle over longer periods of SSRI administration.

Besides differences between groups, the magnitude of changes in psychometric assaultiveness, irritability, negative affect, and behavioral affiliation was correlated with plasma levels of SSRI among SSRI-treated volunteers. Indeed, plasma SSRI predicted functional changes more robustly than did group assignment. This association is somewhat surprising, given that plasma SSRI levels do not consistently predict antidepressant response in clinically depressed patients (34). On the other hand, depressed patients who eventually respond to tricyclic antidepressants do show early changes in negative affect (e.g., at 10 days) that are more strongly associated with subsequent shifts in cerebrospinal serotonin metabolites than with depressive status per se (35). Thus, our measures may be tapping a continuum of early subsyndromal changes that either presage or bear no relation to later therapeutic responses in psychiatric patients. Others have recently reported that 6 weeks of SSRI (fluoxetine) administration did not alter the affect of normal volunteers (36), but these investigators sampled a smaller number of subjects (N = 6) and did not include individual difference measures of SSRI metabolism. Verification of the utility of these measures in predicting affective change awaits further replication.

Clearly, volunteers were not all equally affected by SSRI administration. An open-ended interview at the study's conclusion revealed that SSRI effects were often manifested in subtle and seemingly idiosyncratic ways. For example, SSRI-treated volunteers' responses to the question "What did you experience during the experiment?" ranged from "I used to think about good and bad, but now I don't; I'm in a good mood" (highest plasma SSRI level) to "The side effects were intense at first but then tapered off" (lowest plasma SSRI level). Individual differences in responsiveness to the manipulation may have arisen from several sources including (but not limited to) peripheral metabolic differences (e.g., enzymatic breakdown in the liver), central neurochemical differences (e.g., efficacy of the reuptake mechanism, postsynaptic receptor sensitivity), preexisting personality differences (e.g., baseline levels of chronic negative affect), or a combination of these factors. Unfortunately, the current design did not allow us to test for predisposing predictors of change, since correlation of change scores with the baseline scores used in their calculation invokes collinearity. Future studies might address these questions through repeated measures of relevant constructs at baseline.

In sum, this is the first empirical demonstration that chronic administration of a selective serotonin reuptake blockade can have significant personality and behavioral effects in normal humans in the absence of baseline depression or other psychopathology. These findings concur with the recent discovery of an association between a genetic polymorphism that regulates the efficacy of serotonin reuptake and negative affective components of the trait neuroticism. No such association has been observed between the polymorphism and other traits, including positive affective components of extraversion (37). While the primary application of SSRIs lies within the realm of treating psychiatric disorders, the present work indicates that these agents may provide psychological researchers with powerful tools for the "pharmacological dissection" of distinct phenomenological aspects of normal personality (38). Studies of normal volunteers with other pharmacologically selective agents may help to further delineate the specificity of serotonergic mechanisms in modulating affect and thereby may enable researchers to elucidate other psychobiological substrates of personality.

References

1. Digman JM: Personality structure: emergence of the five-factor model. Annu Rev Psychol 1990; 41:417–440.

2. Costa PT Jr, McCrae RR: Set like plaster: evidence for the stability of adult personality, in Can Personality Change? Edited by Heatherton TF, Weinberger JL. Washington, DC, American Psychological Association, 1994, pp 21–40.

3. Bouchard TJ Jr: Genes, environment, and personality. Science 1994; 264:1700–1701.

4. Cloninger CR: A systematic method for clinical description and classification of personality variants: a proposal. Arch Gen Psychiatry 1987; 44:573–588.

5. Depue RA, Luciana M, Arbisi P, Collins P, Leon A: Dopamine and the structure of personality: relation of agonist-induced dopamine activity to positive emotionality. J Pers Soc Psychol 1994; 67:485–498.

6. Zuckerman M: Good and bad humors: biochemical bases of personality and its disorders. Psychol Science 1995; 6:325–332.

7. Virkkunen M, Rawlings R, Tokola R, Poland RE, Guidotti A, Nemeroff C, Bissette G, Kalogeras K, Karonen SL, Linnoila M: CSF biochemistries, glucose metabolism, and diurnal activity rhythms in alcoholic, violent offenders, fire setters, and healthy volunteers. Arch Gen Psychiatry 1994; 51:20–27.

8. Coccaro EF, Kavoussi RJ: Neurotransmitter correlates of impulsive aggression, in Aggression and Violence: Genetic, Neurobiological, and Biosocial Perspectives. Edited by Stoff DM, Cairns RB. Hillsdale, NJ, Lawrence Erlbaum Associates, 1996, pp 67–85.

9. Fuller RW: The influence of fluoxetine on aggressive behavior. Neuropsychopharmacology 1996; 14:77–81.

10. Ellenbogen MA, Young SN, Dean P, Palmour RM, Benkelfat C: Mood response to acute tryptophan depletion in healthy volunteers: sex differences and

temporal stability. Neuropsychopharmacology 1996; 15:465–474.

11. Smith SE, Pihl RO, Young SN, Ervin FR: A test of possible cognitive and environmental influences on the mood lowering effect of tryptophan depletion in normal males. Psychopharmacology (Berl) 1987; 91: 451–457.

12. Moeller FG, Dougherty DM, Swann AC, Collins D, Davis CM, Cherek DR: Tryptophan depletion and aggressive responding in healthy males. Psychopharmacology (Berl) 1996; 126:97–103.

13. Cleare AJ, Bond AJ: The effect of tryptophan depletion and enhancement on subjective and behavioral aggression in normal male subjects. Psychopharmacology (Berl) 1995; 118:72–81.

14. Higley JD, Mehlman PT, Higley SB, Fernald B, Vickers J, Lindell SG, Taub DM, Suomi SJ, Linnoila M: Excessive mortality in young free-ranging male nonhuman primates with low cerebrospinal fluid 5-hydroxyindoleacetic acid concentration. Arch Gen Psychiatry 1996; 53:537–543.

15. Higley JD, King ST Jr, Hasert MF, Champoux M, Suomi SJ, Linnoila M: Stability of interindividual differences in serotonin function and its relationship to severe aggression and competent social behavior in rhesus macaque females. Neuropsychopharmacology 1996; 14:67–76.

16. Mehlman PT, Higley JD, Faucher I, Lilly AA, Taub DM, Vickers J, Suomi SJ, Linnoila M: Correlation of CSF 5-HIAA concentration with sociality and the timing of emigration in free-ranging primates. Am J Psychiatry 1995; 152:907–913.

17. Raleigh MJ, Brammer GL, Ritvo ER, Geller E, McGuire MT, Yuwiler A: Effects of chronic fenfluramine on blood serotonin, cerebrospinal fluid metabolites, and behavior in monkeys. Psychopharmacology (Berl) 1988; 90:503–508.

18. Raleigh MJ: Differential behavioral effects of tryptophan and 5-hydroxytryptophan in vervet monkeys: influence of catecholaminergic systems. Psychopharmacology (Berl) 1987; 93:44–50.

19. Raleigh MJ, McGuire MT, Brammer GL, Pollack DB, Yuwiler A: Serotonergic mechanisms promote dominance acquisition in adult male vervet monkeys. Brain Res 1991; 559:181–190.

20. Hyttel J: Pharmacological characterization of selective serotonin reuptake inhibitors (SSRIs). Int Clin Psychopharmacol 1994; 9(suppl 1):19–26.

21. Carlson JN, Visker KE, Nielsen DM, Keller RW Jr, Glick SD: Chronic antidepressant drug treatment reduces turning behavior and increases dopamine levels in the medial prefrontal cortex. Brain Res 1996; 707:122–126.

22. Spitzer RL, Williams JBW, Gibbon M, First MB: Structured Clinical Interview for DSM-III-R—Non-Patient Edition (SCID-NP, Version 1.0). Washington, DC, American Psychiatric Press, 1990.

23. Buss AH, Durkee A: An inventory for assessing different kinds of hostility. J Consult Psychol 1957; 21:343–349.

24. Siever L, Trestman RL: The serotonin system and aggressive personality disorder. Int Clin Psychopharmacol 1993; 8(suppl 2):33–39.

25. Watson D, Clark LA, Tellegen A: Development and validation of brief measures of positive and negative affect: the PANAS scales. J Pers Soc Psychol 1988; 54:1063–1070.

26. Brett MA, Dierdorf HD, Zussman BD, Coates PE: Determination of paroxetine in human plasma, using high-performance liquid chromatography with fluorescence detection. J Chromatogr 1987; 419:438–444.

27. Rogosa DR, Willett JB: Understanding correlates of change by modeling individual differences in growth. Psychometrika 1985; 50:203–208.

28. Baron RM, Kenny DA: The moderator-mediator variable distinction in social psychological research: conceptual, strategic, and statistical considerations. J Pers Soc Psychol 1986; 51:1173–1182.

29. Coccaro EF: Impulsive aggression and central serotonergic system function in humans: an example of a dimensional brain-behavior relationship. Int J Psychopharmacol 1992; 7:3–12.

30. Tellegen A: Structures of mood and personality and their relevance to assessing anxiety, with an emphasis on self-report, in Anxiety and the Anxiety Disorders. Edited by Tuma AH, Maser J. Hillsdale, NJ, Lawrence Erlbaum Associates, 1985, pp 681–706.

31. Depue RA, Luciana M, Arbisi P, Collins P, Leon A: Dopamine and the structure of personality: relation of agonist-induced dopamine activity to positive emotionality. J Pers Soc Psychol 1994; 67:485–498.

32. Raleigh MJ, Brammer GL, McGuire MT, Yuwiler A: Dominant social status facilitates the behavioral effects of serotonergic agonists. Brain Res 1985; 348:274–282.

33. Knutson B, Panksepp J: Effects of fluoxetine treatment on play dominance in juvenile rats. Aggressive Behavior 1996; 22:297–307.

34. van Harten J: Clinical pharmacokinetics of selective serotonin reuptake inhibitors. Clin Pharmacokinet 1993; 24:203–220.

35. Katz MM, Maas JW, Frazer A, Koslow SH, Bowden CL, Berman N, Swann AC, Stokes PE: Drug-induced actions on brain neurotransmitter systems and changes in the behaviors and emotions of depressed patients. Neuropsychopharmacology 1994; 11:89–100.

36. Barr LC, Heninger GR, Goodman W, Charney DS, Price LH: Effects of fluoxetine administration on mood response to tryptophan depletion in healthy subjects. Biol Psychiatry 1997; 41:949–954.

37. Lesch K-P, Bengel D, Heils A, Sabol SZ, Greenberg BD, Petri S, Benjamin J, Muller CR, Hamer DH, Murphy DL: Association of anxiety-related traits with a polymorphism in the serotonin transporter gene regulatory region. Science 1996; 274:1527–1531.

38. Klein DF: Anxiety reconceptualized: gleaning from pharmacological dissection: early experience with imipramine and anxiety. Mod Probl Pharmacopsychiatry 1987; 22:1–35.

70

Dopamine and the Structure of Personality: Relation of Agonist-Induced Dopamine Activity to Positive Emotionality

Richard A. Depue, Monica Luciana, Paul Arbisi, Paul Collins, and Arthur Leon

The structure of personality appears to be composed of a limited number, typically varying from three to five, of higher-order personality superfactors. Several of these superfactors have been conceived of as major emotional-motivational dispositional traits with respect to particular classes of eliciting stimuli. Almost every trait model of personality includes one such emotional trait that encompasses the elicitation of positive affect, desire, and incentive–reward motivation by signals of reward (Depue, in press; Digman, 1990; Eysenck, 1981; Gray, 1973, 1982; Tellegen & Waller, 1992; Zuckerman, 1983). That is, the emotional experience is thought to be activated by, and to motivate approach to, rewarding stimuli. Thus, from the standpoint of individual differences, this trait may represent an underlying dimension of *sensitivity* to signals of incentive reward (Depue, in press; Eysenck, 1981; Gray, 1973, 1982; Tellegen & Waller, 1992). Although numerous labels have been used to characterize this trait, including *extraversion*, because of the emotional aspects of the trait, we prefer *positive emotionality* (PE).

Interestingly, a behavioral system analog of PE is consistently observed in animals across phylogeny (Schneirla, 1959). It is variously described as an approach system, expectancy system, and behavioral facilitation system (BFS; Blackburn, Phillips, Jakubovic, & Fibiger, 1989; Collins & Depue, 1992; Depue, in press; Depue & Zald, 1993; Panksepp, 1986). All of these descriptions converge on the same basic theme: The BFS is an emotional system that has evolved to motivate forward locomotion and search behavior as a means of approaching and acquiring rewarding goals. That is, both primary and conditioned incentive stimuli elicit at least three core BFS processes: (a) an internal, subjective state of incentive–reward motivation, (b) forward locomotion as a means of supporting goal acquisition, and (c) cognitive processes, because active goal seeking facilitated by the BFS will increase interaction with, and hence the need to evaluate, the environment (Collins & Depue, 1992; Depue, in press; Depue & Iacono, 1989; Depue & Zald, 1993; Luciana, Depue, Arbisi, & Leon, 1992).

The descriptive similarity between the BFS and PE constructs suggests a strategy whereby basic animal research on BFS processes may help to further define the nature of the PE construct that has evolved from research on the structure of personality. Because of the difficulty in directly assessing central neurobiological function in humans, one particularly important extension of this strategy concerns the understanding of neurobiological bases of PE. Animal research demonstrates that BFS processes are strongly associated with activity in ascending dopamine projection systems arising from cell groups located in the ventral tegmental area (VTA) of the midbrain (Depue, in press; Le Moal & Simon, 1991; Louilot, Taghzouti, Deminiere, Simon, & Le Moal, 1987; Oades, 1985). These neurons give rise to two major ascending projection systems, termed the *mesolimbic* and *mesocortical* dopamine systems (Oades & Halliday, 1987). In innervating forebrain structures related to emotional functions, the mesolimbic dopamine system has been shown to facilitate the basic BFS components of (a) incentive–reward motivation and (b) initiation of forward locomotion by means of gating of emotional information to the motor system. Moreover, there is substantial support for mesolimbic dopamine's facilitatory role in a host of specific goal-directed affective behaviors (Le Moal & Simon, 1991; Louilot et al., 1987; Oades, 1985). On the other hand, mesocortical dopamine projections innervate the entire cortex (Le Moal & Simon, 1991; Oades & Halliday, 1987). Behavioral, neurochemical lesion, and single-cell studies demonstrate that mesocortical dopamine activity facilitates complex cognitive functions in animals and humans that would adaptively relate goal-directed behavior to changing environmental contingencies (Brozoski, Brown, Rosvold, & Goldman, 1979; Luciana, Depue, Arbisi, & Leon, 1992; Sawaguchi & Goldman-Rakic, 1991; Sawaguchi, Matsumura, & Kubota, 1990). Of importance, many of the behavioral and hormonal effects of dopamine activation are significantly influenced by genetic variation in dopamine cell number, including those dopamine cell groups in the VTA (Fink & Reis, 1981; Oades, 1985; Sved, Baker, & Reis, 1984, 1985), indicating a genetic source of individual differences in dopamine function.

Methodological Issues

Investigation of the central neurobiological basis of the PE construct in humans is faced with three complex methodological issues related to (a) the measurement of PE as representing a BFS construct, (b) assessment of central dopamine function, and (c) sampling subjects in relation to several potentially interacting personality traits. Considering personality measurement first, numerous inventories have been constructed that measure traits that conceptually relate to the BFS construct, including the Eysenck Personality Questionnaire Extraversion scale (EPQ E). Because of the emotional aspects of the PE and BFS constructs, however, Tellegen's Multidimensional Personality Questionnaire Positive Emotionality scale (MPQ PE) appeared to have ideal characteristics (Tellegen & Waller, 1992). MPQ PE, which correlates strongly ($r = .62$, $p < .01$) with EPQ E and is subject to strong genetic influence (Tellegen et al., 1988), assesses the general tendency to experience feelings of incentive–reward, effectance motivation, excitement, ambition, behavioral potency, positive affects, and a sense of well-being. An affective interpretation of higher-order MPQ PE, as well as EPQ E, is supported by convergent-discriminant relations to the state dimension of positive affect (Zevon & Tellegen, 1982), which

dominates measures of current mood (Watson & Tellegen, 1985). Most important, the MPQ PE scale was purposefully developed to assess an emotional system based on sensitivity to signals of reward by systematically incorporating in the item pool several subdomains that make up positive emotional experience with strong incentive–reward motivational components. Each of these subdomains was developed into empirically determined independent first-order dimensions, indicating that each subdomain has gained an independent contribution in the assessment of the overall PE construct. Although the most likely alternative scale is EPQ E, it was never derived in a manner to systematically define the subdomains of extraversion or the BFS construct. Extraversion on the original Maudsley Personality Inventory was a combination of sociability and impulsivity, but, in developing the EPQ, impulsivity was moved to the Psychoticism scale (Eysenck, 1981; Zuckerman, 1983). EPQ E was left basically as a sociability or gregariousness scale, tapping social activity more than social effectance, which is less in keeping with the strong motivational aspect of the BFS construct. This suggests that the MPQ PE scale is a more comprehensive measure of the BFS construct than EPQ E. Therefore, MPQ PE would appear to offer distinct advantages in determining whether there is differential association between certain subdomains of the PE construct and central dopamine function. It is also important that the MPQ PE scale is constructed in a manner that is in keeping with the nature of biologic systems. PE is unipolar, not bipolar, affectively: At the high extreme is high positive affect, at the low extreme is, *not* negative affect, as in some other factor solutions, but rather a lack of positive affect. Thus, MPQ PE could potentially map the range of low to high activity in a biological system.

Assessment of central dopamine functioning related to BFS processes poses another set of problems. First, in animals, relatively precise indices of the reactivity of the mesolimbic dopamine system are obtained through assessment of self-administration of dopamine agonists, or by the locomotor-activating effects of injected dopamine agonists, into the nucleus accumbens, the site of a major mesolimbic innervation where incentive–reward motivation and initiation of forward locomotion are strongly modulated by dopamine activity (Le Moal & Simon, 1991; Oades, 1985). Measurement of mesolimbic-induced behavioral variation to dopamine agonists in humans is not yet established, especially at the reasonably low doses of agonist likely to be used in studies of normal volunteers. This indicates that peripheral indicators reflecting the activity of other, nonmesolimbic dopamine projection systems will need to be considered in human studies. Unfortunately, it is not always clear whether the activity of dopamine systems influencing such indicators will covary with mesolimbic dopamine-induced behavioral effects, or, more simply, with BFS processes, and whether individual differences correlate across dopamine systems. Behavioral genetic research on mice has demonstrated that some forms of individual differences do correlate across dopamine systems. For example, individual differences in the number of dopamine neurons within a dopamine cell group are maintained across all dopamine cell groups, including those in the substantia nigra, VTA, and hypothalamus. Importantly, this common genetic influence on dopamine neuron number is reflected in the strongly correlated reactivity of separate indicators of different dopamine cell groups, including hormonal and behavioral indicators (Fink & Reis, 1981; Le Moal & Simon, 1991; Oades, 1985; Sved et al., 1984, 1985). This type of work requires extension to humans, and the current study represents, in part, an initial attempt in this direction.

At least two peripheral indicators of central dopamine functioning serve as potential correlates of mesolimbic dopamine function. First, prolactin secretion was assessed because dopamine is the primary substance of hypothalamic origin involved in the tonic inhibition of prolactin secretion (Ben-Jonathan, 1985). Two interdependent dopamine systems, tuberoinfundibular (TIDA) and tuberohypophyseal (THDA), exert significant inhibitory effects on prolactin secretion by way of D_2 receptors, which is the only type of dopamine receptor found in the pituitary gland (Arbogast, Murai, & Ben-Jonathan, 1989; Ben-Jonathan, 1985; Moore, 1987; Murai, Garris, & Ben-Jonathan, 1989). A correlation between hypothalamic dopamine control of prolactin secretion and of mesolimbic dopamine processes is suggested by the behavior genetics research on dopamine neuron number described above: Individual differences in dopamine neuron number found in both hypothalamic and VTA dopamine cell groups are reflected in the correlated reactivity of dopamine agonists of prolactin secretion (hypothalamic dopamine cell group) and exploratory behavior and locomotor activity (VTA mesolimbic dopamine cell group) in inbred mouse strains (Fink & Reis, 1981; Oades, 1985; Sved et al., 1984, 1985). Second, central dopamine activity, through its action on D_2 postsynaptic receptors, appears to modulate the rate of spontaneous, as opposed to reflex, eyeblinking in nonhuman primates and man (Karson, 1983). Dopamine agonists effect a dose-related increase up to 400% in the spontaneous blink rates of nonhuman primates and humans, whereas a specific D_2 receptor blocker obliterated the agonist-induced increase when administered before an agonist (Karson, 1983; Karson, Staub, Keinman, & Wyatt, 1981). Dose-related effects were not found for other transmitter agonists nor for dopamine itself (which does not cross the blood–brain barrier), the latter finding suggesting that the dopamine effect on blinking is of central origin (Karson, 1983). The neurocircuitry of spontaneous eyeblinks is complex (Karson, in press), although the nigrostriatal, and perhaps the VTA-nucleus accumbens, dopamine projections are implicated (Karson, in press). Covariation of blink modulation and mesolimbic processes is suggested by the fact that blink rates differ remarkably between bipolar depressed and manic states (Karson, in press), conditions that may reflect extreme state decreases and increases, respectively, in mesolimbic dopamine function (Depue & Iacono, 1989). Thus, blink rate and prolactin indicators of central dopamine activity are modulated by separate dopamine projection systems and, in that sense, provide method-independent replications of a dopamine–personality association.

A problem in the use of such peripheral indicators is that they are typically modulated by other neurotransmitters as well as dopamine, although not usually in the same direction. Therefore, specific-transmitter interpretations of resting values is problematic, because no transmitter has been manipulated and, thus, the relative contribution of the different transmitters to the resting value is not certain. One means of substantially increasing interpretative power is the use of a challenge protocol, where an agonist (activator) of the transmitter of interest is administered so that the functional reactivity of that transmitter can be assessed. The cleanest challenge strategy is use of a direct receptor agonist (Oades, 1985), because it reduces error variance in dopamine reactivity associated with agonists operating on release and/or reuptake processes. Accordingly, we adopted a receptor agonist challenge strategy in the current study.

A final methodological problem in a biology and personality trait study concerns subject sampling in terms of relevant combinations of personality traits. A sampling strategy was applied to cover the PE dimension as adequately as possible. However, models of the BFS relying on dopamine mechanisms generally emphasize a counterbalancing effect of serotonin, because dopamine and serotonin serve to oppose each other in the control of many biologic and behavioral variables (Depue & Spoont, 1986; Depue & Zald, 1993). This is true, for example, for prolactin secretion (dopamine inhibits and serotonin activates prolactin). An important question, then, is whether serotonin function relates to a personality trait. We have argued on the basis of

animal and human data on serotonin and behavior that (a) serotonin modulates, in a tonic inhibitory manner, the facilitation of emotional behavior by dopamine (Depue & Spoont, 1986; but particularly in Depue & Zald, 1993) and (b) that this function is related behaviorally to constraint or stability of emotional expression rather than to negative emotionality or anxiety per se, as others have suggested (Gray, 1982). The implication of this discussion for sampling in small-sample studies, which are typical of behavioral neurobiology work with humans, is that this interaction needs to be either assessed or controlled when the biology of either the BFS or constraint system is being studied. This is because not only do the BFS and constraint systems potentially interact to affect overt behavior, but also because their underlying biological systems (dopamine and serotonin?) may interact to influence biological indicators, such as prolactin. Therefore, we obtained estimates of the BFS and constraint systems through the use of Tellegen's MPQ, which defines both PE (BFS?) and Constraint (C) dimensions, where the latter is not related to negative emotionality. As shown in Figure 70.1, a two-dimensional plot of subjects on the MPQ PE (vertical axis) and C (horizontal axis) dimensions was constructed, where the diagonal from the upper left quadrant (high PE, low C) to the lower right quadrant (low PE, high C) in this two-dimensional space represents the hypothesized line of greatest behavioral (and perhaps biological) variation (see Gray, 1973, for a full discussion of a conceptually similar rationale). This is because, on the basis of our theoretical assumptions, PE represents the behavioral facilitation mechanism, whereas C, representing the constraint system, inhibits facilitation (Depue & Spoont, 1986; Depue & Zald, 1993). In the upper left quadrant, facilitation in response to rewarding stimuli would be highest (because PE is high and C is low), whereas in the lower right quadrant, facilitation would be lowest (because PE is low and C is high). Because this was an initial study of a biology–personality associa-

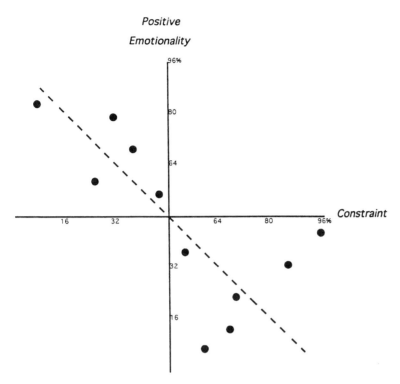

Figure 70.1
Individual plot of all subjects on the basis of a two-dimensional trait assessment. MPQ Positive Emotionality (PE) and MPQ Constraint (C) were used to construct the two-dimensional plot illustrated. Percentiles are shown along each of the two dimensions. The dashed diagonal from the upper left quadrant (high PE, low C) to the lower right quadrant (low PE, high C) represents the hypothesized line of greatest behavioral (and perhaps biological) variation. Subjects in the upper left and lower right quadrants were selected for the study to maximize differentiation along the MPQ PE dimension.

tion, we wished to maximize effects by assessing subjects who fell along the diagonal between two traits while attempting to maintain biologic specificity through direct challenge of dopamine systems. Therefore, only subjects who fell into the upper left and lower right quadrants were sampled.

In sum, then, we assessed the effects of a specific dopamine D_2 receptor agonist on two indices of central dopamine activity in subjects widely distributed along the dimension of PE. Two indices of dopamine response, prolactin and

spontaneous eyeblink, serve as a within-study replication of a PE–dopamine association, because the two indices are innervated by separate dopamine projection systems.

Method

Subjects

Subjects were recruited by distribution of notices to female graduate students and staff of two large departments at the university; all respondents completed Tellegen's MPQ. Of the 25 subjects who attended an initial group meeting, 23 (92%) agreed to be in the study. The remaining 23 subjects were then screened by use of a modified Schedule for Affective Disorders and Schizophrenia—Lifetime version interview, a process that we have used reliably in clinical studies of affective disorders: Our kappa values for agreement between independently assigned diagnoses are typically—major depression, .90; hypomania, .78; substance abuse, .90; panic disorder, .84; generalized anxiety disorder, .78; and antisocial personality, .88 (Depue et al., 1990). Subjects meeting standard psychiatric criteria for Axis I disorders (American Psychiatric Association, 1987) were excluded from the study (no subject manifested severe personality disorder), leaving 20 (89%) normal subjects.

Potential subjects who reported postmenopausal status; pregnancy; use of birth control pills during the previous 4 months; use of any prescribed medication during the past 6 months; any form of substance abuse; menstrual cycle irregularities or significant mood and physical symptoms suggestive of premenstrual syndrome; endocrinopathies or other relevant medical conditions, such as an eating disorder, obesity, oculomotor disorders, or epilepsy were excluded from study. This left 17 (88%) subjects. The sampling strategy described in the introduction was applied to these 17 subjects, whereby all subjects falling into the upper left and lower right quadrants formed by the intersection of MPQ PE and C dimensions were selected (see Figure 70.1). The remaining subjects were excluded. This provided 11 Caucasian premenopausal women, all of whom completed the protocol, who ranged in age from 20 to 36 years ($M = 28.3$, $SD = 3.1$) and in weight from 46.8 to 64.1 kg ($M = 54.1$, $SD = 3.8$).

Bromocriptine: A Dopamine Receptor Agonist

Challenge of the dopamine system was effected by the use of bromocriptine mesylate (Parlodel).

Bromocriptine is a potent agonist at D_2 receptor sites, binding with high affinity, but has little or no agonistic effect at D_1 sites or in releasing dopamine (Barton, Moore, & Demerest, 1987; Burki, Asper, Ruch, & Zuger, 1978; Fuxe et al., 1981; Jackson & Hashizume, 1987; Lieberman, 1989). Conversely, bromocriptine-induced stimulatory effects are completely blocked by the selective D_2 antagonist sulpiride (Jackson & Hashizume, 1987). It is apparently bromocriptine itself, rather than an active metabolite of the drug, that is responsible for its agonist effects. Most agonist effects occur immediately upon application of bromocriptine in in vitro models, long before an active metabolite could be formed (see Jackson & Hashizume, 1987, for a review). At sufficiently high doses, bromocriptine can potentiate the locomotor stimulant effects of other dopamine agonists (Jackson & Hashizume, 1986; Jenkins & Jackson, 1987), and this potentiation is particularly effective when both substances are coadministered into the nucleus accumbens, suggesting that bromocriptine activates dopamine terminals involved in initiating behaviors (locomotor activity) relevant to the BFS construct (Jackson & Hashizume, 1986; Jenkins & Jackson, 1987; Joyce, 1983).

Bromocriptine binds to both presynaptic D_2 autoreceptors and to postsynaptic D_2 receptors (Fuxe et al., 1981), binding preferentially at low doses to presynaptic receptors because of their greater affinity for dopamine agonists (Skirboll, Grace, & Bunney, 1978). Because of having both pre- and postsynaptic effects, bromocriptine has a time-dependent biphasic effect. Behaviorally, the biphasic effect may be seen in an initial dose-dependent immobility or hypomotility in rats, followed some time later, depending on dose, by hyperlocomotion. The biphasic effects have been ascribed to an initial agonist effect of the drug on presynaptic D_2 autoreceptors that inhibit dopamine function (Barton et al., 1987; Burki et al., 1978; Di Chiara, Porceddu, Vargiu, Argiolas, & Gessa, 1976), followed by a subsequent postsynaptic D_2 effect as bromocriptine concentration rises in blood (Gianutsos & Moore, 1980;

Joyce, 1983). The reason that low levels of plasma bromocriptine concentration have an initial presynaptic effect is thought to be the higher affinity of D_2 autoreceptors for agonists relative to postsynaptic D_2 receptors (Bannon, Grace, Bunney, & Roth, 1980; Markey, Colburn, Kopin, & Aamodt, 1979; Skirboll et al., 1978).

Although it appears that bromocriptine is a direct D_2 receptor agonist, its mode of action is complex, because its effect on D_2 receptors may require the presence of other dopamine agonists that affect either D_1 receptors or both D_2 and D_1 receptors, as dopamine does itself (Barton et al., 1987; Jackson & Hashizume, 1986, 1987; Jenkins & Jackson, 1987; Robertson & Robertson, 1986). This complexity is unlikely a concern to the present study, because administration of bromocriptine by itself has strong agonistic effects in animals with intact dopamine systems (Jackson & Hashizume, 1986, 1987), as of course is the case in our normal subjects. Bromocriptine can increase adrenergic and serotonergic metabolites after 4 hr, which may be due to a weak interaction with alpha-adrenergic and serotonin receptors (Joyce, 1983) or to compensatory increases in these transmitters due to increased dopamine activity. However, bromocriptine's effects on the dependent measures used herein (inhibition of prolactin secretion and activation of eyeblink rate) are due to its dopamine agonist properties.

In terms of influencing these dependent variables, bromocriptine effects a dose-related increase by way of D_2 receptors in the spontaneous blink rates of nonhuman primates (Karson, 1983) and has strong inhibitory effects on prolactin secretion by way of D_2 receptors in animals and man (Barton et al., 1987; Jackson & Hashizume, 1987). Bromocriptine's biphasic effect also appears to occur in blink rate, where the drug initially had no effect but later increased blink rate significantly in monkeys 1 hr after injection (Karson, 1983). The existence of autoreceptor regulation in the nigrostriatal dopamine system, which is thought to substantially affect blink rate, could provide an anatomical basis for such

an initial presynaptic effect on spontaneous blinking (Barton et al., 1987). Moreover, the biphasic effect of bromocriptine is evident in prolactin secretion, where although the TIDA system is not regulated by dopamine receptor-mediated mechanisms due to an apparent lack of presynaptic autoreceptors (Ben-Jonathan, 1985; Moore, 1987; Murai et al., 1989), the THDA system does appear to be strongly regulated by autoreceptor mechanisms (Arbogast et al., 1989; Ben-Jonathan, 1985; Murai et al., 1989). Bromocriptine induces a time-dependent biphasic effect in glucose utilization in the arcuate nucleus, the origin for the THDA and TIDA systems (Pizzolato, Soncrant, & Rappoport, 1985), and this biphasic course is temporally correlated in the same animals with bromocriptine's hypomotility–hypermotility effects (Pizzolato et al., 1985).

Finally, bromocriptine dose correlates highly with serum bromocriptine concentration in man ($r = .83$, $p = .005$; Lieberman, 1989), and this correlation would have been higher except for incomplete compliance with the protocol in two subjects. This means that serum concentration will generally reflect dose quite well, as indicated by strong correlations between both dose and serum concentration and prolactin inhibition ($r = -.93$, $p = .001$; and $r = -.76$, $p = .02$, respectively; Lieberman, 1989).

Challenge Protocol

Each protocol began at 11 A.M. with the insertion into the forearm of a 22-gauge indwelling intravenous catheter kept open by use of a heparin lock. In a randomized, crossover design under double-blind conditions, identical bromocriptine (2.5 mg, resulting in a narrow range of 0.04 to 0.05 mg/kg doses) or placebo (2.5 mg lactose) capsules were ingested at 12 noon. The two drug conditions were separated by no less than 3 days. Our pilot data demonstrated that, compared with predrug placebo values, the effects of bromocriptine on prolactin were evident 1 but not

2 days after drug ingestion. To be conservative, we instituted a 3-or-more-day interval between conditions, which was found to be an adequate washout period by others (Lieberman, 1989). The protocol ended at 6 P.M. The period of noon to 6 P.M. was selected because our pilot data showed that placebo prolactin values during this time interval are relatively flat; thereby we avoided an increasing or decreasing placebo series that might interact with drug effects.

Subjects remained awake, were not allowed to sleep, and reclined with head elevated for the entire protocol in a temperature- and humidity-controlled room with an overhead illumination of 500 lux that was measured at eye level. They stood only to go to the bathroom, which occurred on the average once per subject per day, but this did not require alteration of the catheter. Subjects were allowed to read nonemotional material or to do academic work during the protocol, except between 2:30 P.M. and 3:30 P.M., when a cognitive task was administered as part of another study. Subjects fasted from 10 P.M. the previous night until 12 noon on the day of the study, with the exception of an 8-ounce glass of 2% milk at 9 A.M. to prevent extreme hunger. Subjects fasted throughout the remainder of the protocol with the exception of water and an 8-ounce glass of 2% milk taken at the time of medication (or placebo) to prevent nausea. Subjects abstained from caffeine, nonprescription medications, and alcoholic beverages for no less than 24 hr before test days.

Prolactin Assessment

Samples for baseline serum prolactin taken before 12 noon medication were obtained at 11:45 A.M. and 11:55 A.M. and averaged (i.e., no less than 40 min after venapuncture and after adopting a reclined position); 10 samples after the noon medication were obtained every 30 min starting at 1 P.M. and ending at 5:30 P.M. No samples were taken before 1 P.M. because many studies, plus our pilot data, indicated that little or no

prolactin suppression by bromocriptine occurred in the first hour after administration. Timing of prolactin assessment was controlled by testing subjects during only January and February, and only in the early-to-middle follicular phase of the menstrual cycle, when all subjects were tested between 2 and 7 days into the menstrual cycle (the menstrual phase was determined by subject self-reports that were obtained throughout three consecutive menstrual cycles, including the cycle occurring at the time of the study).

Blood samples were spun down immediately, and serum samples were assayed in duplicate within 1 to 2 days by using a double-antibody radioimmunoassay. The assay sensitivity was 1.0 ng/mL, the interassay coefficient of variation was 7.2%, and the intraassay coefficient of variation was 6.1%. Retest stability of basal, early follicular prolactin secretion over a 6-month period was found to be $r = .71$ by Depue et al. (1990).

Spontaneous Eyeblink Assessment

Two-minute samples of spontaneous eyeblink were recorded with lights on by use of close-up lens videotaping just before prolactin samples (and not before 40 min of adaptation to the experimental room). Subjects sat upright and silent and wore noise-damping headphones to prevent auditory elicitation of blinking. Subjects were told to keep their eyes open and to not read or visually fixate on the camera; they were not instructed in any manner about blinking. Subjects did not wear contact lenses during the recordings, did not have acute eye infections, and were instructed not to sleep (which was verified in recordings). No study personnel were present, nor were other activities ongoing, in the experimental room during blink recordings.

The dependent variable was the total number of blinks that occurred in the 2-min period. A 2-min blink assessment period was selected on the basis of our earlier studies (Depue et al., 1990), which showed that the number of blinks per minute during the first 3 min of recording did not vary. However, after 3 min, the rate of blinking became variable and, hence, a less reliable estimate of a subject's blink rate. Two raters independently counted eyeblinks by use of slowed or frame-by-frame replay technology and achieved an interrater agreement ($r = .96$) similar to that found in previous studies using nonrecorded blink ratings (Karson, 1983). Retest stability of resting, nondrug blink rates across 6 months was $r = .70$ (Depue et al., 1990).

Personality Assessment

The MPQ is a factor analytically developed self-report instrument (Tellegen & Waller, 1992). Its scales represent 11 primary personality dimensions and 3 higher-order traits; alpha coefficients range from .76 to .89, with a median of .85; 30-day test–retest correlations range from .82 to .92, with a median of .89. Particular care was taken during the development of the MPQ to achieve relatively independent primary scales. Factor 1 is PE described above. Factor 2, Negative Emotionality (NE), is the extent to which one feels anxiety, anger, hostility, alienation, sadness, tension, stress, and upset. It is primarily associated with the MPQ Stress-Reaction, Alienation, and Aggression scales. This dimension shares important features with Eysenck's EPQ Neuroticism ($r = .67$, $p < .01$) and Norman–Goldberg's (reversed) Agreeability and (reversed) Emotional Stability factors. The third higher-order MPQ dimension, C, is nonaffective and assesses the extent to which someone is impulsive, cautious, and traditional. It is most strongly associated with the MPQ Control, Harm Avoidance, and Traditionalism scales. C is most clearly related to Eysenck's EPQ (reversed) Psychoticism ($r = .54$, $p < .03$) and the Norman–Goldberg Conscientiousness factor. Analysis of the MPQ in twins reared apart suggests that scores on all three higher-order scales are influenced by moderate to strong genetic influences (Tellegen et al., 1988).

Self-Rated Mood and Behavior

Subjects rated six mood and behavior items at the same times as prolactin and blink assessment. The items had 7-point scales, where each point was associated with a statement describing the specific characteristic of the respective state. Five of the items (energy, mood, incentive motivation and ambition, optimism, and speed of thought processes) load heavily ($>.45$) on one single factor that accounted for 67% of the common variance (Krauss, Depue, Arbisi, & Spoont, in press). The sixth item assessed irritability. We have used these items in prior research on daily ratings of behavior (Krauss et al., in press) and have found the items to be quite sensitive to differences between mood states within an individual over time and in mean mood state between individuals.

Interview Assessment of Depression

Because depression can affect prolactin and blink variables (Depue et al., 1990), the Hamilton Depression Rating Scale (HDRS) was administered covering the prior week on the first day of the protocol. The interrater agreement for our group on the HDRS by the use of an audiotape is adequate (intraclass correlation = .86; Depue et al., 1990).

Blood Pressure

Blood pressure was assessed by a registered nurse at the same times as prolactin while the subject was in a reclined position. Standing pressure was assessed as well at the end of the protocol.

Statistical Analysis

To use the full range of PE scores across all subjects, the bulk of the analyses relied on the Pearson product–moment correlational technique. The statistical significance for the Pearson correlations was determined according to Bonferroni's correction for multiple correlations between variables, in most cases being .01 (Kirk, 1969). It may be emphasized that our use of a dopamine receptor agonist challenge protocol means that correlations reflect an association between PE and the functional responsivity of the dopamine system. Other analyses included repeated measures analysis of variance (ANOVA) and post-hoc testing using the Newman–Keuls procedure.

The study was approved by the University Human Subjects Committee, and subjects gave informed voluntary written consent before the study.

Results

Table 70.1 shows the means and standard deviations for all variables, and Table 70.2 displays the intercorrelations between the dependent variables, grouped into maximum and temporal drug effects, and MPQ factors. Two aspects of the data reflect the effects of bromocriptine: the rate at which bromocriptine effects first appear and then reach a maximum, and the maximum bromocriptine effect.

Prolactin Secretion

Analyses began with an assessment of the efficacy of bromocriptine's inhibition of prolactin secretion. A 2 (drug: placebo or bromocriptine) × 11 (time) repeated measures ANOVA (with repeated measures on both factors) on the raw prolactin values revealed highly significant main effects of Drug, $F(1, 10) = 105.4$, $p < .0001$, and Time, $F(10, 100) = 6.72$, $p < .0001$, and a significant Drug × Time interaction, $F(10, 100) = 27.8$, $p < .001$. Post-hoc analysis of the significant interaction indicated that prolactin values were lower in the bromocriptine than in the placebo series of prolactin values, significantly so ($ps < .0001$) for all time comparisons from 2 P.M. to 5:30 P.M., a time course that is typical of bromocriptine's postsynaptic receptor effects (Pizzolato et al., 1985).

Table 70.1
Means and standard deviations for prolactin, spontaneous eyeblink, and multidimensional personality questionnaire variables

Prolactin								Spontaneous eyeblink						MPQ					
Max (ng/mL)		TMax (hr)		Descent (hr)		Baseline (ng/mL)		Max blinks/min		TMax (hr)		Placebo blinks/min		PE		NE		Constraint	
M	SD	M	SD	M	SD	M	SD	M	SD	M	SD	M	SD	M	SD	M	SD	M	SD
5.2	2.7	3.3	1.1	2.2	1.2	6.86	3.1	25.2	16	3.1	1.4	14.55	9.2	150	10	110	6	162	14

Note. MPQ = Multidimensional Personality Questionnaire; PE = Positive Emotionality; NE = Negative Emotionality; Max = maximum inhibitory (prolactin) or activatory (blink rate) effect of bromocriptine; TMax = time to Max; Descent = time to first consistent reduction in prolactin secretion due to bromocriptine; Baseline = mean of two pre-bromocriptine prolactin values; Placebo = mean of all spontaneous eyeblink values during placebo condition.

Table 70.2

Intercorrelations (alpha) between MPQ factors and the dependent variables (categorized by bromocriptine effects)

Factors	Maximum drug effect		Time to drug effect		
	PRL Max	Blink Max	PRL TMax	PRL Descent	Blink TMax
MPQ Factors					
C	.02 (.95)	.08 (.82)	−.11 (.75)	−.18 (.59)	−.24 (.48)
NE	.39 (.24)	.27 (.43)	.43 (.19)	.33 (.33)	.21 (.54)
PE	.75 (.01)	.47 (.15)	.89 (.0001)	.79 (.004)	.83 (.001)
Maximum Drug Effect					
PRL Max	—	.58 (.06)	.88 (.0001)	.68 (.02)	.58 (.06)
Blink Max		—	.54 (.09)	.18 (.59)	.19 (.59)
Time of Drug Effect					
PRL TMax			—	.71 (.01)	.78 (.004)
PRL Descent				—	.54 (.08)
Blink TMax					—

Note. MPQ = Multidimensional Personality Questionnaire; C = Constraint; NE = Negative Emotionality; PE = Positive Emotionality; PRL = prolactin; PRL Max = maximum inhibitory effect of bromocriptine; Blink Max = maximum activatory effect of bromocriptine; PRL TMax = time to PRL Max; PRL Descent = time to first consistent reduction in prolactin secretion due to bromocriptine; Blink TMax = time to Blink Max.

More detailed assessment of drug effects required the use of several corrections. Because each subject and each drug (drug or placebo) day could vary in terms of predrug basal (baseline) prolactin values, interpretation of prolactin values uncorrected for baseline after administration of bromocriptine or placebo could be confounded. Therefore, each raw prolactin value in a subject's placebo and bromocriptine prolactin series (see Figure 70.2A) was expressed as a deviation from its respective mean baseline value (see Figure 70.2B). None of the prolactin dependent variables described below correlated significantly with baseline prolactin (rs = Max .27, Descent .33, TMax .27, Descent-Max Slope .12; all $ps > .25$). Thus, each series was represented by 10 prolactin deviation values (Figure 70.2B). To determine the effect of bromocriptine, each bromocriptine deviation value was subtracted from its respective placebo deviation value (see Figure 70.2C). This corrected each bromocriptine

prolactin value for the natural diurnal variation in prolactin values manifested in the placebo series. This yielded a deviation-from-placebo score or, more simply, a series of drug effect values (Figure 70.2C). A similar method of calculation was also found to be the best representation of drug challenge prolactin values by others (Coccaro et al., 1989). These latter authors found, as did we, that a percentage of baseline calculation correlated with baseline and therefore was unsatisfactory.

These calculations yielded a series of 10 values that more precisely reflects the effect of bromocriptine on prolactin secretion from 1:00 P.M. to 5:30 P.M. Using these adjusted prolactin values, three variables can be defined, as illustrated for idealized conditions in Figure 70.3 and for one actual subject in Figure 70.2A, B, and C above. The first is the maximum postsynaptic D_2 receptor effect of bromocriptine (prolactin Max), which is defined as the maximum drug effect

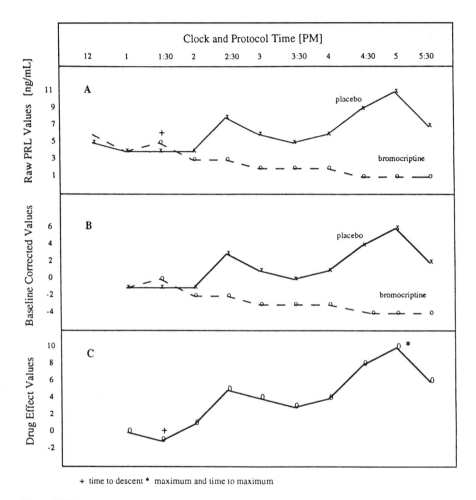

Figure 70.2
Data of an actual subject illustrating calculations used to derive dependent variables. (A) raw prolactin (PRL) values; (B) baseline-corrected PRL values; (C) drug effect values which take diurnal rhythm of placebo PRL values into account. See text for details concerning these calculations.

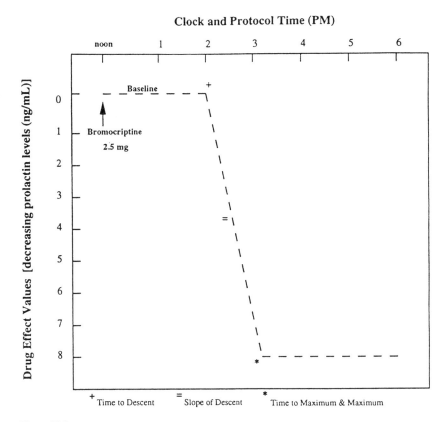

Figure 70.3

Schematic representation of the effects of bromocriptine, administered at 12 noon, on prolactin secretion as a function of protocol time (noon–6 P.M.). After corrections for baseline differences across days and for placebo values (see text for details), yielding prolactin drug effect values represented vertically in the figure, four dependent variables were calculated: time to descent (+), slope of descent (=), time to maximum (time to *), and maximum (*). See text for details concerning the definition of these variables.

value (ng/mL) derived from the adjusted values as described above. The two other prolactin variables assessed the presynaptic D_2 receptor effects of bromocriptine on prolactin secretion. We reasoned that two variables, each reflecting the time to bromocriptine's postsynaptic inhibition of prolactin secretion, would assess the efficacy of presynaptic activation: (a) time until the first, consistent reduction in prolactin drug effect values (i.e., time of first value in a series of continually decreasing values to prolactin Max without ever returning to the predecrease baseline value; prolactin descent) and (b) time until the point of maximum inhibition of prolactin secretion (prolactin TMax). Under this reasoning, presynaptic receptor effects should manifest as longer prolactin descent and prolactin TMax values with lower bromocriptine doses, because the lower dose will have more prolonged effects on the more sensitive presynaptic receptors before a postsynaptic effect. To test this possibility, five subjects were tested on two doses of bromocriptine and placebo in a design exactly as in the current study. Concordant with our hypothesis, relative to a 2.5-mg dose, a 1.25-mg dose resulted in mean increases of 1.25 (171% increase) hr for prolactin descent and of 1.25 (133% increase) hr for prolactin TMax, suggesting that these dependent variables reflect presynaptic effects of bromocriptine. Both variables seem to be influenced by a similar process in that prolactin descent correlates highly with prolactin TMax ($r = .71$, $p < .01$).

In the left column of Graphs A, B, and C of Figure 70.4, the correlational findings between MPQ PE alone (without MPQ C) and the three prolactin variables are shown. Both prolactin descent and prolactin TMax were strongly related to MPQ PE (Figure 70.4, A and B), suggesting the MPQ PE is related to the "sensitivity" of presynaptic D_2 autoreceptors to bromocriptine's agonist effects. These relations were specific to MPQ PE (see Table 70.2), as shown by the absence of significant correlations with MPQ

NE (rs $= .33$ and $.43$, respectively, ps $> .25$) and MPQ C (rs $= -.18$, $-.11$, respectively, ps $> .50$). The possibility that both prolactin descent and prolactin TMax reflect variation in the time that is required for bromocriptine to be metabolized to an active metabolite is unlikely, because most agonist effects occur immediately upon application of bromocriptine in in vitro models, long before an active metabolite could be formed (Jackson & Hashizume, 1987). Moreover, it is the dose and plasma concentration of bromocriptine per se that correlates highly with plasma prolactin inhibition in man ($r = -.93$, $p < .001$; $r = -.76$, $p = .02$, respectively [Lieberman, 1989]). In addition, to assess whether prolactin TMax was affected by the rate of bromocriptine's postsynaptic receptor action, the slope of prolactin values from prolactin time of descent to prolactin Max was calculated for each subject (Slope of Descent, as shown in Figure 70.2), but these rate values were not significantly related to MPQ PE ($r = -.37$, $p < .26$). Thus, results related to the temporal effects of bromocriptine indicate that MPQ PE is significantly correlated with presynaptic drug effects, that is, initial inhibition of prolactin secretion (prolactin descent) and time to reach maximum inhibition of prolactin secretion (prolactin TMax), but not with the rate of the postsynaptic drug effect once that effect has begun (slope of descent). Finally, to assess whether a consistent bias in the trend in prolactin values preceded the drug effect, the degree to which prolactin values before the point of prolactin descent (i.e., the average of the prolactin values occurring 30 and 60 min before the point of descent) were higher or lower than the prolactin value at the point of descent was calculated: This value was not significantly correlated with MPQ PE ($r = -.15$).

We next assessed postsynaptic D_2 receptor effects of bromocriptine on prolactin secretion. Prolactin Max was strongly related to MPQ PE (Figure 70.4C) but not to MPQ NE ($r = .39$, $p < .25$) or MPQ C ($r = .02$, $p > .50$). More-

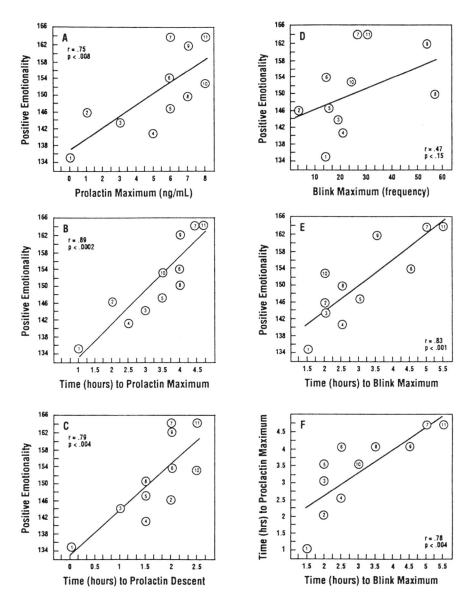

Figure 70.4

Individual subject plots of correlations between MPQ PE scores and (A) time to reach the initial point of consistent reduction in prolactin secretion due to bromocriptine (time to prolactin descent), (B) time to reach the maximum inhibition of prolactin secretion by bromocriptine (time to prolactin maximum), (C) maximum inhibitory effect of bromocriptine on prolactin secretion (prolactin maximum), (D) maximum activating effect on spontaneous eyeblink rate (blink maximum), and (E) time to reach maximum increase in spontaneous eyeblink by bromocriptine (time to blink maximum). Graph F represents the correlation between time to prolactin maximum (B) and time to blink maximum (E). Subjects are represented by the same number of each graph. See text for details concerning the definition of these variables.

over, bromocriptine's postsynaptic receptor index (PRL Max) was significantly related to both presynaptic receptor indices (prolactin TMax, $r = .88$, $p < .0004$; prolactin descent, $r = .68$, $p < .02$). Thus, pre- and postsynaptic prolactin indices of bromocriptine's D_2 receptor effects were highly correlated, and both types of index were specifically related to MPQ PE.

Finally, neither age, weight, nor height correlated significantly with prolactin Max ($rs = 0.11$, 0.12, and 0.21, respectively) or prolactin TMax ($rs = 0.13$, 0.18, and 0.19, respectively).

Spontaneous Eyeblink

A 2 (drug: placebo or bromocriptine) X 11 (time) repeated measures ANOVA (with repeated measures on both factors) on the blink values revealed a nonsignificant main effect of drug, $F(1, 10) = 1.45$, $p > .05$, and a significant main effect for time, $F(10, 100) = 2.02$, $p < .04$, but not a significant Drug × Time interaction, $F(10, 100) = 1.16$, $p > .05$. Although not significant, blink values were higher overall in the bromocriptine than in the placebo series of blink values, especially for all time comparisons from 3:00 P.M. to 5:00 P.M.

Predrug baseline blink rates did not differ significantly between the placebo and bromocriptine series. Within a series, blink rates varied greatly, with no diurnal pattern in rates within the placebo series being evident. Indeed, a one-way repeated measures ANOVA on the placebo data alone did not reveal a significant Time main effect, $F(10, 100) = 1.63$, $p > .11$. Preliminary analyses indicated that the best way to express drug effects on blinking was a simple maximum rate within the bromocriptine series and the time (in hours) to that maximum value, shown in the right column of graphs in Figure 70.4 (D and E). The correlation of MPQ PE with blink maximum (Figure 70.4D) was not significant but yielded a weak trend of $r = .47$, $p < .15$. Observation of the data showed that the drug-induced

increase in blink rate was too variable between subjects to produce significant differences. On the other hand, time to reach a blink maximum was highly significantly related to MPQ PE ($r = .83$, $p < .001$; Figure 70.4E), and again specificity was indicated by the absence of significant associations between blink TMax and MPQ NE ($r = .21$, $p > .30$) and MPQ C ($r = -.24$, $p > .30$). Neither maximum nor time to maximum blink variables correlated significantly with the mean of the placebo blink values ($rs = .11$ and $.23$, respectively). Neither age, weight, nor height correlated significantly with maximum ($rs = .03$, $.15$, $.11$, respectively) or time to maximum ($rs = .08$, $.12$, $.04$, respectively) blink variables.

As shown in graph F of Figure 70.4, the time to maximum for blinks and prolactin values is highly related ($r = .78$, $p < .004$), which suggests that the temporal effects of bromocriptine are similar and are similarly related to MPQ PE (Figure 70.4, B and E) across two variables that are influenced by separate dopamine systems.

Mood Response to Bromocriptine

The mean afternoon placebo values in self-rated mood state did not differ significantly from the mean afternoon bromocriptine values, $t(10) = 1.01$, $p > 0.20$, indicating no significant drug effect on subjective mood state (such an effect is associated with higher doses, Depue & Iacono, 1989). Maximum and time to maximum values in mood state, calculated the same as prolactin maximum and time to prolactin maximum, did not reveal significant correlations with MPQ PE ($rs = 0.10$ and 0.14, respectively). In addition, no subject reported any clinically significant somatic side effects due to bromocriptine challenge.

Level of Depression

HDRS scores ranged from 0 to 4, indicating no clinically significant depression in any subject during the week before or at the time of testing.

Blood Pressure

Blood pressure responses to bromocriptine were unreliable across subjects, showing either no consistent change or relatively episodic decreases. Maximum systolic blood pressure change (maximum − baseline) due to bromocriptine was not significantly related to MPQ PE ($r = .21$, $p > .30$).

Discussion

This initial study of an association between the structure of personality and central dopamine activity indicates that the personality dimension of positive emotionality, as measured by Tellegen's MPQ PE factor scales, is highly related to the effects of a specific D_2 receptor agonist on prolactin secretion and on the rate of spontaneous eyeblink. In terms of prolactin secretion, the strong relation of bromocriptine's D_2 receptor effects with MPQ PE was evident for both presynaptic as well as postsynaptic D_2 receptor indices. This suggests the possibility that the sensitivity of the D_2 receptor to a specific dopamine agonist is reflected equally well by both autoreceptors and postsynaptic receptors, a finding confirmed in within-animal analyses in rodents (Le Moal & Simon, 1991), and that both types of receptor relate equally well, and equally specifically, to the structure of personality. These results indicate that dopamine functional activity is positively related to PE and argue against an interpretation that low dopamine functioning, creating elevated postsynaptic receptor sensitivity, is related inversely to PE. Were the latter finding the case, which has only been demonstrated in the unusual physiologic case of dopamine denervation, then presynaptic receptor sensitivity should be reduced to increase dopamine release (Le Moal & Simon, 1991), which was not found in the current study. Furthermore, the lack of correlation of basal prolactin levels with MPQ PE suggests that direct prolactin

effects on dopamine function do not likely account for the relation between agonist-induced prolactin effects and MPQ PE.

Blink variables were consistent with the former interpretation of prolactin results, but this was only significantly so for the presynaptic association (i.e., time to blink maximum and MPQ PE). Blink rate is so variable across subjects that the sample size may have been insufficiently powerful to detect a significant relation with the postsynaptic index, blink maximum (which showed a weak trend in relation to MPQ PE). Importantly, time to maximum for blinks and time to maximum for prolactin are also highly related, indicating that two distinctly different dopamine indicators strongly reflect a common temporal drug process in relation to PE. It is important that there was no significant correlation between MPQ PE and the slope of prolactin values from time of descent to maximum, indicating that variation in PE is highly related to the time course of presynaptic autoreceptor effects, but not to the rate of the postsynaptic effect once it has begun. Moreover, the time course of drug effect is not likely to be related to the time that is required for bromocriptine to be metabolized to an active metabolite, because evidence reviewed above indicates that bromocriptine itself, rather than an active metabolite, is responsible for its agonist effects.

The strong associations of prolactin and blink rate variables, both of the pre- and postsynaptic type, with MPQ PE appear to be specific to PE. MPQ NE and C superfactors did not correlate significantly with any of the prolactin or blink rate dependent measures (see Table 70.2). The lack of association with MPQ C, despite the fact that subjects were sampled along a dimension reflecting the interaction of MPQ PE and MPQ C, is probably due to the fact that we manipulated dopamine directly. This pattern of results suggests the existence of a specific relation between dopamine and the structure of personality.

Several points of interpretative complexity are noteworthy. First, it is not certain whether blood levels of bromocriptine varied with PE because the latter were not measured. However, substantial individual differences in drug absorption are unlikely, because in humans bromocriptine dose and blood levels are highly related ($r = .83$, $p < .005$; Lieberman, 1989), and both correlate with prolactin inhibition quite highly ($r = -.93$, $p = .001$; and $r = -.76$, $p = .02$, respectively; Lieberman, 1989). Nevertheless, this issue requires analysis.

Second, because the sample was small, and because it was selected evenly along the diagonal of greatest behavioral variation between MPQ PE and MPQ C, the correlations between MPQ PE and the dopamine indices will likely be smaller in unrestricted samples. Indeed, it is important to emphasize that the goal of the current study was not to estimate the PE–dopamine relation in the population. Rather, in view of the fact that the entire paradigm used in the study is new to the area of biology and the structure of personality, the goal was to demonstrate a specific and potentially important relation between the personality construct of PE and central dopamine function, if such an association exists. We believe that this initial study demonstrates such an association, but the limits of the association still need to be determined.

Third, because prolactin and spontaneous eyeblink are regulated by a variety of neurotransmitters and neuropeptides, associations between dopamine indices and PE may be obscured under *basal* conditions, as indicated in our data by the lack of association between MPQ PE and baseline prolactin ($r = .21$, $p > .30$), baseline eyeblink ($r = .19$, $p > .30$), and pre-Descent prolactin ($r = -.15$, $p > .30$) values. Interpretative clarity is increased in this study because the response to a dopamine receptor agonist was assessed. Thus, a PE–dopamine association emerged only after reactivity of dopamine systems was induced. Fourth, interpretation of the effects of bromocriptine on prolactin and eyeblink as due solely to nonspecific processes unrelated to dopamine functioning seems unlikely, because we have observed no significant magnitude or temporal effects ($ps > .30$) of bromocriptine on biletter cancellation (attention) and nonmemory spatial location tasks or on blood pressure (general arousal; Luciana et al., 1992, and this study).

And, fifth, models of personality traits based on only one neurotransmitter are clearly too simplistic, and they will require the addition of other modulating factors. There is, however, good reason to entertain such models when the biogenic amines (dopamine, norepinephrine, and serotonin) are involved. None of the amines appear to serve primarily a mediating role in the central nervous system. Rather, they each have a particular modulatory role in influencing the flow of information in neural networks (Depue, in press; Depue & Zald, 1993; Le Moal & Simon, 1991; Oades, 1985). This fact, taken together with their broad distribution patterns in the brain (Depue & Spoont, 1986; Oades & Halliday, 1987), indicates that variation in a single amine can have widespread effects on behavior, as the animal research clearly shows experimentally (Le Moal & Simon, 1991). Thus, variation in the biogenic amines may come to provide a powerful predictor of behavioral variation. And because the amines are very old from a phylogenetic perspective, they modulate brain structures associated with very basic forms of behavior relevant to personality, including emotions, incentive reward, and motor propensity, as well as important cognitive functions (Le Moal & Simon, 1991; Luciana et al., 1992). Therefore, the currently simplistic biogenic amine models of behavior may be viewed as important building blocks for more complex future modeling of neurobehavioral systems.

What is significant is that prolactin and eyeblink variables, reflecting the action of dopamine in the hypothalamic and nigrostriatal dopamine systems, respectively, were so strongly related to a set of personality behaviors (PE) that most likely reflect dopamine function in ascending projections arising from VTA dopamine cells (Depue, in press; Le Moal & Simon, 1991;

Louilot et al., 1987; Oades, 1985). Significantly, Coccaro et al. (1989) also demonstrated strong correlation between inventory trait measures of irritability ($r = -.68$, $p < .002$); and impulsive aggressive behavior ($r = -.65$, $p < .002$; Buss-Durkee scale) and the magnitude of prolactin response to a serotonin agonist (which increases the secretion of prolactin). Because the serotonergic influence on prolactin secretion is thought to arise from ascending projections from dorsal raphe neurons to the hypothalamus (Coccaro et al., 1989), and because the dorsal raphe projections to the limbic forebrain also appear to influence affective behavior (Depue & Spoont, 1986), it is possible that characteristics of dorsal raphe function are manifested in both prolactin and behavioral variables, as suggested for the VTA above. It appears, then, that the prolactin system holds considerable promise in the study of the relation among dopamine, serotonin, and emotional behavior.

The reason that the prolactin system relates strongly to certain personality traits is not completely clear. As noted above, dopamine cell groups, including those in the substantia nigra, VTA, and hypothalamus, can manifest a common genetic influence that is reflected in their functional properties. For instance, dopamine agonist effects are correlated across prolactin secretion, exploratory behavior, and locomotor activity in inbred strains of mice that differ in dopamine neuron number in all dopamine cell groups (Fink & Reis, 1981; Oades, 1985; Sved et al., 1984, 1985). It is possible, therefore, that the heritability of MPQ PE (Tellegen et al., 1988) is related to genetic influences on dopamine cell groups and that unmeasured genetic variance in our subjects contributed substantially to the observed correlations between MPQ PE and drug response indices controlled by separate (i.e., hypothalamic and nigrostriatal) dopamine projection systems. In any case, the consistently strong and specific PE–dopamine associations found in this study indicate that the emotional–behavioral functions of dopamine derived from

animal research may hold for humans as well and that further study of BFS neurobiology within the higher-order structure of personality is clearly warranted.

References

American Psychiatric Association (1987). *Diagnostic and Statistical Manual of Mental Disorders* (3rd ed., rev.) Washington, DC: Author.

Arbogast, L., Murai, I., & Ben-Jonathan, N. (1989). Differential alterations in dopamine turnover rates in the stalk-median eminence and posterior pituitary during the preovulatory prolactin surge. *Neuroendocrinology,* 49, 525–530.

Bannon, M., Grace, A., Bunney, B., & Roth, R. (1980). Evidence for an irreversible interaction of bromocriptine with central dopamine receptors. *Naunyn-Schmiedeberg's Archives of Pharmacology,* 312, 37–41.

Barton, A., Moore, K., & Demarest, K. (1987). Differential action of bromocriptine on nigrostriatal versus mesolimbic dopaminergic neurons. *Journal of Neural Transmission,* 68, 25–39.

Ben-Jonathan, N. (1985). Dopamine: A prolactin-inhibiting hormone. *Endocrinology Review,* 6, 564–589.

Blackburn, J. R., Phillips, A. G., Jakubovic, A., & Fibiger, H. C. (1989). Dopamine and preparatory behavior: II. A neurochemical analysis. *Behavioral Neuroscience,* 103, 15–23.

Brozoski, T. J., Brown, R. M., Rosvold, H. E., & Goldman, P. S. (1979). Cognitive deficit caused by regional depletion of dopamine in prefrontal cortex of rhesus monkey. *Science,* 205, 929–931.

Burki, H., Asper, H., Ruch, W., & Zuger, P. (1978). Bromocriptine, dihydroergotoxine, methysergide, d-LSD, CF 25-397, and 29-712: Effects on the metabolism of the biogenic amines in the brain of the rat. *Psychopharmacology* 57, 227–237.

Collins, P., & Depue, R. (1992). A neurobehavioral systems approach to developmental psychopathology: Implications for disorders of affect. In D. Cichetti (Ed.), *Developmental psychopathology (Vol. 4).* Hillsdale, NJ: Erlbaum.

Coccaro, E., Siever, L., Klar, H., Maurer, G., Cochrane, K., Cooper, T., Mohs, R., & Davis, K. (1989). Serotonergic studies in patients with affective and personality disorders. *Archives of General Psychiatry, 46,* 587–599.

Depue, R. A. (in press). *Neurobehavioral systems, personality, and psychopathology.* New York: Springer-Verlag.

Depue, R. A., Arbisi, P., Krauss, S., Iacono, W., Leon, A., & Allen, J. (1990). Seasonal independence of low basal prolactin concentration and high spontaneous eye-blink rate in unipolar and bipolar seasonal affective disorder. *Archives of General Psychiatry, 47,* 356–364.

Depue, R. A., & Iacono, W. G. (1989). Neurobehavioral aspects of affective disorders. *Annual Review of Psychology, 40,* 457–492.

Depue, R. A., & Spoont, M. R. (1986). Conceptualizing a serotonin trait: A behavioral dimension of constraint. *Annals of the New York Academy of Sciences, 487,* 47–62.

Depue, R. A., & Zald, D. (1993). Biological and environmental processes in nonpsychotic psychopathology: A neurobehavioral system perspective. In C. Costello (Ed.), *Basic issues in psychopathology.* New York: Guilford Press.

Di Chiara, G., Porceddu, M., Vargiu, L., Argiolas, A., & Gessa, G. (1976). Evidence for dopamine receptors in the mouse brain mediating sedation. *Nature, 264,* 564–567.

Digman, J. (1990). Personality structure: Emergence of the five-factor model. *Annual Review of Psychology, 41,* 417–440.

Eysenck, H. J. (1981). *A model for personality.* New York: Springer-Verlag.

Fink, J. S., & Reis, D. J. (1981). Genetic variations in midbrain dopamine cell number: Parallel with differences in responses to dopaminergic agonists and in naturalistic behaviors mediated by dopaminergic systems. *Brain Research, 222,* 335–349.

Fuxe, K., Agnati, L., Kohler, C., Kuonen, D., Ogren, S., Andersson, F., & Hokfelt, T. (1981). Characterization of normal and supersensitive dopamine receptors: Effects of ergot drugs and neuropeptides. *Journal of Neural Transmission, 51,* 3–37.

Gianutsos, G., & Moore, K. (1980). Differential behavioral and biochemical effects of four dopaminergic agonists. *Psychopharmacology, 68,* 139–146.

Gray, J. A. (1973). Causal theories of personality and how to test them. In J. R. Royce (Ed.), *Multivariate analysis and psychological theory* (pp. 409–463). San Diego, CA: Academic Press.

Gray, J. A. (1982). *The neuropsychology of anxiety.* New York: Oxford Press.

Jackson, D., & Hashizume, M. (1986). Bromocriptine induces marked locomotor stimulation in dopamine-depleted mice when D-1 dopamine receptors are stimulated with SKF 38393. *Psychopharmacology, 90,* 147–149.

Jackson, D., & Hashizume, M. (1987). Bromocriptine-induced locomotor stimulation in mice is modulated by dopamine D-1 receptors. *Journal of Neural Transmission, 69,* 131–145.

Jenkins, O., & Jackson, D. (1987). Bromocriptine enhances the behavioral effects of apomorphine and dopamine after systemic or intracerebral injection in rats. *Neuropharmacology, 2,* 5–15.

Joyce, J. (1983). Multiple dopamine receptors and behavior. *Neuroscience and Behavioral Reviews, 7,* 227–256.

Karson, C. (1983). Spontaneous eye-blink rates and dopaminergic systems. *Brain, 106,* 643–653.

Karson, C. (in press). Neurocircuitry of spontaneous eye blinking. *Schizophrenia Bulletin.*

Karson, C., Staub, R. A., Keinman, J. E., & Wyatt, R. J. (1981). Drug effect on blink rates in rhesus monkeys: Preliminary studies. *Biological Psychiatry, 16,* 249–254.

Kirk, R. (1969). *Statistical procedures for the behavioral sciences.* New York: McGraw-Hill.

Krauss, S., Depue, R., Arbisi, P., & Spoont, M. (in press). Behavioral instability in seasonal affective disorder. *Psychiatry Research.*

Le Moal, M., & Simon, H. (1991). Mesocorticolimbic dopaminergic network: Functional and regulatory roles. *Physiological Reviews, 71,* 155–234.

Lieberman, J. (1989). Bromocriptine sensitivity in schizophrenia. *Archives of General Psychiatry, 46,* 908–913.

Louilot, A., Taghzouti, K., Deminiere, J. M., Simon, H., & Le Moal, M. (1987). Dopamine and behavior: Functional and theoretical considerations. In M. Sandler, *Neurotransmitter interactions in the basal ganglia* (pp. 193–204). New York: Raven Press.

Luciana, M., Depue, R. A., Arbisi, P., & Leon, A. (1992). Facilitation of working memory in humans by a D2 dopamine receptor agonist. *Journal of Cognitive Neuroscience,* 4, 58–68.

Markey, S., Colburn, R., Kopin, I., & Aamodt, R. (1979). Distribution and excretion in the rat and monkey of [^{82}Br]bromocriptine. *Journal of Pharmacology and Experimental Therapeutics,* 211, 31–35.

Moore, K. (1987). Interactions between prolactin and dopaminergic neurons. *Biology of Reproduction,* 36, 47–58.

Murai, I., Garris, P., & Ben-Jonathan, N. (1989). Time-dependent increase in plasma prolactin after pituitary stalk section: Role of posterior pituitary dopamine. *Endocrinology,* 124, 2343–2349.

Oades, R. D. (1985). The role of noradrenaline in tuning and dopamine in switching between signals in the CNS. *Neuroscience and Biobehavioral Reviews,* 9, 261–282.

Oades, R. D., & Halliday, G. M. (1987). Ventral tegmental (A10) system: Neurobiology. 1. Anatomy and connectivity. *Brain Research Reviews,* 12, 117–165.

Panksepp, J. (1986). The anatomy of emotions. In E. Plutchik & H. Kellerman (Eds.), *Emotion: Theory, research, and experience. Vol. 3: Biological foundations of emotion* (pp. 91–124). San Diego, CA: Academic Press.

Pizzolato, G., Soncrant, T. T., & Rapoport, S. I. (1985). Time-course and regional distribution of the metabolic effects of bromocriptine in the rat brain. *Brain Research,* 341, 303–312.

Robertson, G., & Robertson, H. (1986). Synergistic effects of D1 and D2 dopamine agonists on turning behaviour in rats. *Brain Research,* 384, 387–390.

Sawaguchi, T., & Goldman-Rakic, P. S. (1991). D1 dopamine receptors in prefrontal cortex: Involvement in working memory. *Science,* 251, 947–950.

Sawaguchi, T., Matsumura, M., & Kubota, K. (1990). Effects of dopamine antagonists on neuronal activity related to a delayed response task in monkey prefrontal cortex. *Journal of Neurophysiology,* 63, 1401–1412.

Schneirla, T. (1959). An evolutionary and developmental theory of biphasic processes underlying approach and withdrawal. In M. Jones (Ed.), *Nebraska Symposium on Motivation* (pp. 27–58). Lincoln: University of Nebraska Press.

Skirboll, L., Grace, A., & Bunney, B. (1978). Dopamine auto- and postsynaptic receptors: Electrophysiological

evidence for differential sensitivity to dopamine agonists. *Science,* 206, 80–82.

Sved, A. F., Baker, H. A., & Reis, D. J. (1984). Dopamine synthesis in inbred mouse strains which differ in numbers of dopamine neurons. *Brain Research,* 303, 261–266.

Sved, A. F., Baker, H. A., & Reis, D. J. (1985). Number of dopamine neurons predicts prolactin levels in two inbred mouse strains. *Experientia,* 41, 644–646.

Tellegen, A., Lykken, D. T., Bouchard, T. J., Wilcox, K. J., Segal, N. L., & Rich, S. (1988). Personality similarity in twins reared apart and together. *Journal of Personality and Social Psychology,* 54, 1031–1039.

Tellegen, A., & Waller, N. G. (1992). Exploring personality through test construction: Development of the Multidimensional Personality Questionnaire. To appear in S. R. Briggs & J. M. Cheek (Eds.), *Personality measures: Development and evaluation (Vol. 1)*. Greenwich, CT: JAI Press.

Watson, D., & Tellegen, A. (1985). Toward a consensual structure of mood. *Psychological Bulletin,* 92, 426–457.

Zevon, M. A., & Tellegen, A. (1982). The structure of mood change: An idiographic/nomothetic analysis. *Journal of Personality and Social Psychology,* 43, 111–122.

Zuckerman, M. (1983). *Biological bases of sensation seeking, impulsivity, and anxiety.* Hillsdale, NJ: Erlbaum.

VI SOCIAL INFLUENCES ON BIOLOGY AND HEALTH

A. Basic Processes

71

Socioeconomic Status and Health: The Challenge of the Gradient

Nancy E. Adler, Thomas Boyce, Margaret A. Chesney, Sheldon Cohen, Susan Folkman, Robert L. Kahn, and S. Leonard Syme

Throughout history, socioeconomic status (SES) has been linked to health. Individuals higher in the social hierarchy typically enjoy better health than do those below; SES differences are found for rates of mortality and morbidity from almost every disease and condition (Antonovsky, 1967; Illsley & Baker, 1991). Despite recognition for decades of this fundamental association, the reasons for its existence remain largely obscure. Because SES is such a powerful risk factor, a search for other etiologic factors in disease end points is often regarded as suspect unless the influence of SES is controlled. As a result, SES has been almost universally relegated to the status of a control variable and has not been systematically studied as an important etiologic factor in its own right. As Marmot, Kogevinas, and Elston (1987) noted, it is generally included "with as much regularity but with as little thought as ... gender" (p. 111).

Socioeconomic status is "a composite measure that typically incorporates economic status, measured by income; social status, measured by education; and work status, measured by occupation" (Dutton & Levine, 1989, p. 30). The three indicators are interrelated but not fully overlapping variables. Often researchers use one or another of the indicators as the measure of SES. The fact that associations between SES and health are found with each of the indicators suggests that a broader underlying dimension of social stratification or social ordering is the potent factor. In this chapter we consider SES effects broadly and examine studies using a variety of specific indicators.

Of those studies that have examined the health effects of SES, most have compared the health of individuals at the very bottom of the SES hierarchy either with those above the poverty level or with those at the top of the hierarchy (for reviews, see Antonovsky, 1967; Haan, Kaplan, & Syme, 1989). The effects of severe poverty on health may seem obvious through the impact of poor nutrition, crowded and unsanitary living conditions, and inadequate medical care. As important as these variables are, such an analysis underestimates the potent and pervasive effects of SES on biological outcomes. There is evidence that the association of SES and health occurs at every level of the SES hierarchy, not simply below the threshold of poverty. Not only do those in poverty have poorer health than those in more favored circumstances, but those at the highest level enjoy better health than do those just below (Adelstein, 1980; Kraus, Borhani, & Franti, 1980; Marmot et al., 1991; Marmot, Shipley, & Rose, 1984). This poses a challenge to understand the mechanisms by which SES affects health because factors associated with low SES are not likely to account for differences in health status at upper levels. Identifying factors that can account for the link to health all across the SES hierarchy may shed light on new mechanisms that have heretofore been ignored because of a focus on the more readily apparent correlates of poverty.

The goals of this chapter are threefold. First, we review evidence that the relationship of SES to health is not simply a threshold effect in which morbidity and mortality increase only at severe levels of deprivation, but is a graded relationship occurring at all levels within the spectrum of social position. Second, we begin the exploration of the gradient by considering factors that could account for this SES–health gradient. This exploration highlights the potential importance of psychosocial variables. Finally, we present a challenge to develop and apply new conceptual and statistical approaches to help understand the nature of the SES–health gradient.

Evidence for the Gradient

Although most studies of SES and health dichotomize individuals on SES or present a single correlation between gross levels of SES and a health outcome, some researchers have become aware of "finely stratified mortality differences running from the top to the bottom of the social hierarchy" (Smith & Egger, 1992, p. 1080). Figure 71.1 illustrates the findings of a representative subset of studies that have examined mortality rates for at least four levels of SES, and Figure 71.2 illustrates this for disease prevalence by SES. Because the SES indicators and the cutoff points used to define levels are not standardized, it is not possible to make direct comparisons across studies. However, these figures demonstrate that the SES differences in health occur at every level of SES, no matter what the SES indicator or cutoff point.

The most notable of the studies demonstrating the SES–health gradient is the Whitehall study of mortality (Marmot et al., 1984), which covered 17,350 British civil servants over a period of 10 years. The British Civil Service has ranked grades of employment. The lowest grade consists of unskilled workers (e.g., messengers). The next lowest consists of clerical workers, followed by the professional and executive levels, up to the top administrators. Relative risk of mortality over 10 years significantly increased as employment grade decreased. Compared to mortality risk of the top administrators and controlling for age, relative risk of mortality was 1.6 for the professional–executive grades, 2.2 for the clerical grades, and 2.7 for the lowest grades. Because the sample was relatively homogeneous, with all sharing employment in the Civil Service and having access to nationalized health care, these differences in mortality are all the more striking.

Similar findings emerge from census data in the United Kingdom. Susser, Watson, and Hopper (1985) documented a gradient between five levels of occupational status and standardized

mortality rates (SMR, the ratio of observed to expected deaths) in a range of diseases including malignant neoplasms, infectious and parasitic diseases, and diseases of the respiratory, digestive, and circulatory systems. Similarly, Adelstein (1980), using census data, found that SMRs for all causes of death decreased at each of six increasing levels of SES based on occupational status. The SES gradient emerged not only in SMRs but also in the prevalence rates for most, although not all, specific diseases.[1]

The SES–health gradient has been shown in U.S. studies as well.[2] For example, Kitagawa and Hauser (1973) found a graded relationship between mortality and years of education. The ratio of observed to expected deaths within subgroups among White men aged 25 to 64 years was .70 for those with a college education or better, .85 for those with some college, .91 for high school graduates, 1.03 for those with some high school, 1.07 for those completing eight years of schooling, 1.13 for those with five to seven years of education, and 1.15 for those with four years or less. Comparable ratios for White women of this age were .78, .82, .87, .91, 1.08, 1.18, and 1.60 for each of the education levels. In brief, the more years of education, the lower is the ratio of observed to expected deaths. The gradient for both income and education also emerged in more recent analyses of a national sample reported by Pappas, Queen, Hadder, and Fisher (1993). Pappas et al. compared the degree of association of mortality with education and with income in their data, collected in 1986, with that in the data analyzed by Kitagawa and Hauser (1973), collected in 1960. In the 26 years between the two studies, death rates declined, but the decreases were greater in more versus less educated groups. The resulting SES–health gradient was, thus, steeper in 1986 than it had been in 1960.

Socioeconomic status is also linked to prevalence and course of disease. Pincus, Callahan, and Burkhauser (1987) examined reports of health problems for individuals at four levels of educational attainment in a national sample and

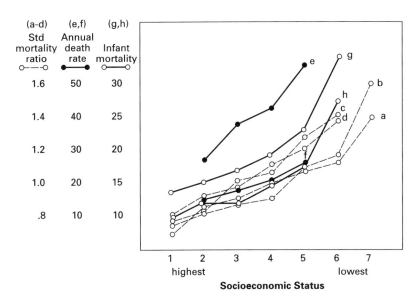

Figure 71.1
Mortality rate by socioeconomic status level.

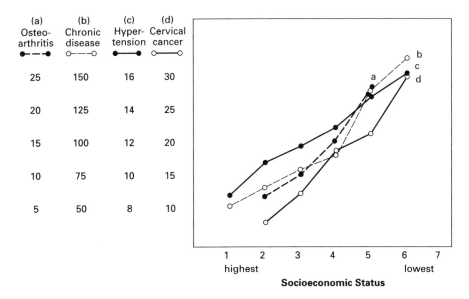

Figure 71.2
Morbidity rate by socioeconomic status level.

tested for a linear trend across educational levels. The frequency of 32 of 37 conditions assessed was greater the lower the educational level. The individual conditions were grouped into eight disease categories, and differences by education were analyzed separately in each of three age groups: 18–44, 45–54, and 55–64 years. There was a significant linear trend for almost all of the diseases in all three groups. The only disease category that was unrelated to education in all age groups was neoplastic disease.[3] Among a group of patients with rheumatoid arthritis, Pincus and Callahan (1985) found that the lower a patient's educational level, the greater was the chance of subsequent mortality or major decline in functional capacity over a 9-year period, even when controls were entered for age, sex, smoking, functional status at baseline, treatments indicative of more severe disease, or duration of disease.

Possible Mechanisms

Having reviewed the substantial evidence for a graded association between socioeconomic position and health, we next examine three possible explanations for the basis of the association. First, the empirical link between SES and health might represent a spurious association, arising from the relationships of both SES and health outcomes to underlying, genetically based factors. For example, physical size or intellectual capacity might lead concurrently to lower social position and poorer health. This explanation is plausible but improbable. As noted in both the Whitehall I and Whitehall II studies (Marmot et al., 1984; Marmot et al., 1991), although job status is inversely related to physical height, the association between job status and health persists even after adjustments for height and body mass index. As noted by Kohn and Schooler (1978), intelligence and cognitive flexibility are important correlates of job status; but it is less clear, beyond the known relationship of mental retardation to greater disease risk, that intelli-

gence in a normative population is reliably linked to health. Indeed, there is evidence that health behaviors such as compliance with medical advice are unrelated to intelligence or education (Becker, Drachman, & Kirscht, 1974; Stimson, 1974). A biologically driven predisposition to both lower SES and poorer health status appears unlikely, given the evidence at hand, to offer a sound explanation for the SES–health association. Furthermore, if genetic predispositions that we have not accounted for are involved in the SES–health link, they are very likely, as are most complex genetic influences, to become important only when environmental and behavioral factors impinge on them.

A second possible explanation for the SES–health gradient, known as the *drift hypothesis*, suggests that the association reflects the influence of illness on SES, rather than of SES on illness. There is evidence, for example, that individuals with schizophrenia follow a trajectory of descending socioeconomic resources as the natural history of their disease unfolds (Goldberg & Morrison, 1963). Nonetheless, two thorough recent reviews have concluded that, although some downward drift in social position accompanies poorer health status, the phenomenon is unlikely to play an important role in accounting for the SES–health relationship (Haan et al., 1989; Wilkinson, 1986). Deteriorating health status among older adults, which has been linked to educational levels, cannot logically affect past education (Haan et al., 1989). Furthermore, if illness principally influenced SES, then no association would be expected for family members when SES is determined by income or occupation of the head of the household, or for retired individuals for whom income is no longer dependent on health. However, such SES–health associations are generally as strong as those found for working heads of households.

Finally, the third explanation for the association is that SES affects biological functions that, in turn, influence health status. Surprisingly, we know little about how SES operates to influence biological functions that determine health status. Part of the problem may be the way in which SES is conceptualized and analyzed. It is usually treated as a main effect, operating independently of other variables to predict health. In reality, however, components of SES, including income, education, and occupation, shape one's life course and are enmeshed in key domains of life, including (a) the physical environment in which one lives and works and associated exposure to pathogens, carcinogens, and other environmental hazards; (b) the social environment and associated vulnerability to interpersonal aggression and violence as well as degree of access to social resources and supports; (c) socialization and experiences that influence psychological development and ongoing mood, affect, and cognition; and (d) health behaviors.

Within these domains, many specific candidate variables may contribute to the SES–health gradient. In this review we have selected those variables that could operate at the upper as well as at the lower end of the hierarchy, although the mechanisms or their relative impact may well differ at different levels. We have focused on variables for which there is empirical evidence of a linear relationship both with SES and with important health outcomes. This review is not exhaustive, but rather it is suggestive of the types of variables and approaches that can be taken to understanding the SES–health gradient. Elsewhere, we have considered the role of access to care in explaining the SES–health gradient and concluded that access alone could not explain the gradient (Adler, Boyce, Chesney, Folkman, & Syme, 1993). Here, we place particular emphasis on psychological and behavioral variables that have largely been overlooked because of the predominant focus on material aspects of SES differences.

Health Behaviors

Health risk behaviors such as cigarette smoking, physical inactivity, poor diet, and substance abuse are closely tied to both SES and health outcomes. Despite the close ties, the association of SES and health is reduced but not eliminated when these behaviors are statistically controlled (Marmot et al., 1984).

Smoking

Cigarette smoking is strongly linked to indexes of SES, including education, income, and employment status, and it is significantly associated with morbidity and mortality, particularly from cardiovascular disease and cancer (Adelstein, 1980; Centers for Disease Control, 1987; Devesa & Diamond, 1983; Escobedo, Anda, Smith, Remington, & Mast, 1990; Kraus et al., 1980; Marmot et al., 1991; Pugh, Power, Goldblatt, & Arber, 1991; Remington et al., 1985; Seccareccia, Menotti, & Prati, 1991; U.S. Department of Health, Education, and Welfare [DHEW], 1979; Winkleby, Fortmann, & Barrett, 1990). Smoking rates vary inversely with SES. In a U.S. community-based survey of 3,349 adults, approximately 41% of men with 12 years' education or less smoked, versus 30% of those with 13–15 years' education, 25% of those with 16 years' education, and 18% of those with more than 16 years' education. Comparable rates of smoking among women at each educational level were 36%, 24%, 15%, and 17%, respectively (Winkleby et al., 1990). A linear gradient between education and smoking prevalence was also shown in a community sample of middle-aged women: Forty-three percent of women with less than a high school education were current smokers, versus 30% of those with some college, 23% of those with a college degree, and 19% of those with advanced degrees. Additionally, among current smokers the number of cigarettes smoked was related to SES (Matthews, Kelsey, Meilahn, Kuller, & Wing, 1989).

Significant employment grade differences in smoking were found in the Whitehall II study, which examined a new cohort of 10,314 subjects from the British Civil Service beginning in 1985 (Marmot et al., 1991). Moving from the lowest to the highest employment grades, the prevalence of current smoking among men was 33.6%, 21.9%, 18.4%, 13.0%, 10.2%, and 8.3%, respectively. For women, the comparable figures were 27.5%, 22.7%, 20.3%, 15.2%, 11.6%, and 18.3%, respectively. Social class differences in smoking are likely to continue because rates of smoking initiation are inversely related to SES and because rates of cessation are positively related to SES (Escobedo et al., 1990; Kaprio & Koskenvuo, 1988; Pugh et al., 1991).

Physical Activity

Involvement in physical activity has both a direct association with health outcomes and an indirect effect insofar as it is associated with obesity. Both lack of physical activity and obesity are positively associated with poor health outcomes (U.S. Department of Health and Human Services [DHHS], 1989; Bouchard, Shepard, Stephens, Sutton, & McPherson, 1990) and are inversely related to SES (Cauley, Donfield, LaPorte, & Warhaftig, 1991; Ford et al., 1991; Kahn, Williamson, & Stevens, 1991; Marmot et al., 1991; Sobel & Stunkard, 1989).

The association of both obesity and lack of physical activity with SES emerged in the Whitehall II study for men but less strongly for women. Among the men but not among the women, those at lower employment grades were significantly more likely to report getting no moderate to vigorous exercise. In a U.S. study, Ford et al. (1991) found an association of physical activity and SES in an urban community sample. Higher SES women spent significantly more time than did their lower SES counterparts in leisure time, job-related, and household physical activity. The men showed qualitative differences in physical activity by SES: Lower SES men spent significantly more time doing household chores and walking, whereas higher SES men spent more time engaged in leisure physical activity.

Alcohol

Alcohol consumption shows the opposite pattern to smoking and other risk behaviors. Several studies (Cauley et al., 1991; Marmot et al., 1991; Matthews et al., 1989) have found a positive correlation of alcohol consumption with SES as measured by education or job status. The relationship between alcohol consumption and health outcomes, however, is not uniform across diseases. For example, although alcohol may increase risk of some cancers (e.g., cancer of the larynx) and alcohol abuse increases risk of cirrhosis of the liver, moderate levels of alcohol consumption are associated with lower risk for coronary heart disease, the leading cause of death for both men and women in the United States. In this context, the interpretation of alcohol intake as a risk factor is unclear.

Psychological Characteristics

There has been increasing evidence that psychological characteristics of the individual contribute to risk of morbidity and mortality. Of these variables, depression and hostility have shown the most consistent relationship with both SES and physical health outcomes.

Depression

Depression has been studied both as a pathological state of major depression and in terms of general depressive symptoms. Socioeconomic status is inversely related to both major depression and depressive symptoms. In a Canadian community sample, the prevalence of major depression was 1.9%, 4.5%, and 12.4% in high, average, and low SES groups, respectively. Over 16 years, the inverse gradient repeated itself in annual incidence of new depression (Murphy et al., 1991). Kaplan, Roberts, Camacho, and Coyne (1987) found higher rates of new reports of depressive symptoms over a nine-year period among those lower in income and education.

Depression is linked to health outcomes, particularly coronary heart disease. Within a sample of patients with coronary artery disease, twice as many of those with a major depressive disorder experienced at least one major cardiac event (e.g., myocardial infarction (MI), bypass surgery) in the subsequent year compared with nondepressed patients (77.8% vs. 34.9%; $p < .02$; Carney et al., 1988). In a meta-analysis of 15 studies of psychological predictors of coronary heart disease, depression was found to have a combined effect size of .21 ($p < .001$); the strongest association was with MI (combined effect size of .26, $p < .001$; Booth-Kewley & Friedman, 1987).

Hostility

Hostility—a disposition reflecting anger-proneness; a cynical, distrusting view of others; and antagonistic behavior (Barefoot, Dodge, Peterson, Dahlstrom, & Williams, 1989)—also relates both to SES and to disease risk. For example, in a national sample in the United States, hostility was inversely related to five levels of education ($p < .001$), occupational status ($p < .001$), and income ($p < .003$; Barefoot et al., 1991). Similarly, Scherwitz, Perkins, Chesney, and Hughes (1991) found greater hostility among less educated than among more educated adults in four urban areas ($p < .001$).

Several prospective studies have linked hostility to risk of coronary heart disease (CHD) and premature mortality. Dembroski, MacDougall, Costa, and Grandits (1989) found that among men under age 47, greater hostility measured on entry into the Multiple Risk Factor Intervention Trial (Multiple Risk Factor Intervention Group, 1976) conferred an adjusted relative risk of 2.1 for subsequent MI or coronary heart disease (CHD) or both ($p = .001$) controlling for cigarette smoking, diastolic blood pressure, and serum cholesterol. In a 25-year follow-up of a sample of medical students, Barefoot, Dahlstrom, and Williams (1983) found CHD incidence density to be .9 per 1000 person-years of follow-up for those with hostility scores at or below the median versus 4.5 for those above the median. And in a 10-year follow-up of a male sample, Shekelle, Gale, Ostfeld, and Paul (1983) found the relative odds of an initial CHD event to be .68 for low versus high hostility groups after adjustment for age, systolic blood pressure, serum cho-

lesterol, cigarette smoking, and alcohol intake ($p < .01$). In addition, cross-sectional studies have found associations between hostility and peripheral arterial disease (Joesoef, Wetterhal, DeStafano, Stroup, & Fronek, 1989), essential hypertension (reviewed in Diamond, 1982), and CHD (reviewed in Diamond, 1982; Barefoot et al., 1983).

Psychological Stress

Associations between SES and health may stem in part from differential exposure to and experience of greater stress. Stress has been characterized in two ways: (a) as exposure to life events that require adaptation, generally measured by a checklist of major events (e.g., divorce, death of a relative, job loss), or (b) as a state that occurs when persons perceive that demands exceed their abilities to cope, usually measured by self-reports of subjective experience. There is evidence for the role of both types of stress indicators in the SES–health link.

Life events presumably trigger perceptions of stress and negative emotion. These perceptions are known to alter neuroendocrine response and immune responses that may put persons at greater risk for a range of illnesses. Persons experiencing recent stressful life events have been found to be at greater risk for gastrointestinal disorders (Harris, 1991), menorrhagia and secondary amenorrhea (Harris, 1989), heart attacks (Theorell, 1974), and susceptibility to infectious agents (Cohen, Tyrrell, & Smith, 1991, 1993; Stone et al., 1992). Perceptions of stress and negative effect have been similarly linked to heart disease (Byrne & Whyte, 1980; Tofler et al., 1990), stroke (Harmsen, Rosengren, Tsipogianni, & Wilhelmsen, 1990), and susceptibility to infectious agents (Cohen et al., 1991, 1993).

Higher placement in the SES hierarchy can reduce stress and its somatic correlates in two ways. First, higher SES diminishes the likelihood that individuals will encounter negative events. In a community survey, lower income respondents were exposed to more stressful life events beyond their control than were higher income respondents (Dohrenwend & Dohrenwend, 1970). Similarly, Dohrenwend (1973) found that families whose head of the household had less than a high school education reported more stressful life events than did those headed by a high school graduate or better. This relation held both for events whose occurrences were within respondent control and for those outside of their control. McLeod and Kessler (1990) found small but consistent associations between SES and exposure to negative life events. A second way in which higher SES placement can reduce stress results because as individuals descend the SES hierarchy, they may have fewer social and psychological resources to cope with stressful life events and thus will be more susceptible to the subjective experience of stress. Those lower in the hierarchy may have less opportunity to form, maintain, and access social networks that can buffer the effects of stressful life events (Cohen & Wills, 1985; House et al., 1991; McLeod & Kessler, 1990). In an analysis of 720 persons interviewed in a New Haven mental health catchment area, Kessler (1979) found that persons of lower SES were exposed to more stressful events than were upper SES persons and that, given equal exposure, emotional functioning was more affected among lower than among upper SES individuals.

Evidence for a gradient relation between SES and appraisals of life as stressful was reported in an analysis of a national probability sample collected by the Harris Poll; perceptions of stress decreased in a dose–response fashion in relation to both increased household income and education (Cohen & Williamson, 1988). In summary, higher social economic status is associated with decreases in stressful events and stress perceptions, both of which may affect risk for illness.

Only one study has examined associations among education, stress, and mortality. Ruberman, Weinblatt, Goldberg, and Chaudhary (1984) examined mortality among 2,572 male survivors of MI who were assigned to the treat-ment condition in a clinical trial of a beta blocker for prevention of subsequent attacks. Educational level, social isolation, and life stress (as measured by questions involving occurrence and evaluation of events or circumstances such as experiencing major financial difficulties, not enjoying one's work, being in a low-status occupation, experiencing a divorce or violent event and reacting by being very upset, etc.) each showed an inverse gradient with mortality over a three-year period. Educational level itself was inversely related to life stress and to social isolation. Moreover, when both life stress and social isolation were high or low, education was no longer linked to differential mortality, suggesting that the zero-order association was due to the linkage of education with stress and social isolation. However, the measure of stress included measures of occupational status, which may have confounded the association with education, and replication of these findings with a better measure of stress is needed.

Effects of Social Ordering

Hierarchical position may have a direct effect on health as well as indirect effects through SES-related differences in the physical and social environment, health behaviors, or personality. In other words, one's relative position in the SES hierarchy, apart from the material implications of one's position, may affect risk of disease. Wilkinson (1992) has shown that among developed countries, per capita income is not as strongly related to life expectancy as is income distribution, with longer life expectancy associated with a greater proportion of income received by the least well-off 70% of the population. Effects of SES hierarchies are most strongly shown within countries rather than across countries, particularly in terms of life satisfaction, suggesting that relative status as opposed to absolute status may be most critical. Provocative research findings in both animals and humans provide evidence for this proposition.

Hierarchical social structures emerge in virtually all human social groups and serve to reduce intragroup aggression (LaFreniere & Charlesworth, 1983). These structures are stable over time and are present as early as the second year of life (Strayer, 1989; Strayer & Trudel, 1984; Vaughn & Waters, 1978). Dominance hierarchies in primate and subprimate groups have been inferred from observations of antagonistic, aggressive behaviors and were initially assumed to be driven primarily by survival-related competition for limited resources (e.g., food; Bernstein, 1976). More recently, evidence for stable, observable patterns of social dominance has appeared even within primate groups artificially constructed in laboratory settings with universal availability of food and other resources (Manuck, Kaplan, Adams, & Clarkson, 1988).

Hierarchical status in animal models in the laboratory and the natural environment relates to health end points and risk factors for disease. Sapolsky and Mott (1987), for example, found decreased levels of high density lipoprotein cholesterol—a protective factor in CHD—among subordinate wild baboons. Other work in the same laboratory (Sapolsky, 1989) has revealed significant associations between social rank and serum cortisol levels, secretion of gonadal steroids, and immune function.

Conditions in the larger social environment will affect the direction and magnitude of status-related health effects. Manuck and colleagues (Kaplan, Manuck, Clarkson, Lusso, & Taub, 1982; Manuck et al., 1988) found decreased coronary atherosclerosis in socially dominant cynomolgus macaques, but only under stable social conditions. Under unstable conditions that presented recurrent threats to dominance status, dominant animals showed more atherosclerosis than did submissive animals. The atherogenic effects of dominance under unstable social conditions were reversed with a beta antagonist, propranolol, implying that autonomic arousal and cardiovascular reactivity may underlie the observed association. Similarly, Sapolsky (1989)

showed that high social rank was protective in the context of a stable hierarchy but was a risk factor for disease under conditions of instability. This work has also produced limited evidence that profiles of protective versus pathogenic physiology change over time with changes in rank, suggesting that physiologic status is a function of hierarchical position rather than the reverse.

The possibility that dominance status can affect physiological and anatomic characteristics is further supported by research on the African cichlid fish, *Haplochromic burtoni*. Davis and Fernald (1990) showed that young, submissive male fish displayed slower phenotypic maturation, hypogonadism, and undersized neuronal cell bodies among the preoptic neurons responsible for secretion of gonadotropin-releasing hormone. Delayed phenotypic and anatomic maturation was found, however, only under rearing conditions in which older, territorial males were also present; in peer-rearing conditions, earlier maturation occurred as a result of more accelerated neuronal development in the preoptic area. These results suggest that the timing of central nervous system (CNS) maturational events are under social control and that dominance status within a given social context can exert profound influences on neurobiologic function.

Taken together, the studies on social order suggest the following general and preliminary observations regarding possible health effects of social dominance status per se: First, responses to hierarchical position may be encoded into the behavioral repertoire of individual organisms to protect the survival of the group and may be expressed at times even at the expense of individual well-being. Second, hierarchical position may have direct effects on physiological processes and neuroanatomic structures, which may in turn influence an individual's biologic vulnerability to agents of disease. Finally, the health effects of dominance status may be largely dependent on characteristics—particularly stability—of the larger social context in which position is assigned.

Issues of Methodology and Analysis

Research on SES and health has been limited by several conceptual and methodological constraints. First, as noted earlier, the vast majority of studies of SES and health have failed to examine the whole range of the SES hierarchy. Differentiations at upper as well as lower levels need to be examined.

Second, SES is typically measured by a single variable, such as income or education. Although various components of SES are intercorrelated, they are not identical. Socioeconomic status may function most powerfully in terms of combinations of variables. In studying psychiatric disorders, Rutter (1985) found that no single adverse condition affected risk but that "psychiatric risk went up sharply when several adversities co-existed" (p. 601). In many studies, moreover, race is used as a proxy for SES. Yet there is evidence that SES may operate differently within racial groups and may interact with race to affect health. For example, the association of race and health appears to be particularly strong among low SES Blacks, for whom the burden of discrimination may be more powerful (Klag, Whelton, Coresh, Grim, & Kuller, 1991).

Third, SES indicators have generally been measured at only one level. For example, income has generally been assessed either at the individual level (e.g., family income) or the aggregate level (e.g., mean income within a census tract). We know little about how these levels may function together to affect health outcomes. It may be that the health implications of low income are quite different for individuals living in relatively more affluent areas than in those residing in poorer areas. For example, Haan, Kaplan, and Camacho (1987) found that residing in a neighborhood that was federally designated as a poverty area (characterized by a high proportion of low-income families, substandard housing, many unskilled male laborers, etc.) was a risk factor for subsequent mortality above and be-

yond the characteristics of the individual. Using data from the Alameda County study, they found that residing in a poverty area predicted nine-year mortality rates even controlling for the individual's own socioeconomic characteristics (e.g., income or education). Similarly, neighborhood residence continued to predict subsequent mortality when controls were entered for access to health care, for health behaviors, or for social isolation. Similarly, Krieger (1992) has shown that "contextual analyses" in which neighborhood (block group, a subdivision of a census tract, encompassing about 1,000 individuals) and census tract information is used in addition to individual data provides a better understanding of health behaviors and outcomes.

Fourth, almost all studies have used either simple correlation or regression analysis to examine the main effects of SES on a health outcome. Regression analysis is severely limited in its ability to disentangle the SES–health gradient. Only a small set of variables can be analyzed in a regression model, particularly if the goal is to evaluate the interactions as well as the separate effects of the variables. For example, Haan et al. (1987), cited above, examined individual and neighborhood data as independent predictors, assessing the contribution of the latter once a given individual-level variable was controlled for. However, this does not inform us about the joint and individual functioning of these factors. Because of the complexity of the expression of SES, we need more complete measures and use of statistical procedures to analyze complex, interrelated variables. One such approach is use of tree-structured regression that examines combinations of conditions associated with poorer health outcomes (Segal & Bloch, 1989). This approach partitions populations into subgroups and then identifies different paths to given outcomes. It may be that individuals who have less than a high school education *and* who smoke *and* who are depressed *and* who live in poor neighborhoods show dramatically worse health outcomes. Taken individually these factors may have relatively weak associations with health outcomes, but their combination may be strongly associated.

Alternatively, "grade of membership" (GOM) analysis provides a way to deal with large numbers of variables. Clive, Woodbury, and Siegler (1983) demonstrated that this technique, which uses "fuzzy sets," better portrayed health status over time than did conventional models. GOM analyses develop profiles or "ideal types" either theoretically or empirically. Individuals can then be classified in terms of how closely they match these profiles. For example, Berkman, Singer, and Manton (1989) identified four profiles based on multiple indicators of health and functioning in a community sample of elderly individuals and compared how well Blacks and Whites were characterized by these profiles. An advantage of GOM analysis is that it becomes more precise as more variables are added, rather than becoming more unstable, as in regression.

A deeper understanding of the SES–health gradient may emerge if we examine how variables across multiple dimensions and levels co-occur and interact. Ideally, we would assess variables that characterize various aspects of SES, including education, income, and occupational status; individual-level variables, such as depression, hostility, sense of control, and health behaviors; and social-level variables, such as characteristics of one's residential neighborhood (e.g., % poverty, air quality), communities (health access, community norms regarding health-relevant behaviors), and work environments. Data analytic strategies that can accommodate multiple correlated variables would allow us to determine which profiles or combinations of variables were associated with better health and lower morbidity and mortality.

Conclusion

Individuals in lower social status groups have the highest rates of morbidity and mortality within most human populations. Moreover, studies of the entire SES hierarchy show that differences in social position relate to morbidity and mortality even at the upper levels of the hierarchy. This observation calls into question traditional explanations for the relationship between SES and health, which pertain primarily to the lower SES levels and the health effects of poverty.

The review presented in this chapter suggests a series of analytic and conceptual steps that should be taken in an effort to elucidate the impact of SES on health. As a first step in increasing our understanding of the SES gradient, SES should be examined in terms of a set of variables beyond the standard SES indicators. On the basis of existing studies, we have suggested several domains of such factors, which include health behaviors, psychological factors, and perceptions of social ordering. Although not reviewed here, variables in the physical and social environments, such as crowding, pollution, and access to health care, should also be included (Stokols, 1992). The range of individual variables should be broad and should include those that may lower as well as increase risk of morbidity and mortality. It is very likely that some variables and domains will be more potent at lower levels, whereas others may be more relevant to the SES–health association at the upper levels. For example, Margolis et al. (1992) found that the prevalence of both acute and persistent respiratory symptoms in infants showed dose–response relationships with SES. When risk factors such as crowding and exposure to smoking in the household were adjusted for, relative risk associated with SES was reduced but still remained significant. The data further suggest that risk factors operated differently for different SES levels; being in day care was associated with somewhat reduced incidence in lower SES families but with increased incidence among infants from high SES families.

Many of the variables linking SES to health may be dynamically intertwined. Standard analytic methods such as linear regression cannot do justice to the complex relationships among these variables. Their impact on the SES–health gradient may therefore be best described by statistical methods such as regression trees and GOM that can disentangle the effects of variables that co-occur and interact. The application of these methods will enable us to build on the foundation provided by the analysis of individual factors and increase knowledge of the ways these factors directly and in interaction affect health outcomes at different points along the SES–health gradient.

We should not expect, however, that the results of these first stages of analysis will exhaustively explain the SES gradient. Alternatively, they may point to higher order variables, which will account for aspects of the gradient not explained by the subordinate variables that interact and co-occur. The concept of individual control over existing life circumstances, for example, might be a higher order variable that synthesizes or renders coherent a number of the factors reviewed here. There is evidence, largely from older populations, that the experience of control contributes to lower morbidity and mortality (Rodin, 1986a, 1986b). Individuals higher on the socioeconomic ladder may have more frequent or more significant opportunities to influence the events that affect their lives, compared with people at lower levels. This sense of control could affect education, occupation, housing, nutrition, health behaviors, medical care, and other aspects of social class experience not previously discussed. New conceptualizations and measures of control will be needed to capture this type of cross-domain influence.

Social class is among the strongest known predictors of illness and health and yet is, paradoxically, a variable about which very little is known. Psychologists have an important role to play in unraveling the mystery of the SES–health gradient. Several plausible explanations for the puzzling and challenging gradient, including the role of stress, have been proposed, and it will be important to explore these possibilities in more depth in future research. Resolution of the conceptual and analytic dilemmas that have been the focus of this review will be key elements in the continuing, and we hope advancing, efforts to improve health and prevent disease.

Notes

1. In a few diseases such as malignant melanoma and breast cancer, a reverse gradient is found. In addition, the gradient may not emerge in every country or epoch. Although beyond the scope of this chapter, study of the variation in the direction and degree of association of SES with specific diseases across time and countries would be valuable.

2. In the United States, research has tended to focus on health differences by race rather than by SES. Research has been hampered by limitations on national data. Although the census provides data on SES, this allows only for analyses of aggregate rather than individual data. Until last year, death certificates provided information only on race; they will now also include years of education. In contrast, Britain provides a ranking of occupational status, which provides a more uniform indicator of social standing (Smith & Egger, 1992).

3. It is interesting to note that a recent review of the contribution of psychosocial factors to disease etiology (Adler & Matthews, 1993) concluded that the evidence for the role of such factors in the etiology of cancer was much weaker than for other diseases, particularly cardiovascular disease.

References

Adelstein, A. M. (1980). Life-style in occupational cancer. *Journal of Toxicology and Environmental Health,* 6, 953–962.

Adler, N. E., Boyce, T., Chesney, M., Folkman, S., & Syme, L. (1993). Socioeconomic inequalities in health: No easy solution. *Journal of the American Medical Association,* 269, 3140–3145.

Adler, N. E., & Matthews, K. (1993). Health psychology: Why do some people get sick and some stay well? *Annual Review of Psychology,* 45, 229–259.

Antonovsky, A. (1967). Social class, life expectancy and overall mortality. *Milbank Memorial Fund Quarterly,* XLV, 31–73.

Barefoot, J. C., Dahlstrom, W. G., & Williams, R. B., Jr. (1983). Hostility, CHD incidence, and total mortality: A 25-year follow-up study of 255 physicians. *Psychosomatic Medicine,* 45(1), 59–63.

Barefoot, J. C., Dodge, K. A., Peterson, B. L., Dahlstrom, W. G., & Williams, R. B., Jr. (1989). The Cook-Medley Hostility Scale: Item content and ability to predict survival. *Psychosomatic Medicine,* 51, 46–57.

Barefoot, J. C., Peterson, B. L., Dahlstrom, W. G., Siegler, I. C., Anderson, N. B., & Williams, R. B. (1991). Hostility patterns and health implications: Correlates of Cook-Medley Hostility Scale scores in a national survey. *Health Psychology,* 10, 18–24.

Becker, M. H., Drachman, R. H., & Kirscht, J. P. (1974). A new approach to explaining sick-role behavior in low-income populations. *American Journal of Public Health,* 64, 205–216.

Berkman, L., Singer, B., & Manton, K. (1989). Black/White differences in health status and mortality among the elderly. *Demography,* 26, 661–678.

Bernstein, I. S. (1976). Dominance, aggression and reproduction in primate societies. *Journal of Theoretical Biology,* 60, 459–472.

Booth-Kewley, S., & Friedman, H. S. (1987). Psychological predictors of heart disease: A quantitative review. *Psychological Bulletin,* 101, 343–362.

Bouchard, C., Shepard, R. J., Stephens, T., Sutton, J. R., & McPherson, B. D. (Eds.). (1990). *Exercise, fitness and health: A consensus of current knowledge.* Champaign, IL: Human Kinetics Books.

Byrne, D. G., & Whyte, H. M. (1980). Life events and myocardial infarction revisited: The role of measures of individual impact. *Psychosomatic Medicine,* 42, 1–10.

Carney, R. M., Rich, M. W., Freedlan, K. E., Sarni, J., TeVelde, A., Sineone, C., & Clark, K. (1988). Major depressive disorder predicts cardiac events in patients with coronary artery disease. *Psychosomatic Medicine,* 50, 627–633.

Cauley, J. A., Donfield, S. M., LaPorte, R. E., & Warhaftig, N. E. (1991). Physical activity by SES in two population-based cohorts. *Medicine and Science in Sports and Exercise,* 23, 343–352.

Centers for Disease Control. (1987). *Smoking, tobacco and health: A fact book.* Rockville, MD: U.S. Department of Health and Human Services, Public Health Service, Office on Smoking and Health.

Clive, J., Woodbury, M. A., & Siegler, I. A. (1983). Fuzzy and crisp set-theoretic-based classification of health and disease: A qualitative and quantitative comparison. *Journal of Medical Systems,* 7, 317–332.

Cohen, S., Tyrrell, D. A. J., & Smith, A. P. (1991). Psychological stress in humans and susceptibility to the common cold. *New England Journal of Medicine,* 325, 606–612.

Cohen, S., Tyrrell, D. A. J., & Smith, A. P. (1993). Negative life events, perceived stress, negative affect, and susceptibility to the common cold. *Journal of Personality and Social Psychology,* 64, 131–140.

Cohen, S., & Williamson, G. M. (1988). Stress and infectious disease in humans. *Psychological Bulletin,* 109, 5–24.

Cohen, S., & Wills, T. A. (1985). Stress, social support and the buffering hypothesis. *Psychological Bulletin,* 98, 310–357.

Cunningham, L. S., & Kelsey, J. L. (1984). Epidemiology of musculoskeletal impairments and associated disability. *Journal of Public Health,* 74, 574–579.

Davis, M. R., & Fernald, R. D. (1990). Social control of neuronal soma size. *Journal of Neurobiology,* 21, 1180–1188.

Dembroski, T. M., MacDougall, J. M., Costa, P. T., Jr., & Grandits, G. A. (1989). Components of hostility as predictors of sudden death and myocardial infarction in the Multiple Risk Factor Intervention Trial. *Psychosomatic Medicine,* 51, 514–522.

Devesa, S. S., & Diamond, E. L. (1983). Socioeconomic and racial differences in lung cancer incidence. *American Journal of Epidemiology,* 118, 818–831.

Diamond, E. L. (1982). The role of anger and hostility in essential hypertension and coronary heart disease. *Psychological Bulletin,* 92, 410–433.

Dohrenwend, B. P. (1973). Social status and stressful life events. *Journal of Personality and Social Psychology,* 28, 225–235.

Dohrenwend, B. S., & Dohrenwend, B. P. (1970). Class and race as status-related sources of stress. In S. Levine & N. A. Scotch (Eds.), *Social stress* (pp. 111–140). Chicago: Aldine.

Dutton, D. B., & Levine, S. (1989). Overview, methodological critique, and reformulation. In J. P. Bunker, D. S. Gomby, & B. H. Kehrer (Eds.), *Pathways to health* (pp. 29–69). Menlo Park, CA: The Henry J. Kaiser Family Foundation.

Escobedo, L. G., Anda, R. F., Smith, P. F., Remington, P. L., & Mast, E. E. (1990). Sociodemographic characteristics of cigarette smoking initiation in the United States. *Journal of the American Medical Association,* 264, 1550–1555.

Feldman, J., Makuc, D., Kleinman, J., & Cornoni-Huntley, J. (1989). National trends in educational differentials in mortality. *American Journal of Epidemiology,* 129, 919–933.

Ford, E. S., Merritt, R. K., Heath, G. W., Powell, K. E., Washburn, R. A., Kriska, A., & Haile, G. (1991). Physical activity behaviors in lower and higher socioeconomic status populations. *American Journal of Epidemiology,* 133, 1246–1256.

Goldberg, E. M., & Morrison, S. L. (1963). Schizophrenia and social class. *British Journal of Psychiatry,* 109, 785–802.

Haan, M. N., Kaplan, G. A., & Camacho, T. (1987). Poverty and health: Prospective evidence from the Alameda County study. *American Journal of Epidemiology,* 125, 989–998.

Haan, M. N., Kaplan, G. A., & Syme, S. L. (1989). Socioeconomic status and health: Old observations and new thoughts. In J. P. Bunker, D. S. Gomby, & B. H. Kehrer (Eds.), *Pathways to health* (pp. 76–135). Menlo Park, CA: The Henry J. Kaiser Family Foundation.

Harmsen, P., Rosengren, A., Tsipogianni, A., & Wilhelmsen, L. (1990). Risk factors for stroke in middle-aged men in Goteborg, Sweden. *Stroke,* 21, 23–29.

Harris, T. O. (1989). Physical illness: An introduction. In G. W. Brown & T. O. Harris (Eds.), *Life events and illness* (pp. 199–212). New York: Guilford Press.

Harris, T. O. (1991). Life stress and illness: The question of specificity. *Annals of Behavioral Medicine,* 13, 211–219.

House, J. S., Kessler, R., Herzog, A. R., Mero, R., Kinney, A., & Breslow, M. (1991). Social stratification, age, and health. In K. W. Scheie, D. Blazer, & J. S. House (Eds.), *Aging, health behaviors, and health outcomes* (pp. 1–32). Hillsdale, NJ: Erlbaum.

Illsley, R., & Baker, D. (1991). Contextual variations in the meaning of health inequality. *Social Science and Medicine,* 32, 359–365.

Joesoef, M. R., Wetterhal, S. F., DeStafano, F., Stroup, N. E., & Fronek, A. (1989). The association of peripheral arterial disease with hostility in a young,

healthy veteran population. *Psychosomatic Medicine,* 51, 285–289.

Kahn, H. S., Williamson, D. F., & Stevens, J. A. (1991). Race and weight change in U.S. women: The roles of socioeconomic and marital status. *American Journal of Public Health,* 81, 319–323.

Kaplan, G. A., Roberts, R. E., Camacho, T. C., & Coyne, J. C. (1987). Psychosocial predictors of depression: Prospective evidence from the Human Population Laboratory studies. *American Journal of Epidemiology,* 125, 206–220.

Kaplan, J. R., Manuck, S. B., Clarkson, T. B., Lusso, F. B., & Taub, D. M. (1982). Social status, environment, and atherosclerosis in cynomolgus monkeys. *Arteriosclerosis,* 2, 359–368.

Kaprio, J., & Koskenvuo, M. (1988). A prospective study of psychological and socioeconomic characteristics, health behavior and morbidity in cigarette smokers prior to quitting compared to persistent smokers and non-smokers. *Journal of Clinical Epidemiology,* 41, 139–150.

Kessler, R. C. (1979). Social status and psychological distress. *Journal of Health and Social Behavior,* 20, 259–272.

Kitagawa, E. M., & Hauser, P. M. (Eds.). (1973). *Differential mortality in the United States: A study in socioeconomic epidemiology.* Cambridge, MA: Harvard University Press.

Klag, M., Whelton, P., Coresh, J., Grim, C., & Kuller, L. (1991). The association of skin color with blood pressure in U.S. Blacks with low socioeconomic status. *Journal of the American Medical Association,* 265, 599–602.

Kohn, M., & Schooler, C. (1978). The reciprocal effects of the substantive complexity of work and intellectual flexibility: A longitudinal assessment. *American Journal of Sociology,* 84, 24–52.

Kraus, J. F., Borhani, N. O., & Franti, C. E. (1980). Socioeconomic status, ethnicity, and risk of coronary heart disease. *American Journal of Epidemiology,* 111, 407–414.

Krieger, N. (1992). Overcoming the absence of socioeconomic data in medical records: Validation and application of a census-based methodology. *American Journal of Public Health,* 82, 703–710.

LaFreniere, P. J., & Charlesworth, W. R. (1983). Dominance, attention and affiliation in a preschool group: A nine-month longitudinal study. *Ethology and Sociobiology*, 4, 55–67.

Manuck, S. B., Kaplan, J. R., Adams, M. R., & Clarkson, T. B. (1988). Studies of psychosocial influences on coronary artery atherogenesis in cynomolgus monkeys. *Health Psychology*, 7, 113–124.

Margolis, P. A., Greenberg, R. A., Keyes, L. L., Lavange, L. M., Chapman, R. S., Denny, F. W., Bauman, K. E., & Boat, B. W. (1992). Lower respiratory illness in infants and low socioeconomic status. *American Journal of Public Health*, 82, 1119–1126.

Marmot, M. G., Kogevinas, M., & Elston, M. A. (1987). Social/economic status and disease. *Annual Review of Public Health*, 8, 111–135.

Marmot, M. G., Smith, G. D., Stansfeld, S., Patel, C., North, F., Head, J., White, I., Brunner, E., & Feeney, A. (1991). Health inequalities among British civil servants: The Whitehall II study. *Lancet*, 337, 1387–1393.

Marmot, M. G., Shipley, M. J., & Rose, G. (1984). Inequalities in death: Specific explanations of a general pattern? *Lancet*, 1, 1003–1006.

Matthews, K., Kelsey, S., Meilahn, E., Kuller, L., & Wing, R. (1989). Educational attainment and behavioral and biologic risk factors for coronary heart disease in middle-aged women. *American Journal of Epidemiology*, 129, 1132–1144.

McLeod, J. D., & Kessler, R. C. (1990). Socioeconomic status differences in vulnerability to undesirable life events. *Journal of Health and Social Behavior*, 31, 162–172.

Multiple Risk Factor Intervention Group. (1976). The Multiple Risk Factor Intervention Trial (MRFIT): A national study of primary prevention of coronary heart disease. *Journal of the American Medical Association*, 235, 825–827.

Murphy, J. M., Olivier, D. C., Monson, R. R., Sobol, A. M., Federman, E. B., & Leighton, A. H. (1991). Depression and anxiety in relation to social status. *Archives of General Psychiatry*, 48, 223–229.

Pappas, G., Queen, S., Hadden, W., & Fisher, G. (1993). The increasing disparity in mortality between socioeconomic groups in the United States, 1960 and 1986. *The New England Journal of Medicine*, 329(2), 103–109.

Pincus, T., & Callahan, L. F. (1985). Formal education as a marker for increased mortality and morbidity

in rheumatoid arthritis. *Journal of Chronic Diseases*, 38, 973–984.

Pincus, T., Callahan, L. F., & Burkhauser, R. V. (1987). Most chronic diseases are reported more frequently by individuals with fewer than 12 years of formal education in the age 18–64 U.S. population. *Journal of Chronic Diseases*, 40, 865–874.

Pugh, H., Power, C., Goldblatt, P., & Arber, S. (1991). Women's lung cancer mortality, socio-economic status and changing smoking patterns. *Social Science and Medicine*, 32, 1105–1110.

Remington, P. L., Forman, M. R., Gentry, E. M., Marks, J. S., Hogelin, G. C., & Trowbridge, F. L. (1985). Current smoking trends in the United States: The 1981–1983 behavioral risk factor surveys. *Journal of the American Medical Association*, 253, 2975–2978.

Rodin, J. (1986a). Aging and health: Effects of the sense of control. *Science*, 233, 1271–1276.

Rodin, J. (1986b). Health, control, and aging. In M. Baltes & P. Baltes (Eds.), *Aging and control* (pp. 139–165). Hillsdale, NJ: Erlbaum.

Ruberman, W., Weinblatt, E., Goldberg. J., & Chaudhary, B. (1984). Psychosocial influences on mortality after myocardial infarction. *The New England Journal of Medicine*, 311, 552–559.

Rutter, M. (1985). Resilience in the face of adversity: Protective factors and resistance to psychiatric disorder. *British Journal of Psychiatry*, 147, 598–611.

Sapolsky, R. M. (1989). Hypercortisolism among socially subordinate wild baboons originates at the CNS level. *Archives of General Psychiatry*, 46, 1047–1051.

Sapolsky, R. M., & Mott, G. E. (1987). Social subordination in wild baboons is associated with suppressed high density lipoprotein-cholesterol concentrations: The possible role of chronic social stress. *Endocrinology*, 121, 1605–1610.

Scherwitz, L., Perkins, L., Chesney, M., & Hughes, G. (1991). Cook-Medley Hostility Scale and subsets: Relationship to demographic and psychosocial characteristics in young adults in the CARDIA study. *Psychosomatic Medicine*, 53, 36–49.

Seccareccia, F., Menotti, A., & Prati, P. L. (1991). Coronary heart disease prevention: Relationship between socio-economic status and knowledge, motivation and behavior in a free-living male, adult population. *European Journal of Epidemiology*, 7(6), 166–170.

Segal, M. R., & Block, D. A. (1989). A comparison of estimated proportional hazards models and regression trees. *Statistics in Medicine, 8,* 539–550.

Shekelle, R. B., Gale, M., Ostfeld, A., & Paul, O. (1983). Hostility, risk of coronary heart disease, and mortality. *Psychosomatic Medicine, 45,* 109–114.

Smith, G. D., & Egger, M. (1992). Socioeconomic differences in mortality in Britain and the U.S. *American Journal of Public Health, 82,* 1079–1080.

Sobel, J., & Stunkard, A. J. (1989). Socioeconomic status and obesity: A review of the literature. *Psychological Bulletin, 105,* 260–271.

Stimson, G. V. (1974). Obeying doctor's orders: A view from the other side. *Social Science and Medicine, 8,* 97–104.

Stokols, D. (1992). Establishing and maintaining healthy environments: Toward a social ecology of health promotion. *American Psychologist, 47,* 6–22.

Stone, A. A. L., Bovbjerg, D. H., Neale, J. M., Napoli, A., Valdimarsdottir, H., Cox, D., Hayden, F. G., & Gwaltney, J. M., Jr. (1992). Development of the common cold symptoms following experimental rhinovirus infection is related to prior stressful life events. *Behavioral Medicine, 13,* 70–74.

Strayer, F. F. (1989). Co-adaptation within the early peer group: A psychobiological study of social competence. In B. H. Schneider (Ed.), *Social competence in developmental perspective* (pp. 145–172). Norwell, MA: Kluwer Academic.

Strayer, F. F., & Trudel, M. (1984). Developmental changes in the nature and function of social dominance among young children. *Ethology and Sociobiology, 5,* 279–295.

Susser, M., Watson, W., & Hopper, K. (1985). *Sociology in medicine* (3rd ed.). Oxford, England: Oxford University Press.

Theorell, T. (1974). Life events before and after the onset of a premature myocardial infarction. In B. S. Dohrenwend & B. P. Dohrenwend (Eds.), *Stressful life events: Their nature and effects* (pp. 101–117). New York: Wiley.

Tofler, G. H., Stone, P. H., Maclure, M., Edelman, E., Davis, V. G., Robertson, T., Antman, E. M., Muller, J. E., & The MILIS Study Group. (1990). Analysis of possible triggers of acute myocardial infarction (The MILIS Study). *The American Journal of Cardiology, 66,* 22–27.

Townsend, P. (1974). Inequality and the health service. *Lancet, 1,* 1179–1189.

U.S. Department of Health, Education and Welfare. (1979). *Smoking and health: A report of the Surgeon General 1979* (USDHEW Publication No. 79-50066). Washington, DC: U.S. Government Printing Office, Public Health Service.

U.S. Department of Health and Human Services. (1989). *Promoting health/preventing disease: Year 2000 objectives for the nation.* Washington, DC: United States Department of Health and Human Service, Public Health Service.

Vaughn, B., & Waters, E. (1978). Social organization among preschooler peers: Dominance, attention and sociometric correlates. In D. R. Omark, F. F. Strayer, & D. Freedman (Eds.), *Dominance relations: An ethological view of human conflict and social interaction* (pp. 359–380). New York: Garland STPM Press.

Wilkinson, R. G. (Ed.). (1986). *Class and health: Research and longitudinal data.* London: Tavistock Publications.

Wilkinson, R. G. (1992). Income distribution and life expectancy. *British Medical Journal, 304,* 165–168.

Winkleby, M., Fortmann, S., & Barrett, D. (1990). Social class disparities in risk factors for disease: Eight-year prevalence patterns by level of education. *Preventive Medicine, 19,* 1–12.

72 Psychological Influences on Surgical Recovery: Perspectives from Psychoneuroimmunology

Janice K. Kiecolt-Glaser, Gayle G. Page, Phillip T. Marucha, Robert C. MacCallum, and Ronald Glaser

Surgery is a threatening experience, with multiple stressful components—concerns about one's physical condition, admission to a hospital, anticipation of painful procedures, worries about survival and recovery, and separation from family. Accordingly, it is not surprising that even operations that physicians consider "minor" can provoke strong emotional reactions in patients (Johnston, 1988). If these psychological responses are sufficiently intense, they can have important consequences: The weight of the evidence suggests that greater distress or anxiety prior to surgery is associated with a slower and more complicated postoperative recovery (Johnston & Wallace, 1990; Mathews & Ridgeway, 1981). Moreover, researchers who have assessed the impact of psychosocial interventions administered before surgery have generally demonstrated positive effects on postsurgical psychological and physical function (see reviews by Contrada, Leventhal, & Anderson, 1994; Devine, 1992; Johnston & Vögele, 1993; Johnston & Wallace, 1990; Mumford, Schlesinger, & Glass, 1982; Suls & Wan, 1989).

Although anxiety presumably interferes with recovery through both behavioral and physiological mechanisms, the pathways for such effects have been unclear. Recent work in psychoneuroimmunology (PNI) has provided evidence that stress delays wound repair (Kiecolt-Glaser, Marucha, Malarkey, Mercado, & Glaser, 1995; Marucha, Kiecolt-Glaser, & Favagehi, 1998; Padgett, Marucha, & Sheridan, 1998). In addition, a second line of research has illustrated the adverse effects of pain on immune and endocrine function (Liebeskind, 1991). Thus, viewing the psychological literature on postsurgical recovery within a PNI context suggests a new conceptual framework, illustrated in Figure 72.1.

The model suggests that psychological variables could influence wound healing, a key variable in short-term postsurgical recovery, through several pathways: (a) Emotions have direct effects on "stress" hormones, and they, in turn, can modulate immune function. (b) The patient's emotional response to surgery can influence the type and amount of anesthetic, and anesthetics vary in their effects on the immune and endocrine systems. (c) Certain health behaviors may dictate differences in choice of anesthetic (e.g., alcohol intake), or extent of surgery (e.g., obesity). In addition, health habits such as smoking that are themselves stress-responsive can have direct deleterious consequences for immune function and wound healing. (d) Individuals who are more anxious are also more likely to experience greater postsurgical pain, and pain can down-regulate immune function. Thus, immune function, already poorer as a consequence of presurgical stress, could decline even further.

After providing a brief overview of key events in wound healing, we discuss the model's components and paths. Literature addressing psychological influences on recovery from surgery is viewed within the context of our framework. Underscoring fundamental methodological concerns that emerge as a consequence of our conceptualization, we suggest that researchers need to consider each of the pathways to maximize the signal-to-noise ratio. We end by highlighting clinical issues and applications.

Wound Healing: Immune and Neuroendocrine Influences

Wound repair progresses through several overlapping stages (Hübner et al., 1996). In the initial inflammatory stage, vasoconstriction and blood coagulation are followed by platelet activation and the release of platelet-derived growth factors (Van De Kerkhof, Van Bergen, Spruijt,

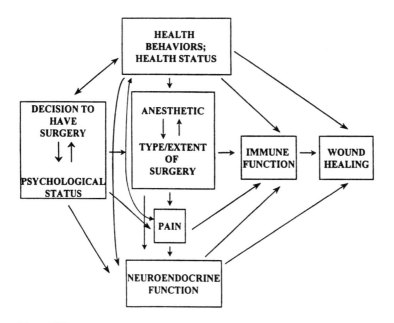

Figure 72.1
A biobehavioral model of the psychological, behavioral, and biological pathways that influence wound healing: the central short-term outcome in recovery from surgery.
Note. This figure is intended to illustrate our conceptual framework for understanding the complex relationships among relevant domains rather than providing a formal testable model. For simplicity, most paths are described as moving in one causal direction, and all possible connections are not illustrated (e.g., psychological variables such as stress and appraisal may influence the relationship between the extent of surgery and immune function). Psychological appraisals of the resulting physical stressor may modulate immune function and wound healing. In addition, direct connections between the central nervous system (CNS) and immune function are also possible, through direct CNS innervation of lymphoid tissue (Felten & Felten, 1991).

& Kuiper, 1994). The factors act as chemo-attractants for the migration of phagocytes (neutrophils and monocytes) to the site, starting the proliferative phase that involves the recruitment and replication of cells necessary for tissue regeneration and capillary regrowth. Wound re-modeling, the final step, may continue for weeks or months. The healing process is a cascade, and success in the later stages of wound repair is highly dependent on initial events (Hübner et al., 1996).

Immune function plays a key role early in this cascade. Proinflammatory cytokines such as in-

terleukin 1 (IL-1) and tumor necrosis factor (TNF) are essential to this effort; they help to protect a person from infection and prepare injured tissue for repair by enhancing phagocytic cell recruitment and activation (Lowry, 1993). Furthermore, cytokines released by recruited cells regulate the ability of fibroblasts and epithelial cells to remodel the damaged tissue (Lowry, 1993).

A number of hormones and neuropeptides can influence this immunological cascade (Hübner et al., 1996; Zwilling, 1994). For example, mice treated with glucocorticoids showed impairments in the induction of IL-1 and TNF, as well as defects in wound repair (Hübner et al., 1996). Human studies have also demonstrated that stress-induced elevations in glucocorticoids can transiently suppress both IL-1 and TNF production (DeRijk et al., 1997). Accordingly, dysregulation of glucocorticoid secretion provides one obvious mechanism by which stress can alter wound healing.

In contrast to the generally negative effects of glucocorticoids, growth hormone (GH) can enhance wound healing (Veldhuis & Iranmanesh, 1996). GH serves as a macrophage activator (Zwilling, 1994); among its activities, it stimulates monocyte migration. GH also amplifies superoxide anion generation and bacterial killing by macrophages, influential mechanisms for protection from infection after wounding (Zwilling, 1994).

Although acute stressors can provoke transient increases in GH (Kiecolt-Glaser, Malarkey, Cacioppo, & Glaser, 1994), deep sleep is the normal stimulus for release of much of our daily GH release (Veldhuis & Iranmanesh, 1996); thus, stressors that modify the architecture of sleep can also lessen GH secretion. Moreover, aging decreases GH secretion, and this steep decline may be further accelerated by a chronic stressor (Veldhuis & Iranmanesh, 1996; Malarkey et al., 1996). Although only a few of the paths have been highlighted here, it is obvious that stress-related alterations in the hypothalamic-pituitary-adrenal (HPA) axis can have important repercussions for the wound-healing cascade.

Stress and Wound Healing

Considerable data from animal and human studies have demonstrated that stress can alter multiple aspects of immune function (Glaser & Kiecolt-Glaser, 1994). For example, family members who provide care for a relative with Alzheimer's disease are typically more distressed than well-matched controls; a number of studies

suggest that caregivers also have poorer immune function (Kiecolt-Glaser et al., 1994; Kiecolt-Glaser, Glaser, Gravenstein, Malarkey, & Sheridan, 1996). Consistent with these differences in immune function, further work showed that caregivers took an average of 9 days or 24% longer than controls to completely heal a small, standardized wound. Importantly, photographic data demonstrated that the largest differences in wound size were most apparent early in the process.

Analyses of the production of IL-1β in response to lipopolysaccharide (LPS) stimulation showed that caregivers' peripheral blood leukocytes (PBLs) produced less than those of controls (Kiecolt-Glaser et al., 1995). IL-1β produced early after tissue injury can regulate the production, release, and activation of metalloproteinases, which are important in the destruction and remodeling of the wound; IL-1 also regulates fibroblast chemotaxis and production of collagen (Lowry, 1993). Moreover, IL-1 stimulates production of other cytokines important for wound healing, including IL-2, IL-6, and IL-8 (Lowry, 1993). Accordingly, these IL-1β data provide evidence of one immunological mechanism that may underlie caregivers' deficits in wound repair.

A subsequent study confirmed and extended the data obtained with caregivers. Mice subjected to restraint stress healed a punch biopsy wound an average of 27% more slowly than unstressed mice (Padgett et al., 1998). In addition, analysis of the dermal and epidermal layers surrounding wounds revealed less cellular infiltration in restraint-stressed mice than controls one to three days after wounding. To test the hypothesis that the delayed wound healing in restrained mice reflected HPA activation, Padgett et al. (1998) assessed serum corticosterone; levels in the stressed group averaged 162.5 ng/ml, compared with 35.7 ng/ml in the controls. Blocking glucocorticoid receptors in restraint-stressed animals with RU40555 resulted in healing rates comparable to control animals. Accordingly, these data provided good evidence that disruption of neuroendocrine homeostasis modulates wound healing.

Further research assessed the impact of a brief commonplace stressor, academic examinations, on alterations in mucosal wound repair. Prior work has demonstrated that medical students' cellular immune responses during examinations were poorer than those measured in the same individuals during lower stress periods (Kiecolt-Glaser & Glaser, 1991); thus, we were interested in whether the distress associated with exams would modulate mucosal wound healing among a group of 11 dental students (Marucha et al., 1998). Wounds placed three days before a major test healed an average of 40% more slowly than those made during summer vacation, and the differences were quite reliable: No student healed as rapidly during this stressful period as during vacation, and no student produced as much IL-1. Although this study demonstrated differences in mucosal wounds, the critical early events in the wound healing process are virtually identical for oral and dermal wounds (Wikesjö, Nilveus, & Selvig, 1992). These data confirmed and extended our prior findings in several important ways.

Perhaps the most notable finding was the demonstration of how a relatively mild stressor impacted wound repair. Like most professional students, these dental students were experts at taking tests—they had long histories of performing well under these very conditions. The fact that something as transient, predictable, and relatively benign as examination stress can have significant consequences for wound healing suggests that other everyday stressors may produce similar deficits in wound repair.

It is clear that each of the three studies that assessed the repair of standardized wounds found marked stress-related reductions in healing, with delays from 24% to 40%. Figure 72.2 shows effect sizes for these studies, using a simple correlation as a measure of the relationship between stress and two key outcome variables, healing

time and production of IL-1. Unquestionably, the effects are not just statistically significant, but large in a substantive sense. Of interest is the fact that the effect sizes for IL-1 and wound healing parallel each other within the two human studies, consistent with the importance of early events in the immunological cascade for subsequent healing (as described earlier, greater stress is associated with lower IL-1 levels, but correlations are shown as positive to simplify the figure). In addition, the effect sizes for wound healing were largest and almost identical in the two paradigms that afforded the greatest control over extraneous influences, that is, the Padgett et al. (1998) study in which mice had been randomly assigned to treatment groups, and the within-subject design whereby each student served as his or her own control (Marucha et al., 1998). These stress-related deficits in wound repair have broad implications for surgical recovery.

Pain: Influences on Neuroendocrine and Immune Function

The impact of painful stress on neuroendocrine and immune function has been studied both in laboratory animals and humans. Animal models of painful stress include acute stimuli that do not cause tissue damage such as footshock and tail-shock (e.g., Pezzone, Dohanics, & Rabin, 1994). Such painful stressors have been shown to suppress natural killer cell activity (NKCA), lymphocyte proliferative responses to mitogens, specific antibody production, and mixed lymphocyte reaction (Liebeskind, 1991). Several reports of stress-induced immune suppression that also incorporated neuroendocrine measures demonstrated elevated plasma beta-endorphin (Sacerdote, Manfredi, Bianchi, & Panerai, 1994) and corticosterone levels (Pezzone et al., 1994).

The neuroendocrine and immune consequences of tissue-damaging stimuli such as surgery have been well documented in both animals and humans. Postoperative elevations in

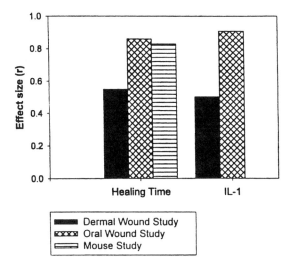

Figure 72.2
Effect sizes for three studies that employed a standardized wound (Kiecolt-Glaser et al., 1995; Marucha et al., 1998; Padgett et al., 1998).
Note. IL-1 = interleukin 1. In each case a simple correlation expresses the relationship between stress and two key outcome variables, healing time and IL-1; stress is associated with longer healing times and lower IL-1 production.

plasma levels of epinephrine, cortisol, and beta-endorphin reflect sympathetic nervous system (SNS) and HPA axis activation (e.g., Salomaki, Leppaluoto, Laitinen, Vuolteenaho, & Nuutinen, 1993). Immune suppression during surgery is evidenced by suppression of NKCA (e.g., Pollock, Lotzova, & Stanford, 1991), lymphocyte proliferative responses to mitogens, and changes in lymphocyte populations (Tonnessen, Brinklov, Christensen, Olesen, & Madsen, 1987). Further supporting the connections among the SNS, the HPA axis, and the immune system, coincidental surgery-induced changes in these systems also have been demonstrated (Koltun et al., 1996).

The above mentioned findings cannot confirm the role of pain per se in these neuroendocrine and immune consequences of painful stress; however, there is evidence to support such a suggestion. First, several studies have shown that anesthetic techniques that block transmission of nociceptive impulses either locally (Pasqualucci et al., 1994) or at the level of the spinal cord (Koltun et al., 1996) also significantly reduce neuroendocrine or immune responses affected by surgery. Moreover, when Pasqualucci et al. (1994) assessed visual analog scale (VAS) pain scores, they found that the local anesthetic infiltration group also exhibited significantly lower pain scores as well. Second, two prospective studies found that, compared with inhalational anesthesia, epidural anesthesia was associated with a significant reduction in the incidence of postoperative infections, a biologically significant immune outcome (Cuschieri, Morran, Howie, & McArdle, 1985; Yeager, Glass, Neff, & Brinck-Johnsen, 1987). Cuschieri et al. (1985) also documented significantly lower postoperative VAS pain scores in the epidural group. Third, narcotic anesthesia has been shown to suppress the hormonal response to surgery (Lacoumenta et al.,

1987). Fourth, effective postoperative pain management with systemic opioids has been associated with reductions in plasma cortisol levels (Moller, Dinesen, Sondergard, Knigge, & Kehlet, 1988). Finally, it was recently shown that providing analgesic doses of morphine in rats significantly attenuates surgery-induced increases in the metastasis of a tumor cell line that is controlled by natural killer cells, providing further evidence of the potential negative immune consequences of pain with implications for the whole organism (Page, Ben-Eliyahu, & Liebeskind, 1994; Page, McDonald, & Ben-Eliyahu, in press).

The inflammatory response is an important mechanism to consider for its contributions to pain, immunity, and the initiation of wound healing. Tissue damage from surgical procedures causes the local release of factors including substance P, bradykinin, prostaglandins, and histamine. Cytokines such as IL-1 are released from indigenous tissue cells and early recruited cells, such as the neutrophil (Hübner et al., 1996). Together, these factors initiate the inflammatory response marked by vasodilation, increased capillary permeability, and the sensitization of peripheral afferent nerve fibers. In addition to its immune-related roles, IL-1 contributes to local hyperalgesia (Schweizer, Feige, Fontana, Muller, & Dinarello, 1988), as well as a systemic hyperalgesic state and illness symptoms such as fever and malaise (Watkins et al., 1995). The sensitization of nociceptive fibers manifests as a decrease in the threshold necessary to initiate nociceptive impulse transmission, resulting in hyperalgesia (Woolf, 1994). Prostaglandin E participates in the local sensitization of nociceptive fibers (Martin, Basbaum, Kwiat, Goetzl, & Levine, 1987), as well as in the suppression of NKCA (Leung, 1989). Faist et al. (1990) showed that inhibiting prostaglandin synthesis with indomethacin treatment reversed surgery-induced depression of postoperative delayed type hypersensitivity responses and lymphocyte prolifera-

tion and also resulted in a significant reduction in the incidence of infection.

It is clear that pain, like other stressors, adversely affects immune function; anesthetics that block transmission of nociceptive impulses are also associated with better immune function, as well as reductions in postoperative infections. As will be discussed shortly, more anxious patients experience greater postsurgical pain (Johnston, 1988). Thus, more distressed individuals could ultimately be doubly disadvantaged: Immune function, already poorer as a consequence of presurgical stress, could decline even further as a consequence of enhanced postsurgical pain.

Health Status and Health Behaviors

Aging is associated with an increased risk for surgery. Immune function declines with age, particularly functional aspects of the cellular immune response (Verhoef, 1990); these age-related declines are related to infectious complications, one factor in the increased surgical mortality in the elderly (Thomas & Ritchie, 1995). Moreover, age and distress appear to interact to promote immune down-regulation: Older adults show greater immunological impairments related to stress or depression than younger adults (Herbert & Cohen, 1993; Kiecolt-Glaser, Glaser, et al., 1996).

Some evidence suggests that surgical stress may also interact with both age and psychological stress to heighten risk for older adults. In work from Linn and Jensen (1983), older and younger adults did not differ immunologically prior to elective surgery for hernia repair; however, the former had significantly lower proliferative responses to two mitogens five days after the operation. In a related study, Linn, Linn, and Jensen (1983) divided older and younger patients on the basis of their preoperative anxiety; high anxious older patients had significantly more complications than the other three groups. Thus, morbidity and mortality following surgery are already substantially greater among older adults (Thomas & Ritchie, 1995); further suppression of the immune response by psychological stress may put older adults at even greater risk.

Key behavioral risk factors for surgery include smoking, alcohol and drug abuse, and nutrition (Kehlet, 1997). It is important to note that heightened distress is associated with riskier behavior on all of these dimensions (Steptoe, Wardle, Pollard, Canaan, & Davies, 1996), and each of these health habits can alter wound healing through their effects on immune function; additional paths for influence include effects on anesthetic choices and changes in levels of stress hormones. Moreover, these behaviors interact with one another; for example, heavy alcohol use is linked to poorer nutrition (Benveniste & Thut, 1981).

In addition to nutrition, other consequences of preoperative alcohol abuse include alcohol-related immunosuppression, subclinical cardiac dysfunction, and amplified endocrine changes in response to surgery (Kehlet, 1997). Alcohol also appears to retard wound healing directly via delays in cell migration and deposition of collagen at the wound site (Benveniste & Thut, 1981). Furthermore, individuals who are depressed or anxious are more likely to self-medicate with alcohol or other drugs, and alcohol abuse can potentiate distress (Grunberg & Baum, 1985).

Smoking, another surgical risk behavior, diminishes proliferation of fibroblasts and macrophages, reduces blood flow to the skin through vasoconstriction, and can inhibit enzyme systems for oxidative metabolism and oxygen transport (Silverstein, 1992). In addition to demonstrably slower healing, smokers have higher rates of postoperative infections, perhaps related to the fact that nicotine and other toxins in cigarette smoke depress both primary and secondary immune responses by reducing the chemotactic and phagocytic activities of leukocytes (Silverstein, 1992).

Distressed individuals are more likely to experience sleep and appetite disturbances. As noted earlier, deep sleep is associated with secretion of GH, a hormone that facilitates wound healing, and fragmented sleep results in reduced GH secretion; even partial sleep loss one night results in elevated cortisol levels the next evening (Leproult, Copinschi, Buxton, & Cauter, 1997). Postoperative sleep is typically disturbed as a function of the physiological stress of surgery, pain, opioid use, noise, and awakenings from monitoring and nursing procedures (Kehlet, 1997). Thus, postsurgical sleep deprivation may itself be a significant stressor (Johnston, 1988), and distress may exacerbate or prolong sleep difficulties through such mechanisms as intensified pain sensitivity.

Certainly, individuals who experience greater pain are likely to modify other health behaviors besides sleep in response to this stressor. In addition, some health behaviors may in turn influence pain perception, for example, smoking is associated with greater pain tolerance (Lane, Lefebvre, Rose, & Keefe, 1995).

The assessment of health behaviors is an important component of PNI studies (Kiecolt-Glaser & Glaser, 1988). Moreover, the surgical literature provides clear evidence for the importance of certain health habits for recovery (Kehlet, 1997). Accordingly, the assessment of key risk factors (e.g., smoking and alcohol and drug use) would seem to be an important component of psychological studies addressing surgical recovery—and yet such data are frequently omitted. For example, few studies mention any assessment of smoking in the analysis of outcomes. Similarly, few researchers have systematically discussed relevant indexes of preoperative health status, even though many postsurgical outcomes of interest are undoubtedly colored by chronic health problems such as diabetes. Our model suggests that the assessment of health behavior should be an important component of studies addressing behavioral influences on postsurgical morbidity.

Psychological Influences on Surgical Recovery

Conceptualizing surgery as a short-term stressor, considerable research has focused on how patients' emotional responses influence postoperative recovery. In general, high preoperative fear or stress is predictive of a variety of poorer outcomes, including greater pain, longer hospital stays, more postoperative complications, and poorer treatment compliance (Johnston, 1988; Mathews & Ridgeway, 1981).

Some of the postoperative repercussions of distress may be mediated through variables such as anesthetic intake; highly anxious patients require more anesthesia than those who are less distressed (Abbott & Abbott, 1995; Gil, 1984; Johnston, 1988; Markland & Hardy, 1993). As one consequence, endocrinological and immunological changes secondary to anesthesia could be greater among more fearful individuals. In addition, Abbott and Abbott (1995) noted that the side effects of various anesthetics, muscle relaxants, and narcotics may include a number of the postoperative behaviors that are sometimes used as outcome measures (e.g., vomiting, nausea, headache, and pain at the incisional site). Higher doses could presumably increase the severity of symptoms.

Across a number of studies, greater self-reported anxiety and stress are typically related to more severe postoperative pain (Johnston, 1988; Mathews & Ridgeway, 1981). In addition to direct effects on endocrine and immune function, the greater pain sensitivity of more anxious patients may also have further consequences for recovery because of differences in compliance. For example, breathing exercises can reduce the risk of pneumonia, and ambulation decreases the risk of phlebitis and may improve wound healing (Kehlet, 1997). However, individuals who are more distressed may be more cautious about following recommendations for walking, coughing, or deep breathing because of pain (Mathews & Ridgeway, 1981).

Linn, Linn, and Klimas (1988) assessed the relevance of differences in preoperative pain tolerance and stress to postoperative immune function; physiological responses to a cold pressor test were measured the day before surgery in 24 men undergoing hernia repair. After controlling for preoperative immunological values (as well as age and social support), lymphocytes from men who reported more recent stressful life events had lower proliferative responses to phytohemagglutinin (PHA). In addition, high responders to the cold pressor stress (i.e., a lower pain threshold) had significantly lower proliferative responses to pokeweed mitogen after surgery; they also required more pain medication and had more complications.

Personality variables may moderate postsurgical outcomes via their influences on stress, mood, and coping (Mathews & Ridgeway, 1981). In an excellent study that assessed the effect of dispositional optimism on recovery from coronary artery bypass surgery, initial analyses showed that optimism was unrelated to severity of disease or to other relevant medical variables (Scheier et al., 1989). Subsequent analyses controlled for extensiveness of surgery, severity of disease, and a triad of risk factors (smoking, hypertension, high cholesterol) before assessing the contribution of optimism to various recovery indexes. Given the rigor of these efforts, the findings are of particular note: Compared with pessimistic men, optimistic men fared better on perioperative physiological indexes—they began walking faster after surgery, and rehabilitation staff rated them as showing a more favorable physical recovery.

Research from another population has provided evidence of possible mechanisms that may underlie optimists' enhanced postoperative recuperation. Among law students in their first year of study, optimism was associated with more positive moods, coping, and differences in response to stress, and these differences appeared to mediate optimists' better immune function during examinations (Segerstrom, Taylor, Kemeny, & Fahey, 1998).

The optimism data are consistent with evidence that interventions that alter appraisal, coping, and/or mood may also modulate immune and endocrine function, thereby enhancing surgical recovery (Kiecolt-Glaser et al., 1985; Kiecolt-Glaser & Glaser, 1992; Manyande et al., 1995). In fact, intervention studies provide some of the best evidence for the role of psychological factors in surgical recovery. In one of the earliest of such studies (Egbert, Battit, Welch, & Barlett, 1964), anesthesiologists paid brief visits to patients the night before surgery to provide information about typical postsurgical physical sensations and to teach them a relaxation technique designed to reduce pain. Those patients who received this additional visit left the hospital an average of 2.7 days earlier and required roughly half as much morphine as individuals receiving routine care. Among the more than 200 treatment studies that have followed Egbert et al.'s (1964) work (see reviews by Contrada et al., 1994; Devine, 1992; Gil, 1984; Johnston & Vögele, 1993; Johnston & Wallace, 1990; Mumford et al., 1982; Suls & Wan, 1989), beneficial outcomes have included decreased anxiety and stress, reductions in hospital stay, fewer postoperative complications, better treatment compliance, less pain and lower use of analgesics, and alterations in physiological indexes (primarily cardiovascular and respiratory measures).[1] Several studies have suggested that presurgical psychological status can influence physiological responses during the surgery itself (Abbott & Abbott, 1995; Greene, Zeichner, Roberts, Callahan, & Granados, 1989; Markland & Hardy, 1993; Scheier et al., 1989) as well as speed of physical recovery (time to open eyes) following the discontinuation of anesthesia (Liu, Barry, & Weinman, 1994).

A meta-analysis by Johnston and Vögele (1993) addressed relationships between the major types of interventions (procedural intervention, sensory information, behavioral instruction, cognitive intervention, relaxation, hypnosis, or emotion-focused intervention) and outcome variables (negative affect, pain, pain medication, length of stay, behavioral and clinical indexes of recovery, physiological indexes, and satisfaction). Using both published and unpublished studies, they concluded that each of the outcomes showed significant benefit. Among the interventions, procedural information and behavioral instruction produced the most ubiquitous improvements across all outcomes, whereas relaxation studies showed benefits for all indexes except behavioral recovery.

Summarizing results from several meta-analyses of presurgical intervention studies, Contrada et al. (1994) argued that the association between surgical preparation and outcome is clinically meaningful. Depending on the meta-analysis, two thirds to three quarters of intervention patients had better outcomes than controls, and the size of the improvement was 20% to 28%. Moreover, the effect sizes for interventions with two or three content categories (information, coping skills training, and psychosocial support) were larger than those that had only a single thrust (Contrada et al., 1994).

In contrast to their efficacy, most presurgical interventions have been remarkably brief. For example, the psychoeducational treatments included in Devine's (1992) meta-analysis took 7 to 90 minutes, with a median length of 30 minutes; the great majority were limited to a single session. Moreover, delivery was frequently not individualized; some studies used a group format, whereas others relied on such low-cost alternatives as booklets, manuals, audiotapes, and videotapes. Nonetheless, 79% to 84% of the studies showed beneficial effects (depending on the outcome) for pain, psychological distress, and various indexes of recovery. In fact, 79% of the studies showed that these interventions were associated with a shorter length of hospital stay: Compared with controls, treatment patients spend an average of 1.5 fewer days in the hospital.

Indeed, positive effects are not limited to formal interventions; one study suggested that even small environmental differences may be beneficial. Hospital records of gall bladder surgery from 1972 to 1981 were examined to determine whether assignment to a room with a view from a window made a difference (Ulrich, 1984). Consistent with studies that have documented the utility of distraction or attention redirection as a coping strategy to reduce distress and pain (Gil, 1984), comparisons of well-matched patient pairs showed that those with a view had shorter hospital stays (7.96 vs. 8.70 days) and that they took fewer potent analgesics than those without a view.

How do such modest interventions produce such differences? Recall the magnitude of the effect sizes for stress and wound healing (Figure 72.2); those data suggest that even treatments that have relatively small consequences for psychological distress could translate into faster repair through the direct and indirect routes suggested by our model.

The positive effects of interventions are even more striking in view of the significant limitations of many studies. These have included heterogeneity in patient groups, in surgical and anesthetic procedures, and in the types of outcomes assessed; failure to assess and control for patients' prior experience with surgery or other invasive medical procedures; differential treatment of comparison groups on variables other than those being manipulated; and the absence of manipulation checks to demonstrate that interventions were delivered in a uniform manner, or that patients actually acquired or utilized new skills or implemented cognitive or behavioral strategies (see critiques by Anderson & Masur, 1983; Gil, 1984; Johnston & Vögele, 1993; Ludwick-Rosenthal & Neufield, 1988). In addition, we suggest that many of the published studies may also have underestimated effect sizes because they failed to consider relevant health behaviors that can make sizable contributions to error variance.

In the same vein, differences in pain and analgesic use should also be assessed. Our model highlights the importance of effective pain control, particularly in the immediate postoperative period. As discussed earlier, the healing process is a cascade, with success in the later stages of wound repair highly dependent on initial events (Hübner et al., 1996); it is important to note that effective postoperative pain management with systemic opioids has been associated with reductions in plasma cortisol, a hormone strongly associated with poorer wound healing (Moller et al., 1988). Although most of the researchers studying psychological influences on postsurgical outcomes have conceptualized pain as an outcome, it also contributes to the process: Poorly controlled acute pain could retard wound healing and prolong the recovery period (Liebeskind, 1991; Page et al., 1994, in press).

Implications for Research and Practice

In the United States, 80% of all surgeries are considered "elective" in the sense that the patient can choose when to have the operation (Sobel & Ornstein, 1996). Early assessment of psychological predictors of outcome provides the opportunity to identify those patients who might be at greater risk (e.g., Block, 1996). However, to provide maximally effective interventions, further information about the impact of individual differences in coping style and level of anticipatory anxiety would be valuable. For example, "monitors," patients with a vigilant coping style, scan for threat-relevant cues, whereas "blunters" rely more on avoidant coping (Miller, 1992). The two groups appear to show better adjustment in health-related contexts when interventions are tailored to their coping style. Monitors fare better with voluminous sensory and procedural information; blunters show the opposite response (Miller, 1992; Prokop, Bradley, Burish, Anderson, & Fox, 1991). Such data are particularly important precisely because there is less opportunity to provide care for patients following surgery (Deardorff & Reeves, 1997).

As a consequence of technical advances, many surgeries are less invasive than in the past and thus are now performed on an outpatient basis, or with a greatly reduced hospital stay (Macho & Gable, 1994). In addition, managed care guidelines are increasingly constraining the length of hospitalization. With any extended convalescence at home, family members play more prominent roles. The self-regulatory model proposed by Contrada et al. (1994) provides guidance regarding intervention content that explicitly addresses the patient, the patient's spouse or partner, and the patient–partner relationship. In this context, the demands that at-home recuperation may place on family members who provide care should not be overlooked, and neither should the potential toll for caregivers (see also Kiecolt-Glaser et al., 1994).

Our knowledge of how psychological interventions are actually translated into faster physical recovery is limited by the range of measures used in most studies. Despite the fact that reduction of anxiety or stress is a goal of many of the interventions, the kinds of outcomes assessed do not typically include data from each of the relevant domains: self-report, behavioral, and physiological. Although the addition of endocrine and immune measures both pre- and postoperatively would be worthwhile for psychological studies, appending psychological measures to biologically oriented studies would also be quite valuable. For example, researchers who used an indwelling catheter to collect blood samples every 20 minutes for 24 hours found that presurgical patients showed remarkable increases in cortisol secretion as they were being prepared preoperatively (body shaving, wash, and enema), with values that spiked 6.9 to 10.5 standard deviations above the mean for control patients for that time of day (Czeisler et al., 1976). The interdisciplinary study of such phenomena could amplify our understanding of psychological and behavioral influences on health.

Indeed, surgery offers an attractive paradigm for examining the responses of patients to a distinctive naturalistic stressor (Johnston, 1988). One innovative study addressed social comparison and affiliation under threat among coronary-bypass patients (Kulik, Mahler, & Moore, 1996). The men were assigned preoperatively to a room alone, or they shared a semiprivate room with a roommate who was either cardiac or noncardiac, and either preoperative or postoperative. Those patients assigned a postoperative roommate were less anxious before surgery. In addition, those who either roomed with a cardiac patient or a postoperative patient walked more after their operation, and had shorter hospital stays. The no-roommate patients had the slowest recoveries.

The Kulik et al. (1996) data illustrate an important theme in this literature: Whatever their content, many presurgical interventions may benefit recovery in part because they provide additional interpersonal support during a stressful time (Contrada et al., 1994; Johnston, 1988). There is certainly ample evidence that social support can moderate the effects of psychological stress; in addition, a number of studies have shown relationships between social support and dimensions of autonomic, endocrine, and immune function, with family ties appearing to be a key source of support related to physiological functioning (Kiecolt-Glaser, Newton et al., 1996; Uchino, Cacioppo, & Kiecolt-Glaser, 1996). Consistent with this literature, male coronary bypass patients who received greater spousal support used less pain medication, had a more rapid discharge from the surgical intensive care unit, and spent fewer total days in the hospital (Kulik & Mahler, 1989).

Indeed, one factor that should spur research in this arena is its obvious and immediate practical applicability. Compared with the costs of hospitalization, psychological interventions are clearly cost-effective (Contrada et al., 1994; Devine, 1992; Mumford et al., 1982).

As described earlier, dental students took an average of 40% longer to heal a small, standardized wound made prior to examinations, compared with an identical wound made during vacation (Marucha et al., 1998). In contrast to the relatively mild and predictable stress of academic examinations, surgery is a high-stakes stressor, with possible consequences that include death, pain, disfigurement, economic losses, alterations in social roles, and uncertainty about both the outcome and the time course for recovery (Contrada et al., 1994). Given the multiple threats embodied in an approaching surgery, it is not surprising that patients may display marked elevations in anxiety for at least six days prior to surgery, with clearly heightened distress persisting for five to six days afterward, dropping back to normal levels only after a period of weeks (Johnston, 1980). Stressors that are perceived as unpredictable and uncontrollable can continue to be associated with elevated stress hormones (Baum, Cohen, & Hall, 1993). The ability to "unwind" after stressful encounters, that is, quicker return to one's neuroendocrine baseline, influences the total burden that stressors place on an individual (Frankenhaeuser, 1986). Accordingly, interventions that promote early adaptation can produce substantial benefits for mental and physical health.

Note

1. Because most surgical wounds are sutured, direct assessments of healing are not possible. In addition, although infection is a highly relevant complication within our PNI context, it usually occurs at base rates too low to be useful for research purposes.

References

Abbott, J., & Abbott, P. (1995). Psychological and cardiovascular predictors of anaesthesia induction, operative and postoperative complications in minor gynecological surgery. *British Journal of Clinical Psychology, 34*, 613–625.

Anderson, K. O., & Masur, F. T., III. (1983). Psychological preparation for invasive medical and dental procedures. *Journal of Behavioral Medicine, 6*, 1–40.

Baum, A., Cohen, L., & Hall, M. (1993). Control and intrusive memories as possible determinants of chronic stress. *Psychosomatic Medicine, 55*, 274–286.

Benveniste, K., & Thut, P. (1981). The effect of chronic alcoholism on wound healing. *Proceedings of the Society for Experimental Biology and Medicine, 166*, 568–575.

Block, A. R. (1996). *Presurgical psychological screening in chronic pain syndromes*. Hillsdale, NJ: Erlbaum.

Contrada, R. J., Leventhal, E. A., & Anderson, J. R. (1994). Psychological preparation for surgery: Marshaling individual and social resources to optimize self-regulation. In S. Maes, H. Leventhal, & M. Johnson (Eds.), *International Review of Health Psychology* (Vol. 3, pp. 219–266). New York: Wiley.

Cuschieri, R. J., Morran, C. G., Howie, J. C., & McArdle, C. S. (1985). Postoperative pain and pulmonary complications: Comparison of three analgesic regimens. *British Journal of Surgery, 72*, 495–498.

Czeisler, C. A., Ede, M. C., Regestein, Q. R., Kisch, E. S., Fang, V. S., & Ehrlich, E. N. (1976). Episodic 24-hour cortisol secretory patterns in patients awaiting elective cardiac surgery. *Journal of Clinical Endocrinology and Metabolism, 42*, 273–283.

Deardorff, W. W., & Reeves, J. R. (1997). *Preparing for surgery: A mind–body approach to enhance healing and recovery*. Oakland, CA: New Harbinger Publications.

DeRijk, R., Michelson, D., Karp, B., Petrides, J., Galliven, E., Deuster, P., Paciotti, G., Gold, P. W., & Sternberg, E. M. (1997). Exercise and circadian rhythm-induced variations in plasma cortisol differentially regulate interleukin-1? (IL-1?), IL-6, and tumor necrosis factor-a (TNF-?) production in humans: High sensitivity of TNF-? and resistance of IL-6. *Journal of Clinical Endocrinology and Metabolism, 82*, 2182–2192.

Devine, E. C. (1992). Effects of psychoeducational care for adult surgical patients: A meta-analysis of 191 studies. *Patient Education and Counseling, 19*, 129–142.

Egbert, L. D., Battit, G. E., Welch, C. E., & Barlett, M. K. (1964). Reduction of postoperative pain by encouragement and instruction of patients. *New England Journal of Medicine, 270*, 825–827.

Faist, E., Ertel, W., Chonert, T., Huber, P., Inthorn, D., & Heberer, G. (1990). Immunoprotective effects of cyclooxygenase inhibition in patients with major surgical trauma. *Journal of Trauma, 3*, 8–18.

Felten, D. L., & Felten, S. Y. (1991). Innervation of lymphoid tissue. In R. Ader, D. L. Felten, & N. Cohen (Eds.), *Psychoneuroimmunology* (pp. 87–101). San Diego, CA: Academic Press.

Frankenhaeuser, M. (1986). A psychobiological framework for research on human stress and coping. In M. H. Appley (Ed.), *Dynamics of stress: Physiological, psychological, and social perspectives* (pp. 101–116). New York: Plenum.

Gil, K. M. (1984). Coping effectively with invasive medical procedures: A descriptive model. *Clinical Psychology Review, 4,* 339–362.

Glaser, R., & Kiecolt-Glaser, J. K. (Eds.). (1994). *Handbook of human stress and immunity.* San Diego, CA: Academic Press.

Greene, P. G., Zeichner, A., Roberts, N. L., Callahan, E. J., & Granados, J. L. (1989). Preparation for cesarean delivery: A multicomponent analysis of treatment outcome. *Journal of Consulting and Clinical Psychology, 57,* 484–487.

Grunberg, N. E., & Baum, A. (1985). Biological commonalities of stress and substance abuse. In S. Shiffman & T. A. Wills (Eds.), *Coping and substance use* (pp. 25–62). San Diego, CA: Academic Press.

Herbert, T. B., & Cohen, S. (1993). Stress and immunity in humans: A meta-analytic review. *Psychosomatic Medicine, 55,* 364–379.

Hübner, G., Brauchle, M., Smola, H., Madlener, M., Fassler, R., & Werner, S. (1996). Differential regulation of pro-inflammatory cytokines during wound healing in normal and glucocorticoid-treated mice. *Cytokine, 8,* 548–556.

Johnston, M. (1980). Anxiety in surgical patients. *Psychological Medicine, 10,* 142–152.

Johnston, M. (1988). Impending surgery. In S. Fisher & J. Reason (Eds.), *Handbook of life stress, cognition and health* (pp. 79–100). New York: Wiley.

Johnston, M., & Vögele, C. (1993). Benefits of psychological preparation for surgery: A meta-analysis. *Annals of Behavioral Medicine, 15,* 245–256.

Johnston, M., & Wallace, L. (Eds.). (1990). *Stress and medical procedures.* Oxford, England: Oxford University Press.

Kehlet, H. (1997). Multimodal approach to control postoperative pathophysiology and rehabilitation. *British Journal of Anaesthesia, 78,* 606–617.

Kiecolt-Glaser, J. K., & Glaser, R. (1988). Methodological issues in behavioral immunology research with humans. *Brain, Behavior, and Immunity, 2,* 67–78.

Kiecolt-Glaser, J. K., & Glaser, R. (1991). Stress and immune function in humans. In R. Ader, D. Felten, & N. Cohen (Eds.), *Psychoneuroimmunology II* (pp. 849–867). San Diego, CA: Academic Press.

Kiecolt-Glaser, J. K., & Glaser, R. (1992). Psychoneuroimmunology: Can psychological interventions modulate immunity? *Journal of Consulting and Clinical Psychology, 60,* 569–575.

Kiecolt-Glaser, J. K., Glaser, R., Gravenstein, S., Malarkey, W. B., & Sheridan, J. (1996). Chronic stress alters the immune response to influenza virus vaccine in older adults. *Proceedings of the National Academy of Sciences, 93,* 3043–3047.

Kiecolt-Glaser, J. K., Glaser, R., Williger, D., Stout, J., Messick, G., Sheppard, S., Ricker, D., Romisher, S. C., Briner, W., Bonnell, G., & Donnerberg, R. (1985). Psychosocial enhancement of immunocompetence in a geriatric population. *Health Psychology, 4,* 25–41.

Kiecolt-Glaser, J. K., Malarkey, W., Cacioppo, J. T., & Glaser, R. (1994). Stressful personal relationships: Endocrine and immune function. In R. Glaser & J. K. Kiecolt-Glaser (Eds.), *Handbook of human stress and immunity* (pp. 321–339). San Diego, CA: Academic Press.

Kiecolt-Glaser, J. K., Marucha, P. T., Malarkey, W. B., Mercado, A. M., & Glaser, R. (1995). Slowing of wound healing by psychological stress. *Lancet, 346,* 1194–1196.

Kiecolt-Glaser, J. K., Newton, T., Cacioppo, J. T., MacCallum, R. C., Glaser, R., & Malarkey, W. B. (1996). Marital conflict and endocrine function: Are men really more physiologically affected than women? *Journal of Consulting and Clinical Psychology, 64,* 324–332.

Koltun, W. A., Bloomer, M. M., Tilberg, A. F., Seaton, J. F., Ilahi, O., Rung, G., Gifford, R. M., & Kauffman, G. L. (1996). Awake epidural anesthesia is associated with improved natural killer cell cytotoxity and a reduced stress response. *American Journal of Surgery, 171,* 68–73.

Kulik, J. A., & Mahler, H. I. (1989). Social support and recovery from surgery. *Health Psychology, 8,* 221–238.

Kulik, J. A., Mahler, H. I., & Moore, P. J. (1996). Social comparison and affiliation under threat: Effects on recovery from major surgery. *Journal of Personality and Social Psychology, 71,* 967–979.

Lacoumenta, S., Yeo, T. H., Burrin, J. M., Bloom, S. R., Paterson, J. L., & Hall, G. M. (1987). Fentanyl and the beta-endorphin, ACTH, and glucoregulatory hormonal response to surgery. *British Journal of Anaesthesia, 59,* 713–720.

Lane, J. D., Lefebvre, J. C., Rose, J. E., & Keefe, F. J. (1995). Effects of cigarette smoking on perception of thermal pain. *Experimental and Clinical Psychopharmacology, 3,* 140–147.

Leproult, R., Copinschi, G., Buxton, O., & Cauter, E. V. (1997). Sleep loss results in an elevation of cortisol levels the next evening. *Sleep, 20,* 865–870.

Leung, K. H. (1989). Inhibition of human NK cell and LAK cell cytotoxicity and differentiation by PGE2. *Cellular Immunology, 123,* 384–395.

Liebeskind, J. C. (1991). Pain can kill. *Pain, 44,* 3–4.

Linn, B. S., & Jensen, J. (1983). Age and immune response to a surgical stress. *Archives of Surgery, 118,* 405–409.

Linn, B. S., Linn, M. W., & Jensen, J. (1983). Surgical stress in the healthy elderly. *Journal of the American Geriatric Society, 31,* 544–568.

Linn, B. S., Linn, M. W., & Klimas, N. G. (1988). Effects of psychophysical stress on surgical outcome. *Psychosomatic Medicine, 50,* 230–244.

Liu, R., Barry, J. E. S., & Weinman, J. (1994). Effect of background stress on postoperative recovery. *Anaesthesia, 49,* 382–386.

Lowry, S. F. (1993). Cytokine mediators of immunity and inflammation. *Archives of Surgery, 28,* 1235–1241.

Ludwick-Rosenthal, R., & Neufield, R. W. J. (1988). Stress management during noxious medical procedures: An evaluative review of outcome studies, *Psychological Bulletin, 104,* 326–342.

Macho, J., & Gable, G. (1994). *Everyone's guide to outpatient surgery.* Toronto, Ontario, Canada: Somerville.

Malarkey, W. B., Wu, H., Cacioppo, J. T., Malarkey, K. L., Poehlmann, K. M., Glaser, R., & Kiecolt-Glaser, J. K. (1996). Chronic stress down regulates growth hormone gene expression in peripheral blood mononuclear cells of older adults. *Endocrine, 5,* 33–39.

Manyande, A., Simon, B., Gettins, D., Stanford, S. C., Mazhero, S., Marks, D. F., & Salmon, P. (1995). Preoperative rehearsal of active coping imagery influences subjective and hormonal responses to abdominal surgery. *Psychosomatic Medicine, 57,* 177–182.

Markland, D., & Hardy, L. (1993). Anxiety, relaxation, and anaesthesia for day-case surgery. *British Journal of Clinical Psychology, 32,* 493–504.

Martin, H. A., Basbaum, A. I., Kwiat, G. C., Goetzl, E. J., & Levine, J. D. (1987). Leukotriene and prostaglandin sensitization of cutaneous high-threshold C- and A-delta mechanonociceptors in the hairy skin of rat hindlimbs. *Neuroscience, 22,* 651–659.

Marucha, P. T., Kiecolt-Glaser, J. K., & Favagehi, M. (1998). Mucosal wound healing is impaired by examination stress. *Psychosomatic Medicine, 60,* 362–365.

Mathews, A., & Ridgeway, V. (1981). Personality and surgical recovery: A review. *British Journal of Clinical Psychology, 20,* 243–260.

Miller, S. (1992). Monitoring and blunting in the face of threat: Implications for adaptation and health. In L. Montada, S. Filipp, & M. J. Lerner (Eds.), *Life crises and experiences of loss in adulthood* (pp. 255–273). Hillsdale, NJ: Erlbaum.

Moller, I. W., Dinesen, K., Sondergard, S., Knigge, U., & Kehlet, H. (1988). Effect of patient-controlled analgesia on plasma catecholamine, cortisol and glucose concentrations after cholecystectomy. *British Journal of Anaesthesia, 61,* 160–164.

Mumford, E., Schlesinger, H. J., & Glass, G. V. (1982). The effect of psychological intervention on recovery from surgery and heart attacks: An analysis of the literature. *American Journal of Public Health, 72,* 141–151.

Padgett, D. A., Marucha, P. T., & Sheridan, J. F. (1998). Restraint stress slows cutaneous wound healing in mice. *Brain, Behavior, and Immunity, 12,* 64–73.

Page, G. G., Ben-Eliyahu, S., & Liebeskind, J. C. (1994). The role of LGL/NK cells in surgery-induced promotion of metastasis and its attenuation by morphine. *Brain, Behavior, and Immunity, 8,* 241–250.

Page, G. G., McDonald, J. S., & Ben-Eliyahu, S. (in press). Pre- versus postoperative administration of morphine: Impact on the neuroendocrine, behavioral, and metastatic-enhancing effects of surgery. *British Journal of Anaesthesia.*

Pasqualucci, A., Contardo, R., Da Broi, U., Colo, F., Terrosu, G., Donini, A., Sorrentino, M., Pasetto, A., & Bresadola, F. (1994). The effects of intraperitoneal local anesthetic on analgesic requirements and endocrine response after laparoscopic cholecystectomy: A randomized double-blind controlled study. *Journal of Laparoendoscopic Surgery, 4,* 405–412.

Pezzone, M. A., Dohanics, J., & Rabin, B. S. (1994). Effects of footshock stress upon spleen and peripheral blood lymphocyte mitogenic responses in rats with lesions of the paraventricular nucleus. *Journal of Neuroimmunology, 53,* 39–46.

Pollock, R. E., Lotzova, E., & Stanford, S. D. (1991). Mechanism of surgical stress impairment of human perioperative natural killer cell cytotoxicity. *Archives of Surgery, 126,* 338–342.

Prokop, C. K., Bradley, L. A., Burish, T. G., Anderson, K. O., & Fox, J. E. (1991). Psychological preparation for stressful medical and dental procedures. In C. K. Prokop & L. A. Bradley (Eds.), *Health psychology: Clinical methods and research* (pp. 159–196). New York: Macmillan.

Sacerdote, P., Manfredi, B., Bianchi, M., & Panerai, A. E. (1994). Intermittent but not continuous inescapable footshock stress affects immune responses and immunocyte beta-endorphin concentrations in the rat. *Brain, Behavior, and Immunity, 8,* 251–260.

Salomaki, T. E., Leppaluoto, J., Laitinen, J. O., Vuolteenaho, O., & Nuutinen, L. S. (1993). Epidural versus intravenous fentanyl for reducing hormonal, metabolic, and physiologic responses after thoracotomy. *Anesthesiology, 79,* 672–679.

Scheier, M. F., Matthews, K. A., Owens, J. F., Magovern, G. J., Sr., Lefebvre, R. C., Abbott, R. A., & Carver, C. S. (1989). Dispositional optimism and recovery from coronary artery bypass surgery: The beneficial effects on physical and psychological well-being. *Journal of Personality and Social Psychology, 57,* 1024–1040.

Schweizer, A., Feige, U., Fontana, A., Muller, K., & Dinarello, C. A. (1988). Interleukin-1 enhances pain reflexes: Mediation through increased prostaglandin E2 levels. *Agents and Actions, 25,* 246–251.

Segerstrom, S. C., Taylor, S. E., Kemeny, M. E., & Fahey, J. L. (1998). Optimism is associated with mood, coping, and immune change in response to stress. *Journal of Personality and Social Psychology, 74,* 1646–1655.

Silverstein, P. (1992). Smoking and wound healing. *American Journal of Medicine, 93,* 22S–24S.

Sobel, D. S., & Ornstein, R. (1996). *The healthy mind, healthy body handbook.* New York: Patient Education Media.

Steptoe, A., Wardle, J., Pollard, T. M., Canaan, L., & Davies, G. J. (1996). Stress, social support and health-related behavior: A study of smoking, alcohol consumption and physical exercise. *Journal of Psychosomatic Research, 41,* 171–180.

Suls, J., & Wan, C. K. (1989). Effects of sensory and procedural information on coping with stressful medical procedures and pain: A meta-analysis. *Journal of Consulting and Clinical Psychology, 57,* 372–379.

Thomas, D. R., & Ritchie, C. S. (1995). Preoperative assessment of older adults. *Journal of the American Geriatrics Society, 43,* 811–821.

Tonnessen, E., Brinklov, M. M., Christensen, N. J., Olesen, A. S., & Madsen, T. (1987). Natural killer cell activity and lymphocyte function during and after coronary artery bypass grafting in relation to the endocrine stress response. *Anesthesiology, 67,* 526–533.

Uchino, B. N., Cacioppo, J. T., & Kiecolt-Glaser, J. K. (1996). The relationship between social support and physiological processes: A review with emphasis on underlying mechanisms. *Psychological Bulletin, 119,* 488–531.

Ulrich, R. S. (1984). View from a window may influence recovery from surgery. *Science, 224,* 420–421.

Van De Kerkhof, P. C. M., Van Bergen, B., Spruijt, K., & Kuiper, J. P. (1994). Age-related changes in wound healing. *Clinical and Experimental Dermatology, 19,* 369–374.

Veldhuis, J. D., & Iranmanesh, A. (1996). Physiological regulation of the human growth hormone (GH)-insulin-like growth factor type I (IGF-I) axis: Predominant impact of age, obesity, gonadal function, and sleep. *Sleep, 19,* S221–S224.

Verhoef, J. (1990). Transient immunodepression. *Journal of Antimicrobial Chemotherapy, 26,* 23–29.

Watkins, L. R., Goehler, L. E., Relton, J. K., Tartaglia, N., Silbert, L., Martin, D., & Maier, S. F. (1995). Blockade of interleukin-1 induced hyperthermia by subdiaphragmatic vagotomy: Evidence for vagal mediation of immune–brain communication. *Neuroscience Letters, 183,* 27–31.

Wikesjö, U. M. E., Nilveus, R. E., & Selvig, K. A. (1992). Significance of early healing events on periodontal repair: A review. *Journal of Periodontology, 63*, 158–165.

Woolf, C. J. (1994). A new strategy for treatment of inflammatory pain: Prevention or elimination of central sensitization. *Drugs, 47*, 1–9.

Yeager, M. P., Glass, D. D., Neff, R. K., & Brinck-Johnsen, T. (1987). Epidural anesthesia and analgesia in high-risk surgical patients. *Anesthesiology, 66*, 729–736.

Zwilling, B. S. (1994). Neuroimmunomodulation of macrophage function. In J. K. Kiecolt-Glaser & R. Glaser (Eds.), *Handbook of human stress and immunity* (pp. 53–76). San Diego, CA: Academic Press.

Bruce S. McEwen

Over 60 years ago, Selye[1] recognized the paradox that the physiologic systems activated by stress can not only protect and restore but also damage the body. What links these seemingly contradictory roles? How does stress influence the pathogenesis of disease, and what accounts for the variation in vulnerability to stress-related diseases among people with similar life experiences? How can stress-induced damage be quantified? These and many other questions still challenge investigators.

This chapter reviews the long-term effect of the physiologic response to stress, which I refer to as allostatic load.[2] Allostasis—the ability to achieve stability through change[3]—is critical to survival. Through allostasis, the autonomic nervous system, the hypothalamic–pituitary–adrenal (HPA) axis, and the cardiovascular, metabolic, and immune systems protect the body by responding to internal and external stress. The price of this accommodation to stress can be allostatic load,[2] which is the wear and tear that results from chronic overactivity or underactivity of allostatic systems.

The Physiologic Response to Stress

Stressful experiences include major life events, trauma, and abuse and are sometimes related to the environment in the home, workplace, or neighborhood. Acute stress (in the sense of "fight or flight" or major life events) and chronic stress (the cumulative load of minor, day-to-day stresses) can both have long-term consequences. The effects of chronic stress may be exacerbated by a rich diet and the use of tobacco and alcohol and reduced by moderate exercise.

Genetic factors do not account for all the individual variability in sensitivity to stress, as evinced by the lack of concordance between identical twins in many disorders.[4,5] Moreover, genetic factors do not explain the gradients of health across socioeconomic levels in Western societies.[6] Two factors largely determine individual responses to potentially stressful situations: the way a person perceives a situation[7] and a person's general state of physical health, which is determined not only by genetic factors but also by behavioral and lifestyle choices (Fig. 73.1). Whether one perceives a situation as a threat, either psychological or physical, is crucial in determining the behavioral response—whether it is fleeing, fighting, or cowering in fear—and the physiologic response—calmness or heart palpitations and elevated cortisol levels.

The ability to adjust or habituate to repeated stress is also determined by the way one perceives a situation. For example, most people react initially to the challenge of public speaking with activation of the HPA axis. After repeated public speaking, however, most people become habituated and their cortisol secretion no longer increases with the challenge. But approximately 10 percent of subjects continue to find public speaking stressful, and their cortisol secretion increases each time they speak in public.[8] Others are prone to a cardiovascular stress response, as shown by a recent study of cardiovascular responses to a stressful arithmetic test. Blood-pressure responses to this experimental stress predicted elevated ambulatory blood pressure during periods of perceived stress in everyday life.[9] Genetics may also have a role in susceptibility to cardiovascular stress; many people whose blood pressure remains elevated for several hours after the stress of an arithmetic test have a parent with hypertension.[10]

One's physical condition has obvious implications for one's ability to mount an appropriate physiologic response to stressful stimuli, and there may be a genetic component to the response as well. In inbred BioBreeding (BB) rats, an animal model of insulin-dependent diabetes,

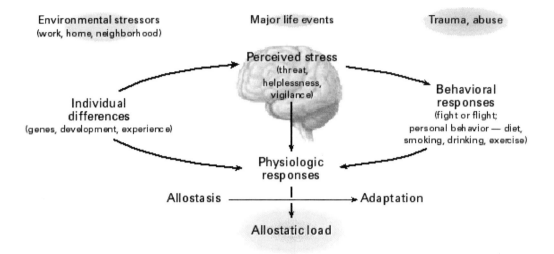

Figure 73.1
The stress response and development of allostatic load. The perception of stress is influenced by one's experiences, genetics, and behavior. When the brain perceives an experience as stressful, physiologic and behavioral responses are initiated, leading to allostasis and adaptation. Over time, allostatic load can accumulate, and the overexposure to mediators of neural, endocrine, and immune stress can have adverse effects on various organ systems, leading to disease.

exposure to repeated stress increased the incidence of diabetes.[11] In children, family instability increases the incidence and severity of insulin-dependent diabetes.[12] Chronic stress, defined as feelings of fatigue, lack of energy, irritability, demoralization, and hostility, has been linked to the development of insulin resistance,[13] a risk factor for non-insulin-dependent diabetes. Deposition of abdominal fat, a risk factor for coronary heart disease and diabetes,[14] is increased by the psychosocial stress of colony reorganization in nonhuman primates[15] and may also be increased by stress in humans.[16]

Allostasis and Allostatic Load

In contrast to homeostatic systems such as blood oxygen, blood pH, and body temperature, which must be maintained within narrow ranges, allo-

static (adaptive) systems have much broader boundaries. Allostatic systems enable us to respond to our physical states (e.g., awake, asleep, supine, standing, exercising) and to cope with noise, crowding, isolation, hunger, extremes of temperature, danger, and microbial or parasitic infection.

The core of the body's response to a challenge—whether it is a dangerous situation, an infection, living in a crowded and unpleasant neighborhood, or a public-speaking test—is twofold, turning on an allostatic response that initiates a complex adaptive pathway, and then shutting off this response when the threat is past. The most common allostatic responses involve the sympathetic nervous systems and the HPA axis. For these systems, activation releases catecholamines from nerves and the adrenal medulla and leads to the secretion of corticotropin from the pituitary. The corticotropin, in turn, mediates

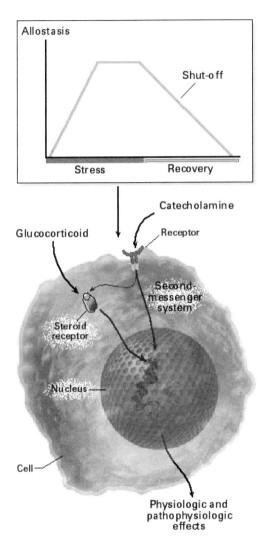

the release of cortisol from the adrenal cortex. Figure 73.2 shows how catecholamines and glucocorticoids affect cellular events. Inactivation returns the systems to base-line levels of cortisol and catecholamine secretion, which normally happens when the danger is past, the infection is contained, the living environment is improved, or the speech has been given. However, if the inactivation is inefficient (see below), there is overexposure to stress hormones. Over weeks, months, or years, exposure to increased secretion of stress hormones can result in allostatic load[2] and its pathophysiologic consequences.

Four situations are associated with allostatic load (Fig. 73.3). The first and most obvious is frequent stress. For example, surges in blood pressure can trigger myocardial infarction in susceptible persons,[17] and in primates repeated elevations of blood pressure over periods of weeks and months accelerate atherosclerosis,[18] thereby increasing the risk of myocardial infarction.

In the second type of allostatic load (Fig. 73.3), adaptation to repeated stressors of the same type is lacking, resulting in prolonged exposure to stress hormones, as was the case for some of the people subjected to the repeated-public-speaking challenge.[8]

In the third type of allostatic load (Fig. 73.3) there is an inability to shut off allostatic responses after a stress is terminated. As we have noted, the blood pressure in some people fails to recover after the acute stress of an arithmetic test,[10] and hypertension accelerates atherosclerosis.[18] Women with a history of depressive illness have decreased bone mineral density, because the

Figure 73.2
Allostasis in the autonomic nervous system and the HPA axis. Allostatic systems respond to stress (upper panel) by initiating the adaptive response, sustaining it until the stress ceases, and then shutting it off (recovery). Allostatic responses are initiated (lower panel) by an increase in circulating catecholamines from the autonomic nervous system and glucocorticoids from the adrenal cortex. This sets into motion adaptive processes that alter the structure and function of a variety of cells and tissues. These processes are initiated through intracellular receptors for steroid hormones, plasma-membrane receptors, and second-messenger systems for catecholamines. Cross-talk between catecholamines and glucocorticoid-receptor signaling systems can occur.

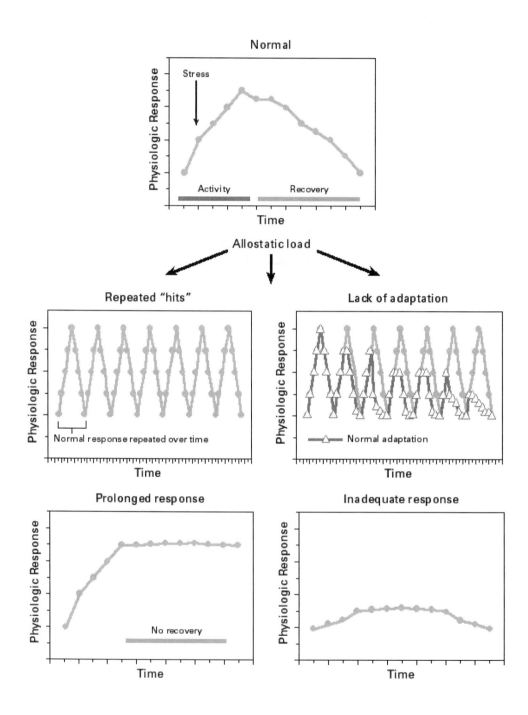

allostatic load of chronic, moderately elevated serum cortisol concentrations inhibits bone formation.[19] Intense athletic training also induces allostatic load in the form of elevated sympathetic and HPA-axis activity, which results in weight loss, amenorrhea, and the often-related condition of anorexia nervosa.[20,21]

The failure to turn off the HPA axis and sympathetic activity efficiently after stress is a feature of age-related functional decline in laboratory animals,[22-24] but the evidence of this in humans is limited.[25,26] Stress-induced secretion of cortisol and catecholamines returns to base line more slowly in some aging animals with other signs of accelerated aging,[22-24] and the negative-feedback effects of cortisol are reduced in elderly humans.[26] One other sign of age-related impairment in rats is that the hippocampus fails to turn off the release of excitatory amino acids after stress,[27] and this may accelerate progressive structural damage and functional impairment (see below).

One speculation is that allostatic load over a lifetime may cause the allostatic systems to wear out or become exhausted.[25] A vulnerable link in the regulation of the HPA axis and cognition is the hippocampal region. According to the "glucocorticoid-cascade hypothesis," wear and tear on this region of the brain leads to dysregulation of the HPA axis and cognitive impairment.[23,28] Indeed, some but not all aging rats have impairment of episodic, declarative, and spatial memory and hyperactivity of the HPA axis, all of which can be traced to hippocampal damage.[29] Recent data suggest that similar events may occur in humans.[30,31]

In the fourth type of allostatic load (Fig. 73.3), inadequate responses by some allostatic systems trigger compensatory increases in others. When one system does not respond adequately to a stressful stimulus, the activity of other systems increases, because the underactive system is not providing the usual counterregulation. For example, if cortisol secretion does not increase in response to stress, secretion of inflammatory cytokines (which are counterregulated by cortisol) increases.[32] The negative consequences of an enhanced inflammatory response are seen, for example, in Lewis rats; these animals are very susceptible to autoimmune and inflammatory disturbances, because of a genetically determined hyporesponsiveness of the HPA axis.[33]

In another model, rats that become subordinate in a psychosocial living situation called the "visible-burrow system" have a stress-induced state of HPA hyporesponsiveness.[34,35] In these rats, the response to stressors applied by the experimenter is very limited, and concentrations of corticotropin-releasing hormone messenger RNA in the hypothalamus are abnormally low.[36] Human counterparts with HPA hyporesponsiveness include adults with fibromyalgia[37,38] and chronic fatigue syndrome[39,40] and children with atopic dermatitis.[41] In post-traumatic stress disorder, basal HPA activity is also low,[42,43] although reactivity to stress may not be blunted.

Feelings of anticipation and worry can also contribute to allostatic load.[44] Anticipation participates in the reflex that prevents us from blacking out when we get out of bed in the morning[3] and is also part of worry, anxiety, and cognitive preparation for a threat. Anticipatory

Figure 73.3
Three types of allostatic load. The top panel illustrates the normal allostatic response, in which a response is initiated by a stressor, sustained for an appropriate interval, and then turned off. The remaining panels illustrate four conditions that lead to allostatic load: repeated "hits" from multiple stressors; lack of adaptation; prolonged response due to delayed shutdown; and inadequate response that leads to compensatory hyperactivity of other mediators (e.g., inadequate secretion of glucocorticoids, resulting in increased concentrations of cytokines that are normally counterregulated by glucocorticoids).

anxiety can drive the secretion of mediators like corticotropin, cortisol, and epinephrine, and for this reason, prolonged anxiety and anticipation are likely to result in allostatic load.[44] For example, salivary cortisol concentrations increase within 30 minutes after waking in people who are under considerable psychological stress due to work or family matters.[45] In a related fashion, intrusive memories of a traumatic event (as in post-traumatic stress disorder) can produce a form of chronic stress and can drive physiologic responses.[46]

Allostasis and allostatic load are also affected by the consumption of tobacco and alcohol, dietary choices, and the amount of exercise (Fig. 73.1). These forms of behavior are integral to the overall notion of allostasis—the way people cope with a challenge—and also contribute to allostatic load by known pathways (e.g., a high-fat diet accelerates atherosclerosis and progression to non-insulin-dependent diabetes by increasing cortisol secretion, leading to fat deposition and insulin resistance;[47] smoking elevates blood pressure and accelerates atherogenesis;[48] and exercise protects against cardiovascular disease[49]).

Examples of Allostatic Load

Cardiovascular and Metabolic Systems

The best-studied system of allostasis and allostatic load is the cardiovascular system and its links to obesity and hypertension. In nonhuman primates, the incidence of atherosclerosis is increased among the dominant males of unstable social hierarchies and in socially subordinate females.[50,51] In humans, lack of control on the job increases the risk of coronary heart disease,[52] and job strain (high psychological demands and lack of control) results in elevated ambulatory blood pressure at home and an increased left-ventricular-mass index,[53] as well as increased progression of atherosclerosis.[54] Chronic stress (feelings of fatigue, lack of energy, irritability,

and demoralization) and hostility are linked to increased reactivity of the fibrinogen system and of platelets, both of which increase the risk of myocardial infarction.[55,56]

Quantifying allostatic load, a major challenge, has been attempted with the use of measures of metabolic and cardiovascular pathophysiology. In a recent analysis,[57] data from the MacArthur Studies of Successful Aging were used to assess eight measures of increased activity of allostatic systems between 1988 and 1991. Allostatic load was approximated by determining the number of measures for which a person had values in the highest quartile from among the following: systolic blood pressure, overnight urinary cortisol and catecholamine excretion, the ratio of the waist to the hip measurement, the glycosylated hemoglobin value, and the ratio of serum high-density lipoprotein in the total serum cholesterol concentration; and the number of the following for which the person had values in the lowest quartile: serum concentration of dehydroepiandrosterone sulfate and serum concentration of high-density lipoprotein cholesterol. In cross-sectional analyses of base-line data, subjects with higher levels of physical and mental functioning had lower allostatic-load scores and a lower incidence of cardiovascular disease, hypertension, and diabetes. During the three years of follow-up (1988 to 1991), people in this higher-functioning group with higher allostatic-load scores at base line were more likely to have incident cardiovascular disease and were significantly more likely to have declines in cognitive and physical functioning. Among women in this group, increased cortisol secretion predicted a decline in memory.[31]

The Brain

Repeated stress affects brain function, especially in the hippocampus, which has high concentrations of cortisol receptors.[58] The hippocampus participates in verbal memory and is particularly important for the memory of "context," the time and place of events that have a strong emotional bias.[59,60] Moreover, glucocorticoids are involved in remembering the context in which an emotionally laden event took place.[61] Impairment of the hippocampus decreases the reliability and accuracy of contextual memories. This may exacerbate stress by preventing access to the information needed to decide that a situation is not a threat.[62] The hippocampus also regulates the stress response and acts to inhibit the response of the HPA axis to stress.[63,64]

The mechanism for stress-induced hippocampal dysfunction and memory impairment is twofold. First, acute stress increases cortisol secretion, which suppresses the mechanisms in the hippocampus and temporal lobe that subserve short-term memory.[65,66] Stress can impair memory in the short term, but fortunately these effects are reversible and relatively short-lived.[67] Second, repeated stress causes the atrophy of dendrites of pyramidal neurons in the CA3 region of the hippocampus through a mechanism involving both glucocorticoids and excitatory amino acid neurotransmitters released during and after stress.[68] This atrophy is reversible if the stress is short-lived, but stress lasting many months or years can kill hippocampal neurons.[23,69] Magnetic resonance imaging has shown that stress-related disorders such as recurrent depressive illness, post-traumatic stress disorder, and Cushing's disease are associated with atrophy of the hippocampus.[70,71] Whether this atrophy is reversible or permanent is not clear.

Long-term stress also accelerates the appearance of several biologic markers of aging in rats, including the loss of hippocampal pyramidal neurons and the excitability of pyramidal neurons in the CA1 region by a calcium-dependent mechanism.[72] Glucocorticoids may mediate these effects by enhancing calcium currents in the hippocampus,[73] since calcium ions have a key role in destructive as well as plastic processes in hippocampal neurons.[74-76] The persistent release of the excitatory amino acid glutamate in the hippocampus after stress in aged rats may

also contribute to age-related neuronal damage[27] and may potentiate atrophy and possibly even neuronal loss.

Early stress and neonatal handling influence the course of aging and age-related cognitive impairment in animals. Early experiences are believed to set the level of responsiveness of the HPA axis and autonomic nervous system. These systems overreact in animals subjected to early unpredictable stress and underreact in animals exposed to neonatal handling.[77] In the former condition, aging of the brain is accelerated, whereas in the latter, aging of the brain is reduced.[29,77]

The Immune System

The immune system responds to pathogens or other antigens with its own form of allostasis that may include an acute-phase response as well as the formation of an immunologic "memory." At the same time, other allostatic systems, such as the HPA axis and the autonomic nervous system, tend to contain acute-phase responses and dampen cellular immunity.[78] However, not all the effects are suppressive. Acute stress causes lymphocytes and macrophages to be redistributed throughout the body and to "marginate" on blood-vessel walls and within certain compartments, such as the skin, lymph nodes, and bone marrow. This "trafficking" is mediated in part by glucocorticoids.[78-82] If an immune challenge is not encountered and the hormonal-stress signal ceases, immune cells return to the bloodstream. When a challenge occurs, however, as is the case in delayed-type hypersensitivity, acute stress enhances the traffic of lymphocytes and macrophages to the site of acute challenge.[83,84]

The immune-enhancing effects of acute stress depend on adrenal secretion and last for three to five days. Acute stress has the effect of calling immune cells to their battle stations, and this form of allostasis enhances responses for which there is an established immunologic "memory."[83-85] If the immunologic memory is of a pathogen or a tumor cell, the result of stress is presumably beneficial. If, on the contrary, the immunologic memory leads to an autoimmune or allergic response, then stress is likely to exacerbate a pathologic state. When allostatic load is increased by repeated stress, the outcome is completely different; the delayed hypersensitivity response is substantially inhibited[86] rather than enhanced. The consequences of suppressed cellular immunity resulting from chronic stress include increased severity of the common cold, accompanied by increased titers of cold-virus antibody.[87] In laboratory animals, repeated stress also leads to recurrent endotoxemia, which decreases the reactivity of the HPA axis to a variety of stimuli and decreases production of the cytokine tumor necrosis factor α.[88]

Implications of Allostatic Load in Human Society

The gradients of health across the range of socioeconomic levels[6] relate to a complex array of risk factors that are differentially distributed in human society.[89,90] Perhaps the best example is offered by the Whitehall studies of the British civil service, in which mortality and morbidity were found to increase stepwise from the lowest to the highest of the six grades of the British civil service.[91] Hypertension was a sensitive index of job stress,[92] particularly among factory workers, other workers with repetitive jobs and time pressures,[93] and workers whose jobs were unstable because of departmental privatization (Marmot MG: personal communication). Plasma fibrinogen concentrations, which predict an increased risk of death from coronary heart disease, are elevated among men in the lower British civil-service grades.[56] In less stable societies, conflict and social instability have been found to accelerate pathophysiologic processes and increase morbidity and mortality. For example, cardiovascular disease is a major contributor to the increase of almost 40 percent in the death rate among Russian men during the social collapse that followed the fall of Communism.[94] Blood-

pressure surges and sustained elevation are linked to accelerated atherosclerosis[18] as well as to an increased risk of myocardial infarction.[17]

Another stress-linked change is abdominal obesity (see above), measured as an increased waist-to-hip ratio. The waist-to-hip ratio is increased at the lower end of the socioeconomic-status gradient in Swedish men[95] and in the lower civil-service grades in the Whitehall studies.[96] Immune-system function is also a likely target of psychosocial stress,[97] increasing vulnerability to such infections as the common cold.[87,98]

Therapeutic Implications

A consideration of allostatic load is increasingly important in the diagnosis and treatment of many illnesses. Allostatic load is also important in illuminating the relation between disease and social instability, job loss, dangerous living environments, and other conditions that are chronically stressful. Medical illness itself is a source of stress, producing anxiety about prognosis, treatment, disability, and interference with social roles and relationships.

Physicians and other health care providers can help patients reduce allostatic load by helping them learn coping skills, recognize their own limitations, and relax. Patients should also be reminded of the interactions of a high-fat diet and stress in atherosclerosis, the role of smoking in cardiovascular disease and cancer, and the beneficial effects of exercise. But the patients themselves must change their behavior patterns appropriately.[99,100]

Beyond these obvious steps, other types of interventions must be considered. Two important causes of allostatic load appear to be isolation[101] and lack of control in the work environment.[52] Interventions that increase social support and enhance coping prolong the life spans of patients with breast cancer,[102] lymphomas,[103] and malignant melanoma.[104] Interventions designed to increase a worker's control over his or her job, such as the reorganization of auto production at

Volvo, have also improved health and attitudes toward work.[93]

Discussion

Dr. Jeffrey Flier: Is there any known correlation between lifelong stress (and therefore allostatic load) and Alzheimer's disease?

Dr. McEwen: There are a few anecdotes from admissions personnel at Veterans Affairs hospitals but nothing concrete. It is interesting, however, that education appears to have a "protective" role against the development of Alzheimer's disease.[105] It is not clear, though, whether education protects against the disease or provides more redundancy in the brain, which delays the symptoms.[106]

Dr. Barbara B. Kahn: What are the important differences between men and women in the biology of stress?

Dr. McEwen: Estrogens appear to protect the cardiovascular system, and at menopause, women's risk of cardiovascular disease increases to that of age-matched men. The decline in estrogen secretion at menopause also increases the activity of the HPA axis,[107] a development that has been linked to greater cognitive decline among elderly women than among elderly men.[31] A decline in androgen secretion in older men may affect HPA function, although to a lesser extent. In rats, castration increases HPA activity.[108] Finally, there are structural and functional differences between the sexes in hippocampal formation in rodents,[109–111] and behavioral evidence suggests functional and possibly structural sex differences in humans, as well.[112] We do not yet know whether these differences influence the vulnerability of the hippocampus to severe stress, although a number of studies now suggest that female rodents and primates may be less vulnerable than males.[69,113]

Dr. Flier: Is there any evidence that humans are more susceptible to the effects of stress than animals because of the greater human capacity for cognition and insight, as well as the human ability to feel guilt?

Dr. McEwen: I believe that humans are more at risk for allostatic load than animals, because of the enormous individual differences in stress responsiveness and aging among humans, which relate to life experiences, personality, and physiologic phenotype. However, stress responsiveness and aging also differ among rats, so I don't think we can be definitive about the importance of cognition in our own species.

A Physician: What mechanisms underlie the differences between immune responses to acute stress and those to chronic stress?

Dr. McEwen: These mechanisms are just beginning to be understood. One key process is the redistribution, or trafficking, of immune cells. Acute stress enhances this response to delayed-type hypersensitivity. Chronic stress impairs delayed-type hypersensitivity, with the result that the blood is depleted of fewer lymphocytes. The greater the impairment of delayed-type hypersensitivity, the less the blood is depleted of lymphocytes (Dhabhar FS: unpublished data). Glucocorticoids are responsible for the trafficking of lymphocytes and for the stress enhancement of delayed-type hypersensitivity, but they do not act alone. Various cytokines function as more-local signals, emanating from a site of infection or challenge, and Dr. Firdaus Dhabhar at Rockefeller University is investigating their involvement. Beyond that, it is well known that stress hormones modulate immune function and influence the class of the immune response by their ability to increase the expression of some cytokines and decrease the expression of others.[78]

References

1. Selye H. Syndrome produced by diverse nocuous agents. Nature 1936; 138:32.

2. McEwen BS, Stellar E. Stress and the individual: mechanisms leading to disease. Arch Intern Med 1993; 153:2093–101.

3. Sterling P, Eyer J. Allostasis: a new paradigm to explain arousal pathology. In: Fisher S, Reason J, eds. Handbook of life stress, cognition and health. New York: John Wiley, 1988:629–49.

4. Berg K. Genetics of coronary heart disease. Prog Med Genet 1983; 5:35–90.

5. Plomin R. The role of inheritance in behavior. Science 1990; 248:183–8.

6. Adler NE, Boyce T, Chesney MA, et al. Socioeconomic status and health: the challenge of the gradient. Am Psychol 1994; 49:15–24.

7. Lazarus RS, Folkman S. Stress, appraisal and coping. New York: Springer-Verlag, 1984.

8. Kirschbaum C, Prussner JC, Stone AA, et al. Persistent high cortisol responses to repeated psychological stress in a subpopulation of healthy men. Psychosom Med 1995; 57:468–74.

9. Matthews KA, Owens JF, Allen MT, Stoney CM. Do cardiovascular responses to laboratory stress relate to ambulatory blood pressure levels? Yes, in some of the people, some of the time. Psychosom Med 1992; 54:686–97.

10. Gerin W, Pickering TG. Association between delayed recovery of blood pressure after acute mental stress and parental history of hypertension. J Hypertens 1995; 13:603–10.

11. Lehman C, Rodin J, McEwen BS, Brinton R. Impact of environmental stress on the expression of insulin-dependent diabetes mellitus. Behav Neurosci 1991; 105:241–5.

12. Hagglof B, Blom L, Dahlquist G, Lonnberg G, Sahlin B. The Swedish childhood diabetes study: indications of severe psychological stress as a risk factor for type 1 (insulin-dependent) diabetes mellitus in childhood. Diabetologia 1991; 34:579–83.

13. Raikkonen K, Keltikangas-Jarvinen L, Adlercreutz H, Hautenen A. Psychosocial stress and the insulin resistance syndrome. Metabolism 1996; 45:1533–8.

14. Bjorntorp P. "Portal" adipose tissue as a generator of risk factors for cardiovascular disease and diabetes. Arteriosclerosis 1990; 10:493–6.

15. Jayo JM, Shively CA, Kaplan JR, Manuck SB. Effects of exercise and stress on body fat distribution in male cynomolgus monkeys. Int J Obes Relat Metab Disord 1993; 17:597–604.

16. Moyer AE, Rodin J, Grilo CM, Cummings N, Larson LM, Rebuffe-Scrive M. Stress-induced cortisol response and fat distribution in women. Obes Res 1994; 2:255–61.

17. Muller JE, Tofler GH, Stone PH. Circadian variation and triggers of onset of acute cardiovascular disease. Circulation 1989; 79:733–43.

18. Kaplan JR, Pettersson K, Manuck SB, Olsson G. Role of sympathoadrenal medullary activation in the initiation and progression of atherosclerosis. Circulation 1991; 84:Suppl VI:VI-23–VI-32.

19. Michelson D, Stratakis C, Hill L, et al. Bone mineral density in women with depression. N Engl J Med 1996; 335:1176–81.

20. Boyar RM, Hellman LD, Roffwarg H, et al. Cortisol secretion and metabolism in anorexia nervosa. N Engl J Med 1977; 296:190–3.

21. Loucks AB, Mortola JF, Girton L, Yen SSC. Alterations in the hypothalamic-pituitary-ovarian and the hypothalamic-pituitary-adrenal axes in athletic women. J Clin Endocrinol Metab 1989; 68:402–11.

22. McCarty R. Sympathetic-adrenal medullary and cardiovascular responses to acute cold stress in adult and aged rats. J Auton Nerv Syst 1985; 12:15–22.

23. Sapolsky RM. Stress, the aging brain and the mechanisms of neuron death. Cambridge, Mass.: MIT Press, 1992.

24. McEwen BS. Re-examination of the glucocorticoid hypothesis of stress and aging. In: Swaab DF, Hofman MA, Mirmiran M, Ravid R, van Leeuwen FW, eds. Progress in brain research. Vol. 93. The human hypothalamus in health and disease. Amsterdam: Elsevier Science, 1992:365–83.

25. Seeman TE, Robbins RJ. Aging and hypothalamic-pituitary-adrenal response to challenge in humans. Endocr Rev 1994; 15:233–60.

26. Wilkinson CW, Peskind ER, Raskind MA. Decreased hypothalamic-pituitary-adrenal axis sensitivity to cortisol feedback inhibition in human aging. Neuroendocrinology 1997; 65:79–90.

27. Lowy MT, Wittenberg L, Yamamoto BK. Effect of acute stress on hippocampal glutamate levels and spectrin proteolysis in young and aged rats. J Neurochem 1995; 65:268–74.

28. Sapolsky RM, Krey LC, McEwen BS. The neuroendocrinology of stress and aging: the glucocorticoid cascade hypothesis. Endocr Rev 1986; 7:284–301.

29. Meaney MJ, Aitken DH, van Berkel C, Bhatnagar S, Sapolsky RM. Effect of neonatal handling of age-related impairments associated with the hippocampus. Science 1988; 239:766–8.

30. Lupien S, Lecours AR, Lussier I, Schwartz G, Nair NPV, Meaney MJ. Basal cortisol levels and cognitive deficits in human aging. J Neurosci 1994; 14:2893–903.

31. Seeman TE, McEwen BS, Singer BH, Albert MS, Rowe JW. Increase in urinary cortisol excretion and memory declines: MacArthur studies of successful aging. J Clin Endocrinol Metab 1997; 82:2458–65.

32. Munck A, Guyre PM, Holbrook NJ. Physiological functions of glucocorticoids in stress and their relation to pharmacological actions. Endocr Rev 1984; 5:25–44.

33. Sternberg EM, Young WS III, Bernardini R, et al. A central nervous system defect in biosynthesis of corticotropin-releasing hormone is associated with susceptibility to streptococcal cell wall-induced arthritis in Lewis rats. Proc Natl Acad Sci U S A 1989; 86:4771–5.

34. Blanchard DC, Sakai RR, McEwen BS, Weiss SM, Blanchard RJ. Subordination stress: behavioral, brain, and neuroendocrine correlates. Behav Brain Res 1993; 58:113–21.

35. McKittrick CR, Blanchard DC, Blanchard RJ, McEwen BS, Sakai RR. Serotonin receptor binding in a colony model of chronic social stress. Biol Psychiatry 1995; 37:383–93.

36. Albeck DS, McKittrick CR, Blanchard DC, et al. Chronic social stress alters expression of corticotropin-releasing factor and arginine vasopressin mRNA in rat brain. J Neurosci 1997; 17:4895–903.

37. Crofford LJ, Pillemer SR, Kalogeras KT, et al. Hypothalamic-pituitary-adrenal axis perturbations in patients with fibromyalgia. Arthritis Rheum 1994; 37:1583–92.

38. Heim C, Ehlert U, Hanker J, Hellhammer DH. Abuse-related posttraumatic stress disorder and alterations of the hypothalamo-pituitary adrenal axis in women with chronic pelvic pain. Psychosom Med (in press).

39. Poteliakhoff A. Adrenocortical activity and some clinical findings in acute and chronic fatigue. J Psychosom Res 1981; 25:91–5.

40. Ur E, White PD, Grossman A. Hypothesis: cytokines may be activated to cause depressive illness and chronic fatigue syndrome. Eur Arch Psychiatry Clin Neurosci 1992; 241:317–22.

41. Buske-Kirschbaum A, Jobst S, Psych D, et al. Attenuated free cortisol response to psychosocial stress in children with atopic dermatitis. Psychosom Med 1997; 59:419–26.

42. Yehuda R, Giller EL, Southwick SM, Lowy MT, Mason JW. Hypothalamic-pituitary-adrenal dysfunction in posttraumatic stress disorder. Biol Psychiatry 1991; 30:1031–48.

43. Yehuda R, Teicher MH, Trestman RL, Levengood RA, Siever LJ. Cortisol regulation in posttraumatic stress disorder and major depression: a chronobiological analysis. Biol Psychiatry 1996; 40:79–88.

44. Schulkin J, McEwen BS, Gold PW. Allostasis, amygdala, and anticipatory angst. Neurosci Biobehav Rev 1994; 18:385–96.

45. Schulz P, Kirschbaum C, Pruessner J, Hellhammer DH. Increased free cortisol secretion after wakening in chronically-stressed individuals due to work overload. Stress Med (in press).

46. Baum A, Cohen L, Hall M. Control and intrusive memories as possible determinants of chronic stress. Psychosom Med 1993; 55:274–86.

47. Brindley DN, Rolland Y. Possible connections between stress, diabetes, obesity, hypertension and altered lipoprotein metabolism that may result in atherosclerosis. Clin Sci 1989; 77:453–61.

48. Verdecchia P, Schillaci G, Borgioni C, et al. Cigarette smoking, ambulatory blood pressure and cardiac hypertrophy in essential hypertension. J Hypertens 1995; 13:1209–15.

49. Bernadet P. Benefits of physical activity in the prevention of cardiovascular diseases. J Cardiovasc Pharmacol 1995; 25:Suppl 1:S3–S8.

50. Manuck SB, Kaplan JR, Adams MR, Clarkson TB. Studies of psychosocial influences on coronary artery atherogenesis in cynomolgus monkeys. Health Psychol 1988; 7:113–24.

51. Shively CA, Clarkson TB. Social status and coronary artery atherosclerosis in female monkeys. Arterioscler Thromb 1994; 14:721–6.

52. Bosma H, Marmot MG, Hemingway H, Nicholson AC, Brunner E, Stansfeld SA. Low job control

and risk of coronary heart disease in Whitehall II (prospective cohort) study. BMJ 1997; 314:558–65.

53. Schnall PL, Schwartz JE, Landsbergis PA, Warren K, Pickering TG. Relation between job strain, alcohol, and ambulatory blood pressure. Hypertension 1992; 19:488–94.

54. Everson SA, Lynch JW, Chesney MA, et al. Interaction of workplace demands and cardiovascular reactivity in progression of carotid atherosclerosis: population based study. BMJ 1997; 314:553–8.

55. Raikkonen K, Lassila R, Keltikangas-Jarvinen L, Hautanen A. Association of chronic stress with plasminogen activator inhibitor-1 in healthy middle-aged men. Arterioscler Thromb Vasc Biol. 1996; 16: 363–7.

56. Markowe HLJ, Marmot MG, Shipley MJ, et al. Fibrinogen: a possible link between social class and coronary heart disease. BMJ 1985; 291:1312–4.

57. Seeman TE, Singer BH, Rowe JW, Horwitz RI, McEwen BS. Price of adaptation—allostatic load and its health consequences: MacArthur studies of successful aging. Arch Intern Med 1997; 157:2259–68.

58. McEwen BS, De Kloet ER, Rostene W. Adrenal steroid receptors and actions in the nervous system. Physiol Rev 1986; 66:1121–88.

59. Eichenbaum H, Otto T, Cohen NJ. The hippocampus—what does it do? Behav Neural Biol 1992; 57:2–36.

60. LeDoux JE. In search of an emotional system in the brain: leaping from fear to emotion and consciousness. In: Gazzaniga M, ed. The cognitive neurosciences. Cambridge, Mass.: MIT Press, 1995:1049–61.

61. Pugh CR, Tremblay D, Fleshner M, Rudy JW. A selective role for corticosterone in contextual-fear conditioning. Behav Neurosci 1997; 111:503–11.

62. Sapolsky RM. Stress in the wild. Sci Am 1990; 262:116–23.

63. Jacobson L, Sapolsky R. The role of the hippocampus in feedback regulation of the hypothalamic-pituitary-adrenocortical axis. Endocr Rev 1991; 12: 118–34.

64. Herman JP, Cullinan WE. Neurocircuitry of stress: central control of the hypothalamo-pituitary-adrenocortical axis. Trends Neurosci 1997; 20:78–84.

65. Kirschbaum C, Wolf OT, May M, Wippich W, Hellhammer DH. Stress- and treatment-induced elevations of cortisol levels associated with impaired declarative memory in healthy adults. Life Sci 1996; 58:1475–83.

66. McEwen BS, Sapolsky RM. Stress and cognitive function. Curr Opin Neurobiol 1995; 5:205–16.

67. Lupien SJ, McEwen BS. The acute effects of corticosteroids on cognition: integration of animal and human model studies. Brain Res Rev 1997; 24:1–27.

68. McEwen BS, Albeck D, Cameron H, et al. Stress and the brain: a paradoxical role for adrenal steroids. Vitam Horm 1995; 51:371–402.

69. Uno H, Tarara R, Else JG, Suleman MA, Sapolsky RM. Hippocampal damage associated with prolonged and fatal stress in primates. J Neurosci 1989; 9:1705–11.

70. Sapolsky RM. Why stress is bad for your brain. Science 1996; 273:749–50.

71. McEwen BS, Magarinos AM. Stress effects on morphology and function of the hippocampus. Ann N Y Acad Sci 1997; 821:271–84.

72. Kerr DS, Campbell LW, Applegate MD, Brodish A, Landfield PW. Chronic stress-induced acceleration of electrophysiologic and morphometric biomarkers of hippocampal aging. J Neurosci 1991; 11:1316–24.

73. Kerr DS, Campbell LW, Thibault O, Landfield PW. Hippocampal glucocorticoid receptor activation enhances voltage-dependent Ca2+ conductances: relevance to brain aging. Proc Natl Acad Sci U S A 1992; 89:8527–31.

74. Choi DW. Calcium-mediated neurotoxicity: relationship to specific channel types and role in ischemic damage. Trends Neurosci 1988; 11:465–9.

75. Mills LR, Kater SB. Neuron-specific and state-specific differences in calcium homeostasis regulate the generation and degeneration of neuronal architecture. Neuron 1990; 4:149–63.

76. Mattson MP. Calcium as sculptor and destroyer of neural circuitry. Exp Gerontol 1992; 27:29–49.

77. Meaney MJ, Tannenbaum B, Francis D, et al. Early environmental programming; hypothalamic-pituitary-adrenal responses to stress. Semin Neurosci 1994; 6:247–59.

78. McEwen BS, Biron CA, Brunson KW, et al. The role of adrenocorticoids as modulators of immune function in health and disease: neural, endocrine and immune interactions. Brain Res Rev 1997; 23:79–113.

79. Dhabhar FS, Miller AH, Stein M, McEwen BS, Spencer RL. Diurnal and acute stress-induced changes in distribution of peripheral blood leukocyte subpopulations. Brain Behav Immun 1994; 8:66–79.

80. Dhabhar FS, Miller AH, McEwen BS, Spencer RL. Effects of stress on immune cell distribution: dynamics and hormonal mechanisms. J Immunol 1995; 154:5511–27.

81. Miller AH, Spencer RL, Hassett J, et al. Effects of selective type I and II adrenal steroid agonists on immune cell distribution. Endocrinology 1994; 135:1934–44.

82. Herbert TB, Cohen S. Stress and immunity in humans: a meta-analytic review. Psychosom Med 1993; 55:364–79.

83. Dhabhar FS. Stress-induced enhancement of antigen-specific cell-mediated immunity: the role of hormones and leukocyte trafficking. New York: Rockefeller University, 1996.

84. Dhabhar FS, McEwen BS. Stress-induced enhancement of antigen-specific cell-mediated immunity. J Immunol 1996; 156:2608–15.

85. Dhabhar FS, Miller AH, McEwen BS, Spencer RL. Stress-induced changes in blood leukocyte distribution: role of adrenal steroid hormones. J Immunol 1996; 157:1638–44.

86. Dhabhar FS, McEwen BS. Moderate stress enhances, and chronic stress suppresses, cell-mediated immunity in vivo. Soc Neurosci 1996; 22:1350, abstract.

87. Cohen S, Tyrrell DAJ, Smith AP. Psychological stress and susceptibility to the common cold. N Engl J Med 1991; 325:606–12.

88. Hadid R, Spinedi E, Giovambattista A, Chautard T, Gaillard RC. Decreased hypothalamo-pituitary-adrenal axis response to neuroendocrine challenge under repeated endotoxemia. Neuroimmunomodulation 1996; 3:62–8.

89. Taylor SE, Repetti RL, Seeman T. Health psychology: what is an unhealthy environment and how does it get under the skin? Annu Rev Psychol 1997; 48:411–47.

90. Lynch JW, Kaplan GA, Cohen RD, Tuomilehto J, Salonen JT. Do cardiovascular risk factors explain the relation between socioeconomic status, risk of all-cause mortality, cardiovascular mortality, and acute myocardial infarction? Am J Epidemiol 1996; 144:934–42.

91. Marmot MG, Smith GD, Stansfeld S, et al. Health inequalities among British civil servants: the Whitehall II study. Lancet 1991; 337:1387–93.

92. Pickering TG, Devereux RB, James GD, et al. Environmental influences on blood pressure and the role of job strain. J Hypertens Suppl 1996; 14:S179–S185.

93. Melin B, Lundberg U, Soderlund J, Granqvist M. Psychological and physiological stress reactions of male and female assembly workers: a comparison between two different forms of work organization. J Organizat Psychol (in press).

94. Bobak M, Marmot M. East-West mortality divide and its potential explanations: proposed research agenda. BMJ 1996; 312:421–5.

95. Larsson B, Seidell J, Svardsudd K, et al. Obesity, adipose tissue distribution and health in men—the study of men born in 1913. Appetite 1989; 13:37–44.

96. Brunner EJ. The social and biological basis of cardiovascular disease in office workers. In: Blane D, Brunner EJ, Wilkinson RG, eds. Health and social organization. London: Routledge, 1996:272–313.

97. Cohen S, Kaplan JR, Cunnick JE, Manuck SB, Rabin BS. Chronic social stress, affiliation and cellular immune response in nonhuman primates. Psychol Sci 1992; 3:301–4.

98. Cohen S, Doyle WJ, Skoner DP, Rabin BS, Gwaltney JM Jr. Social ties and susceptibility to the common cold. JAMA 1997; 277:1940–4.

99. Redelmeier DA, Rozin P, Kahneman D. Understanding patients' decisions: cognitive and emotional perspectives. JAMA 1993; 270:72–6.

100. Horwitz RI, Horwitz SM. Adherence to treatment and health outcomes. Arch Intern Med 1993; 153:1863–8.

101. Seeman TE, McEwen BS. The impact of social environment characteristics on neuroendocrine regulation. Psychosom Med 1996; 58:459–71.

102. Spiegel D, Bloom JR, Kraemer HC, Gottheil E. Effect of psychosocial treatment on survival of patients with metastatic breast cancer. Lancet 1989; 2:888–91.

103. Richardson JL, Shelton DR, Krailo M, Levine AM. The effect of compliance with treatment on survival among patients with hematologic malignancies. J Clin Oncol 1990; 8:356–64.

104. Fawzy FI, Fawzy NW, Hyun CS, et al. Malignant melanoma: effects of an early structured psychiatric intervention, coping, and affective state on recurrence and survival 6 years later. Arch Gen Psychiatry 1993; 50:681–9.

105. Stern Y, Alexander GE, Prohovnik I, et al. Relationship between lifetime occupation and parietal flow: implications for a reserve against Alzheimer's disease pathology. Neurology 1995; 45:55–60.

106. Stern Y, Alexander GE, Prohovnik I, Mayeux R. Inverse relationship between education and parietotemporal perfusion deficit in Alzheimer's disease. Ann Neurol 1992; 32:371–5.

107. Van Cauter E, Leproult R, Kupfer DJ. Effects of gender and age on the levels and circadian rhythmicity of plasma cortisol. J Clin Endocrinol Metab 1996; 81:2468–73.

108. Handa RJ, Nunley KM, Lorens SA, Louie JP, McGivern RF, Bollnow MR. Androgen regulation of adrenocorticotropin and corticosterone secretion in the male rat following novelty and foot shock stressors. Physiol Behav 1994; 55:117–24.

109. Juraska JM, Fitch JM, Henderson C, Rivers N. Sex differences in the dendritic branching of dentate granule cells following differential experience. Brain Res 1985; 333:73–80.

110. Gould E, Westlind-Danielsson A, Frankfurt M, McEwen BS. Sex differences and thyroid hormone sensitivity of hippocampal pyramidal cells. J Neurosci 1990; 10:996–1003.

111. Roof RL. The dentate gyrus is sexually dimorphic in prepubescent rats: testosterone plays a significant role. Brain Res 1993; 610:148–51.

112. Kimura D. Sex differences in the brain. Sci Am 1992; 267:118–25.

113. Mizoguchi K, Kunishita T, Chui DH, Tabira T. Stress induces neuronal death in the hippocampus of castrated rats. Neurosci Lett 1992; 138:157–60.

74 Cytokines for Psychologists: Implications of Bidirectional Immune-to-Brain Communication for Understanding Behavior, Mood, and Cognition

Steven F. Maier and Linda R. Watkins

In this chapter we argue that a variety of behavioral, affective, and cognitive phenomena are driven by events in the immune system. These events occur in response to infection, injury, and even harmless foreign substances of which the organism (animal or human) is unaware. Furthermore, we argue that appreciation of the pathways involved and appreciation of their evolution provide new perspectives for understanding both the nature of stress and a variety of stress-related phenomena including behavioral, affective, and cognitive sequelae of exposure to stressors. It is argued that the immune system, in addition to its well-known functions of recognizing foreign substances and arranging for their destruction and removal, functions as a *diffuse sense organ* distributed throughout the body. In this sensory role, it provides the central nervous system with information concerning a variety of processes occurring in the periphery. This view of the immune system is not new to researchers (e.g., Blalock, Smith, & Meyer, 1985), but the implications of this view for psychology have not previously been well developed. It should be noted at the outset that parts of this view that are presented are speculative and extend beyond well-accepted facts. Our goal is to present a broad model that will stimulate interest and research; as a result, some "reaching" and "selective ignoring" is unavoidable. However, we feel that these extensions are rational, and we attempt to indicate when points that we make would be regarded in this manner.

The relatively new field of psychoneuroimmunology is devoted to the study of behavior–brain–immune interrelationships. However, until recently the focus has been on a flow of causation that proceeds from psychological and behavioral events, to changes in the brain, to consequent alterations in autonomic and endocrine outflow from the brain, to the cells and organs of the immune system. This is schema-tized in Figure 74.1 by Pathways A and B. The brain has two major outflow pathways by which it can control peripheral organs such as those of the immune system. One is the autonomic nervous system, and the figure shows sympathetic nervous system innervation of immune organs, with catecholamines (norepinephrine and epinephrine) released from the terminals of sympathetic nerves controlling the activity of organs such as the spleen (Felten & Felten, 1991). The other pathway involves synthesis and release of *releasing factors* by cells in the hypothalamus that are secreted into the bloodstream at the hypothalamus and travel to the pituitary gland. The pituitary gland in turn secretes and releases hormones that lead to the production of further hormones that can influence many peripheral organs and cells such as those of the immune system. The particular neuroendocrine system shown in the figure is the hypothalamo-pituitary-adrenal (HPA) axis. The hypothalamus manufactures and releases corticotropin releasing hormone (CRH) in response to a wide variety of stimuli including "stressors," which lead cells in the anterior pituitary to produce and release into the blood corticotropin releasing hormone (ACTH), which in turn leads the adrenal cortex to produce and release into the blood glucocorticoids (cortisol in humans and corticosterone in the rat).

Organs and cells of the immune system express receptors for these hormones and are regulated by them (Plaut, 1987). The topic of how stress affects immune function is an example of this direction of causation. Stressors activate the HPA axis and the sympathetic nervous system, and the products of these systems then alter the function of immune organs and cells. However, it is now clear that the brain and immune system form a bidirectional communication network (Pathway C), with products of the immune system communicating to the brain. The purpose of this chapter

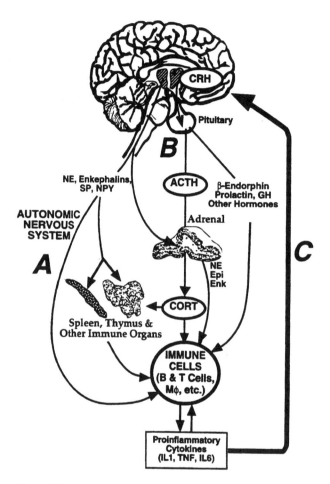

Figure 74.1
Schematic representation of brain-immune system connections. CRH, coricotropin releasing hormone; ACTH, adrenocorticotropic hormone; CORT, corticosterone; NE, norepinephrine; Epi, epinephrine; Enk, enkephalin; SP, substance P; NPY, neuropeptide Y; GH, growth hormone; Mϕ, macrophages; IL1, interleukin-1; TNF, tumor necrosis factor; IL6, interleukin-6.

is to elaborate on the implications of immune-to-brain communication for psychology.

The plan of the chapter is to first review some basic information concerning the immune system and its communication to the brain. This is not an exhaustive or detailed review, but it is intended only to provide the reader with the necessary background. We ask the reader to bear with us through this preliminary description because we feel that the rest is not intelligible unless these descriptions are provided. We then attempt to provide some insight into the functions that these pathways serve in fighting infection and injury. The major point is that activation of these pathways produces a constellation of adaptive behavioral and physiological changes that we call "sickness." These function in a variety of ways, but we argue that one function is to produce energy and conserve its use for processes such as fever, which combat the growth of infectious agents. Again, this may not seem relevant to psychological issues, but the role of bidirectional immune-to-brain communication in mediating psychological phenomena and its functional meaning cannot be understood unless the original functions of the communication pathway and its evolution are understood. Next, we relate these pathways and functions to psychological phenomena not previously understood to be connected to these pathways. The central argument is that physical and psychological stressors activate the same bidirectional immune–brain circuits, which have previously been described in the chapter, although their "entry point" into the loop is argued to be at the brain rather than at peripheral immune cells. Because the circuitry is bidirectional, the ultimate outcome is similar to that produced by infection or injury, and so the consequence is that many of the sequelae of exposure to stressors are products of these circuits and can better be understood by viewing them as reactions that originally evolved to combat infection and injury. We argue that stressors activate these circuits because fight–flight evolved later than the immune machinery and coopted its

use because fight–flight also requires the production of energy and because this allowed the system to anticipate injury or infection consequent to defensive actions. Thus, we argue that many of the sequelae of stressors that have been viewed as maladaptive or pathophysiological may actually be better understood as adaptive anticipatory reactions to promote recuperation from the stressor. We further argue that many phenomena often associated with stress including depression, learned helplessness, suppression of the specific immune response, and cognitive disturbances may be partial consequences of the immune processes to be discussed. Finally, we attempt to provide an evolutionary perspective that we hope provides insight into the adaptiveness of the phenomena discussed.

Some Considerations Concerning the Immune System

Specific Immunity

The reader is likely to be familiar with the basics of what is called *specific immunity* or the *specific immune response,* which is shown in Figure 74.2. The process begins when foreign substances (bacteria, viruses, or proteins not part of "self") enter the body. This initiates a long cascade of events culminating with the production of antibody. Indeed, foreign substances that trigger this cascade are called *antigens,* meaning antibody generators. The cascade leading to antibody production begins when the foreign substances are engulfed by antigen presenting cells (APCs; for example, macrophages and dendritic cells). The engulfed foreign substance is processed inside the APC, and then specific parts of the invader are moved to the external surface of the APC, where they are displayed. Specific molecular sites (called *antigenic sites*) on the displayed piece of foreign invader are recognized by a class of white blood cell called *T cells.* Each T cell has receptors on their external surfaces that serve in antigen rec-

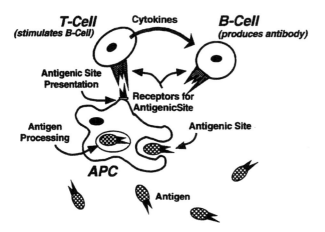

Figure 74.2
Aspects of the specific immune response. APC = antigen presenting cells.

ognition. Each individual T cell has receptors that allow it to bind to (recognize) only a single antigenic site. Of course, there are a large number of different foreign substances that can enter the body, so there is a huge diversity of antigenic sites that the immune system needs to be able to recognize. In turn, this means that to recognize all of these antigenic sites there must be an equally huge diversity in the T-cell population. Indeed, humans are estimated to have about a million different T cells, with only a very small number of T cells capable of recognizing the same antigenic site. This means that when a foreign substance enters the body, leading to its antigenic sites being displayed by APCs, only a very few T cells can recognize and respond to this invader. When the APCs displaying the antigenic site are finally encountered by the few T cells expressing receptors for it, this binding causes these few T cells to activate and differentiate. The T cells then undergo a series of cell divisions (proliferation) resulting in an increasing number of T cells with receptors specific for the foreign substance that has entered the body.

The responding T cells are not a homogenous group. For example, one class of these T cells is

called *cytotoxic T cells,* which can kill certain kinds of antigens. The class of T cell directly relevant for antibody formation is called *T-helper cells.* T-helper cells secrete substances that help a second class of white blood cell, *the B cells,* to expand their number. B cells also have specific receptors on their surface for antigens, and the B cells that proliferate are the ones with the receptor for the antigen because only these have been activated by the antigen. Thus, a large number of B cells are made with receptors for the antigen, and it is these B cells that secrete the antibody directed against the antigen. In fact, antibodies are actually soluble forms of the antigen-recognizing receptor on the surface of the B cell for the antigen. An antibody can destroy or arrange for the destruction of the invader in a variety of ways. In addition, a class of white blood cell with a receptor for the antigen, which is called a *memory cell,* is ultimately formed. These cells persist and respond much more rapidly to the antigen if it again enters the body. This is the basis of immunization. It is worth noting here that the APC, the T-helper cell, and the B cell secrete substances that coordinate and stimulate the complex cellular interactions leading to antibody production and memory cell formation. These substances are called *cytokines,* with the interleukins being prominent examples. They are called cytokines because their primary role has been thought to be to communicate between cells, and the name "interleukins" reflects their role in communication between leukocytes (white blood cells).

Nonspecific Immunity

The reason for providing this level of detail is so that the reader can understand why the specific immune response is a slow process. The specificity of the response entails a cost—a large number of cell divisions are needed to generate enough cells with the required receptor before an effective response can be mounted, and each cell cycle requires 8–12 hr. Indeed, an antibody to an antigen cannot even be detected for 3–5 days after entry into the body and is not at high levels for many more days. This suggests that the specific immune response cannot be the initial line of defense following infection. Indeed, it has been suggested that the specific immune response is most useful the second time an antigen is encountered because then the much more rapid memory response can occur.

The actual initial line of defense is provided by a set of processes that is likely to be less familiar to the reader and is often given less attention in psychoneuroimmunology; namely, *innate* or *nonspecific immunity.* This form of defense against infectious agents and tissue injury operates to restrict tissue damage and infection to the site of the wound or the point of entry of the infectious agent into the body. It involves a number of quite different mechanisms, but here we focus on the action of phagocytes (literally, "eating cells") such as the macrophage (literally "big eater") and the neutrophil. Note that cells such as macrophages serve a dual role as APCs in the specific immune response and now as phagocytes in the nonspecific immune response. Phagocytes recognize foreign substances, but they do so in a non-

specific way. They do not recognize just a single antigenic site but rather respond to general features of "nonself." Because a large population of these cells can respond to a particular invader, this is a much more rapid response than the specific immune response. The proliferation of immune cells is not required, and a response can be observed within 1–2 hr of entry of the foreign substance into the body. Macrophages can also respond to a number of products of injured "self" cells, and so macrophages are key players in the response to injury as well as to infection.

Recognition of a foreign substance or injured cells by phagocytes such as the macrophage is followed by a number of different processes. The macrophage contains enzymes that can kill foreign cells such as bacteria and may engulf and thus destroy them directly. In addition, the macrophage becomes activated and synthesizes and releases a number of products that function in defense. For example, the activated macrophage synthesizes nitric oxide. Nitric oxide is a gas and so diffuses from the macrophage into the region surrounding the macrophage. It can alter the function of other cells in this region and, in particular, is capable of interfering with the proliferation of cells via a number of mechanisms (e.g., nitric oxide interferes with mitochondrial respiration). If the macrophages are activated by bacteria, for example, then the nitric oxide would interfere with the growth of the bacteria. Activated macrophages also synthesize and release proinflammatory cytokines called *interleukin-1* (IL-1), *interleukin-6* (IL-6), and *tumor necrosis factor alpha* (TNFα). These proteins exert local actions that facilitate the development of an inflammatory reaction and attract other immune cells that will participate in healing at a wound site.

The Acute-Phase Response

In addition to their local actions, the proinflammatory cytokines orchestrate a complex set of widespread changes throughout the entire organism that also function to combat infection and injury. These defenses are not local, as is the case for phagocytosis and nitric oxide inhibition of growth of foreign cells, but rather are global in nature. This global reaction to infection or injury is often called the *acute-phase response* (Baumann & Gauldie, 1994) or sickness (Kent, Bluthé, Kelley, & Dantzer, 1992), and its components are summarized in the Appendix. Physiological adjustments include fever, increased slow-wave sleep, alterations in plasma ions, shifts in protein synthesis by the liver toward the production of acute-phase proteins and away from proteins that the liver normally produces such as albumin and carrier proteins, increased levels of circulating white blood cells (leukocytosis), and so forth. In addition, there are behavioral changes that include increased responsiveness to pain as well as reductions in activity, exploration, social interaction, aggression, and sexual behavior (see Kent et al., 1992). There are also less well-defined mood changes that have been described as depressed mood (Hart, 1988) and cognitive alterations described as loss of attention and interference with certain types of memory (Aubert, Vega, Dantzer, & Goodall, 1995). More is said about these later. There is also a classic "stress response" as defined by the activation of the sympathetic nervous system leading to the release of plasma catecholamines and activation of the HPA system leading to the release of ACTH and glucocorticoids (Dunn, 1995).

Why These Global Alterations During Infection and Injury: The Adaptiveness of Sickness

How is this syndrome to be understood? It is important to recognize that this pattern is widespread throughout phylogeny and can be observed in various forms throughout the vertebrates (Kluger, 1978). Conservation through evolution suggests that the set of responses to infection and injury is adaptive, and it has been argued that the sickness pattern is an *evolved*

strategy to combat infection and injury (Hart, 1988). That is, the symptoms of sickness are not pathological or a sign of debilitation produced by microbial or viral infection but rather are defensive responses that evolved long before medicine to control the infection. Furthermore, the behavioral alterations that are part of the pattern are not reflexive reactions to illness but rather are motivated behaviors. They are motivated in the sense that organisms will learn responses to be allowed to engage in the behaviors (Dantzer, Bluthé, Kent, & Goodall, 1993) and will choose conditions in which they can occur (Bernheim & Kluger, 1976). For example, fever occurs during infection in mammals, birds, reptiles, amphibians, and fish. Fever is a "defended increase" in core body temperature in that animals will choose conditions that allow core body temperature to rise (Kluger, Kozak, Conn, Leon, & Sozynski, 1996). This is most clearly revealed in ectotherms that can only raise core body temperature by behavioral means. Ectotherms such as lizards will choose an environment with a temperature that produces elevated body temperature following infection (Kluger et al., 1996), and goldfish have been shown to perform a shuttlebox response to gain access to a water temperature that produces a fever (Covert & Reynolds, 1977). As a result, sickness has been argued to represent a *central motivational state* (Dantzer et al., 1993). Some of the physiological alterations are straightforward in that they play well-defined roles in combating infection. For example, microorganisms require iron for efficient reproduction, and so the reduction in plasma iron is adaptive, acute-phase proteins modulate the inflammatory response, and so forth. However, others are less obvious.

Fever

Fever is likely to be the key to understanding these consequences of infection and injury. Fever occurs even in primitive organisms and is highly adaptive (Kluger, 1979). There are several reasons. First, a variety of microbial organisms grows best at or below the body temperature of the host and reproduces poorly at even slightly elevated temperatures. For example, in humans, some of the infectious agents that cause syphilis and gonorrhea are suppressed by the febrile response, and before the advent of modern antibiotics these were treated by inducing malaria and its consequent high fever, and then treating the malaria with quinine (Merritt, Adams, & Soloman, 1946). This does not mean that all infectious agents grow more slowly during fever, but only that this is often enough true that the response is adaptive (Blatteis, 1986). Second, fever increases the intensity of immunological responses to infection. It can potentiate both nonspecific and specific immunity. For example, white blood cells divide more rapidly at elevated temperatures (Manzella & Roberts, 1979), and phagocytes may kill more efficiently because some of the enzymatic processes involved proceed at a greater intensity (Sebag, Reed, & Williams, 1977).

In summary, increases in body temperature can retard the development of infectious agents and augment immune defenses. Indeed, there are many experimental demonstrations that inhibiting fever is detrimental to survival (Hart, 1988). However, fever entails a large metabolic cost. As for other aspects of sickness, the febrile process is initiated by the proinflammatory cytokines. The cytokines lead to an increase in the hypothalamic set point for body temperature so that an organism feels cold at previous normal, external temperatures. This will lead the organism to attempt to arrive at a new thermal equilibrium by reducing heat loss and by increasing heat production. To conserve heat, animals and humans shift blood flow away from the periphery, curl up, huddle, seek warm places, and so forth. To produce heat they increase muscle contractions by shivering and increase metabolism. The total increase in metabolism required for each 1°C rise in body temperature has been estimated to be 10–13% (Kluger, 1979). Shivering is the most

important involuntary method of heat production in many mammals including humans, and this raises the metabolic rate by a factor of 3 to 5 (Hart, 1988). This is an enormous cost, and so it would be adaptive to reduce the need for shivering as much as possible. It is much more energy efficient to reduce heat loss than it is to produce more heat.

Sickness

The pattern of changes observed during sickness can be understood in this context. Arguments about function are hazardous, but the changes that occur can be argued to function to (a) reduce the energetic cost of behavior so that the available energy stores can be used to produce fever, (b) reduce heat loss, and (c) produce energy. The roles of increased sleep and depressed activity, exploration, social interaction, sexual behavior, and mood should be apparent in this context. These all function to reduce the energy used in behavior and also reduce the amount of exposed bodily surface area because it is not readily possible to both move about engaging in normal activities and stay huddled or under covers.

However, the anorexia (decreased feeding) and the adipsia (decreased drinking) that occur during infection require special comment because they do not fit as obviously. After all, the intake of calories and nutrients should be beneficial. Several factors can be noted in this regard. First, it is important to allow the levels of plasma iron to be reduced, and food intake would counter this adaptive process. Second, an organism that is not hungry or thirsty will not move about in search of food and water—a tendency that can save energy usage for fever as well as reduce heat loss produced by exposure of the body surface during movement. Foraging for food and water would also expose the organism to possible predation at a time during which its resources are directed toward defense against the infectious agent rather than being available to defend against a predator.

Finally, the physiological stress response can be understood by considering the physiological functions of the end points of the sympathetic response and the HPA response. Both plasma catecholamines and glucocorticoids function to liberate energy from body stores. They catalyze the conversion of glycogen to glucose and break down muscle proteins into amino acids. Thus, these responses are capable of mobilizing energy for use in fever, as well as for cellular proliferation associated with immune activation.

Immune-to-Brain Communication

The foregoing demonstrates indirectly that the immune system must communicate to the brain and also provides some insight into why it must do so. The responses to infection begin with activation of peripheral immune cells such as macrophages, but many of the responses summarized as sickness are mediated by the brain rather than by peripheral organs. Thus, products of these immune cells must be capable of providing a signal to the brain. Fever, sleep, and pituitary adrenal and sympathetic activation are mediated by discrete nuclei in the hypothalamus. Furthermore, mood and behavior are products of the brain. Thus, the bulk of the adaptive changes observed after infection and injury is directly mediated by the brain. The sickness syndrome involves a mobilization of the entire resources of the organism in the service of defense against infection and tissue injury. After all, these are life and death situations and should preempt all other activities. The fact that animals and humans before the advent of modern medicine have survived through eons of evolutionary history attests to the efficacy of these mechanisms. Only the central nervous system is capable of orchestrating such a diverse and widespread pattern of changes that involve coordinated changes in numerous organ systems as well as in behavior.

We have already suggested that the proinflammatory cytokines released by activated macrophages and other cells are the critical signals to the central nervous system provided by the immune system. To summarize an enormous amount of literature, it is known that this complex set of events that we are calling sickness is initiated by the proinflammatory cytokines released by macrophages and related cell types because (a) blocking the effects of these cytokines with antagonists for their receptors or antiserum that neutralizes them prevents these sickness reactions during infection, and (b) administration of the cytokines in the absence of infection produces the full syndrome of responses (see Dinarello, 1991; Dinarello & Thompson, 1991, for reviews). It should be noted here that IL-1 is the most potent of the cytokines with regard to initiating the responses mediated by the brain. Thus, blocking only IL-1 blunts much of the sickness reaction to infection, and administering IL-1 peripherally produces most of the syndrome. For example, Bluthé, Dantzer, and Kelley (1992) reported that the antagonist acting at the IL-1 receptor substantially blunts the reduction in social exploration and weight loss produced by administration of lipopolysaccharide (LPS; a component of the cell wall of gram negative bacteria, which is also called *endotoxin*).

The foregoing suggests that it ought to be possible to observe directly neural alterations in response to the activation of peripheral immune cells by infectious agents or by the administration of cytokines such as IL-1 and that these responses should be blocked by peripheral administration of antagonists to IL-1. Again, a large amount of literature can only be summarized here. A variety of agents that activate macrophages have been administered, but the endotoxin (LPS) has been by far the most frequent. LPS leads to the release of proinflammatory cytokines from macrophages and other immune cells and is followed by a series of discrete and specific changes in the brain. The most pronounced changes are in norepinephrine in the hypothalamus (Dunn, 1992) and in serotonin in the hippocampus (Linthorst, Flachskamm,

Holsboer, & Reul, 1994). Large increases in the release of these transmitters as measured by in vivo microdialysis are observed within 30–90 min following the peripheral administration of LPS, other agents such as Newcastle's disease virus, or IL-1 itself (Lavicky & Dunn, 1995). We return to the importance of these specific neurochemical responses later. Changes in the electrical activity of the brain can be detected as well (Saphier, 1992). Also, as expected, these responses of the brain to peripheral immune activation can be attenuated by blocking peripheral receptors for IL-1 or by neutralizing peripheral IL-1 with antiserum to IL-1 (Dunn, 1993).

How Does the Signal Get to the Brain?

It is clear that the proinflammatory cytokines released from immune cells communicate to the brain and alter neural activity, thereby producing the behavioral, affective, and cognitive changes involved in sickness. How do they communicate with cells in the brain? The most obvious possibility is that they accumulate in the blood, travel to the brain in the bloodstream, and cross the blood–brain barrier to act on neurons and other cells in the brain. This pathway is especially sensible when three further facts are considered: (a) There are specific receptors for IL-1, IL-6, and TNF in the brain. These receptors have a discrete distribution and are not present in a nonselective fashion. Although there is some controversy concerning the exact localization of IL-1 receptors in the brain (see Schöbitz, de Kloet, & Holsboer, 1994, for review), in all species examined the receptors are especially dense in discrete cell layers of the hippocampus (E. T. Cunningham & de Souza, 1993). There is also debate concerning the cell type(s) on which the receptors are localized. It is clear that IL-1 receptors are on glial cells (Ban, Sarlieve, & Haour, 1993) and neurons (Takao, Tracey, Mitchell, & de Souza, 1990). (b) Blocking IL-1 receptors in the brain can prevent some of the sickness responses to peripheral administration of infectious agents or cytokines

(Rothwell & Hopkins, 1995). (c) Administration of IL-1 (and other cytokines) directly into the brain produces many or all of the sickness responses (Rothwell & Hopkins, 1995).

These facts are consistent with the idea that cytokines cross into the brain from the bloodstream to communicate to the brain. Otherwise, why would the brain have receptors for them, why would blocking these brain receptors block sickness responses, and why should putting cytokines into the brain reproduce the sickness syndrome? However, there is a significant problem with this scenario. The proinflammatory cytokines are relatively large (e.g., IL-1β is 17.5 kD) lipophobic molecules and so are unlikely to be able to cross the blood–brain barrier and enter the brain. The term blood–brain barrier refers to the fact that the walls of the capillaries that supply the brain are specialized, forming "tight" intercellular endothelial cell junctions. This renders the extracellular space of the central nervous system impermeable from the blood to even relatively small molecules. Of course, the brain requires certain substances to enter such as glucose and amino acids, and there are a number of specific active transport mechanisms (mechanisms that have an energy source to move the molecule in question across the barrier) to bring these substances into the extracellular space of the brain. We return to the blood–brain barrier later.

The difficulties raised by the existence of the blood–brain barrier have led a number of investigators to propose the existence of specialized mechanisms to allow blood-borne cytokines access to the brain (see Watkins, Maier, & Goehler, 1995b, for review). These specialized mechanisms are that (a) there are active transport mechanisms that are specific to the cytokines that bring them into the brain (Banks, Oritz, Plotkin, & Kastin, 1991), (b) the cytokines enter regions of the brain where the blood–brain barrier is weak (Saper & Breder, 1994), and (c) the cytokines bind to receptors on the inside of the blood vessels in the brain and activate secondary messengers that then enter the brain (Van Dam, Brown, Man-A-Hing, & Berkenbosch, 1993). The question is not whether there is some transport, some entry, or some binding to receptors in blood vessels. These all occur to some extent. However, it is doubtful that a sufficient quantity of cytokine enters to produce the physiological and behavioral changes discussed here (Watkins, Maier, & Goehler, 1995a). In addition, there are a variety of facts that are inconsistent with all of these specific mechanisms as causes of sickness responses as well as with the general idea that the cytokines communicate to the brain via the blood or by entry into the brain. As an example, the administration of quantities of LPS or cytokines too small to produce measurable blood levels nevertheless can induce central nervous system changes and sickness responses such as fever, under conditions in which potential insensitivity of the assays cannot be invoked as an explanation (reviewed in Watkins et al., 1995a).

These and other considerations led us and other investigators to inquire into alternative communication pathways. If the immune system is conceived of as a diffuse sense organ that communicates the status of infection- and injury-related events to the brain, it is then sensible to inquire how sense organs generally communicate to the brain. They do not generally do so by accumulating chemical signals in the blood that then cross into the brain. Rather, they do so by activating peripheral nerves that go to the brain. Indeed, there is a nerve that innervates regions of the body in which immune responses occur (the gut, spleen, thymus, lymph nodes, etc.) and provides afferent input to the brain from these regions, which is called the *vagus nerve*. Although the vagus has traditionally been viewed as an efferent nerve providing parasympathetic input from the brain to visceral organs, modern anatomy has revealed that many of the vagal fibers (roughly 70%) are actually sensory, sending afferent messages from the innervated organs to the brain.

The obvious way to determine whether the vagus nerve carries the message from peripheral immune activation to the brain is to cut the vagus and determine whether sickness responses still occur—they do not. We have found that fever (Watkins et al., 1994a), increases in pain responsivity (Watkins et al., 1994b), brain norepinephrine changes (Fleshner, Goehler, et al., 1995), glucocorticoid increases (Fleshner, Goehler, et al., 1995), and conditioned taste aversions (Goehler et al., 1995) produced by cytokines no longer occur. It has also been found that reductions in activity (Layé et al., 1995), social interaction (Bluthé et al., 1994), and food intake (Bret-Dibat, Bluthe, Kent, Kelley, & Dantzer, 1995) fail to occur. These and other data (for review see Maier, Goehler, Fleshner, & Watkins, in press) suggest that cytokines communicate to the brain via the vagus nerve.

How could this happen? The most obvious possibility is that there might be receptors for IL-1 on the terminals of the vagus nerve. IL-1 released by immune cells would then bind to these receptors at their local site of release in the gut, lymph nodes, and so forth, and this would activate the vagal fibers that terminate in the brain. This led us to examine the vagus for the presence of IL-1 receptors with immunohistochemical procedures (Goehler et al., in press). We were unable to detect the presence of IL-1 binding sites on vagal terminals. However, we found very dense binding sites for IL-1 on structures that surround vagal terminals called *paraganglia*. These paraganglia have the structural features of chemoreceptors when examined microscopically, and they synapse onto the vagal fibers where they release a number of different neurotransmitters (Berthoud, Kressel, & Neuhaiber, 1995). Thus, the available evidence suggests the scheme shown in Figure 74.3. IL-1 released by activated immune cells such as macrophages binds to IL-1 receptors on paraganglia in the nearby vicinity. This causes the paraganglia to release the transmitter (we are cur-

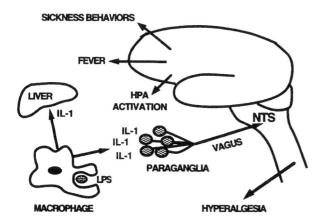

Figure 74.3
Schematic representation of pathway of immune-to-brain communication. LPS, lipopolysaccharide; HPA, hypothalamo-pituitary-adrenal; NTS, nucleus tractus solitarius; IL-1, interleukin-1.

rently identifying the specific transmitter(s) used) onto the vagal terminals, thereby activating afferent vagal fibers. Afferent vagal fibers terminate in a brain-stem nucleus called the *nucleus tractus solitarius* (NTS) and the connected *area postrema,* and this is where the neural cascade then begins. This schema, if correct, suggests that the view that the immune system is a sense organ is more than an analogy. This does not mean that cytokines cannot also accumulate in blood if released in sufficient quantity and travel to the brain. It means that there is a neural route of communication that is sufficient to signal the brain.

Brain IL-1 and Neural Circuitry

If IL-1 (and other cytokines) communicate to the brain via activation of peripheral nerves, then a number of facts become difficult to understand. Why do cells in the brain have IL-1 receptors, why does blockade of these receptors blunt sickness responses to peripheral infection and cytokines, and why does IL-1 injected into the brain produce illness responses? These findings that

suggested that IL-1 communicates to the brain via the blood now become riddles. A potential solution to the riddle is provided by the presence of IL-1 in brain cells; that is, cells in the brain synthesize and release IL-1, as well as IL-6 and TNF (see Schöbitz et al., 1994, for review). The evidence is quite good that glial cells can synthesize IL-1, and neurons probably do so as well (Hopkins & Rothwell, 1995). This is not an essential issue because glia are similar to neurons in many regards. They have receptors for numerous neurotransmitters and hormones and release a variety of neuroactive substances on stimulation. Indeed, virtually every synapse in the brain is encapsulated by glia, and so glia release transmitters onto neurons and are receiving, thereby increasing attention as a source of neural signals (Meller, Dykstra, Grzbycki, Murphey, & Gebhart, 1994). Interestingly, certain types of glial cells are actually immune cells in that they derive from the monocyte macrophage lineage.

The conditions under which cells in the brain are led to manufacture IL-1 and other cytokines are not certain and there is considerable debate

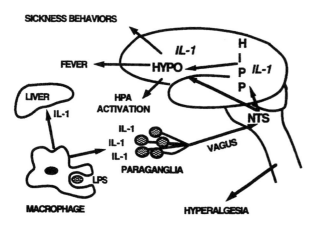

Figure 74.4
Schematic representation of further elaborated pathway of immune-to-brain communication. HYPO, hypothalamus; HIPP, hippocampus; LPS, lipopolysaccharide; HPA, hypothalamo-pituitary-adrenal; NTS, nucleus tractus solitarius; IL-1, interleukin-1.

about this (Quan, Zhang, Emery, Bonsall, & Weiss, 1996). However, it is clear that the peripheral administration of LPS, other infectious agents, and IL-1 itself induces IL-1 production in brain as measured by increases in IL-1 immunoreactivity (Van Dam, Bauer, Tilders, & Barkenbosch, 1995), bioactivity (Quan, Sundar, & Weiss, 1994) and mRNA (Layé et al., 1995). The hypothalamus and hippocampus are brain regions in which this increase in IL-1 has most clearly been demonstrated. We argue that it is this IL-1 (or other cytokines), not the IL-1 synthesized and released at the periphery, that acts within the brain (see Layé et al., 1995, for the same argument). That is, peripheral IL-1 begets new central IL-1, and the centrally produced IL-1 is the IL-1 that acts on IL-1 receptors in the brain to mediate sickness. This scenario in which a molecule released in the periphery leads to the production of the very same molecule in the brain is quite unusual although not unique, and we comment later on why it might have evolved.

A final step here concerns the pathway by which peripheral IL-1 begets brain IL-1—it is

the vagus nerve. Layé et al. (1995) have shown that severing the vagus nerve prevents the induction of IL-1 in hypothalamus and hippocampus following the peripheral administration of LPS.

Figure 74.4 summarizes what researchers know of the organization of the system to this point. To repeat, IL-1 is released by macrophages after they are activated by an infectious or inflammatory agent such as LPS in the figure. The vagus nerve is widely distributed throughout body sites at which such immune responses occur (the gut, lymph nodes, liver, spleen, etc.), and the IL-1 then binds to receptors on paraganglia that surround vagal nerve fibers at the local site where the IL-1 is released. The paraganglia in turn release neurotransmitters onto the vagus, thereby activating vagal fibers. Specific vagal fibers then carry a neural signal to the NTS, which then sends projections to other regions of the brain such as hypothalamus and hippocampus where IL-1 is induced and where other neural events in the cascade are initiated, which then result in the individual responses that are collectively called sickness.

As an example of the brain part of this proposed circuit, consider fever. Fever occurs because of alterations in the activity of temperature-sensitive neurons in the anterior preoptic region of the hypothalamus (Saper & Breder, 1994). Catecholaminergic fibers project to the anterior preoptic region from the NTS, and when catecholamines are released there they, in turn, produce the synthesis and release of prostaglandins. The induction of IL-1 may be involved in this process of prostaglandin production. The prostaglandins then act on the temperature-sensitive neurons. Indeed, prostaglandins are released in this brain region when peripheral immune cells are stimulated, and prostaglandin inhibitors microinjected into this region prevent fever (Sehic, Székely, Ungar, Oladehin, & Blatteis, 1996). Sehic and Blatteis (1996) have shown that severing the vagus prevents this prostaglandin release in the preoptic region, as well as fever, thereby supporting this scheme. Similarly, catecholaminergic projections from the NTS to the paraventricular nucleus of the hypothalamus are responsible for the outflow from the brain that activates the pituitary and adrenal to secrete their hormones, and knife cuts of the catecholamine connections between this nucleus and the NTS prevent its activation following peripheral immune stimulation (Ericcson, Kovacs, & Sawchenko, 1994).

Outflow from the Brain

We have indicated that IL-1 in the brain is involved in the mediation of the central nervous system changes that follow peripheral immune stimulation. What about the peripheral organ changes such as shifts in liver metabolism? The scheme illustrated in Figure 74.4 is not fully bidirectional, yet we began with the idea that brain–immune communication is bidirectional. Indeed, a variety of data indicate that IL-1 in brain initiates an outflow of signaling from brain that feeds back to and alters the functioning of peripheral organs. For example, the administra-

tion of small amounts of IL-1 into the brain leads to the production of acute-phase proteins by the liver (Hagan, Poole, & Bristow, 1993) and increases in the levels of cytokines in the periphery (DeSimoni et al., 1990). The identity of the messenger from the brain to the periphery in response to brain IL-1 is not known, but the available data justify the addition of the arrows shown in Figure 74.5. Thus, the system involving the activation of innate immunity and the brain is a fully closed loop.

Counterregulation

The circuit shown in Figure 74.5 is a positive feedback system, and so there must be restraining counterregulatory forces. To this point we have treated IL-1 in a very loose fashion, but actually, there are seven different proteins in the IL-1 family. There are two forms of IL-1 (IL-1α and IL-1β), two types of IL-1 receptors (Type I and Type II), a prohormone from which IL-1 is cleaved, a converting enzyme that catalyzes the cleavage of IL-1 from the prohormone (IL-1 converting enzyme; ICE), and an endogenous IL-1 receptor antagonist (IL-1ra). The existence of an endogenous receptor antagonist (Eisenberg et al., 1990) is worthy of comment. A receptor antagonist is a substance that binds to a receptor but does not act on the receptor to initiate the receptor processes that ultimately alter the activity of the cell on which the receptor is located. The antagonist competes with the agonist for the receptor and so prevents the agonist from binding to the receptor and producing its normal outcomes. We know of no other instance in which there exists a naturally occurring receptor antagonist for a neuroactive substance. The fact that an antagonist for IL-1 has evolved suggests the extreme potency and importance of this cytokine. Of course, IL-1ra is a counterregulatory force. If levels of IL-1ra are increased, then the actions of IL-1 would be restrained.

In addition, the Type II IL-1 receptor appears to be a "decoy" receptor (Colotta et al., 1993).

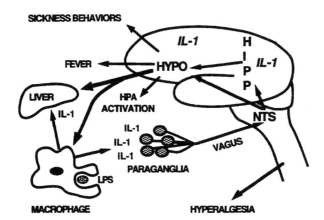

Figure 74.5
Bidirectional immune-to-brain circuitry. HYPO, hypothalamus; HIPP, hippocampus; LPS, lipopolysaccharide; HPA, hypothalamo-pituitary-adrenal; NTS, nucleus tractus solitarius; IL-1, interleukin-1.

That is, this receptor is not coupled to intracellular signaling systems, and so binding of IL-1 to this receptor does not initiate or alter neural activity. All of the signaling seems to be carried out by the Type I receptor. Thus, the Type II receptor operates as a kind of sponge for IL-1, the more IL-1 that binds to the Type II receptor, the less is available to bind to the active Type I receptor. If Type II receptor numbers are increased following some event (e.g., infection), then IL-1 action would again be restrained. Finally, the production of IL-1 requires ICE, and so reductions in ICE would reduce IL-1 action. Thus, there are three mechanisms within the IL-1 system itself that are capable of counterregulating IL-1.

Furthermore, there are restraining forces outside of the IL-1 system. At least two other peptides in the brain, alpha melanocyte stimulating hormone and arginine vasopressin, oppose IL-1 action (Dantzer, Bluthé, & Kelley, 1991; Lipton, 1990). Here the restraint is not produced because the substance binds to the IL-1 receptor and competes with IL-1, but probably because counteracting neural circuitry is activated. The existence of these multiple levels of restraint on IL-1

action supports the idea that IL-1 plays an absolutely pivotal role in the brain and periphery and that the system is a positive feedback circuit, thereby requiring strong control.

Stress

The discussion thus far has focused on immune-to-brain-to-immune circuits that mediate and organize the organism's defense against infection and injury. Here we begin to discuss potential implications for psychology and begin with stress. The focus is on acute exposure to a stressor or a series of stressors extending over at most hours rather than chronic stress or repetitive exposure to an acute stressor extending over days. This is because our primary interest in this chapter is physiological function rather than pathology. It has often been argued that the stress response evolved to aid fight–flight emergencies and is adaptive in the short run (Sapolsky, 1992). When activated for many days, quite different outcomes, often pathophysiological in nature, may result. In addition, this initial discussion is restricted to the nonspecific immune processes that have been under discussion. Specific immunity, most often suppressed by stress, is discussed later.

Consider the sequelae of exposure to acute stressors. The question is not what occurs during exposure to a stressor: During stressors the organism engages in defensive behavior (discussed later). For a period of time after exposure to a stressor there are reductions in food and water intake (Weiss, 1968), decreases in activity (Weiss & Simpson, 1985), exploration (van Dijken, Van der Heyden, Mos, & Tilders, 1992), social interaction (Short & Maier, 1993), and aggression (Maier, Anderson, & Lieberman, 1972). Of course, there is also activation of the HPA axis and the sympathetic nervous system. Indeed, many would define a stressor as something that activates these two systems. Depressed mood (Brown, 1993) and interference with various forms of cognitive activity (Steckler & Sahgal, 1995) are also often held to be consequences of exposure to a stressor and occur during a post-stressor period.

Clearly, the behavioral and endocrine changes produced by stressors are very similar to those produced by immune activation. However, this could easily be no more than a superficial resemblance. After all, stressors are not known to shift liver metabolism, produce fever, alter white blood cell counts, and so forth. However, do they? Figure 74.6 shows data from our laboratory in which we measured core body temperature by telemetry in home cage controls and in rats exposed to a session of inescapable tailshock with the identical parameters to those used in learned helplessness experiments (e.g., Maier, Grahn, & Watkins, 1995). It is perhaps not surprising that temperature was increased during the session as this may simply reflect hyperthermia induced by restraint and exercise. However, there is a substantial fever for at least 45 hr after the session has ended. Thus, inescapable shock produces fever. Together with T. Deak and M. Fleshner, we measured the white blood cell count, levels of seromucoid and haptoglobin

(these are acute-phase protein produced by the liver during illness), and corticosteroid binding globulin (a carrier protein normally produced by the liver but which decreases during sickness)—24 hr after inescapable shock or control treatment (Figure 74.7). This is the classic pattern produced by infection or immune activation—increased white cells and shifts in liver metabolism away from carrier proteins toward production of acute-phase proteins. Lest it be thought that such effects are restricted to inescapable tailshock, simply placing a rat in a novel environment produces fever (LeMay, Vander, & Kluger, 1990). Thus psychological as well as physical stressors seem capable of producing outcomes similar to those produced by infection (also discussed later). Indeed, in humans, situations such as public speaking and an impending athletic contest produce fever (Marazziti, Di Muro, & Castrogiovanni, 1992; Renbourn, 1960).

This pattern of peripheral changes following infection is easy to understand. Microbial and inflammatory agents lead to the production of cytokines because they directly contact and activate macrophages and other peripheral cells (fibroblasts, mast cells, endothelial cells, etc.). For some infectious agents the cytokine production is induced by phagocytosis of the agent consequent to contact with and attachment to the macrophage surface, whereas other agents such as LPS contain products that can directly bind to membrane receptor proteins on the macrophage surface (Ulevitch, 1993). However, stressors are not microbial products and cannot somehow make this physical contact with macrophages or other peripheral cells. Nevertheless, stressors lead to increases in the levels of cytokines circulating in the blood, with IL-6 being the most frequently measured. As indicated earlier, the stressor does not have to be physical—merely placing a rat in a novel environment (LeMay et al., 1990), or exposing it to a previously neutral cue that had been paired with footshock (Zhou, Kusnecov, Shurin, DePaoli, &

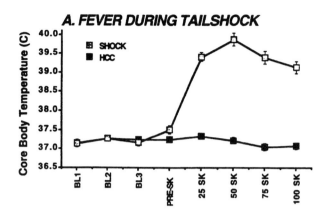

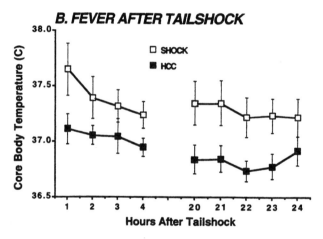

Figure 74.6
Core body temperature during and after exposure to inescapable shock (SHOCK) or home cage control treatment (HCC). BL, baseline; SK, shocks. Bars: SEM.

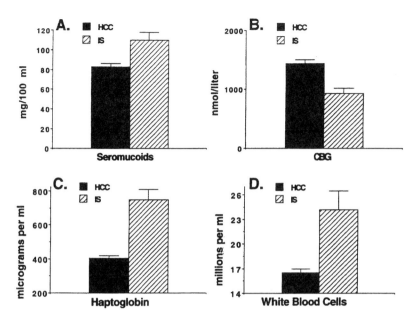

Figure 74.7
White blood cell count, serum levels of seromucoid, haptoglobin, and corticosteroid binding globulin (CBG), 24 h after inescapable shock (IS) or home cage control treatment (HCC). Bars: SEM.

Rabin, 1993), increases plasma levels of IL-6. It is interesting to note that IL-6 is the most important of the cytokines with regard to mediating the shifts in liver metabolism that occur during sickness and so could be responsible for the acute-phase responses observed after inescapable shock. In addition, the proinflammatory cytokines induce each other's synthesis by cells such as macrophages, and so the observed increases in IL-6 would be likely to produce increases in IL-1 and TNF as well.

The source of the stress-induced IL-6 is not likely to be macrophages (van Gool, van Vugt, Helle, & Aarden, 1990). Nevertheless, with M. Fleshner and K. Nguyen we have studied macrophages after exposure to inescapable shock. We measured nitric oxide production in cells taken from the spleens of inescapably shocked and control subjects 0, 48, or 96 hr after treat-

ment. None of the cells produced nitric oxide unless stimulated with a substance such as LPS. However, as can be seen in Figure 74.8, after stimulation, the cells from the stressed animals produced excess quantities of nitric oxide 48 hr after inescapable tailshock, an effect that was still present 4 days after exposure to the stressor. Thus the stressor seems to "prime" the macrophage so that it is very ready to respond to its normal stimuli and does so in an exaggerated fashion. Again, the stressor does not have to be physical. Coe, Rosenberg, and Levine (1988) were among the first to suggest that stressors might activate macrophages, and the stressor used in their experiments was a 24-hr separation of a mother and an infant squirrel monkey. Again, the effect was observed long after the stressor was terminated. Thus stressors do lead to the priming and activation of macrophages

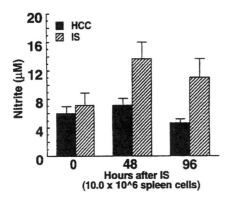

Figure 74.8
Nitric oxide levels (Nitrite) produced by spleen cells taken 0, 48, or 96 h after inescapable shock (IS) or home cage control treatment (HCC). Bars: SEM.

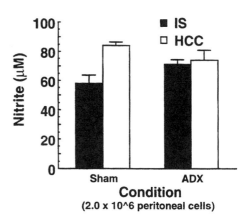

Figure 74.9
Nitric oxide levels (Nitrite) produced by peritoneal cells taken immediately after inescapable shock (IS) or home cage control treatment (HCC). Animals had received either sham surgery (Sham) or bilateral adrenalectomy (ADX). Bars: SEM.

at a time distant from the stressor. Clearly, stressors cannot do so directly but instead must stimulate the brain to produce the release of a messenger in the periphery that acts on macrophages. We do not yet know the identity of this messenger.

It should be noted that here is a case in which chronic stressor exposure is known to produce a different outcome. Chronic stressors such as 10 days of 18 hr/day restraint suppress a variety of measures of macrophage function (Zwilling, 1994). This suppression is mediated by adrenal corticosteroid release produced by the stressor (Zwilling, Brown, Feng, Sheridan, & Pearl, 1993). Because acute stressors also increase levels of corticosteroids, macrophage function might also be expected to be suppressed during or shortly after the stressor session. Figure 74.8 shows that nitric oxide production failed to be enhanced shortly after the stressor, but it was not suppressed. In a different population of macrophages (peritoneal macrophages) we have found that nitric oxide production is indeed suppressed when cells are taken immediately after the stressor and that this was blocked by adrenalectomy (Figure 74.9). Furthermore, other measures (in-

terferon production and IL-1 production) indicated suppression immediately after the stressor in both populations of macrophages. In addition, the sickness measures shown in Figure 74.7 were for blood samples taken 24 hr after the inescapable shock and do not emerge until 6–12 hr after the stressor. It is some time after the stressor session that peripheral responses similar to sickness seem to occur. Finally, chronic stressors could still produce parts of the sickness pattern that are not dependent on macrophage products. There is simply not enough known to draw a firm conclusion here.

Brain IL-1

This earlier discussion suggests that stressors are capable of activating some aspects of innate immunity and priming others. How could this be? As described earlier, infectious agents physically contact macrophages and other cells and activate them. A stressor cannot do this. An alternative is provided by the hypothesis depicted in

Figure 74.5, that there is a closed loop system with IL-1 playing pivotal roles in both the periphery and the brain. A stressor could not initiate the loop by releasing IL-1 or any other substance in the periphery as does an infectious agent, but what if a stressor could induce IL-1 production in the brain? After all, there is no reason why there can be only one pathway to brain IL-1 induction. If inescapable shock, and perhaps other stressors, do act to increase brain levels of IL-1, then of course the behavioral and physiological symptoms of sickness would follow.

Three kinds of experiments would be required to test this hypothesis. There are not much data yet, but the results so far are powerful.

1. Does blocking IL-1 receptors in the brain block the effects of exposure to stressors? IL-1 receptors in the brain were blocked by injecting a recombinant form of the endogenous IL-1ra directly into the brain, and Maier and Watkins (1995) have found this to block completely behavioral learned helplessness effects. That is, inescapably shocked animals do not fail to learn to escape, do not show exaggerated fear, and so forth. Furthermore, Shintani et al. (1995) reported that IL-1ra administered into the brain prevented the normal changes in brain neurotransmitters produced by restraint, as well as blunting the pituitary–adrenal response. However, there has not been much work here, and further research will be required to determine definitively the impact of IL-1ra.

2. Does administering IL-1 into the brain reproduce the effects of stressors? All of the usual sequelae of stressors have not been examined, but the available evidence does suggest the classic stress pattern (Plata-Salaman, Oomura, & Kai, 1988; Sapolsky, Rivier, Yamamoto, Plotsky, & Vale, 1987; Shintani et al., 1993; Sundar et al., 1989). Importantly, IL-1 administered into the brain produces large increases in plasma IL-6 (DeSimoni et al., 1990)—a potential key mediator of the peripheral sickness changes observed after exposure to stressors. As noted previously,

the outflow product from the brain that activates peripheral immune processes has not clearly been identified, and so the mediator of the IL-6 response is not conclusively known.

3. Do stressors increase brain levels of IL-1? This is a question researchers are just beginning to explore. However, it can be noted that restraint has been shown to increase mRNA for IL-1 in the hypothalamus (Minami et al., 1991).

However, it should be noted that the scheme that we are presenting does not depend on stressors entering the bidirectional immune–brain loop by inducing IL-1. Stressors could enter by activating any of the central nervous system steps involved in the loop (discussed later).

Neural Circuitry

The theory being proposed is that events in the environment categorized as stressors activate the same circuitry as is activated by infectious agents, they just enter the loop at a different location. The evidence discussed earlier suggests that both types of events do increase levels of brain IL-1, but what of the remainder of the known circuitry? There is a very large amount of literature examining the neural changes that follow exposure to stressors. This is complex literature, and all stressors do not produce the identical pattern. It would require an entire review paper to compare the patterns produced by stressors and immune activation in detail. However, stressors do activate the same regions and produce the release of the same neurotransmitters as does immune activation. For example, stressors activate the NTS, the catecholaminergic projections from the NTS, hypothalamic nuclei, and regions within the hippocampus (e.g., Cullinan, Herman, Battaglea, Akil, & Watson, 1995; Helmreich, Cullinan, & Watson, 1996). Furthermore, as with immune activation, norepinephrine is released in the hypothalamus (Pacok et al., 1992) and serotonin in the hippocampus (Kirby, Allen, & Lucki, 1995). This is not to argue that stressors and immune activation produce identical changes. Stressors often produce neural alterations in addition to those produced by immune activation, and different stressors can produce different effects rather than leading to a generic response. For example, stressors activate dopaminergic projections to the frontal cortex, and immune activation does not (Dunn, 1992). The conclusion is that stressors activate the same neural circuitry as immune activation, plus additional changes dependent on the nature of the stressor.

A final issue here concerns how stressors access the sickness circuit. The neural cascade following immune activation begins in the NTS (Ericcson et al., 1994), the site of termination of incoming vagal nerves. It can be noted that afferent input from laminae I, IV–VII, and X of the spinal cord terminates in regions of the NTS, close to the sites of vagal termination. These laminae of the spinal cord receive sensory input from physical stressors such as inescapable shock and convey the input to the brain. Thus, stressors such as inescapable shock also begin their neural cascade in the NTS. Psychological stressors do not provide direct sensory input to the NTS. However, it is possible that these stressors activate regions of the brain that send descending input to the NTS, thereby activating the NTS. Indeed, simply exposing a rat to an environmental cue that has previously signaled electric shock (Pezzone, Lee, Hoffman, Pezzone, & Rabin, 1993) or a taste previously paired with sickness (Schafe, Seeley, & Bernstein, 1995) activates the NTS.

Evolution of the Immune and Stress Responses

We have thus far argued that stimulation of the innate immune response by infectious agents and stressors activates the same immune–brain circuits. Why should this be so, and how does it help in the understanding of stress? If the meaning of what has been presented is that infection and immune activation activate what is con-

ceptualized as a stress response, thereby adding one more class of events to the list of stressors, not much has been gained. Instead, we argue that the situation is the reverse—that stressors "make animals and humans sick" and that this view illuminates many difficult-to-understand aspects of stress. Our argument is that the bidirectional immune-to-brain machinery first evolved to mediate defense against infectious agents and sickness and was then later coopted to mediate stress. The behavioral, affective, cognitive, and physiological products of exposure to stressors have often been viewed as pathological because they serve no obvious function and even seem maladaptive. Why should exposure to stressors be followed by reductions in food and water intake, decreased aggressiveness, depressed mood, and so forth? Why not the opposite? Why not increased food and water intake, increased aggressiveness, and so forth? Indeed, these would often seem more adaptive. We argue that stress-induced changes are indeed adaptive, but in the context of sickness. Our argument here is speculative and other constructions could doubtlessly be made. However, we feel that it is consistent with current knowledge and rationalizes the facts that we have presented.

The function or adaptiveness of a set of mechanisms is often best appreciated in the context of the evolution of the mechanisms in question. The stress response as it is typically conceived is a fight–flight response and is involved with defense against a predator, an aggressive conspecific, and so forth. The usual defining conditions of HPA and sympathetic activation are viewed as providing energy for fight or flight (Sapolsky, 1992). Indeed, as briefly described earlier, glucocorticoids and catecholamines do function to liberate energy. However, the fight–flight response is a much more recent adaptation than is innate immunity. A fight–flight response requires the sensory ability to detect a predator at a distance, the motor capacity to flee or fight, and the sensorimotor integration to direct the motor activity in relation to the distal sensory stimulation.

However, even the most primitive organisms require defense against infection and tissue injury and contain immune cells and processes (Beck, Cooper, Hobicht, & Harchonis, 1994). All animals are capable of the recognition, processing, and elimination of nonself by means of phagocytosis and wound healing. Even sponges (the most primitive multicellular creatures) contain phagocytes, which recognize infectious agents and participate in wound healing (Johnston & Heldemann, 1982). The most primitive phagocytes are amoebocytes, which can move throughout the invertcbrate body by means of active migration or by passive transport via circulation with body fluids. They contain enzymes that are quite similar to those in mammalian macrophages and are analogous to macrophages in most regards (Bayne, 1990). Importantly, even in animals as primitive as mollusks, amoebocytes synthesize and release IL-1, TNF, and IL-6, and do so in response to agents such as LPS (Hughes, Smith, Barnett, Charles, & Stefano, 1991). Furthermore, the cytokines appear to have similar local functions in attracting amoebocytes to sites of infection and tissue injury.

However, the analogy does not stop at local action. IL-1 has been localized in neural tissue in mollusks (Paeman et al., 1992), and neural tissue in mollusks has receptors for the cytokines (Sawada, Hara, & Maeno, 1991). Furthermore, amoebocytes contain many of the substances that are traditional neurotransmitters in mammals—norepinephrine, epinephrine, dopamine, serotonin, endogenous opioids such as met-enkephalin, substance P, somatostatin, neurotensin, and so forth (e.g., reviewed in Ottaviani & Franceschi, 1996). These substances are also in neurons in mollusks, and so amoebocytes use the same extracellular signals to perform immune defense as is used by the nervous system in these animals. Indeed, the cytokines released by amoebocytes can alter neural excitability in mollusks (see Clatworthy, 1996, for a review). The point is that even as early in evolution as the mollusks (pre-Cambrian era), with animals that do not have a discrete brain but rather a series of separate ganglia, there was bidirectional immune-to-neural communication. Thus, from the beginning, immune cells communicated with the nervous system to organize defense against infectious agents and tissue injury. There is a danger in assuming that modern-day representatives of primitive phyla are identical to their ancestral progenitors (Hodos & Campbell, 1969). However, the presence of IL-1 and other cytokines in immune cells and neural tissue in a widely diverse range of species (Pestarino, De Anna, Masini, & Sturla, 1997) is consistent with the argument made here.

Primitive organisms such as mollusks identify predators or external threat via contact with its body surface, rather than by vision or audition. Contact elicits withdrawal reflexes and locomotion that can move the organism or the affected part of the organism from the threat (see Walters, 1994, for a review). The amoebocytes appear to participate in this process, with the proinflammatory cytokines sensitizing the neurons involved in the withdrawal reflexes (Clatworthy, 1996). Thus, immune cells analogous to the macrophage have participated in defense against even distal threat from early in evolution and sent signals carried by cytokines to neural elements involved in defensive withdrawal reflexes.

One more point needs to be made. In mammals, the hormones produced by the HPA response (corticotropin releasing hormone, adrenocorticotropin, and glucocorticoids) and the catecholamines released by sympathetic nervous system terminals function to release energy from bodily stores. These hormones and the catecholamines are present in amoebocytes, and even there they function in energy metabolism (see Ottaviani & Franceschi, 1996, for review). That is, before the hypothalamus, pituitary, and adrenal existed, the products now contained in these structures in mammals functioned in energy metabolism and were in communication with cytokines. Thus, from early in evolution, immune cells and cytokines were involved in energy production and were in close contact with what today are thought of as stress hormones. Furthermore, the cytokines themselves are involved with energy balance both in these primitive organisms and in mammals. For example, administration of IL-1 either peripherally (Flores, Istfan, Blackburn, & Bistrian, 1990) or into the brain (Petit et al., 1994) increases the production of glucose by the liver. Interleukin-1 also is a key initiator of proteolysis, breaking down muscle into amino acids that can be used in tissue repair and immune cell proliferation.

The points to be taken from this discussion are that from the earliest times in evolution, before the concept of fight–flight would have meaning, immune activation in the service of defense against infection and injury involved cytokines in bidirectional communication with nerve cells and in orchestrating the regulation of energy balance. These immune processes were also involved in primitive forms of defense against external threat. As organisms evolved and behavior came to play a more prominent role, behavioral adjustments came to be required in the service of fighting infection and recuperating from injury. Bidirectional cytokine communication between immune cells and nerve cells in cellular defense already existed, and so it would be only natural that the cytokines would coordinate the behavioral adjustments involved in sickness.

Now consider fight–flight. The evolution of more elaborate defenses against predators and other threats that could be identified at a distance by sense organs required mediating mechanisms. Fight–flight requires the mobilization of energy stores just as innate immune defense does. Cooptation of existing solutions to solve a related problem is a frequent occurrence in evolution because it is easier to refine an existing mechanism than it is to create a new one (Gould, 1982). There already existed mechanisms to create energy and to defend against proximal threat, and so it is reasonable to argue that these processes involving cytokines in communication with neural tissue were coopted to function as a substrate for fight–flight (see Ottaviani & Franceschi,

1996, for a related argument). Of course, there is always a cost, and here the cost may be the appearance of other adaptations during or after fight–flight that function to combat infection and injury, rather than distal threat. This may be why stressors produce subsequent reactions that appear more reasonable during sickness than as a defense against threat. It may also be that the appearance of these reactions serves an adaptive function under some circumstances. Perhaps they function in an anticipatory fashion, preparing the organism to engage in immune defense against infection and injury that can occur during fight–flight defense. Because the proinflammatory cytokines are not expressed constitutively in cells such as macrophages but must first be synthesized before they can be released (Dinarello, 1991), and because many of the peripheral changes such as shifts in liver metabolism are slow even after they are initiated, several hours or more are required to produce a full acute-phase response to injury and infection. It may therefore be adaptive to initiate or prime the response before injury when the threat is present. Indeed, as noted earlier, some aspects of the response such as macrophage alterations are primed by stressors rather than being fully activated. Furthermore, glucocorticoids, released during a fight–flight response, suppress these and many other aspects of immune function, thereby preventing them from being fully expressed during the fight–flight emergency.

Finally, this evolutionary discussion may also help to rationalize a number of peculiar features of the mammalian immune-to-brain circuitry described earlier. We have noted that the peripheral release of IL-1 induces the brain to manufacture the very same molecule. However, primitive organisms such as the lower mollusks do not have a blood–brain barrier (Abbott, Lane, & Bundgaard, 1986). Indeed, these organisms do not possess a discrete "brain," and cytokines released by amoebocytes have direct access to neural tissue, and neural products have direct access to amoebocytes. As nervous systems became more complex they required a more stable ionic environment, leading to the development of the blood–brain barrier (Cserr & Bandgaard, 1988). However, now the cytokines released by immune cells could no longer reach target nerve cells. Obviously, one solution to this problem would be to develop mechanisms by which the release of the cytokines outside the blood–brain barrier leads to signals that reach cells inside the brain parenchyma that can now manufacture the cytokines and release them. Thus, the cytokine signal could reach the target nerve cells, it is just newly synthesized cytokine inside the brain rather than the cytokine outside. Of course, neural signals had always had direct access to the immune cells, and the blood–brain barrier blocks access of substances released in the brain from reaching the body as well. Thus, outflow mechanisms were also needed, explaining why IL-1 in the brain in mammals leads to outflow from the brain that feeds back to the immune cells. This picture also makes good sense of the fact that stressors may tap into the circuit by inducing brain IL-1. This allows a stressor to send messages that can activate peripheral immune cells.

In summary, bidirectional immune-to-neural tissue communication existed long before discrete brains and fight–flight in the sense in which it occurs in mammals. Furthermore, the hormones that are traditionally viewed as stress hormones in mammals were intimately involved in this process. Part of the function of this machinery was to release energy from bodily stores, and it may be that it was coopted to produce energy during fight–flight in mammals, thereby leading to the overlap between sickness and stress that we argue exists. In addition, this cooptation would have allowed immune defense to be sensitized during a fight–flight emergency.

Functional-Behavior System

Another way to view the current proposed scheme is in relation to the perceptual-defensive-recuperation model first proposed by Bolles and Fanselow (1980). The essential features of this model are that threat activates defensive behavior and inhibits recuperative behavior. This was proposed because defense against predators or attack is of foremost importance for survival, and recuperative behaviors such as licking wounds, decreased motor output, and so forth would interfere with defense. Injury and the termination of threat were then argued to activate recuperative behavior. Furthermore, both defense and recuperation were viewed as functional-behavior systems. Timberlake and Lucas (1989) have defined a functional-behavior system as a "complex control structure related to a particular function or need of the organism such as feeding, reproduction, defense, or body care" (p. 241). It has been argued that there are four criteria that must be identified to define a functional-behavior system (Fanselow & Sigmundi, 1987). These are (a) the observable behaviors must be described, (b) the evolutionary benefit or adaptive function of the behaviors must be detailed, (c) the initiating conditions in the environment or organism must be specified, and (d) a neural substrate must be provided.

However, the overwhelming majority of the research conducted within this context has been directed at exploring the structure of defensive behavior (e.g., Blanchard, Blanchard, & Hori, 1989) and the neural circuitry that mediates defensive behavior (e.g., Fanselow, 1994). The study of recuperative behavior as a functional-behavior system has relatively been ignored. The scheme developed in this article can be viewed as a functional-behavior system model of recuperative behavior. We have indeed met the four criteria described earlier, at least in broad outline.

The present model differs from the perceptual-defensive-recuperation model (Bolles & Fanselow, 1980) in that the threat itself is argued to activate the circuitry that underlies both types of processes. The perceptual-defensive-recuperation model suggested that threat activates defense and that recuperative processes would only be initiated if injury actually occurred during defense.

If injury occurred while the threat was still present recuperative processes were held to be inhibited. This scheme makes good sense. However, as noted earlier, the recuperative circuit has inherent time delays, and so it may well be adaptive to initiate or prime these processes in an anticipatory fashion so that injury and infection consequent to injury can more rapidly be dealt with. Our model also differs in that we have argued that the system evolved to combat infection and can be understood in those terms, and only later did it take over the function of recuperation following distal threat.

Within this context, shifts in pain reactivity and sensitivity require comment because they have played an important role in the development of the perceptual-defensive-recuperation model (Bolles & Fanselow, 1980). The peripheral administration of LPS or IL-1 results in an increase in pain sensitivity (Watkins et al., 1995b). Such *hyperalgesia* during recuperation has been argued to be potentially adaptive, directing attention and behaviors such as licking to wound sites, as well as decreasing movement. As such, hyperalgesia has been viewed as a part of sickness behavior (Maier, Watkins, & Fleshner, 1994). However, the consequence of exposure to a threat or stressor is generally a decrease in pain sensitivity and reactivity (Amir & Galena, 1986). Stress-induced *analgesia* has been thought to be adaptive in that defensive fight–flight behavior would be protected from disruption by interfering recuperative activities elicited by pain (Bolles & Fanselow, 1980). However, if stressors and infectious agents activate shared circuitry, why do they produce opposite modulation of pain?

It may be that this is an instance in which stressors or threats activate a circuit, here a pain inhibition circuit, that is distinct and unique to stressors rather than illness-inducing events. In keeping with its hypothesized function, stress-induced analgesia is a very rapid response, appearing as quickly on exposure to a stressor as pain testing can be accomplished (Maier, 1989). This is far too rapid to involve the induction of

brain IL-1 or any similar process. The hyperalgesia that follows infectious or inflammatory agents is much slower to develop, requiring many minutes (Watkins et al., 1995b). Thus, there is again a delay in the recuperative circuit. However, even here there may be overlap. In experiments in which the hyperalgesia to immune stimuli was blocked with pharmacological agents that interfere with the spinal mechanisms that enhance pain reactivity, the result has been the unmasking of an analgesic reaction rather than a simple return to baseline pain sensitivity (e.g., Wiertelak, Furness, Watkins, & Maier, 1994). That is, immune stimulation activates both analgesia and hyperalgesia circuitry, with the hyperalgesic effect predominating, resulting in behavioral hyperalgesia. There is even some evidence that hyperalgesia can be observed after the analgesia to a stressor has dissipated if testing is continued for a long enough period of time (Hendrie, 1989).

In summary, it is possible to view the present model as providing the circuitry that underlies recuperative motivation and behavior. Finally, it can be noted that investigators interested in the behavioral and physiological consequences of stress typically study the organism after the stressor has been applied and not during the threat, as is the focus of those interested in defensive behavior. Thus, a stressor (e.g., restraint, shock, an aggressive conspecific, or public speaking) is provided, and food intake, social behavior, brain neurotransmitters, and so forth are studied for the next several days after the stressor. From the present perspective, the phenomena measured are actually recuperative activities and can be understood in this context.

Stress-Related Phenomena

The idea that stressors activate circuitry that evolved to mediate defense against infection and produce sickness behaviors may help in the understanding of a variety of phenomena related to stress. Here we can only provide a brief sampling.

Depression

Researchers who have studied infection and immune activation in animals have often described the behavioral state observed during sickness as depression or depressed mood (Hart, 1988). Indeed, the behavioral sequelae of immune activation that we have described do resemble the characteristics of depression. The essential features of depression as described in the *Diagnostic and Statistical Manual of Mental Disorders* (4th ed.; American Psychiatric Association, 1994) are depressed mood and the loss of interest in, or the pleasure derived from, most of the individual's usual activities (anhedonia). To be diagnosed as depressed, the individual must also exhibit at least five of a cluster of symptoms that are (a) disturbance in appetite or weight loss, (b) psychomotor disturbance, (c) sleep disturbances, (d) fatigue or loss of energy, (e) difficulty in thinking or maintaining attention, (f) thoughts of suicide or attempts at suicide, and (g) feelings of worthlessness or excessive guilt. We have already reviewed research that indicates that infection, inflammation, or the administration of peripheral cytokines such as IL-1 produces reduced food intake and weight loss, reduced activity, and alterations in sleep characterized by increased slow-wave sleep. Obviously, Symptoms f and g cannot be assessed in animals. We return to cognitive effects of immune activation later.

This leaves for discussion whether animals given peripheral inflammatory or infectious agents show depressed mood and anhedonia. We have already noted that animals given immune-activating stimuli show reduced exploration, social interaction, and sexual behavior and do not engage in normal grooming activities. However, is this anhedonia? A number of animal models have been developed to assess anhedonia. Perhaps the best validated model involved testing an animals' preference for a sweet-tasting sucrose or saccharin solution. Rats normally prefer a sweet solution to plain water and will work to obtain sucrose or saccharin. However, chronic exposure to stressors leads to a reduction in the preference for the sweet taste (Katz, 1982). It is not that the subjects no longer drink, it is that they have become indifferent to the sweet taste and no longer choose it in preference to plain water nor do they drink exaggerated amounts of it if given only the sweet solution. This loss of preference for a sweet solution produced by chronic stress has been argued to represent anhedonia—the rat no longer cares about one of its normal pleasures (see Dess, Minor, & Brewer, 1989, for a different interpretation). As with depression, the reduction in preference for sweet solutions produced by chronic stress can be reversed by chronic but not acute administration of tricyclic antidepressant drugs (Willner, Towell, Sampson, Sophokleous, & Muscat, 1987). Yirmiya (1996a) has shown that a single administration of the immune-stimulating compound LPS produces the same reduction in preference for a sweet solution as is produced by chronic stress and that chronic but not acute administration of a tricyclic antidepressant abolishes this effect of LPS. Yirmiya (1996b) has also found chronic administration of both the tricyclic antidepressant imipramine and the selective serotonin reuptake inhibitor Prozac to prevent LPS from reducing social interaction, exploration, and food intake. That is, the single administration of a substance that activates macrophages to release cytokines and therefore activates the immune-to-brain circuit under discussion here produces anhedonia, and this is reversed by antidepressant drugs.

Finally, it should be noted that depression is often associated with a dysregulation of the HPA axis characterized by increases in basal levels of adrenal glucocorticoids and a reduced potency of dexamethasone to suppress adrenal glucocorticoids (for review see Gold, Wong, Chroesos, & Licinio, 1996). Glucocorticoid receptors in the hippocampus, hypothalamus, and pituitary exert negative feedback action on the HPA axis, and dexamethasone (a synthetic glucocorticoid) therefore normally suppresses glucocorticoid secreted from the adrenal. As we have already described, the proinflammatory cytokines are potent stimulators of the HPA axis. In addition, LPS reduces the ability of dexamethasone to suppress adrenal glucocorticoid levels (Yirmiya, 1996b). Furthermore, a single administration of IL-1 can produce long-lasting changes in the HPA axis (Tilders, Schmidt, & de Goeji, 1993). Finally, depression has often been argued to involve alterations in brain noradrenergic and serotonergic activity, effects we have already described following immune activation.

In summary, the animal literature strongly supports the contention that immune activation and the proinflammatory cytokines induce a state that is "depressive-like." Perhaps this should not be surprising because immune-to-brain circuitry has been argued here to be a key mediator of stress effects, and stress has often been related to depression (Gold et al., 1996). Despite the fact that depression is associated with interference with specific immunity and increased disease susceptibility (Herbert & Cohen, 1993), there do exist numerous intriguing findings that are consistent with the argument that nonspecific immune activation and cytokines are involved in the etiology or symptomology of depression. A number of investigators have studied the psychological changes that occur during and following infectious diseases. Infectious diseases obviously involve immune activation and cytokine release, and depression has been the most consistently reported psychological disturbance (e.g., Meijer, Zakay-Rones, & Morag, 1988). Interestingly, R. Yirmiya (personal communication, June 1997) has found that vaccination for rubella produces an increase in depressive symptomology 2 weeks after administration of the vaccine, a time at which immune responding to the vaccine should be high. There are also a number of poorly understood conditions such as chronic fatigue syndrome that are associated with elevated levels of circulating cytokines (Patarca, Klimas, Lug-

tendorf, Antoni, & Fletcher, 1994), and depression has been reported to occur in 75–80% of the individuals diagnosed with these conditions (Abbey & Garfinkel, 1991). Finally, cytokines have been administered to humans, and depressed mood has frequently been observed as a consequence (e.g., Fent & Zbinden, 1987).

Clearly, the argument being entertained requires that innate immunity should be activated in depressed individuals. Indeed, this would appear to be the case. There is evidence that blood monocytes and macrophages taken from depressed populations are activated as measured by increased IL-1 and IL-6 production in stimulated cultures of mononuclear cells (Seidel et al., 1995), and plasma levels of circulating IL-6 are even elevated in depressed individuals (Sluzewska et al., 1995). This is not inconsistent with the hypercortisolism often observed in depression. Glucocorticoids do suppress macrophage function (Zwilling, 1994), but the elevated levels of glucocorticoids that occur during depression are far below the levels used in the macrophage experiments. In addition, just as in a classic acute-phase response occurring during inflammation and infection, white blood cell counts are elevated during depression (Maes et al., 1992), and circulating levels of positive acute-phase proteins such as haptoglobin and alpha1-acid-glycoprotein are elevated (Maes, 1993). Also as in infection, negative acute-phase reactants are reduced (Maes, 1993). These changes are most prominent in melancholic depression and correlate most closely with the vegetative symptoms of depression such as anorexia, weight loss, lethargy, and sleep disturbances (Maes, 1993). Consistent with the idea that there is chronic immune activation during depression, depressed individuals have recently been reported to show a blunted response to LPS (Heninger, Price, Malison, & Pelton, 1996)—a blunted response being a frequent adaptation to overstimulation.

Finally, Schweiger et al. (1994) have reported that depression is associated with a large reduction in bone mineral density and is thus a major risk factor in osteoporosis. Although a number of factors (e.g., hypercortisolism) could be responsible, it can be noted that IL-1 and other cytokines stimulate osteoclast development, thereby producing bone resorption (Manolagas, 1995). Indeed, the IL-1 receptor antagonist can decrease bone loss (Kimble et al., 1995). The activation of innate immunity associated with depression may well be responsible for this important consequence of depression.

Thus, depression does appear to be associated with the activation of innate immunity, just as is stress. The data are not sufficient to decide whether this apparent peripheral inflammatory response is involved in the etiology of depression, a consequence of depression that is involved in mediating some of the symptomology of depression, or is only epiphenomenally related to depression. However, the pattern produced by immune activation that is called sickness and the syndrome called depression bear such a striking similarity that speculation is tempting. Why do the particular symptoms and characteristics of depression cluster together, rather than there being some other combination? Is the constellation of characteristics merely accidental or pathological, or is there an adaptive function that has been served through evolution? Perhaps the essential features of what we call depression served to decrease energy usage during periods of sickness or injury, helping to promote recuperation. These adaptive responses then became part of the bidirectional immune-to-brain circuitry, and as organisms became more complex they then came to be elicited by more and more complex events. In rats this circuitry appears to be accessible by simple stressors, and perhaps in humans it is accessible by more complex social and ideational events. Intriguingly, however, the essential underlying circuitry may be the same. Finally, depression has also sometimes been related to a conservation–withdrawal reaction occurring during periods of prolonged threat (Engel & Schmale, 1972). The notion is that it would be adaptive to conserve energy during threats be-

yond the organism's ability to cope, and this same circuitry might have been cooptable to serve this important function.

The argument is not that depression is caused by immune activation. The argument is that whatever does cause depression (e.g., negative cognitions about the self or loss of a loved one) may have access to the same neural circuitry that evolved to mediate sickness and activate that circuitry. Some of the symptoms of depression, particularly the vegetative symptoms, may then be the result of this process and represent essentially sickness responses. In addition, as noted earlier, the circuit is bidirectional, and so peripheral immune cells should also become activated, and the products of these activated immune cells in turn provide signals to the brain. It is conceivable that this positive feedback circuit could help to maintain depression.

Specific Immunity

We have argued that acute stressors lead to the delayed activation or priming of nonspecific immune processes and that depression is associated with activated nonspecific immune processes. However, stress has most often been viewed as suppressing or interfering with immune function (see Solomon, 1969, for an excellent early study), and depression has also been most often reported to be associated with decreased immune function (Herbert & Cohen, 1993). Furthermore, stress is frequently associated with increased disease progression (Cohen & Williamson, 1991). Indeed, these sorts of findings have been a major focus of psychoneuroimmunology and are largely responsible for the development and recent interest in this field.

How can these seeming discrepancies be reconciled? With regard to studies of stress and disease, the huge majority has used chronic stressors (e.g., Sheridan & Dobbs, 1994) that also appear to inhibit rather than prime aspects of innate immunity (Zwilling, 1994). Indeed, there are few reports of consistent effects of acute stressors on disease progression or induction. Furthermore, many investigations of stress and specific immunity, particularly at the human level, have used chronic stress conditions (e.g., Kiecolt-Glaser, Dura, Speicher, Trask, & Glaser, 1991). Studies of chronic stress are surely important and are doubtlessly better models for understanding impacts on human disease than are acute-stress experiments. However, our goal in this article has been to attempt to understand function and adaptiveness rather than pathophysiology, and so we have focused on acute stress because we believe that this is where the stress response is adaptive.

However, acute stressors also frequently interfere with specific immune function. It can first be noted that there is no incompatibility between activated innate immunity and retarded specific immunity. Indeed, the very same stressor conditions can produce both at the same time (Jiang, Morrow-Tesch, Beller, Levy, & Black, 1990). It is possible that these are independent effects of acute stressors. It is also possible that some of the interference with specific immunity produced by an acute stressor is, at least partially, a by-product of activated and primed nonspecific immunity.

To understand this possibility, recall that the nonspecific (innate) immune response is the first line of defense against infectious agents. Infectious agents activate phagocytes such as macrophages that combat the infectious agent by releasing enzymes that destroy them, by engulfing them, and by releasing products such as nitric oxide that interfere with the ability of the infectious agent to multiply. The infectious agent or antigen is also presented to T cells (i.e., T-helper cells), which bear the surface receptor for that antigen, leading that specific T-helper cell population to divide, thereby beginning the specific immunity cascade that will ultimately produce cytotoxic T cells that can destroy the infectious agent and B-cell generated antibody directed against the antigen. This process of T-helper cell expansion and B-cell expansion is ini-

tiated a few hours after infection and continues for 2–4 days. However, the innate immune response with macrophage activation and the production of macrophage products occur during some of this time that T- and B-cell development is occurring, particularly during the early phases. Importantly, macrophage products such as nitric oxide, which interfere with the multiplication of infectious agents, also interfere with the multiplication of the antigen-specific T-helper cells and B cells (Albina & Henry, 1991). This is because the processes that underlie the cell division of microbes and other cells such as T cells and B cells are similar. Thus, the very mechanisms that allow nitric oxide to slow the growth of infectious agents also of necessity slow specific immune cell growth. This is simply the cost that the mechanism entails. That is, the very same mechanisms that allow macrophage products to protect the organism by slowing the growth of infectious agents must slow T- and B-cell growth. Of course, this is only a relative effect and T cells and B cells still divide and antibody is still produced, it is just that fewer T cells, B cells, and antibodies are produced than if the macrophage processes did not occur.

Although this might seem to be a peculiar situation, it may be inevitable. Rather than evolving a new mechanism for the cellular proliferation of immune cells, a simpler solution may have been a system that produces antibodies and other products in excess of those required for efficient defense so that a reduction is not deleterious. In any case, there is extensive evidence that the scenario described here is indeed present. Thus, inactivation or killing of macrophages has been shown to enhance specific immunity. For example, inactivation of macrophages with gadolinium chloride has been shown to increase the formation of antibody to an antigen (Souhami, Addison, & Bradfield, 1975). Conversely, simply activating macrophages interferes with antibody formation to an antigen, and the activation of innate immunity by a variety of means has been shown to interfere with T-cell function (Abrahamsohn & Coffman, 1995; Araneo, Dowell, Moon, & Daynes, 1989). As already noted, it should not be concluded that it would then be adaptive to suppress macrophage function. This is clearly an issue of balance, and on balance the rapid protection offered by the innate immune defense may more than compensate for the reduction in specific immunity that is a necessary outcome. This may well not be true when the reactions become chronic, as in depression. The combination of effects here has been most often reported to facilitate disease processes (Herbert & Cohen, 1993).

Now consider stress and specific immunity experiments. For example, consider experiments in which an antigen is administered, a stressor or control treatment then given, and antibody is measured some time later, say 7–21 days. The frequent result is that the stressor reduces the level of antibody to the antigen that is observed (Laudenslager et al., 1988). The antigen will, of course, activate macrophages and other phagocytes. However, if, as argued here, the stressor also initiates processes in the brain that lead to an outflow from the brain that also primes or activates macrophages in a delayed fashion, then the macrophage will be more activated in the group that has received the stressor some time after stressor termination. Macrophage products such as nitric oxide should be greater in the stressor group 1–4 days after the stressor, just the time at which antigen-specific T cells expand. Interference with specific immunity should therefore occur.

There is abundant evidence to support this argument. A full consideration of this evidence is beyond the scope of this article. However, here it can be noted that the removal of macrophages prevents stressors from interfering with T-cell function. For example, Fleshner, Bellgrau, Watkins, Laudenslager, and Maier (1995) gave rats inescapable shock or control treatment. One day later white blood cells were removed, and the ability of T cells to divide was measured. As would be expected, the T cells taken from the inescapably shocked group divided poorly on stimulation. However, macrophages were part of the blood sample. In a separate assay the macrophages were removed from the culture before the T-cell division was assessed. Now the T cells from the inescapably shocked rats divided normally. Furthermore, the addition of macrophages taken from inescapably shocked rats to T cells from controls suppressed the ability of the control T cells to divide in response to stimulation. Clearly, it was the macrophages from the shocked animals that were responsible for the suppression. Furthermore, there is evidence that stressors can increase the proportion of a macrophage subpopulation that is especially suppressive to T-cell proliferation (Kizaki et al., 1996). Similarly, blocking the ability of the macrophages to make nitric oxide blocks the effects of stress on specific immunity (Coussons-Read, Maslonek, Fecho, Perez, & Lysle, 1994). The suppression of specific immunity in depression can be viewed similarly. Alternatively, suppression of specific immunity in depression may have other causes.

We are not arguing that all interactions between stress and specific immunity can be explained in this manner. It is clear that both the autonomic nervous system and pituitary–adrenal hormones have direct effects on immune cells and organs and that stress effects on specific immunity can be mediated in this fashion. The points that we are making are that there is no incompatibility between a stressor simultaneously enhancing innate immunity while interfering with specific immunity and that some instances of suppressed specific immunity might actually be caused by products of activated innate immunity. In addition, this view provides a different perspective on findings that acute stressors reduce the specific immune response. Rather than representing a pathophysiologic effect, some instances may simply be the outcome of an adaptive process. These processes may no longer be beneficial when stressors become chronic.

Learned Helplessness

The degree of behavioral control that an organism has over a stressor determines many of the outcomes of exposure to stressors (Maier, 1993). A number of outcomes follow only if the stressor is uncontrollable, and these have been termed *learned helplessness effects* (Maier & Seligman, 1976). Although stressor controllability modulates numerous consequences of stressor exposure, and this has been the focus in most controllability research, it should be noted that not all sequelae of stressors are sensitive to the controllability of the stressor. For example, both escapable (controllable) and yoked inescapable (uncontrollable) shock lead to the same level of HPA activation as measured by plasma ACTH and plasma corticosterone (Maier, Ryan, Barksdale, & Kalin, 1986). This is not to say that conditions cannot be found that might not lead to differential activation by escapable and inescapable shock (Dess, Linwick, Patterson, Overmier, & Levine, 1983). However, the very same paradigm that produces behavioral differences following escapable and inescapable shock in our laboratory does not lead to different levels of pituitary ACTH or adrenal corticosterone. The effects of shock on specific immunity also often do not vary with controllability. We have found that both escapable and inescapable shock produce equal suppression of T-cell proliferation on stimulation (Maier & Laudenslager, 1988), and we have conducted numerous unpublished experiments in which these two types of shock have had equal effects on the development of antibody to an antigen. Furthermore, there are behavioral products of stressors that also do not differ after escapable and inescapable shock (Grahn & Maier, 1995; Woodmansee, Silbert, & Maier, 1993).

The position developed in the present chapter may help in understanding why some consequences of stressors such as electric shock are sensitive to controllability and some are not. We have argued that the bidirectional circuitry depicted in Figure 74.5 is of primitive origin, and, indeed, it does involve brainstem and subcortical structures. These may well not be sensitive to controllability, a dimension that must be extracted from sensory input and that may require higher brain structures for its computation. Physical stressors such as shock have direct access to the NTS, the area of the brain argued to be the initiating point of the neural cascade. This is because spinal cord pathways that carry somatosensory pain input from stimuli like shock (laminae I, IV–VII, and X) terminate in the NTS (Esteves, Lima, & Coimbra, 1993). Thus, the sensory input from shock is itself sufficient to activate the NTS and, indeed, does so (Pezzone et al., 1993), as does input from other stressors (Cullinan et al., 1995). Thus the NTS should be activated by shock, regardless of whether it is controllable or uncontrollable. We are not arguing that the NTS cannot be activated by descending cognitive influences but only that the sensory aspects of the stressor are by themselves sufficient to activate the NTS. Thus, sequelae of stressors that depend on the activation of the NTS and the bidirectional immune–brain circuit depicted in Figure 74.5 should be insensitive to controllability. For example, not only should HPA activity not differ but neither should other aspects of sickness such as the acute-phase response as described earlier. T. Deak in our laboratory has assessed the level of plasma corticosteroid binding globulin, a negative acute-phase reactant, after escapable and inescapable shock. Both inescapable and escapable shock produce the same level of reduction.

However, stressors do more than duplicate the effects of infection by activating this circuit. As already argued, less primitive parts of the brain should be sensitive to controllability and other cognitive variables and mediate learned helplessness effects. We have cited experiments earlier showing that blocking IL-1 receptors in the brain blocks learned helplessness effects such as debilitated escape learning (Maier & Watkins, 1995). Thus, action at brain IL-1 receptors is necessary for learned helplessness. However, we have been unable to produce learned helplessness effects such as poor escape learning by administering IL-1 into the brain—IL-1 is not sufficient. It is sufficient to produce the outcomes of stressors that are part of the sickness circuit but not other outcomes such as poor escape learning. Thus the bidirectional immune–brain circuitry proposed here may mediate "primitive" outcomes of stressor exposure, but more recently evolved neural structures may mediate more cognitive outcomes.

Cognition

Common experience suggests that cognitive alterations occur during sickness. Unfortunately, we have been unable to locate systematic study of this issue with humans. However, the precise location of IL-1 and IL-1 receptors in the brain, and some of the neurophysiological effects of IL-1, suggest that changes should be demonstrable and that they should be specific rather than general.

IL-1 receptors are especially abundant in the hippocampus (E. T. Cunningham & de Souza, 1993), and peripheral immune stimulation produces a large increase in IL-1 in the hippocampus (Layé et al., 1995). The hippocampus has often been implicated in learning, memory, and cognition (Cohen & Eichenbaum, 1993), with a phenomenon called *long-term potentiation (LTP)* within the hippocampus appearing to play a key role (Bliss & Collingridge, 1993). LTP refers to the observation that in some neural circuits a few seconds of intense electrical stimulation to input fibers can produce a long-lasting increase in synaptic efficacy in the circuit such that later input leads to an exaggerated response. This phenomenon is especially prevalent in the hippocampus and has been argued to be a mechanism involved in certain forms of learning and memory (Bear & Malenka, 1994). This is noted because IL-1 has been shown to interfere with LTP in the hippocampus (Bellinger, Madamba,

& Siggins, 1993). IL-1 does so in part because it interferes with the entry of calcium (A. J. Cunningham, Murray, O'Neill, Lynch, & O'Connor, 1996), a critical step in producing LTP. In addition, peripheral immune stimulation leads to the release of large amounts of serotonin (5-HT) in the hippocampus (Linthorst et al., 1994), with this release being dependent on IL-1 induction within the hippocampus (Linthorst et al., 1994). This is noted because 5-HT increases inhibition within the hippocampus (by acting on neurons containing inhibitory neurotransmitters) and also interferes with LTP (Stäubli & Otaky, 1994) and other processes within the hippocampus more generally (Rada et al., 1991).

The foregoing suggests that infection or injury should interfere with cognitive processes that depend on the hippocampus and LTP. A large body of research has been directed at determining the classes of learning and memory that are dependent on hippocampal function and LTP. This is a topic that is still unresolved, but spatial learning (Morris, Garrud, Rawlins, & O'Keefe, 1982) and learning involving contextual cues (Kim & Fanselow, 1992) have clearly been linked to the hippocampus. Spatial learning has often been studied by using the Morris water maze task (Morris, 1984). In the spatial form of this task a mouse or a rat is placed in a circular pool of opaque water with a platform located slightly below the water level so that it is not visible. The platform is always in the same location, but the starting location of the rat is varied from trial to trial. The rat or mouse can escape the water by finding the platform, and normal animals learn to do so quite readily. Because the platform is not visible and because the rat begins different trials at different locations in the maze, the rat can only learn the location of the platform by using spatial cues provided by the surrounding environment. There is also a nonspatial version of this task in which the platform is above the water and visible. Here the subject does not have to use spatial cues to learn to escape efficiently. The general result in which this task is used is that manipulations of the hippocampus alter performance on the spatial but not on the non-spatial form of the task (Morris et al., 1982).

This discussion would suggest that infection, inflammation, and the like should interfere with performance of the spatial but not of the non-spatial form of the Morris water maze task (Morris, 1984). In an interesting series of experiments Gibertini and colleagues infected mice with *Legionella pneumophilia,* the bacterium responsible for Legionnaires' disease in humans. This interfered with performance on the spatial form of the task, and the mice were very poor at learning and remembering the location of the hidden platform (Gibertini, Newton, Klein, & Friedman, 1995). However, this deficit was specific and did not represent a general debilitation, lack of motivation to escape the water, and so forth. The bacterium had no effect whatsoever on learning and performance on the visible platform version of the task. Importantly, Gibertini, Newton, Friedman, and Klein (1995) demonstrated that the effect on spatial learning and memory was mediated by IL-1. In a set of infected mice they administered an antibody directed against IL-1 2 hr before testing in the maze. The infected animals in which the IL-1 had been neutralized learned as rapidly as did the uninfected controls. Consistent with these findings, Oitzl, van Oers, Schöbitz, and de Kloet (1993) reported that IL-1 injected directly into the brain interferes with spatial learning.

The Morris water maze (Morris, 1984) is only one task, but Aubert et al. (1995) have found both LPS and IL-1 to interfere with performance on a different learning task, and in collaboration with M. Fleshner, R. Pugh, and J. Rudy we have begun to explore context learning. Indeed, we have found peripheral administration of LPS to interfere with fear conditioning to contextual cues but not to discrete cues. Clearly, the body of research reviewed is not large. However, there do appear to be suggestions that peripheral immune stimulation will interfere with some cognitive processes, and perhaps there will be some spe-

cificity to cognitive processes that depend on the hippocampus.

In keeping with the general orientation of this chapter, it is reasonable to ask whether there is any adaptive value to sickness interfering with cognitive processes such as spatial learning that depend on the hippocampus. Why would it be adaptive to be deficient at learning about spatial and contextual cues during illness but not about discrete cues? We are unable to provide an answer. However, it may be that there is no real adaptive purpose. The hippocampus is a very large structure, and it is unlikely that it would serve only one function. Investigators interested in cognition tend to view the hippocampus as a cognitive structure, a structure primarily serving cognition. However, the hippocampus is also a major site of neuroendocrine integration providing input to the hypothalamus that regulates the activity of the HPA axis (De Kloet, 1991). It also appears to be a major site of integration for sickness and sickness behaviors, and microinjecting IL-1 into the hippocampus produces most or all of the symptoms of sickness (Linthorst et al., 1994). It is not at all unusual for the same set of neurons to participate in different circuits that serve different functions, and it may simply be that the same hippocampal neurons participate in some aspects of both learning and memory and the organization of sickness. To the extent that these neurons are demanded by peripheral immune stimulation to participate in the organization of sickness, these neurons may be less able to participate in their cognitive functions. We argue that infection and injury are life threatening and command the attention of the relevant circuitry.

These considerations may also aid in the understanding of interactions between stress and learning, memory, and cognitive functions. The many and complex relationships between stress and cognitive function cannot be reviewed here, and we do not propose that the bidirectional immune-to-brain circuit reviewed here is important for all of them. However, there are instances in which these circuits may play an important role. For example, we have found that stressors such as inescapable shock induce IL-1 in the hippocampus as well as in the hypothalamus. It is thus interesting to note that stressors have been reported to interfere with both LTP in the hippocampus (Shors, Siet, Levine, & Thompson, 1989) and the memory for spatial learning (Healy & Drugan, 1996). It is not known whether brain IL-1 is, in fact, responsible for these. Nevertheless, this possibility as well as the general importance of brain IL-1 in mediating the effects of stress on learning and memory is worthy of study.

Conclusion

We have argued that the brain and the immune system form a bidirectional network that functions to defend the organism against infection and to promote tissue repair. The brain is required in this process because many of the component processes that operate to control infection, inflammation, and injury are either behavioral adjustments or physiological adjustments that are mediated by the central nervous system. The brain can only organize and control this defense if it both receives input from the periphery informing it as to the occurrence of infection and the progress of the immune responses against the invading infectious agent and has output mechanisms to the periphery that can regulate critical organs involved in defense such as the liver. Activation of peripheral immune cells by microbes therefore signals the brain, resulting in physiological, behavioral, affective, and cognitive changes. We have further argued that a variety of psychological phenomena can be understood as being products of this functional system. Many of these phenomena are related to what is often termed stress, and we have suggested that many stressors may access this bidirectional immune–brain circuitry via neural connections. We suggested that this may have evolved because defense against distal threat

such as a predator requires many of the same functions and because this would allow a recuperative system that has an inherent time delay of several hours to anticipate the possibility of infection and injury.

We have focused on experiments that have administered agents such as LPS that potently stimulate immune cells and thereby result in dramatic changes in behavior. Are there more subtle influences? Consider the following experiment conducted by Besedovsky, Sorkin, Keller, and Muller (1975). Rats were given a small injection of sheep red blood cells. Sheep red blood cells are harmless proteins, but because they are foreign to the rat they will produce an immune response. We have emphasized products of the rapidly occurring innate immune response as signaling the brain. Recall that the specific immune response is much slower, with antibody production being at its peak roughly 7 days after antigen administration. Besedovsky et al. acquired daily blood samples from the rats, and they observed a dramatic rise in plasma glucocorticoids and catecholamines 7 days after the sheep red blood cells had been injected. That is, a classic stress response was observed at the time of the peak specific immune response to the harmless sheep red blood cells. Furthermore, brain neurotransmitter systems such as norepinephrine in the hypothalamus have been shown to be activated at roughly this time (Carlson, Felten, Livnat, & Felten, 1987). Thus, products of the specific immune response must also be capable of signaling the brain. It can be noted that cytokines such as IL-1 are also produced by T cells and B cells and not just by macrophages.

Potential behavioral, affective, and cognitive alterations at different stages of the specific immune response have not yet been studied. However, the implications of these experiments are intriguing because here the measured neural and physiological changes are occurring 5–9 days after the organism has encountered a harmless protein. We often encounter such proteins in our daily lives and are likely to be unaware that we have done so. Could this type of immune stimulation play a role in causing the variations in behavior, mood, and cognition that people all experience from day to day? Psychologists have focused on the study of variables and mechanisms that are responsible for differences between individuals but have given relatively little attention to mechanisms that produce within-individual differences across time. Events in the immune system may play an important and neglected role.

Finally, we suggest that bidirectional interactions between the central nervous system and peripheral organ systems are not restricted to the immune system and that as a discipline researchers have underestimated the extent to which the roots of psychological phenomena are embedded in this sort of matrix. The understanding of many psychological phenomena may elude researchers if inquiry is restricted to the central nervous system as a disembodied entity and psychological phenomena as if they are disconnected from other systems and levels. Processing information about external events is only one function of the central nervous system and may not have been of the greatest importance for much of evolution. After all, survival has required the central nervous system to control and respond to the pipes, plumbing, and housekeeping operations that are essential for life.

References

Abbey, S. E., & Garfinkel, P. E. (1991). Chronic fatigue syndrome and depression: Cause, effect, or covariate. *Review of Infectious Diseases,* 13, S73–S83.

Abbott, N. J., Lane, N. J., & Bundgaard, M. (1986). The blood–brain interface in invertebrates. *Annals of the New York Academy of Sciences,* 481, 20–42.

Abrahamsohn, I. A., & Coffman, R. L. (1995). Cytokine and nitric oxide regulation of the immunosuppression in *Trypanosoma cruzi* infection. *Journal of Immunology,* 155, 3955–3963.

Albina, J. E., & Henry, W. L. (1991). Suppression of lymphocyte proliferation through the nitric oxide syn-

thesizing pathway. *Journal of Surgical Research,* 50, 403–409.

American Psychiatric Association. (1994). *Diagnostic and statistical manual of mental disorders* (4th ed.). Washington, DC: Author.

Amir, Z., & Galena, H. (1986). Stress-induced analgesia: Adaptive pain suppression. *Physiological Reviews,* 66, 1091–1119.

Araneo, B. A., Dowell, T., Moon, H. B., & Daynes, R. A. (1989). Regulation of murine lymphokine production in vivo: Ultraviolet radiation exposure depresses IL-2 and enhances IL-4 production by T cells through an ILK-1-dependent mechanism. *Journal of Immunology,* 143, 1737–1744.

Aubert, A., Vega, C., Dantzer, R., & Goodall, G. (1995). Pyrogens specifically disrupt the acquisition of a task involving cognitive processing in the rat. *Brain, Behavior, and Immunity,* 9, 129–148.

Ban, E. M., Sarlieve, L. L., & Haour, F. (1993). Interleukin-1 binding sites on astrocytes. *Neuroscience,* 52, 725–733.

Banks, W. A., Oritz, L., Plotkin, S. R., & Kastin, A. J. (1991). Human interleukin (IL) 1 alpha, murine IL-1 alpha, and murine IL-1 beta are transported from blood to brain in the mouse by a shared saturable mechanism. *Journal of Pharmacology and Experimental Therapeutics,* 259, 988–996.

Baumann, H., & Gauldie, J. (1994). The acute phase response. *Immunology Today,* 15, 74–81.

Bayne, C. J. (1990). Phagocytosis and non-self recognition in invertebrates. *Bio Science,* 40, 723–731.

Bear, M. F., & Malenka, R. C. (1994). Synaptic plasticity: LTP and LTD. *Current Opinion in Neurobiology,* 4, 389–400.

Beck, G., Cooper, E. L., Hobicht, G. S., & Harchonis, J. J. (1994). *Primordial immunity: Foundations for the vertebrate immune system. Annals of the New York Academy of Sciences,* 712.

Bellinger, F. P., Madamba, S., & Siggins, G. R. (1993). Interleukin-1b inhibits synaptic strength and long-term potentiation in the rat CA1 hippocampus. *Brain Research,* 628, 227–234.

Bernheim, H. A., & Kluger, M. J. (1976). Fever and antipyresis in the lizard *Vipsosaurus dorsalis. American Journal of Physiology,* 231, 198–203.

Berthoud, H. R., Kressel, M., & Neuhaiber, W. L. (1995). Vagal afferent innervation of rat abdominal paraganglia as revealed by anterograde D.I. tracing and confocal microscopy. *Acta Anatomica,* 152, 127–132.

Besedovsky, H. O., Sorkin, E., Keller, M., & Muller, J. (1975). Changes in blood hormone levels during immune response. *Proceedings of the Society for Experimental Biology and Medicine,* 150, 466–470.

Blalock, J. E., Smith, E. M., & Meyer, W. J. (1985). The pituitary–adrenocortical axis and the immune system. *Clinics in Endocrinology and Metabolism,* 14, 1021–1038.

Blanchard, R. J., Blanchard, D. C., & Hori, K. (1989). *An ethoexperimental approach to the study of defense* (NATO ASI Series D ed., Vol. 48). Norwell, MA: Kluwer Academic.

Blatteis, C. M. (1986). Fever: Is it beneficial? *Yale Journal of Biology and Medicine,* 59, 107–116.

Bliss, T. V. P., & Collingridge, G. L. (1993). A synaptic model of memory: Long-term potentiation in the hippocampus. *Nature,* 361, 31–39.

Bluthé, R.-M., Dantzer, R., & Kelley, K. W. (1992). Effects of interleukin-1 receptor antagonist on the behavioral effects of lipopolysaccharide in rat. *Brain Research,* 573, 318–320.

Bluthé, R.-M., Walter, V., Parnet, P., Layé, S., Lestage, J., Verrier, D., Poole, S., Stenning, B. E., Kelley, K. W., & Dantzer, R. (1994). Lipopolysaccharide induces sickness behaviour by a vagal mediated mechanism. *C. R. Acad. Sci. Ser. III Sci. Vie,* 317, 499–503.

Bolles, R. C., & Fanselow, M. S. (1980). A perceptual–defensive–recuperative model of fear and pain. *Behavioral and Brain Sciences,* 3, 291–301.

Bret-Dibat, J. L., Bluthe, R. M., Kent, S., Kelley, K. W., & Dantzer, R. (1995). Lipopolysaccharide and interleukin-1 depress food-motivated behavior in mice by a vagal-mediated mechanism. *Brain, Behavior, and Immunity,* 9, 242–246.

Brown, G. W. (Ed.). (1993). *The role of life events in the aetiology of depressive and anxiety disorders.* London: Academic Press.

Carlson, S. L., Felten, D. L., Livnat, S., & Felten, S. Y. (1987). Alterations of monoamines in specific central autonomic nuclei following immunization in mice. *Brain, Behavior, and Immunity,* 1, 52–64.

Clatworthy, A. L. (1996). A simple systems approach to neural–immune communication. *Comparative Biochemistry and Physiology,* 115A, 1–10.

Coe, C. L., Rosenberg, L. T., & Levine, S. (1988). Prolonged effect of psychological disturbance on macrophage chemiluminescence in the squirrel monkey. *Brain, Behavior, and Immunity,* 2, 151–161.

Cohen, N. J., & Eichenbaum, H. (1993). *Memory, amnesia, and the hippocampal system.* Cambridge, MA: MIT Press.

Cohen, S., & Williamson, G. (1991). Stress and infectious disease in humans. *Psychological Bulletin,* 109, 5–24.

Colotta, R., Re, F., Muzio, M., Bertini, R., Polentarutti, N., Sironi, M., Giri, J. G., Dower, S. K., Sims, J. E., & Mantovani, A. (1993). Interleukin-1 type II receptor: A decoy target for IL1-1 that is regulated by IL-4. *Science,* 261, 472–474.

Coussons-Read, M. E., Maslonek, K. A., Fecho, K., Perez, L., & Lysle, D. T. (1994). Evidence for the involvement of macrophage-derived nitric oxide in the modulation of immune status by a conditioned aversive stimulus. *Journal of Neuroimmunology,* 50, 51–58.

Covert, J. B., & Reynolds, W. W. (1977). Behavioral fever in anuran amphibian larvae. *Life Sciences,* 20, 593–596.

Cserr, H. F., & Bandgaard, M. (1988). The neuronal microenvironment: A comparative view. *Annals of the New York Academy of Sciences,* 481, 1–7.

Cullinan, W. E., Herman, J. B., Battaglea, D. F., Akil, H., & Watson, S. J. (1995). Pattern and time course of immediate early gene expression in rat brain following acute stress. *Neuroscience,* 64, 477–505.

Cunningham, A. J., Murray, C. A., O'Neill, L. A. J., Lynch, M. A., & O'Connor, J. J. (1996). Interleukin-1b (IL-1b) and tumour necrosis factor (TNF) inhibit long-term potentiation in the rat dentate gyrus in vitro. *Neuroscience Letters,* 203, 17–20.

Cunningham, E. T., Jr., & De Souza, E. B. (1993). Interleukin-1 receptors in the brain and endocrine tissues. *Immunology Today,* 14, 171–176.

Dantzer, R., Bluthé, R.-M., & Kelley, K. W. (1991). Androgen-dependent vasopressinergic neurotransmission attenuates interleukin-1-induced sickness behavior. *Brain Research,* 557, 115–120.

Dantzer, R., Bluthé, R.-M., Kent, S., & Goodall, G. (1993). Behavioral effects of cytokines: An insight into mechanisms of sickness behavior. In E. B. De Souza (Ed.), *Neurobiology of cytokines* (pp. 130–151). San Diego, CA: Academic Press.

De Kloet, E. R. (1991). Brain corticosteroid receptor balance and homeostatic control. *Frontier Neuroendocrinology,* 12, 95–164.

DeSimoni, M. G., Seroni, M., DeLuigi, A., Manfridi, A., Mantovani, A., & Ghezzi, P. (1990). Intracerebroventricular injection of IL-1 induces high circulating levels of IL-6. *Journal of Experimental Medicine,* 171, 1773–1778.

Dess, N. K., Linwick, D., Patterson, J., Overmier, J. B., & Levine, S. (1983). Immediate and proactive effects of controllability and predictability on plasma cortisol responses to shocks in dogs. *Behavioral Neuroscience,* 97, 1005–1016.

Dess, N. K., Minor, T. R., & Brewer, J. (1989). Suppression of feeding and body weight after inescapable shock: Modulation by quinine adulteration, stressor reinstatement, and controllability. *Physiology and Behavior,* 45, 975–983.

Dinarello, C. A. (1991). Interleukin-1 and interleukin-1 antogenism. *Blood,* 77, 1627–1652.

Dinarello, C. A., & Thompson, R. C. (1991). Blocking IL-1: Interleukin-1 receptor antagonist in vivo and in vitro. *Immunology Today,* 12, 404–410.

Dunn, A. J. (1992). Endotoxin-induced activation of cerebral catecholamine and serotonin metabolism: Comparison with interleukin-1. *Journal of Pharmacology and Experimental Therapeutics,* 261, 964–969.

Dunn, A. J. (1993). Role of cytokines in infection-induced stress. *Annals of the New York Academy of Sciences,* 697, 189–202.

Dunn, A. J. (1995). Interactions between the nervous system and the immune system: Implications for psychopharmacology. In F. E. Bloom & D. J. Kupfer (Eds.), *Psychopharmacology: The fourth generation of progress* (pp. 719–733). New York: Raven Press.

Eisenberg, S. P., Evans, R. J., Arend, W. P., Verderber, E., Brewer, M. T., Hannum, C. H., & Thompson, R. C. (1990). Primary structure and functional expression from complementary DNA of a human interleukin-1 receptor antagonist. *Nature,* 343, 341–346.

Engel, G. L., & Schmale, A. H. (1972). Conservation-withdrawal: A primary regulatory process for organismic homeostasis. *CIBA Foundation Symposium,* 8, 57–75.

Ericcson, A., Kovacs, K. J., & Sawchenko, P. E. (1994). A functional anatomical analysis of central pathways subserving the effects of interleukin-1 on stress-related neuroendocrine neurons. *Journal of Neuroscience,* 14, 897–913.

Esteves, F., Lima, D., & Coimbra, A. (1993). Structural types of spinal cord marginal neurons projecting in the NTS of the rat. *Somatosensory Motor Research,* 10, 203–216.

Fanselow, M. S. (1994). Neural organization of the defensive behavior system responsible for fear. *Psychonomic Bulletin and Review,* 1, 429–438.

Fanselow, M. S., & Sigmundi, R. A. (1987). Functional behaviorism and aversively motivated behavior: A role for endogenous opioids in the defensive behavior of the rat. *Psychological Record,* 37, 317–334.

Felten, S. Y., & Felten, D. L. (1991). *Innervation of lymphoid tissue* (2nd ed.). San Diego, CA: Academic Press.

Fent, K., & Zbinden, G. (1987). Toxicity of interferon and interleukin. *Trends in Pharmacological Sciences,* 8, 100–105.

Fleshner, M., Bellgrau, D., Watkins, L. R., Laudenslager, M. L., & Maier, S. F. (1995). Stress-induced reduction in the rat mixed lymphocyte reaction is due to macrophages and not changes in T-cell phenotypes. *Neuroimmunology,* 56, 45–52.

Fleshner, M., Goehler, L. E., Hermann, J., Relton, J. K., Watkins, L. R., & Maier, S. F. (1995). Interleukin-1b induced corticosterone elevation and hypothalamic NE depletion is vagally mediated. *Brain Research Bulletin,* 37, 605–610.

Flores, E. A., Istfan, N., Blackburn, G. L., & Bistrian, B. R. (1990). Effects of interleukin-1 and tumor necrosis factor on glucose turnover in the rat: *Metabolism,* 39, 738–743.

Gibertini, M., Newton, C., Friedman, H., & Klein, T. W. (1995). Spatial learning impairment in mice infected with *Legionella pneumophila* or administered exogenous interleukin-1-b. *Brain, Behavior, and Immunity,* 9, 113–128.

Gibertini, M., Newton, C., Klein, T. W., & Friedman, H. (1995). *Legionella pneumophila*-induced visual learning impairment reversed by anti-interleukin-1b. *Proceedings of the Society of Experimental Behavioral Medicine,* 210, 7–12.

Goehler, L. E., Busch, C. R., Tartaglia, N., Relton, J., Sisk, D., Maier, S. F., & Watkins, L. R. (1995). Blockade of cytokine induced conditioned taste aversion by subdiaphragmatic vagotomy: Further evidence for vagal mediation of immune–brain communication. *Neuroscience Letters,* 185, 163–166.

Goehler, L. E., Relton, J. K., Dripps, D., Kiechle, R., Tartaglia, N., Maier, S. F., & Watkins, L. R. (in press). Vagal paraganglia bind biotinylated interleukin-1 receptor antagonist (IL-1ra) in the rat: A possible mechanism for immune-to-brain communication. *Brain Research Bulletin.*

Gold, P. W., Wong, M. L., Chroesos, G. P., & Licinio, J. (1996). Stress system abnormalities in melancholic and atypical depression: Molecular, pathophysiological, and therapeutic implications. *Molecular Psychiatry,* 1, 257–265.

Gould, S. J. (1982). Darwinism and the expansion of evolutionary theory. *Science,* 216, 380–387.

Grahn, R. E., & Maier, S. F. (1995). The elevated plus-maze is not sensitive to the effects of stressor controllability in rats. *Pharmacology, Biochemistry, and Behavior,* 52, 565–570.

Hagan, P. M., Poole, S., & Bristow, A. F. (1993). Corticotrophin-releasing factor as a mediator of the acute-phase response in rats, mice and rabbits. *Journal of Endocrinology,* 136, 207–216.

Hart, B. L. (1988). Biological basis of the behavior of sick animals. *Neuroscience and Biobehavioral Reviews,* 12, 123–137.

Healy, D. J., & Drugan, R. C. (1996). Escapable stress modulates retention of spatial learning in rats: Preliminary evidence for involvement of neurosteroids. *Psychobiology,* 24, 110–117.

Helmreich, D. L., Cullinan, W. E., & Watson, S. J. (1996). The effect of adrenolectomy on stress-induced c-fos mRNA expression in the rat brain. *Brain Research,* 706, 137–144.

Hendrie, C. A. (1989). Naloxone-sensitive hyperalgesia follows analgesia induced by morphine and environmental stimulation. *Pharmacology, Biochemistry, and Behavior,* 32, 961–966.

Heninger, G. R., Price, L. H., Malison, R. T., & Pelton, G. (1996). Neural-immune abnormalities in depressed patients and healthy controls. *Society for Neuroscience Abstracts,* 1456.

Herbert, I., & Cohen, S. (1993). Depression and immunity: A meta-analytic review. *Psychological Bulletin,* 113, 472–486.

Hodos, W., & Campbell, C. B. G. (1969). Scala naturae: Why there is no theory in comparative psychology. *Psychological Review,* 76, 337–350.

Hopkins, S. J., & Rothwell, N. J. (1995). Cytokines and the nervous system: I. Expression and recognition. *Trends in Neuroscience,* 18, 83–88.

Hughes, T. K., Smith, E. M., Barnett, J. A., Charles, R., & Stefano, G. B. (1991). LPS stimulated invertebrate hemocytes: A role for immunoreactive TNF and IL-1. *Developmental and Comparative Immunology,* 15, 117–122.

Jiang, C. G., Morrow-Tesch, J. L., Beller, D. I., Levy, E. M., & Black, P. H. (1990). Immunosuppression in mice induced by cold water stress. *Brain, Behavior, and Immunity,* 4, 278–291.

Johnston, I. S., & Heldemann, W. H. (1982). *Cellular defense systems in the porifera* (Vol. 3). New York: Plenum Press.

Katz, R. M. (1982). Animal model of depression: Pharmacological sensitivity of a hedonic deficit. *Pharmacology, Biochemistry, and Behavior,* 16, 965–968.

Kent, S., Bluthé, R.-M., Kelley, K. W., & Dantzer, R. (1992). Sickness behavior as a new target for drug development. *Trends in Pharmacological Sciences,* 13, 24–28.

Kiecolt-Glaser, J. K., Dura, J. R., Speicher, C. E., Trask, O. J., & Glaser, R. (1991). Spousal caregivers of dementia victims: Longitudinal changes in immunity and health. *Psychosomatic Medicine,* 53, 345–362.

Kim, J. J., & Fanselow, M. S. (1992). Modality specific retrograde amnesia of fear. *Science,* 256, 675–677.

Kimble, R. B., Matayoshi, A. B., Vannice, J. L., Kung, V. T., Williams, C., & Pacifici, R. (1995). Simultaneous block of interleukin-1 and tumor necrosis factor is required to completely prevent bone loss in the early postovariectomy period. *Endocrinology,* 136, 3054–3061.

Kirby, L. G., Allen, A. R., & Lucki, I. (1995). Regional differences in the effects of forced swimming on extracellular levels of 5-HT and 5-HIAA. *Brain Research,* 682, 189–196.

Kizaki, T., Oh-Ishi, S., Ookawara, T., Yamamoto, M., Izawa, T., & Ohno, H. (1996). Glucocorticoid-mediated generation of suppressor macrophages with high density FcγRII during acute cold stress. *Endocrinology,* 137, 4260–4267.

Kluger, M. J. (1978). The evolution and adaptive value of fever. *American Scientist,* 66, 38–43.

Kluger, M. J. (1979). *Fever: Its biology, evolution and function.* Princeton, NJ: Princeton University Press.

Kluger, M. J., Kozak, W., Conn, C. A., Leon, L. R., & Soszynski, D. (1996). The adaptive value of fever. *Infectious Disease Clinics of North America*, 10, 1–21.

Laudenslager, M. L., Fleshner, M., Hofstader, P., Held, P. E., Simons, L., & Maier, S. F. (1988). Suppression of specific antibody production by inescapable shock: Stability under varying conditions. *Brain, Behavior, and Immunity*, 2, 92–101.

Lavicky, J., & Dunn, A. J. (1995). Endotoxin stimulates cerebral catecholamine release in freely moving rats as assessed by microdialysis. *Journal of Neuroscience Research*, 40, 407–413.

Layé, S., Bluthé, R.-M., Kent, S., Combe, C., Médina, C., Parnet, P., Kelley, K., & Dantzer, R. (1995). Subdiaphragmatic vagotomy blocks induction of IL-1b mRNA in mice brain in response to peripheral LPS. *American Journal of Physiology*, 268, R1327–R1331.

LeMay, L. G., Vander, A. J., & Kluger, M. J. (1990). The effects of psychological stress on plasma interleukin-6 activity in rats. *Physiology and Behavior*, 47, 957–961.

Linthorst, A. C. E., Flachskamm, C., Holsboer, F., & Reul, J. M. H. M. (1994). Local administration of recombinant human interleukin-1b in the rat hippocampus increases serotonergic neurotransmission, hypothalamic–pituitary–adrenocortical axis activity, and body temperature. *Endocrinology*, 135, 520–532.

Lipton, J. M. (1990). Modulation of host defense by the neuropeptide a-MSH. *Yale Journal of Biology and Medicine*, 63, 173–182.

Maes, M. (1993). A review on the acute phase response in major depression. *Reviews in the Neurosciences*, 4, 407–416.

Maes, M., Van der Planken, M., Stevens, W., Peeters, D., DeClerck, K., & Bridts, C. (1992). Leukocytosis, monocytosis and neurotrophilia: Hallmarks of severe depression. *Journal of Psychiatric Research*, 26, 125–134.

Maier, S. F. (1989). Determinants of the nature of environmentally induced hypoalgesia. *Behavioral Neuroscience*, 103, 131–143.

Maier, S. F. (1993). *Learned helplessness, fear, and anxiety*. London: Academic Press.

Maier, S. F., Anderson, C., & Lieberman, D. (1972). The influence of control of shock on subsequent shock-elicited aggression. *Journal of Comparative and Physiological Psychology*, 81, 94–101.

Maier, S. F., Goehler, L. E., Fleshner, M., & Watkins, L. R. (in press). The role of the vagus nerve in cytokine-to-brain communication. *Annals of the New York Academy of Sciences*.

Maier, S. F., Grahn, R. E., & Watkins, L. R. (1995). 8-OH-DPAT microinjected in the region of the dorsal raphe nucleus blocks and reverses the enhancement of fear conditioning and the interference with escape produced by exposure to inescapable shock. *Behavioral Neuroscience*, 109, 404–413.

Maier, S. F., & Laudenslager, M. L. (1988). Commentary: Inescapable shock, shock controllability, and mitogen stimulated lymphocyte proliferation. *Brain, Behavior, and Immunity*, 2, 87–91.

Maier, S. F., Ryan, S. M., Barksdale, C. M., & Kalin, N. H. (1986). Stressor controllability and the pituitary–adrenal system. *Behavioral Neuroscience*, 100, 669–678.

Maier, S. F., & Seligman, M. E. P. (1976). Learned helplessness: Theory and evidence. *Journal of Experimental Psychology: General*, 105, 3–46.

Maier, S. F., & Watkins, L. R. (1995). Intracerebroventricular interleukin-1 receptor antagonist blocks the enhancement of fear conditioning and interference with escape produced by inescapable shock. *Brain Research*, 695, 279–286.

Maier, S. F., Watkins, L. R., & Fleshner, M. (1994). Psychoneuroimmunology: The interface between behavior, brain, and immunity. *American Psychologist*, 49, 1004–1017.

Manolagas, S. C. (1995). Role of cytokine in gene resorption. *Bone*, 17, 63–67.

Manzella, J. P., & Roberts, N. J., Jr. (1979). Human macrophage and lymphocyte responses to mitogen stimulation after exposure to influenza virus, ascorbic acid, and hyperthermia. *Journal of Immunology*, 123, 940–1044.

Marazziti, D., Di Muro, A., & Castrogiovanni, P. (1992). Psychological stress and body temperature changes in humans. *Physiological Behavior*, 52, 393–395.

Meijer, A., Zakay-Rones, Z., & Morag, A. (1988). Post-influenzal psychiatric disorder in adolescents. *Acta Psychiatrica Scandinavia*, 78, 176–181.

Meller, S. T., Dykstra, C., Grzybycki, D., Murphey, S., & Gebhart, G. C. (1994). The possible role of glia in nociceptive processing and hyperalgesia in the rat. *Neuropharmacology*, 33, 1471–1478.

Merritt, H. H., Adams, R. D., & Soloman, H. C. (1946). *Neurosyphilis.* New York: Oxford University Press.

Minami, M., Kuraishi, Y., Yamaguchi, T., Nakai, S., Hirai, Y., & Satoh, M. (1991). Immobilization stress induces interleukin-1 mRNA in the rat hypothalamus. *Neuroscience Letters, 123,* 254–256.

Morris, R. G. M. (1984). Development of a water maze procedure for studying spatial learning in the rat. *Journal of Neuroscience Methods, 11,* 47–60.

Morris, R. G. M., Garrud, P., Rawlins, J. N. P., & O'Keefe, J. (1982). Place navigation impaired in rats with hippocampal lesions. *Nature, 297,* 681–683.

Oitzl, M. S., van Oers, H., Schöbitz, B., & de Kloet, E. R. (1993). Interleukin-1b, but not interleukin-6, impairs spatial navigation learning. *Brain Research, 613,* 160–163.

Ottaviani, E., & Franceschi, C. (1996). The neuro-immunology of stress from invertebrates to man. *Progress in Neurobiology, 48,* 421–440.

Pacok, K., Armando, I., Fukuhara, K., Koetansky, R., Palkovitz, M., Kopin, I. J., & Goldstein, D. S. (1992). Noradrenergic activation in the paraventricular nucleus during acute and chronic immobilization stress in rats: An in vivo microdialysis study. *Brain Research, 589,* 91–96.

Paeman, L. R., Porchet-Hennere, E., Masson, M., Leung, M. K., Hughes, T. K., & Stefano, G. B. (1992). Glial localization of interleukin-1 in invertebrate ganglia. *Cellular and Molecular Neurobiology, 12,* 463–472.

Patarca, R., Klimas, N. G., Lugtendorf, S., Antoni, M., & Fletcher, M. A. (1994). Dysregulated expression of tumor necrosis factor in chronic fatigue syndrome: Interrelations with cellular sources and patterns of soluble immune mediator expression. *Clinical and Infectious Diseases, 18,* S147–S153.

Pestarino, M., De Anna, E., Masini, M., & Sturla, M. (1997). Localization of interleukin-1β mRNA in the cerebral ganglion of the protochordate, *Styela plicata. Neuroscience Letters, 222,* 151–154.

Petit, F., Jarous, A., Dickinson, R. D., Molina, P. E., Abumrad, N. N., & Lang, C. H. (1994). Contribution of central and peripheral adrenergic stimulation to IL-1-mediated glucoregulation. *American Journal of Physiology, 267,* E49–E56.

Pezzone, M. A., Lee, W.-S., Hoffman, G. E., Pezzone, K. M., & Rabin, B. S. (1993). Activation of brainstem catecholaminergic neurons by conditioned and unconditioned aversive stimuli as revealed by c-Fos immunoreactivity. *Brain Research, 608,* 310–318.

Plata-Salaman, C. R., Oomura, Y., & Kai, Y. (1988). Tumor necrosis factor and interleukin-1b: Suppression of food intake by direct action in the central nervous system. *Brain Research, 448,* 106–114.

Plaut, M. (1987). Lymphocyte hormone receptors. *Annual Review of Immunology, 5,* 621–669.

Quan, N., Sundar, S. K., & Weiss, J. M. (1994). Induction of interleukin-1 in various brain regions after peripheral and central injections of lipopolysaccharide. *Journal of Neuroimmunology, 49,* 125–134.

Quan, N., Zhang, Z., Emery, M., Bonsall, R., & Weiss, J. M. (1996). Detection of interleukin-1 bioactivity in various brain regions of normal healthy rats. *Neuroimmunomodulation, 3,* 47–55.

Rada, P., Mark, G. P., Vitek, M. P., Mangano, R. M., Blume, A. J., Beer, B., & Hoebel, B. G. (1991). Interleukin-1b decreases acetylcholine measured by microdialysis in the hippocampus of freely moving rats. *Brain Research, 550,* 287–290.

Renbourn, E. T. (1960). Body temperature and pulse rate in boys and young men prior to sporting contests. A study in emotional hyperthermia: With a review of the literature. *Journal of Psychosomatic Research, 4,* 149–175.

Rothwell, N. J., & Hopkins, S. J. (1995). Cytokines and the nervous system: II. Actions and mechanisms of action. *Trends in Neuroscience, 18,* 130–136.

Saper, C. B., & Breder, C. D. (1994). The neurologic basis of fever. *New England Journal of Medicine, 330,* 1880–1886.

Saphier, D. (1992). Electrophysiological studies of the effects of interleukin-1 and a-interferon on the EEG and pituitary–adrenocortical activity. In J. J. Rothwell & R. D. Dantzer (Eds.), *Interleukin-1 in the brain* (pp. 51–75). Oxford, England: Pergamon Press.

Sapolsky, R., Rivier, C., Yamamoto, G., Plotsky, P., & Vale, W. (1987). Interleukin-1 stimulates the secretion of hypothalamic corticotropin-releasing factor. *Science, 238,* 522–524.

Sapolsky, R. M. (1992). *Stress: The aging brain and the mechanisms of neuron death.* Cambridge, MA: MIT Press.

Sawada, M., Hara, N., & Maeno, T. (1991). Ionic mechanism of the outward current induced by extracellular ejection of interleukin-1 onto identified neurons of aplysia. *Brain Research,* 545, 248–256.

Schafe, G. E., Seeley, R. J., & Bernstein, I. L. (1995). Forebrain contribution to the induction of a cellular correlate of conditioned taste aversion in the nucleus of the solitary tract. *Journal of Neuroscience,* 15, 6789–6795.

Schleifer, S. J., Keller, S. E., Meyerson, A. T., Raskin, M. J., Davis, K. L., & Stein, M. (1984). Lymphocyte function in major depressive disorder. *Archives of General Psychiatry,* 41, 484.

Schöbitz, B., de Kloet, E. R., & Holsboer, F. (1994). Gene expression and function of IL-1, IL-6 and TNF in the brain. *Progress in Neurobiology,* 44, 397–432.

Schweiger, U., Deuschle, M., Korner, A., Lammers, C. H., Schmider, J., Gotthardt, U., Holsboer, F., & Heuser, I. (1994). Low lumbar bone mineral density in patients with major depression. *American Journal of Psychiatry,* 151, 1691–1693.

Sebag, J., Reed, W. P., & Williams, R. C. (1977). Effect of temperature on bacterial killing by serum and by polymorphonuclear leukocytes. *Infection and Immunity,* 10, 947–954.

Sehic, E., & Blatteis, C. M. (1996). Blockade of lipopolysaccharide-induced fever by subdiaphragmatic vagotomy in guinea pigs. *Brain Research,* 726, 160–166.

Sehic, E., Székely, M., Ungar, A. L., Oladehin, A., & Blatteis, C. M. (1996). Hypothalamic prostaglandin E$_2$ during lipopolysaccharide-induced fever in guinea pigs. *Brain Research Bulletin,* 39, 391–399.

Seidel, A., Arolt, V., Hunstiger, M., Rink, L., Behnisch, A., & Kirchner, H. (1995). Cytokine production and serum proteins in depression. *Scandinavian Journal of Immunology,* 41, 534–538.

Sheridan, J. F., & Dobbs, C. M. (1994). Stress, viral pathogenesis, and immunity. In R. Glaser & J. K. Kiecolt-Glaser (Eds.), *Handbook of human stress and immunity* (pp. 101–123). San Diego, CA: Academic Press.

Shintani, F., Kanba, S., Nakaki, T., Nibuya, M., Kinoshita, N., Suzuki, E., Yagi, G., Kato, R., & Asai, M. (1993). Interleukin-1b augments release of norepinephrine, dopamine and serotonin in the rat hypothalamus. *Journal of Neuroscience,* 12, 3574–3581.

Shintani, F., Nakaki, T., Kanba, S., Sato, K., Yagi, G., Shiozawa, M., Aiso, S., Kato, R., & Asai, M. (1995). Involvement of interleukin-1 in immobilization stress-induced increase in plasma adrenocorticotropic hormone and in release of hypothalamic monamines in the rat. *Journal of Neuroscience,* 15(3), 1961–1970.

Shors, T. J., Siet, T. B., Levine, S., & Thompson, R. F. (1989). Inescapable versus escapable shock modulates long-term potentiation in the rat hippocampus. *Science,* 244, 224–226.

Short, K. R., & Maier, S. F. (1993). Stressor controllability, social interaction, and benzodiazepine systems. *Pharmacology, Biochemistry, and Behavior,* 45, 1–9.

Sluzewska, A., Rybakowski, M., Laciak, M., Mackiewicz, A., Sobieska, M., & Wiktorowicz, K. (1995). IL-6 serum levels in depressed patients before and after treatment with fluoxetine. *Annals of the New York Academy of Sciences,* 762, 474–476.

Solomon, G. (1969). Stress and antibody responses in rats. *Archives of Allergy,* 35, 97–104.

Souhami, R. L., Addison, I. E., & Bradfield, J. W. B. (1975). Increased antibody production following depression of hepatic phagocytosis. *Clinical Experimental Immunology,* 20, 155–159.

Stäubli, U., & Otaky, N. (1994). Serotonin controls the magnitude of LTP induced by theta bursts via an action on NMDA-receptor-mediated responses. *Brain Research,* 643, 10–16.

Steckler, A., & Sahgal, A. (1995). The role of serotonergic–cholinergic interactions in the mediation of cognitive behavior. *Behavioral Brain Research,* 67, 165–199.

Sundar, S. K., Becker, K. J., Cierpial, M. A., Carpenter, M. D., Rankin, L. A., Fleener, S. L., Ritchie, J. C., Simson, P. E., & Weiss, J. M. (1989). Intracerebroventricular infusion of interleukin 1 rapidly decreases peripheral cellular immune responses. *Proceedings. National Academy of Sciences (United States of America),* 86, 6398–6402.

Takao, T., Tracey, D. E., Mitchell, W. M., & de Souza, E. B. (1990). Interleukin-1 receptors in mouse brain: Characterization and neuronal localization. *Endocrinology,* 127, 3070–3078.

Tilders, F. J., Schmidt, E. D., & de Goeji, D. C. (1993). Phenotypic plasticity of CRF neurons during stress.

Annals of the New York Academy of Sciences, 697, 39–52.

Timberlake, W., & Lucas, G. A. (1989). *Behavior systems and learning: From misbehavior to general principles.* Hillsdale, NJ: Erlbaum.

Ulevitch, R. J. (1993). Recognition of bacterial endotoxin by receptor-dependent mechanisms. *Advances in Immunology, 53,* 267–289.

Van Dam, A.-M., Bauer, J., Tilders, F. J., & Barkenbosch, F. (1995). Endotoxin-induced appearance of immunoreactive interleukin-1 beta in ramified microglia in rat brain: A light and electron microscopic study. *Neuroscience, 65,* 815–828.

Van Dam, A.-M., Brown, M., Man-A-Hing, W., & Berkenbosch, F. (1993). Immunocytochemical detection of prostaglandin E2 in microvasculature and in neurons of rat brain after administration of bacterial endotoxin. *Brain Research, 613,* 331–336.

van Dijken, H. H., Van der Heyden, J. A. M., Mos, J., & Tilders, F. (1992). Inescapable footshocks induce progressive and long-lasting behavioral deficits resulting from one short stress experience in male rats. *Physiology and Behavior, 51,* 787–794.

van Gool, J., van Vugt, H., Helle, M., & Aarden, L. A. (1990). The relation among stress, adrenalin, interleukin 6 and acute phase proteins in the rat. *Clinical Immunology and Immunopathology, 57,* 200–210.

Walters, E. T. (1994). Injury-related behavior and neuronal plasticity: An evolutionary perspective on sensitization, hyperalgesia, and analgesia. *International Review of Neurobiology, 36,* 325–427.

Watkins, L. R., Goehler, L. E., Relton, J. K., Tartaglia, N., Silbert, L., Martin, D., & Maier, S. F. (1994). Blockade of interleukin-1 induced fever by subdiaphragmatic vagotomy: Evidence for vagal mediation of immune–brain communication. *Neuroscience Letters, 183,* 1–5.

Watkins, L. R., Maier, S. F., & Goehler, L. E. (1995a). Cytokine-to-brain communication: A review and analysis of alternative mechanisms. *Life Sciences, 57,* 1011–1027.

Watkins, L. R., Maier, S. F., & Goehler, L. E. (1995b). Immune activation: The role of proinflammatory cytokines in inflammation, illness responses, and pathological pain states. *Pain, 63,* 289–302.

Watkins, L. R., Wiertelak, E. P., Goehler, L., Mooney-Heiberger, K., Martinez, J., Furness, L., Smith, K. P., Iadorola, M. J., & Maier, S. F. (1994). Neurocircuitry of illness-induced hyperalgesia. *Brain Research, 639,* 283–299.

Weiss, J. M. (1968). Effects of coping responses on stress. *Journal of Comparative Physiological Psychology, 65,* 251–260.

Weiss, J. M., & Simpson, P. G. (1985). *Neurochemical mechanisms underlying stress-induced depression.* Hillsdale, NJ: Erlbaum.

Wiertelak, E. P., Furness, L. E., Watkins, L. R., & Maier, S. F. (1994). Illness-induced hyperalgesia is mediated by a spinal NMDA-nitric oxide cascade. *Brain Research, 664,* 9–16.

Willner, P., Towell, A., Sampson, D., Sophokleous, S., & Muscat, R. (1987). Reduction of sucrose preference by chronic unpredictable mild stress, and its restoration by a tricyclic antidepressant. *Psychopharmacology, 93,* 358–364.

Woodmansee, W. W., Silbert, L. H., & Maier, S. F. (1993). Factors that modulate inescapable shock-induced reductions in daily activity in the rat. *Pharmacology, Biochemistry, and Behavior, 45,* 553–559.

Yirmiya, R. (1996a). Effects of antidepressant drugs on endotoxin and IL-1 induced sickness behavior. *International Society for Neuroimmodulation Abstracts,* 101.

Yirmiya, R. (1996b). Endotoxin produces a depressive-like episode in rats. *Brain Research, 711,* 163–174.

Zhou, D., Kusnecov, A. W., Shurin, M. R., DePaoli, M., & Rabin, B. S. (1993). Exposure to physical and psychological stressors elevates plasma interleukin 6: Relationship to the activation of hypothalamic-pituitary–adrenal axis. *Endocrinology, 133(6),* 2523–2530.

Zwilling, B. S. (1994). Neuroimmunomodulation of macrophage function. In R. Glaser & J. K. Kiecolt-Glaser (Eds.), *Handbook of human stress and immunity* (pp. 53–76). San Diego, CA: Academic Press.

Zwilling, B. S., Brown, D., Feng, N., Sheridan, J., & Pearl, D. (1993). The effect of adrenalectomy on the restraint stresses induced suppression of MHC Class II expression by murine peritoneal macrophages. *Brain, Behavior, and Immunity, 7,* 29–35.

Appendix: Sickness and the Acute-Phase Response

Physiological adjustments	Behavioral adjustments	Stress response
Fever	Reduced food and water intake	Increased sympathetic nervous system activity
Shift in liver metabolism	Reduced activity and exploration	Increased hypothalamo-pituitary-adrenal activity
Reduced albumin	Reduced social behavior, sexual behavior, and aggression	
Reduced carrier proteins	Increased pain sensitivity and reactivity	
Increased acute-phase proteins	Depressed mood	
Alterations in plasma iron, zinc, and copper	Cognitive alterations	
Leukocytosis (increased white cell count)		
Increased sleep		
Increased slow wave sleep		

VI SOCIAL INFLUENCES ON BIOLOGY AND HEALTH

B. Social Applications

i. Deleterious Influences

David A. Padgett, John F. Sheridan, Julianne Dorne, Gary G. Berntson, Jessica Candelora, and Ronald Glaser

There is compelling evidence that the nervous, endocrine, and immune systems communicate by means of a common biochemical language (1). The sharing of ligands (hormones, neurotransmitters, and cytokines) and their receptors constitute a biochemical information circuit between each of these systems to maintain physiological homeostasis (2). Good health, whether physical or psychological, is predicated on a highly integrated repertoire of defensive responses against external pathogens and stimuli that threaten homeostasis. Disruption of homeostasis, by engagement of either the immune, nervous, or endocrine systems by an external or internal stimulus, will alter the production of signaling molecules in one system, resulting in the modulation of the other systems.

When demands imposed by life events compromise an organism's ability to cope, a psychological stress response composed of negative cognitive and emotional states and associated physiological adjustments is elicited. It is now known that stressful life events can suppress several components of the immune response and that these effects are large enough to have biological and health consequences.

Data from studies with human subjects have been modeled using animals to explore the effects of stress on the immune system and the implications of these effects on the pathophysiology of infectious agents. These include studies in mice with influenza virus, herpes simplex virus type 1 (HSV-1), and *Mycobacterium tuberculosis* (3, 4). There are also a series of studies in rats that demonstrate that stress can modulate the metastatic spread of mammary tumor cells (5, 6). Because the immune system is modulated by nervous system/endocrine system interactions (1–2), it is probable that the ability of the immune system to defend against an external challenge is a homeostatic process regulated not only from within the immune system, but also modulated by the central nervous and endocrine systems (7, 8).

There are now several reports that support the hypothesis that the interactions among these physiological systems are influenced by psychological stress and that stress-associated immune modulation has implications for illness. The changes in the immune response that have been linked to psychological stress include innate immunity, e.g., natural killer cells, and specific T and B lymphocyte functions, including specific reactions against infectious agents (9–11). For example, it was shown that psychological stress can impact the appearance and severity of clinical symptoms of five different strains of cold viruses in a dose-response relationship (12). It also has been shown that stress can influence the virus-specific antibody and T cell responses to hepatitis B and influenza virus vaccines (13–15) and that stress can affect wound healing (16). Furthermore, there are studies that correlate reactivation of labial or ocular latent HSV infections after stressful life events (17–20). For example, Schmidt et al. (18) demonstrated that traumatic life experiences such as the death of a family member, the stress of interpersonal problems, or work-related difficulties were more common in individuals with frequent recurring oral HSV infection than in individuals with infrequent episodes. Similar relationships between psychological stress and reactivation of other herpesviruses, including Epstein–Barr virus and varicella zoster virus, also have been reported (21, 22).

Several animal models have been developed to study the pathogenic aspects of recurrent HSV-1-associated keratitis (23–27). A stable model of HSV-1 latency with an extremely low spontaneous reactivation rate has been established in mice (27). In these latently infected mice, UV irradiation alone, or in combination with ocular or systemic corticosteroid treatment, has been shown to result in the reactivation of latent HSV-1 and recurrent herpes keratitis with viral shedding in up to 80% of the animals (27). Although the resulting lesions appear similar to the disease state in humans, the mechanism of reactivation is not known. Immune suppression, perhaps in combination with the direct effect of one or more stress hormones (e.g., glucocorticoids), are theorized to be factors in recrudescence (17–19, 28). However, there are no reliable animal models in which a behavioral stressor has been shown to induce reactivation of latent HSV-1 that parallels the stress-associated reactivation of the virus that is clinically recognized in humans.

In previous work from our laboratory, we explored the relationship between stress-induced immune modulation, innate immunity, and the virus-specific T cell response to HSV-1 after a primary infection of the virus; we also studied the impact of stress on the virus-specific memory immune response (3, 9, 29). Restraint (RST)-stressed mice showed a depression in natural killer cell lysis and a decrease in the generation of virus-specific cytotoxic T lymphocytes to HSV-1 after primary infection; these stress-induced changes were accompanied by an increase in the replication of the virus (29). We now report on the development of a model to study the impact of psychological and social stress on the recrudescence of HSV-1.

Methods

Virus and Cells

In each experiment, HSV-1 McKrae strain (kindly provided by Jay Pepose, Washington University School of Medicine, St. Louis) was used for ocular infections. Virus stock was grown and assayed on VERO cells in modified Eagle's medium containing 10% fetal bovine serum and $4 \times$ penicillin/streptomycin. Material from eye swabs was similarly cultured on VERO cell

monolayers for determination of viral cytopathic effect. Cells were cultured at $36°C$ in a humidified incubator containing 5% CO_2.

Mice and Virus Infection

HSV-1 antibody-negative BALB/c male mice at 4–6 weeks of age were obtained from Charles River Breeding Laboratories and allowed to acclimate to their surroundings for 7–10 days before initiation of any experimental procedures. BALB/c mice were chosen because of their susceptibility to reactivation of latent HSV-1. All mice were housed five per cage and provided free access to food and water. The American Association for the Accreditation of Laboratory Animal Care-accredited facility was maintained on a 12-hr light/dark cycle (lights on at 6 A.M.). Before experimentation, the eyes of all mice were examined; only mice with no apparent abnormalities were included. Before infection, all mice were anesthetized with an intramuscular injection (0.1 ml) of 10% Rompun (Haver-Lockhart, Shawnee, KS) plus 10% Ketaset (Bristol Laboratories). The surface of the right cornea was scarified in a grid pattern with a 25-gauge needle. A 5:1 drop of DMEM media containing 10^6 plaque-forming units of HSV-1 McKrae strain was placed on the scarified cornea. At the time of infection, 0.5 ml of pooled human serum containing antibodies to HSV-1 (effective dose for 100% viral neutralization, of a 1:320 dilution) was injected i.p. to limit the spread of virus in the nervous system during the acute phase of infection. On days 2, 3, 4, and 5 postinoculation, the eyes of infected mice were swabbed with type 1 sterile dacron swabs (Spectrum Laboratories, Houston) to detect infectious virus and confirm infection. The animals were left for 5 weeks to permit the virus to establish latency.

UV Sources and Irradiation Procedure

To irradiate the animals, mice were anesthetized as described above and placed on a UV light source. To ensure that only the infected eye was exposed during the irradiation procedure, a shield with an eye hole was placed between the mouse and the UV source. Mice received a total UV dosage of 250–260 mJ/cm (2).

RST Stress Paradigm

After viral latency had been established (4–5 weeks postinfection), mice were RST-stressed by being placed in well-ventilated 50-ml centrifuge tubes for 16 hr each day, beginning 3 days before irradiation (or mock irradiation) and RST-stressed for an additional 5 days (3, 4). Each day, individual mice were placed in tubes at 5 P.M. (lights out at 6 P.M.) and removed at 9 A.M. (lights on at 6 A.M.). Control mice were deprived of food and water during the same time period; however, they were free to move about in their cages.

Social Reorganization Paradigm

After their acclimation period, "aggressor" mice were identified in each cage by using behavioral observations (30, 31). All observations were made during 15-min periods in the dark phase. Each group was observed for 3×15-min periods at arbitrary intervals during a 3-hr period. During observation, the number of social investigatory (sniffing), aggressive (chase, bite, tail-rattle, allogroom, and aggressive upright and aggressive sideways postures) and defensive (flee and submissive upright or sideways postures) behaviors were assessed for each individual animal. In addition, a fur score was assigned ranging from 1 (no bald, damaged, or disheveled patches, fur well groomed) to 5 (reflecting increasing incidence of damage to, or deterioration in, the apparent condition of the fur). Individuals within groups were ranked according to the ratio of the number of investigatory/aggressive interactions initiated and the number of defensive interactions (31). Top-ranked aggressor males had the highest attack ratio. Subsequently, for social reorganization, aggressor mice were switched between cages at the beginning of the 12-hr dark cycle (6 P.M.). Social reorganization was performed every second day for four cycles.

Determination of Serum Corticosterone Levels

To guard against fluctuations in serum corticosterone levels caused by circadian rhythm, blood samples were obtained at 10 A.M. each day of assessment. Mice were briefly restrained (less than 2 min) in polystyrene tubes, and blood was taken from the tail vein. Sera was stored at $-70°C$ until assayed for corticosterone by RIA. [^{125}I]Corticosterone kits for rats and mice (ICN) were used to determine serum corticosterone levels. Levels were determined from individual mice by using a standard curve and expressed in ng/ml.

Detection of Viral Shedding

To detect infectious virus at the ocular surface, the cornea was swabbed with a sterile dacron swab soaked in 0.5 ml of DMEM. Swab material was plated on confluent monolayers of VERO cells in 24-well tissue culture plates. If infectious virus was present on the ocular surface, visible cytopathic effect was noted in the VERO cultures within 2–5 days.

Results

The Influence of RST Stress on HSV-1 Reactivation

In a series of studies from our laboratory, we demonstrated the impact of RST stress on HSV-1-specific primary and memory immune responses as discussed above (3, 9, 29). Applying this approach to reactivation of latent HSV-1, we used a well-defined model for latent ocular herpesvirus infection (27). Male BALB/c mice were inoculated with HSV-1 by corneal scarification to establish a latent infection in the trigeminal and superior cervical ganglia.

Before our attempts at modulating reactivation of latent HSV-1, it was important to first establish that the expression of the latent HSV-1 genome was sufficiently repressed to rule out that recovery of infectious virus in a stress protocol was not caused by spontaneous reactivation. Sixteen male 5- to 6-week-old BALB/c mice were infected with HSV-1 as described; all mice showed evidence of being infected with HSV-1. Eye swabs were taken and assayed for infectious virus once per week for 3 weeks starting 5–6 weeks postinfection. None of the mice (0/16) showed evidence of spontaneous reactivation of latent HSV-1.

Eight consecutive daily 16-hr cycles of RST stress then were used to activate the hypothalamic-pituitary-adrenal (HPA) axis. Evidence for reactivation of the virus was characterized by the presence of infectious virus shed in the area of the eye. RST-stressed mice were compared with the home-caged control animals as well as a group of animals that were exposed to UV irradiation to induce reactivation of the latent virus.

As shown in Fig. 75.1, RST-stressed mice showed a significant rise in serum corticosterone induced as a result of the activation of the HPA axis by the stressor. After six cycles of RST, corticosterone levels among RST-stressed BALB/c mice increased greater than 5-fold (222.9 ± 29.8 ng/ml) as compared with control animals, (48.8 ± 7.3 ng/ml) (Fig. 75.1). None of the animals in the home-cage controls showed evidence for viral shedding or eye lesions over a 10-day period, 4–5 weeks after latency was established (Table 75.1). Seven of 16 mice in the UV-irradiated group in experiment 1 and five of 10 mice in experiment 2 (total 46.2%) demonstrated reactivation of latent HSV-1 as measured by the presence of infectious virus [compared with controls, χ^2 (df $= 1, n = 16$) $= 8.96$, $P < 0.005$]. The reactivation of latent HSV-1 was only 8% in the RST-stressed mice. Further, the use of RST did not increase reactivation within the UV-irradiated group as compared with the UV-

irradiated alone group (Table 75.1). We conclude that RST stress can activate the HPA axis and down-regulate the HSV-1-specific immune response to primary infection (and memory response) (3, 9, 29), but does not induce (significantly) the necessary physiological pathway(s) to reactivate latent HSV-1.

The Effect of a Social Stressor on the Reactivation of HSV-1

Additional groups of latently infected mice were stressed by using an established protocol that results in social stress. Established social hierarchies were disrupted by moving dominant animals from one cage to another. This disruption resulted in increased investigative, offensive, and defensive behaviors. The next morning, at 10 A.M., serum corticosterone levels were measured by RIA. Corticosterone levels among reorganized mice increased almost 2-fold (89.6 ± 25.1 ng/ml) as compared with control animals (46.3 ± 6.4 ng/ml) (Fig. 75.2). Subsequent social reorganization events resulted in further increases in serum corticosterone to 195.8 ± 34.8 ng/ml after four cycles of reorganization (Fig. 75.2).

Mice in the home-cage control groups showed no signs of viral shedding over a 10-day period, 4–5 weeks after latency was established, confirming the data obtained in the previous two studies. Seven of 16 mice in two separate experiments (43.7%) in the groups that were exposed to UV radiation alone showed evidence of shedding of infectious HSV-1 (Table 75.2). Animals that were in the social reorganization group showed evidence of reactivation of latent HSV-1 by the presence of infectious virus in eye swabs in 15 of 37 animals (41.7%) [compared with controls, χ^2 (df $= 1, n = 16$) $= 9.05$, $P < 0.003$] in three separate experiments. Animals that were both UV-irradiated and socially reorganized showed viral shedding in 21 of 37 animals (56.7%). Seven of 16 (43.7%) mice exposed to UV irradiation alone showed reactivation of HSV-1. The data show that social reorganization stress activated

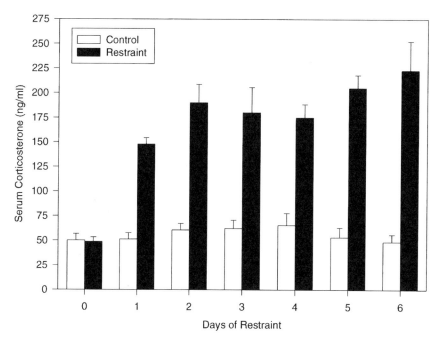

Figure 75.1
Influence of RST stress on serum corticosterone levels. Data represent 10 A.M. serum corticosterone as measured by RIA. Baseline samples were obtained 2 days before initiation of any experimental manipulations. Mice were restrained for 16 hr on sequential evenings. Control mice were deprived of food and water for the same period of time. $n = 5$ animals per group at each time point.

Table 75.1
Influence of RST stress on ocular HSV-1 reactivation

Treatment group	Experiment 1	Experiment 2	Total
Control	0/16	0/10	0/26 (0%)
UV (250 mJ/cm^2)	7/16	5/10	12/26 (46.2%)
RST	1/15	1/10	2/25 (8%)
RST + UV	6/15	7/15	13/30 (43.3%)

Data are represented as the number of mice positive for replicating virus in eye swabs within 10 days of reactivation per the total numbers of animals within that group.

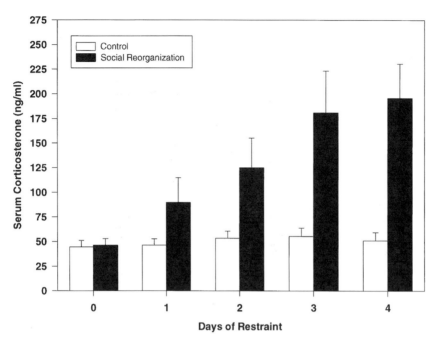

Figure 75.2
Influence of social reorganization on serum corticosterone. Data represent 10 A.M. serum corticosterone as measured by RIA. Baseline samples were obtained 2 days before initiation of any experimental manipulations. For social reorganization, dominant animals were identified and placed in new cages at 6 P.M. the evening before blood sampling. $n = 5$ animals per group at each time point.

Table 75.2
Influence of social reorganization on ocular HSV-1 reactivation

Treatment group	Experiment 1	Experiment 2	Experiment 3	Total
Control	NA	0/7	0/8	0/15 (0%)
UV (250 mJ/cm^2)	NA	4/8	3/8	7/16 (43.7%)
Social reorganization	6/17	5/10	4/10	15/37 (40.5%)
Social reorganization + UV	9/18	6/9	6/10	21/37 (56.75)

Data are represented as the number of mice positive for replicating virus in eye swabs within 10 days of reactivation per the total number of animals within that group. NA = not available.

the HPA axis, raised serum corticosterone levels comparable to levels observed in RST-stressed mice, and reactivated latent HSV-1 in a significant number of mice.

Social Dominance and HSV-1 Reactivation

During social reorganization in mice, three basic forms of behavior were observed: offensive, defensive, and submissive. Offensive behaviors consisted of physical assaults of one animal on another. Defensive behaviors consisted of actual attacks, but more often took the form of threats (postures, gestures) that warned an adversary to leave or become the target of an attack. Alternatively, the threatened or attacked animal might show submissive behavior that indicated that it would not challenge the other animal. Dominant animals were more likely to be involved in confrontations among cohorts, and it was often dominant individuals that experienced aggression and the greatest risk of injury, at least while maintaining their dominant status. Therefore, if the social environment and the behavioral interactions that establish a social hierarchy are sources of stress, animals involved in the most numerous and severe interactions may be the ones most affected by the detrimental influences of those social interactions.

In this experiment we determined whether the benefits of dominance (e.g., access to food, reproduction, shelter) were offset by the increase in stressful social interactions. After identifying the dominant mouse in each group over the course of the experiment, we determined the frequency of reactivation of latent HSV-1. As shown in Table 75.3, we found that the dominant mouse in each stressed group was more likely than subordinate mice to show signs of HSV-1 reactivation as measured by the ability to isolate infectious HSV-1 from the eye. These preliminary data suggest that increased social conflict leads to a greater chance of reactivation of latent HSV-1 in the animals involved in the greatest

Table 75.3

Influence of dominance and social stress on ocular HSV-1 reactivation

Treatment group	Subordinate	Dominant
Social reorganization	9/30 (30%)	6/7 (85.7%)
Social reorganization +UV	13/29 (44.9%)	8/8 (100%)

Data are represented as the number of mice positive for replicating virus in eye swabs within 10 days of reactivation per the total numbers of animals within that group.

number of potentially dangerous social interactions, i.e., the dominant mouse.

Discussion

In this study, we demonstrated that the use of an ocular model of HSV-1 latency enabled the establishment of a latent infection within a month after inoculation of HSV-1. Expression of the latent HSV-1 genome was restricted because we found no evidence of spontaneous reactivation of the latent virus. We confirm a previous report (27) that the exposure of the eyes of the mice latently infected with HSV-1 to UV irradiation results in reactivation of latent HSV-1. There was little evidence for reactivation of latent HSV-1 in animals that were RST-stressed, even in the presence of high serum levels of corticosterone. One putative link for stress effects on immune function and virus reactivation is glucocorticoid hormones (3, 28). These levels are high enough to result in the down-regulation of the immune response, including the specific immune response to HSV-1, and to enhance the pathophysiology of an HSV-1 infection (3, 9, 29). However, mice whose hierarchy and social interactions were disrupted showed significant evidence of reactivation of latent HSV-1.

The impact of psychological stress on immune function is well documented in the literature. The data support the hypothesis that both physical and psychological stressors can impact the pathophysiology of disease (3–6, 9–22). With the significant progress in the field of psychoneuroimmunology because of recent advances in molecular biology, immunology, neuroendocrinology, and psychophysiology, researchers are getting a better understanding of the underlying molecular mechanisms of altered disease susceptibility that result from stress-induced changes in the immune response. We believe that the social stress model described in this chapter may provide an approach to study and delineate the mechanisms that underlie the neuroendocrine influence of stress and HPA activation on HSV-1 reactivation. As with all animal models, it may not be possible to directly relate our results to stress-induced reactivation of latent herpesviruses like HSV-1 to humans. However, it is possible that the basic underlying mechanisms may be applicable to humans who are latently infected with HSV-1.

In sum, it has been shown that social stress has the ability to modulate the reactivation/replication of latent herpesviruses. Activation of the HPA axis by stress results in increases in corticosterone. However, the data show that corticosterone is itself insufficient to reactivate latent HSV-1 as the high levels of serum corticosterone induced by RST stress did not lead to viral shedding. Different stressors can lead to distinct neuroendocrine, neurobehavioral, and neuroimmunological consequences, and the data show that social stress is unique in activating systems involved in reactivating latent HSV-1. Although the present study does not define the underlying link, it offers important directions for further investigations of those mechanisms. For example, stress also activates the sympathetic nervous system with the subsequent release of catecholamines into the circulation and into innervated tissue (32, 33). The mechanism(s) underlying the interactions among products of the nervous, endocrine, and immune systems are complex and not completely understood. How-

ever, it is possible that under certain circumstances, the individual products may not be sufficient to modulate the expression of a latent virus, but that in combination, they may act synergistically to alter the control of the restriction of the endogenous latent virus genome and/or its replication after reactivation. The use of social stress to model reactivation of latent HSV-1 provides an experimental model that will allow us to explore the complex relationships among behavior, stress-associated immune modulation, and the reactivation of latent herpesviruses.

Acknowledgments

We thank Marco Vasquez for excellent technical assistance. This study was supported by the Gilbert and Kathryn Mitchell Endowment, Ohio State University Comprehensive Cancer Center Core Grant CA16058 (R.G.), and grants from the National Institute of Mental Health (MH46801) to J.F.S. and the MacArthur Foundation Mind-Body Network (J.F.S. and D.A.P.).

References

1. Blalock, J. E. (1984) *J. Immunol.* 132, 1067–1070.

2. Chrousos, G. P. & Gold, P. W. (1992) *J. Am. Med. Assoc.* 267, 1244–1252.

3. Bonneau, R. H., Sheridan, J. F., Feng, N. & Glaser, R. (1993) *J. Neuroimmunol.* 42, 167–176.

4. Brown, D. H., Sheridan, J., Pearl, D. & Zwilling, B. S. (1993) *Infect. Immun.* 61, 4793–4800.

5. Stefanski, V. & Ben-Eliyahu, S. (1996) *Physiol. Behav.* 60, 277–282.

6. Ben-Eliyahu, S., Yirmiya, R., Liebeskind, J. C., Taylor, A. N. & Gale, R. P. (1991) *Brain Behav. Immun.* 5, 193–205.

7. Sterling, P. & Eyer, J. (1988) in *Handbook of Life Stress, Cognition, and Health,* eds. Fisher, S. & Reason, J. (Wiley, New York), pp. 629–649.

8. McEwen, B. S. & Stellar, E. (1993) *Arch. Intern. Med. (Moscow)* 153, 2093–2101.

9. Bonneau, R. H., Sheridan, J. F., Feng, N. & Glaser, R. (1991) *Brain Behav. Immun.* 5, 274–295.

10. Sheridan, J. F., Feng, N., Bonneau, R. H., Allen, C. M., Hunnicutt, B. S. & Glaser, R. (1992) *J. Neuroimmunol.* 47, 83–94.

11. Hermann, G., Tovar, C. A., Beck, F. M., Allen, C. & Sheridan, J. F. (1993) *J. Neuroimmunol.* 47, 83–94.

12. Cohen, S., Tyrrell, D. A. & Smith, A. P. (1991) *N. Engl. J. Med.* 325, 606–612.

13. Glaser, R., Kiecolt-Glaser, J. K., Bonneau, R., Malarkey, W., Kennedy, S. & Hughes, J. (1992) *Psychosom. Med.* 54, 22–29.

14. Jabaaij, L., van-Hattum, J., Vingerhoets, J. J., Oostveen, F. G., Duivenvoorden, H. J. & Ballieux, R. E. (1996) *J. Psychosom. Res.* 41, 129–137.

15. Kiecolt-Glaser, J. K., Glaser, R., Gravenstein, S., Malarkey, W. B. & Sheridan, J. (1996) *Proc. Natl. Acad. Sci. USA* 93, 3043–3047.

16. Kiecolt-Glaser, J. K., Marucha, P. T., Malarkey, W. B., Mercado, A. M. & Glaser, R. (1995) *Lancet* 346, 1194–1196.

17. Longo, D. & Koehn, K. (1993) *Int. J. Psychol. Med.* 23, 99–117.

18. Schmidt, D. D., Schmidt, P. M., Crabtree, B. F., Hyun, J., Anderson, P. & Smith, C. (1991) *Family Med.* 23, 594–599.

19. Silver, P. S., Auerbach, S. M., Vishniavsky, N. & Kaplowitz, L. G. (1986) *J. Psychosom. Res.* 30, 163–171.

20. Kemeny, M. E., Cohen, F., Zegans, L. A. & Conant, M. A. (1989) *Psychosom. Med.* 51, 195–208.

21. Glaser, R., Rice, J., Sheridan, J., Fertel, R., Stout, J., Speicher, C. E., Pinsky, D., Kotur, M., Post, A., Beck, M. & Kiecolt-Glaser, J. K. (1987) *Brain Behav. Immun.* 1, 7–20.

22. Schmader, K., Studenski, S., MacMillan, J., Grufferman, S. & Cohen, H. J. (1990) *J. Am. Geriatr. Soc.* 38, 1188–1194.

23. Beyer, C. F., Hill, J. M., Reidy, J. J. & Beuerman, R. W. (1990) *Invest. Ophthalmol. Visual Sci.* 31, 925–932.

24. Shimeld, C., Hill, T. J., Blyth, W. A. & Easty, D. L. (1990) *J. Gen. Virol.* 71, 681–687.

25. Gordon, J. Y., Romanowski, E. & Araullo-Cruz, T. (1990) *Invest. Ophthalmol. Visual Sci.* 31, 921–924.

26. Stanberry, L. R. (1989) *J. Med. Virol.* 28, 125–128.

27. Laycock, R. A., Lee, S. F., Brady, R. H. & Pepose, J. S. (1991) *Invest. Ophthalmol. Visual Sci.* 32, 2741–2746.

28. Glaser, R., Kutz, L. A., MacCallum, R. C. & Malarkey, W. B. (1995) *Neuroendocrinology* 62, 356–361.

29. Bonneau, R. H., Sheridan, J. F., Feng, N. G. & Glaser, R. (1991) *Brain Behav. Immun.* 5, 170–192.

30. Adams, H. E. (1986) in *Handbook of Behavioral Assessment,* eds. Ciminero, A. R., Calhoun, K. S. & Adams, H. E. (Wiley, New York), pp. 496–525.

31. Barnard, C. J., Behnke, J. M. & Sewell, J. (1993) *Parasitology* 107, 183–192.

32. Madden, K. S. & Livnat, S. (1991) in *Psychoneuroimmunology,* eds., Ader, R., Felten, D. L. & Cohen, N. (Academic, New York), 2nd Ed., pp. 283–310.

33. Kvetnansky, R., Fukuhara, K., Pacak, K., Cizza, G., Goldstein, D. S. & Kopin, I. J. (1993) *Endocrinology* 133, 1411–1419.

76 Hostile Attitudes Predict Elevated Vascular Resistance during Interpersonal Stress in Men and Women

Mary C. Davis, Karen A. Matthews, and Claire E. McGrath

Introduction

Over the past two decades, accumulating evidence has pointed to the role of dispositional hostility as an independent and robust risk factor for CHD (see Ref. 1 for a review). Available data suggest that scores generated from one measure of the cynical outlook associated with hostility, the Cook-Medley Hostility Scale (2), predict CHD incidence and severity (3–7). Several potential mechanisms have been proposed to explain the association between hostility and CHD, including physiological responsivity to environmental stress. This model draws on data implicating exaggerated or prolonged sympathetic nervous system responses to behavioral challenge in the initiation and progression of CHD and in the precipitation of acute coronary events in individuals with underlying atherosclerosis (8). Thus, a propensity of hostile individuals to respond to stress with pronounced neuroendocrine and/or cardiovascular elevations might account in part for their greater risk for CHD relative to their nonhostile counterparts.

Numerous empirical reports have documented that cynical hostility is positively related to heightened BP adjustments to behavioral challenge (e.g., Refs. 9–11). However, hostile individuals are not overly reactive to all types of events; rather, they seem especially responsive to social situations (see Ref. 11 for a review). The types of social stressors selected for study have varied to some degree, but the majority have included anger provocation, often involving overt harassment of the participant by a stranger. The provocation typically elicits increased negative affect in both hostile and nonhostile individuals but heightened BP reactivity only in those who are hostile. This pattern of findings has held for both men (9, 10, 12) and women (12–14). In addition, high hostile men exhibit decreased forearm vascular resistance and increased blood flow in response to harassment (see Refs. 9 and 10; cf. Ref. 15), a pattern suggesting that heightened myocardial responsivity accounts for the BP elevations.

Less empirical attention has been directed toward understanding the relationship between hostility and cardiovascular arousal in stressful social contexts that are not deliberately provocative. Examining the physiological responses of hostile individuals to situations other than harassment is important because the majority of daily experiences are not marked by deliberate provocation, even among those who are hostile (e.g., Ref. 16). In that regard, Smith et al. have demonstrated that hostility is related to elevated BP responses in men when they engage in conflictual role playing (17), arguing from an assigned position (18), and self-disclosure of personal information to a confederate (19). Because the strongest and most consistent physiological correlate of hostility was DBP, with no HR effects (17, 19), the authors postulated that the enhanced BP increases were attributable to increased peripheral resistance (19). Indeed, subsequent work demonstrated that men high in hostility who also reported that they expressed their anger outwardly tended to show smaller CO increases and larger TPR increases to a public speaking task than did their low hostile counterparts, with no differences based on hostility among men who did not express their anger outwardly or during an asocial task (20).

Thus, the limited data available suggest that hostile individuals respond to social stressors with enhanced BP responses, but the hemodynamic response patterns underlying BP elevations may depend on the presence of provocation. Anger-provoking interactions seem to enhance myocardial activity, whereas more ambiguous social interactions seem to enhance vascular responding. Williams et al. (21) were among the first to suggest that perception of the demands of the task is a key determinant of physiological response patterns and also proposed that two qualitatively distinct response patterns are evident. The defense or "fight/flight" response is characterized by enhanced CO and occurs when an individual senses danger or the need for continuing mental effort, conditions likely to exist in social situations involving harassment. The vigilance response, on the other hand, is characterized by increased peripheral vasoconstriction and occurs when an individual feels uncertain and needs to be watchful of the environment, conditions likely to exist in ambiguous social interactions.

The literature is limited in at least three respects. First, the majority of investigations have included only measures of BP and HR in the study of ambiguous social contact. As a result, little is known about the hemodynamic response patterns underlying the stress-related BP increases among high and low hostile individuals during social stress that lacks deliberate provocation. A second concern is that the majority of research exploring the association between hostility and reactivity is based on male samples. Among the exceptions to this trend are two studies reporting that high hostile women showed greater BP increases during stress than low hostile women (13, 14). Several additional investigations have included both men and women, which permits evaluation of the extent to which the association between hostility and reactivity varies by sex. The results yielded by these studies have been inconsistent. Some suggest that hostility is associated with enhanced BP stress responses in both sexes (22, 23), in men but not women (12, 24, 25) or in neither sex (26, 27). Of note, no investigation has reported that the effects of hostility are more pronounced in women than in men. More comprehensive assessment of cardiovascular reactivity, including measures of TPR and CO, in a sample that includes both sexes would permit determination of the nature and extent of sex differences in the hostility-reactivity association. Finally, some

findings point to the likely importance of task perception and affective arousal as determinants of the association between hostility and physiological responses to mild social stress (e.g., Ref. 19), but these data are few and were obtained primarily from men.

The primary purpose of the present investigation was to examine the association between hostility and hemodynamic patterns underlying BP increases during a social stressor without deliberate anger provocation. Consistent with the only other investigation examining hemodynamic responses to social stress in a nonprovocative context (20), we hypothesized that individuals high in hostility would exhibit more marked increases in TPR and smaller increases in CO in response to the stress relative to low hostile individuals. In addition, we tested whether the relationship between hostility and physiological responses to interpersonal stress were similar for women and men. Finally, we explored the association between affective arousal and task perception, and hemodynamic response patterns.

Methods

Participants

Data for the current study were derived from a project that was designed to examine gender-relevant stress and reactivity (28). Forty-two male and 42 female white undergraduates, ranging in age from 18 to 30 years (mean = 19.9 years, SD = 2.86 years), participated for course credit or $10. Participants completed questionnaires during a screening session to determine that they met the following eligibility criteria: (a) in good health; (b) free from use of medication (including oral contraceptives); (c) <20% overweight according to Metropolitan Life tables; (d) non-smoking; and (e) for females, regular menstrual cycles during the previous 3 months. To be eligible for participation in the original study, individuals also had to endorse primarily either instrumental or expressive gender role attributes, based on scores derived from the Personality Attributes Questionnaire (29). Instrumental attributes include competitiveness and dominance, whereas expressive attributes include attunement to others and empathy. For the present investigation, individuals were categorized as high or low hostile based on sex-specific median splits of scores on the Cook-Medley Hostility Scale.[1]

Data from two female participants were discarded before analyses, one because of equipment failure and the second because of a marked cardiac arrhythmia that distorted the impedance waveform. Additionally, two male subjects did not complete the hostility measure. Therefore, statistical analyses were based on data from 20 participants in each sex by hostility group.

Psychological Measures

Hostility

The Cook-Medley Hostility Scale (2) consists of 50 items that assess suspiciousness, resentment, and cynical mistrust. Each item is rated on a four-point scale (from "strongly agree" $= 4$ to "strongly disagree" $= 1$), resulting in a possible range of scores from 50 to 200. Scores on this measure (Ho scores) were normally distributed and were similar for males (mean $= 118.4$, SD $= 14.0$) and females (mean $= 115.3$, SD $= 16.2$) ($t(78) = 0.90$, $p = .37$). These values are akin to those reported in other studies of college undergraduates (e.g., Ref. 23). Individuals were identified as high or low hostile by median splits, performed separately for men and women to maintain equal cell size. A 2×2 (sex by hostility group) analysis of variance did not yield a significant sex by hostility group interaction, indicating that males and females within each hostility group had similar Ho scores.

Affect and task perception

A questionnaire completed immediately after the baseline rest period and again after the task asked participants to indicate the extent to which they felt anxious or angry. The questionnaire comprised three items assessing anger and four items assessing anxiety, each rated on a four-point scale (ranging from "not at all" $= 1$ to "very much so" $= 4$). Both the anger and anxiety items were internally consistent (Cronbach's α values $= 0.74$) and were summed to yield separate scores for anger and anxiety at both baseline and immediately after task completion.

After the task, participants completed a questionnaire assessing their perception of the task and of their own performance. Items were rated on a five-point scale (ranging from "not at all" $= 1$ to "very much so" $= 5$). Three items were summed to yield a score labeled "effort," which reflected the extent to which participants reported that they tried hard and found the task difficult and challenging (Cronbach's $\alpha = 0.61$). An additional six items assessing the extent to which participants felt the task required them to be persuasive, competitive, dominant, and aggressive and to show a lack of both attunement and understanding were summed to generate a score termed "interpersonal control" (Cronbach's $\alpha = 0.87$).

Procedure

To determine eligibility, individuals attended a screening session during which they provided information regarding their health and completed psychological measures, including the Cook-Medley Hostility Scale. They were subsequently contacted by telephone, told that they were being recruited to participate in a study examining heart functioning during speaking, and scheduled for a laboratory session. Participants were instructed to abstain from caffeine and exercise for 15 hours, and from medication and alcohol for 3 days, before their sessions. Female participants were scheduled to participate during the follicular phase of their menstrual cycles, between days 4 and 11, to control for the effects of menstrual cycle phase on hemodynamic stress responses (30).

When participants arrived for a session, they found a same-sex confederate sitting quietly in a reception area. A female experimenter escorted the participant to the laboratory, briefly described the protocol, and obtained written informed consent. All participants were told that the confederate was undergoing an identical procedure in an adjacent laboratory. HR and impedance electrodes were positioned, a BP cuff was placed on the nondominant arm, and the participant was seated in a comfortable chair.

Physiological measures began with a 10-minute baseline period, during which participants relaxed while sitting quietly. After the prestress baseline period, participants completed the mood questionnaire and then were instructed that they would engage for 6 minutes in a videotaped discussion with the confederate regarding capital punishment. Participants were told that they were matched with the confederate because they held opposite positions on this topic and were randomly assigned either to persuade the confederate that their own view was correct or to empathize with the confederate's view of capital punishment.

Participants were told that their effectiveness would be evaluated immediately after the task by the confederate and later by raters watching the videotape. They were instructed that the confederate knew he or she would be engaging in a discussion about capital punishment with another individual but did not know the purpose of the task. Confederates were trained to maintain a neutral tone and demeanor throughout the discussion while establishing a position on capital punishment opposite of the position held by the participant. They were explicitly instructed to avoid provoking the participant and to respond to comments made by the participant with calmly delivered statements regarding their own position. Confederates remained resolute in their position on capital punishment throughout the discussion.

After instructions were given to the participant, the confederate was escorted into the experimental room wearing band electrodes. A BP cuff was placed on the confederate's arm, and bogus leads were attached to the electrodes. Directions regarding the discussion were given, and discussants were reminded that they would be videotaped for later evaluation. The task began with a 1.5-minute preparation period, during which the discussants were allowed to prepare for the subsequent discussion. After the preparation period, participants engaged in 4.5 minutes of structured talk with the confederate. The participant and confederate alternated speaking and listening for three 45-second periods, with participants initiating the discussion when signaled to begin the task. At the conclusion of the structured talk period, participants and confederates continued the discussion for 1.5 additional minutes with no constraints regarding taking turns.

After completing the discussion, the participant and the confederate filled out questionnaires regarding their mood and impressions of the task. The confederate was excused, and the participant relaxed for a final 10-minute period. After the rest period, the participant was debriefed, given a credit slip or $10, and excused.

Physiological Measures

SBP and DBP were measured with an IBS (model SD-700A) automated BP monitor using a standard inflatable BP cuff placed on the participant's nondominant arm. The IBS assesses BP using the auscultatory method and is equipped to detect artifact caused by movement or poor cuff placement and correlates highly ($r > 0.90$) with BP measured with a mercury sphygmomanometer. Impedance cardiography, performed with the Minnesota Impedance Cardiograph (model 304B) in conjunction with a tetrapolar configuration, was used to measure cardiac performance. Disposable Mylar band electrodes (M6001, Contact Products, Inc., Dallas, TX) were applied with one voltage electrode encircling the base of the neck and one encircling the thorax over the tip of the xiphisternal junction. One current electrode was placed around the neck and one was placed around the thorax, at a minimum distance of 3 cm above and below the upper and lower voltage electrodes, respectively.

HR was detected using silver or silver chloride electrodes placed on the right arm and abdomen below the impedance electrodes, and a ground electrode was placed beside the navel. The electrocardiogram and impedance cardiogram were processed by using the Cardiac Output Program, an online computerized system developed by Bio-Impedance Technology (distributed by Instrumentation for Medicine, Inc., Greenwich, CT). A continuous sample of impedance waveforms was processed to generate an ensemble-averaged cardiac cycle for each 60-second unit of interest during baseline and recovery periods and each 45-second unit of interest during the task periods. The impedance cardiogram was used to derive measures of CO and HR. TPR was calculated by the Cardiac Output Program from a formula adapted from Guyton (31):

$$TPR = \{[(SBP - DBP)/3] + DBP\}/Q \times 80$$

where TPR is total peripheral resistance (dynes–s $\cdot$ cm^{-5}) and Q is CO (liters/min).

Data Reduction

BP was monitored at minutes 5, 7, and 9 of the baseline and recovery periods, once during the 45-second preparation period, and once during each of the three 45-second speaking turns of the participant. During the task and rest periods throughout the session, HR and impedance measures were monitored continuously. Using the Cardiac Output Program ensemble averaging technique, HR and CO values were averaged across each of the last 5 minutes of the 10-minute baseline and recovery periods and across each

45-second period of each phase of the discussion task. The BP readings were matched with appropriate values for CO to derive estimates of TPR for the last 5 minutes of the baseline and recovery periods and during the discussion task. For the present study, we examined hemodynamic stress responses during the preparation and structured talk phases of the task, because these periods were highly similar across the persuasion and empathy task conditions. Furthermore, task condition was not included as a variable of interest in the current analyses.[2]

Data collected during the last 5 minutes of the baseline and recovery periods were used to compute prestress baseline and poststress recovery means, respectively, for each physiological variable. Mean values were computed for the task periods for each physiological variable by averaging values collected within the preparation and structured talk periods. Mean change from baseline during the task and recovery periods for all physiological measures were calculated by subtracting the mean level at prestress baseline from the mean level during the task and recovery periods (32).

Results

Baseline Cardiovascular Levels

Table 76.1 displays the baseline levels and unadjusted change scores during the task and recovery periods of each cardiovascular measure by hostility group. ANOVAs (2 × 2, hostility group by sex) conducted with baseline values as the dependent measure did not yield effects involving hostility for any variable. Sex differences in resting SBP were observed (sex main effect, $F(1, 76) = 28.13$, $p < .0001$), with men showing higher levels (mean = 114.64 mm Hg, SD = 8.64) than women (mean = 104.88 mm Hg, SD = 6.93). No other terms emerged for SBP, nor were there any significant findings for baseline levels of DBP, TPR, HR, or CO.

Table 76.1
Cardiovascular baseline levels and unadjusted change (SD) during task according to hostility group

Variable	Hostility group		Hostility effects[a] F
	Low ($N = 40$)	High ($N = 40$)	
SBP (mm Hg)			Hostility group $\times$ sex $\times$ trial, $F(2, 152) = 3.95^*$
Baseline	108.89 (9.86)	110.07 (8.16)	
ΔPreparation	16.93 (9.75)	17.88 (10.67)	
ΔTalk	28.37 (11.63)	28.02 (9.49)	
ΔRecovery	3.38 (5.00)	3.38 (5.10)	
DBP (mm Hg)			Hostility, $F(1, 75) = 6.81^{**}$
			Hostility group $\times$ trial, $F(2, 152) = 3.67^*$
Baseline	66.44 (8.09)	68.42 (8.48)	
ΔPreparation	6.23 (9.05)[A]	10.39 (9.30)[B]	
ΔTalk	14.44 (9.77)[A]	18.98 (10.49)[B]	
ΔRecovery	2.93 (3.67)	2.67 (5.21)	
HR (beats/min)			Hostility group $\times$ sex, $F(1, 75) = 7.68^{**}$
Baseline	72.02 (9.62)	72.57 (11.13)	
ΔPreparation	16.25 (10.71)	15.07 (11.44)	
ΔTalk	25.74 (11.37)	24.12 (12.60)	
ΔRecovery	1.97 (3.07)	3.02 (4.15)	
CO (liter/min)			Hostility group $\times$ trial, $F(2, 152) = 3.82^*$
Baseline	6.54 (1.19)	6.34 (1.11)	
ΔPreparation	1.62 (1.66)[A]	1.05 (1.13)[B]	
ΔTalk	1.87 (1.71)[A]	1.33 (1.21)[B]	
ΔRecovery	0.15 (0.39)	0.25 (0.45)	
TPR (dynes–s·cm^{-5})			Hostility group $\times$ trial, $F(2, 152) = 3.56^*$
Baseline	1028.15 (252.14)	1073.45 (211.86)	
ΔPreparation	−64.86 (213.44)[A]	9.43 (172.64)[B]	
ΔTalk	−7.43 (224.58)	49.69 (194.38)	
ΔRecovery	15.60 (84.64)	−3.97 (91.25)	

a. Different uppercase superscripts within a trial denote hostility group difference at $p < .05$. Baseline level was included as a covariate for SBP and DBP analyses.
* $p < .05$.
** $p < .01$.

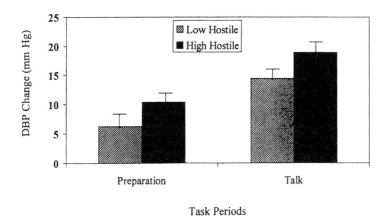

Figure 76.1
Unadjusted change in DBP (mm Hg) ± SEM during task preparation and talk periods as a function of hostility group.

Hostility and Sex Effects on Physiological Arousal

The primary analyses were $2 \times 2 \times 3$ (hostility group by sex by trial, i.e., preparation, talk or recovery) repeated-measures ANCOVAs, with physiological change scores serving as the dependent measures and baseline levels serving as the covariate. Huynh-Feldt corrections were applied to control for violation of the assumption of homogeneity of variance common in trial data. Comparison among means was accomplished with the Tukey honestly significant difference procedure (33), and a significance value of .05 was adopted unless otherwise noted.

Blood Pressure
Analyses for SBP, covarying baseline, revealed a significant sex by hostility group by trial interaction (see Table 76.1). Inspection of the adjusted means revealed that the hostility effects were apparent only among men during the talk period. High hostile men showed smaller increases in SBP during the talk period than did their low hostile counterparts (mean values = 26.50 vs.

32.72 mm Hg, respectively; $p < .05$) but showed comparable changes during the preparation (means = 19.93 vs. 18.84 mm Hg, respectively) and recovery periods (mean = 4.37 vs. 4.44 mm Hg, respectively; $p > .05$). In contrast, high and low hostile women showed comparable changes during the preparation period (mean = 16.76 vs. 14.20 mm Hg, respectively), talk period (mean = 29.35 vs. 24.52 mm Hg, respectively), and recovery period (mean = 2.44 vs. 2.27 mm Hg, respectively) ($p > .05$).

Hostility group also affected DBP stress responses. The analyses yielded a significant main effect for hostility and a significant hostility by trial interaction. Follow-up comparisons of adjusted means revealed that high hostile relative to low hostile individuals exhibited greater DBP increases during the preparation and talk periods ($p < .05$) but not the recovery period ($p > .05$) (see Table 76.1 and Figure 76.1). Additionally, as reported previously (28), results revealed a main effect for sex ($F(1, 75) = 5.62$, $p = .02$) and a significant sex by trial interaction ($F(2, 152) = 5.74$, $p = .004$). Examination of adjusted means indicated that DBP reactivity was more

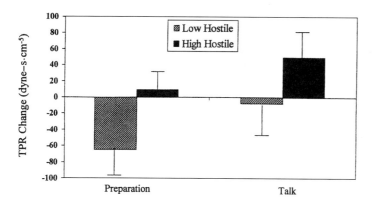

Figure 76.2

Unadjusted change in TPR (dynes–s · cm^{-5}) ± SEM during task preparation and talk periods as a function of hostility group.

pronounced in women relative to men during the preparation period (mean = 11.35 vs. 5.22 mm Hg, respectively; $p < .05$) but not during the talk (mean = 18.46 vs. 14.97 mm Hg, respectively) or recovery period (mean = 2.65 vs. 2.96 mm Hg, respectively) ($p > .05$).

Total Peripheral Resistance

As expected, the analyses for TPR yielded a significant hostility by trial interaction (see Table 76.1 and Figure 76.2). Follow-up analyses indicated that high hostile individuals showed enhanced TPR responses during the preparation period compared with low hostile individuals ($p < .05$), with no group differences evident during the talk or recovery periods ($p > .05$). Also apparent was a sex by trial interaction ($F(2, 152) = 6.00$, $p = .003$), which we noted in a prior report (28). Post hoc probing showed that TPR in women increased and in men decreased during the preparation (mean = 31.08 vs. −79.68 dynes–s · cm^{-5}, respectively; $p < .05$) and talk periods (mean = 61.76 vs. −19.92 dynes–s · cm^{-5}, respectively; $p < .05$), with no sex dif-

ference during recovery (mean = 0.36 vs. 7.80 dynes–s · cm^{-5}, respectively; $p > .05$).

Cardiac Output

CO change varied over the course of the session according to hostility group, reflected in a hostility by trial interaction (see Table 76.1 and Figure 76.3). Examination of mean adjusted changes indicated that low hostile individuals showed larger increases in CO during both the preparation and talk periods of the session than their high hostile counterparts ($p < .05$) but that groups did not differ during the recovery period ($p > .05$).

Heart Rate

Evaluation of HR changes indicated that HR increases during the session were moderated by both hostility group and sex, as indicated by a hostility by sex interaction (see Table 76.1). Follow-up analyses indicated that among men, high hostile individuals showed less marked HR increases than did low hostile individuals over the course of the session (mean = 21.29 vs. 30.36,

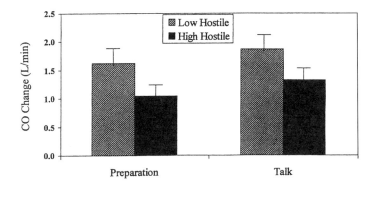

Figure 76.3
Unadjusted change in CO (liter/min) ± SEM during task preparation and talk periods as a function of hostility group.

respectively; $p < .05$). In contrast, high and low hostile women showed comparable changes in HR during the session (mean $= 27.60$ vs. 20.65 beats/min, respectively; $p > .05$).

No other effects involving sex or hostility emerged in the analyses.

Affect and Task Perception Measures

Sex by hostility ANOVAs of baseline anger and anxiety scores yielded no significant effects, indicating that groups reported low and comparable levels of anger and anxiety at rest. Anger and anxiety change scores served as dependent variables in subsequent 2×2 (sex by hostility) ANCOVAs, controlling for baseline anger or anxiety. Results yielded a significant interaction between sex and hostility for anxiety ($F(1, 75) = 5.43$, $p = .02$). Post hoc comparisons within each sex revealed only that hostile women tended to report greater increases in anxiety than did nonhostile women ($p < .07$), with no difference between hostile and nonhostile men. In the current study, the effect size reflecting pre- to posttask change in anger was approximately 0.33. In

contrast, studies comparing the anger levels of harassed vs. nonharassed groups yield much larger effect sizes, typically >1.0 (e.g., 14). The small anger effect that we observed, particularly when compared with those observed in studies of harassment, suggests that the interaction task did not elicit substantial anger in participants. With regard to task perception, sex by hostility ANOVAs of posttask scores yielded no main effects or interaction terms. Thus, the extent to which participants felt angry, effortful, and a need to exert interpersonal control over the interaction did not vary by sex or hostility group.

Internal Analyses

We were interested in evaluating whether task perception or affective arousal was associated with different response patterns in hostile and nonhostile individuals. Individuals were first categorized separately by hostility group as high or low in effort, need for interpersonal control, or change in negative affect based on median splits of these scores. Next, a series of $2 \times 2 \times 2 \times 2$ (sex by hostility group by perception group by trial, i.e., preparation or talk) repeated-measures ANOVAs was conducted, with TPR and CO change scores serving as dependent variables.

Task Perception

Analyses examining effort ratings yielded significant main effects of effort for both CO and TPR ($F(1, 72) > 4.83$, $p < .03$) and significant interactions between hostility and effort ($F(1, 72) > 5.76$, $p < .02$). Follow-up comparisons indicated that among low hostile individuals, those high in effort showed enhanced CO and dampened TPR responses during the task relative to those low in effort ($p < .05$). In contrast, effort ratings were unrelated to CO and TPR responses among high hostile individuals.

With regard to need for interpersonal control, findings revealed a significant interaction between hostility and control perception for TPR ($F(1, 72) = 4.94$, $p = .03$). Post hoc comparisons showed that among hostile individuals, those who perceived a high need to control the confederate exhibited greater TPR increases relative to those who perceived a low need for interpersonal control ($p < .05$). Among low hostile individuals, those high in control perception showed dampened TPR responses relative to those low in control perception ($p < .05$). No other main effects or interaction terms involving control perception emerged in the analyses.

Affective Arousal

None of the main effects or interaction terms involving anger or anxiety groups achieved significance, indicating that the relationships between affect arousal and CO and TPR responses were similar for high and low hostility groups.

Discussion

Only rarely in the course of daily life are we forced to confront misbehavior that is so flagrant as to be irrefutable. Rather, social dynamics are usually intricate, complex, and deeply nuanced.

Yet we know relatively little about how these more common and subtle interpersonal exchanges influence an individual's perception and physiological responding. In the present study, we examined the relationship between hostility and hemodynamic response patterns in the context of a subtle social challenge. Consistent with our expectations based on earlier work in men (20), high hostile individuals showed greater TPR and smaller CO responses than did low hostile individuals during a mild social stressor. Enhanced vascular responsivity among high hostile participants was evident not only during the actual discussion but also during the preparation period of the task, a finding that has two important implications. First, it suggests that hostile individuals were not more physiologically reactive simply because they behaved differently during the discussion. Second, it points to the likelihood that those characterized by high levels of mistrust and suspicion anticipate trouble in interpersonal situations, even before they have any overt indication that there is cause for alarm. In an ambiguous social interaction, then, hostile individuals were more likely to exhibit the vigilance response described by Williams et al. (21).

What can account for the heightened vascular stress responses of hostile relative to nonhostile individuals? Some investigators have posited that the relationship between hostility and reactivity is mediated by arousal of negative affect (10). For example, high levels of hostility are associated with more self-reported anger after conflictual social interactions (15) and frustrating cognitive tasks (22). Moreover, arousal of negative affect among hostile men (9, 10) and women (14) is positively related to BP and HR responses during harassment, a relationship that is not evident among low hostile individuals. However, in the current study and others including nonprovocative social stress (e.g., Refs. 17 and 19), hostile and nonhostile individuals generally reported comparable levels of low anger and moderate anxiety in response to the social task and showed comparable associations between physiological and affective arousal. Thus, negative affect arousal may be likely to account for the hostility-reactivity association only in social contexts involving extreme provocation.

The current findings suggest that in less provocative, more ambiguous social contexts, subtle perceptions of the situational demands may determine responsivity. Hostile and nonhostile participants perceived the interaction with an unchangeable confederate similarly in terms of the degree of effort and the amount of interpersonal control required to perform well. However, the associations between task perception and physiological responding varied by hostility level. Greater perceived effort was related to heightened myocardial responsivity in low hostile individuals, and a greater perceived need to control was related to heightened vascular responsivity in high hostile individuals. Stated differently, nonhostile individuals appear to be more physiologically responsive to effort perceptions, and hostile individuals to control perceptions, during mild interpersonal stress. Thus, hostile individuals did not exhibit a propensity to perceive that they needed to control the interaction but did show a propensity to respond to a control perception with heightened vascular responsivity relative to their nonhostile counterparts. Christensen and Smith (19) reported compatible findings in their study of self-disclosure in men. High and low hostile men did not differ in how open they intended to be with a confederate regarding a stressful event they had experienced; however, the association between intent to be open and BP reactivity was positive for high hostile and negative for low hostile men (19). Together, these findings suggest that even when high and low hostile individuals report that their perceptions of and intentions to behave in uncertain social circumstances are similar, their perceptions and intentions are differentially related to physiological responses. Future research that includes more detailed assessment and/or manipulation of participants' perception of social stressors and

evaluation of neuroendocrine parameters may elaborate the extent to which the processes linking perception and physiological reactivity vary by hostility.

The present findings also showed that hostility was related to stress-related changes in cardiovascular measures in both sexes. Hostility was associated with enhanced DBP in both men and women, consistent with earlier findings (e.g., Refs. 22 and 23). Moreover, hostile men and women showed elevated TPR and dampened CO changes underlying the BP increases relative to their nonhostile counterparts. To our knowledge, this is the first study to document that the hemodynamic responses underlying BP increases to social stress are generally comparable among hostile men and women.

Although some investigations have noted hostility effects in men but not women (e.g., Refs. 12, 24, and 25), no study that has included both sexes has reported that reactivity is enhanced among hostile women but not among hostile men. Together, the data in this literature point to the possibility that hostile women respond with exaggerated physiological reactivity to a narrower range of social stimuli than do hostile men. For example, hostile individuals of both sexes respond excessively to stressful interpersonal interactions with a stranger (e.g., Refs. 13 and 21), but only hostile men show enhanced responses to challenging discussions with their spouses (25). Thus, hostile women may make finer distinctions than do hostile men between the threats posed by stimulus situations, distinctions reflected in their more variable cardiovascular arousal. Recent data gleaned from ambulatory assessments point to this possibility. Hostility was associated with higher levels of DBP in men but not women when examining BP levels assessed throughout the entire work or school day (34, 35). However, hostility was related to elevations in SBP in *both* men and women during periods of social interaction (34). The possibility that the sexes differ in terms of the range of stimuli that elicits reactivity remains speculative, however, until additional research comparing response patterns in hostile men and women broadens to include a variety of social interactions with strangers, acquaintances, and familiar others.

Caution is warranted in interpreting the present findings, particularly with regard to generalizability. We examined a sample of white undergraduates who were originally recruited because they endorsed either an instrumental or expressive gender role orientation. Although instrumentality and expressivity scores in this sample were not extreme and were unrelated to hostility, the current results may not generalize to other ethnic, racial, age, or gender role groups. Additionally, because we included only a highly structured social interaction task involving a same-sex stranger in the laboratory, we cannot comment on the extent to which the patterns we observed are also apparent in routine daily interactions in naturalistic settings. Finally, our hypotheses regarding the impact of nonprovocative interpersonal stress on hemodynamic responses of hostile individuals were theoretically driven, but a stronger test of the hypotheses would have involved experimental manipulation of the social stressor. Still, the results of this study suggest that high levels of hostility are associated with enhanced vascular and dampened cardiac reactivity to nonprovocative social stress in both men and women and that experiencing a high need to control the interaction exacerbates the responding of hostile but not nonhostile individuals. The findings not only highlight the utility of social psychophysiological methods but also point to the need for further elaboration of the salient features of social context as a means of refining our understanding of the hostility-reactivity association.

Notes

1. To assure that hostility was not confounded with sex role attributes, we computed first-order correlations between instrumentality and communality scores from the Personality Attributes Questionnaire and Ho scores. In the sample as a whole, sex role attributes were unrelated to hostility (r values < 0.14, p values $> .21$). Moreover, categorization into instrumental and communal groups was unrelated to categorization into high and low hostility groups ($\chi^2(1) = 0.205$, $p = .66$). The same nonsignificant associations were apparent when these analyses were repeated separately by sex.

2. The persuasion and empathy versions of the task were included in the original study to examine gender-relevant stress. Approximately half of high and low hostile individuals participated in each task condition. However, because task condition was not expected to interact with hostility group to predict reactivity, and because individuals were not randomly assigned to task condition on the basis of hostility group, task condition was not evaluated in the primary analyses. When we repeated the analyses, including task condition as an independent variable, no effects involving condition emerged, and the pattern of findings reported remains intact.

References

1. Miller TQ, Smith TW, Turner CW, Guijarro ML, Hallet AJ. A meta-analytic review of research on hostility and physical health. Psychol Bull 1996; 119:322–48.

2. Cook WW, Medley DM. Proposed hostility and pharisaic-virtue scales for the MMPI. J Appl Psychol 1954; 38:414–8.

3. Dembroski TM, MacDougall JM, Costa PT, Grandits GA. Components of hostility as predictors of sudden death and myocardial infarction in the Multiple Risk Factor Intervention Trial. Psychosom Med 1989; 51:514–22.

4. Dembroski TM, MacDougall JM, Williams RB, Haney TL, Blumenthal J. Components of type A, hostility, and anger-in: relationship to angiographic findings. Psychosom Med 1985; 47:219–33.

5. Hecker MHL, Chesney MA, Black GW, Frautschi N. Coronary-prone behaviors in the Western Collaborative Group Study. Psychosom Med 1988; 50:153–64.

6. Matthews KA, Glass DC, Rosenman RH, Bortner RW. Competitive drive, pattern A, and coronary heart disease: a further analysis of some data from the Western Collaborative Group Study. J Chronic Dis 1977; 30:489–98.

7. Shekelle RB, Gale M, Ostfeld AM, Paul O. Hostility, risk of coronary heart disease, and mortality. Psychosom Med 1983; 45:109–14.

8. Krantz DS, Manuck SB. Acute psychophysiologic reactivity and risk of cardiovascular disease: a review and methodological critique. Psychol Bull 1984; 96:535–64.

9. Suarez EC, Williams RB. The relationships between dimensions of hostility and cardiovascular reactivity as a function of task characteristics. Psychosom Med 1990; 52:558–70.

10. Suarez EC, Kuhn CM, Schanberg SM, Williams RB, Zimmerman EA. Neuroendocrine, cardiovascular, and emotional responses of hostile men: the role of interpersonal challenge. Psychosom Med 1998; 60:78–88.

11. Suls J, Wan CK. The relationship between trait hostility and cardiovascular reactivity: a quantitative review and analysis. Psychophysiology 1993; 30:615–26.

12. Lawler KA, Harralson TL, Armstead CA, Schmied LA. Gender and cardiovascular responses: what is the role of hostility? J Psychosom Res 1993; 37:603–13.

13. Powch IG, Houston BK. Hostility, anger-in, and cardiovascular reactivity in white women. Health Psychol 1996; 15:200–8.

14. Suarez EC, Harlan E, Peoples MC, Williams RB. Cardiovascular and emotional responses in women: the role of hostility and harassment. Health Psychol 1993; 12:459–68.

15. Miller SB, Dolgoy L, Friese M, Sita A. Parental history of hypertension and hostility: moderate cardiovascular responses to interpersonal conflict. Int J Psychophysiol 1998; 28:193–206.

16. Raikkonen K, Matthews KA, Flory JD, Owens JF. Effects of hostility on ambulatory blood pressure and mood during daily living in healthy adults. Health Psychol 1999; 18:44–53.

17. Hardy JD, Smith TW. Cynical hostility and vulnerability to disease: social support, life stress, and physiological response to conflict. Health Psychol 1988; 7:447–59.

18. Smith TW, Allred KD. Blood-pressure responses during social interaction in high- and low-cynically hostile males. J Behav Med 1989; 12:135–43.

19. Christensen AJ, Smith TW. Cynical hostility and cardiovascular reactivity during self-disclosure. Psychosom Med 1993; 55:193–202.

20. Bongard S, al'Absi M, Lovallo WR. Interactive effects of trait hostility and anger expression on cardiovascular reactivity in young men. Int J Psychophysiol 1998; 28:181–91.

21. Williams RB, Barefoot JG, Shekelle RB. The health consequences of hostility. In: Chesney MA, Rosenman RH, editors. Anger and hostility in cardiovascular and behavioral disorders. New York: Hemisphere; 1985; 173–85.

22. Lepore SJ. Cynicism, social support, and cardiovascular reactivity. Health Psychol 1995; 14:210–6.

23. Weidner G, Friend R, Ficarrotto TJ, Mendell NR. Hostility and cardiovascular reactivity to stress in women and men. Psychosom Med 1989; 51:36–45.

24. Rasmussen PR, Willingham JK, Glover TL. Self-esteem stability, cynical hostility, and cardiovascular reactivity to challenge. Pers Individual Differences 1996; 5:711–8.

25. Smith TW, Brown PC. Cynical hostility, attempts to exert social control, and cardiovascular reactivity in married couples. J Behav Med 1991; 14:581–92.

26. Burns JW, Katkin ES. Psychological, situational, and gender predictors of cardiovascular reactivity to stress: a multivariate approach. J Behav Med 1993; 16:445–65.

27. Durel LA, Carver CS, Spitzer SB, Llabre M, Weintraub JK, Saab PG, Schneiderman N. Associations of blood pressure with self-report measures of anger and hostility among black and white men and women. Health Psychol 1989; 8:557–75.

28. Davis MC, Matthews KA. Do gender-relevant characteristics determine cardiovascular reactivity? Match versus mismatch of traits and situation. J Pers Soc Psychol 1996; 71:527–35.

29. Spence JT, Helmreich R, Stapp J. Ratings of self and peers on sex-role attributes and their relation to self-esteem and conceptions of masculinity and femininity. J Pers Soc Psychol 1975; 32:29–39.

30. Girdler SS, Pedersen CA, Stern RA, Light KC. Menstrual cycle and premenstrual syndrome: modifiers of cardiovascular reactivity in women. Health Psychol 1993; 12:180–92.

31. Guyton AC. Textbook of medical physiology. Philadelphia: WB Saunders; 1981.

32. Llabre MM, Spitzer SB, Saab PG, Ironson GH, Schneiderman N. The reliability and specificity of delta versus residualized change as measures of cardiovascu-

lar reactivity to behavioral challenges. Psychophysiology 1991; 28:701–11.

33. Kirk RE. Experimental design: procedures for the behavioral sciences. Belmont (CA): Wadsworth; 1968.

34. Guyll M, Contrada RJ. Trait hostility and ambulatory cardiovascular activity: responses to social interaction. Health Psychol 1998; 17:30–9.

35. Linden W, Chambers L, Maurice J, Lenz JW. Sex differences in social support, self-deception, hostility, and ambulatory cardiovascular activity. Health Psychol 1993; 12:376–80.

77 Hostility and the Metabolic Syndrome in Older Males: The Normative Aging Study

Raymond Niaura, Sara M. Banks, Kenneth D. Ward, Catherine M. Stoney, Avron Spiro III, Carolyn M. Aldwin, Lewis Landsberg, and Scott T. Weiss

Introduction

Considerable evidence links hostility and CHD as well as other adverse health outcomes. Hostility has been associated, in cross-sectional studies, with angiographically determined coronary artery disease severity (1–3) and peripheral artery disease (4). In prospective studies, hostility has predicted CHD incidence (4–8), hypertension (4), and premature mortality from all causes (4, 5, 8, 9). Although the results of some studies have been negative (10–13), the majority of studies have pointed to hostility as a probable risk factor for CHD and mortality from all causes.

Not only has hostility been found to directly predict CHD and other adverse health outcomes, but there is also abundant evidence to suggest a relationship between hostility and various sociodemographic, behavioral, and physiological risk factors for these disease outcomes. For instance, studies investigating the relationship between hostility and sociodemographic variables have consistently found a pattern of relationships that mimics the pattern found between these variables and morbidity and mortality. That is, higher hostility scores have been found in nonwhites, men, and those of lower socioeconomic status (i.e., lower education and income) (14, 15). Likewise, most studies investigating the associations between hostility and behavioral risk factors have found relationships in the expected direction. Hostility has been positively associated with alcohol consumption (8, 16–19), cigarette use (7, 9, 19), current smoking status and caffeine consumption (19), and caloric intake (18).

In addition to sociodemographic and behavioral risk factors, several physiological correlates of CHD, stroke, diabetes, and premature death have been investigated for their relationship with hostility. Findings in this area, however, have

been less consistent. Positive relationships have been identified between hostility and WHR (18, 20), BMI (16, 19), hypertension (4, 19, 21), total cholesterol (22–24), and the ratio of total cholesterol divided by HDL-C (19). One study, however, failed to find a relationship with BMI, total cholesterol, HDL-C, or LDL-C (18). Yet, although there have been other studies that failed to find an association between hostility and one or more CHD risk factors (6, 8, 11, 12, 16, 25), no studies have reported that high levels of hostility are associated with reduced risk. Overall, the preponderance of data suggests that hostility is associated with many of the risk factors of CHD and other adverse health outcomes.

Observation of a statistical association among abdominal obesity/upper body fat distribution (usually measured by WHR), insulin resistance, hyperglycemia, dyslipidemia (i.e., elevated VLDL-C and TRG levels and by low HDL-C levels), and hypertension on one hand, and their ability to independently predict atherosclerotic cardiovascular disease, stroke, non–insulin-dependent diabetes mellitus, and premature death on the other (26–31), has led to a recent medical hypothesis of a common pathogenic "metabolic syndrome" underlying these disease outcomes and premature death (26, 27, 32). The metabolic syndrome, or "Syndrome X," has come to refer to this cluster of metabolic disorders and disease end points. The metabolic syndrome has become the focus of much recent empirical investigation into the pathogenesis of cardiovascular disease and non–insulin-dependent diabetes mellitus. Yet, although hostility clearly seems to play an important role in the development of cardiovascular disease, little empirical attention has been given to the role that hostility may play in the development of the metabolic syndrome. Ravaja et al. (32) found that high baseline aggression in male adolescents and young adults predicted elevations of serum TRG and insulin concentrations and increased BMI at 3-year follow-up examination. Vitaliano et al. (33) found that women who had high anger-out/hostility *and* high hassles and men who had high anger-out/hostility *or* high hassles had elevated fasting insulin levels. Furthermore, anger-out/hostility was positively associated with elevated fasting glucose levels in both men and women.

The present study augments prior studies (32, 33) in a number of ways. First, hostility was measured using the Cook-Medley Hostility Scale (34). This scale is the most commonly used measure of hostility and has well-established psychometric properties, facilitating comparisons across studies. Second, because hostility has been conceptualized as a multidimensional construct (35), two different methods, one statistical (36) and the other conceptual (9), were used to divide this construct into its subcomponents. Third, upper-body fat distribution was measured by the WHR, which has been associated extensively with the metabolic syndrome (30), and a more comprehensive assessment of physiological correlates of the metabolic syndrome was included. Unique aspects of this study were the simultaneous examination of associations among Ho scores and variables representing aspects of the metabolic syndrome among older males and the application of path analysis to describe more completely the structure of these associations.

The aims of the present study, then, were twofold: 1) to comprehensively examine the relationship between hostility and the most important constituents of the metabolic syndrome, including insulin resistance, hyperglycemia, upper-body fat distribution, dyslipidemia, and hypertension; and 2) to clarify and extend previous findings of an association between hostility and sociodemographic and health behavior variables. To achieve these aims, we analyzed data obtained in the Normative Aging Study, which offers unique opportunities for investigation of the relationship between hostility and the metabolic syndrome because of its large sample size and extensive range of sociodemographic, behavioral, and physiological measures.

Methods

Sample

The data used in this study were collected as part of the Normative Aging Study, a prospective study of 2280 men begun in 1963 to characterize the biomedical and psychosocial parameters of normal aging (37). Details of sample selection have been described previously (38) and are briefly summarized here. Between 1961 and 1970, more than 6000 men from the Boston, Massachusetts, area were recruited through newspaper advertisements, physician referrals, flyers, and word of mouth to participate in the Normative Aging Study. Applicants were screened for good health (only during the initial enrollment period) in three phases (39), which included completion of a medical history form, laboratory and radiographic workup, and physical examination. Applicants were ineligible to participate if they had service-related disability, orthopedic defects, cataracts, loss of hearing, chronic illness (e.g., asthma, bronchitis, or diabetes), hypertension (blood pressure >140/90 mm Hg), prior heart attacks, peptic ulcer, gout, or other major illnesses requiring hospitalization or physician visits. Applicants assessed as geographically unstable (i.e., unlikely to remain in the Boston area for follow-up) were also excluded (40). On the basis of this screening process, the initial cohort consisted of 2280 men in good health and aged 21 to 80 years. Ninety-eight percent of the initial sample were white; 2% were black or another race. Sixty-six percent of the men had high school diplomas; 26% were college graduates. About 44% were classified as working in white-collar occupations (i.e., professionals, managers, and proprietors). Originally, participants reported every 3 years (age 52 or older) or 5 years (younger than age 52) for examination. Since 1986, a

3-year interval has been used for all men. Men were excluded according to the aforementioned criteria only at study entry; during follow-up examinations, they were followed for progression of, among other things, risk factors for CHD.

For inclusion in the present analyses, participants had to have completed the MMPI (41). The MMPI was completed in 1986 by 1548 participants. In addition, only participants who were examined between the years 1987 and 1991, during which time serum insulin and WHR measures were collected, were included in the present analyses. The final sample consisted of 1081 men.

Procedures

On the night before examination, participants refrained from eating or drinking after midnight and refrained from smoking after 8:00 PM. The examination included blood pressure measurement, blood work (serum levels of glucose, insulin, and lipids), anthropometric evaluation, and assessment of health behaviors (diet, alcohol intake, and smoking) by standardized questionnaires. Blood was drawn at 8:00 AM while the participant was fasting. Sociodemographic data, including educational attainment, were obtained on entry into the study.

Measures

Blood Lipids

Serum samples were drawn the morning after an overnight fast and analyzed for total cholesterol, HDL-C, TRG, and (calculated) LDL-C. Serum cholesterol was assayed enzymatically (SCALVO Diagnostics, Wayne, NJ). The HDL-C fraction was measured in the supernatant after precipitation of the LDL-C and VLDL-C fractions with dextran sulfate and magnesium, using the Abbott Biochromatic Analyzer 100 (Abbott Laboratories, South Pasadena, CA). TRG concentration was measured using the Dupont ACA discrete clinical analyzer (Dupont Company, Biomedical Products Department, Wilmington, DE). LDL-C

concentration was estimated using the formula of Friedewald et al. (42).

Fasting Blood Glucose

Serum glucose concentration was measured in duplicate on an autoanalyzer by the hexokinase method (43).

Fasting Insulin

Serum insulin concentration was determined by a solid phase [^{125}I]-radioimmunoassay (Diagnostic Products Corporation, Los Angeles, CA).

Blood Pressure

Blood pressure was measured using a standard mercury sphygmomanometer with a 14-cm cuff. SBP and fifth-phase DBP were measured to the nearest 2 mm Hg. Both left and right arm pressures were measured with the subject sitting; right arm pressures were then taken with the subject in a supine position, and 30 seconds later a second reading of right arm pressures was taken with the subject standing. The palpatory method was used to check auscultatory systolic readings. The means of all systolic and all diastolic readings were used in analyses. There were no methodological differences in assessing blood pressure from one examination to another.

Medication Use

During the laboratory examination, current use of prescription and over-the-counter medication was assessed by the examining physician. In addition, diagnosed conditions were also noted (e.g., hypertension and hypercholesterolemia).

Body Mass Index

Weight was taken on a standard hospital scale with the participant dressed in undershorts and socks. Weight was measured to the nearest 0.5 lb and then converted to kilograms. Height was measured with the participant standing in bare feet against a wall to the nearest 0.1 inch and then converted to meters. Body mass index was computed as kilograms per squared meters (kg/m^2).

Waist-to-hip Ratio

With the participant standing, abdomen circumference was measured in centimeters at the level of the umbilicus, and hip circumference was measured in centimeters at the greatest protrusion of the buttocks. WHR was calculated as abdomen circumference divided by hip circumference.

Health Behaviors

Behavioral risk factors assessed included alcohol and tobacco consumption and diet. Dietary data were obtained by means of a semiquantitative food frequency questionnaire (44), which was mailed to each participant and completed before the examination. The food frequency questionnaire lists food items with serving sizes and elicits information on frequency of intake during the past year. Nutrient scores are computed by multiplying the frequency of intake by the nutrient content of the food items. Macronutrients examined in the present analyses were total energy intake (kcal/day) and alcohol (drinks/week). Information was obtained on number of cigarettes currently smoked per day. Smoking status was categorized into never or ex-smokers vs. current smokers (≥ 1 cigarettes/day).

Hostility

Hostility was measured with the Cook-Medley Hostility Scale (34) taken from the MMPI. Form AX (41) of the MMPI was administered, which includes items from both the MMPI and MMPI-2. Nine different scores were derived from the Cook-Medley scale, including a total hostility score (Ho), scores for paranoid alienation and cynicism based on the factor structure of Costa et al. (36), and scores for the six subcategories of hostility (cynicism, hostile attributions, hostile affect, aggressive responding, social avoidance, and other) based on the scheme of Barefoot et al. (9).

Demographic Risk Factors

Education was divided into four categories: less than high school, high school graduate (includ-ing attainment of a general education diploma), some college or college graduate (2 years of technical school or 4 years of college), and postcollege (some postgraduate or postgraduate). Age (in years) was assessed at the time of the laboratory examination.

Data Analysis

Data analysis was conducted using the following strategy. First, bivariate relationships among the variables were examined using correlational procedures (Spearman's r). Next, based on the initial bivariate results and hypotheses concerning whether hostility was directly related to variables representing the metabolic syndrome or whether the influence of hostility on the metabolic syndrome was mediated by BMI and WHR, multivariate relationships were explored using multiple linear regression. Finally, on the basis of these initial results, a path model was developed in which Ho indirectly predicts TRG, HDL-C, SBP, and DBP through the mediating effects of BMI, WHR, and fasting insulin. This model was then constructed and evaluated using structural equation modeling procedures (45). Structural equation modeling offers a unique opportunity to examine simultaneously the relationship among multiple variables, to estimate path coefficients or relative weights of the paths among the variables, and to test the directionality of such paths.

Results

Sample Characteristics

Demographic, personality, and behavioral characteristics of the sample are presented in Table 77.1. Study participants ranged in age from 44 to 92 years and had an average Ho score of 17.1 (SD = 7.8). Almost 11% currently smoked, about 69.1% had smoked at some point in their lives, and 79.8% were drinkers (operationalized as ≥ 1

Table 77.1
Demographic, personality, and behavioral characteristics of sample

Variable[a]	Mean or percentage	SD	Range
Age (yr)	63.1	7.9	44–92
Total hostility	17.1	7.8	1–44
Cynicism-C	10.1	5.0	0–24
Cynicism-B	5.7	2.9	0–13
Hostile attributions	2.8	2.1	0–12
Hostile affect	1.8	1.4	0–5
Aggressive responding	3.7	1.9	0–9
Paranoid alienation	3.0	2.4	0–13
Social avoidance	1.2	1.1	0–4
Other	1.9	1.4	0–7
Cigarettes per day	2.7	8.7	0–60
Drinks per week	10.5	15.9	0–169
Total caloric intake (kcal/day)	1972	614	803–4194
Education			
Less than high school	9.5%		
High school	24.3%		
Some college	38.9%		
College or postgraduate study	27.3%		
Current smoker	11.0%		

a. $N = 989$–1081. Cynicism C = cynicism subscale derived by Costa et al. (36); Cynicism B = cynicism subscale derived by Barefoot et al. (9).

drinks/year). Participants reported smoking an average of 2.7 cigarettes/day and drank a mean of 10.5 alcoholic beverages/week.

Table 77.2 presents statistics on the anthropometric and physiological characteristics of the sample. Study participants had an average WHR of 0.98 and BMI of 26.8. Average total cholesterol for the sample was 235 mg/dl, and SBP and DBP averaged 129 and 78 mm Hg, respectively. Although subjects had been free of medical illness on entry into the Normative Aging Study, at the time of laboratory assessment, 42.6% were found to be hypertensive, and 26.0% were taking medications for hypertension, 3.3% for hypercholesterolemia, and 2.7% for diabetes mellitus.

Bivariate Relationships among Hostility and Other Variables

Total Ho and the eight derived subcomponents were examined for their relationships with demographic, behavioral, anthropometric, and physiological variables. Table 77.3 displays selected Spearman correlations among hostility, demographic, and behavioral measures. The total Ho score was associated negatively with educational level and positively with total calories consumed. Three of the four Barefoot et al. (9) subcategories (cynicism, hostile attributions, and aggressive responding) were also associated negatively with educational level. Both aggressive responding

Table 77.2
Physiological characteristics of sample

Variable[a]	Mean	SD	Range
BMI	26.8	3.6	17–46
WHR	0.98	0.05	0.79–1.18
Total cholesterol (mg/dl)	235	39	121–406
LDL-C (mg/dl)	157	35	57–278
HDL-C (mg/dl)	48	12	17–104
TRG (mg/dl)	155	106	32–1335
Lipid ratio	5.2	1.4	2.0–13.7
SBP (mm Hg)	129	16	83–197
DBP (mm Hg)	78	9	45–112
Insulin (mU/ml)	11.9	8.5	1–81
Glucose (mg/dl)	105	24	66–414

a. $N = 989$–1081. Lipid ratio = total cholesterol/HDL-C.

and hostile affect correlated positively with total calories consumed. Additionally, aggressive responding was associated positively with number of cigarettes smoked per day and number of alcoholic drinks per week.

Table 77.4 displays Spearman correlations of total Ho and subscales with the physiological and anthropometric variables. The total Ho score and all subscales were associated positively with BMI and WHR. Ho and all subscales, except hostile affect, correlated positively with TRG, lipid ratio, and fasting insulin and correlated negatively with HDL-C. Total Ho and most of the subscales were not significantly correlated with fasting glucose; only aggressive responding was found to correlate positively with this variable. None of the measures of hostility were associated with LDL-C, SBP, or DBP.

Bivariate Relationships among Anthropometric and Physiological Variables

Table 77.5 presents the correlation matrix for the anthropometric and physiological variables.

WHR, fasting insulin, fasting glucose, SBP, DBP, and TRG all correlated positively, with the exception of glucose and DBP, which were not significantly correlated with each other. Furthermore, HDL-C correlated negatively with all physiological variables except SBP and DBP.

Multivariate Relationships

Given that bivariate analyses identified significant correlations for Ho with fasting insulin, HDL-C, and TRG, the next step was to examine whether Ho directly predicted these physiological measures or whether such relationships were mediated by anthropometric parameters such as BMI and WHR, because BMI and WHR bear significant independent relationships with these variables (30). A series of preliminary hierarchical multiple linear regression analyses were conducted using TRG, fasting insulin, HDL-C, SBP, and DBP as the criterion variables and Ho, WHR, BMI, and fasting insulin as the predictor variables, entered in order. Ho was chosen for these analyses over the hostility subscales because it has been more extensively studied in terms of its relationship with CHD morbidity and mortality. Before entering fasting insulin and TRG into the regression equation, these variables were log-transformed to normalize the distribution of the data. Hierarchical regression analyses revealed that in all cases, the effects of Ho on a given criterion variable disappeared when one or more additional predictors was entered into the regression equation, suggesting that the relationship between Ho and the given physiological measure was being mediated by the other variable. Specifically, the relationships of Ho with fasting insulin, TRG, and HDL-C were found to be mediated by both BMI and WHR. Furthermore, the relationships of Ho with TRG and HDL-C were found to be mediated by fasting insulin. Age, disease status, use of medications, smoking status, and alcohol consumption (drinks per week, log-transformed) did not significantly

Table 77.3
Correlations of subscales of hostility with demographic and behavioral variables

Variable[a]	Ho	Cynicism C[b]	Cynicism B[c]	Hostile attributions	Hostile affect	Aggressive responding	Paranoid alienation	Social avoidance	Other
Age	0.010	.027	.046	-.023	-.029	-.054	-.027	.026	.049
Education	-.160***	-.146***	-.170***	-.154***	-.037	-.134***	-.133***	-.117***	-.023
Cigarettes per day	.059	.055	.039	.043	.032	.093**	-.046	.021	.040
Alcoholic drinks per week	-.003	-.012	-.028	-.031	-.022	.069*	.003	-.079*	.072*
Total caloric intake (kcal/day)	.096**	.096**	.052	.054	.087**	.094**	.062	.011**	.085**

a. $N = 989$–1081.
b. Cynicism C = cynicism subscale derived by Costa et al. (36).
c. Cynicism B = cynicism subscale derived by Barefoot et al. (9).
d. * $p < .05$; ** $p < .01$; *** $p < .001$.

Table 77.4
Correlations of subscales of hostility with anthropometric and physiological variables

Variable[a]	Ho	Cynicism C[b]	Cynicism B[c]	Hostile attributions	Hostile affect	Aggressive responding	Paranoid alienation	Social avoidance	Other
BMI	.132***	.143***	.081**	.151***	.094**	.166***	.073**	-.005	.016
WHR	.108***	.107****	.073**	.124***	.070*	.095**	.074**	.022	.052
Total cholesterol	.036	.032	.042	-.019	.032	.019	.047	.036	.034
LDL-C	.011	.011	.033	-.046	.025	-.007	.033	.027	.011
HDL-C	-.067*	-.075*	-.080**	-.080**	-.020	-.065*	-.042	-.015	-.011
TRG	.089**	.096**	.075*	.088**	.055	.084**	.057	.036	.053
Lipid ratio	.081**	.089**	.097†	.061*	.034	.067*	.039	.031	.022
Insulin	.094**	.10**	.075**	.106***	.059	.085**	.043	.006	.025
Fasting glucose	.051	.045	.055	.009	.048	.060*	.046	.002	.038
SBP	.011	.016	.018	.014	.024	.006	.007	.009	-.030
DBP	-.012	-.016	-.026	.003	-.019	.037	-.016	-.001	-.040

* $p < .05$; ** $p < .01$; *** $p < .001$.
a. $N = 989$–1081.
b. Cynicism C = cynicism subscale derived by Costa et al. (36).
c. Cynicism B = cynicism subscale derived by Barefoot et al. (9).

Table 77.5
Intercorrelation matrix of selected physiological variables

Variable[a]	WHR	Insulin	Fasting glucose	SBP	DBP	TRG	HDL-C
BMI	0.459***	.437***	.212***	.122***	.205***	.245***	−.254***
WHR		.337***	.134***	.124***	.131***	.263***	−.200***
Insulin			.271***	.143***	.182***	.301***	−.206***
Fasting glucose				.146***	.024	.234***	−.143***
SBP					.573***	.149***	−.042
DBP						.131***	−.003
TRG							−.477***

a. $N = 989–1081$.
*** $p < .001$.

affect the relationships among hostility and the anthropometric and physiological measures.

On the basis of these initial regression results, a path model was developed in which Ho indirectly predicts TRG, HDL-C, SBP, and DBP through the mediating effects of BMI, WHR, and fasting insulin (see Figure 77.1).[1] Fasting insulin was hypothesized, on the basis of prior empirical and theoretical work (30), to mediate the effects of BMI and WHR on HDL-C and TRG. An initial model was tested and then revised by dropping paths that were not significant. The final model is presented in Figure 77.1. Parameter estimates were calculated using maximum likelihood methods. F1 and F2 represent latent constructs that underlie two variable pairs (TRG with HDL-C and SBP with DBP) and indicate that the variables are correlated. The variances of the F1 and F2 factors were fixed at 1 so that the fixed path from each factor to its measured variable indicator could be set free to be estimated (45). The overall fit of the model was good ($\chi^2(12) = 50.23$, $p < .001$; comparative fit index $= 0.957$).

This analysis confirmed that BMI mediated the relationships of Ho with fasting insulin, TRG, and HDL-C. WHR was found to mediate the relationship between Ho and fasting insulin.

Furthermore, BMI was found to be associated with TRG, HDL-C, SBP, and DBP directly and indirectly by way of fasting insulin. In separate models, we tested whether the effects of Ho on BMI and WHR were mediated by education level, age, and calories consumed. These variables did not explain (mediate) the relationships between Ho, BMI, and WHR, nor did they alter substantially the final model path parameter estimates or goodness of fit. In addition, the sample was divided at the median age of 63 years, and separate models were evaluated for men falling above and below the median age. The parameter estimates remained the same for both age groups. Another model was constructed in which antihypertensive medication use was entered as a covariate for blood pressure. Use of antihypertensive medications was associated positively with blood pressure, but inclusion of this variable in the model did not substantially alter parameter estimates. Finally, the effects of diabetes were evaluated in two ways: by excluding men who were taking medication to control diabetes and by also excluding men whose fasting glucose was ≥140 mg/dl. In both instances, the parameter estimates and model fit did not differ materially from the final model, which included diabetic men.

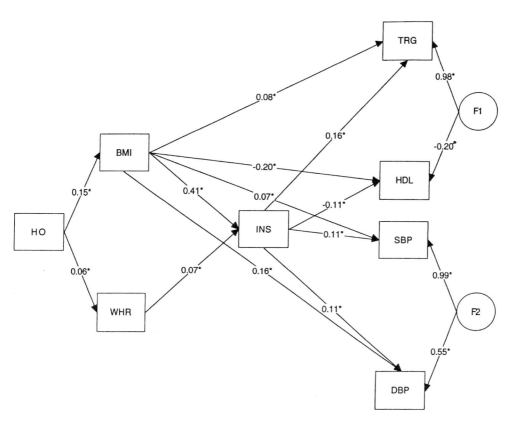

Figure 77.1
Path model illustrating relationships among hostility (HO), BMI, WHR, insulin (INS), blood pressure, and lipids.
* $P < .05$ for standardized path coefficients. Error terms are omitted for ease of presentation.

Discussion

Relationships among total Ho scores with socio-demographic and behavioral variables noted in prior research were largely confirmed in the present study. For instance, our finding of a negative association between Ho and education has been consistently observed in earlier research (14, 15). In terms of behavioral risk factors, a positive association between Ho and total caloric intake has also been previously found (18). Al-though total Ho in this study was not related to alcohol consumption or cigarette use, subscale scores on aggressive responding were related to these two behavioral risk factors.

Also consistent with prior studies were the findings that total Ho scores were associated positively with both BMI (16, 19) and WHR (18, 20). Furthermore, we were able to demonstrate that Ho was *not* significantly associated with serum total cholesterol or with serum LDL-C but *was* associated with higher serum TRG, a higher lipid ratio, and lower serum HDL-C. Although the relationships of hostility and serum lipid levels have been inconsistent in the literature as a whole, these findings are consistent with results from several earlier studies. For example, at least three studies found no relationships between Ho and total cholesterol or LDL-C (4, 8, 18). Siegler et al. (19) observed a positive association between Ho and the lipid ratio, and Ravaja et al. (32) found that a baseline measure of aggression predicted elevations in serum TRG 3 years later.

Another contribution of this study was the simultaneous examination of Ho subscales and their relationships with sociodemographic, behavioral, anthropometric, and physiological variables representing the metabolic syndrome. Consistent with the findings reported by Scherwitz et al. (15), we found inverse associations for Barefoot et al.'s subscales of cynicism, hostile attributions, and aggressive responding with education; however, we failed to find a significant relationship between hostile affect and education. The cynicism subscale derived by Costa et al. (36) was also inversely related to years of education. Regarding the behavioral variables, Costa et al.'s cynicism subscale and Barefoot et al.'s hostile affect and aggressive responding subscales were associated positively with caloric intake. However, Barefoot et al.'s cynicism and hostile attributions subscales were not associated with calories consumed. Of note, correlations of the five subscales with demographic and behavioral variables were largely of similar magnitude. No one subscale stood out as particularly associated with these variables except aggressive responding, which was positively associated with cigarette use and alcohol consumption, in addition to education and total caloric intake.

Except for social avoidance, and other, the remaining hostility subscales behaved similarly to the total Ho score with regard to their relationships with BMI and WHR. That is, higher scores on these subscales were associated with greater BMI and greater WHR. Correlations of the subscales with anthropometric and physiological variables varied to some degree but were gener-

ally similar in magnitude and direction compared with the total Ho score. Only hostile affect stood out, because it was consistently unrelated to all physiological measures of the metabolic syndrome.

We also replicated earlier observations of a bivariate association between hostility and fasting insulin concentrations (32, 33). Our study, however, examined the hostility-insulin relationship using Ho, which has been shown to be related to CHD and total mortality in several studies (1, 2, 4, 6, 9, 14), whereas previous studies have used a measure of aggression (32) and a measure of anger-out proneness (33) as proxies for hostility. Moreover, in the latter study, the relationship between anger-out proneness and insulin remained significant after controlling for BMI. Thus, more work is needed to determine the degree to which related, but not entirely overlapping, constructs of hostility and anger expression may be associated with insulin and other aspects of the metabolic syndrome, independent of their relationships with obesity and body fat distribution. At least two studies have reported that higher hostility is associated with increased incidence of hypertension (4, 21). We failed, however, to find a relationship between hostility and either SBP or DBP. Similarly, although higher hostility was found to be associated with elevated fasting glucose levels in a recent study (33), we did not confirm this finding.

The most important contribution of this study was the construction of a multivariate path model, which demonstrated that Ho does not have direct effects on the physiological variables of the metabolic syndrome. Rather, its effects are mediated by BMI and WHR. Specifically, Ho was found to have indirect effects on fasting insulin by way of both BMI and WHR and to predict indirectly both serum TRG and HDL-C by way of BMI. Hostility, however, was more strongly associated with BMI compared with WHR. Therefore, BMI may be relatively more important in determining the indirect relationships between Ho and other variables which define the metabolic syndrome. Furthermore, BMI was found to exert its influence on TRG, HDL-C, SBP, and DBP both directly and indirectly by way of fasting insulin; WHR, on the other hand, exerted its effects on TRG, HDL-C, SBP, and DBP only indirectly through its effects on fasting insulin. These relationships were not influenced by age, educational level, caloric intake, use of antihypertensive medications, or diabetes or clinically elevated glucose concentrations. That the relationships among Ho and other variables in the path model were not affected by excluding diabetics suggests that these associations fall more along a continuum rather than being influenced by development of a diabetic state. Others have noted consistent, positive relationships among the variables that define the metabolic syndrome (fasting insulin, TRG, HDL-C, and blood pressure) among adults and even children who are not diabetic, dyslipidemic, or hypertensive (46).

The path model suggests that insulin is antecedent to and exerts its effects on blood pressure and serum lipid values. This directional relationship is consistent with what is currently known about the pathogenesis of the metabolic syndrome, namely, that fasting insulin concentrations, which may signal insulin resistance, drive hypertension and dyslipidemia (e.g., Refs. 29, 32, and 47–49).

Some limitations to this study must be noted. First, although Ho was measured 1 to 4 years before the anthropometric and physiological variables, the data were analyzed cross-sectionally; therefore, causality cannot be inferred. Second, the sample used in this study was drawn from an older, male, predominantly white population. Therefore, generalizability to other populations, such as females, younger adults, or nonwhites may be limited. Third, the magnitude of the associations between Ho and demographic, behavioral, and physiological variables may be viewed as small; however, this is generally consistent with the results of other studies (e.g., Ref. 20). Thus, the clinical implications of the findings (e.g.,

whether hostile men who keep their BMI and WHR low may decrease their health risk) are not immediately apparent. It is possible, though, that there exist subgroups of high hostility men for whom these relationships are stronger and for whom CHD risk factors may be reduced in a clinically significant way by weight loss and reduction in the WHR. Finally, we did not include measures of perceived stress, stress hormones, other CHD risk factors, and morbidity or mortality outcomes, the significance of which is discussed below.

The results of this study may have implications for interpreting findings from other studies, past and future, which examine the association between hostility, CHD risk factors, and CHD morbidity and mortality. The finding that Ho does not have direct effects on metabolic dysfunction raises questions about the relationship of Ho with CHD risk factors and CHD. Our findings suggest that if one controls for the influence of BMI and WHR, the association observed between hostility and CHD risk factors may be attenuated or eliminated. However, this may not be true in every instance (e.g., Ref. 33), and further work is needed to explore in which populations and under what conditions these relationships hold. One could also interpret the findings of the path model to suggest that Ho will not be related to CHD morbidity or mortality if one adjusts for CHD risk factors. This interpretation should be viewed with caution because the results of the present study portrayed cross-sectional associations, and we did not assess CHD morbidity or mortality. However, longitudinal studies that did control for CHD risk factors (e.g., lipids) nevertheless found positive associations between Ho and CHD morbidity and mortality (4, 5, 8). Moreover, it is entirely possible that Ho predisposes toward CHD not only through its associations with risk factors but also independently through other mechanisms (e.g., cardiac arrhythmia; imbalance in sympathetic and parasympathetic nervous system activity; cardiovascular, endocrine, and neuroendocrine responses to stress; coronary artery va-sospasm; and clotting factors). The question also remains whether Ho is causally related to CHD or whether it is just a correlate of metabolic dysfunction. Prospective studies examining Ho in relation to the development of metabolic dysfunction, other CHD risk factors, and incidence of CHD are needed to answer these questions.

Future studies should focus on the mechanisms underlying the observed relationships of hostility with BMI and WHR. A number of studies have revealed associations of centrally distributed body fat with socioeconomic, psychosocial, and behavioral correlates of low socioeconomic status (20, 50–54). These findings have led Björntorp (28) to hypothesize that abdominal fat distribution is the end result of a series of physiological responses to psychosocial stress. The chronic stress associated with low socioeconomic status leads to chronic stimulation of the adrenal-cortical system, causing elevated levels of adrenal corticosteroids, which in turn direct the storage of fat to central adipose tissue depots. Related findings come from studies observing associations between WHR and depression and anxiety symptoms (55, 56). The observed relationship between hostility and WHR suggests that hostility may be part of the cognitive/emotional/behavioral response to the chronic stress of low socioeconomic status. Therefore, future studies may do well to incorporate measurements of socioeconomic, psychosocial, and behavioral correlates of low socioeconomic status, as well as measurement of perceived stress and stress hormones, in an attempt to elucidate psychosocial and physiological mechanisms for the relationship between hostility, obesity, and distribution of body fat. For example, stressful challenges may potentiate physiological reactions in individuals with high Ho scores. Examination of interactions with socioeconomic status, race, and sex is also in order, given some evidence that associations of BMI and WHR with psychosocial factors differ across race and sex groups (20). Research should also consider the possibil-ity that hostility might be associated with clinical or subclinical eating disorders (57), increasing BMI and WHR, given that hostility appears to be associated with greater caloric intake (although, in this study, caloric intake did not mediate the association between Ho and BMI or WHR).

In conclusion, this study replicated previous findings of a negative association between Ho and education, a positive association between Ho and total caloric intake, and positive correlations between Ho and both BMI and WHR. Furthermore, Ho was found to be related to constituents of the metabolic syndrome, in particular higher serum TRG, a higher lipid ratio, and lower serum HDL-C. However, multivariate analyses demonstrated that Ho was associated with the metabolic syndrome variables only indirectly through its influence on BMI and WHR.

Note

1. Because sample size varied according to variable ($N = 989-1081$), the covariance matrix was constructed using pairwise selection of variables.

References

1. Dembroski TM, MacDougall JM, Williams RB, Haney TL, Blumenthal JA. Components of type A, hostility, and anger-in: relationship to angiographic findings. Psychosom Med 1989; 47:219–33.

2. MacDougall JM, Dembroski TM, Dimsdale JE, Hackett TP. Components of type A, hostility, and anger-in: further relationships to angiographic findings. Health Psychol 1985; 4:137–52.

3. Williams RB, Haney TL, Lee KL, Kong Y, Blumenthal JA, Whalen R. Type A behavior, hostility, and coronary atherosclerosis. Psychosom Med 1980; 42:539–49.

4. Barefoot JC, Dahlstrom WG, Williams RB. Hostility, CHD incidence, and total mortality: a 25-year follow-up study of 255 physicians. Psychosom Med 1983; 45:59–64.

5. Barefoot JC, Larsen S, von der Lieth L, Schroll M. Hostility, incidence of acute myocardial infarction, and

mortality in a sample of older Danish men and women. Am J Epidemiol 1995; 142:477–84.

6. Dembroski TM, MacDougall JM, Costa PT, Grandits GA. Components of hostility as predictors of sudden death and myocardial infarction in the Multiple Risk Factor Intervention Trial. Psychosom Med 1989; 51:514–22.

7. Matthews KA, Glass DC, Rosenman RH, Bortner RW. Competitive drive, pattern A, and coronary heart disease: a further analysis of some data from the Western Collaborative Group Study. J Chronic Dis 1977; 30:489–98.

8. Shekelle RB, Gale M, Ostfeld AM, Paul O. Hostility, risk of coronary heart disease, and mortality. Psychosom Med 1983; 45:109–14.

9. Barefoot JC, Dodge KA, Peterson BL, Dahlstrom WG, Williams RB. The Cook-Medley Hostility Scale: item content and ability to predict survival. Psychosom Med 1989; 51:46–57.

10. Leon GR, Finn SE, Murray D, Bailey JM. The inability to predict cardiovascular disease from hostility scores or MMPI items related to type A behavior. J Consult Clin Psychol 1988; 56:597–600.

11. Hearn MD, Murray DM, Luepker RV. Hostility, coronary heart disease, and total mortality: a 33-year follow-up study of university students. J Behav Med 1989; 12:105–21.

12. McCranie EW, Watkins LO, Brandsma JM, Sisson BD. Hostility, coronary heart disease (CHD) incidence, and total mortality: lack of association in a 25-year follow-up study of 478 physicians. J Behav Med 1986; 9:119–25.

13. Seeman TE, Syme SL. Social networks and coronary artery disease: a comparison of the structure and function of social relations as predictors of disease. Psychosom Med 1987; 49:341–54.

14. Barefoot JC, Peterson BL, Dahlstrom WG, Siegler IC, Anderson NB, Williams RB. Hostility patterns and health implications: correlates of Cook-Medley Hostility Scale scores in a national survey. Health Psychol 1991; 10:18–24.

15. Scherwitz L, Perkins L, Chesney M, Hughes G. Cook-Medley Hostility Scale and subsets: relationship to demographic and psychosocial characteristics in young adults in the CARDIA study. Psychosom Med 1991; 53:36–49.

16. Houston BK, Vavak CR. Cynical hostility: developmental factors, psychosocial correlates, and health behaviors. Health Psychol 1991; 10:9–17.

17. Leiker M, Hailey BJ. A link between hostility and disease: poor health habits. Behav Med 1988; 14:129–33.

18. Scherwitz L, Perkins L, Chesney M, Hughes GH, Sidney ST, Manolio TA. Hostility and health behaviors in young adults: the CARDIA study. Am J Epidemiol 1992; 136:136–45.

19. Siegler IC, Peterson BL, Barefoot JC, Williams RB. Hostility during late adolescence predicts coronary risk factors at midlife. Am J Epidemiol 1992; 136:146–54.

20. Kaye SA, Folsom AR, Jacobs DR Jr, Hughes GH, Flack JM. Psychosocial correlates of body fat distribution in black and white young adults. Int J Obes 1993; 17:271–7.

21. Irvine J, Garner DM, Craig HM, Logan AG. Prevalence of type A behavior in untreated hypertensive individuals. Hypertension 1991; 18:72–8.

22. Dujovne VF, Houston BK. Hostility-related variables and plasma lipid levels. J Behav Med 1991; 14:553–63.

23. Lundberg U, Hedman M, Melin B, Frankenhaeuser M. Type A behavior in healthy males and females as related to physiological activity and blood lipids. Psychosom Med 1989; 51:112–22.

24. Weidner G, Sexton G, McLellarn R, Conner SL, Matarazzo JD. The role of type A behavior and hostility in an elevation of plasma lipids in adult women and men. Psychosom Med 1987; 49:136–45.

25. Barefoot JC, Smith RH, Dahlstrom WG, Williams RB. Personality predictors of smoking behavior in a sample of physicians. Psychol Health 1989; 3:37–43.

26. Björntorp P. Obesity and adipose tissue distribution as risk factors for the development of disease: a review. Infusionstherapis 1990; 17:24–7.

27. Björntorp P. "Portal" adipose tissue as a generator of risk factors for cardiovascular disease and diabetes [editorial]. Arteriosclerosis 1990; 10:493–6.

28. Björntorp P. Hypothesis: visceral fat accumulation. The missing link between psychosocial factors and cardiovascular disease. J Intern Med 1991; 230:195–201.

29. DeFronzo RA, Ferrannini E. Insulin resistance: a multifacted syndrome responsible for NIDDM, obesity, hypertension, dyslipidemia, and atherosclerotic cardiovascular disease. Diabetes Care 1991; 14:173–94.

30. Kissebah AH, Krakower GR. Regional adiposity and morbidity. Physiol Rev 1994; 74:761–811.

31. Wing RR, Matthews KA, Kuller LH, Meilahn EN, Plantinga P. Waist to hip ratio in middle-aged women: associations with behavioral and psychosocial factors and with changes in cardiovascular risk factors. Arterioscler Thromb 1991; 11:1250–7.

32. Ravaja N, Keltikangas-Järvinen L, Keskivaara P. Type A factors as predictors of changes in the metabolic syndrome: precursors in adolescents and young adults. A 3-year follow-up study. Health Psychol 1996; 15:18–29.

33. Vitaliano PP, Scanlan JM, Krenz C, Fujimoto W. Insulin and glucose: relationships with hassles, anger, and hostility in nondiabetic older adults. Psychosom Med 1996; 58:489–99.

34. Cook WW, Medley DM. Proposed hostility and pharisaic-virtue scales from the MMPI. J Appl Psychol 1954; 38:414–8.

35. Smith TW. Hostility and health: current status of a psychosomatic hypothesis. Health Psychol 1992; 11:139–50.

36. Costa PT, Zonderman AB, McCrae RR, Williams RB. Cynicism and paranoid alienation in the Cook and Medley HO Scale. Psychosom Med 1986; 48:283–5.

37. Bossé R, Ekerdt DJ, Silbert JE. The Veterans Administration Normative Aging Study. In: Mednick SA, Harway M, Finello KM, editors. Handbook of longitudinal research. Vol 2: Teenage and adult cohorts. New York: Praeger; 1984. p. 273–95.

38. Spiro A III, Aldwin CM, Ward KD, Mroczek DK. Personality and the incidence of hypertension among older men: longitudinal findings from the Normative Aging Study. Health Psychol 1995; 6:563–9.

39. Dawber TR, Thomas HE. Clinical evaluation in the Normative Aging Study. Int J Aging Hum Dev 1972; 3:63–9.

40. Rose CL, Bell B. Selection of geographically stable subjects in longitudinal studies of aging. J Am Geriatr Soc 1965; 13:143–51.

41. Butcher JN, Dahlstrom WG, Graham JR, Tellegen A, Kaemmer B. MMPI-2: Minnesota Multiphasic Personality Inventory-2. Manual for administration and scoring. Minneapolis (MN): University of Minnesota; 1989.

42. Friedewald WT, Levy RI, Fredrickson DS. Estimation of the concentration of low-density lipoprotein cholesterol in plasma, without use of the preparative ultracentrifuge. Clin Chem 1972; 18:449–52.

43. Leon LP, Chu DK, Stasiw RP. New, more specific methods for the SMA 12/60 multichannel biochemical analyzer: advances in automated analysis. Tarrytown (NY): Mediad; 1977.

44. Willett WC, Sampson L, Stampfer MJ, Rosner B, Bain C, Witschi J, Hennekens CH, Speizer FE. Reproducibility and validity of a semi-quantitative food frequency questionnaire. Am J Epidemiol 1985: 122:51–65.

45. Bentler PM. EQS structrual equations program manual. Encino (CA): Multivariate Software; 1995.

46. Bao W, Srinivasan S, Wattingney W, Berenson GS. Persistence of multiple cardiovascular risk clustering related to syndrome X from childhood to young adulthood: the Bogalusa Heart Study. Arch Intern Med 1994; 154:1842–7.

47. Ward KD, Sparrow D, Vokonas PS, Willett WC, Landsberg L, Weiss ST. The relationships of abdominal obesity, hyperinsulinemia and saturated fat intake to serum lipid levels: the Normative Aging Study. Int J Obes Relat Metab Disord 1994; 18:137–44.

48. Ward KD, Sparrow D, Landsberg L, Young JB, Vokonas PS, Weiss ST. The relationship of epinephrine excretion to serum lipid levels: the Normative Aging Study. Metabolism 1994; 43:509–13.

49. Ward KD, Sparrow D, Landsberg L, Young JB, Vokonas PS, Weiss ST. Influence of insulin, sympathetic nervous system activity, and obesity on blood pressure: the Normative Aging Study. J Hypertens 1996; 14:301–8.

50. Björntorp P. The associations between obesity, adipose tissue distribution and disease. Acta Med Scand Suppl 1988; 723:121–34.

51. Björntorp P. Regional fat distribution: potential mechanisms for metabolic and clinical consequences. Environmental-neurological-stress influences. Proceedings of the National Institutes of Health Workshop on Basic and Clinical Aspects of Regional Fat Distribution; 1989 Sept; Bethesda, MD. Bethesda (MD): National Institutes of Health; 1989. p. 123–7.

52. Georges E, Mueller WH, Wear ML. Body fat distribution in men and women of the Hispanic Health and Nutrition Examination Survey of the United States: associations with behavioral variables. Ann Hum Biol 1993; 20:275–91.

53. Lapidus L, Bengtsson C, Hällström T, Björntorp P. Obesity, adipose tissue distribution and health in women: results from a population study in Gothenburg, Sweden. Appetite 1989; 12:25–35.

54. Rosmond R, Lapidus L, Björntorp P. The influence of occupational and social factors on obesity and body fat distribution in middle-aged men. Int J Obes 1996; 20:599–607.

55. Lloyd EC, Wing RR, Orchard TJ. Waist to hip ratio and psychosocial factors in adults with insulin-dependent diabetes mellitus: the Pittsburgh Epidemiology of Diabetes Complications Study. Metabolism 1996; 45:268–72.

56. Rosmond R, Lapidus L, Mårin P, Björntorp P. Mental distress, obesity and body fat distribution in middle-aged men. Obes Res 1996; 4:245–52.

57. Williams GJ, Chamove AS, Millar HR. Eating disorders, perceived control, assertiveness and hostility. Br J Clin Psychol 1990; 29:327–35.

Types of Stressors That Increase Susceptibility to the Common Cold in Healthy Adults

Sheldon Cohen, Ellen Frank, William J. Doyle, David P. Skoner, Bruce S. Rabin, and Jack M. Gwaltney Jr.

On exposure to an infectious agent, only a proportion of people develop illness. The possibility that psychological stress contributes to this variability in response has received considerable attention (e.g., S. Cohen, Tyrrell, & Smith, 1991; Glaser et al., 1987; Stone et al., 1993; Turner Cobb & Steptoe, 1996). Probably because of their very high incidence, upper respiratory infections (URIs) have served as the primary model in the study of stress and susceptibility to infectious disease. Although there is a large literature on the relation between stress and self-reported episodes of colds and influenza (review in S. Cohen & Williamson, 1991), the most convincing work in this area provides biological verification of illness. This work includes three prospective epidemiological studies that found that family conflict and disorder predicted serologically verified URIs (Clover, Abell, Becker, Crawford, & Ramsey, 1989; Graham, Douglas, & Ryan, 1986; Meyer & Haggerty, 1962). It also includes virus-challenge studies in which volunteers who completed stressful life event or emotional distress scales were subsequently exposed to a cold or influenza virus. The development of upper respiratory illness was verified by viral shedding and increases in virus-specific antibody titers. Although early work with this paradigm provided mixed support for a relation between stress and susceptibility to URIs (Totman, Kiff, Reed, & Craig, 1980, and Broadbent, Broadbent, Phillpotts, & Wallace, 1984, found effects; Greene, Betts, Ochitill, Iker, & Douglas, 1978, and Locke & Heisel, 1977, did not), studies using large samples and more sophisticated methodologies provide strong evidence for a dose–response relation between psychological stress and risk of developing a cold (S. Cohen et al., 1991; Stone et al., 1993). There is, however, some variability in how different stress measures are associated with colds. Emotional distress is associated with

a greater risk of infection (S. Cohen, Tyrrell, & Smith, 1993), whereas stressful life events are associated with the risk of infected participants developing illness (S. Cohen, Tyrrell, & Smith, 1993; Stone et al., 1993).

Although existing evidence has increasingly supported a link between life stressors and susceptibility to URIs, we know little about the specific types of stressors that place people at increased risk. For example, are acute stressful events as important as ongoing chronic stressors? Are educational or reproductive events as important as losing a job or an interpersonal conflict? Moreover, up until now, we have been unable to establish the behavioral or biological pathways that link psychological stress to greater risk. Although earlier research has examined the potential role of health practices such as smoking, alcohol consumption, and exercise (S. Cohen et al., 1991; Turner Cobb & Steptoe, 1996) and of limited (quantitative) measures of immune status such as numbers of various types of white blood cells (S. Cohen et al., 1991), no evidence for mediation has been found.

This study uses the virus-challenge paradigm in an attempt to learn about the nature (duration and domain) of life stressors that compromise host resistance to URIs and to identify the behavioral and biological pathways that link stressors to disease susceptibility. We assessed acute and chronic stressors with an intensive interview technique *before* experimentally exposing healthy participants to one of two common cold viruses. We then carefully monitored participants for the development of infection and clinical illness. By intentionally exposing people to an upper respiratory virus, we were able to control for the possible effects of life stressors on exposure to infectious agents (as opposed to their effects on host resistance). We also evaluated behavioral, endocrinological, and immunological pathways through which stressors might influence susceptibility to infectious disease. Behavioral pathways we examined included smoking, drinking alcohol, diet, exercise, and sleep habits. Endocrine pathways included basal (prechallenge) urinary levels of epinephrine, norepinephrine, and cortisol. Finally, immune pathways included quantitations of white blood cell populations and natural killer (NK) cell activity. Control variables included demographic factors as well as prechallenge levels of virus-specific antibody, body mass, season, social network ties, and personality characteristics.

Method

Participants

The participants were 125 men and 151 women who responded to newspaper advertisements and were judged to be in good health after a medical examination. Ages ranged from 18 to 55 years; 19.5% had a high school education or less, 58% had some college, and 22.5% had completed a bachelor's degree; 81.2% were White, 15.2% African American, 2.2% Asian, and 1.4% Hispanic. Volunteers were studied in six groups (four in the spring and two in the fall); $ns = 40$–60). Volunteers were paid $800 for their participation.

Experimental Plan

All volunteers came to the hospital for medical eligibility screenings. Participants were required to be free of disease based on examination and laboratory testing (see S. Cohen, Doyle, Skoner, Rabin, & Gwaltney, 1997). They also could not be pregnant or currently lactating or on a regular medication regimen. Social networks, health practices (except diet), age, education, race, gender, body weight, and height were also assessed at the screening and used as baseline data for those who were deemed eligible.

Eligible volunteers returned to the hospital both 4 and 5 weeks after screening to have blood drawn for assessment of NK cell activity (based on both blood draws) and antibody to the challenge virus (based on second blood draw). A personality questionnaire was administered twice, once at each blood draw. Participants also returned to the hospital during the 4th or 5th week after screening for the life stressor interview.

After completing life stressor, social network, personality, health practice, immune, and prechallenge antibody measures, participants entered quarantine. During the first 24 hr of quarantine (before viral exposure), they received a nasal examination (including a nasal wash culture for rhinovirus) and were excluded if there was any indication of recent or current URI or illness. An update life stressor interview was administered at this time to identify events occurring between the initial interview and quarantine. Baseline respiratory symptoms, nasal mucociliary clearance, and nasal mucus production were assessed at this time. Urine samples for endocrine assessment and information on dietary intake were also collected.

At the end of the first 24 hr of quarantine, participants were given nasal drops containing a low infectious dose of one of two types of rhinovirus (RV39 [$n = 147$] or Hanks [$n = 129$]). The quarantine continued for 5 days after exposure. During this period, they were housed individually but were allowed to interact with each other at a distance of 3 feet or more. Nasal secretion samples for virus culture were collected on each of the 5 days. Participants were also tested each day for respiratory symptoms, nasal mucociliary clearance, and nasal mucus production with the same procedures as used at baseline. Approximately 28 days after challenge, another blood sample was collected for serological testing. All investigators were unaware of participants' status on psychosocial, endocrine, health practice, immune, and prechallenge antibody measures.

Standard Control Variables

We used eight control variables that might provide alternative explanations for the relation between life stressors and colds. These included prechallenge antibody to the virus to which they were exposed, age, body mass index (weight in kilograms divided by height in meters squared), season (fall or spring), race (White or not), gender, education (high school graduate or less, some college, and bachelor's degree or greater), and virus type (RV39 or Hanks).

Life Stressor Assessment

Life stressors were assessed by a standardized semistructured interview, the Bedford College Life Events and Difficulties Schedule (LEDS; Brown & Harris, 1989; Harris, 1991). The LEDS provides a number of significant advantages over the checklist approach to the assessment of life events, including strict criteria for what constitutes a stressful life event; classification of each event on the basis of severity of threat, emotional significance, and domain of life experience in which it occurred (e.g., work, relationship); identification of the temporal course (onset and offset) of each event; and information on the extent to which persons of various levels of intimacy with the respondent are involved in the event. The LEDS has been found to have acceptable levels of reliability and validity (Brown & Harris, 1989; Wethington, Brown, & Kessler, 1995).

The LEDS diverges from other life stressor measures in providing consensually defined contextual ratings of threat. For example, although loss of employment receives a uniform score within many checklist approaches, the LEDS differentiates leaving an unsatisfying job because of lack of financial need from being fired after 20 years of dedicated and fulfilling service. Raters who are unaware of the individual's subjective response to an event are provided with extensive information regarding each event and the context in which it occurred, and then rely on thorough "dictionaries" of precedent examples to rate several scales, including long-term threat, timing of the event (onset and offset), and extent to which the event is focused on the participant or on others. The dictionary ratings are based on the likely response of an average person to an event occurring in the context of the participant's particular set of biographical circumstances.

The two primary scores provided by the LEDS indicate whether a severe acute event and whether a severe chronic difficulty was experienced during the last year. Acute events have durations of less than 1 month, and indeed most last only minutes or hours (e.g., a severe reprimand at work or a fight with a spouse). Difficulties typically last a month or more and involve the disruption of everyday routines (e.g., ongoing marital problems or unemployment). We use the LEDS terminology in referring to "acute stressful life events" but, to maintain consistency with common terminology in the field, refer to "chronic difficulties" as "chronic stressors."

Although the duration of an acute event is short, the impact may last months or years, and it is the long-term threat of the event that is thought to determine its implications for health. For this reason, we focused on those events that are rated as having marked or moderate long-term threat. After LEDS practice, we also included only those events in which the participant alone or together with a significant other is the major focus (e.g., excludes events focused on pets and possessions and events with sole focus on another person). We calculated two versions of acute events: one based on events that occurred during the previous year and the other limited to events that occurred during the previous 6 months.

We similarly focused on chronic stressors that are rated as having a high moderate or marked long-term threat. They also must not have ended more than 6 months before assessment (beginning of quarantine in our study). In calculating chronic stressors, we also excluded physical illness stressors in the volunteer to avoid confounding a chronic health condition with susceptibility. In our analyses, we compared three duration criteria for chronic stressors: 1, 3, and 6 months. The interview also classifies each chronic stressor into 1 of 10 domains: work, marital–partner relationship, other relationships, money–possessions, housing, crime–legal, education, reproduction, bereavement, and miscellaneous. Because of insufficient numbers of chronic stressors in some domains in our sample, we collapsed these into three categories: work, marital–partner or other relationships, and other stressors.

LEDS interviews were conducted by trained interviewers between 1 and 14 days before virus challenge with a short update interview on the first day of quarantine, just before challenge. Interviews were rated by a consensus group consisting of no fewer than four persons. Interviewing and rating were conducted in an independent laboratory with all staff unaware of other measures the study.

Pathways Linking Life Stressors to Susceptibility

Health practices and markers of endocrine and immune function were assessed before virus challenge as possible factors linking life stressors to susceptibility. Smokers were defined as those smoking cigarettes, cigars, or a pipe on a daily basis (S. Cohen, Tyrrell, Russell, Jarvis, & Smith, 1993). In calculating the average number of alcoholic drinks consumed per day, a bottle or can of beer, glass of wine, and shot of whiskey were each treated as a single drink (S. Cohen, Tyrrell, Russell, et al., 1993). Exercise was assessed by a question asking the number of times per week that the participant engaged in an activity long enough to work up a sweat, get the heart thumping, or get out of breath (Paffenbarger, Blair, Lee, & Hyde, 1993). Quality of sleep was measured by scales assessing subjective sleep quality, sleep latency, disturbance, and efficiency (percentage of time in bed sleeping; Buysse, Rey-

nolds, Monk, Berman, & Kupfer, 1989). Dietary intake of vitamin C and zinc was also assessed by standard questionnaire (Block, Hartman, & Naughton, 1990). Analyses including diet variables are limited to 228 participants who completed the questionnaire according to standard criteria (Block, Thompson, Hartman, Larkin, & Guire, 1992).

Epinephrine, norepinephrine, and cortisol were assessed as biological markers of stress at the time of viral exposure (Baum & Grunberg, 1995). These hormones were measured in 24-hr urine samples collected the day before virus challenge. High-performance liquid chromatography with electrochemical detection was used for measurement of the urinary catecholamines. Urinary cortisol assays were performed by a double-antibody competitive radioimmunoassay.

NK cell activity is thought to play an important role in limiting viral infection (Whiteside, Bryant, Day, & Herberman, 1990). NK cell activity was measured in the two blood samples drawn before virus challenge. We conducted a whole blood NK cell assay (Fletcher, Baron, Ashman, Fischl, & Klimas, 1987). The results of the two blood draws ($r = .50$, $p < .001$) were averaged to estimate cytotoxicity. We also assessed total number of white blood cells as well as total number of monocytes, neutrophils, eosinophils, and lymphocytes by a complete blood count with differential. Numbers of T (CD3+), B (CD19+), T helper (CD4+), cytotoxic/suppressor T (CD8+), and NK (CD16+CD56+) cells were determined with flow cytometry with appropriate monoclonal antibodies. Again, the cell counts were based on the average of the two blood samples. Correlations between cell counts from the two blood draws ranged from .62 to .82 ($p < .001$ for all correlations).

Alternative Explanations

We present data on personality characteristics and social network ties to assess whether associations between stress and the incidence of colds might be attributable to other individual or social factors.

Personality

The Big Five personality factors are thought to represent the basic structure of personality. The factors are commonly described as extraversion, agreeableness, conscientiousness, emotional stability, and openness. We used a modified version of Goldberg's (1992) adjective scale measure of the Big Five. Our version includes 50 adjectives, 10 for each factor. The scale was administered twice (at each blood draw), and we averaged the two scores. Correlations between the same subscales at the two administrations were .86 for extraversion, .84 for agreeableness, .87 for conscientiousness, .79 for emotional stability, and .81 for openness. Average of Cronbach's α for the two assessments ranged from .79 to .86.

Social Network Ties

We also examined the potential overlap between measures of stress and social networks. The Social Network Index assesses participation in 12 types of social relationships (S. Cohen et al., 1997). These include relationships with a spouse, parents, parents-in-law, children, other close family members, close neighbors, friends, coworkers, schoolmates, fellow volunteers, members of groups without religious affiliations (e.g., social, recreational, professional), and members of religious groups. One point was assigned for each type of relationship (possible score of 12) for which respondents indicate that they speak (in person or on the telephone) to someone in that relationship at least once every 2 weeks.

Infection and Illness

Infectious diseases result from the growth and action of microorganisms or parasites in the body (see S. Cohen & Williamson, 1991). Infection is the multiplication of an invading microorgan-

ism. Clinical disease occurs when infection is followed by the development of symptoms characteristic of the disease.

We used two common procedures for detecting infection by a specific virus. In the viral isolation procedure, nasal secretions were inoculated into cell cultures. If the virus is present in nasal secretions, it grows in the cell cultures and can be detected. Alternatively, one can indirectly assess the presence of a replicating virus by looking at changes in serum antibody levels to that virus. An invading microorganism (i.e., infection) triggers the immune system to produce antibody. Because each antibody recognizes only a single type of microorganism, the production of antibody to a specific infectious agent is evidence for the presence and activity of that agent.

Nasal washes were performed daily during quarantine to provide samples of nasal secretions for virus culture (Gwaltney, Colonno, Hamparian, & Turner, 1989). Neutralizing antibodies to the challenge virus were tested in pre- and 28-day postchallenge serum samples (Gwaltney et al., 1989). Serum antibody titers are reported as reciprocals of the initial dilution of serum.

On each day of quarantine, we collected two objective signs of disease—mucus weights and mucociliary clearance function—and one subjective measure—self-reported symptoms. Mucus weights were determined by collecting used tissues in sealed plastic bags (Doyle, McBride, Swarts, Hayden, & Gwaltney, 1988). The bags were weighed, and the weight of the tissues and bags was subtracted. To adjust for baseline, mucus weight on the day before challenge (mode = 0) was subtracted from each daily mucus weight after virus challenge. The adjusted postchallenge weights were summed to create an adjusted total mucus weight score.

Nasal mucociliary clearance function refers to the effectiveness of nasal cilia in clearing mucus from the nasal passage toward the nasopharynx. Clearance function was assessed as the time required for a dye administered into the nose to reach the nasopharynx (Doyle et al., 1988). Each daily time was adjusted (by subtracting) for baseline, and the adjusted average time in minutes was calculated across the postchallenge days of the trial.

On each day of quarantine, participants rated the severity of eight symptoms (congestion, runny nose, sneezing, cough, sore throat, malaise, headache, and chills) during the previous 24-hr period (Farr et al., 1990). Ratings ranged from 0 (*none*) to 4 (*very severe*) for each symptom. The symptom scores were summed within each day. The baseline (24 hr before challenge) score (mode = 0) was subtracted from each daily score. Finally, adjusted daily symptoms were summed across the 5 postchallenge days to create a total symptom score. Participants were also asked each day whether they had a cold.

Volunteers were considered to have a cold if they were both infected and met illness criteria. They were classified as infected if the challenge virus was isolated on any of the 5 postchallenge study days or there was a fourfold or greater rise in virus-specific serum neutralizing antibody titer. The illness criterion was based on selected objective indicators of illness: a total adjusted mucus weight of at least 10 g or an adjusted average mucociliary nasal clearance time of at least 7 mins. By basing the definition of a cold entirely on objective indicators, we are able to exclude interpretations of our data based on psychological influences on symptom reporting.

There is substantial evidence for the validity of the objective criterion. Those participants with colds by this criterion had higher mean total adjusted symptom scores ($M = 19.28$, $SD = 14.7$) than those without ($M = 5.67$, $SD = 8.1$), $t(274) = -9.88$, $p < .001$. The percentage of those developing colds decreased with increasing prechallenge antibody titers (63% for <2; 40% for 2, 4; 15% for 8, 16; 9% for 32, 64; $p < .001$). There was also reasonable concordance between the objective criterion and traditional criteria based on self-reported symptoms (80% agree-

ment for RV39 and 74% for Hanks). Finally, only 3.6% of those meeting either clearance time or mucus weight criteria were not infected based on viral culture or antibody response.

Statistical Analyses

We used stepwise logistic regression to predict the binary outcome incidence of a cold (Hosmer & Lemeshow, 1989) and multiple linear regression to predict continuous outcomes (J. Cohen & Cohen, 1975). To provide an estimate of relative risk, we present odds ratios (ORs) and 95% confidence intervals (CIs) based on a comparison of persons with and without acute events and with and without chronic stressors. These ORs provide an estimate of how much more likely it is that an outcome (e.g., colds) would occur in those with versus those without events or those with versus those without chronic stressors. We sequentially added variables to the first step of regression analyses to determine whether the association between acute stressful events or chronic stressors (entered in second step) and susceptibility to colds is substantially reduced after controlling for the contribution of other variables.

Results

Rates of Infections and Colds

Participants can be infected (replicate virus) without developing a cold. Ninety-nine percent who entered the trial without antibody (titer of ≤2) to the virus to which they were exposed were infected, whereas 69% of those with antibody (titer of ≥4) were infected. This resulted in a total infection rate of 84%. Fifty-eight percent of those without antibody developed colds, whereas only 19% of those with antibody developed colds. This resulted in a total of 40% of participants with colds.

Table 78.1

Percentages (and numbers) of persons with colds for chronic stressors lasting at least 1 month, 3 months, and 6 months, stratified by prechallenge antibody titer and virus

Prechallenge antibody titer and virus type	≥1 month		≥3 months		≥6 months	
	No chronic stressor	Chronic stressor	No chronic stressor	Chronic stressor	No chronic stressor	Chronic stressor
≤2						
RV39	60.4 (32/53)	72.2 (13/18)	58.2 (32/55)	81.3 (13/16)	59.6 (34/57)	78.6 (11/14)
Hanks	46.4 (26/56)	76.5 (13/17)	46.4 (26/56)	76.5 (13/17)	48.3 (29/60)	76.9 (10/13)
Both viruses	53.2 (58/109)	74.3 (26/35)	52.3 (58/111)	78.8 (26/33)	53.8 (63/117)	77.8 (21/27)
≥4						
RV39	20.4 (10/49)	33.3 (9/27)	19.2 (10/52)	37.5 (9/24)	21.4 (12/56)	35.0 (7/20)
Hanks	9.3 (4/43)	15.4 (2/13)	9.3 (4/43)	15.4 (2/13)	8.9 (4/45)	18.2 (2/11)
Both viruses	15.2 (14/92)	27.5 (11/40)	14.7 (14/95)	29.7 (11/37)	15.8 (16/101)	29.0 (9/31)
Total	35.8 (72/201)	49.3 (37/75)	35.0 (72/206)	52.9 (37/70)	36.2 (79/218)	51.7 (30/58)

Note. The first number in each set of parentheses is the number of people with colds, and the second number is the number of participants.

Standard Controls and Susceptibility

As we have reported elsewhere (S. Cohen et al., 1997), when the eight standard controls were entered into the regression simultaneously to test the independent contribution of each control variable, incidence of colds decreased with increased antibody titers ($p < .001$) and increased with age ($p < .03$) and exposure to RV39 as opposed to Hanks ($p < .03$). Unexpectedly, the most colds occurred among those with high school diplomas or less education followed by college graduates; the fewest colds occurred among those with some college education ($p < .04$).

Acute Stressful Life Events, Chronic Stressors, and Susceptibility

A total of 179 participants had at least one event occurring within 1 year of study onset, and 119 had at least one event occurring within 6 months. Neither acute events during the 12 months (43%

colds for those with events vs. 33% for those without; adjusted OR = 1.4; CI = .76, 2.55) or 6 months (40% colds for those with events vs. 39% for those without; adjusted OR = 1.0; CI = .54, 1.74) preceding quarantine were associated with the likelihood of developing a cold.

A total of 75 participants had a chronic stressor lasting 1 month or longer, 70 had a chronic stressor lasting 3 months or longer, and 58 had a chronic stressor lasting 6 months or longer. Table 78.1 presents rates of colds for those with and without chronic stressors stratified by virus type and by prechallenge antibody status. As apparent from Table 78.1, those with chronic stressors were at higher risk for colds than those without irrespective of the duration criterion applied (1-month adjusted OR = 2.2, CI = 1.08, 4.34; 3-month adjusted OR = 2.9, CI = 1.39, 5.88; 6-month adjusted OR = 2.3, CI = 1.10, 4.94). Moreover, there were no interactions between any of the standard control variables and chronic stressors in predicting colds. Hence, the relations were similar for the two virus types, for

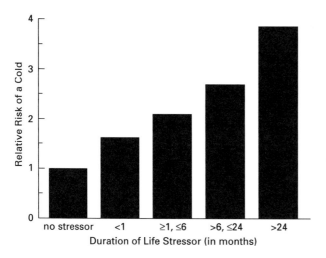

Figure 78.1
Relative risk (odds ratio adjusted for standard controls) of developing a cold contrasting persons with stressors of varying duration with those without any stressor. Participants are grouped by their longest stressor.

different levels of serological status, age, gender, race, education, and body mass and across the two seasons. Of special note for interpretation of our data is the similar association between chronic stressors and rates of colds across virus types and across prechallenge seropositive and seronegative results (observed [unadjusted] rates are presented in Table 78.1).

In an additional analysis, we compared the risk of developing colds among persons with stressors of different durations. Each participant was assigned to a group based on his or her longest stressor (including acute and chronic stressors as determined by the LEDS). The groups were as follows: no acute or chronic stressor ($n = 83$), a stressor lasting less than 1 month ($n = 118$), a stressor lasting at least 1 month but not exceeding 6 months ($n = 17$), a stressor lasting more than 6 months but not exceeding 2 years ($n = 32$), and a stressor lasting more than 2 years ($n = 26$). As depicted in Figure 78.1, there was a linear increase in the relative risk for colds with increased duration of the

stressor. However, when broken into these small groups, only the last OR (more than 2 years) was reliably greater than 1.0.

To assess the independent association of chronic stressors and acute events and the possibility that chronic stressors and acute events might interact, we fit a regression equation in which the standard controls were entered in the first step, whether or not the participant (a) had a chronic stressor lasting at least 3 months and (b) had an acute event during the last 12 months in the second step, and the interaction of chronic stressors and acute events in the last. Again, the occurrence of a chronic stressor (OR = 2.8, CI = 1.32, 5.74) was associated with developing a cold, but the occurrence of an event was not (OR = 1.2, CI = .62, 2.21). There was a marginal interaction ($\beta = 1.4$, $p < .13$) suggesting that having a chronic stressor without an event (69% colds) was associated with greater risk for colds than a chronic stressor accompanied by an event (49%), and event alone (40%), or neither a chronic stressor nor an event (27%). Identical

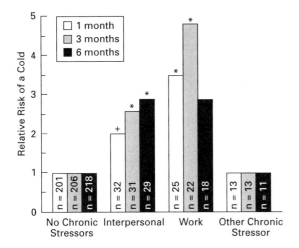

Figure 78.2
Relative risk (odds ratio adjusted for standard controls) of developing a cold contrasting persons with interpersonal, work, and other chronic stressors with those with no chronic stressors. The odds ratios are derived from separate analyses using the "at least 1 month," "at least 3 months," and "at least 6 months" criteria for chronic stressors. Sample sizes are indicated inside each bar. * $P < .05$; + $P < .15$.

analyses using the 1- and 6-month duration criteria for chronic stressors yielded similar results (interaction with 1 month, $\beta = 1.5$, $p < .09$; with 6 month, $\beta = 1.7$, $p < .08$).

We were also interested in examining whether the type (domain) of the chronic stressor mattered in predicting susceptibility. Chronic stressors were categorized into three domains: interpersonal, work, and other. Seventeen people had more than one stressor lasting 1 month or longer. For the purpose of these analyses, those with a work or interpersonal stressor were assigned to those categories irrespective of whether or not they had another type of chronic stressor (six overlaps with work and six with interpersonal stressors). However, the 5 persons with both work and interpersonal stressors were excluded. (Three of these 5 persons developed colds.) We then fit logistic regression equations, including standard control variables, in which each of the three domains (work, interpersonal, other) was contrasted with the group of

participants not experiencing a chronic stressor (OR = 1). Three separate equations were fit: 1-, 3-, and 6-month criteria for a chronic stressor. As apparent from Figure 78.2, having either a work or interpersonal chronic stressor was associated with greater risk for colds in comparison with those with no chronic stressor. The effect of a chronic work stressor is attenuated (and drops below statistical significance) when a 6-month criterion is applied. Having other types of chronic stressors was not associated with greater risk for colds.

We considered the possibility that chronic stressors at work were in fact interpersonal stressors as well. To pursue this issue, we had each of the 30 (1-month criterion) chronic stressors coded by two coders for interpersonal content (criteria from Johnson, Monroe, Simons, & Thase, 1994). Only 2 of the 30 were found to be interpersonal conflicts at work. However, 27 were attributable to unemployment or underemployment.

Finally, we considered the possibility that those with a work or an interpersonal stressor had more chronic stressors than those with another type of stressor. The differences between groups did not approach significance (1.2 chronic stressors for work, 1.3 for relationships, and 1.1 for other). Nor was there an association between number of chronic stressors (for those with at least one stressor) and colds.

Pathways Linking Chronic Stressors to Colds

Because the association between chronic stressors and incidence of colds was greatest using a 3-month criterion, we used 3-month or longer stressors in testing potential pathways.

Pathogenic Mechanisms

Amount of viral replication (over the 5 days after exposure) was assessed as a possible mechanism responsible for greater incidence of colds among persons with chronic stressors. Greater replication was associated with a greater likelihood of developing a cold (adjusted $\beta = 1.04 \pm .18$, $p < .001$ for all participants; $\beta = .93 \pm .19$, $p < .001$ for infected participants only). Although higher mean replication was found in persons with chronic stressors, this relation was only marginal: mean for chronic stressors, $1.76 \log_{10}$ titer, and mean for no stressors, $1.62 \log_{10}$ titer; $F(1, 263) = 2.02$, $p < .16$, for all participants; mean for chronic stressors, $2.17 \log_{10}$ titer, and mean for no stressors, $1.89 \log_{10}$ titer; $F(1, 220) = 2.82$, $p < .10$, for infected participants only. When we added total viral replication as an additional control variable, it had little effect on the relation between chronic stressors and colds (Table 78.2).

Health Practices

As we have reported earlier (S. Cohen et al., 1997), smokers (adjusted for standard controls $OR = 3.0$, $CI = 1.48, 6.06$), persons exercising two or fewer times a week (adjusted $OR = 1.8$, $CI = 1.01, 3.24$), those with sleep efficiency of

Table 78.2
Odds of developing a cold for persons with chronic stressors (3-month criterion) in comparison to those without chronic stressors when different explanatory variables are controlled for

Explanatory variables in equation	Odds ratio (95% CI)
Eight standard control variables (SC)	2.9 (1.39–5.88)
Testing pathways	
SC and total viral replication	2.5 (1.16–5.56)
SC and health practices	2.2 (1.02–4.61)
SC and endocrine and immune markers	2.7 (1.26–5.70)
Testing alternative explanations	
SC and personality (extraversion/ introversion)	2.7 (1.30–5.60)
SC and social network diversity	2.6 (1.27–5.48)

Note. The explanatory variables are added to the first step of the equation, and chronic stressors are entered into the second step. CI = confidence interval.

.80 or less (adjusted $OR = 2.6$, $CI = 1.16, 5.78$), those drinking one or fewer drinks per day (adjusted $OR = 2.0$, $CI = 1.02, 3.84$), and those who ingest 85 mg or less of vitamin C a day (adjusted $OR = 2.0$, $CI = 1.04, 3.82$) were all at greater risk for developing colds. There were no associations between zinc ingestion and colds or between the other sleep measures and colds. Table 78.3 presents the relation between each of these health practices and having a chronic stressor lasting 3 months or longer. Those with chronic stressors were more likely to be smokers. There were also marginal associations between having a stressor and less exercise and poorer sleep efficiency.

To determine whether health practices might operate as pathways through which chronic stressors were related to colds, smoking status, exercise frequency, sleep efficiency, vitamin C, and alcohol consumption were entered along with the standard controls in the first step of the

Table 78.3
Percentages of persons with health practice and endocrine risk factors for colds stratified by experience of a chronic stressor lasting 3 months or longer

Variable	Chronic stressor	No chronic stressor	Odds ratio	CI
Health practices				
Smokers	51.4	28.6	2.95	1.49–5.85
Exercising ≤ 2 times/week	62.9	49.0	1.57	0.86–2.86
With sleep efficiency ≤ .80	27.1	16.5	1.87	0.91–3.85
Drinking ≤ 1 drink/day	71.4	69.1	0.94	0.48–1.84
Ingesting ≤ 85 mg vitamin C per day	39.0	37.9	1.01	0.52–1.94
Endocrine measures				
≥ 3.78 μg/24 hr[a] of epinephrine	47.8	51.0	0.90	0.46–1.77
≥ 29.7 μg/24 hr[a] of norepinephrine	58.0	47.6	1.05	0.57–1.95
≥ 33 μg/24 hr[a] of cortisol	52.2	50.5	1.25	0.67–2.34

Note. Odds ratios adjusted for standard control variables are reported along with 95% confidence intervals (CI). The odds ratios indicate the likelihood that the specific risk factor would be present among those with chronic stressors as opposed to those without. Analysis of vitamin C was done on a subsample of 228 participants who completed the diet questionnaires accurately.
a. Median value.

regression equation. Simultaneous addition of all of these health practices to the regression equation slightly reduced the association between chronic stressors and susceptibility to colds (OR = 2.1, CI = 0.92, 4.84, $n = 226$ compared with OR = 2.7, CI = 1.23, 5.86 with the same reduced sample standard controls only). Similar results were obtained when diet was dropped from this analysis and the entire sample of 274 (with complete data on all variables in equation) was used (see Table 78.2).

Hormones and Immune Markers
We have reported elsewhere (S. Cohen et al., 1997) that persons with levels of norepinephrine above the median level (29.6 μg/total volume) were at greater risk for developing colds than those with levels below the median (OR = 1.9, CI = 1.04, 3.50). A similar but weaker relation was found for epinephrine (median = 3.78 μg/ total volume; OR = 1.8, CI = 0.94, 3.58. Cortisol levels, NK cell cytotoxicity, and the blood cell counts were not associated with colds.

None of the endocrine measures were associated with experiencing a chronic stressor (see Table 78.3). Among those with chronic stressors, helper T cells (750 ± 232/mm³) were higher than in those without (638 ± 227/mm³), $F(1, 262) = 5.38$, $p < .03$. There was also a marginal association between having a stressor and greater numbers of neutrophils (with chronic stressor 4,160 ± 1,374/mm³; without stressor 3,714 ± 1,345/mm³), $F(1, 263) = 2.39$, $p < .13$.

We entered as controls any endocrine or immune measure we found to be even marginally associated with either chronic stressors or with colds. Hence, epinephrine, norepinephrine, number of helper T cells, and number of neutrophils were entered along with the standard controls in the first step of the regression equation. Simultaneous addition of all of these hormone and immune measures to the regression equation did not substantially alter the association between chronic stressors and susceptibility to colds (see Table 78.2). Hence, none of these variables were primary contributors to the association between chronic stressors and colds in this study.

Alternative Explanations

Personality
We have reported that only extraversion was associated with susceptibility; those with low scores ("introverts," below median of 28.5) were at greater risk for colds (adjusted OR = 2.7, CI = 1.45, 4.92) in this sample (S. Cohen et al., 1997). Extraversion scores were not associated with having a chronic stressor (28.2 for those with stressor vs. 26.8 for those without), adjusted for standard controls, $F(1, 263) = 1.86$, $p < .18$. Moreover, adding extraversion to the regression equation, including standard controls and chronic stressors lasting 3 months or longer, did not substantially reduce the relation between chronic stressors and incidence of colds (see Table 78.2). The interaction between chronic stressors and extraversion did not reach significance, suggesting that the stressor effect is relatively similar across introverts and extraverts.

Social Network Ties
We have reported elsewhere that greater social network diversity was associated with less susceptibility in this sample (adjusted OR = 4.2 [1.34, 13.29] comparing those with one to three roles with those with six or more; S. Cohen et al., 1997). Social network diversity was marginally associated with having a chronic stressor (5.5 ± 1.9 roles for those with stressors and 5.8 ± 1.7 roles for those without), adjusted for standard controls, $F(1, 263) = 2.91$, $p < .09$. However, adding network diversity to the regression equation only slightly reduced the relation between chronic stressors and incidence of colds (see Table 78.2). There was also no interaction between chronic stressors and network diversity, suggesting that the chronic stressor effect was similar across levels of social network diversity.

Discussion

This study provides additional supporting evidence for the role of psychological stress in susceptibility to upper respiratory infectious disease (see, e.g., virus-challenge studies by S. Cohen et al., 1991; Stone et al., 1993; epidemiologic studies by Graham, Douglas, & Ryan, 1986; Meyer & Haggerty, 1962). It also furthers our understanding of the types of stressors that alter host resistance. Although acute (lasting less than 1 month) stressful events did not alter susceptibility to colds, enduring chronic stressors (lasting 1 month or longer) were associated with greater susceptibility to rhinovirus-induced colds. Moreover, there was some indication that the longer the duration of the stressor, the greater was the risk for colds. These relations were unaffected by controls for prechallenge virus-specific antibody, age, education, race, gender, body mass, season, and virus type. They also occurred equally across demographic characteristics and variations in body mass, season, virus type, and prechallenge serostatus. Persons experiencing chronic stressors associated with marked or severe long-term threats were between two and three times more likely to develop colds than those without such an experience. This result supports the generally held (but seldom tested) hypothesis that chronic stressors are a more important determinant of disease risk than are acute stressful events (e.g., Lepore, Miles, & Levy, 1997). This may be viewed as inconsistent with some of the self-reported illness epidemiology studies that suggest that acute dips in positive daily events in the days just before the onset of an illness are markers of risk (Evans & Edgerton, 1991; Evans, Pitts, & Smith, 1988; Stone, Bruce, & Neale, 1984). This discrepancy may be attributable to limitations of the epidemiological studies, including the possibility of premorbid influences of infection on daily events, and to influences of daily events on self-report of illness. Alternatively, the difference may be attributable to the kinds of events being studied: the acute events that constitute marked or severe long-term threats as assessed by the LEDS in contrast to the minor day-to-day events and associated acute affective changes assessed in the epidemiological studies.

Chronic stressors based on interpersonal conflicts (relative risk as high as 2.9) and problems concerning work (relative risk as high as 4.8; mostly attributable to under- and unemployment) were primarily responsible for the associations found in this study. Because many types of chronic stressors had low (or no) frequencies in our sample, this result should not be interpreted as meaning that these are the only types of enduring stressors that place people at risk. Instead, it indicates that these stressors, when they occur, are potent. These results are, however, consistent with other evidence that both interpersonal conflicts (Bolger, DeLongis, Kessler, & Schilling, 1989; Brown & Harris, 1989; Kiecolt-Glaser et al., 1993) and unemployment (Kasl, 1978) are detrimental to health.

Although the association (Chronic Stressors × Acute Events interaction) was marginal, the finding that having a concurrent event was protective for persons with chronic stressors is provocative. It is consistent with some evidence from the mental health literature (McGonagle & Kessler, 1990), and suggests the possibility that events distract from chronic stressors rather than accumulate to create greater impact.

Altered host susceptibility for those experiencing a chronic stressor could be a manifestation of a more virulent course of infection as indicated by greater viral replication. Although those with chronic stressors shed marginally greater amounts of virus than those without, amount of viral shedding accounted for only a small proportion of the relation between chronic stressors and the development of colds. These results suggest that chronic stressors may be associated with more than one disease process (i.e., extent of viral replication and a process or processes that modulate the production of cold signs and symptoms).

Although chronic stressors were associated with several behavioral risk factors for colds (including being a smoker, exercising fewer than two times a week, and poor sleep quality) together these accounted for only a small part of the relation between experiencing a chronic stressor and developing a cold. These results are consistent with our failure in an earlier virus-challenge study to explain the relation between psychological stress and colds by differences in health practices (S. Cohen et al., 1991) as well as a similar failure in an epidemiological study of psychological stress and self-reported URI (Turner Cobb & Steptoe, 1996). In the context of finding associations between smoking, alcohol consumption, sleep quality, diet, and exercise and colds, the failure of these health practices to explain the relation between stress and colds increases our confidence that this relation is not primarily mediated by health practices.

We were surprised that chronic stressors were not associated with elevated epinephrine, norepinephrine, or cortisol, hormones whose elevation is generally associated with chronic psychological stress (Baum & Grunberg, 1995). Elevated levels of epinephrine and norepinephrine were associated with greater risk for colds. These hormones are sensitive to relatively low levels of psychological stress as well as to the severe threats that are represented by chronic stressors (difficulties) in the LEDS (Baum & Grunberg, 1995). Hence, it is possible that any association with chronic stressors might be obscured by other less severe stressful experiences that are not picked up by the LEDS. For example, it might be variations in the acute elevation of epinephrine and norepinephrine in response to anxiety about the virus challenge or quarantine period that is responsible for the variation in catecholamines that is associated with susceptibility to colds.

We can only speculate on what mechanisms might mediate the association of chronic stressors and colds. Our data suggest eliminating a number of possibilities. At least for those who were seronegative before viral inoculation, the relation was attributable to increased colds among infected persons (99% were infected) and not increased incidence of infection. This result is consistent with those of earlier studies of stressful life events (S. Cohen et al., 1991; Stone et al., 1993). The similarity of the association across serostatus also suggests that the mechanism is not primarily mediated by a memory antibody response. In addition, we found little evidence here for the role of either numbers of circulating white blood cell populations or NK cell activity. It is possible, however, that other characteristics of immune status operate as pathways. For example, behavioral effects on cytokine release in the nasal passage may effect the triggering of symptoms (Akira & Kishimoto, 1992). It is also possible that these associations are mediated not by the immune system but rather by effects of chronic stressors on the nasal mucosa with resultant changes in airflow, ciliary movement, and local membrane defense that might increase susceptibility (Swartz, 1991).

Acknowledgments

This work was supported by National Institute of Mental Health Grant MH50429, Research Scientist Development and Senior Scientist Awards from the National Institute of Mental Health (MH00721), National Institutes of Health Grant NCRR/GCRC 5M01 RR00056 to the University of Pittsburgh Medical Center General Clinical Research Center, and National Institute of Mental Health Grant MH30915 to the Mental Health Research Center for Affective Disorder. Supplemental support was also provided by the Fetzer Institute and the John D. and Catherine T. MacArthur Foundation.

We are indebted to Janet Schlarb, James Seroky, Pat Fall, Susan Strelinski, Darleen Noah, Barbara Anderson, the staff of the General Clinical Research Center, the LEDS interviewers from the Depression and Manic-Depression Prevention Program, Theresa Whiteside and Robert McDonald and their laboratory staffs, and the volunteers for their contributions to the research. We also thank Stephen Lepore for his comments on an earlier draft of this chapter.

References

Akira, S., & Kishimoto, T. (1992). IL-6 and NF-IL6 in acute phase response and infection. *Immunological Reviews, 127,* 25–50.

Baum, A., & Grunberg, N. (1995). Measurement of stress hormones. In S. Cohen, R. C. Kessler, & L. Underwood Gordon (Eds.), *Measuring stress* (pp. 175–192). New York: Oxford University Press.

Block, G., Hartman, A. M., & Naughton, D. (1990). A reduced dietary questionnaire: Development and validation. *Epidemiology, 1,* 58–64.

Block, G., Thompson, F. E., Hartman, A. M., Larkin, F. A., & Guire, K. E. (1992). Comparison of two dietary questionnaires validated against multiple dietary records collected during a 1-year period. *Journal of the American Dietetic Association, 92,* 686–693.

Bolger, N., DeLongis, A., Kessler, R. C., & Schilling, E. A. (1989). Effects of daily stress on negative mood. *Journal of Personality and Social Psychology, 57,* 808–817.

Broadbent, D. E., Broadbent, M. H. P., Phillpotts, R. J., & Wallace, J. (1984). Some further studies on the prediction of experimental colds in volunteers by psychological factors. *Journal of Psychosomatic Research, 28,* 511–523.

Brown, G. W., & Harris, T. O. (Eds.). (1989). *Life events and illness.* New York: Guilford Press.

Buysse, D. J., Reynolds, C. F., Monk, T. H., Berman, S. R., & Kupfer, D. J. (1989). The Pittsburgh Sleep Quality Index. *Psychiatry Research, 28,* 193–213.

Clover, R. D., Abell, T., Becker, L. A., Crawford, S., & Ramsey, C. N. (1989). Family functioning and stress as predictors of influenza B infection. *The Journal of Family Practice, 28,* 536–539.

Cohen, J., & Cohen, P. (1975). *Applied multiple regression/correlation analysis for the behavioral sciences.* Hillsdale, NJ: Erlbaum.

Cohen, S., Doyle, W. J., Skoner, D. P., Rabin, B. S., & Gwaltney, J. M., Jr. (1997). Social ties and susceptibility to the common cold. *Journal of the American Medical Association, 277,* 1940–1944.

Cohen, S., Tyrrell, D. A. J., Russell, M. A. H., Jarvis, M. J., & Smith, A. P. (1993). Smoking, alcohol consumption and susceptibility to the common cold. *American Journal of Public Health, 83,* 1277–1283.

Cohen, S., Tyrrell, D. A. J., & Smith, A. P. (1991). Psychological stress and susceptibility to the common cold. *New England Journal of Medicine, 325,* 606–612.

Cohen, S., Tyrrell, D. A. J., & Smith, A. P. (1993). Life events, perceived stress, negative affect and susceptibility to the common cold. *Journal of Personality and Social Psychology, 64,* 131–140.

Cohen, S., & Williamson, G. M. (1991). Stress and infectious disease in humans. *Psychological Bulletin, 109,* 5–24.

Doyle, W. J., McBride, T. P., Swarts, J. D., Hayden, F. G., & Gwaltney, J. M., Jr. (1988). The response of the nasal airway, middle ear and Eustachian tube to provocative rhinovirus challenge. *American Journal of Rhinology, 2,* 149–154.

Evans, P. D., & Edgerton, N. (1991). Life-events and mood as predictors of the common cold. *British Journal of Medical Psychology, 64,* 35–44.

Evans, P. D., Pitts, M. K., & Smith, K. (1988). Minor infection, minor life events and the four day desirability dip. *Journal of Psychosomatic Research, 32,* 533–539.

Farr, B. M., Gwaltney, J. M., Hendley, J. O., Hayden, F. G., Naclerio, R. M., McBride, T., Doyle, W. J., Sorrentino, J. V., & Proud, D. (1990). A randomized controlled trial of glucocorticoid prophylaxis against experimental rhinovirus infection. *Journal of Infectious Diseases, 162,* 1173–1177.

Fletcher, M. A., Baron, G. C., Ashman, M. R., Fischl, M. A., & Klimas, N. G. (1987). Use of whole blood methods in assessment of immune parameters in immunodeficiency. *Diagnostic and Clinical Immunology, 5,* 68–91.

Glaser, R., Rice, J., Sheridan, J., Fertel, R., Stout, J., Speicher, C. E., Pinsky, D., Kotur, M., Post, A., Beck, M., & Kiecolt-Glaser, J. K. (1987). Stress-related immune suppression: Health implications. *Brain, Behavior, and Immunity, 1,* 7–20.

Goldberg, L. R. (1992). The development of markers for the Big-Five factor structure. *Psychological Assessment, 4,* 26–42.

Graham, N. M. H., Douglas, R. B., & Ryan, P. (1986). Stress and acute respiratory infection. *American Journal of Epidemiology, 124,* 389–401.

Greene, W. A., Betts, R. F., Ochitill, H. N., Iker, H. P., & Douglas, R. G. (1978). Psychosocial factors and immunity: Preliminary report. *Psychosomatic Medicine, 40,* 87.

Gwaltney, J. M., Jr., Colonno, R. J., Hamparian, V. V., & Turner, R. B. (1989). Rhinovirus. In N. J. Schmidt & R. W. Emmons (Eds.), *Diagnostic procedures for viral, rickettsial and chlamydial infections* (6th ed., pp. 579–614). Washington, DC: American Public Health Association.

Harris, T. O. (1991). Life stress and illness: The question of specificity. *Annals of Behavioral Medicine, 13,* 211–219.

Hosmer, D. W., Jr., & Lemeshow, S. (1989). *Applied logistic regression.* New York: Wiley.

Johnson, S. L., Monroe, S., Simons, A., & Thase, M. E. (1994). Clinical characteristics associated with interpersonal depression: Symptoms, course and treatment response. *Journal of Affective Disorders, 31,* 97–109.

Kasl, S. V. (1978). Epidemiological contributions to the study of work stress. In C. I. Cooper & R. Payne (Eds.), *Stress at work* (pp. 3–48). New York: Wiley.

Kiecolt-Glaser, J. K., Malarkey, W. B., Chee, M., Newton, T., Cacioppo, J. T., Mao, H.-Y., & Glaser, R. (1993). Negative behavior during marital conflict is associated with immunological down-regulation. *Psychosomatic Medicine, 55,* 395–409.

Lepore, S. J., Miles, H. J., & Levy, J. S. (1997). Relation of chronic and episodic stressors to psychological distress, reactivity, and health problems. *International Journal of Behavioral Medicine, 4,* 39–59.

Locke, S. E., & Heisel, J. S. (1977). The influence of stress and emotions on the human immune response. *Biofeedback and Self-Regulation, 2,* 320.

McGonagle, K. A., & Kessler, R. C. (1990). Chronic stress, acute stress, and depressive symptoms. *American Journal of Community Psychology, 18,* 681–706.

Meyer, R. J., & Haggerty, R. J. (1962). Streptococcal infections in families. *Pediatrics, 29,* 539–549.

Paffenbarger, R. S., Jr., Blair, S. N., Lee, I., & Hyde, R. T. (1993). Measurement of physical activity to assess health effects in free-living populations. *Medicine and Science in Sports and Exercise, 25,* 60–70.

Stone, A. A., Bovbjerg, D. H., Neale, J. M., Napoli, A., Valdimarsdottir, H., & Gwaltney, J. M., Jr. (1993). Development of common cold symptoms following experimental rhinovirus infection is related to prior stressful life events. *Behavioral Medicine, 8*, 115–120.

Stone, A. A., Bruce, R., & Neale, J. M. (1984). Changes in daily event frequency precede episodes of physical symptoms. *Journal of Human Stress, 46*, 892.

Swartz, M. N. (1991). Editorial: Stress and the common cold. *New England Journal of Medicine, 325*, 654–655.

Totman, R., Kiff, J., Reed, S. E., & Craig, J. W. (1980). Predicting experimental colds in volunteers from different measures of recent life stress. *Journal of Psychosomatic Research, 24*, 155–163.

Turner Cobb, J. M., & Steptoe, A. (1996). Psychosocial stress and susceptibility to upper respiratory tract illness in an adult population sample. *Psychosomatic Medicine, 58*, 404–412.

Wethington, E., Brown, G. W., & Kessler, R. C. (1995). Interview measurement of stressful life events. In S. Cohen, R. C. Kessler, & L. Underwood Gordon (Eds.), *Measuring stress* (pp. 59–79). New York: Oxford University Press.

Whiteside, T. L., Bryant, J., Day, R., & Herberman, R. B. (1990). Natural killer cytotoxicity in the diagnosis of immune dysfunction: Criteria for a reproducible assay. *Journal of Clinical Laboratory Analysis, 4*, 102–114.

Sarah S. Knox and Kerstin Uvnäs-Moberg

Introduction

Accumulating data from longitudinal epidemiological research has provided evidence that social isolation can increase risk of morbidity and mortality from all causes (Berkman and Syme, 1979; Blazer, 1982; House et al., 1982; Kaplan et al., 1988; Orth-Gomer and Johnson, 1987; Schoenback et al., 1986; Seeman et al., 1993; Welin et al., 1985). The strength of this research is that these studies have utilized prospective, population-based cohorts, have had few losses to follow-up, and have controlled for relevant covariates (Berkman, 1995).

Although the increased relative risk for mortality from social isolation includes a broad range of diseases, the present chapter will be confined to a discussion of the relationship between social ties and cardiovascular disease (CVD) risk. Since CVD kills more men and women than any other disease, including all malignant neoplasms combined (Kochanek and Hudson, 1994), and since evidence for a connection between social isolation and primary and secondary CVD endpoints is now strong, a deeper understanding of mediating mechanisms will hopefully improve our efforts at treatment and prevention.

There are three types of studies which have shown a relationship between low social affiliation and cardiovascular risk: prospective and cross-sectional epidemiological studies, studies of post myocardial infarction patients and cardiovascular reactivity studies. With respect to prospective epidemiological data, there is evidence for a significant independent association between low social support and subsequent cardiovascular morbidity (Hedblad et al., 1992; Orth-Gomer et al., 1993; Seeman and Syme, 1987; Woloshin et al., 1997) and mortality (Berkman and Syme, 1979; House et al., 1982; Kaplan et al., 1988; Kawachi et al., 1996; Welin et al., 1992). Research in post myocardial infarction patients

also provides strong evidence that patients with high social support have fewer rehospitalizations (Helgeson, 1991) and survive longer (Berkman et al., 1992; Case et al., 1992; Oxman et al., 1995) than patients who are more socially isolated.

With respect to cardiovascular reactivity to acute psychological stressors, several studies report attenuated responses in conditions with a supporting other present. Lepore et al. (1993) reported lower increases in systolic blood pressure in both sexes during a condition with a supportive other in comparison to being alone or with a non-supportive other before and during a speech stressor. The same tendency was shown for diastolic pressure but was significant only between conditions of supportive versus non-supportive other. These effects were not moderated by gender. Kamarck et al. (1990) found reduced heart rate and blood pressure responses in women to two laboratory tasks under conditions with a friend present as opposed to being alone. In another study on women (Kamarck et al., 1995), he again found attenuated blood pressure responses to challenges but only under conditions of "high threat." Finally, Gerin et al. (1992) and Gerin et al. (1995) reported two experiments on women who were exposed to psychological challenge in the presence or absence of a supportive other. In the first study, heart rate and blood pressure reactivity were lower in the support condition. In the second study, which investigated the interaction with level of stress, diastolic blood pressure was lower in the support condition under "high" stress but not during "low" stress. A study by Kirschbaum et al. (1995) that tested the influence of social support on cortisol response showed gender specific responses with respect to cortisol reactivity. Men but not women had an attenuated cortisol response in a partner support condition during anticipation of public speaking. While the results of reactivity studies are not totally consistent (three others found no differences between the friend and alone condition and one reports higher reactivity in the presence of a friend), a review of reactivity and social support literature (Uchino et al., 1996) points out that these latter studies may have been confounded by interactions involving performance pressure (as evidenced by a faster rate of response) in the presence of a friend and gender of the experimenter in relation to participants.

To understand the way in which psychosocial influences are linked to CVD, it is important to see them in a context. Genetic predisposition explains a significant amount of the variance in major CVD risk factors such as lipid metabolism, hypertension, obesity and diabetes. However, the interaction of the genotype with the environment determines the extent to which these factors are expressed. It is in this phenotypical context that psychosocial factors can play a crucial role. There are primarily two types of interactions which mediate these influences. The first, or behavioral pathway, involves the association between psychosocial factors and health behaviors (e.g. smoking, diet, exercise, alcohol consumption) which influence risk. The second, or neuroendocrine pathway, includes feedback loops between the brain and CVD relevant physiological systems. Though the present chapter gives a short summary of the data concerning behavioral mediators of social support and CVD outcome, these are fairly self-evident. Its major focus will be on possible neuroendocrine pathways linking the experience of social isolation to the etiology and progression of coronary heart disease.

Social Support and Cardiovascular Functioning

Influence of Social Support on Health Behaviors

There are a number of behaviors that serve to enhance cardiovascular health. These include regular physical exercise, moderate alcohol consumption, a diet low in saturated fats and regular medical check-ups. There are others, such as smoking, which promote disease. It is not surprising to learn that social support has often been found to enhance health-promoting behaviors. Cohen (1988) summarizes various psychosocial models which have been developed to explain the nature of psychosocial mediation on behavior. These involve supply of information, social norms and tangible resources. Here, we will limit our discussion to examples of these influences. In the Edgecombe County Blood Pressure Study (Williams et al., 1985), it was reported that women who dropped out of treatment could be characterized as having less social support on the job, less perceived spousal approval (if married) and a lower level of perceived access to supportive resources. Treiber et al. (1991) reported two studies in which social support for exercise was positively correlated with physical activity. In men who were considered to have inadequate diet (Hanson et al., 1987), no differences in social class or marital status were found; however, low social anchorage was an independent risk factor along with low physical activity and high body mass index. With respect to smoking, Hanson et al. (1990) found that emotional support had a significant association with successful smoking cessation, even after adjustments for social class, marital status, alcohol consumption, physical activity, smoking of spouse and different medical conditions. In the Lung Health Study, Murray et al. (1995) reported gender differences in the efficacy of social support. Men but not women who were supported in their attempts to quit were more likely to be successful. However, type of support was important. Participants who were supported by a smoker were less than half as likely to have quit after 1 year as those who were supported by an ex-smoker who had also attended the group program. The importance of type of support may be the reason for negative results with respect to smoking cessation reported by Conn et al. (1992). In that study, social support did predict exercise and medication behavior but was not related to smoking. However, only a scale score was used to define support, and no information was given about the smoking status of the supportive persons. The importance of this issue has been demonstrated by Landrine et al. (1994), who showed that smoking among peers was the best predictor of smoking for white adolescents.

The fact that psychosocial factors can influence health behaviors challenges the common practice of statistically controlling for certain CVD related covariates in analyses of the effects of social support on morbidity and mortality. If social support influences smoking and dietary habits, for instance, then controlling for these in social support analyses eliminates some of the effect one is proposing to investigate. This problem can be circumvented by using structural equation modeling to describe the differing types of relationships.

Neuroendocrine Mechanisms

Coronary Artery Disease: Onset and Progression

In order to understand the second pathway concerning neuroendocrine factors as mediators of the effect of social support/isolation on coronary heart disease risk, we must first understand something about its onset and progression. The primary cause of myocardial infarction and stroke is atherosclerosis, which accounts for 50% of all mortality in the USA, Europe and Japan (Ross, 1993a). The most widely held view is that atherosclerosis begins as a response to injury (Ross, 1993b), which can be caused by mechanical (e.g. sheer stress) and immunologic factors, toxins, viruses or homocysteine.

The inflammatory response to endothelial injury has been extensively reviewed by Ross (1993a) and Ross (1993b) and will only be summarized here. With the initial injury to the endothelium comes a change in its structure and or function, such that adhesive glycoproteins begin to attach to it. T lymphocytes and monocytes attach to these glycoproteins and are then actively moved into the subendothelial matrix through

a process of chemotaxis. The transmigration through the endothelium is facilitated by growth regulatory molecules and chemotactic factors, one of which may be oxidized LDL. The monocytes differentiate to macrophages, and by ingestion of lipids become foam cells. Accumulating together with the lymphocytes, these foam cells form fatty streaks. This is followed by smooth muscle cell proliferation, which is regulated by a number of cytokines and growth factors. One of these is platelet derived growth factor (PDGF), which is released by platelets adhering to the site of injury and then degranulating to release their contents. The lesion progresses by adding more layers of foam cells and smooth muscle cells and often breaking through the endothelium to attract more platelet interactions and form thrombi.

Non-local Factors Influencing Lesion Formation

Genetic

The process as it has thus far been described is localized to the blood vessel. However, this is only part of the story. There are also interactions with genetic and environmental factors. An example of a genetic interaction is homocystinuria, an autosomal recessive trait characterized by excessive homocystine in plasma and urine, which is associated with increased incidence of arteriosclerosis (Ross, 1993a). Homocystine can cause injury to the endothelium and increased utilization of platelets. Another form of endothelial injury stems from elevated cholesterol levels. These are partially influenced by diet but also by genetic predisposition (Berg et al., 1986; Dzau et al., 1995).

Pituitary-adrenocortical

There is now also evidence that the central nervous system is intricately involved in the development of arterial lesions. Fingerle et al. (1992) demonstrated that pituitary factors are necessary for smooth muscle cell proliferation to occur. Their work on hypophysectomized (hypox) rats showed that muscle cells will not proliferate in response to injury in animals without a pituitary. Two important stimulants of smooth muscle cell proliferation, PDGF and insulin-like growth factor (IGF-I) mRNA, were present in the hypox rats but the cells did not proliferate. Basic fibroblast growth factor (bFGF), now considered to be the main mitogen for smooth muscle proliferation (Fingerle et al., 1992; Schwartz and Liaw, 1993), can only be activated after injury. When the injured (non proliferating) arteries from the hypox rats were transplanted into normal rats, the smooth muscle cells showed abundant proliferation. These results indicate that the locally produced growth factors responsible for smooth muscle cell proliferation were present but were not sufficient to initiate a proliferative response without circulating factors derived from or dependent upon pituitary function. Identification of these pituitary interactions requires further research.

However, Sanchez et al. (1994) have shown that the hypothalamo-pituitary-adrenocortical axis (HPA) is disturbed in rats that have been socially isolated. This study found that rats isolated from all social contact have reduced basal plasma corticosterone concentrations and a selective decrease in the spontaneous electrical activity of neurons within the hypothalamic paraventricular nucleus and preoptic areas. There was a reduction in excitatory responses and an increase in inhibition and nonresponsiveness. Their conclusion was that these rats either have an altered synaptology of these regions or a disruption of glucocorticoid feedback mechanisms. In addition, Shively et al. (1997) reported hypersecretion of cortisol in subordinate female monkeys (Macaca fascicularis) with significantly greater coronary artery atherosclerosis than dominants. These monkeys were characterized as engaging in less affiliation and spending more time alone than dominants.

Sympathetic-adrenomedullary
Kaplan et al. (1991) summarize a series of separate experiments by the authors which show a link

between the sympatho-adrenal-medullary system and atherosclerosis. These experiments were performed on cynomolgus monkeys (Macaca fascicularis), whose cardiovascular systems resemble that of humans. Research from this group had previously demonstrated that a socially unstable environment exacerbates coronary artery atherosclerosis in dominant (cholesterol fed) monkeys who must continually defend their position in the hierarchy (Kaplan et al., 1982). In the new set of experiments, specific mechanisms were examined. The first tested the effect of treating one group of monkeys in a socially unstable environment with propranolol HCL (a β-adrenergic blocker) on a daily basis for the 2 years of the experiment, while leaving the other group untreated. In the monkeys treated with β-blocker, there was a significant reduction of heart rate and blood pressure. In the treated dominant monkeys, there was significantly less coronary artery atherosclerosis than in the dominant untreated monkeys. There were no significant group differences in lipid concentrations. These data indicate a β-adrenergic influence on lesion formation in a subset of monkeys (dominants) in a chronically stressful situation.

In another experiment described in this series, the effect of sympathetic nervous stimulation on cell death as defined by IgG incorporation was examined. Rabbits were treated with chloralose anesthesia, which induces stable increases in heart rate, blood pressure and plasma norepinephrine. Half the group was pretreated with the β-blocker, metoprolol. A 5-fold increase in cell death was found in the chloralose treated group without metoprolol. But the group pretreated with β-blocker could not be distinguished from the control group. There was more injury in areas of high shear stress (circumostial) than in areas of low shear stress (unbranched aorta). In a similar experiment, rabbits were treated with chloralose anesthesia, one group with and one without metoprolol pretreatment. The chloralose caused significant platelet accumulation in the group that was not pretreated with metoprolol. Again, intercostal and coronary artery orifices showed more accumulation than unbranched aorta, demonstrating the interaction with shear stress location.

In the fourth experiment described by Kaplan et al. (1991), social stress was manipulated (not just observed). Half the socially stressed monkeys were treated with daily doses of metoprolol via a subcutaneous osmotic minipump and half were left untreated. All monkeys had the same diet. The untreated, socially stressed group had significantly more endothelial injury, but again, only at the branching sites. Together, this group of experiments demonstrates sympatho-adrenal-medullary influence in lesion formation and associates this with a psychosocial stressor. One such stressor is social isolation. Shively et al. (1989) reported that the extent of coronary artery atherosclerosis in female cynomolgus monkeys in single cages was four times greater than monkeys housed in social groups, though there was no difference in plasma lipid concentrations.

Manuck et al. (1995) reviewed the research on CAD in chronically stressed monkeys and concluded that animals exhibiting a heightened cardiac responsivity to stress also develop the most extensive coronary lesions. The exacerbation of atherosclerosis in stressed monkeys can be blocked by β-blockade, indicating that it is of sympathetic origin. One probable mechanism is that increased heart rate causes an increase in turbulent flow and shear stress on the artery wall, resulting in endothelial injury.

In summary, these experiments present strong evidence of β-adrenergic influence on lesion formation, most probably through the mechanism of injury caused by increased shear stress on the vessel wall. The reactivity experiments mentioned earlier demonstrate that in humans, the presence of a "supporting other" during acute stress in the laboratory, reduces β-adrenergic responsivity to the stressor. It has also been demonstrated in the monkey model that social isolation causes an increase in heart rate that is not associated with increased activity. Watson et al. (1998) measured heart rate in 12 female cynomolgus monkeys that were first socially housed and then individually housed so that they had visual but not physical contact with each other. Afternoon heart rates were significantly increased during social separation, despite the fact that activity levels were actually lower. This demonstrates that social isolation is, of itself, physiologically stressful to the cardiovascular system.

Platelet Function and Psychological Stress
The series of animal studies just described establishes that both the hypothalamic-pituitary-adrenocortical axis and the sympatho-adrenal-medullary system interact with local factors in lesion formation in the coronary arteries. Studies of platelet function in humans have been more difficult to interpret. Summarizing in vivo and in vitro experiments on human platelet function, Hjemdahl et al. (1991) concluded that the literature has yielded contradictory results due to a number of methodological problems, but that there is support for the hypothesis that stress related sympathoadrenal activation could enhance platelet aggregability. One of the major methodological hurdles was analysis of platelet rich plasma (PRP) in aggregation experiments in vitro. This preparation can destroy platelets in greatly varying amounts, confounding interpretation of results. In 1992, Hjemdahl's group (Larsson et al., 1992) published a study trying to elucidate the functional significance of β-adrenoceptor responses in vivo and in vitro, using whole blood for the in vitro experiments. Previous in vitro studies had indicated that activation of the α-adrenoceptors carried by platelets stimulated, whereas activation of β-adrenoceptors inhibited platelet aggregation (Abdulla, 1969; Kerry and Scrutton, 1983; Yu and Latour, 1977). The 1992 study utilized in vivo infusions of the non-selective β-adrenoceptor agonist isoprenaline and infusions of adrenaline with and without β-blockade by propranolol. It compared these results to in vitro platelet aggregability in whole blood using propranolol on

adrenaline-induced platelet activation. The purpose of the in vitro experiments was to isolate aggregability from other in vivo β-adrenoceptor mediated effects. Their conclusion was that von Willebrand factor (necessary for the adhesion of platelets to the glycoprotein on the endothelium) antigen levels were increased by both adrenaline and high dose isoprenaline. β-blockade with propranolol did not alter platelet aggregability during rest or adrenaline infusion but did inhibit adrenaline-induced increases in von Willebrand antigen levels.

Despite the methodological problems with platelet aggregability studies, Thaulow et al. (1991) reported that men with the most rapid platelet aggregability response (PRP preparation) to ADP stimulation had significantly increased coronary heart disease mortality after 13.5 years of follow-up. This was the first prospective evidence of a link between platelet aggregability in healthy men and fatal coronary heart disease.

Because of the problems involved with the methodology of platelet aggregability, another review article published in 1991 (Markovitz and Matthews, 1991) emphasized the importance of platelet secretion as an indication of platelet function, specifically levels of beta thromboglobulin (βTG) and platelet factor 4 (PF4). This review acknowledges that there are also problems with these assays. The main problem, also discussed by Hjemdahl et al. is that platelets are easily activated by stasis and contact with foreign surfaces, so that the analysis process itself can influence the results and cause a great deal of variability. However, ten of the 14 studies reviewed in this article involving patients with stable coronary artery disease showed elevated levels of βTG and PF4 compared with controls.

Three later studies on laboratory stress reactivity have also reported an increase in platelet activation as measured by platelet secretion. Two of these studies also measured in vitro platelet aggregability but found no significant increases. Malkoff et al. (1993) found an increase in plate-

let dense granule secretion but not aggregability in response to laboratory stress, even though the analyses were performed on whole blood. Naesh et al. (1993) found an increase in post stress βTG but not platelet aggregability using the PRP preparation. Patterson et al. (1994) found an increase in PF4 to mental stress but did not measure aggregability. The finding of increases in platelet secretion but lack of in vitro aggregability in these latter studies mirrors the results by Larsson et al. (1992) and may be a result of problems with the in vitro methodology. In summary, these studies support the conclusion that platelet function is influenced by sympathetic stimulation and that psychological factors may serve as a trigger. It is not yet clear whether social isolation functions as one of these triggers.

Psychosocial Factors and Endothelial Dysfunction

Platelets interact with the endothelium, and endothelial dysfunction is an important manifestation of coronary artery disease. Coronary arteries of CAD patients respond differently to vasodilatory stimuli than those of people without lesions. Arteries of patients without coronary disease show moderate vasodilation in response to acetylcholine infusion (Drexler et al., 1989), whereas even smooth arteries in patients with lesions elsewhere in the coronary circulation vasoconstrict to the same stimulation (Werns et al., 1989). In addition, patients with angina and positive exercise tests but angiographically normal coronary arteries show significantly less vasodilation to acetylcholine than controls (Egashira et al., 1993). This would suggest that endothelial dysfunction may precede lesion formation. A confirmation of this can be found in an in vivo study by Drexler and Zeiher (1991), showing that hypercholesterolemia, known to be causally associated with lesion formation in primates, elicits endothelial dysfunction in coronary arteries without (e.g. prior to) angiographically visible atherosclerotic lesions. Galle et al. (1994) confirmed that oxidized low-density lipoproteins

(LDL) could inhibit endothelium-dependent vasodilation to acetylcholine under high (but not low) pressure in rabbit arteries in vitro, effects which were prevented by high-density lipoproteins. The authors' explanation is that endothelial dysfunction is caused by pressure dependent arterial infiltration with lipid.

Comparing these studies of endothelial function in humans to those of endothelial function in chronically stressed monkeys provides some interesting insight about mechanisms. Williams et al. (1991) published a study demonstrating that the coronary arteries of monkeys consuming a high cholesterol diet and living in unstable (stressful) social conditions, vasoconstricted in response to intracoronary infusion of acetylcholine, whereas arteries of monkeys fed the same diet but living in stable (not stressful) conditions, vasodilated. This same study also showed that the vasoconstriction in the unstable group continued even on a cholesterol lowering diet. Examination of intimal wall thickness at necropsy showed that monkeys on a cholesterol lowering diet showed similar wall thickness across the social group, indicating endothelial impairment independent of lesion size. Since previous work in their laboratory had shown that social disruption resulted in modest heart rate increases and damage to the endothelium, which could be reduced by β-blockade, the authors speculated that repeated episodes of sympathetic stimulation in the chronically stressful living condition may have damaged the endothelium, thus impairing endothelial-dependent vasomotion. In a later study, Williams et al. (1993) demonstrated that psychosocial stress impairs endothelium mediated dilation through receptor (acetylcholine)—and non-receptor—mediated mechanisms and that it is mediated through endothelium-derived relaxing factor (EDRF), later shown to be identical to nitric oxide (Ignarro et al., 1987). This study also showed that current but not previous stress resulted in endothelial dysfunction. Based on these data and results of previous research, the authors concluded that the release or breakdown

of EDRF was impaired due to endothelial damage caused by repeated sympathetic stimulation.

These experiments indicate a disturbance of vagal function which may precede lesion formation in coronary artery disease. Although this dysfunction has been demonstrated in the psychologically stressed monkeys, no experiments to date have tested endothelial function as a result of social isolation. It is hypothesized based on the oxytocin literature (see below) that vagal disturbances also result from social isolation, but this will remain speculative until further research is performed.

Neuroendocrine Changes Associated with Lack of Social Support

Research on chronic lack of social support has shown that it is also associated with an increase in sympathetic activation. Fleming et al. (1982) showed an increase of urinary norepinephrine in people with low social support, independent of their level of stress. Knox et al. (1985), showed that two social support factors: lack of attachment (intimate contacts) and a low number of regular contacts with acquaintances were associated with high resting plasma adrenaline levels, which in turn explained a significant amount of the variance in resting systolic blood pressure in men who were only 28 years old. A low number of contacts with acquaintances was also associated with higher heart rate, which in turn explained a significant amount of the variance in resting diastolic blood pressure. In a later study, Knox (1993) showed that young normotensive men with low social support had significantly higher resting diastolic blood pressure than normotensive men with high social support, and that they also had higher diastolic blood pressure during laboratory stress. The high and low support groups showed no significant differences in parental history of hypertension, body mass index, state anxiety, anger inhibition or ongoing stress as measured by financial hardship and living conditions. The reactivity studies mentioned earlier showed a relationship between sympathetic activation and lack of social support during acute stress. The latter two studies reveal that chronic sympathetic activation is also associated with a chronic lack of social support at a very young age, before the onset of CAD manifestation.

In summary, available data strongly support the conclusion that sympathetic activation is associated with both lesion formation and endothelial dysfunction, and that both of these can be caused by chronic stress. It has been demonstrated that social support reduces cardiovascular reactivity to acute stress and that ongoing lack of social support is associated with increased resting levels of sympathetic activation, i.e. that lack of social support is itself a stressor.

Social Isolation versus Social Support—Are There Different Mechanisms?

Thus far, the focus has been on the deleterious effects of social isolation, but little has been said about the apparent buffering effects of social support. Epidemiological data suggest that people with social support live longer and laboratory data show lower cardiovascular reactivity to stressful situations in people accompanied by a "supporting other." Does having social support simply mean that one does not suffer the deleterious physiological consequences of social isolation, or does social support trigger specific physiological mechanisms which could have a protective effect with respect to cardiovascular risk? Although there have been no studies specifically designed to investigate this question, there are some tantalizing hints in the literature. A number of studies have examined the physiology involved in the establishment of bonding relationships between mother and young and between partners, as well as in sexual behavior (Carter, 1990; Carter et al., 1992). These studies suggest that mechanisms involving oxytocin are central to the physiology of bonding.

Oxytocin—A Neuroendocrine Buffer?

Oxytocin is a neuropeptide secreted from the magnocellular supraoptic and paraventricular nuclei of the hypothalamus to the posterior pituitary and then into the systemic circulation (Sawchenko, 1991). It differs by only two amino acids from arginine vasopressin (AVP), which is produced and secreted through the same pathways (Berecek, 1992). Hypothalamic oxytocin and AVP neurons have projections to the peripheral vasculature causing vasoconstriction and dilation of different vessels. Oxytocin fibers can also be found in many areas in the brain associated with emotion and cardiovascular control (Sofroniew, 1985). In addition to the neuroanatomical evidence that oxytocin is involved in cardiovascular regulation, experimental studies show that exogenous administration of oxytocin lowers blood pressure and cardiac output via central nervous mechanisms (Berecek, 1992; Petersson et al., 1996; Uvnäs-Moberg, 1997).

Although oxytocin is most well known for its association with lactation in females, its secretion can also be induced in both males and females by stimuli such as touch, light pressure, warm temperature and massage (Stock and Uvnäs-Moberg, 1988; Uvnäs-Moberg et al., 1993a,b). The psychological importance of touch in affiliative relationships, whether they be between parent and child or between sexual partners, is readily apparent. That touch may also have positive physiological consequences is less well known. However, stimulation of somatosensory afferents by nonnoxious stimulation such as touch in anaesthetized animals leads to an effect pattern characterized by an inhibited activity in the sympathoadrenal system (lowering of pulse rate and blood pressure, reduced firing activity in the adrenal nerve and lowered plasma levels of catecholamines), as well as enhanced activity of the vagus nerve (Uvnäs-Moberg, 1997). Afferent stimulation of somatosensory afferents can trigger oxytocin release, and the administration of oxytocin can induce sedation, lowering of pulse rate and blood pressure, elevation of pain threshold and lowering of tail-skin temperature (Uvnäs-Moberg, 1997). Oxytocin is reduced by behavioral stress (Kalin et al., 1985). Since elevated heart rate and blood pressure are associated with an increase in shear stress, which at high chronic levels can cause endothelial injury and initiate coronary lesions, the lowering of blood pressure and heart rate by oxytocin may be an important buffer against lesion development. It is interesting to note that in the earlier discussion of chronic stress in monkeys, one of the distinguishing behavioral characteristics of those (the dominants) with the least coronary artery disease is that they received a lot of grooming (Shively et al., 1997). Not only does grooming cause oxytocin release (Stock and Uvnäs-Moberg, 1988), but oxytocin release facilitates bonding and attachment (Carter et al., 1995; Witt et al., 1992). In the experiment with single caged monkeys (Shively et al., 1989) who had four times the atherosclerosis as socially caged monkeys, the primary difference was that although the socially isolated monkeys could see, hear and smell each other, they could not touch each other. The effect of oxytocin on blood pressure has been shown to last for weeks in animals, much longer than the circulating levels themselves since the half-life is 2–3 min (Uvnäs-Moberg, 1997). This could explain why there are positive effects of ongoing social support on resting levels of blood pressure even when a supporting other is not present (Knox, 1993; Knox et al., 1985). Though oxytocin mechanisms are not fully understood, they are consistent with inhibited activity in the sympathoadrenal system and an enhanced vagal nerve tone enhancing anabolic metabolism.

It is thus likely that touch plays an important role in the protective effects of social support in close or intimate relationships. However, this does not explain the data which supports a buffering or protective effect of regular contact (including telephone contact) with more casual acquaintances. Clearly, instrumental support, e.g. help with everyday needs, may explain part of the association. But Knox et al. (1985) have also shown an inverse relationship between regular, casual (non touching) contacts and resting plasma adrenaline and heart rate levels, which would be difficult to explain solely on the basis of instrumental support. Although there is no direct evidence, we speculate that oxytocin may also be released by warm, positive, psychological contacts devoid of tactile stimulation. In support of this are several studies (Uvnäs-Moberg et al., 1990, 1991, 1993a) which show that oxytocin is correlated with personality traits such as attachment, calm and social dependency. It has also been shown by Sanchez et al. (1994) that the paraventricular nucleus which produces oxytocin is affected in rats that are isolated from all social contact.

Conclusion

In addition to the data showing an association between social support and health behaviors, there is evidence that lack of social support may be etiologically related to coronary lesion development through two mechanisms: sympathetic-adrenomedullary influences on heart rate and blood pressure in the initial endothelial injury; and pituitary-adrenal cortical factors involved in smooth muscle cell proliferation during progression of the lesion after injury has taken place. We speculate that sympathetic activation associated with lack of social support also contributes adversely to platelet function but this has yet to be demonstrated. We suggest that the buffering effects of social support are primarily mediated through mechanisms associated with the release of oxytocin. A reduction of oxytocin release in socially isolated people may adversely affect endothelial function through a disturbance in autonomic nervous tone leading to enhanced sympathetic and decreased vagal tone. We believe that the epidemiological and laboratory evidence relating social isolation to cardiovascular disease strongly supports a causal connection with coronary artery atherosclerosis. The clinical implications of these findings warrant an emphasis on future research designed to elucidate them.

Acknowledgements

This study was supported by a National Heart, Lung, and Blood Institute collaboration investigating "Biobehavioral Mechanisms of Cardiovascular Disease in Women." The collaborators were the National Heart, Lung, and Blood Institute in the US and the Karolinska Institute and the Institute of Psychosocial Factors and Health in Stockholm, Sweden.

References

Abdulla, Y. H. (1969) Adrenergic receptors in human platelets. *Journal of Atherosclerotic Research* 9, 113–117.

Berecek, K. H. (1992) Role of vasopressin in central cardiovascular regulation. In: Kunos, G. and Ciriello, J. (Eds.). *Central Neural Mechanisms in Cardiovascular Regulation*, Vol. 1. Birkhauser, Basel, pp. 1–34.

Berg, K., Powell, L. M., Wallis, S. C., Pease, R., Knott, T. J. and Scott, J. (1986) Genetic linkage between the antigenic group (Ag) variation and the apolipoprotein gene: assignment of the Ag locus. *Proceedings of the National Academy of Sciences USA* 83, 7367–7370.

Berkman, L. F. (1995) The role of social relations in health promotion. *Psychosomatic Medicine* 57, 245–254.

Berkman, L. F. and Syme, S. L. (1979) Social networks, host resistance and mortality: a 9 year follow-up study of Alameda County residents. *American Journal of Epidemiology* 109, 186–204.

Berkman, L. F., Leo-Sumers, L. and Horwitz, R. I. (1992) Emotional support and survival after myocardial infarction. *Annals of Internal Medicine* 117, 1003–1009.

Blazer, D. (1982) Social support and mortality in an elderly community population. *American Journal of Epidemiology* 115, 684–694.

Carter, C. S. (1990) Oxytocin and sexual behavior. *Neuroscience Biobehavior* 16, 11–144.

Carter, C. S., Williams, J. R., Witt, D. M. and Insel, T. R. (1992) Oxytocin and social bonding. *Annals of New York Academy of Science* 652, 204–211.

Carter, C. S., DeVries, A. C. and Getz, I. L. (1995) Physiological substrates of mammalian monogamy: the prairie vole model. *Neuroscience Biobehavior Review* 19, 303–313.

Case, R. B., Moss, A. J., Case, N., McDermott, M. and Eberly, S. (1992) Living alone after myocardial infarction. *Journal of the American Medical Association* 267, 515–519.

Cohen, S. (1988) Psychosocial models of the role of social support in the etiology of physical disease. *Health Psychology* 7, 269–297.

Conn, V. S., Taylor, S. G. and Hayes, V. (1992) Social support, self-esteem, and self-care after myocardial infarction. Health values. *Journal of Health Behavior, Education and Promotion* 16, 25–31.

Drexler, H. and Zeiher, A. M. (1991) Endothelial function in human coronary arteries in vivo. Focus on hypercholesterolemia. *Hypertension* 189 (Suppl II), 90–99.

Drexler, H., Zeihe, A. M., Wolschlager, H., Meinertz, T., Just, H. and Bonzel, T. (1989) Flow-dependent coronary artery dilation in humans. *Circulation* 80, 466–474.

Dzau, V. J., Gibbons, G. H., Kobilka, B. K., Lawn, R. M. and Pratt, R. E. (1995) Genetic models of human vascular disease. *Circulation* 91, 521–531.

Egashira, K., Inou, T., Hirooka, Y., Yamada, A., Urabe, Y. and Takeshita, A. (1993) Evidence of impaired endothelium-dependent coronary vasodilation in patients with angina pectoris and normal coronary angiograms. *New England Journal of Medicine* 328, 1659–1664.

Fingerle, J., Faulmuller, A., Muller, G., Bowen-Pope, D. F., Clowes, M. M., Reidy, M. A. and Clowes, A. W. (1992) Pituitary factors in blood plasma are necessary for smooth muscle cell proliferation in response to injury in vivo. *Arteriosclerosis and Thrombosis* 12, 1488–1495.

Fleming, R., Baum, A., Gisriel, M. M. and Gatchel, R. J. (1982) Mediating influences of social support on stress at three mile island. *Journal of Human Stress* 8, 14–22.

Galle, J., Ochslen, M., Schollmeyer, P. and Wanner, C. (1994) Oxidized lipoproteins inhibit endothelium-dependent vasodilation. Effects of pressure and high-density lipoprotein. *Hypertension* 23, 556–564.

Gerin, W., Pieper, C., Levy, R. and Pickering, T. G. (1992) Social support insocial interaction: a moderator of cardiovascular reactivity. *Psychosomatic Medicine* 54, 324–336.

Gerin, W., Milner, D., Chawla, S. and Pickering, T. G. (1995) Social support as a moderator of cardiovascular reactivity in women: a test of the direct effects and buffering hypotheses. *Psychosomatic Medicine* 57, 16–22.

Hanson, B. S., Mattisson, I. and Steen, B. (1987) Dietary intake and psychosocial factors in 68-year-old men. *Comprehensive Gerontology* 62–67.

Hanson, B. S., Isacsson, S. O., Janzon, L. and Lindell, S. E. (1990) Social support and quitting smoking for good. Is there an association? Results from the population study, "Men born in 1914," Malmo, Sweden. *Addictive Behavior* 15, 221–233.

Hedblad, B., Ostergren, P. O., Hanson, B. S. and Janzon, L. (1992) Influence of social support on cardiac event rate in men with ischaemic type ST segment depression during ambulatory 24 h long-term ECG recording. *European Heart Journal* 13, 433–439.

Helgeson, V. S. (1991) The effects of masculinity and social support on recovery from myocardial infarction. *Psychosomatic Medicine* 53, 621–633.

Hjemdahl, P., Larsson, T. and Wallen, N. H. (1991) Effects of stress and β-blockade on platelet function. *Circulation* 84, 44–62.

House, J. S., Robbins, C. and Metzner, H. L. (1982) The association of social relationships and activities with mortality: prospective evidence from the Tecumseh community health study. *American Journal of Epidemiology* 116, 123–140.

Ignarro, L. J., Burns, R. E., Buga, G. M. and Wood, K. S. (1987) Endothelium-derived relaxing factor from pulmonary artery and vein possesses pharmacologic and chemical properties identical to those of nitric oxide radical. *Circulation Research* 61, 866–879.

Kalin, N. H., Gibbs, D. M., Barksdale, C. M., Shelton, S. E. and Carnes, M. (1985) Behavioral stress decreases plasma oxytocin concentrations in primates. *Life Sciences* 36, 1275–1280.

Kamarck, T. W., Manuck, S. B. and Jennings, J. R. (1990) Social support reduces cardiovascular reactivity to psychological challenge: a laboratory model. *Psychosomatic Medicine* 52, 42–58.

Kamarck, T. W., Annunziato, B. A. and Amateau, L. M. (1995) Affiliation moderates the effects of social threat on stress-related cardiovascular responses: boundary conditions for a laboratory model of social support. *Psychosomatic Medicine* 57, 183–1994.

Kaplan, J. R., Manuck, S. B., Clarkson, T. B., Lusso, F. M. and Taub, D. M. (1982) Social status, environment and atherosclerosis in cynomolgus monkeys. *Arteriosclerosis* 2, 359–368.

Kaplan, J. R., Salonen, J. T., Cohen, R. D., Brand, R. J., Syme, S. L. and Puska, P. (1988) Social connections and mortality from all causes and cardiovascular disease: prospective evidence from eastern Finland. *American Journal of Epidemiology* 128, 370–380.

Kaplan, J. R., Pettersson, K., Manuck, S. B. and Olsson, G. (1991) Role of sympathoadrenal medullary activation in the initiation and progression of atherosclerosis. *Circulation* 84 (Suppl. VI), 23–32.

Kawachi, I., Colditz, G. A., Ascherio, A., Rimm, E. B., Giovannucci, E., Stampfer, M. J. and Willett, W. C. (1996) A prospective study of social networks in relation to total mortality and cardiovascular disease in men in the USA. *Journal of Epidemiology and Community Health* 50, 245–251.

Kerry, R. and Scrutton, M. C. (1983) Platelet β-adrenoceptors. *British Journal of Pharmacology* 79, 681–691.

Kirschbaum, C., Klauer, T., Flipp, S. H. and Hellhammer, D. H. (1995) Sex-specific effects of social support on cortisol and subjective responses to acute psychological stress. *Psychosomatic Medicine* 57, 23–31.

Knox, S. S. (1993) Perception of social support and blood pressure in young men. *Perceptual and Motor Skills* 77, 132–134.

Knox, S. S., Theorell, T., Svensson, J. and Waller, D. (1985) The relation of social support and working environment to medical variables associated with elevated blood pressure in young males: a structural model. *Social Science and Medicine* 21, 525–531.

Kochanek, K. D., and Hudson, B. L. for the Division of Vital Statistics (1994). Advance report of final mortality statisics, 1992. *Monthly Vital Statistics Report* 43, 6S.

Landrine, H., Richardson, J. L., Klonoff, E. A. and Flay, B. (1994) Cultural diversity in the predictors of adolescent cigarette smoking: the relative influence of peers. *Journal of Behavioral Medicine* 17, 331–346.

Larsson, P. T., Wallen, N. H., Martinsson, A., Egberg, N. and Hjemdahl, P. (1992) Significance of platelet β-adrenoceptors for platelet responses in vivo and in vitro. *Thrombosis Haemostasis* 68, 687–693.

Lepore, S. J., Allen, K. A. M. and Evans, G. W. (1993) Social support lowers cardiovascular reactivity to an acute stressor. *Psychosomatic Medicine* 55, 518–524.

Malkoff, S. B., Muldoon, M. F., Zeigler, Z. R. and Manuck, S. B. (1993) Blood platelet responsivity to acute mental stress. *Psychosomatic Medicine* 55, 477–482.

Manuck, S. B., Marsland, A. L., Marsland, M. A., Kaplan, J. R. and Williams, J. K. (1995) The pathogenicity of behavior and its neuroendocrine mediation: An example from coronary artery disease. *Psychosomatic Medicine* 57, 275–283.

Markovitz, J., and Matthews. (1991). Platelets and coronary heart disease: potential psychophysiologic mechanisms. *Psychosomatic Medicine* 53, 643–668.

Murray, R. P., Johnston, J. J., Dolce, J. J., Lee, W. W. and O'Hara, P. (1995) Social support for smoking cessation and abstinence. *The Lung Health Study* 20, 159–170.

Naesh, O., Haerdersdal, C., Hindberg, I., and Trap-Jensen. (1993). Platelet activation in mental stress. *Clinical Physiology* 13, 299–307.

Orth-Gomer, K. and Johnson, J. (1987) Social network interaction and mortality: a 6 year follow-up of a random sample of the Swedish population. *Journal of Chronic Disorders* 40, 949–957.

Orth-Gomer, K., Rosengren, A. and Wilhelmsen, L. (1993) Lack of social support and incidence of coronary heart disease in middle-aged Swedish men. *Psychosomatic Medicine* 55, 37–43.

Oxman, T. E., Freeman, H. H. D. H. and Manheimer, E. D. (1995) Lack of social participation or religious strength and comfort as risk factors for death after cardiac surgery in the elderly. *Psychosomatic Medicine* 57, 5–15.

Patterson, S. M., Zakowski, S. G., Hall, M. H., Cohen, L., Wollman, K. and Baum, A. (1994) Psychological stress and platelet activation: differences in platelet reactivity in healthy men during active and passive stressors. *Health Psychology* 113, 34–38.

Petersson, M., Alster, P., Lundeberg, T. and Uvnäs-Moberg, K. (1996) Oxytociin causes a long-term decrease of blood pressure in female and male rats. *Physiology and Behavior* 60, 1311–1315.

Ross, R. (1993a) The pathogenesis of atherosclerosis: a perspective for the 1990's. *Nature* 362, 801–809.

Ross, R. (1993b) Atherosclerotic coronary heart disease. In: Hurst, J. W., Schlant, R. C., Rackley, C. E., Sonnenblick, E. H. and Wenger, N. K. (Eds.). *The Heart*, 8th. McGraw-Hill, New York, pp. 977–991.

Sanchez, M. M., Aguado, F., Sanchez-Toscano, F. and Saphier, D. (1994) Effects of prolonged social isolation on responses of neurons in the bed nucleus of the stria terminalis, preoptioc area, and hypothalamic paraventricular nucleus to stimulation of the medial amygdala. *Psychoneuroendocrinology* 20, 525–541.

Sawchenko, P. E. (1991) Tale of three peptides: corticotropin-releasing factor-, oxytocin-, and vasopressin-containing pathways mediating integrated hypothalamic responses to stress. In: McCubbin, J. A., Kaufmann, P. G. and Nemeroff, C. B. (Eds.). *Stress, Neuropeptides and Systemic Disease*. Academic Press, New York, pp. 3–17.

Schoenback, V. J., Kaplan, B. G., Freedman, L. and Kleinbaum, D. G. (1986) Social ties and mortality in Evans County, Georgia. *American Journal of Epidemiology* 123, 577–591.

Schwartz, S. M. and Liaw, L. (1993) Growth control and morphogenesis in the development and pathology of arteries. *Journal of Cardiovascular Pharmacology* 21 (Suppl. 1), 31–49.

Seeman, T. E. and Syme, S. L. (1987) Social networks and coronary artery disease: a comparison of the structure and function of social relations as predictors of disease. *Psychosomatic Medicine* 49, 341–354.

Seeman, T. E., Berkman, L. F., Kohout, F., LaCroix, A., Glynn, R. and Blazer, D. (1993) Intercommunity variations in the association between social ties and mortality in the elderly: a comparative analysis of three communities. *Annals of Epidemiology* 3, 325–335.

Shively, C. A., Clarkson, T. B. and Kaplan, J. R. (1989) Social deprivation and coronary artery atherosclerosis in female cynomolgus monkeys. *Atherosclerosis* 77, 69–76.

Shively, C. A., Laber-Laird, K. and Anton, R. F. (1997) Behavior and physiology of social stress and depression in female cynomolgus monkeys. *Biological Psychiatry* 41, 871–882.

Sofroniew, M. V. (1985) Vassopressin, oxytocin and their related neurophysins. In: Bjorklund, A. and Hokfelt, T. (Eds.). *Handbook of Chemical Neuroanatomy, GABA and Neuropeptides in the CNS,* Vol. 4 (part I). Elsevier Science, pp. 93–149.

Stock, S. and Uvnäs-Moberg, K. (1988) Increased plasma levels of oxytocin in response to afferent electrical stimulation of the sciatic and vagal nerves and in response to touch and pinch in anaesthetized rats. *Acta Physiologica Scandanavia* 132, 29–34.

Thaulow, E., Erikssen, J., Sandvik, L., Stormorken, H. and Cohn, P. F. (1991) Blood platelet count and function are related to total and cardiovascular death in apparently healthy men. *Circulation* 84, 613–617.

Treiber, F. A., Batanowski, T., Braden, D. S., Strong, W. B., Levy, M. and Knox, W. (1991) Social support for exercise: relationship to physical activity in young adults. *Preventive Medicine* 20, 737–750.

Uchino, B. N., Cacioppo, J. T. and Kiecolt-Glaser, J. K. (1996) The relationship between social support and physiological processes: a review with emphasis on underlying mechanisms and implications for health. *Psychology Bulletin* 119, 488–531.

Uvnäs-Moberg, K. (1997) Physiological and endocrine effects of social contact. *Annals of the New York Academy of Sciences* 807, 146–163.

Uvnäs-Moberg, K., Widstrom, A. M., Nissen, E. and Bjorvell, H. (1990) Personality traits in women 4 days postpartum and their correlation with plasma levels of oxytocin and prolactin. *Journal of Psychosomatics in Obstetrics and Gynecology* 11, 261–273.

Uvnäs-Moberg, K., Arn, I., Theorell, T. and Jonsson, C. O. (1991) Personality traits in a group of individuals with functional disorders of the gastrointestinal tract and their correlation with gastrin, somatostatin and oxytocin levels. *Journal of Psychosomatic Research* 35, 515–523.

Uvnäs-Moberg, K., Arn, I., Jonsson, C. O., Ek, S. and Nilsonne, A. (1993a) The relationships between personality traits and plasma gastrin, cholecystokinin, somatostatin, insulin, and oxytocin levels in healthy women. *Journal of Psychosomatic Research* 37, 581–588.

Uvnäs-Moberg, K., Bruzelius, G., Alster, P. and Lundeberg, T. (1993b) The antinociceptive effect of non-noxious sensory stimulation is partly mediated through oxytocinergic mechanisms. *Acta Physiologica Scandanavia* 149, 199–204.

Watson, S. L., Shively, C. A., Kaplan, J. R. and Line, S. W. (1998) The effects of chronic social separation on cardiovascular disease risk in female cynomolgus monkeys. *Atherosclerosis* 137, 259–266.

Welin, L., Tibblin, G., Svardsudd, K., et al. (1985) Prospective study of social influences on mortality. The Study of Men Born in 1913 and 1923. *Lancet* 1 (8434), 915–918.

Welin, L., Larsson, B., Svardsudd, K., Tibblin, B. and Tibblin, G. (1992) Social network and activities in relation to mortality from cardiovascular diseases, cancer and other causes: a 12 year follow up of the Study of Men Born in 1913 and 1923. *Journal of Epidemiology and Community Health* 46, 127–132.

Werns, S. W., Walton, J. A., Hsia, H. H., Nabe, E. G., Sanz, M. L. and Pitt, B. (1989) Evidence of endothelial dysfunction in angiographically normal coronary arteries of patients with coronary artery disease. *Circulation* 79, 287–291.

Williams, C. A., Beresford, S. S. A., James, S. A., LaCroix, A. Z., Strogatz, D. S., Wagner, E. H., Kleinbaum, D. G., Cutchin, L. M. and Ibrahim, M. A. (1985) The Edgecombe County High Blood Pressure Control Program: II. Social support, social stressors, and treatment dropout. *American Journal of Public Health* 75, 483–486.

Williams, J. K., Vita, J. A., Manuck, S. B., Selwyn, A. P. and Kaplan, J. R. (1991) Psychosocial factors impair vascular responses of coronary arteries. *Circulation* 84, 2146–2153.

Williams, J. K., Kaplan, J. R. and Manuck, S. B. (1993) Effects of psychosocial stress on endothelium-mediated dilation of atherosclerotic arteries in cynomolgus monkeys. *Journal of Clinical Investigation* 92, 1819–1823.

Witt, D. M., Winslow, J. T., and Insel, T. R. (1992). Physiological substrates of mammalian monogamy: the prairie vole model. *Neuroscience and Biobehavioral Review* 19.

Woloshin, S., Schwartz, L. M., Tosteson, A. N., Chang, C. H., Wright, B., Plohman, J. and Fisher, E. S. (1997) Perceived adequacy of tangible social support and health outcomes in patients with coronary artery disease. *Journal of General Internal Medicine* 10, 613–618.

Yu, S. K. and Latour, J. G. (1977) Potentiation of α and inhibiition by β-adrenergic stimulations of rat platelet aggregation. A comparative study with human and rabbit platelets. *Thrombosis and Haemostasis* 37, 413–421.

VI SOCIAL INFLUENCES ON BIOLOGY AND HEALTH

B. Social Applications

ii. Salubrious Influences

80 Emotional Support and Survival after Myocardial Infarction: A Prospective, Population-Based Study of the Elderly

Lisa F. Berkman, Linda Leo-Summers, and Ralph I. Horwitz

Prognostic indicators based on illness severity are strong predictors of survival after acute myocardial infarction. Yet, much variability in survival is seen among patients with similar severity of disease. Several studies have recently documented that patients with myocardial infarction who lived alone (1) or who were not married and lacked a confidant (2) were at increased risk for death after myocardial infarction, and several others have indicated the importance of several psychosocial conditions in predicting survival and recovery of patients who have had a myocardial infarction (3–7).

Few studies have provided detailed information on social support assessed prospectively, that is, before the onset of myocardial infarction. In many studies, psychosocial features were measured retrospectively (1, 3, 7). Such retrospective data may be distorted by recall bias because subjects' memories of circumstances may be affected by the severity or clinical course of their illness. Further, most studies in which psychosocial conditions were rigorously assessed have inadequately measured and controlled for the effects of the severity of the myocardial infarction and comorbid diseases (8). Conversely, many studies that have supplied excellent data on clinical conditions have provided much weaker data on psychosocial conditions (1, 3). Finally, although many studies have documented a strong relation between psychosocial conditions and increased mortality from cardiovascular disease, rarely have investigators been able to identify whether psychosocial factors influence the risk for disease onset or survival after acute myocardial infarction. This is especially important in view of evidence (9–11) that pathophysiologic processes leading to coronary disease may differ from those that are related to recovery from myocardial infarction.

We examined the effect of psychosocial conditions on survival in a cohort of men and women who were hospitalized for acute myocardial infarction and who were participating in a longitudinal, community-based study of elderly persons living in New Haven, Connecticut. The important features of our study include the rigorous collection of data on psychosocial conditions before the occurrence of acute myocardial infarction; the collection of important clinical data; and the presence of a study sample drawn from a representative population.

Methods

Established Populations for the Epidemiologic Study of the Elderly Program

Data for our study come from the New Haven, Connecticut, site of the Established Populations for the Epidemiologic Study of the Elderly (EPESE) program. The study was designed as a longitudinal, community-based cohort study of noninstitutionalized men and women 65 years and older and living in New Haven in 1982. The New Haven cohort of 2806 subjects was drawn from a probability sample stratified by housing type, with an oversampling of men.

Details of our stratified sampling design have been described previously (12). The baseline response rate was 82%, resulting in an enrollment of 1165 men and 1641 women. The cohort is heterogeneous and includes men and women from different ethnic, racial, and social backgrounds (13).

Since assembling the cohort in 1982, respondents have been interviewed annually and monitored regularly for mortality, hospitalizations, and entry into nursing homes. To date, only 14 of the 2806 subjects have been lost to follow-up.

New Haven Cohort of Elderly Patients with Myocardial Infarction

We enrolled elderly men and women from the EPESE cohort who were hospitalized for an acute myocardial infarction. To accomplish this, we monitored, on a weekly basis, two New Haven hospitals (Saint Raphael's and Yale-New Haven) where we had previously determined that 90% to 95% of EPESE respondents would be hospitalized for myocardial infarction. Patients who were hospitalized between the start of the EPESE project in 1982 and 31 October 1988 and who received a final discharge diagnosis of acute myocardial infarction were identified for inclusion in the study ($n = 211$). We excluded 17 patients who did not meet standard clinical and laboratory criteria for myocardial infarction (that is, enzyme and electrocardiographic findings did not indicate such as diagnosis) (14). All records were reviewed by one of the investigators (RIH), who was blinded to other patient characteristics. Death within 6 months of hospital admission for the infarction was the main end point. Mortality status was known, and data were complete for all 194 enrolled men and women. Death within 6 months was selected as the major mortality end point because deaths occurring in this period would most likely be attributable to the infarction rather than to comorbid disorders. Mortality data were derived from death certificates. Cause of death was determined by a single nosologist who classified cause of death for all EPESE sites.

Social and Psychological Assessments

All social and psychological data were collected by trained EPESE interviewers. Social and psychological information was collected in 1982 and in 1985, and our analysis was based on patient information collected during the interview closest in time to but preceding the myocardial infarction. Annual interviews in intervening years were done by telephone and did not cover areas related to psychosocial conditions.

The measures of social ties we used covered two dimensions of social relations. The first was the extent to which a person received emotional support from the social network. Emotional sup-

port was measured by responses to the following items: "Can you count on anyone to provide you with emotional support? (talking over problems or helping you make a difficult decision)." We then asked who provided this support. The measure we used is a count of the sources of support (0, 1, or ≥ 2). Detailed information on network and support measures used in our study have been reported previously (15).

We were also interested in the structure of the individual's social network (16, 17). This measure covers four components: marital status; contacts with friends and relatives; membership in religious organizations; and activities in voluntary groups.

Depressive symptoms were measured by the Center for Epidemiologic Study Depressive Symptomatology Questionnaire, a 20-item, self-report measure. This measure of depressive symptoms taps feelings of psychological distress, is scored on a scale ranging from 0 to 60, and is a reliable indicator of depressive symptoms in elderly populations (12, 18). Education was divided into tertiles: those having less than a high school education, those completing a high school education, and those having more than a high school education. Regarding race, subjects were categorized as white and nonwhite.

Functional Status and Other Health-related Conditions

Information on functional ability and health practices was collected from the EPESE interview preceding the myocardial infarction. A scale of physical functioning is based on self-report items related to basic activities of daily living, physical performance, and gross mobility (12). Scoring ranged from 1 (no impairment) to 4 (major impairment in at least one activity of daily living as well as in other areas of physical performance and mobility). Data from interviews were available on smoking history, alcohol consumption, and obesity.

Myocardial Infarction and Comorbidity

The presence and severity of the myocardial infarction was determined from review of hospital records. Severity of the infarction was measured using several variables. First, we used the Killip classification (19), which is based on four ordinal categories: 1 = no failure, that is, the absence of any clinical signs of cardiac decompensation; 2 = heart failure, defined by the presence of rales, S_3 gallop, and venous hypertension; 3 = pulmonary edema; and 4 = cardiogenic shock, defined by a systolic blood pressure of less than 90 mm Hg, with associated peripheral hypoperfusion.

Second, we abstracted information related to left ventricular ejection fraction for respondents (approximately 50%) who had had either an echocardiographic evaluation or a radionuclide study. Respondents were assigned to one of the five following categories: 1) ejection fraction of less than 35%; 2) ejection fraction of 35% or greater but less than 45%; 3) ejection fraction of 45% or greater but less than 55%; 4) ejection fraction of 55% or more; and 5) "no procedures assessing left ventricular function."

We determined whether patients had had a previous myocardial infarction as well as the position of the index infarction (anterior, inferior, subendocardial, or other). We also abstracted information about the presence during hospitalization of complications such as reinfarction, atrial fibrillation, and ventricular tachycardia.

Comorbidity was assessed by adapting an index developed by Charlson and colleagues (20) that is based on the history of eight conditions: cerebrovascular accident, diabetes mellitus, chronic obstructive pulmonary disease, congestive heart failure, dementia, peripheral arterial disease, chronic renal failure, and cancer. The comorbidity score, based on medical records, was weighted, with the first six conditions receiving 1 point and the last two conditions receiving 2 points.

Statistical Analysis

To test our hypotheses about the association of social support and social networks and other potential covariates with the outcome variable of 6-month survival, we initially conducted a bivariate analysis. We used a chi-square technique to conduct tests of significance for all variables. We then stratified by covariates of importance to examine the effects of emotional support on the risk for death within risk strata. Finally, variables for which statistically significant differences in 6-month survival were found and those of special clinical or psychosocial importance were identified for inclusion in further multivariate models.

We conducted two series of multivariate analyses using multiple logistic regression and proportional hazards models (21). Because these two multivariate analyses identified similar predictors of survival and because length of survival time over the 6-month period was shown not to be an important factor, we present only results from the multiple logistic regression analyses.

Results

Of the 194 men and women hospitalized for a myocardial infarction, 76 died during the first 6 months (Table 80.1). Of these 76 deaths, 59 (78%) were clearly attributable to cardiovascular disorders.

Two characteristics were associated with an increased risk for death. Men and women who were 75 years of age or more had nearly twice the risk for death as those 65 to 74 years of age ($P = 0.01$). Patients who had no one on whom to rely for emotional support also had twice the risk for death compared with those who had two or more sources of support ($P = 0.02$). Although not statistically significant, results showed that patients with many social network ties had a decreased risk for death compared with all other patients. Survival was unrelated to symptoms

Table 80.1
Percentage of patients who died, by demographic and social characteristics

Characteristic	Total patients n	Patients who died within 6 months n (%)	P value	Characteristic	Total patients n	Patients who died within 6 months n (%)	P value
Age at time of myocardial infarction, y				*Social Network Index*			
				No or few ties	52	22 (42)	0.09
				Some ties	85	35 (41)	
65–74	77	20 (26)	0.01	More ties	28	13 (46)	
75–84	85	40 (47)		Many ties	25	4 (16)	
85 or greater	32	16 (50)		*Emotional support*			
Gender				No sources	53	28 (53)	0.02
Male	100	44 (44)	0.16	One source	111	40 (36)	
Female	94	32 (34)		Two or more sources	26	6 (23)	
Race				*Depressive symptoms†*			
White	158	65 (41)	>0.2	<16	155	60 (37)	>0.2
Nonwhite	36	11 (31)		≥16	32	13 (40)	
Education, y				*Living alone*			
<12	132	58 (44)	0.07	Yes	97	36 (37)	>0.2
12	28	6 (21)		No	97	40 (41)	
>12	29	10 (35)		*Marital status*			
Functional ability				Married	69	26 (38)	>0.2
No disability	39	13 (33)	0.07	Not married	124	50 (40)	
Minor disability	42	14 (33)					
Moderate disability	61	19 (31)					
ADL limitations*	44	24 (55)					
Cigarette smoking							
Current	37	14 (38)	>0.2				
Past	67	27 (41)					
Never	90	35 (39)					

* ADL = activities of daily living.
† Based on Center for Epidemiologic Study Depressive Symptomatology Questionnaire (*see* Methods).

Table 80.2

Percentage of patients who died, by clinical characteristics

Characteristic	Total patients *n*	Patients who died within 6 months *n* (%)	*P* value
Killip class			
No heart failure	123	34 (28)	<0.001
Congestive heart failure	37	20 (54)	
Pulmonary edema	23	13 (57)	
Cardiogenic shock	11	9 (82)	
Previous myocardial infarction			
Yes	67	35 (53)	0.007
No	127	41 (32)	
Ejection fraction			
Not done	100	47 (47)	<0.001
<35%	29	17 (59)	
35% to <55%	41	6 (15)	
≥55%	24	6 (25)	
Position of infarction			
Anterior	59	24 (41)	0.01
Inferior	52	19 (37)	
Subendocardial	70	23 (33)	
Other	10	9 (90)	
Reinfarction during hospitalization			
Yes	10	8 (80)	0.007
No	184	68 (37)	
Atrial fibrillation during hospitalization			
Yes	27	12 (44)	>0.2
No	167	64 (38)	
Ventricular tachycardia during hospitalization			
Yes	37	22 (60)	0.005
No	157	54 (34)	

Table 80.2
(continued)

Characteristic	Total patients *n*	Patients who died within 6 months *n* (%)	*P* value
Comorbidity score			
0	50	11 (22)	0.001
1	46	17 (37)	
2	43	15 (35)	
3	28	14 (50)	
≥4	27	19 (70)	

of depression, marital status, or living arrangements. In contrast to demographic and social characteristics, all measured clinical characteristics (with the exception of atrial fibrillation) were significantly associated with the risk for death within 6 months (Table 80.2).

Figure 80.1 shows the risk for death in relation to the degree of emotional support after adjustments for age, gender, severity of myocardial infarction (Killip class), and comorbidity. The number of sources of emotional support was a predictor of mortality in the younger and older age groups, for both men and women, and across varying levels of severity of myocardial infarction and comorbidity. With only one exception, a clear dose-response relation was observed.

Lack of emotional support was related to both early, in-hospital mortality and later mortality over the 6-month period (Table 80.3). Thirty-eight percent of patients who reported having no support died in the hospital compared with 12% of those who reported having two or more sources of support. The pattern continued throughout the follow-up period. By the end of 1 year, 55% of those with no sources of support had died compared with 27% of those with two or more sources. Further, if the analysis is lim-

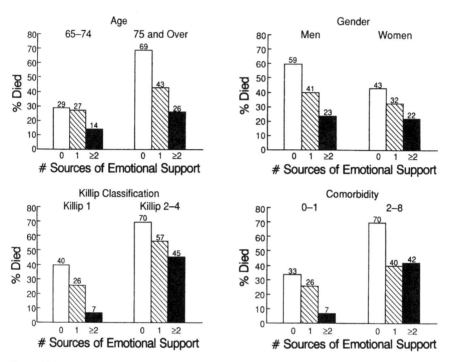

Figure 80.1
Percentage of patients with myocardial infarction who died within 6 months by level of social support. Adjustments were made for age (top left), gender (top right), severity of myocardial infarction as defined by Killip class (bottom left), and comorbidity (bottom right).

ited to those whose deaths were clearly cardiac-related (78%), the pattern was similar. The percent of patients with a cardiac cause of death was 45% among those with no sources of support, 27% among those with one source of support, and 19% among those with two or more sources of support ($P = 0.02$).

To test for selection bias, we examined the relation between risk for death from coronary heart disease and support among persons not hospitalized for a myocardial infarction. During the same 6-month period, approximately 150 deaths occurred in this group (ICD codes 410–414). The risk for experiencing such a death was not significantly associated with emotional sup-

port among persons who were not hospitalized for myocardial infarction ($P > 0.2$).

Table 80.4 shows the results of the final regression model combining clinical and psychosocial conditions predicting all-cause, 6-month mortality. Lack of emotional support emerged as the principal psychosocial condition that was independently associated with an increased risk for death at 6 months. Controlling for clinical prognostic indicators of survival, we found that patients who reported having no emotional support had almost three times the risk for death as those who reported at least one source of support (odds ratio, 2.9; 95% CI, 1.2 to 6.9). Most measures of network and support showed similar

Table 80.3

Cumulative mortality among elderly persons hospitalized for myocardial infarction compared with the number of sources of emotional support

Time to death	Percentage Dying		
	No source of emotional support ($n = 53$)	One source of emotional support ($n = 111$)	Two or more sources of emotional support ($n = 26$)
In-hospital	38	23	12
≤30 days	40	31	15
≤60 days	43	32	19
≤90 days	47	34	23
≤180 days	53	36	23
≤360 days	55	42	27

Table 80.4

Predictors of 6-month mortality after hospitalization for myocardial infarction, as determined by multiple logistic regression*

Variable	Odds ratio (95% CI)
Gender (male versus female)	1.3 (0.6 to 2.9)
Age at time of myocardial infarction (per year)	1.1 (1.0 to 1.1)
Emotional support (no support compared with one or more sources)	2.9 (1.2 to 6.9)
Killip class†	
Killip 1 versus Killip 2	2.2 (0.8 to 5.7)
Killip 1 versus Killip 3	5.0 (1.4 to 17.4)
Killip 1 versus Killip 4	29.4 (3.8 to 227.8)
Ejection fraction	
≥45% versus "evaluation not done"	3.5 (1.1 to 11.5)
≥45% versus < 35%	5.3 (1.3 to 22.2)
≥45% versus 35% to 45%	0.2 (0.0 to 1.6)
Reinfarction (Yes versus no)	34.9 (3.6 to 341.8)
Comorbidity (per unit, 0 to 4+)	1.4 (1.0 to 1.8)
Functional disability (per unit, 0 to 3)	1.2 (0.9 to 1.6)
Previous myocardial infarction (yes versus no)	1.2 (0.4 to 3.1)
Ventricular tachycardia (yes versus no)	1.8 (0.7 to 5.1)

* The analysis included 182 patients.
† *See* Methods for explanation of the Killip classification system.

trends, but they were not as powerful or consistent as those related to emotional support.

The most important clinical variables were the Killip class and reinfarction during hospitalization. Comorbidity also showed a strong, linear association with 6-month survival after acute myocardial infarction. The per-unit odds ratio was 1.4, and patients who scored 4 or more had a risk for death 3.6 times that of patients with no comorbidity.

Three variables (functional disability, previous myocardial infarction, and ventricular tachycardia) that were only significant in bivariate analyses were retained in the multivariate model to confirm the independent effects of emotional support on mortality. Gender was entered as an additional control. A best-fit model with only statistically significant variables did not change the magnitude of the effects for significant variables. Several factors were not included in the final model because they were not related to the risk for death in either bivariate or multivariate models: These included cigarette smoking, history of hypertension, presence of angina pectoris, symptoms of depression, and marital status.

Table 80.5 shows the results of four multiple logistic models in which we sequentially added significant sociodemographic features, clinical conditions related to severity of disease, comorbidity, and functional status to models in which emotional support was included. The odds ratio for lack of support alone in a model was 2.2 (CI, 1.1 to 4.1). With additional covariates added to

Table 80.5
Relation of emotional support to 6-month mortality after sequential adjustment for sociodemographic characteristics, clinical severity, and functional status*

Model	Odds ratio (95% CI)
1. No support only	2.2 (1.2 to 4.2)
2. No support, with adjustment for sociodemographic characteristics	2.1 (1.1 to 4.0)
3. No support, with adjustment for sociodemographic characteristics, and clinical severity	2.6 (1.1 to 5.8)
4. No support, with adjustment for sociodemographic characteristics, clinical severity, comorbidity, and functional status	2.9 (1.2 to 6.9)

* Sociodemographic characteristics = age and gender. Clinical severity = ejection fraction, Killip class, ventricular tachycardia, reinfarction, and previous history of myocardial infarction. Comorbidity = presence of a cerebrovascular accident, diabetes, chronic obstructive pulmonary disease, congestive heart failure, dementia, peripheral arterial disease, chronic renal failure, or cancer. Functional status = limitations in activities of daily living, gross mobility, or physical performance.

the model, the odds ratios tend to increase, indicating that the clinical features tend to mask, rather than reduce, the magnitude of the association. These results suggest that the association between lack of emotional support and increased risk for death is not the result of more severe underlying disease or comorbidity among those with less support.

Discussion

Our results indicate that the level of emotional support reported by elderly persons before their myocardial infarction is related to subsequent risk for death in the 6-month period after infarction. In multiple logistic regression analysis, lack of emotional support was significantly associated with 6-month mortality (odds ratio, 2.9; CI, 1.2 to 6.9), even after controlling for the severity of the myocardial infarction, comorbidity, and diverse sociodemographic features including socioeconomic status. Depression, marital status, and education were not associated with an increased risk for death in these multivariate models. Our investigation is one of the first to show this effect in a prospective, population-based, epidemiologic study. It is also important to note that emotional support is related to risk for death in both men and women.

Although other community-based studies have shown social isolation or lack of social ties to be related to the risk for death (16, 17, 22–27), most have used relatively simple measures of social ties and have not been able to control carefully for severity of disease or comorbidity. In such studies, more global measures of ties have consistently predicted risk for death over periods ranging from 3 to 17 years; however, these studies have not clarified where in the spectrum of disease social factors might have their greatest effect. For instance, these studies do not indicate whether social factors are related to incidence of disease or death after the event.

More recently, researchers have begun to address these questions. Investigators observed an increased risk for death in persons who were isolated (3), not married and lacking a confidant (2), or living alone (1). Our study indicates that a critical factor among such persons may be the lack of emotional support they experience. Other measures of networks and support (for example, the Social Network Index and contacts with friends and relatives) showed trends in which those who lacked ties were at increased risk; however, emotional support appeared to be the most powerful and consistent predictor of survival after myocardial infarction. Further, in our study of elderly patients, the effects associated with lack of emotional support were much stronger than those associated with either living alone or being unmarried. In fact, among elderly persons, especially women, living alone is a normative experience and not particularly associated with lack of support or social isolation.

The New Haven study has several methodologic strengths. Our findings are based on the prospective assessment of emotional support and are therefore unlikely to be influenced by the severity of the episode; moreover, our study cohort was derived from a large, random sample of the elderly population of New Haven and is representative of older men and women hospitalized with myocardial infarctions in that population.

Our study had several limitations. First, although our study population was derived from a representative population-based cohort, it included only persons hospitalized with a myocardial infarction. Excluded were persons who had a silent or undiagnosed infarction and those who had a severe infarction and died out of the hospital. Our study is directed toward understanding the recovery of persons who are hospitalized with documented myocardial infarction and is not well suited to studying these other end points. Second, in our study, we were unable to examine whether the association between lack of emotional support and risk for death is mediated by direct biologic pathways presumably involving neurohormonal and stress responses or by some indirect pathways involving differential access to care, delay in treatment, or adherence to treatment regimens (28, 29). The possibility that persons who lack emotional support have higher rates of out-of-hospital death or wait longer to come to the hospital after the onset of symptoms of myocardial infarction is worthy of careful consideration. Although we could not test this hypothesis conclusively, emotional support was not related to risk for death from coronary heart disease among those members of the cohort not hospitalized for a myocardial infarction nor to severity of myocardial infarction.

The processes by which such social factors might be related to the pathogenesis of coronary heart disease remains unclear (30). Available data indicate that the effects of social relationships, in general, may operate at several stages in the disease process. For instance, in laboratory animals, social factors such as living in a stable social environment (31) and handling of laboratory animals by humans (32), protect against the development of coronary atherosclerosis in healthy animals. In an angiographic study of men and women (33), those who felt loved and who had adequate instrumental support (help with daily tasks) had less coronary occlusion than others. In a large cohort of Israeli men, those who reported that their wives loved them had less angina pectoris (34). One community study has shown measures of social ties to be related to death from coronary heart disease and to be independent of standard risk factors (24). In addition, several investigators have speculated that stressful circumstances that involve neuroendocrine responses may influence endothelial injury and platelet function and may increase the risk for ventricular fibrillation in susceptible persons (35–38).

Our findings emphasize the importance of emotional support, along with clinically relevant prognostic indicators of severity of myocardial infarction and comorbidity, as a risk factor for mortality in patients who experience myocardial infarction. Much research needs to be directed toward identifying different aspects of network structure and the support provided by the persons who make up the network and toward uncovering the pathways by which network structure and support might influence health status.

References

1. Case RB, Moss AJ, Case N, McDermott M, Eberly S. Living alone after myocardial infarction. Impact on prognosis. JAMA. 1992; 267:515–9.

2. Williams RB, Barefoot JC, Califf RM, Haney TL, Saunders WB, Pryor DB, et al. Prognostic importance of social and economic resources among medically treated patients with angiographically documented coronary artery disease. JAMA. 1992; 267:520–4.

3. Ruberman W, Weinblatt E, Goldberg JD, Chaudhary BS. Psychosocial influences on mortality after

myocardial infarction. N Engl J Med. 1984; 311:552–9.

4. Ruberman W, Weinblatt E, Goldberg JD, Chadhary BS. Education, psychosocial stress and sudden cardiac death. J Chron Dis. 1983; 36:151–60.

5. Krantz DS. Cognitive processes and recovery from heart attack: a review and theoretical analysis. J Human Stress. 1980; 6:27–38.

6. Mayou R. Prediction of emotional and social outcome after a heart attack. J Psychosom Res. 1984; 28:17–25.

7. Powell L, Thoresen CE. Behavioral and physiologic determinants of long-term prognosis after myocardial infarction. J Chron Dis. 1985; 38:253–63.

8. Croog SH, Levine S. The Heart Patient Recovers: Social and Psychological Factors. New York: Human Sciences Press; 1977.

9. Henning H, Gilpin EA, Covell JW, Swan EA, O'Rourke RA, Ross J. Prognosis after acute myocardial infarction: a multivariate analysis of mortality and survival. Circulation. 1979; 59:1124–36.

10. Sanz G, Castaner A, Betriu A, Magrina J, Roig E, Coll S, et al. Determinants of prognosis in survivors of myocardial infarction: a prospective clinical angiographic study. N Engl J Med. 1982; 306:1065–70.

11. Sokolow M, McIlroy MB. Clinical Cardiology. Los Altos, California: Lange Medical Publications; 1987.

12. Berkman LF, Berkman CS, Kasl S, Freeman DH Jr, Leo L, Ostfeld AM, et al. Depressive symptoms in relation to physical health and functioning in the elderly. Am J Epidemiol. 1986; 124:372–88.

13. Berkman L, Singer B, Manton K. Black/white differences in health status and mortality among the elderly. Demography. 1989; 26:661–78.

14. Ischemic Heart Disease Registers. Report of the Fifth Working Group on Ischemic Heart Disease Registers. Copenhagen: World Health Organization; 1971.

15. Seeman TE, Berkman LF. Structural characteristics of social networks and their relationship with social support in the elderly: who provides support? Soc Sci Med. 1988; 26:737–49.

16. Berkman LF, Syme SL. Social networks, host resistance, and mortality: a nine-year follow-up study of Alameda County residents. Am J Epidemiol. 1979; 109:684–94.

17. Seeman TS, Kaplan GA, Knudsen L, Cohen R, Guralnik J. Social network ties and mortality among the elderly in the Alameda County Study. Am J Epidemiol. 1987; 126:714–23.

18. Radloff LS. The CES-D scale: a self-report depression scale for research in the general population. J Appl Psychol Meas. 1977; 1:385–401.

19. Killip T, Kimball JT. Treatment of myocardial infarction in a coronary care unit. A two year experience with 250 patients. Am J Cardiol. 1967; 20:467–74.

20. Charlson M, Pompei P, Ales KL, McKenzie CR. A new method of classifying prognostic comorbidity in longitudinal studies: development and validation. J Chron Dis. 1984; 37:369–75.

21. Harrell F. The PHGLM Procedure-SUGI Supplemental Library User's Guide. Fifth edition. Cary, North Carolina: SAS Institute, Inc.; 1986:437–66.

22. Blazer DG. Social support and mortality in an elderly community population. Am J Epidemiol. 1982; 115:684–94.

23. House JS, Robbins C, Metzner HL. The association of social relationships and activities with mortality: prospective evidence from the Tecumseh Community Health Study. Am J Epidemiol. 1982; 116:123–40.

24. Kaplan GA, Salonen JT, Cohen RD, Brand RJ, Syme SL, Puska P. Social connections and mortality from all causes and cardiovascular disease: prospective evidence from eastern Finland. Am J Epidemiol. 1988; 128:370–80.

25. Orth-Gomer K, Johnson JV. Social network interaction and mortality: A six year follow-up of a random sample of the Swedish population. J Chron Dis. 1987; 4:944–57.

26. Welin L, Tibblin G, Svardsudd K, Tibblin B, Ander-Peciva S, Larsson B, et al. Prospective study of social influences on mortality: the study of men born in 1913 and 1923. Lancet. 1985; 1:915–8.

27. Seeman TE, Berkman LF, Kohout F, LaCroix A, Glynn R, Blazer D. Inter-community variations in the association between social ties and mortality in the elderly: a comparative analysis of three communities. Ann Epidemiol. [In press].

28. Mermelstein R, Cohen S, Lichtenstein E, Baer JS, Kamarck T. Social support and smoking cessation and maintenance. J Consult Clin Psychol. 1986; 54:447–53.

29. Ayanian JZ, Epstein AM. Differences in the use of procedures between women and men hospitalized for

coronary heart disease. N Engl J Med. 1991; 325:221–5.

30. Cohen S. Psychosocial models of the role of social support in the etiology of physical disease. Health Psychol. 1988; 7:269–97.

31. Kaplan JR, Manuck SB, Clarkson TB, Lusso FM, Taub DB. Social status, environment, and atherosclerosis in cynomolgus monkeys. Arteriosclerosis. 1982; 2:359–68.

32. Nerem RM, Levesque MJ, Cornhill JF. Social environment as a factor in diet-induced atherosclerosis. Science. 1980; 208:1475–6.

33. Seeman TE, Syme SL. Social networks and coronary artery disease: a comparison of the structure and function of social relationships as predictors of disease. Psychosom Med. 1987; 49:340–53.

34. Medalie JH, Goldbourt V. Angina pectoris among 10,000 men. II. Psychosocial and other risk factors as evidenced by multivariate analyses of five year incidence study. Am J Med. 1976; 60:910–21.

35. Ruberman W. Psychosocial influences on mortality of patients with coronary heart disease. JAMA. 1992; 267:559–60.

36. Lown B. Sudden cardiac death: biobehavioral perspectives. Circulation. 1987; 76(Suppl 1):186–95.

37. Brackett CD, Powell LH. Psychosocial and physiological predictors of sudden cardiac death after healing of acute myocardial infarction. Am J Cardiol. 1988; 61:979–83.

38. Markowe HL, Marmot MG, Shipley MG, Bulpitt CJ, Meade TW, Stirling Y, et al. Fibrinogen: A possible link between social class and coronary heart disease. Br Med J (Clin Res Ed). 1985; 291:1312–4.

81   Social Ties and Susceptibility to the Common Cold

Sheldon Cohen, William J. Doyle, David P. Skoner, Bruce S. Rabin, and Jack M. Gwaltney Jr.

The hypothesis that multiple ties to friends, family, work, and community are beneficial in terms of physical health has gained substantial support over the last decade. Particularly provocative is epidemiologic evidence that those who participate in more diversified social networks—for example, are married, interact with family members, friends, neighbors, and fellow workers, and belong to social and religious groups—live longer than their counterparts with fewer types of social relationships.[1–3] This association has been reported in multiple prospective studies,[1–3] and the relative risk for mortality among those with less diverse networks is comparable in magnitude to the relation between smoking and mortality from all causes.[3] Unfortunately, the behavioral and biological characteristics that link social networks of greater scope to longevity have not been identified. However, evidence implicating social network ties in the regulation of the immune system suggests that social networks may play a role in the ability of the host to resist infection.[4,5]

We report a prospective study assessing the role of social network diversity in susceptibility to upper respiratory tract infections. In theory, participation in a more diverse social network may influence the motivation to care for oneself by promoting feelings of self-worth, responsibility, control, and meaning in life.[6,7] This motivation would be manifest in an increase in health promoting behaviors such as abstaining from smoking, moderating alcohol consumption, and improving diet, exercise regimens, and sleep quality.[7,8] Greater network diversity has also been related to less anxiety, depression, and nonspecific psychological distress.[9] Lower levels of these negative mood states have been associated with lower basal levels of epinephrine, norepinephrine, and cortisol.[10] In turn, these hormones are thought to influence both cellular and humoral immune function and potentially to alter host resistance to infection.[11,12]

Although there is evidence for increased susceptibility to common colds among smokers[13] and decreased risk among moderate drinkers,[13] little is known about the role of other health practices or about levels of catecholamines, cortisol, or normal variations in cellular immune function in susceptibility to the common cold.[14] The study reported here examines the importance of network diversity for susceptibility, the importance of these behavioral and biological markers for susceptibility, and the possible role that these markers might play in linking social network diversity to colds.

Methods

Subjects

The subjects were 125 men and 151 women from the Pittsburgh, Pa., area who responded to newspaper advertisements and were judged to be in good health after a medical examination. Their ages ranged from 18 to 55 years. They were studied in 6 groups (4 in the spring and 2 in the fall) with 40 to 60 subjects in each. Subjects were paid $800 for their participation. The study was approved by the institutional review boards of Carnegie Mellon University, University of Pittsburgh, and Children's Hospital of Pittsburgh, and informed consent was obtained from each subject after the nature and possible consequences of the study were fully explained.

Experimental Plan

All volunteers came to the hospital for medical eligibility screenings. They were not accepted into the study if they had previous nasal or otologic surgery; a history of asthma or cardiovascular disorders; abnormal clinical profiles on urinalysis, complete blood cell count, blood enzymes, or any of 3 nutritional markers (albumin, transferrin, or retinol binding protein); or were pregnant or currently lactating, seropositive for human immunodeficiency virus, or on a regular medication regimen. Social networks, health practices (except diet), age, education, race, sex, and body weight and height were also assessed at the screening and used as baseline data for those who were deemed eligible.

Eligible subjects returned to the hospital both 4 and 5 weeks after screening to have blood drawn for assessment of natural killer (NK) cell activity (based on both blood draws) and antibody to the challenge virus (based on the second blood draw). A personality questionnaire was administered twice, once at each blood draw.

Subjects were quarantined within 1 week following the second blood draw. During the first 24 hours of quarantine (before viral exposure), they received a nasal examination. They were excluded from the study at this point if a nasal wash culture indicated they were infected by a rhinovirus; the nasal examination showed congestion, mucosal edema, or nasal discharge; or they reported symptomatic upper respiratory tract infections within the 30 days before quarantine. Baseline respiratory symptoms, nasal mucociliary clearance, and nasal mucus production were assessed at this time. Urine samples for endocrine assessment and information on dietary intake were also collected.

At the end of the first 24 hours of quarantine, subjects were given nasal drops containing a low infectious dose (100–300 tissue culture infectious dose ($TCID_{50}$)/mL) of 1 of 2 types of rhinovirus—RV39 (n = 147) or Hanks (n = 129). Two viruses were used to assess whether predictors of susceptibility are equivalent across different rhinovirus types. Rhinovirus type RV39 was used in the first 3 groups of subjects and rhinovirus strain Hanks in the last 3.

The quarantine continued for 5 days after exposure. During this period, the subjects were housed individually but were allowed to interact with each other at a distance of 3 ft or more. Nasal secretion samples for virus culture were collected on each of the 5 days. Subjects were also tested on each day for respiratory symptoms, nasal mucociliary clearance, and nasal mucus production with the same procedures as used at baseline. Approximately 28 days after challenge, another blood sample was collected for serological testing. All investigators were blinded to subjects' status on social network, personality, endocrine, health practice, immune, and prechallenge antibody measures.

Standard Control Variables

We used 8 control variables that might provide alternative explanations for the relation between network diversity and illness. Prechallenge antibody titer was categorized into approximate quartiles: less than 2, 2 to 4, 8 to 16, and greater than 16. Age and body mass index (weight in kilograms divided by the square of height in meters) were scored as continuous variables. Whether the trial was conducted in the fall (November) or spring (April and May), race (white [81.2%] or not [18.8%]), sex, and viral type (RV39 or Hanks) were scored as dichotomous variables. Education levels were categorized as high school graduate or less, some college, and bachelor's degree or greater.

Social Network Diversity

The Social Network Index assesses participation in 12 types of social relationships.[15] These include relationships with a spouse, parents, parents-in-law, children, other close family members, close neighbors, friends, workmates, schoolmates, fellow volunteers (e.g., charity or community work), members of groups without religious affiliations (e.g., social, recreational, or professional), and members of religious groups. One point is assigned for each type of relationship (possible score of 12) for which respondents indicate that they speak (in person or on the phone) to someone in that relationship at least once every 2 weeks. The total number of persons with whom they speak at least once every 2 weeks (number of network members) was also assessed.

Pathways Linking Social Networks to Susceptibility

Health practices and markers of endocrine and immune function were assessed before viral challenge as possible pathways linking network diversity to susceptibility. Smokers were defined as those smoking cigarettes, cigars, or a pipe on a daily basis.[13] In calculating the average number of alcoholic drinks per day, a bottle or can of beer, a glass of wine, or a shot of spirits were each treated as a single drink.[13] Exercise was assessed by a question asking the number of times per week that the subject engaged in an activity long enough to work up a sweat, get the heart thumping, or become out of breath.[16] Quality of sleep was assessed by scales assessing subjective sleep quality, sleep latency, disturbance, and efficiency (percentage of time in bed sleeping).[17] Dietary intake of vitamin C and zinc was also assessed by standard questionnaire.[18] Analyses including diet variables are limited to 228 subjects who completed the questionnaire according to standard criteria.[19]

Epinephrine, norepinephrine, and cortisol levels were assessed as markers of stress.[10] These hormones were measured in 24-hour urine samples collected just prior to viral challenge. High-performance liquid chromatography with electrochemical detection was used for measurement of the urinary catecholamines. Urinary cortisol assays were performed by a double-antibody competitive radioimmunoassay.

Natural killer cell activity is thought to play an important role in limiting viral replication.[20] We conducted a whole blood NK assay.[21] The

results of the 2 blood draws were averaged to estimate cytotoxicity.

Personality as an Alternative Explanation

We examined personality factors that might account for both greater network diversity and less susceptibility. We assessed the "Big-Five" characteristics thought to represent the basic structure of personality.[22] These factors are commonly described as extraversion, agreeableness, conscientiousness, emotional stability, and openness. To assess the Big-Five, we used a modified version of Goldberg's[22] adjective scales. Our version includes 50 adjectives, 10 for each factor. We used the average of the scores from the 2 administrations of the scales.

Viral Cultures and Antibody Response

Nasal washes were cultured for virus, and all positive specimens were quantitated.[23] Neutralizing antibody to the challenge virus was measured in serum collected before and 28 days after exposure to the challenge virus.[23] Serum antibody titers are reported as reciprocals of the initial dilution of serum.

Signs and Symptoms

At the end of each day of quarantine, subjects rated the severity of 8 respiratory symptoms (congestion, runny nose, sneezing, cough, sore throat, malaise, headache, and chills) during the previous 24 hours.[24] Ratings ranged from 0 (none) to 4 (very severe) for each symptom. The symptom scores were summed within each day. The score for the day before challenge was subtracted from each daily score after viral challenge. The adjusted postchallenge symptom scores were summed to create an adjusted total symptom score. Subjects were also asked each day if they had a cold.

Mucus production was assessed by collecting used tissues in sealed plastic bags.[25] The bags were weighed and the weight of the tissues and bags subtracted. To adjust for baseline, weight on the day before challenge was subtracted from each daily weight after viral challenge. The adjusted postchallenge weights were summed to create an adjusted total mucus weight score.

Nasal mucociliary clearance function refers to the effectiveness of nasal cilia in clearing mucus from the nasal passage toward the nasopharynx. Clearance function is assessed as the time required for a dye administered in the nostrils to reach the nasopharynx.[25] Each daily time was adjusted (by subtracting) for baseline, and the adjusted average time in minutes was calculated across the postchallenge days of the trial.

Infections and Colds

Volunteers were considered to have a cold if they *both* were infected and met illness criteria. They were classified as infected if the challenge virus was isolated on any of the 5 postchallenge study days or there was a 4-fold or greater rise in viral-specific serum neutralizing antibody titer from before exposure to 28 days after exposure. We examined colds using 3 different illness criteria. The illness criterion used in the primary analyses was based on objective indicators of illness—a total adjusted mucus weight of at least 10 g or adjusted average mucociliary nasal clearance time of at least 7 minutes. The mean ($\pm$SD) total adjusted respiratory symptom score for those with colds defined as infection plus the objective illness criterion was 19.28 ($\pm$14.7) vs 5.67 ($\pm$8.1) for those without colds ($t[274] = -9.88$; $P < .001$). The 2 other illness criteria we used in defining colds were based on subject self-report. The first required subjects reporting (using their own definition) having a "cold." The second, the modified Jackson criterion, is previously validated and requires a total adjusted symptom score of 6 or more in addition to either reporting having a cold or reporting rhinorrhea on 3 or more days of the trial.[17]

Statistical Analyses

We used stepwise logistic regression to predict the binary outcome incidence of a cold[26] and multiple linear regression to predict continuous outcomes.[27] Social network diversity was initially treated as a continuous variable. In these cases, we report the regression coefficient for network diversity, its SE, and probability level. However, to provide an estimate of relative risk, we also present odds ratios (ORs) and 95% confidence intervals (CIs) based on network diversity categorized into low (1–3 types of relationships), moderate (4–5 types), and high ($\geq$6 types). We sequentially added variables to the first step of regression analyses to determine whether the association between network diversity (entered alone in the second step) and susceptibility to colds is substantially reduced after controlling for the contribution of other variables. Finally, when we report mean levels of continuous outcomes, we also report the SEM.

Results

Rates of infections and colds stratified by prechallenge serostatus are presented in Table 81.1. Rates of colds were similar for the objective, self-reported cold, and Jackson illness criteria. The greater protective effects of antibody for rhinovirus strain Hanks is a new observation.

Standard Controls and Susceptibility

When examined as an individual predictor, increasing prechallenge antibody was associated with decreased incidence of colds (objective criterion for illness, $P < .001$). Education was also associated with incidence in an unexpected manner. The highest rate of colds was associated with those with high school degrees or less (52%), the next highest with those with college degrees or more (45%), and the lowest with those with some college (33%, $P = .04$). Other standard

Table 81.1
Rates and numbers of infected persons and of persons with colds stratified by prechallenge antibody titer and virus

Prechallenge antibody titer	Virus type	Challenge, no.	Infection, % (no.)	Colds defined as infection and		
				Objective criterion, % (no.)	Self-reported criterion, % (no.)	Jackson criterion, % (no.)
≤2	RV39	71	99 (70)	63 (45)	55 (39)	59 (42)
	Hanks	73	99 (72)	53 (39)	52 (38)	56 (41)
	Total	144	99 (142)	58 (84)	54 (77)	58 (83)
≥4	RV39	76	82 (62)	25 (19)	29 (22)	24 (18)
	Hanks	56	52 (29)	11 (6)	11 (6)	16 (9)
	Total	132	69 (91)	19 (25)	21 (28)	21 (27)

control variables were not individually associated with the incidence of colds. When the 8 standard controls were entered into the regression simultaneously to test the independent contribution of each control variable, associations with antibody titers $(P < .001)$ and education $(P = .04)$ remained the same. In addition, increasing age was associated with increased incidence $(P = .03)$, as was being exposed to rhinovirus type 39 (44% colds) as opposed to rhinovirus strain Hanks (35% colds; $P = .03$).

Social Networks and Susceptibility

As apparent from Figure 81.1, when we used the objective illness criterion, the rate of colds decreased with increased social network diversity $(\pm SE)$ (b = -0.19 [± 0.08]; $P = .01$ for continuous variable; OR, 3.0 [95% CI, 1.23–7.44] for low, 1.5 [95% CI, 0.87–2.46] for moderate, and 1.0 for high social network diversity). Entering the standard control variables into the equation before social network diversity strengthened this association (b = -0.29 [± 10], $P = .01$; adjusted OR, 4.2 [95% CI, 1.34–13.29] for low, 1.9 [95% CI, 1.00–3.51] for moderate, and 1.0 for high). There were no interactions between the standard control variables and social network diversity in predicting colds. Hence, the relationships were

similar for the 2 virus types, for different levels of serologic status, age, sex, race, education, and body mass index, and across the 2 seasons. Of special note for interpretation of our data is that network diversity and rates of colds are similarly associated across virus types and across prechallenge seropositives and seronegatives (Table 81.2).

Use of the self-reported cold criterion for illness resulted in adjusted ORs similar to those found with the objective illness criterion (adjusted OR, 3.5 [95% CI, 1.18–10.20] for low, 1.9 [95% CI, 1.02–3.50] for moderate, and 1.0 for high social network diversity groups) (Figure 81.1). In the case of the modified Jackson criterion, there was no graded association between network diversity and colds but a difference between the low and high network diversity groups (adjusted OR, 3.2 [95% CI, 1.04–9.77], 1.2 [95% CI, 0.66–2.26], and 1.0) (Figure 81.1). In later analyses, we use the objective criterion in defining colds because this measure of illness is not subject to biases in subjects' symptom reporting.

We also examined whether social network diversity was associated with continuous measures of the 2 objective signs of illness among infected people. Both analyses were adjusted for standard control variables. Increases in network diversity were associated with decreases in mucus weights

Table 81.2
Rates and numbers of persons with colds by number of types of social relationships, stratified by prechallenge antibody titer and virus*

Prechallenge antibody titer	Virus type	Number of types of social relationships	
		1–5, no. (%) with colds	≥6, no. (%) with colds
≤2	RV39	25/33 (76)	20/38 (53)
	Hanks	18/30 (60)	21/43 (49)
	Total	43/63 (68)	41/81 (51)
≥4	RV39	11/34 (32)	8/42 (19)
	Hanks	3/26 (12)	3/30 (10)
	Total	14/60 (23)	11/72 (15)

* Low and moderate levels of social diversity have been combined into 1 category (1–5) so that there are a sufficient number of persons within each cell to provide a reliable estimate of the rates of colds.

(mean, 0.95 [±0.18] $\log_{10}$ grams for low, 0.73 [±0.07] for moderate, and 0.66 [±0.05] for high diversity; $F[1, 216] = 7.65$; $P = .007$) and increases in mucociliary clearance function (mean, 6.3 [±1.4] minutes for low, 5.0 [±0.6] for moderate, and 3.6 [±0.4] for high diversity; $F[1, 218] = 5.75$; $P = .02$).

In contrast to the diversity of the network, the total number of network members was not associated with colds ($P = .12$). Moreover, entering the number of network members into the first step of the regression equation along with standard controls did not reduce the association between diversity and colds (b = −0.36 [±0.13]; $P = .01$).

Social Networks and the Quantity of Viral Replication

Because greater replication of virus during the 5 days following exposure was associated with greater likelihood of developing a cold (b = 1.04

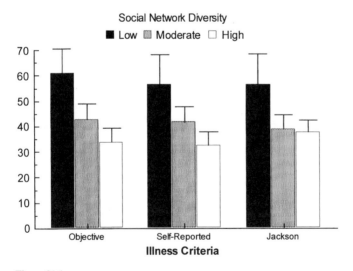

Figure 81.1
Observed incidence of colds by social network diversity using 3 illness criteria. Low diversity is defined as 1–3 types of social relationships; moderate, 4–5; and high, 6 or more. Error bars: SE.

[±0.18], $P < .001$ for all subjects; b = 0.93 [±0.19], $P < .001$ for infected subjects), we thought it might account for the relations between social network diversity and colds. Viral replication as measured by viral concentration in nasal washes decreased with increases in network diversity (adjusted for standard controls, F[1, 263] = 5.76; $P = .02$; for all subjects: mean, 2.23 [±0.30] log$_{10}$ titers for low, 1.74 [±0.12] for moderate, and 1.51 [±0.10] for high; F[1, 220] = 6.19; $P = .02$; for infected subjects: mean, 2.57 [±0.28] log$_{10}$ titers for low, 2.00 [±0.12] for moderate, and 1.83 [±0.10] for high). However, the association between network diversity and the incidence of colds was only slightly reduced when quantity of viral replication was added as a control variable (b = −0.24 [±0.11], $P = .03$ for all subjects; b = −0.25 [±0.10], $P = .02$ for infected subjects; without viral replication in the equation, b = −0.29 [±0.10], $P = .01$ for both infected and all subjects). Overall, these analyses suggest that the relationship between social network diversity and colds was not primarily mediated by quantity of viral replication.

Pathways Linking Social Networks to Susceptibility

We began by testing whether each of the proposed health behavior endocrine and immune pathways was associated with susceptibility to colds. Each was tested individually and then simultaneously with other measures in their category (e.g., smoking independent of other health practices). In all cases, the standard control variables were entered in the first step of the regression, and the variables representing the proposed pathway were entered in the second step. Table 81.3 presents these data for factors that were individually associated with colds.

Smokers, persons exercising 2 times or fewer a week, those with sleep efficiency of 0.80 or less, those drinking 1 drink or fewer per day, and those ingesting 85 mg or fewer of vitamin C a day were all at greater risk for developing colds.

Table 81.3
Adjusted odds ratios (95% confidence intervals) for health practices and endocrine measures associated with the incidence of colds*

	Potential mediators entered in equation	
	Individually	With others
Health practices		
Smoking	3.0 (1.5–6.1)	3.3 (1.5–7.0)
Exercising ≤ 2 times/wk	1.8 (1.0–3.2)	1.5 (0.8–2.7)
Sleep efficiency of ≤0.80	2.6 (1.2–5.8)	2.8 (1.2–4.8)
Drinking ≤ 1 drink/d	2.0 (1.0–3.8)	2.6 (1.3–5.3)
Ingesting ≤ 0.85 mg vitamin C/d	2.0 (1.0–3.8)†	…‡
Endocrine measures		
Norepinephrine	1.9 (1.0–3.5)	1.7 (0.9–3.2)
Epinephrine	1.8 (0.9–3.6)	1.5 (0.8–3.1)

* Odds ratios are adjusted for standard control variables. Separate regressions were fit to examine the association of each individual mediator with colds and a single regression was fit to examine the association of each mediator independent of other variables in its group (simultaneous entry).
† The table is based on the entire sample for all but vitamin C, which is based on the subsample who completed diet questionnaires ($n = 228$).
‡ Analyses of the subsample, controlling for vitamin C intake as well as the other health practices result in identical conclusions. In these analyses, diet is not related to colds after controlling for other health practices (odds ratio, 1.6; 95% confidence interval, 0.80–3.23).

There were no associations between zinc and colds or between the other sleep measures and colds. When the health practices that were individually associated with colds were entered into the regression simultaneously, smoking, drinking 1 drink or fewer per day, and sleep efficiency all made independent contributions.

Persons with levels of norepinephrine above the median level (175 nmol/d) were at greater risk for developing colds than those below the median. A similar but weaker relation was found for epinephrine (median, 21 nmol/d). Neither cortisol levels nor NK cell cytotoxicity was associated with colds. When epinephrine and norepinephrine were entered into the equation simultaneously, the contributions of both were attenuated.

We then conducted a series of logistic regressions to determine whether social network diversity was associated with each of the health practice and endocrine factors that we determined to be risks for colds. All analyses included the standard control variables. Lower levels of network diversity were associated with being a smoker (b = −0.22 [±0.09], P = .02) and with insufficient exercise (b = −0.28 [±0.08], P = .01). However, network diversity was not associated with alcohol consumption, dietary intake of vitamin C, or sleep efficiency or with above-median levels of epinephrine or norepinephrine.

Because smoking and exercise were associated with both social network diversity and with colds, they are the only proposed mediators that could operate as pathways linking network diversity to susceptibility. To determine whether these factors might operate as pathways, they were entered along with the standard controls in the first step of the regression equation, with network diversity entered in the second step. Addition of these health practices to the equation slightly decreased the association between social network diversity and susceptibility to colds (b = −0.24 [±0.10], P = .02 with smoking and exercise; b = −0.29 [±0.10], P = .01 before adding smoking and exercise). Hence the health practices account for a small proportion of the relationship but do not act as primary pathways linking network diversity and colds in this study.

Personality as an Alternative Explanation

We entered each of the Big-Five personality factors into separate equations along with the standard controls predicting colds. Only extraversion was associated with susceptibility with those with low scores (introverts—below the median of 28.5) at greater risk for colds (adjusted OR, 2.7; 95% CI, 1.45–4.92). Moreover, extraversion was associated with higher levels of social network diversity (b = 0.25 [±.08], P = .01). However, adding extraversion to the regression equation including standard controls does not substantially alter the relation between network diversity and incidence of colds (b = −0.24 [±0.10], P = .02 with extraversion; b = −0.29 [±0.10], P = .01 without extraversion).

Comment

The results indicate people who participate in more types of social relationships have less susceptibility to rhinovirus-induced colds. This association is graded, although the risk increases most among those with the fewest types of relationships. Moreover, the adjusted OR is substantial, with those reporting 1 to 3 types of relationships having more than 4 times the risk of those reporting 6 or more types of relationships. The association between network diversity and susceptibility held even after controlling for the number of people in the social network indicating that it is diversity of the network (having multiple types of relationships) that matters not the sheer number of network members.

Although the quantity of viral replication decreased with increased network diversity, the quantity of replication did not act as a primary pathway linking network diversity and the development of colds. These results suggest that social network diversity may be associated with more than 1 disease process, i.e., extent of viral replication and a process or processes that modulate the production of signs and symptoms of illness.

Several health practices and endocrine measures were associated with risk for colds, including replications of previously established risks of smoking,[13] as well as benefits of moderate alcohol consumption.[13] Although not previously reported, the elevated risk associated with high basal levels of catecholamines is consistent with previous reports of an association between psychological stress and increased susceptibility.[28,29] We also found new evidence for increased risk among those exercising 2 times or fewer a week and among those with sleep efficiencies lower than 0.80. Intake of vitamin C below 85 mg/d (this cutoff was empirically derived) were also associated with greater risk, but additional intake was not beneficial. The relative risks associated with health practices ranged from 1.8 to 3.0, while the relative risk associated with elevated catecholamines ranged from 1.8 to 1.9. However, only smoking and exercise met the criteria for pathways linking social network diversity to susceptibility, and together these could account for only a part of this relation. Finally, the personality characteristic extraversion was examined as a factor that might account for increases in network diversity and decreases in susceptibility. Although those with low scores (introverts) had less diverse networks and were at greater risk for colds, this variable was unable to account for the relation between social network diversity and susceptibility.

We can only speculate on what other mechanisms might mediate the association of network diversity and colds. Our data suggest eliminating a number of possibilities. At least for seronegative subjects, the relation was attributable to increased illness among infected persons (99% were infected) and not increased incidence of infection. The similarity of the association across serostatus also suggests that the mechanism is not primarily mediated by serum antibody production in response to the virus among those previously exposed. In addition, we found little evidence for the role of NK cell activity. However, other characteristics of immune status may operate as pathways. For example, there may be behavioral effects on the release of cytokines in the nasal passage that effect the triggering of symptoms.[30]

A relation between network diversity and host resistance may provide a partial explanation for the association between social network diversity and all-cause mortality. Unfortunately, without a better understanding of the underlying mechanisms linking network diversity to colds, we cannot say whether our data have implication for host resistance to other infectious agents that may cause or contribute to mortality.

Acknowledgments

This study was supported by a grant from the National Institute of Mental Health (MH50429), a Research Scientist Development Award to Dr Cohen from the National Institute of Mental Health (MH00721), a grant from the National Institute of Health to the University of Pittsburgh Medical Center General Clinical Research Center (NCRR/GCRC 5M01 RR00056), and support from the Fetzer Institute.

We are indebted to Janet Schlarb, James Seroky, the staff of the General Clinical Research Center, Theresa Whiteside, PhD, and Robert McDonald, Jr, MD, and their laboratory staffs, and the volunteers for their contributions to the research, and to Joel Greenhouse, PhD, for statistical advice, and Kenneth Kotovsky, PhD, and Vicki Helgeson; PhD, for comments on earlier drafts.

References

1. Berkman LF, Syme, SL. Social networks, host resistance, and mortality. *Am J Epidemiol.* 1979; 109: 186–204.

2. Vogt TM, Mullooly JP, Ernst D, Pope CR, Hollis JF. Social networks as predictors of ischemic heart disease, cancer, stroke and hypertension. *J Clin Epidemiol.* 1992; 45:659–666.

3. House JS, Landis KR, Umberson D. Social relationships and health. *Science.* 1988; 241:540–545.

4. Uchino BN, Cacioppo JT, Kiecolt-Glaser JK. The relationship between social support and physiological processes. *Psychol Bull.* 1996; 119:488–531.

5. Kiecolt-Glaser JK, Malarkey WB, Cacioppo JT, Glaser R. Stressful personal relationships: immune and endocrine function. In: Glaser R, Kiecolt-Glaser J, eds. *Handbook of Human Stress and Immunity.* San Diego, Calif: Academic Press Inc; 1994:321–339.

6. Thoits PA. Multiple identities and psychological well-being. *Am Sociol Rev.* 1983; 48:174–187.

7. Cohen S. Psychosocial models of the role of social support in the etiology of physical disease. *Health Psychol.* 1988; 7:269–297.

8. Berkman LF, Breslow L. *Health and Ways of Living: The Alameda County Study.* New York, NY: Oxford University Press; 1983.

9. Cohen S, Wills TA. Stress, social support, and the buffering hypothesis. *Psychol Bull.* 1985; 98:310–357.

10. Baum A, Grunberg N. Measurement of stress hormones. In: Cohen S, Kessler RC, Underwood Gordon L, eds. *Measuring Stress.* New York, NY: Oxford University Press; 1995:175–192.

11. Glaser R, Kiecolt-Glaser J, eds. *Handbook of Human Stress and Immunity.* San Diego, Calif: Academic Press Inc; 1994.

12. Ader R, Cohen N, Felton D, eds. *Psychoneuroimmunology.* San Diego, Calif: Academic Press Inc; 1991.

13. Cohen S, Tyrrell DAJ, Russell MAH, Jarvis MJ, Smith AP. Smoking, alcohol consumption, and susceptibility to the common cold. *Am J Public Health.* 1993; 83:1277–1283.

14. Gwaltney JM Jr. Rhinoviruses. In: Evans AS, ed. *Viral Infections of Humans: Epidemiology and Control.* New York, NY: Plenum Publishing Corp; 1984.

15. Cohen S. Social supports and physical health. In: Greene AL, Cummings M, Karraker KH, eds. *Life-Span Developmental Psychology: Perspectives on Stress and Coping.* Hillsdale, NJ: Erlbaum Associates; 1991.

16. Paffenbarger RS Jr, Blair SN, Lee I, Hyde RT. Measurement of physical activity to assess health effects in free-living populations. *Med Sci Sports Exerc.* 1993; 25:60–70.

17. Buysse DJ, Reynolds CF, Monk TH, Berman SR, Kupfer DJ. The Pittsburgh Sleep Quality Index. *Psychiatry Res.* 1989; 28:193–213.

18. Block G, Hartman AM, Naughton D. A reduced dietary questionnaire. *Epidemiology.* 1990; 1:58–64.

19. Block G, Thompson FE, Hartman AM, Larkin FA, Guire KE. Comparison of two dietary questionnaires validated against multiple dietary records collected during a 1-year period. *J Am Diet Assoc.* 1992; 92:686–693.

20. Whiteside TL, Bryant J, Day R, Herberman RB. Natural killer cytotoxicity in the diagnosis of immune dysfunction. *J Clin Lab Anal.* 1990; 4:102–114.

21. Fletcher MA, Baron GC, Ashman MR, Fischl MA, Klimas NG. Use of whole blood methods in assessment of immune parameters in immunodeficiency. *Diagn Clin Immunol.* 1987; 5:68–91.

22. Goldberg LR. The development of markers for the Big-Five factor structure. *Psychol Assess.* 1992; 4:26–42.

23. Gwaltney JM Jr, Colonno RJ, Hamparian VV, Turner RB. Rhinovirus. In: Schmidt NJ, Emmons RW, eds. *Diagnostic Procedures for Viral, Rickettsial, and Chlamydial Infections.* 6th ed. Washington, DC: American Public Health Association; 1989:579–614.

24. Farr BM, Gwaltney JM Jr, Hendley JO, et al. A randomized controlled trial of glucocorticoid prophylaxis against experimental rhinovirus infection. *J Infect Dis.* 1990; 162:1173–1177.

25. Doyle WJ, McBride TP, Swarts JD, Hayden FG, Gwaltney JM Jr. The response of the nasal airway, middle ear, and eustachian tube to provocative rhinovirus challenge. *Am J Rhinol.* 1988; 2:149–154.

26. Hosmer DW Jr, Lemeshow S. *Applied Logistic Regression.* New York, NY: John Wiley & Sons Inc; 1989.

27. Cohen J, Cohen P. *Applied Multiple Regression/Correlation Analysis for the Behavioral Sciences.* Hillsdale, NJ: Erlbaum Associates, 1975.

28. Cohen S, Tyrrell DAJ, Smith AP. Psychological stress and susceptibility to the common cold. *N Engl J Med.* 1991; 325:606–612.

29. Stone AA, Bovbjerg DH, Neale JM, Napoli A, Valdimarsdottir H, Gwaltney JM Jr. Development of common cold symptoms following experimental rhinovirus infection is related to prior stressful life events. *Behav Med.* 1993; 8:115–120.

30. Akira S, Kishimoto T. IL-6 and NF-IL6 in acute-phase response and viral infection. *Immunol Rev.* 1992; 127:25–50.

Kathleen Stern and Martha K. McClintock

Pheromones are airborne chemical signals that are released by an individual into the environment and which affect the physiology or behaviour of other members of the same species.[1] The idea that humans produce pheromones has excited the imagination of scientists and the public, leading to widespread claims for their existence, which, however, has remained unproven. Here we investigate whether humans produce compounds that regulate a specific neuroendocrine mechanism in other people without being consciously detected as odours (thereby fulfilling the classic definition of a pheromone). We found that odourless compounds from the armpits of women in the late follicular phase of their menstrual cycles accelerated the preovulatory surge of luteinizing hormone of recipient women and shortened their menstrual cycles. Axillary (underarm) compounds from the same donors which were collected later in the menstrual cycle (at ovulation) had the opposite effect: they delayed the luteinizing-hormone surge of the recipients and lengthened their menstrual cycles. By showing in a fully controlled experiment that the timing of ovulation can be manipulated, this study provides definitive evidence of human pheromones.

The existence of human pheromones was first suggested by the demonstration that women living together can develop synchronized menstrual cycles under specific conditions.[2-5] In rats, a similar process of ovarian synchrony occurs and is mediated by the exchange of two different pheromones.[6-7] One, produced before ovulation, shortens the ovarian cycle; the second, produced at ovulation, lengthens the cycle. These two opposing pheromones were predicted by a coupled-oscillator model of ovarian synchrony and shown by computer simulation to be sufficient for producing not only synchrony, but also the other observed effects of ovarian asynchrony and cycle stabilization.[7,8] By applying this model

to humans, we demonstrate the existence of human pheromones and identify a potential pheromonal mechanism for menstrual synchrony, as well as for other forms of social regulation of ovulation.

We found that the recipients had shorter cycles when receiving axillary compounds produced by donors in the follicular phase of the menstrual cycle (-1.7 ± 0.9 days) and longer cycles when receiving ovulatory compounds ($+1.4 \pm 0.5$ days), which represent significantly different opposite effects (Fig. 82.1). The response was manifest within the first cycle, rather than requiring three cycles of exposure as suggested previously,[2,7] and the sequence of compound presentation had no effect. The two types of axillary compounds had effects that were significantly different from each other and from the baseline cycle. The carrier had no effect on cycle lengths of the control recipients. In five of the cycles, women had mid-cycle nasal congestion, which could have prevented their exposure to pheromones; including these cycles in the analysis made the results slightly less robust (follicular compounds: -1.4 ± 0.9 days; ovulatory compounds: $+1.4 \pm 0.5$ days; ANOVA: follicular versus ovulatory compounds $F(1, 18) = 4.32$, $P \leq 0.05$; cycle 1 versus cycle 2 of exposure (not significant, NS); order of presentation (NS); all interactions between factors were not significant).

The finding that axillary compounds changed cycle length indicates that the compounds contain pheromones. The existence of two opposing effects, especially one that accelerates ovulation, makes it unlikely that a simple disruption of ovulation by a chemical produced the observed changes.[9] It also suggests two functionally different ovarian-dependent pheromones in humans, as in rats, with opposing effects. The existence of a phase-advance pheromone and a phase-delay pheromone supports the coupled-oscillator model of menstrual synchrony.[7,8] Women reported that

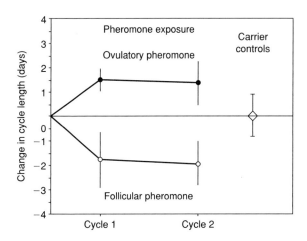

Figure 82.1

Effect of axillary compounds, donated by women during the follicular or ovulatory phases of their menstrual cycle, on the menstrual cycle length of recipients. This was measured as a change in length from the recipient's baseline cycle with a repeated measures analysis of variance: within-subject factors were follicular versus ovulatory compounds ($F(1, 18) = 5.81$, $P \leq 0.03$) and cycle 1 versus cycle 2 of exposure (not significant, NS); the between-subjects factor was: order of presentation (NS); all interactions between factors were not significant). Cycles were shorter than baseline during exposure to follicular compounds ($t = 1.78$, $P \leq 0.05$, 37 cycles) but longer during exposure to ovulatory compounds ($t = 2.7$, $P \leq 0.01$, 38 cycles). Cycles during exposure to the carrier were not different from baseline ($t = 0.05$, $P \leq 0.96$, 27 cycles).

they detected only alcohol (the control odorant, and carrier of the compounds), indicating that these changes were due to pheromones that were not consciously detected.

These results are consistent with another central prediction of the coupled-oscillator model: that there are individual differences in sensitivity to pheromones and therefore in the strength of the response.[8] Although a significant proportion of women in this experiment responded to the pheromones with changes in cycle length in the expected directions (68% of women responded to follicular pheromones, 68% to ovulatory pheromones), some women did not. In addition, the range of response magnitude was considerably more than the variation in cycle length typical for this age group[10]: cycles were shortened from 1 to 14 days and lengthened from 1 to 12 days.

There are three phases of the menstrual cycle that vary and might mediate the effect of pheromones on cycle length; each is controlled by different neuroendocrine mechanisms (menses, follicular and luteal phases). To determine the specific mechanism of pheromone action, we measured the luteinizing hormone (LH) and progesterone glucuronide content from urine samples to pinpoint the time of the preovulatory LH surge and verify the occurrence of ovulation. Previous hypotheses have focused on the menses or luteal phases,[2–7,11,12] although most medical texts report that the normal luteal phase is relatively fixed in length and it is the follicular phase that varies. In our sample, each of these three phases, including the luteal phase, varied significantly in length (indicated by the range of x-axis values in Fig. 82.2) and correlated sufficiently

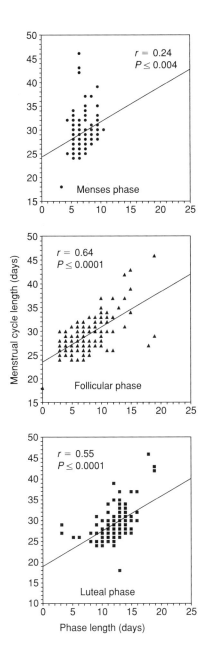

with cycle length for any of the three hypotheses to be correct.

Nonetheless, we traced all the changes caused by the pheromones presented in our study to the follicular phase (Fig. 82.3). For the menses and luteal phases, the distribution during the pheromone and control conditions were the same (indicated by overlapping log-survivor curves). Only the follicular phase was regulated, shortened by follicular compounds and lengthened by ovulatory compounds, suggesting that these ovarian-dependent pheromones have opposite effects on the recipient's ovulation by differentially altering the rate of follicular maturation or hormonal threshold for triggering the LH surge.

This experiment confirms the coupled oscillator model of menstrual synchrony and refocuses attention on the ovarian-dependent pheromones that regulate ovulation, producing either synchrony, asynchrony or cycle stabilization within a social group, namely two distinct pheromones, produced at different times of the cycle, which phase-advance or phase-delay the preovulatory LH surge. From this initial test of human ovarian-dependent pheromones, we do not know whether the phenomenon is fragile—that is,

Figure 82.2

Each of the three phases of the menstrual cycle are variable in length (*x*-axis) and correlate with overall menstrual cycle length (Pearson's *r*), establishing each as a potential mediator of the effects of axillary compounds. Menses phase (●, day 1 to the end of menses); follicular phase (▲, day after menses to the day before the preovulatory LH surge); luteal phase (■, three days after the LH surge to day before menses, verified to be functional by ovulatory levels of progesterone glucuronide (PG) and rise in basal body temperature). The ovulatory phase is a fixed 3-day interval (day of LH surge onset plus 2 subsequent days). Note that the luteal phase of these normal subjects is significantly more variable than the 12–16-day range described in standard medical texts.

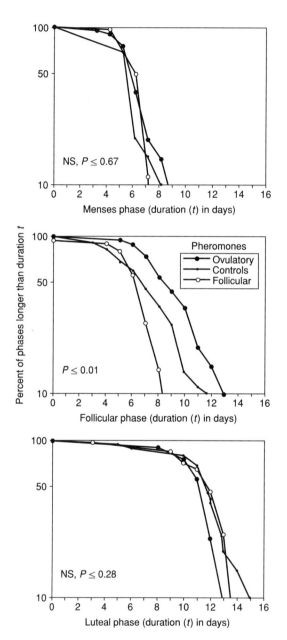

Figure 82.3
Effect of follicular and ovulatory pheromones on the length of each of the three phases that could mediate the observed change in menstrual-cycle length. Log-survivor analysis of the percentage of phases that are longer than a given length (time (t) in days; Mantel-Cox test). The same conclusions were reached with repeated measures analysis of variance on each of these three phases.

limited to modulation of ovulation timing in
healthy young women—or robust, and so capable of modulating ovulation in a diverse
population for either contraception or treatment
of infertility. Moreover, we need to determine
whether humans naturally receive compounds
that have similar effects in the context of everyday life.

There may be other consequences of ovarian-
dependent pheromones in women, in addition
to the alteration of the timing of ovulation. Our
work in rats and with computer simulations
demonstrates that these same ovarian-dependent
pheromones have qualitatively different effects
depending on the initial conditions under which
pheromonal and social interactions begin, as well
as on the point in the reproductive lifespan when
they occur.[7,8,13-15] Further work in this area
may well reveal that, as in rats, social interactions
mediated by ovarian-dependent pheromones affect age of puberty, interbirth intervals, age at
menopause, and level of chronic oestrogen exposure throughout a women's lifetime.

These data demonstrate that humans have
the potential to communicate pheromonally. In
other species there are many other types of pheromones, not dependent on ovarian function,
which enable individuals to regulate diverse aspects of their internal neuroendocrine states on
the basis of information about another's internal
state or environment. For example, pheromones
influence mating preference in hamsters,[16] dominance relationships among male elephants in
musth,[17] timing of weaning in rats[18] and how
rat pups learn to distinguish edible foods from
poisons,[19] how hamsters recognize individual
members of their social group,[20] and the level of
stress experienced by a mouse in a new environment on the basis of the emotional state of the
previous occupant.[21] Well controlled studies of
humans are now needed to determine whether
there are other types of pheromones, with effects
that are as far-reaching in humans as they are in
other species.

Methods

Subjects and Procedures

The experiment involved 29 women aged 20–35,
who were students or staff at a university, used
barrier contraception and had histories of regular and spontaneous ovulation. They were the
first women who met our subject criteria among
those responding to our request for volunteers
and none dropped out once the experiment had
begun. We collected compounds from the axillae
of 9 donor women in hormonally distinct phases
of the menstrual cycle and applied them daily
just under the noses of 20 recipients. All participants were unaware of the experiment's hypothesis and the source of the compounds. The
study was presented as focused primarily on
the development of non-invasive methods for
detecting ovulation, and secondarily on sensitivity to the odour of small amounts of "natural
essences" (consent was obtained for a list of 30
compounds).

Axillary Compounds

As in other species, human pheromones might be
produced by apocrine glands (active only during
reproductive maturity), eccrine glands (which
produce sweat that contains compounds found
also in saliva and urine), exfoliated epithelial
cells or bacterial action.[22-24] We collected compounds from axillae because they contain all
four of these potential sources and because the
two previous, albeit highly criticized, attempts to
study this issue used axillary compounds.[3,4,25-28]
The 9 donors bathed without perfumed products
every day and then wore 4×4 cotton pads in
their axillae for at least eight hours. Each pad
was cut into four sections for distribution to different recipients, treated with 4 drops of 70%
isopropyl alcohol[25] and then frozen immediately
at $-80°C$ in a glass vial.

Menstrual Cycle Assessment

Donors provided urine samples every evening, which we assayed for LH to detect the onset of the LH surge that triggers ovulation.[29] This singular hormonal event unambiguously demarcates the follicular from the ovulatory phases of the cycle. The LH surge was used together with data on vaginal secretions, menses, basal body temperature, and a rise in progesterone glucuronide in the postovulatory luteal phase, to classify each pad as containing compounds produced during the follicular phase (2 to 4 days before the onset of the LH surge) or the ovulatory phase (the day of the LH surge onset and the 2 subsequent days). To ensure a similar stimulus for all recipients regardless of individual differences among donors, all 9 donors contributed equally to the follicular and ovulatory compounds received by each subject.

As it is not yet known when during the menstrual cycle women are physiologically most sensitive to putative pheromones, applying compounds every day ensured covering a potentially sensitive period. However, our computer simulation experiments indicated that in rats this pheromonal-sensitive period occurs mid-cycle, around the time of ovulation[8] (a period when women are particularly sensitive to some olfactory stimuli[30]). Any condition preventing exposure to the compounds, such as nasal congestion anytime during the mid-cycle period from three days before to two days after the preovulatory LH, could weaken the effect. We analysed the data taking this into account.

Experimental Design

All recipients were studied for one baseline cycle without exposure to axillary compounds. Then, in a crossover experimental design during the next four consecutive cycles, axillary compounds were applied daily by wiping a thawed pad above the recipients upper lip. Half of the recipients ($n = 10$) received follicular compounds daily for two menstrual cycles and were then switched to exposure to ovulatory compounds for the next two cycles. The other 10 recipients received the same compounds in the reverse order. After applying the compounds, recipients were free to go about their normal activities but were asked not to wash their faces for the next six hours. All but two subjects, who missed only the last cycle of their second treatment, completed all five cycles of the experiment.

A between-subjects control group was provided by women (the donors) who collected all ovarian-cycle measures, but received only the carrier above their upper lip each day: 70% isopropyl alcohol. In addition, because the two-day change in menstrual cycle length (expected from the initial study[2]) is substantially less than individual variation in cycle length typical for this age group,[10] we created within-subjects controls by measuring the effect on the menstrual cycle in terms of a change in length from each individual subject's cycle preceding each condition. (For experimental subjects this was the cycle that preceded exposure to each type of compound; for control subjects this was the cycle that preceded exposure to the carrier, 70% alcohol).

Acknowledgements

We thank T. Z. Snyder for editing and J. Altmann, J. Charrow, S. Fisher and S. Goldin-Meadow for their comments. This work was supported by the US NIMH and NIH and a grant from the John D. and Catherine T. MacArthur Foundation.

References

1. Beauchamp, G. K., Doty, R. L., Moulton, D. G. & Mugford, R. A. In *Mammalian Olfaction, Reproductive Processes and Behavior* (ed. Doty, R. L.) 144–157 (Academic, New York, 1976).
2. McClintock, M. K. Menstrual synchrony and suppression. *Nature* 291, 244–245 (1971).

3. Graham, C. A. Menstrual synchrony: an update and review. *Human Nature* 2, 293–311 (1992).

4. Weller, L. & Weller, A. Human menstrual synchrony: A critical assessment. *Neurosci. Behav. Rev.* 17, 427–439 (1993).

5. Weller, A. & Weller, L. Menstrual synchrony under optimal conditions: Bedouin families. *J. Comp. Psychol.* 111, 143–151 (1997).

6. McClintock, M. K. Estrous synchrony: Modulation of ovarian cycle length by female pheromones. *Physiol. Behav.* 32, 701–705 (1984).

7. McClintock, M. K. *Pheromones and Reproduction in Mammals* (ed. Vandenbergh, J. G.) 113–149 (Academic, New York, 1983).

8. Schank, J. & McClintock, M. K. A coupled-oscillator model of ovarian-cycle synchrony among female rats. *J. Theor. Biol.* 157, 317–362 (1992).

9. Christian, M. S., Galbraith, W. M., Voytek, P. & Mehlman, M. A. *Advances in Modern Environmental Toxicology III: Assessment of Reproductive and Teratogenic Hazards* (Princeton Scientific, NJ, 1983).

10. Treloar, N. E., Boynton, R. E., Gorghild, G. B. & Brown, B. W. Variation of the human menstrual cycle through reproductive life. *Int. J. Fertil.* 12, 77–126 (1967).

11. Cutler, W. B., Garcia, C. R., Kreiger, A. M. Luteal phase defects: A possible relationship between short hyperthermic phase and sporadic sexual behavior in women. *Horm. Behav.* 13, 214–218 (1979).

12. Ryan, K. D. & Schwartz, N. B. Grouped female mice: demonstration of pseudopregnancy. *Biol. Reprod.* 17, 578–583 (1977).

13. McClintock, M. K. Social control of the ovarian cycle and the function of estrous synchrony. *Am. Zool.* 21, 243–256 (1981).

14. Mennella, J., Blumberg, M., Moltz, H. & McClintock, M. K. Inter-litter competition and communal nursing among Norway rats: Advantages of birth synchrony. *Behav. Ecol. Sociobiol.* 27, 183–190 (1990).

15. LeFevre, J. L. & McClintock, M. K. Isolation accelerates reproductive senescence and alters its predictors in female rats. *Horm. Behav.* 25, 258–272 (1991).

16. Vandenbergh, J. G. (ed.). *Pheromones and Reproduction in Mammals* (Academic, New York, 1983).

17. Rasmussen, L. E. L., Perris, T. E. & Gunawardena, R. Isolation of potential musth-alerting signals from the temporal gland secretions of male Asian elephants (*Elephas maximus*): A new method. *Chemical Senses* 19, 540 (1994).

18. Leon, M. & Moltz, H. The development of the pheromonal bond in the albino rat. *Physiol. Behav.* 8, 683–686 (1972).

19. Galef, G. Social identification of toxic diets by Norway rats (*Rattus norvegicus*). *J. Comp. Psychol.* 100, 331–334 (1986).

20. Johnson, E. Pheromones, the vomeronasal system and communication: From hormonal responses to individual recognition. *Ann. N.Y. Acad. Sci.* (in the press).

21. Rottman, S. J. & Snowdon, C. T. Demonstration and analysis of an alarm pheromone in mice. *J. Comp. Physiol. Psychol.* 81, 483–490 (1972).

22. Nixon, A., Mallet, A. I. & Gower, D. B. Simultaneous quantification of five odorous steroids (16-androstenes) in the axillary hair of men. *J. Ster. Biochem.* 29, 505–510 (1988).

23. Cohn, B. A. In search of human skin pheromones. *Arch. Dermatol.* 130, 1048–1051 (1994).

24. Spielman, A. I., Zeng, X. N., Leyden, J. J. & Preti, G. Proteinaceous precursors of human axillary odor: isolation of two novel odor-binding proteins. *Experimentia* 51, 40–47 (1995).

25. Russell, M. J., Switz, G. M., Thompson, K. Olfactory influences on the human menstrual cycle. *Pharmacol. Biochem. Behav.* 13, 737–738 (1980).

26. Preti, G., Cutler, W. B., Garcia, C. R., Huggins, G. R. & Lawkey, H. J. Human axillary secretions influence women's menstrual cycles: The role of donor extract from females. *Horm. Behav.* 20, 474–482 (1986).

27. Doty, R. Olfactory communication in humans. *Chem. Senses* 6, 351–376 (1981).

28. Wilson, H. C. Female axillary secretions influence women's menstrual cycles: A critique. *Horm. Behav.* 21, 536–546 (1987).

29. Stern, K. & McClintock, M. K. In *Psychopharmacology of Women* (eds. Jensvold, M. F., Halbreich, U. & Hamilton, J.) 393–413 (Am. Psychiatry Press, Washington DC, 1996).

30. Doty, R. L., Snyder, P. J., Huggins, G. R. & Lowry, L. D. Endocrine, cardiovascular and psychological correlates of olfactory sensitivity changes during the human menstrual cycle. *J. Comp. Physiol. Psychol.* 95, 45–60 (1981).

Psychosocial Factors, Sex Differences, and Atherosclerosis: Lessons from Animal Models

Jay R. Kaplan, Michael R. Adams, Thomas B. Clarkson, Stephen B. Manuck, Carol A. Shively, and J. Koudy Williams

Introduction

The use of animals in medical investigation goes back at least two millennia, to Galen's dissections of Barbary macaques and his physiological experiments involving pigs, goats, and sheep (1, 2). The application of animal models to study the psychobiological aspects of disease is a more recent innovation, owing much to the seminal experiments of Cannon (3) and Selye (4) in the first third of the 20th century. Since then, numerous investigators have explored one facet or another of the hypothesis that behaviorally evoked, excessive perturbations of the body's principal axes of neuroendocrine response (i.e., pituitary-adrenocortical or sympathetic-adrenomedullary) may produce pathophysiological consequences (5, 6). However, most researchers generally have ignored the possibility that there might be sex-related differences in the expression of such phenomena. Experimental research in atherosclerosis, the pathological process that underlies much of symptomatic coronary heart disease, is an exception. Here, investigations with chickens, pigeons, and, ultimately, monkeys not only have provided part of the basis for understanding sex differences in the epidemiology of CHD, they also have identified how sex interacts with psychosocial phenomena to influence the disease process. After a brief presentation of relevant background material, we review the data derived from investigations of monkeys and other animals and discuss the public health implications of the findings.

Background

Coronary heart disease (CHD), a disease spectrum subsuming myocardial infarction, angina pectoris, and disturbances in the rhythm, performance, and electrical activity of the heart, became widely recognized as a clinically significant and distinct entity in the 1920s (7). Between 1940 and 1960, CHD reached epidemic proportions in most of the technologically advanced nations of the world (7, 8). Even today, CHD remains among the most significant causes of death in the United States (9). Clinical manifestations of CHD usually occur in conjunction with atherosclerosis, a gruel-like accumulation of lipid (from the Greek *athere*, or mush) in the intima or inner layer of the large muscular and elastic arteries of the body (10, 11). The clinical autopsies performed by Quain and Virchow in the 1850s linked atherosclerotic lesions in the coronary arteries of patients to angina pectoris and to other indications of CHD exhibited by the same individuals while alive (12). Similarly, contemporary autopsy studies have established that the incidence of CHD is closely associated with the extent and severity of underlying atherosclerotic lesions, a relationship that exists both within and among geographic regions (13).

Emotional factors have always figured prominently in the characterization, if not understanding, of CHD (14, 15). Recently, systematic investigation has revealed an association in men between CHD and specific behavioral attributes of individuals, particularly "Type A" behavior and aspects of anger and its expression (16). Studies in animals, especially monkeys, have extended this research by demonstrating that the pathogenesis of coronary artery atherosclerosis is linked to both behavior and particular neuroendocrine mediators (5).

Another prominent feature of CHD and atherosclerosis, yet one that has not attracted significant research effort until recently, is the relative sparing of premenopausal females compared with males (7). Although this phenomenon is sometimes referred to as "female protection," it is more accurately characterized as a delay in disease onset; women actually succumb to CHD in larger numbers than men, although they do so later in life (17). The CHD death rate among 40-year-old men in the United States is approximately 40 per 100,000 persons, compared with 8 per 100,000 persons in women of the same age, a 5 to 1 advantage for women (18). By 60 years of age, mortality rates increase substantially in both sexes, but the mortality ratio is still more than 2 to 1 in favor of women (rates: 400 per 100,000 men vs. 175 per 100,000 women) (18). International investigations reveal that these general relationships persist, without exception, wherever CHD is a major cause of death. Even in Japan, with a relatively low incidence of CHD, the male:female mortality ratio is 3 to 1 (19).

The various effects of estrogen are believed to account for most of the sex difference in CHD incidence and atherosclerosis (20). Not only are premenopausal women "protected" from atherosclerosis and CHD, but the provision of estrogen replacement to postmenopausal women is associated with a significant reduction in CHD risk (relative risk of treated women compared to controls ≈ 0.50) as well as a reduction in angiographically documented coronary artery stenosis (20–23). Conversely, CHD risk is greatly increased among women undergoing early menopause or oophorectomy without estrogen replacement (20, 21, 24–26). From 25% to 50% of the benefit associated with estrogen results from its effects on plasma lipids (27, 28). For example, high-density lipoprotein (HDL) concentrations, which are inversely associated with CHD and atherosclerosis, are higher in women than in men beginning at puberty and persisting at least through menopause (7, 19). The plasma HDL levels of women may fall following menopause, although the data on this point are equivocal (7, 19, 29). Exogenous estrogen affects plasma lipids more demonstrably than do endogenous hormonal variations. Hence, unopposed estrogen given orally to postmenopausal women increases HDL and reduces low-density lipoprotein (LDL)

(30–35), effects probably mediated by estrogen's delivery to the liver (19, 20). High-dose estrogen treatment of men also reduces LDL and increases HDL, although not without adverse effects on hemostasis, breast sensitivity, and libido (7).

Despite the foregoing results, there are reasons to believe that the natural history of CHD and atherosclerosis among women is not solely a function of fluctuations in endogenous estrogen production. First, data from the Nurses Health Study (a cohort of 121,700 women subjected to long-term follow-up) indicate that there is no appreciable increase in CHD risk among non-smoking women having a natural menopause with no estrogen replacement (26). Furthermore, national and international mortality data show a steady increase in age-related CHD mortality rates among women, with no acceleration after menopause (36, 37). The steadily increasing CHD mortality rate in aging women contrasts with the obvious downward shift in the mortality curve associated with breast cancer; this latter outcome reflects the carcinogenic effects of estrogen exposure, which diminish after menopause (7, 19, 38). A shift in the opposite direction would be expected with respect to CHD mortality if variability in endogenous estrogen, alone, was responsible for the pattern of CHD risk among pre- and postmenopausal women (19).

The puzzling absence of a precise association between endogenous estrogen and CHD risk may be due, in part, to the intervening role played by psychosocial factors. Numerous studies of women have shown that emotional distress can result in ovarian dysfunction, affecting the hormonal qualities and perhaps even timing of the menopause (39–42). In fact, ovarian dysfunction that presents as secondary amenorrhea is relatively common, affecting between 5% and 18% of women less than 40 years old (43–46). Up to half the incidence of this premature ovarian failure, in turn, is attributed to undetermined causes, which are often assumed to be environmental or psychogenic (giving rise to the term "functional hypothalamic amenorrhea" [FHA]) (46, 47).

These observations suggest that not all pre-menopausal women have equivalent ("normal") hormonal histories. Women with FHA or other ovarian dysfunctions may experience substantially reduced exposure to estrogen, potentially eliminating a portion of their "female protection" from atherosclerosis and placing them on a high-risk trajectory for CHD. In fact, two studies have linked a history of menstrual irregularity with an increased risk of premature CHD (24, 48). Furthermore, the same psychosocial distress that leads to impaired ovarian function could potentiate atherogenesis directly by means of excessive neuroendocrine, e.g., pituitary-adrenocortical or sympatho-adrenomedullary) activity (49). The preceding observations suggest that CHD mortality rates in women may reflect a combination of high- and low-risk trajectories influenced, in turn, by the premenopausal interaction between psychosocial factors and reproductive function.

Unfortunately, most studies of psychosocial factors and CHD have been conducted in men (50), partly because myocardial infarction is infrequent among premenopausal women and because chest pain—although it often signals angina pectoris in men—frequently is unrelated to CHD in women (50). Furthermore, reproductive data rarely are collected in conjunction with psychosocial investigations of atherosclerosis and CHD in women. As a result, there is only a general understanding of the way in which psychosocial factors may relate to CHD risk in women. For example, increased CHD risk is observed in women with low educational levels, those in low-status occupations (e.g., clerical workers and video display terminal operators), and among individuals with an inability to express or discuss anger (51). It is, however, studies with animal models, not epidemiological investigations, that have provided the greatest insight into how behavioral factors may influence CHD pathogenesis in young and middle-aged women. These studies also identify the most important future directions for investigation.

Initial Development of Animal Models for Investigation of Psychosocial and Sex Hormone Influences on Atherosclerosis

By 1950, the extraordinary resistance of pre-menopausal women to CHD was already well-known. In a remarkable series of studies, Stamler et al. (52) demonstrated that estrogen, given either orally or parenterally, could substantially inhibit the development of coronary artery atherosclerosis in cockerels; estrogen treatment even caused regression of established plaques in these birds. Further studies by these investigators demonstrated that egg-laying hens, in contrast to similarly aged roosters, were resistant to coronary artery atherosclerosis; notably, ovariectomy eliminated this resistance (52). Estrogen at appropriate doses also is cardioprotective in White Carneau pigeons (53). However, this species does not show the male–female difference in susceptibility to lesions demonstrated by chickens (54).

Although early work in avian species was encouraging, attempts to replicate these findings in mammals initially were disappointing (7). For example, rabbits had been used in atherosclerosis research from the time that Ignatowski (in 1909) and Saltykow (in 1908) first showed that milk, meat, and eggs could induce fatty arterial lesions in these animals (cited in [10]). Early studies did not indicate sex differences in atherosclerosis of cholesterol-fed rabbits, nor did these studies reveal a consistent effect of exogenous administration or ovariectomy on the diet-induced lesions of rabbits (7, 10, 55–57). More recently, however, a series of investigations by Christiansen and colleagues (58, 59) has shown that estrogen treatment inhibits atherogenesis in ovariectomized rabbits. Nevertheless, the rabbit's usefulness for investigating sex differences in atherosclerosis is limited by the difference between rabbits and most anthropoid primates in the anatomy of the coronary arteries and in reproductive biology (e.g., female rabbits are induced ovulators without a menstrual cycle) (60).

Finally, cynomolgus macaque monkeys emerged as the model of choice for the investigation of sex-related phenomena in atherosclerosis (61–63). Monkeys offer numerous advantages for investigation of atherosclerosis, particularly when the research focuses on psychosocial factors or sex differences. First, nonhuman primates (especially macaques and baboons) develop diet-induced lesions that are similar in their location and morphological characteristics to those seen in human beings. Also relevant is the elaborate social repertoire of these animals, which subsumes behaviors analogous to those prominent in epidemiological studies of the psychosocial antecedents of CHD (e.g., competitiveness, aggression). Finally, these animals exhibit a 28-day menstrual cycle that is hormonally similar to the cycle in women (64, 65).

Effects of Psychosocial Factors and Variability in Endogenous Estrogen on Atherosclerosis in Monkeys

The first study evaluating sex differences in coronary artery atherosclerosis of cynomolgus monkeys identified psychosocial factors as a significant predictor of lesion extent (66). This study used 16 male and 16 female monkeys, all living in single-gender groupings of four animals each. For 16 months, the animals consumed a diet that was high in fat (45% of calories) and provided the human equivalent of 1140 mg cholesterol per day. This diet resulted in significant hyperlipoproteinemia, with total plasma cholesterol (TPC) concentrations averaging 430 mg/dl. During the latter half of the study, we evaluated the "competitiveness" of each animal nine times using the following procedure. Technicians placed grapes in each pen, noting the number of grapes taken by each animal and the order of animals taking the grapes. For each of the trials, animals in each group were assigned a number from 1 (most successful) to 4 (least successful). We estimated the percentage of lumen occupied

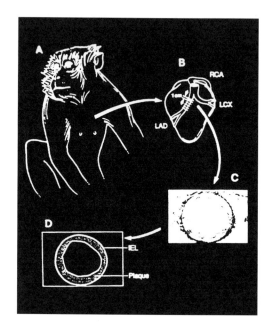

Figure 83.1
Evaluation of atherosclerosis, as depicted for a single section of artery. (A) pressure fixation and removal of heart; (B) 1 cm blocks taken from proximal portions of the major coronary arteries; (C) single sections from each block are mounted, stained and projected on a flat surface; (D) the section evaluated either visually (initial study) or with a computerized digitization system (later studies). The extent of atherosclerosis is the area between the IEL and the lumen. LAD, left anterior descending; RCA, right coronary artery; LCX, left circumflex; IEL, internal elastic lamina, the boundary between the media and intima of the artery.

by plaque in each section of coronary artery ("lumen stenosis"), and then calculated a mean score for each animal based on all 15 sections of coronary artery (Figure 83.1).

Statistical analysis revealed that males were significantly more affected than females, and that competitive animals, both males and females, were significantly less affected than their noncompetitive (submissive) counterparts (Table 83.1).

Table 83.1
Atherosclerosis (% lumen "stenosis") and plasma lipids (mg/dl) in male and female monkeys living in social groups[a]

	Atherosclerosis	TPC[b]	HDLC	TPC/HDLC
Male				
Competitive	23 ± 8	374 ± 45	38 ± 8.8	13.2 ± 2.4
Submissive	44 ± 7	491 ± 29	24 ± 2.1	21.7 ± 1.8
Female				
Competitive	7 ± 3	424 ± 63	48 ± 6.0	10.3 ± 2.1
Submissive	14 ± 7	437 ± 37	28 ± 2.1	16.2 ± 1.7

a. All values represent mean ± SEM. Significant effects: Atherosclerosis: males > females; competitive < submissive. HDLC: males < females; competitive > submissive. TPC/HDLC: males > females; competitive < submissive.
b. TPC, total plasma cholesterol; HDLC, high density lipoprotein cholesterol.

Variability in plasma lipids was concordant with the differences in atherosclerosis. Hence, submissive animals had lower HDL concentrations than did competitive animals, whereas males had lower HDL concentrations than females. However, an analysis of covariance demonstrated that both of the main effects (sex, "competitiveness") were *independent* of the concomitant differences in plasma lipids. This result suggested that other factors, as yet unexplored, must have accounted for the results.

Next, we designed three related experiments to investigate in more detail and with greater sophistication the role of psychosocial and reproductive factors in atherogenesis. The first of these was a 24-month study involving 23 females and 15 males (67). Of the 15 males, 10 lived in two all-male groups of 5. The five remaining males were assigned as "harem" males to groups of females allowed to become pregnant as part of one of the related experiments. The females were divided into groups of 4 or 5, each containing a vasectomized male to simulate a "normal" heterosexual group composition. Animals were fed an atherogenic diet that derived 40% of calories from fat and provided the human equivalent of 860 mg cholesterol per day. In response, TPC concentrations averaged approximately 300 mg/dl for males and females.

We monitored social behavior using focal sampling techniques and an electronic data collection device (68). Each animal was observed for 15 minutes, three times per week for the entire experiment. These data allowed determination of the social ranking or dominance status of each animal. For cynomolgus monkeys, a series of specific facial expressions, postures, and vocalizations indicate readiness for a fight, and an animal's relative social status is based on these indicators. Typically, one animal in a fight signals aggression and the other signals submission. This highly asymmetric pattern allows fight outcomes to be judged in terms of clear winners and losers (69, 70). The animal in each group that defeats all others (as evidenced by an ability to elicit consistently submissive responses) is designated as the first-ranking monkey. The monkey that defeats all but the first-ranking animal is designated as the second-ranking monkey, and so forth. In general, dominance relationships within small groups are transitive; that is, if monkey one is dominant to monkey two, and monkey two is dominant to monkey three, then monkey one is usually dominant to monkey three also (67). Social status was stable in this experiment, allowing us to use rank for each monkey aggregated over the entire experiment in all analyses. Animals that on average ranked one

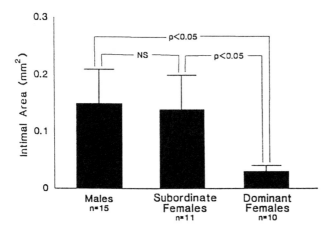

Figure 83.2
The extent of coronary artery atherosclerosis among socially housed male and female monkeys where females are divided on basis of fight wins and losses into dominants (winners) and subordinates (losers). All females are reproductively intact. (Modified with permission from ref. 64.)

or two in their social groups were considered "dominant," and the rest were labeled "subordinate." Such differences in social status most likely determined the patterns of wins and losses in the grape competition used in our first experiment.

In addition to observing social behavior, animals were subjected to daily vaginal swabbing to monitor menses. Furthermore, we collected blood samples for the determination of plasma progesterone concentrations 7 days after onset of menstruation (follicular phase), and at 3-day intervals beginning 12 days after onset of menstruation (luteal phase). These evaluations provided the basis for judging ovarian function in each animal in relation to social factors and atherosclerosis.

At the end of this experiment and all subsequent investigations, we measured the intimal lesions (the area between the internal elastic lamina and lumen) directly with a computerized image analyzer. We also visually graded the coronary sections as an index of intimal changes, with a scale ranging from "0" (no changes) to "3"

(plaque formation). Sex and psychosocial factors again interacted to affect coronary artery atherosclerosis, with female "protection" with respect to plaque development extended only to the dominant animals (Figure 83.2).

The data describing ovarian function (Table 83.2) show that the subordinate females had five times as many anovulatory cycles and three times as many cycles characterized by luteal-phase deficiencies (peak plasma progesterone concentrations between 2.0 and 4.0 ng/dl) as their dominant counterparts (67, 71). Notably, the females with the most extensive coronary artery atherosclerosis were all subordinate and all had marked ovarian endocrine dysfunction. These data suggest that social subordination may increase the risk of coronary artery atherosclerosis in females by inducing a relative ovarian endocrine deficiency state similar to that observed in postmenopausal women, that, in terms of estrogenic stimulation, is not grossly different from that of males.

Further evidence of the potential atherogenic significance of impaired ovarian function was

Table 83.2
Ovarian and adrenal function (median values) in dominant and subordinate monkeys[a]

	Dominant	Subordinate	p value[b]
Luteal-phase peak plasma progesterone (mg/ml)	8.9	4.0	<0.01
% anovulatory cycles	3.5	16.5	<0.01
% cycles with luteal-phase deficiencies	8.9	24.3	<0.01
Adrenal weight (mg/kg body weight)	168	201	<0.05

a. Reprinted with permission from ref. 72. Copyright 1985 American Heart Association.
b. By Mann-Whitney test.

provided by the second investigation in this series, a study involving 21 ovariectomized females placed in social groups for the same amount of time and fed the same diet as the 23 intact females described above (72). The ovariectomized females as a group had significantly more extensive coronary artery atherosclerosis than did the intact females. Figure 83.3 suggests that this effect was due to the loss of protection experienced by the ovariectomized dominant animals compared with their intact counterparts. The subordinates, intact and ovariectomized, were equally affected with atherosclerosis.

The third and final study in this series focused on a hyperestrogenic state, pregnancy (73). In this investigation, animals that experienced repeated pregnancy had less than one-fourth the atherosclerosis of the 23 intact, nonpregnant females described previously (Figure 83.4). Furthermore, atherosclerosis extent among the pregnant animals correlated inversely with the magnitude and duration of the pregnancy-induced elevation in plasma 17β-estradiol. The inhibition of atherosclerosis among pregnant animals occurred irrespective of differences in social status.

Plasma lipid concentrations, especially HDL, are often implicated in the mediation of the sex differential in atherosclerosis. Table 83.3 details the plasma lipids of all of the animals in the preceding set of three related studies. As among human beings, HDL in every study correlated inversely with the extent of atherosclerosis (rs between -0.35 and -0.50, ps < 0.05), whereas

the ratio of TPC to HDL correlated positively with lesion extent (rs between 0.38 and 0.55, ps < 0.05). Also, plasma concentrations of HDL were significantly higher in females than in males ($p < 0.05$). However, plasma lipids did not differ significantly between dominant and subordinate females, and thus could not convincingly account for the relative sparing of the reproductively intact, dominant animals. Moreover, HDL concentrations did not differ significantly between ovariectomized and intact animals, though these monkeys did differ with respect to atherosclerosis extent. Finally, the pregnant animals were characterized by both the lowest plasma concentrations of HDL and the least coronary artery atherosclerosis. The pattern of variability in plasma HDL concentrations argues against linking psychosocial or sex differences to atherosclerosis solely via effects on plasma lipids.

Psychosocial Factors, Oral Contraceptives, and Atherosclerosis

Our most recent investigation extended the foregoing findings by evaluating atherosclerosis among reproductively intact female monkeys that all consumed an atherogenic diet but either did or did not receive exogenous estrogen in the form of the oral contraceptive (OC) Triphasil® (74). The study sought to: a) confirm that low social status enhances the vulnerability of female monkeys to atherosclerosis; and b) evaluate the

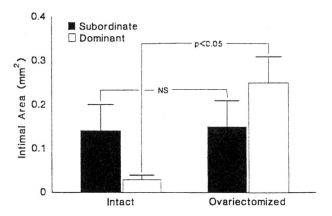

Figure 83.3
The extent of coronary artery atherosclerosis in reproductively intact and ovariectomized monkeys, divided into dominant and subordinate subsets. Ovariectomized animals have more atherosclerosis than intacts, an effect due entirely to the exacerbation of atherosclerosis among dominant ovariectomized monkeys. (Reproduced with permission from ref. 72. Copyright 1985 American Heart Association.)

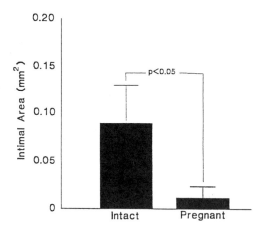

Figure 83.4
The extent of coronary artery atherosclerosis in reproductively intact and repeatedly pregnant monkeys. The extent of atherosclerosis was minimal across all pregnant animals, irrespective of social status. (Reproduced with permission from ref. 73. Copyright 1987 American Heart Association.)

Table 83.3
Plasma lipids (mg/dl, mean ± SEM) in male and female monkeys: results from three experiments[a]

	TPC[b]	HDLC	TPC/ HDLC ratio
Males	271 ± 21	33.4 ± 4.1	8.5 ± 1.3
Females			
Intact dominant	311 ± 24	42.5 ± 3.0	8.1 ± 1.2
Intact subordinate	321 ± 23	41.3 ± 4.3	8.7 ± 1.1
OVX dominant	358 ± 25	34.6 ± 4.7	11.8 ± 1.6
OVX subordinate	380 ± 20	40.3 ± 3.0	10.2 ± 1.1
Pregnant	260 ± 12	36.0 ± 2.0	7.2 ± 1.4

a. All animals consumed the same diet. See text for significant effects in each experiment. Reprinted with permission from ref. 64.
b. TPC, total plasma cholesterol; HDLC, high density lipoprotein cholesterol.

Table 83.4
Plasma lipids (mg/dl, mean ± SEM) of dominant and subordinate female monkeys in a control condition after treatment with oral contraceptive[a]

	TPC		HDLC		TPC/HDLC	
	Control	OC[b]	Control	OC	Control	OC
Dominant	385 ± 18	426 ± 22	47 ± 3	30 ± 2	11.5 ± 1.1	20 ± 1.9
Subordinate	461 ± 16	465 ± 22	37 ± 2	28 ± 2	16.0 ± 1.3	22.4 ± 2.0

a. Reprinted with permission from ref. 74. Copyright 1995 American Heart Association.
b. OC, oral contraceptive.

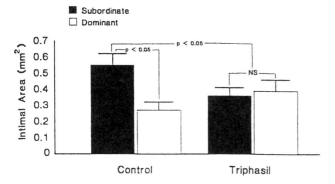

Figure 83.5
The extent of iliac artery atherosclerosis by contraceptive treatment (Triphasil®) and social status. Dominant and subordinate monkeys differed significantly in the untreated but not in the treated condition, and treated animals regardless of status differed from untreated subordinates. (Reproduced with permission from ref. 74. Copyright 1995 American Heart Association.)

hypothesis that contraceptive hormone treatment provides relative protection from the development of atherosclerosis, especially to those animals placed at increased risk of ovarian impairment by subordinate social status. To this end, the experiment contained 193 adult females, all housed in social groups of five or six animals each. The diet consumed by all monkeys derived 43% of calories from fat and provided the human equivalent of 560 mg cholesterol per day. This diet resulted in average TPC concentrations of 434 mg/dl. At the end of 26 months, we measured atherosclerosis in an iliac artery biopsy taken from each monkey (all animals were then ovariectomized and assigned to a postmenopausal study). The social rankings aggregated over the entire period were used in all analyses, with overall median rank used as the cutpoint for determining dominant versus subordinate social status. Table 83.4 shows the plasma lipids of dominant and subordinate female monkeys after OC treatment.

The extent of atherosclerosis, measured as the average intimal lesion size from five sections of iliac artery from each monkey, is depicted in Figure 83.5. Statistical evaluation of these data demonstrated that, as expected, untreated dominant monkeys were protected relative to their

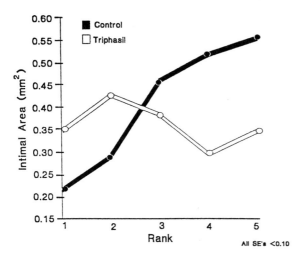

Figure 83.6
The extent of iliac artery atherosclerosis plotted against the average social rank of animals in each of the treatment conditions (control, Triphasil®). Average rank is aggregated into five categories, from high (1) to low (5). In the plot, untreated and low-ranking animals differ significantly in atherosclerosis; there are no significant differences among treated individuals. (Reproduced with permission from ref. 74. Copyright 1995 American Heart Association.)

subordinate counterparts. However, OC treatment eliminated the difference in the extent of atherosclerosis between dominant and subordinate individuals. In addition, we plotted the average ranks of the animals (grouped into five categories, from high to low) against intimal area (Figure 83.6). This plot suggests the presence of a linear association (i.e., a "dose-response" relationship) between social status and atherosclerosis among the control animals; in contrast, there was no association between atherosclerosis and status among OC-treated animals.

Dominant monkeys, both treated and control, exhibited higher HDL and lower TPC concentrations than subordinates. However, this effect was overwhelmed by the effect of OC treatment, which markedly reduced plasma HDL concentrations irrespective of status. After statistical analysis that adjusted for the effects of plasma lipids on atherosclerosis, the original outcome was unchanged—dominant social status was still

protective, as was OC treatment (particularly for subordinates) ($p < 0.05$).

Mechanisms Mediating Effects of Sex and Psychosocial Factors

Sex and psychosocial factors interact to influence atherosclerosis in monkeys and, perhaps, women. The series of experiments reviewed above suggests that such effects are mediated, in part, through non-lipid pathways. One pathway may involve estrogenic interactions with the artery wall (20, 75). For example, subcutaneous implantation of 17β-estradiol inhibits the accumulation of LDL degradation products in the coronary arteries of ovariectomized monkeys (75), whereas OC treatment has a similar effect in premenopausal animals (76). Moreover, 17β-estradiol prevents the oxidative modification of LDL (77). Because the oxidation, uptake, and catabolism of plasma LDL seem to be the primary mechanisms by which cholesterol accumulates in the atherosclerotic lesion, estrogen may influence atherosclerosis initiation and progression by modulating these processes.

Estrogenic effects on vascular function also may be relevant to atherogenesis. Numerous studies have demonstrated that atherosclerosis impairs endothelium-dependent dilation of the coronary arteries and augments endothelium-dependent vasoconstriction, as indicated by vasomotor response to intracoronary infusion of acetylcholine (78). These vasomotor abnormalities, in turn, may result in accelerated progression of atherosclerosis, plaque instability or rupture, thrombosis, and myocardial ischemia or infarction (79–81). Estrogen, administered either acutely or chronically to ovariectomized monkeys, reverses impairment in vasomotor responsiveness resulting from advanced coronary atherosclerosis (82–84). Additionally, socially dominant (with normal ovarian function) premenopausal monkeys exhibit coronary artery dilation in response to acetylcholine infusion, whereas subordinates (with poor ovarian function) vasoconstrict following the same stimulus (85). The dominance-associated variability in endogenous estrogen is itself significantly correlated with the degree of arterial dilation in response to acetylcholine (85).

Other effects of estrogens include potential interference in cellular and/or molecular processes occurring in the arterial intima. Inasmuch as locally mediated immune and inflammatory reactions are implicated in the initiation and progression of atherosclerosis, sex hormones may influence atherogenesis through autocrine, paracrine, or endocrine effects on these processes (86–90). Furthermore, production of extracellular matrix by the cells of the artery wall is altered in atherosclerosis; this represents yet another process that may be modulated by sex hormones and thereby influence atherosclerosis progression.

The foregoing discussion emphasizes the possibility that psychosocial factors may indirectly influence atherosclerosis in females through alterations in endogenous estrogen activity. There is evidence that behavioral effects also are mediated by nonestrogenic phenomena, such as excessive neuroendocrine stimulation. Hypercortisolemia, for example, is positively associated with coronary artery atherosclerosis as determined angiographically (91). Furthermore, infusion of physiological concentrations of cortisol causes marked exacerbation of coronary artery atherosclerosis in rhesus monkeys, an effect that was observed much earlier in cockerels (52, 92, 93). Among premenopausal monkeys, the adrenal glands of subordinates are larger than those of dominants, and subordinate monkeys exhibit a greater cortisol response to exogenous ACTH stimulation than do dominants (93). Also, endogenous variability in luteal-phase plasma progesterone concentrations (an index of ovarian condition) correlates inversely with adrenal weight (94). Taken together, these results suggest that subordinate social status is a stressor that predictably evokes a potentially atherogenic increase in adrenocortical activity in female monkeys. However, in our studies we have not observed significant associations between atherosclerosis extent and any index of adrenocortical function.

Numerous investigators have proposed that excessive sympathetic activation in response to behavioral stimuli also may potentiate increased atherogenesis (16, 48, 94, 95). Such activation has been linked to endothelial injury (an initial stage of atherogenesis) in both monkeys and rabbits (96–98). Current evidence suggests that endothelial injury may be induced via hemodynamic changes (e.g., increases in turbulence and shear stress) that occur as sequelae of the acute alterations in heart rate and blood pressure accompanying sympathetic nervous system activation (99, 100). The preferential location of sympathetically induced endothelial damage in the coronary arteries and at aortic bends and bifurcations seem to support this hemodynamic hypothesis of arterial injury (100). Further evidence for the role of sympathetic activation in atherogenesis is the observation that treatment with a β-adrenergic blocking agent inhibits the development of behaviorally induced coronary artery atherosclerosis (100).

Significantly, there is some evidence that loss of ovarian function in postmenopausal women is accompanied by an increase in sympathetically mediated cardiovascular response to behavioral stimuli (101, 102). Such changes may contribute to the increased risk of CHD in older women (103). Our studies indicate that premenopausal monkeys with exaggerated heart rate responses to a standardized behavioral challenge have significantly lower luteal-phase plasma progesterone concentrations and a somewhat higher frequency of anovulatory menstrual cycles compared with low heart rate responders (104). These individual differences in cardiovascular reactivity to behavioral stress have pathophysiological consequences, as the monkeys with the largest heart rate responses to challenge have the greatest extent of both coronary and carotid atherosclerosis. Furthermore, their hearts are 50% larger than those of low heart rate reactors. If an enhanced cardiovascular response to stress also accompanies chronic ovarian endocrine deficiencies among reproductively intact women, this increased reactivity might account for some of their heightened coronary risk (103).

Among female monkeys, social dominance and individual differences in heart rate response to behavioral challenge are not significantly associated (104). It is possible nonetheless that sympathetic nervous system arousal mediates the accelerated atherosclerosis reliably observed in subordinate females. Repeated exposure of such females to the aggressive intrusions of dominant animals could trigger excessive and prolonged sympathetic responses. This pattern of environmentally induced, sustained emotional stimulation, in turn, could cause arterial damage similar to that observed in individuals ("high heart rate reactors") that are intrinsically hyperresponsive to stimulation of any intensity.

Finally, activation of the renin-angiotensin system (RAS) may also have contributed to the accelerated atherogenesis of subordinate, estrogen-deprived female monkeys. Numerous studies show, for example, that production of renin in the kidney is enhanced by sympathetic stimulation and emotional arousal (105, 106). Reciprocal stimulation of the RAS and sympathetic nervous system occurs in the brain as well as in the kidney and at other peripheral sites (107). Activation of the RAS initiates a cascade (via the activity of renin and angiotensin-converting enzyme [ACE]) that ultimately results in the increased production and circulation of angiotensin II (ANGII), the most potent vasoconstrictor known (108). Recent research suggests that ANGII accelerates atherosclerosis independently of any pressor effects (109). This is because ANGII directly affects smooth muscle cell signal transduction (110) as well as a number of growth factors (transforming growth factor-β, platelet-derived growth factor, and basic fibroblast growth factor) that influence smooth muscle proliferation (111). The observation that treatment with an ACE inhibitor prevents the development of atherosclerosis in normotensive monkeys (109) further supports the contention that ANGII is atherogenic (110) and may comprise part of the mechanism causing excessive lesion development in animals subjected to emotional stress and arousal (e.g., subordinate female monkeys).

Whereas ANGII is potentially atherogenic, estrogen modulates the RAS in ways that could inhibit lesion formation. For example, estrogen attenuates the pressor response to ANGII infusion in ovariectomized, normotensive, and hypertensive rats (Ping et al., unpublished observations). In the same model, estrogen suppresses ACE activity (Ping et al., unpublished observations), an effect also observed in post-menopausal women receiving hormone replacement therapy (112). The estrogen-induced suppression of ACE activity, in turn, is associated experimentally with a decrease in ANGII and an increase in activity of the vasodilator peptide, angiotensin 1–7 (ANG1-7) (113). The stimulatory effects of estrogen on ANG1-7 and inhibitory effects on ACE activity suggest that the increase in renin activity associated with estrogen use (e.g., see reference 112) paradoxically may inhibit, rather than accelerate, atherosclerosis. Thus, variability in endogenous estrogen production, such as is observed between dominant and subordinate monkeys, may also influence the balance between ANGII and ANG1-7 production and by this mechanism affect atherogenesis.

Summary and Conclusions

Premenopausal women are usually considered to be relatively protected from atherosclerosis and CHD (7). However, to the extent that the results from our investigations with female monkeys apply also to women, they highlight the potential importance of behavioral stressors and their effects on estrogen activity in the development of atherosclerosis during the premenopausal period. In fact, numerous lines of investigation suggest that women and monkeys share a common pattern of stress response that may similarly influence premenopausal atherosclerosis risk. As shown in our studies and those of others, socially subordinate female monkeys reliably exhibit adrenocortical hyperactivity and, under both field and laboratory conditions, impaired reproduction (114–119). Behaviorally, social subordination in captive female monkeys is further accompanied by relative social withdrawal and isolation, and a generally reduced freedom of movement and expression (67, 93, 120). Together, these findings indicate that social subordination represents a significant stressor to female monkeys, particularly under conditions of confinement that demand a high rate of social interaction.

Among women, the stress-associated syndrome of FHA (also called "psychogenic" amenorrhea) similarly involves the triad of ovarian dysfunction, adrenal hyperactivity, and behavioral abnormalities (121, 122). These observations suggest that FHA may be one of the manifestations of a multifaceted stress disorder, similar in many respects to the syndrome represented by social subordination in monkeys. In both women and monkeys, the excessive adrenocortical response and disrupted gonadotropin-releasing hormone pacemaker activity are presumably potentiated by a stress-related release of corticotropin-releasing factor (41, 123).

Thus, although there may exist no precise human analogue for subordinate female monkeys, women with FHA seem to share with such animals a profile of neuroendocrine dysfunction that may result in a similar predilection for accelerated atherosclerosis and increased risk of CHD. A related observation of potential importance is that, in the studies involving monkeys, relatively modest impairment of ovarian function is associated with substantial exacerbation of atherosclerosis (72, 74). Such moderate ovarian abnormalities, in women, probably would be occult. If so, the percentage of premenopausal women at risk of accelerated atherosclerosis may be considerably larger than that indicated by the incidence of (diagnosed) FHA.

It is unknown whether there is a behaviorally defined subset of premenopausal women that, as a result of ovarian impairment and neuroendocrine hyperstimulation, is on a high-risk trajectory with respect to atherosclerosis and CHD. As reviewed earlier, there is an increase in CHD risk among women whose occupations involve low control, high demands, and suppressed emotions (51). Yet, virtually no evidence exists regarding their physiological characteristics, particularly with respect to ovarian function. This lack of knowledge suggests a two-tiered research strategy, directed at women as well as monkeys. First, women's ovarian function and atherosclerosis progression (evaluated noninvasively) could both be assessed in a single human trial. Further investigations involving premenopausal monkeys could focus on the specific mechanisms most likely to mediate the hormonal and behavioral effects described in this chapter. These mechanisms could well involve the RAS, which has been generally ignored by biobehavioral investigators.

Finally, an underlying theme of this chapter is that psychosocial stress can impair ovarian function in premenopausal females, with potential adverse effects on the cardiovascular system. However, it could be speculated that stress-mediated suppression of ovarian activity causes deficits in other estrogen-sensitive tissues, such as bone and brain (e.g., see references 124–126). Such deficits might be exacerbated if these other tissues also were susceptible to the prolonged hypercortisolemia or sympathetic arousal that typically accompanies a stress response. The proposed studies alluded to above could well be extended to include for evaluation a much larger array of bodily systems as part of an overall strategy to better understand the determinants of women's health throughout the life cycle.

Acknowledgments

This work was supported, in part, by National Institute of Health Grants P50HL 45666 and R01HL 38964. The editorial assistance of Karen Klein is gratefully acknowledged, as are the efforts of numerous technicians working in the laboratories of the Comparative Medicine Clinical Research Center of the Bowman Gray School of Medicine.

References

1. Sarton G: Galen of Pergamon. Lawrence. University of Kansas, 1954.

2. Prichard RW: Animal models in human medicine. In: Animal Models of Thrombosis and Hemorrhagic Diseases. Proceedings of the Workshop on Animal Models of Thrombosis and Hemorrhagic Diseases, National Academy of Sciences, Washington, DC, 1975, pp 169–172 (DHEW Publication No. (NIH) 76:982).

3. Cannon WB: Bodily Changes in Pain, Hunger, Fear and Rage: An Account of Recent Researches into the Function of Emotional Excitement. New York, Appleton, 1929.

4. Selye H: The Stress of Life, Revised Edition. New York, McGraw-Hill, 1976.

5. Manuck SB, Marsland AL, Kaplan JR, Williams JK: The pathogenicity of behavior and its neuroendocrine mediation: An example from coronary artery disease. Psychosom Med 57:275–283, 1995.

6. Folkow B: Stress, hypothalamic function and neuroendocrine consequences. Acta Med Scand 723:61–69, 1988.

7. McGill HC, Stern NP: Sex and atherosclerosis. Atheroscler Rev 4:157–242, 1979.

8. Moriyama IM, Krueger DE, Stamler J: Cardiovascular Diseases in the United States, Chap 4. Cambridge, MA, Harvard University Press, 1971.

9. American Heart Association: 1992 Heart and Stroke Facts. Dallas, American Heart Association, 1993.

10. Katz LN, Stamler J: Experimental atherosclerosis. Springfield, IL, Charles C Thomas, 1953.

11. McGill HC Jr: Atherosclerosis: Problems in pathogenesis. Atheroscler Rev 2:27–65, 1977.

12. Klemperer P: Franz Groedel Memorial Lecture. The history of coronary sclerosis. Am J Cardiol 1:94–107, 1960.

13. McGill HC Jr: The Geographic Pathology of Atherosclerosis. Baltimore, Williams & Wilkins, 1968.

14. Wolf SG: History of the study of stress and heart disease. In Beamish RE, Singal PK, Dhalla NS (eds.), Stress and Heart Disease. Boston, MA, Martinus Nijhoff Publishing, 1985, 3–16.

15. Prichard RW: Introducing behavioral factors into atherosclerosis research. Am J Pathol 101(Suppl 3S):S171–S176, 1980.

16. Manuck SB, Kaplan JR, Matthews KA: Behavioral antecedents of coronary heart disease and atherosclerosis. Arteriosclerosis 6:2–14, 1986.

17. Higgins M, Thom T: Cardiovascular disease in women as a public health problem. In Wenger NK, Speroff L, Packard B (eds.), Cardiovascular Health and Disease in Women. Greenwich, CT, LeJacq Communications, Inc., 1993, 15–19.

18. Thom TJ: Cardiovascular disease mortality among United States women. In Eaker ED, Packard B,

Wenger NK, Clarkson TB, Tyroler HA (eds), Coronary Heart Disease in Women. New York, Haymarket Doyma, Inc., 1987, 33–41.

19. Godsland IF, Wynn V, Crook D, Miller NE: Sex, plasma lipoproteins, and atherosclerosis: Prevailing assumptions and outstanding questions. Am Heart J 114:1467–1503, 1987.

20. Manson JE: Postmenopausal hormone therapy and atherosclerotic disease. Am Heart J 128:1337–1343, 1994.

21. Stampfer MJ, Colditz GA, Willett WC, Manson JE, Rosner B, Speizer FE: Postmenopausal estrogen therapy and cardiovascular disease. N Engl J Med 325:756–762, 1991.

22. Gruchow HW, Anderson AJ, Barboriak JJ, Sobocinski KA: Postmenopausal use of estrogen and occlusion of coronary arteries. Am Heart J 115:954–963, 1988.

23. Sullivan JM, Vander Zwaag R, Lemp GF, Hughes JP, Maddock V, Kroetz FW, Ramanathan KB, Mirvis DM: Postmenopausal estrogen use and coronary atherosclerosis. Ann Intern Med 108:358–363, 1988.

24. Oliver MF: Ischaemic heart disease in young women. Br Med J 4:253–259, 1974.

25. Bengtsson C: Ischaemic heart disease in women. Acta Med Scand 549(Suppl):1–128, 1973.

26. Colditz GA, Willett WC, Stampfer MJ, Rosner B, Speizer FE, Hennekens CH: Menopause and the risk of coronary heart disease in women. N Engl J Med 316:1105–1110, 1987.

27. Matthews KA, Meilahn E, Kuller LH, Kelsey SF, Caggiula AW, Wing RR: Menopause and risk factors for coronary heart disease. N Engl J Med 321:641–646, 1989.

28. Speroff L: The impact of oral contraception and hormone replacement therapy on cardiovascular disease. In Wenger NK, Speroff L, Packard B (eds), Cardiovascular Health and Disease in Women. Greenwich, CT, LeJacq Communications, Inc., 1993, 37–45.

29. Lobo RA: Hormones, hormone replacement and heart disease. In Douglas PS (ed), Cardiovascular Health and Disease in Women. Philadelphia, Saunders, 1993, 153–173.

30. LaRosa JC: Some aspects of coronary risk and prevention factors in women. In Wenger NK, Speroff L, Packard B (eds), Cardiovascular Health and Disease

in Women. Greenwich, CT, LeJacq Communications, Inc., 1993, 31–35.

31. Bush TL, Miller VT: Effects of pharmacologic agents used during menopause: Impact on lipids and lipoproteins. In Mishell DR (ed), Menopause: Physiology and Pharmacology. Chicago, Year Book Medical Publishers, 1987, 187–208.

32. Barrett-Connor E, Wingard DL, Criqui MH: Postmenopausal estrogen use and heart disease risk factors in the 1980s. JAMA 261:2095–2100, 1989.

33. Bush TL, Barrett-Connor E, Cowan LD, Criqui MH, Wallace RB, Suchindran CM, Tyroler HA, Rifkind BM: Cardiovascular mortality and non-contraceptive estrogen use in women: Results from the Lipid Research Clinics' Program Follow-Up Study. Circulation 75:1002–1009, 1987.

34. McGill HC Jr: Sex steroid hormone receptors in the cardiovascular system. Postgrad Med April:64–68, 1989.

35. Godsland IF, Wynn V, Crook D, Miller NE: Sex, plasma lipoproteins, and atherosclerosis: Prevailing assumptions and outstanding questions. Am Heart J 114:1467–1503, 1987.

36. Heller RF, Jacobs HS: Coronary heart disease in relation to age, sex, and the menopause. Br Med J 1:472–474, 1978.

37. Colditz GA, Hankinson SE, Hunter DJ, Willett WC, Manson JE, Stampfer MJ, Hennekens C, Rosner B, Speizer FE: The use of estrogens and progestins and the risk of breast cancer in postmenopausal women. New Engl J Med 332:1589–1593, 1995.

38. Ballinger S: Stress as a factor in lowered estrogen levels in the early postmenopause. Ann NY Acad Sci 592:95–112, 1990.

39. Seibel MM, Taymor ML: Emotional aspects of infertility. Fertil Steril 37:137–145, 1982.

40. Giles DE, Berga SL: Cognitive and psychiatric correlates of functional hypothalamic amenorrhea: A controlled comparison. Fertil Steril 60:486–492, 1993.

41. Judd SJ: Pathophysiological mechanisms of stress-induced chronic anovulation. In Sheppard KE, Boublik JH, Funder JW (eds), Stress and Reproduction. New York, Raven Press, 1992, 253–265.

42. Kinch RAH, Plunkett ER, Smout MS, Carr DH: Primary ovarian failure. A clinicopathological and cytogenetic study. Am J Obstet Gynecol 91:630–644, 1965.

43. Russell P, Bannatyne P, Shearman RP, Fraser IS, Corbett P: Premature hypergonadotropic ovarian failure. Clinicopathological study of 19 cases. Int J Gynecol Pathol 1:185–201, 1982.

44. Starup J, Sele V: Premature ovarian failure. Acta Obstet Gynecol Scand 52:259–268, 1973.

45. Aiman J, Smentek C: Premature ovarian failure. Obstet Gynecol 66:9–14, 1985.

46. Berga SL, Loucks AB, Rossmanith WG, Kettel LM, Laughlin GA, Yen SSC: Acceleration of luteinizing hormone pulse frequency in functional hypothalamic amenorrhea by dopaminergic blockade. J Clin Endocrinol Metab 72:151–156, 1991.

47. LaVecchia C, Decardi A, Franceschi S, Gentile A, Negri E, Parazzini F: Menstrual and reproductive factors and the risk of myocardial infarction in women under fifty-five years of age. Am J Obstet Gynecol 157:1108–1112, 1987.

48. Schneiderman N: Psychophysiologic factors in atherogenesis and coronary artery disease. Circulation 76(Suppl I):I41–I47, 1987.

49. Blumenthal SJ, Matthews KA: Working group report: Psychosocial aspects of cardiovascular disease in women. In NK Wenger, L Speroff, B Packard (eds), Cardiovascular Health and Disease in Women. Greenwich, CT, LeJacq Communications, Inc., 1993, 213–216.

50. Wenger NK: Coronary heart disease in women: An overview (myths, misperceptions, and missed opportunities). In Wenger NK, Speroff L, Packard B (eds), Cardiovascular Health and Disease in Women. Greenwich, CT, LeJacq Communications, Inc., 1993, 21–29.

51. Haynes SG, Czajkowski SM: Psychosocial and environmental correlates of heart disease. In Douglas PS (ed), Cardiovascular Health and Disease in Women. Philadelphia, Saunders, 1993, 269–282.

52. Stamler J, Pick R, Katz LN: Experiences in assessing estrogen antiatherogenesis in the chick, the rabbit, and man. Ann NY Acad Sci 64:596–619, 1956.

53. Prichard RW, Clarkson TB, Lofland HB: Estrogen in pigeon atherosclerosis. Estradiol valerate effects at several dose levels on cholesterol-fed male white Carneau pigeons. Arch Pathol 82:15–17, 1966.

54. Prichard RW, Clarkson TB, Goodman HO, Lofland HB: Aortic atherosclerosis in pigeons and its complications. Arch Pathol 77:244–257, 1964.

55. Fillios LC, Mann GV: The importance of sex in the variability of cholesteremic response of rabbits fed cholesterol. Circ Res 4:406–412, 1956.

56. Ludden JB, Bruger M, Wright IS: Experimental atherosclerosis IV. Effects of testosterone propionate and estradiol dipropionate on experimental atherosclerosis in rabbits. Arch Pathol 33:58–62, 1942.

57. Lorenzen I: Vascular connective tissue under the influence of oestrogens: 1. Biochemical and morphological studies of aortae of untreated female and male rabbits, and aortae of castrated and sham operated female rabbits. Acta Endocrinol (Kbh) 52:565–572, 1966.

58. Haarbo J, Leth-Espensen P, Stender S, Christiansen C: Estrogen monotherapy and combined estrogen-progestogen therapy attenuate aortic accumulation of cholesterol in ovariectomized cholesterol-fed rabbits. J Clin Invest 87:1274–1279, 1991.

59. Haarbo J, Svendsen OL, Christiansen C: Progestogens do not affect aortic accumulation of cholesterol in ovariectomized cholesterol-fed rabbits. Circ Res 70:1198–1202, 1992.

60. Jayo JM, Schwenke DC, Clarkson TB: Atherosclerosis research. In Manning PJ, Ringler DH, Newcomer CE (eds), The Biology of the Laboratory Rabbit, 2nd Edition. San Diego, Academic Press, 1994, 367–380.

61. Kaplan JR, Manuck SB, Clarkson TB, Prichard RW: Animal models of behavioral influences on atherogenesis. Adv Behav Med 1:115–163, 1985.

62. MacDonald GT: Reproductive patterns of three species of macaques. Fertil Steril 22:373–377, 1971.

63. Mahoney CJ: A study of the menstrual cycle in *Macaca irus* with special reference to the detection of ovulation. J Reprod Fertil 21:153–163, 1970.

64. Kaplan JR, Adams MR, Clarkson TB, Manuck SB, Shively CA: Social behavior and gender in biomedical investigations using monkeys: Studies in atherogenesis. Lab Anim Sci 41:334–343, 1991.

65. Clarkson TB, Williams JK, Adams MR, Wagner JD, Klein KP: Experimental effects of estrogens and progestins on the coronary artery wall. In Wenger NK, Speroff L, Packard B (eds), Cardiovascular Health and Disease in Women. Greenwich, CT, LeJacq Communications, Inc., 1993, 169–174.

66. Hamm TE Jr, Kaplan JR, Clarkson TB, Bullock BC: Effects of gender and social behavior on the de-

velopment of coronary artery atherosclerosis in cynomolgus macaques. Atherosclerosis 48:221–233, 1983.

67. Kaplan JR, Adams MR, Clarkson TB, Koritnik DR: Psychosocial influences on female "protection" among cynomolgus macaques. Atherosclerosis 53:283–295, 1984.

68. Altmann J: Observational study of behavior: Sampling methods. Behaviour 48:1–41, 1974.

69. Sade DS: An ethogram for rhesus monkeys. I. Antithetical contrasts in posture and movement. Am J Phys Anthropol 38:537–542, 1973.

70. Sade DS: Determinants of dominance in a group of free ranging rhesus monkeys. In Altmann S (ed), Social Communication among Primates. Chicago, University of Chicago Press, 1967, 99–114.

71. Adams MR, Kaplan JR, Koritnik DR: Psychosocial influences on ovarian endocrine and ovulatory function in *Macaca fascicularis*. Physiol Behav 35:935–940, 1985.

72. Adams MR, Kaplan JR, Koritnik DR, Clarkson TB: Ovariectomy, social status, and atherosclerosis in cynomolgus monkeys. Arteriosclerosis 5:192–200, 1985.

73. Adams MR, Kaplan JR, Koritnik DR, Clarkson TB: Pregnancy-associated inhibition of coronary artery atherosclerosis in monkeys. Evidence of a relationship with endogenous estrogen. Arteriosclerosis 7:378–384, 1987.

74. Kaplan JR, Adams MR, Anthony MS, Morgan TM, Manuck SB, Clarkson TB: Dominant social status and contraceptive hormone treatment inhibit atherogenesis in premenopausal monkeys. Atheroscler Thromb Vasc Biol 15:2094–2100, 1995.

75. Wagner JD, Clarkson TB, St. Clair RW, Schwenke DC, Shively CA, Adams MR: Estrogen and progesterone replacement therapy reduces LDL accumulation in the coronary arteries of surgically postmenopausal cynomolgus monkeys. J Clin Invest 88:1995–2002, 1991.

76. Wagner JD, Adams MR, Schwenke DC, Clarkson TB: Oral contraceptive therapy decreases arterial low density lipoprotein degradation in female cynomolgus monkeys. Circ Res 72:1300–1307, 1993.

77. Sack MN, Rader DJ, Cannon RO: Oestrogen and inhibition of oxidation of low-density lipoproteins in postmenopausal women. Lancet 343:269–270, 1994.

78. Ludmer PL, Selwyn AP, Shook TL, Wayne RR, Mudge GH, Alexander RW, Ganz P: Paradoxical vasoconstriction induced by acetylcholine in atherosclerotic coronary arteries. N Engl J Med 315:1046–1051, 1986.

79. Maseri A, L'Abbate A, Bardoli G, Chierchia S, Marzilli M, Ballestra AM, Severi S, Paradi O, Biagini A, Distante A, Pestola A: Coronary vasospasm as a possible cause of myocardial infarction: A conclusion derived from the study of "preinfarction" angina. N Engl J Med 299:1271–1277, 1978.

80. Maseri A, Severi S, DeNes M, L'Abbate A, Chierchia S, Marzilli M, Ballestra AM, Paradi O, Biagini A, Distante A: "Variant" angina: One aspect of a continuous spectrum of vasospastic myocardial ischemia: Pathogenetic mechanisms, estimated incidence and clinical and coronary arteriographic findings in 138 patients. Am J Cardiol 42:1019–1035, 1978.

81. Roberts WC, Durry RC, Isner JM: Sudden death in Prinzmetal's angina with coronary spasm documented by angiography: Analysis of three necropsy patients. Am J Cardiol 50:203–210, 1982.

82. Williams JK, Adams MR, Klopfenstein HS: Estrogen modulates responses of atherosclerotic coronary arteries. Circulation 81:1680–1687, 1990.

83. Williams JK, Adams MR, Herrington DM, Clarkson TB: Short-term administration of estrogen and vascular responses of atherosclerotic coronary arteries. J Am Coll Cardiol 20:452–457, 1992.

84. Williams JK, Honoré EK, Washburn SA, Clarkson TB: Effects of hormone replacement therapy on reactivity of atherosclerotic coronary arteries in cynomolgus monkeys. J Am Coll Cardiol 24:1757–1761, 1994.

85. Williams JK, Shively CA, Clarkson TB: Determinants of coronary artery reactivity in premenopausal female cynomolgus monkeys with diet-induced atherosclerosis. Circulation 90:983–987, 1994.

86. Ahmed SA, Penhale WJ, Talal N: Sex hormones, immune responses, and autoimmune diseases: Mechanisms of sex hormone action. Am J Pathol 121:531–551, 1985.

87. Loy RA, Loukides JA, Polan ML: Ovarian steroids modulate human monocyte tumor necrosis factor alpha messenger ribonucleic acid levels in cultured human peripheral monocytes. Fertil Steril 58:733–739, 1992.

88. Polan ML, Loukides J, Nelson P, Carding S, Diamond M, Walsh A, Bottomly K: Progesterone and

estradiol modulate interleukin-1 beta messenger ribonucleic acid levels in cultured human peripheral monocytes. J Clin Endocrinol Metab 69:1200–1206, 1989.

89. Schuurs AHWM, Verheul HAM: Effects of gender
and sex steroids on the immune response. J Steroid
Biochem 35:157–172, 1990.

90. Troxler RG, Sprague EA, Albanese RA, Fuchs R,
Thompson AJ: The association of elevated plasma
cortisol and early atherosclerosis as demonstrated by
coronary angiography. Atherosclerosis 26:151–162,
1977.

91. Sprague EA, Troxler RG, Peterson DF, Schmidt
RE, Young JT: Effect of cortisol on the development
of atherosclerosis in cynomolgus monkeys. In Kalter
SS (ed), The Use of Nonhuman Primates in Cardiovascular Disease. Austin, University of Texas Press,
1980, 261–264.

92. Stamler J, Pick R, Katz LN: Experiences in
assessing estrogen antiatherogenesis in the chick, the
rabbit, and man. Ann NY Acad Sci 64:596–619, 1956.

93. Kaplan JR, Adams MR, Koritnik DR, Rose JC,
Manuck SB: Adrenal responsiveness and social status
in intact and ovariectomized Macaca fascicularis. Am J
Primatol 11:181–193, 1986.

94. Williams RB, Suarez ED, Kuhn CM, Zimmerman
EA, Schanberg SM: Biobehavioral basis of coronary-
prone behavior in middle-aged men. Part I: Evidence
for chronic SNS activation of Type. As. Psychosom
Med 53:517–527, 1991.

95. Kaplan JR, Pettersson K, Manuck SB, Olsson G:
Role of sympathoadrenal medullary activation in the
initiation and progression of atherosclerosis. Circulation 84(Suppl VI):VI-23–VI-32, 1991.

96. Pettersson K, Bejne B, Bjork H, Strawn WB,
Bondjers G: Experimental sympathetic activation
causes endothelial injury in the rabbit thoracic aorta
via B$_1$-adrenoceptor activation. Circ Res 67:1027–
1034, 1990.

97. Strawn WB, Bondjers G, Kaplan JR, Manuck SB,
Schwenke DC, Hansson GK, Shively CA, Clarkson
TB: Endothelial dysfunction in response to psychoso-
cial stress in monkeys. Circ Res 68:1270–1279, 1991.

98. Schwartz S, Gadusek C, Sheldon S: Vascular wall
growth control: The role of endothelium. Arteriosclerosis 1:107–126, 1981.

99. Manuck SB, Kaplan JR, Muldoon MF, Adams
MR, Clarkson TB: The behavioral exacerbation of

atherosclerosis and its inhibition by propranolol. In
McCabe PM, Schneiderman N, Field TM, Skylar JS
(eds), Stress, Coping and Disease. Hillsdale, NJ, Lawrence Erlbaum Associates, 1991, 51–72.

100. Kaplan JR, Manuck SB, Adams MR, Weingand
KW, Clarkson TB: Inhibition of coronary atherosclerosis by propranolol in behaviorally predisposed
monkeys fed an atherogenic diet. Circulation 76:1364–
1372, 1987.

101. Manuck SB, Polefrone JM: Psychophysiologic
reactivity in women. In Eaker ED, Packard B, Wenger
NK, Clarkson TB, Tyroler HA (eds), Coronary Heart
Disease in Women. New York, Haymarket Doyma,
Inc., 1987, 164–171.

102. Owens JF, Stoney CM, Matthews KA: Menopausal status influences ambulatory blood pressure
levels and blood pressure changes during mental stress.
Circulation 88:2794–2802, 1993.

103. Stoney CM, Davis MC, Matthews KA: Sex differences in physiological responses to stress and in
coronary heart disease: A causal link? Psychophysiology 24:127–131, 1987.

104. Manuck SB, Kaplan JR, Adams MR, Clarkson
TB: Behaviorally elicited heart rate reactivity and
atherosclerosis in female cynomolgus monkeys (Macaca
fascicularis). Psychosom Med 51:306–318, 1989.

105. Reid IA, Morris BJ, Ganong WF: The renin-
angiotensin system. Annu Rev Physiol 40:377–410,
1978.

106. Hilgers KF, Veelken R, Kreppner I, Ganten D,
Luft FC, Geiger H, Mann JFE: Vascular angiotensin
and the sympathetic nervous system: Do they interact?
Am J Physiol 267:H187–H194, 1994.

107. Dorward PK, Rudd CD: Influence of brain renin-
angiotensin system on renal sympathetic and cardiac
baroreflexes in conscious rabbits. Am J Physiol
260:H770–H778, 1991.

108. Ganong WF: Review of Medical Physiology,
17th Edition. Norwalk, CT, Appleton & Lange, 1993.

109. Aberg G, Ferrer P: Effects of captopril on atherosclerosis in cynomolgus monkeys. J Cardiovasc
Pharmacol 15(Suppl 5):S65–S72, 1990.

110. Marrero MB, Paxton WG, Duff JL, Berk BC,
Bernstein KE: Angiotensin II stimulates tyrosine
phosphorylation of phospholipase C-γ1 in vascular
smooth muscle cells. J Biol Chem 269:10935–10939,
1994.

111. Rogers TB, Lokuta AJ: Angiotensin II signal transduction pathways in the cardiovascular system. Trends Cardiovasc Med 4:110–116, 1994.

112. Proudler AJ, Ahmed AIH, Crook D, Fogelman I, Rymer JM, Stevenson JC: Hormone replacement therapy and serum angiotensin-converting-enzyme activity in postmenopausal women. Lancet 346:89–90, 1995.

113. Brosnihan KG, Li P, Ferrario CM: Angiotensin-(1–7) elicits nitric oxide-dependent vasodilation in canine coronary arteries [Abstract]. Hypertension 26:544, 1995.

114. Dittus WPJ: The evolution of behaviors regulating density and age-specific sex ratios in a primate population. Behaviour 69:265–302, 1979.

115. Drickamer LC: A ten-year summary of reproductive data for free-ranging Macaca mulatta. Folia Primatol (Basel) 21:61–80, 1974.

116. Sade D, Cushing K, Cushing P, Dunaif J, Figueroa A, Kaplan JR, Lauer C, Rhodes D, Schneider J: Population dynamics in relation to social structure on Cayo Santiago. Yearbook Phys Anthropol 20:253–262, 1976.

117. Silk JB, Clark-Wheatley C, Rodman PS, Samuels A: Differential reproductive success and facultative adjustment of sex ratios among captive female bonnet macaques (Macaca radiata). Anim Behav 29:1106–1120, 1981.

118. Walker ML, Gordon TP, Wilson ME: Menstrual cycle characteristics of seasonally breeding rhesus monkeys. Biol Reprod 29:841–848, 1983.

119. Wilson ME, Gordon TP, Bernstein IS: Timing of births and reproductive success in rhesus monkey social groups. J Med Primatol 7:202–212, 1978.

120. Shively CA, Kaplan JR, Adams MR: Effects of ovariectomy, social instability and social status on female Macaca fascicularis social behavior. Physiol Behav 36:1147–1153, 1986.

121. Reifenstein EC Jr: Psychogenic or "hypothalamic" amenorrhea. Med Clin North Am 30:1103–1104, 1946.

122. Berga SL, Girton LG: The psychoneuroendocrinology of functional hypothalamic amenorrhea. Psychiatric Clin North Am 12:105–116, 1989.

123. Berga SL, Mortola JF, Girton L, Suh B, Laughlin G, Pham P, Yen SSC: Neuroendocrine aberrations in women with functional hypothalamic amenorrhea. J Clin Endocrinol Metab 68:301–308, 1989.

124. Biller BMK, Coughlin JF, Saxe V, Schoenfeld D, Sprat DI, Klibanski A: Osteopenia in women with hypothalamic amenorrhea: A prospective study. Obstet Gynecol 78:996–1001, 1991.

125. Seeman E, Szmukler GI, Formica C, Tsalamandria C, Mestrovic R: Osteoporosis in anorexia nervosa: The influence of peak bone density, bone loss, oral contraceptive use, and exercise. J Bone Miner Res 7:1467–1474, 1992.

126. Ohkura T, Isse K, Akazawa K, Hamomoto M, Yaoi Y, Hagino N: Long-term estrogen replacement therapy in female patients with dementia of the Alzheimer type: 7 case reports. Dementia 6:99–107, 1995.

Sources

2. Crabbe, J. C., Wahlsten, D., and Dudek, B. C. (1999). Genetics of mouse behavior: Interactions with laboratory environment. *Science* 284:1670–1672. Reprinted with permission of *Science*. Copyright 1999 American Association for the Advancement of Science.

3. Cacioppo, J. T., Berntson, G. G., Sheridan, J. F., and McClintock, M. K. (2000). Multilevel integrative analyses of human behavior: Social neuroscience and the complementing nature of social and biological approaches. *Psychological Bulletin,* 126, no. 6, 829–843. Reprinted with permission of the American Psychological Association.

4. Klein, S. B., and Kihlstrom, J. F. (1998). On bridging the gap between social-personality psychology and neuropsychology. *Personality and Social Psychology Review,* 2, 228–242. Reprinted with permission of Lawrence Erlbaum Associates.

5. Dunbar, R. I. M. (1998). The social brain hypothesis. *Evolutionary Anthropology,* 6, 178–190. Reprinted with permission of Wiley-Liss, Inc., a subsidiary of John Wiley & Sons.

6. Anderson, N. B. (1998). Levels of analysis in health science: A framework for integrating sociobehavioral and biomedical research. *Annals of the New York Academy of Sciences,* 840, 563–576. Reprinted with permission of the Annals of the New York Academy of Sciences.

7. Koechlin, E., Basso, G., Pietrini, P., Panzer, S., and Grafman, J. (1999). The role of the anterior prefrontal cortex in human cognition. *Nature,* 399, 149–151. Reprinted with permission of *Nature*. © 1999 Macmillan Magazines Ltd.

8. Schacter, D. L. (1999). The seven sins of memory: Insights from psychology and cognitive neuroscience. *American Psychologist,* 54, 182–203. Reprinted with permission of the American Psychological Association.

9. Bechara, A., Tranel, D., Damasio, H., Adolphs, R., Rockland, C., and Damasio, A. R. (1995). Double dissociation of conditioning and declarative knowledge relative to the amygdala and hippocampus in humans. *Science,* 269, 1115–1118. Reprinted with permission of *Science*. © 1995 American Association for the Advancement of Science.

10. Dehaene, S., Naccache, L., Le Clec'H, G., Koechlin, E., Mueller, M., Dehaene-Lambertz, G., van de Moortele, P., and Le Bihan, D. (1998). Imaging unconscious semantic priming. *Nature,* 395, 597–600.

Reprinted with permission of *Nature*. © 1998 Macmillan Magazines Ltd.

11. Smith, E. E., and Jonides, J. (1999). Storage and executive processes in the frontal lobes. *Science,* 283, 1657–1661. Reprinted with permission of *Science*. © 1999 American Association for the Advancement of Science.

12. McGaugh, J. L. (2000). Memory—a century of consolidation. *Science,* 287, 248–251. Reprinted with permission of *Science*. © 2000 American Association for the Advancement of Science.

13. Craik, F. I. M., Moroz, T. M., Moscovitch, M., Stuss, D. T., Winocur, G., Tulving, E., and Kapur, S. (1999). In search of the self: A positron emission tomographic study. *Psychological Science,* 10, 26–34. Reprinted with permission of Blackwell Publishers.

14. Gazzaniga, M. S. (1998). Brain and conscious experience. *Advances in Neurology,* 77, 181–192. Reprinted with permission of Lippincott Williams & Wilkins.

15. Posner, M. I., and Rothbart, M. K. (1998). Attention, self-regulation and consciousness. *Philosophical Transactions of the Royal Society of London—Series B: Biological Sciences,* 353, 1915–1927. Reprinted with permission of Philip Allen Publishers, Ltd.

16. Sabbagh, M. A., and Taylor, M. (2000). Neural correlates of theory-of-mind reasoning: An event-related potential study. *Psychological Science,* 11, 46–50. Reprinted with permission of Blackwell Publishers.

17. Rizzolatti, G., and Arbib, M. A. (1998). Language within our grasp. *Trends in Neurosciences,* 21, 188–194. Reprinted with permission of Elsevier Science.

18. Kanwisher, N., McDermott, J., and Chun, M. (1997). The fusiform face area: A module in human extrastriate cortex specialized for face perception. *Journal of Neuroscience,* 17, 4302–4311. Reprinted with permission of the Society for Neuroscience.

19. Gauthier, I., Skudlarski, P., Gore, J. C., and Anderson, A. W. (2000). Expertise for cars and birds recruits brain areas involved in face perception. *Nature Neuroscience,* 3, 191–197. Reprinted with permission of Nature. © 2000 Macmillan Magazines Ltd.

20. Belin, P., Zatorre, R. J., LaFaille, P., Ahad, P., and Pike, B. (2000). Voice-selective areas in human auditory cortex. *Nature,* 403, 309–312. Reprinted with permission of *Nature*. © 2000 Macmillan Magazines Ltd.

21. Skuse, D. H., James, R. S., Bishop, D. V. M., Coppin, B., Dalton, P., Aamodt-Leeper, G., Bacarese-Hamilton, M., Creswell, C., McGurk, R., and Jacobs, P. A. (1997). Evidence from Turner's syndrome of an imprinted X-linked locus affecting cognitive function. *Nature,* 387, 705–708. Reprinted with permission of *Nature.* © 1997 Macmillan Magazines Ltd.

22. Adolphs, R. (1999). Social cognition and the human brain. *Trends in Cognitive Sciences,* 3, 469–479. Reprinted with permission of Elsevier Science.

23. Anderson, S. W., Bechara, A., Damasio, H., Tranel, D., and Damasio, A. R. (1999). Impairment of social and moral behavior related to early damage in human prefrontal cortex. *Nature Neuroscience,* 2, 1032–1037. Reprinted with permission of *Nature.* © 1999 Macmillan Magazines Ltd.

24. Adolphs, R., Tranel, D., and Damasio, A. R. (1998). The human amygdala in social judgment. *Nature,* 393, 470–474. Reprinted with permission of *Nature.* © 1998 Macmillan Magazines Ltd.

25. Baron-Cohen, S., Ring, H. A., Wheelwright, S., Bullmore, E. T., Brammer, M. J., Simmons, A., and Williams, S. C. R. (1999). Social intelligence in the normal and autistic brain: An fMRI study. *European Journal of Neuroscience,* 11, 1891–1898. Reprinted with permission of Blackwell Science (UK).

26. Brothers, L. (1990). The social brain: A project for integrating primate behavior and neurophysiology in a new domain. *Concepts in Neuroscience,* 1, 27–51. Reprinted with permission of World Scientific Publishing (HK).

27. LeDoux, J. (1995). Emotion: Clues from the brain. *Annual Review of Psychology,* 46, 209–235. Reprinted with permission of the Annual Review of Psychology, www.annualreviews.org.

28. LeDoux, J. (1998). Fear and the brain: Where have we been, and where are we going? *Biological Psychiatry,* 44, 1229–1238. Reprinted with permission of Elsevier Science. © 1998 by the Society of Biological Psychiatry.

29. Berntson, G. G., Sarter, M., and Cacioppo, J. T. (1998). Anxiety and cardiovascular reactivity: The basal forebrain cholinergic link. *Behavioural Brain Research,* 94, 225–248. Reprinted with permission of Elsevier Science.

30. Lang, P. J., Bradley, M. M., and Cuthbert, B. N. (1992). A motivational analysis of emotion: Reflex-cortical connections. *Psychological Science,* 3, 44–49. Reprinted with permission of Blackwell Publishers.

31. Davidson, R. J., and Irwin, W. (1999). The functional neuroanatomy of emotion and affective style. *Trends in Cognitive Sciences,* 3, 11–21. Reprinted with permission of Elsevier Science.

32. Cacioppo, J. T., Gardner, W. L., and Berntson, G. G. (1999). The affect system has parallel and integrative processing components: Form follows function. *Journal of Personality and Social Psychology,* 76, 839–855. Reprinted with permission of the American Psychological Association.

33. Rogers, R. D., Owen, A. M., Middleton, H. C., Williams, E. J., Pickard, J. D., Sahakian, B. J., and Robbins, T. W. (1999). Choosing between small, likely rewards and large, unlikely rewards activates inferior and orbital prefrontal cortex. *Journal of Neuroscience,* 19, 9029–9038. Reprinted with permission of the Society for Neuroscience.

34. Schultz, W., Dayan, P., and Montague, P. (1997). A neural substrate of prediction and reward. *Science,* 275, 1593–1599. Reprinted with permission of *Science.* © 1997 American Association for the Advancement of Science.

35. Kim, J. J., Shih, J. C., Chen, K., Chen, L., Bao, S., Maren, S., Anagnostaras, S. G., Fanselow, M. S., DeMaeyer, E., Seif, I., and Thompson, R. F. (1997). Selective enhancement of emotional, but not motor, learning in monoamine oxidase A–deficient mice. *Proceedings of the National Academy of Sciences,* 94, 5929–5933. Reprinted with permission of the National Academy of Sciences, U.S.A.

36. Berridge, K. C., and Robinson, T. E. (1995). The mind of an addicted brain: Neural sensitization of wanting versus liking. *Current Directions in Psychological Science,* 4, 71–76. Reprinted with permission of Blackwell Publishers.

37. Ito, T. A., Larsen, J. T., Smith, N. K., and Cacioppo, J. T. (1998). Negative information weighs more heavily on the brain: The negativity bias in evaluative categorizations. *Journal of Personality and Social Psychology,* 75, 887–900. Reprinted with permission of the American Psychological Association.

38. Pizzagalli, D., Lehmann, D., Koenig, T., Regard, M., and Pascual-Marqui, R. D. (2000). Face-elicited ERPs and affective attitude: Brain electrical microstate and tomography analyses. *Clinical Neurophysiology,*

111, 521–531. Reprinted with permission of Elsevier Science.

39. Phelps, E. A., O'Connor, K. J., Cunningham, W. A., Funayama, E. S., Gatenby, J. C., Gore, J. C., and Banaji, M. R. (in press). Performance on indirect measures of race evaluation predicts amygdala activation. *Journal of Cognitive Neuroscience*. Reprinted with permission of MIT Press.

40. Bechara, A., Damasio, H., Tranel, D., and Damasio, A. R. (1997). Deciding advantageously before knowing the advantageous strategy. *Science, 275,* 1293–1295. Reprinted with permission of *Science*. © 1997 American Association for the Advancement of Science.

41. Lieberman, M. D., Ochsner, K. N., Gilbert, D. T., and Schacter, D. L. (in press). Do amnesics exhibit cognitive dissonance reduction? The role of explicit memory and attention in attitude change. *Psychological Science*. Reprinted with permission of Blackwell Publishers.

42. Johnsrude, I. S., Owen, A. M., White, N. M., Zhao, W. V., and Bohbot, V. (2000). Impaired preference conditioning after anterior temporal lobe resection in humans. *Journal of Neuroscience,* 20, 2649–2656. Reprinted with permission of the Society for Neuroscience.

43. Taylor, S. E., Klein, L. C., Lewis, B. P., Gruenwald, T. L., Gurung, R. A. R., and Updegraff, J. A. (in press). Biobehavioral responses to stress in females: Tend-and-befriend, not fight-or-flight. *Psychological Review*. Reprinted with permission of the American Psychological Association.

44. Insel, T. R., O'Brien, D. J., and Leckman, J. F. (1999). Oxytocin, vasopressin, and autism: Is there a connection? *Biological Psychiatry,* 45, 145–157. Reprinted with permission of Elsevier Science. © 1999 by the Society of Biological Psychiatry.

45. LeMarquand, D. G., Pihl, R. O., Young, S. N., Tremblay, R. E., Seguin, J. R., Palmour, R. M., and Benkelfat, C. (1998). Tryptophan depletion, executive functions, and disinhibition in aggressive, adolescent males. *Neuropsychopharmacology,* 19, 333–341. Reprinted with permission of Elsevier Science. © 1998 by the American College of Neuropsychopharmacology.

46. McCrae, R. R., Costa, P. T., Jr., Ostendorf, F., Angleitner, A., Hřebíčková, M., Avia, M. D., Sanz, J., Sanchez-Bernardos, M. L., Kusdil, M. E., Woodfield, R., Saunders, P. R., and Smith, P. B. (2000). Nature

over nurture: Temperament, personality, and life span development. *Journal of Personality and Social Psychology,* 78, 173–186.

47. Maestripieri, D. (in press). Biological bases of maternal attachment. *Current Directions in Psychological Science*. Reprinted with permission of Blackwell Publishers.

48. Liu, D., Diorio, J., Tannenbaum, B., Caldji, C., Francis, D., Freedman, A., Sharma, S., Pearson, D., Plotsky, P. M., and Meaney, M. J. (1997). Maternal care, hippocampal glucocorticoid receptors and HPA responses to stress. *Science,* 277, 1659–1662. Reprinted with permission of *Science*. Copyright 1997 American Association for the Advancement of Science.

49. Francis, D., and Meaney, M. J. (1999). Maternal care and the development of stress responses. *Current Opinion in Neurobiology,* 9, 128–134. Reprinted with permission of Elsevier Science.

50. Suomi, S. (1999). Attachment in rhesus monkeys. In J. Cassidy and P. Shaver (eds.), *Handbook of attachment: Theory, research, and clinical applications* (New York: Guilford Press), pp. 181–197. Reprinted with permission of Guilford Press.

51. Francis, D. D., Diorio, J., Liu, D., and Meaney, M. J. (1999). Nongenomic transmission across generations of maternal behavior and stress responses in the rat. *Science,* 286, 1155–1158. Reprinted with permission of *Science*. © 1999 American Association for the Advancement of Science.

52. Young, L. J., Wang, Z., and Insel, T. R. (1998). Neuroendocrine bases of monogamy. *Trends in Neurosciences,* 21, 71–75. Reprinted with permission of Elsevier Science.

53. Pugh, C. R., Nguyen, K. T., Gonyea, J. L., Fleshner, M., Watkins, L. R., Maier, S. F., and Rudy, J. W. (1999). Role of interleukin-1 beta in impairment of contextual fear conditioning caused by social isolation. *Behavioural Brain Research,* 106, 109–118. Reprinted with permission of Elsevier Science.

54. Schmidt, L. A., Fox, N. A., Sternberg, E. M., Gold, P. W., Smith, C. C., and Schulkin, J. (1999). Adrenocortical reactivity and social competence in seven-year-olds. *Personality & Individual Differences,* 26, 977–985. Reprinted with permission of Elsevier Science.

55. Cacioppo, J. T., Ernst, J. M., Burleson, M. H., McClintock, M. K., Malarkey, W. B., Hawkley, L. C., Kowalewski, R. B., Paulsen, A., Hobson, J. A., Hug-

dahl, K., Spiegel, D., and Berntson, G. G. (2000). Lonely traits and concomitant physiological processes: The MacArthur Social Neuroscience Studies. *International Journal of Psychophysiology*, 35, 143–154. Reprinted with permission of Elsevier Science.

56. Carter, C. S. (1998). Neuroendocrine perspectives on social attachment and love. *Psychoneuroendocrinology*, 23, 779–818. Reprinted with permission of Elsevier Science.

57. Winslow, J. T., Hastings, N., Carter, C. S., Harbaugh, C. R., and Insel, T. R. (1993). A role for central vasopressin in pair bonding in monogamous prairie voles. Nature, 365, 545–548. Reprinted with permission of *Nature*. © 1993 Macmillan Magazines Ltd.

58. Cushing, B. S., and Carter, C. S. (1999). Prior exposure to oxytocin mimics the effects of social contact and facilitates sexual behavior in females. *Journal of Neuroendocrinology*, 11, 765–769. Reprinted with permission of Blackwell Science, UK.

59. Jacob, S., and McClintock, M. K. (2000). Psychological state and mood effects of steroidal chemosignals in women and men. *Hormones and Behavior*, 37, 57–78. Reprinted with permission of Academic Press.

60. Perrett, D. I., Lee, K. J., Penton-Voak, I., Rowland, D., Yoshikawa, S., Burt, D. M., Henzil, S. P., Castles, D. L., and Akamatsu, S. (1998). Effects of sexual dimorphism on facial attractiveness. *Nature*, 394, 884–887. Reprinted with permission of *Nature*. © 1998 Macmillan Magazines Ltd.

61. Wallen, K., (1996). Nature needs nurture: The interaction of hormonal and social influences on the development of behavioral sex differences in rhesus monkeys. *Hormones and Behavior*, 30, 364–378. Reprinted with permission of Academic Press.

62. Tremblay, R. E., Japel, C., Perussew, D., Bolvin, M., Zoccolillo, M., Montplaisir, J., and McDuff, P. (1999). The search for the age of onset of physical aggression: Rousseau and Bandura revisited. *Criminal Behavior and Mental Health*, 9, 8–23. Reprinted with permission of Whurr Publishers.

63. Westergaard, G. C., Suomi, S. J., Higley, J. D., and Mehlman, P. T. (1999). CSF 5-HIAA and aggression in female primates: Species and interindividual differences. *Psychopharmacology*, 146, 440–446. Reprinted with permission of Springer-Verlag.

64. Stribley, J. M., and Carter, C. S. (1999). Developmental exposure to vasopressin increases aggression in adult prarie voles. *Proceedings of the National Academy of Sciences*, 96, 12601–12604. Reprinted with permission of the National Academy of Sciences, U.S.A.

65. Higley, J. D., Mehlman, P. T., Poland, R. E., and Taub, D. M. (1996). CSF testosterone and 5-HIAA correlate with different types of aggressive behaviors. *Biological Psychiatry*, 40, 1067–1082. Reprinted with permission of Elsevier Science. © 1996 by the Society of Biological Psychiatry.

66. Raine, A., Lencz, T., Bihrle, S., LaCasse, L., and Colletti, P. (2000). Reduced prefrontal gray matter volume and reduced autonomic activity in antisocial personality disorder. *Archives of General Psychiatry*, 57, 119–127. Reprinted with permission of the American Medical Association.

67. Kalin, N. H., Larson, C., Shelton, S. E., and Davidson, R. J. (1998). Asymmetric frontal brain activity, cortisol, and behavior associated with fearful temperament in rhesus monkeys. *Behavioral Neuroscience*, 112, 286–292. Reprinted with permission of the American Psychological Association.

68. Schmidt, L. A. (1999). Frontal brain electrical activity in shyness and sociability. *Psychological Science*, 10, 316–320. Reprinted with permission of Blackwell Publishers.

69. Knutson, B., Wolkowitz, O., Cole, S. W., Chan, T., Moore, E., Johnson, R., Terpstra, J., Turner, R. A., and Reus, V. I. (1998). Selective alteration of personality and social behavior by serotonergic intervention. *American Journal of Psychiatry*, 155, 373–379. Reprinted with permission of the American Psychiatric Association.

70. DePue, R. A., Luciana, M., Arbisi, P., Collins, P., and Leon, A. (1994). Dopamine and the structure of personality: Relation of agonist-induced dopamine activity to positive emotionality. *Journal of Personality and Social Psychology*, 67, 485–498. Reprinted with permission of the American Psychological Association.

71. Adler, N. E., Boyce, T., Chesney, M. A., Cohen, S., Folkman, S., Kahn, R. L., and Syme, S. L. (1994). Socioeconomic status and health: The challenge of the gradient. *American Psychologist*, 49, 15–24. Reprinted with permission of the American Psychological Association.

72. Kiecolt-Glaser, J. K., Page, G. G., Marucha, P. T., MacCallum, R. C., and Glaser, R. (1998). Psycho-

logical influences on surgical recovery: Perspectives from psychoneuroimmunology. *American Psychologist,* 11, 1209–1218. Reprinted with permission of the American Psychological Association.

73. McEwen, B. S. (1998). Protective and damaging effects of stress mediators. *New England Journal of Medicine,* 338, 171–179. Reprinted with permission of the Publishing Division of the Massachusetts Medical Society. © 1998 Massachusetts Medical Society, all rights reserved.

74. Maier, S. F., and Watkins, L. R. (1998). Cytokines for psychologists: Implications of bidirectional immune-to-brain communication for understanding behavior, mood, and cognition. *Psychological Review,* 105, 83–107. Reprinted with permission of the American Psychological Association.

75. Padgett, D. A., Sheridan, J. F., Dorne, J., Berntson, G. G., Candelora, J., and Glaser, R. (1998). Social stress and the reactivation of latent herpes simplex virus-type 1. *Proceedings of the National Academy of Sciences,* 95, 7231–7235. Reprinted with permission of the National Academy of Sciences, U.S.A.

76. Davis, M. C., Matthews, K. A., and McGrath, C. E. (1999). Hostile attitudes predict elevated vascular resistance during interpersonal stress in men and women. *Psychosomatic Medicine,* 62, 17–25. Reprinted with permission of *Psychosomatic Medicine.*

77. Niaura, R., Banks, S. M., Ward, K. D., Stoney, C. M., Spiro, A., Aldwin, C. M., Landsberg, L., and Weiss, S. T. (1999). Hostility and the metabolic syndrome in older males: The normative aging study. *Psychosomatic Medicine,* 62, 7–16. Reprinted with permission of *Psychosomatic Medicine.*

78. Cohen, S., Frank, E., Doyle, W. J., Skoner, D. P., Rabin, B. S., and Gwaltney, J. M., Jr. (1998). Types of stressors that increase suscpetibility to the common cold in adults. *Health Psychology,* 17, 214–223. Reprinted with permission of the American Psychological Association.

79. Knox, S. S., and Uvnäs-Moberg, K. (1998). Social isolation and cardiovascular disease: An atherosclerotic pathway? *Psychoneuroendocrinology,* 23, 877–890. Reprinted with permission of Elsevier Science.

80. Berkman, L. F., Leo-Summers, L., and Horwitz, R. I. (1992). Emotional support and survival after myocardial infarction: A prospective, population-based study of the elderly. *Annals of Internal Medicine,* 117, 1003–1009. Reprinted with permission of the American College of Physicians—American Society of Internal Medicine.

81. Cohen, S., Doyle, W. J., Skoner, D. P., Rabin, B. S., and Gwaltney, J. M., Jr. (1997). Social ties and susceptibility to the common cold. *Journal of the American Medical Association,* 277, 1940–1944. Reprinted with permission of the American Medical Association.

82. Stern, K. and McClintock, M. K. (1998). Regulation of ovulation by human pheromones. *Nature,* 392, 177–179. Reprinted with permission of *Nature.* © 1998 Macmillan Magazines Ltd.

83. Kaplan, J. R., Adams, M. R., Clarkson, T. B., Manuck, S. B., Shively, C. A., and Williams, J. K. (1996). Psychosocial factors, sex differences, and atherosclerosis: Lessons from animal models. *Psychosomatic Medicine,* 58, 598–611. Reprinted with permission of *Psychosomatic Medicine.*

Index